Second Edition

Cataract Surgery

Techniques, Complications, and Management

Editor

Roger F. Steinert, MD
Associate Clinical Professor
Department of Ophthalmology
Harvard Medical School
Ophthalmic Consultants of Boston
Boston, Massachusetts

Associate Editors

I. Howard Fine, MD, MPH, FRCSC
Howard V. Gimbel, MD, MPH
Douglas D. Koch, MD
Richard L. Lindstrom, MD
Thomas F. Neuhann, MD
Robert H. Osher, MD

SAUNDERS
An Imprint of Elsevier

Saunders
An Imprint of Elsevier

The Curtis Center
Independence Square West
Philadelphia, Pennsylvania 19106

CATARACT SURGERY: Techniques, Complications, and Management Second Edition ISBN 0-7216-9057-2

NOTICE

Cataract surgery is an ever-changing field. Standard safety precautions must be followed, but as new research and clinical experience broaden our knowledge, changes in treatment and drug therapy may become necessary or appropriate. Readers are advised to check the most current product information provided by the manufacturer of each drug to be administered to verify the recommended dose, the method and duration of administration, and contraindications. It is the responsibility of the treating physician, relying on experience and knowledge of the patient, to determine dosages and the best treatment for each individual patient. Neither the publisher nor the editor assumes any liability for any injury and/or damage to persons or property arising from this publication.

Previous edition copyrighted 1995

International Standard Book Number 0-7216-9057-2

Acquisitions Editor: Natasha Andjelkovic
Developmental Editor: Agnes Byrne
Project Manager: Peggy Fagen
Designer: Amy Buxton

Printed in China

Last digit is the print number: 9 8 7 6 5 4 3 2

Dedication

To our parents
For nurturing our development and imbuing fundamental values

To our families
For your support, your encouragement, your tolerance every day

To our teachers
We try to honor you by building on your foundation

To our residents and fellows
You are the future; learn, then lead

To our patients
In return for entrusting us with the most precious of senses, we commit to an unrelenting pursuit of excellence

CONTRIBUTORS

Robert C. Allen, MD
Department of Ophthalmology
Medical College of Virginia
Richmond, Virginia

David J. Apple, MD
Professor of Ophthalmology and Pathology and Director, David J. Apple Laboratories for Ophthalmic Biodevices Research
John A. Moran Eye Center
University of Utah
Salt Lake City, Utah

Martin S. Arkin, MD, PhD
Active Staff, Munson Medical Center
Bay Eye Associates
Traverse City, Michigan

Stella Arthur, MD
Department of Ophthalmology and Visual Sciences
University of Utah
Salt Lake City, Utah

C. Davis Belcher, III, MD
Harvard Medical School
Tufts Medical School
Ophthalmic Consultants of Boston
Boston, Massachusetts

Hiroko Bissen-Miyajima, MD, PhD
Professor, Department of Ophthalmology
Tokyo Dental College Suidobashi Hospital
Tokyo, Japan

Mark Blumenkranz, MD
Professor and Chairman
Department of Ophthalmology
Stanford University School of Medicine
Stanford, California

Scott Burk, MD, PhD
Clinical Ophthalmologist
Department of Ophthalmology
Yale University
New Haven, Connecticut;
Cincinnati Eye Institute
Cincinnati, Ohio

Leo T. Chylack, Jr., MD
Professor and Vice Chairman (Research)
Department of Ophthalmology
Harvard Medical School;
Director of Research
Center for Ophthalmic Research
Brigham and Women's Hospital
Boston, Massachusetts

Robert J. Cionni, MD
Volunteer Assistant Professor of Ophthalmology
Department of Ophthalmology
University of Cincinnati;
Cincinnati Eye Institute
Cincinnati, Ohio

John S. Cohen, MD
Volunteer Clinical Professor
University of Cincinnati;
Chief, Glaucoma Service
Cincinnati Eye Institute
Cincinnati, Ohio

Alan S. Crandall, MD
Professor of Ophthalmology
Vice Chair of Clinical Services
Director of Glaucoma and Cataract
Department of Ophthalmology and Visual Sciences
University of Utah
Salt Lake City, Utah

Andrea P. Da Mata, MD
Ophthalmologist
Cincinnati Eye Institute
Cincinnati, Ohio

Elizabeth A. Davis, MD, FACS
Clinical Assistant Professor
Department of Ophthalmology
University of Minnesota
St. Paul, Minnesota

Brian M. DeBroff, MD
Associate Professor
Department of Ophthalmology and Visual Science
Yale University School of Medicine
New Haven, Connecticut

Jack M. Dodick, MD, FACS
Professor and Chairman (Acting)
Department of Ophthalmology
New York University School of Medicine
New York, New York

Jay S. Duker, MD
Professor and Chairman
Department of Ophthalmology
Tufts University School of Medicine
Boston, Massachusetts

Jared Emery, MD
Retired

I. Howard Fine, MD, MPH, FRCSC
Clinical Associate Professor of Ophthalmology
Oregon Health and Science University
Portland, Oregon;
Director, Oregon Eye Associates
Eugene, Oregon

William J. Fishkind, MD, FACS
Clinical Professor of Ophthalmology
The University of Utah
Salt Lake City, Utah;
Co-Director
Fishkind & Bakewell Eye Care and Surgery Center
Tucson, Arizona

Robert E. Foster, MD
Staff
Cincinnati Eye Institute
Cincinnati, Ohio

Howard V. Gimbel, MD, MPH
Professor and Chair
Department of Ophthalmology
Loma Linda University
Loma Linda, California;
Medical Director
Gimbel Eye Center
Calgary, Alberta, Canada

Robert C. (Roy) Hamilton, MB, BCh
Clinical Professor, Anesthesiology
University of Calgary
Calgary, Alberta, Canada

Kenneth Hoffer, MD
Clinical Professor of Ophthalmology
University of California at Los Angeles
Los Angeles, California;
St. Mary's Eye Center
Santa Monica, California

Richard S. Hoffman, MD
Clinical Instructor of Ophthalmology
Casey Eye Institute
Oregon Health and Science University
Portland, Oregon

Alex P. Hunyor, MB, BS
VMO, Retina Unit
Sydney Eye Hospital
Sydney, Australia;
Chatswood Retina Service
Chatswood, Australia

Andrea Izak, MD
John A. Moran Eye Center
Department of Ophthalmology and Visual Sciences
University of Utah
Salt Lake City, Utah

Marianne B. Mellem Kairala, MD
Center for Eye Research and Education
Ophthalmic Consultants of Boston
Boston, Massachusetts

Paul H. Kalina, MD
Associate Professor of Ophthalmology
Mayo Medical School
Mayo Graduate School of Medicine
Rochester, Minnesota

Julia D. Katz, MD
Manhattan Eye, Ear and Throat Hospital
New York, New York

Anup K. Khatana, MD
Clinical Assistant Professor of Ophthalmology
University of Cincinnati School of Medicine;
Cincinnati Eye Institute
Cincinnati, Ohio

Douglas D. Koch, MD
Professor and the Allen, Mosbacher, and Law Chair in Ophthalmology
Baylor College of Medicine;
Deputy Chief of Ophthalmology Service
Medical Director, Ophthalmology Operating Rooms
The Methodist Hospital
Houston, Texas

Stephen Lane, MD
Clinical Professor
University of Minnesota
Minneapolis, Minnesota

Richard Lyndon Lindstrom, MD
Adjunct Professor Emeritus
Department of Ophthalmology
University of Minnesota
Minneapolis, Minnesota;
Founder and Managing Partner
Minnesota Eye Consultants

Nick Mamalis, MD
Professor of Ophthalmology
University of Utah;
University Hospital
John A. Moran Eye Center
Salt Lake City, Utah

Tamer A. Mackey, MD
John A. Moran Eye Center
Department of Ophthalmology
University of Utah
Salt Lake City, Utah

Samuel Masket, MD
Clinical Professor of Ophthalmology
Jules Stein Eye Institute
UCLA School of Medicine
Los Angeles, California

David J. McIntyre, MD
McIntyre Eye Clinic & Surgical Center
Bellevue, Washington

Michael G. Morley, MD
Clinical Instructor in Ophthalmology
Harvard Medical School;
Assistant Clinical Professor in Ophthalmology
Tufts University School of Medicine;
Surgeon in Ophthalmology
Boston Eye Surgery & Laser Center
Boston, Massachusetts

Paul Moyer, MD
Good Samaritan Hospital
Kettering Medical Center
VA Medical Center
Dayton, Ohio

Thomas F. Neuhann, MD
Professor
University LMU Munich;
Head Ophthalmologist
Red Cross Hospital
Munich, Germany

Kenneth D. Novak, MD
Clinical Assistant Professor of Ophthalmology
SUNY Upstate Medical Center;
Eye Associates of Utica, PC
Utica, New York

Robert H. Osher, MD
Professor of Ophthalmology
University of Cincinnati
College of Medicine;
Medical Director Emeritus
Cincinnati Eye Institute
Cincinnati, Ohio

Mark Packer, MD
Oregon Eye Associates
Eugene, Oregon

Suresh K. Pandey, MD
John A. Moran Eye Center
Department of Ophthalmology and Visual Sciences
University of Utah
Salt Lake City, Utah

Robert I. Park, MD
University of Arizona
Phoenix, Arizona

Qun Peng, MD
John A. Moran Eye Center
Department of Ophthalmology
University of Utah
Salt Lake City, Utah

Richard Pesavento, MD
Assistant Clinical Professor of Ophthalmology
Loma Linda University
Loma Linda, California

Michael B. Raizman, MD
Associate Professor of Ophthalmology
Tufts University School of Medicine;
Director, Cornea and Anterior Segment Service
New England Eye Center
Boston, Massachusetts

Claudia Richter, MD
Clinical Assistant in Ophthalmology
Harvard Medical School;
Assistant Surgeon in Ophthalmology
Massachusetts Eye and Ear Infirmary
Boston, Massachusetts

Bradford Shingleton, MD
Assistant Clinical Professor of Ophthalmology
Harvard Medical School
Boston, Massachusetts

Richard J. Simmons, MD
Center for Eye Research and Education
Ophthalmic Consultants of Boston
Boston, Massachusetts

Ruthanne B. Simmons, MD†
Ophthalmic Consultants of Boston
Boston, Massachusetts

Michael E. Snyder, MD
Cincinnati Eye Institute
Cincinnati, Ohio

Terrence S. Spencer, MD
Ophthalmology Resident
University Hospital
John A. Moran Eye Center
Salt Lake City, Utah

Roger F. Steinert, MD
Associate Clinical Professor
Department of Ophthalmology
Harvard Medical School;
Ophthalmic Consultants of Boston
Boston, Massachusetts

Gregory M. Sulkowski, BA
Harvard Medical School
Boston, Massachusetts

Trexler Topping, MD
Ophthalmic Consultants of Boston
Boston, Massachusetts

Rupal H. Trivedi, MD
John A. Moran Eye Center
Department of Ophthalmology and Visual Sciences
University of Utah
Salt Lake City, Utah

Carl B. Tubbs, MD
Clinical Assistant Professor
University of Minnesota
Associated Eye Care
Stillwater, Minnesota

†Deceased.

Li Wang, MD, PhD
Cullen Eye Institute
Houston, Texas

Liliana Werner, MD, PhD
John A. Moran Eye Center
Department of Ophthalmology and Visual Sciences
University of Utah
Salt Lake City, Utah

PREFACE

Machiavelli wrote, "There is nothing more difficult to take in hand, more perilous to conduct, or more uncertain in success, than to take the lead in the introduction of a new order of things." In 1974, a bright young ophthalmologist, recognizing the potential of intraocular lenses, undertook the challenge of creating a vehicle for the new order and founded the American Intra-Ocular Implant Society. That man was Kenneth Hoffer, MD, who, in addition to his definitive chapter on IOL power calculation, has contributed a highly personal chapter on the history of IOL implantation. He captured the attention and then the commitment of a group of surgeons whose inspiration, talent, and energy have carried cataract surgery farther and faster than anyone could have imagined a quarter century ago. The group, subsequently renamed the American Society of Cataract and Refractive Surgery, is now the largest and most vigorous specialty society in ophthalmology by a large margin. This text is, in part, a tribute to where these surgeons have brought us.

In creating the Second Edition, we are reaffirming a commitment to excellence in the dominant ophthalmic surgical procedure. Cataract surgery cures the most common cause of vision loss. Because of the inspiration and perspiration of the previous generation of surgeons, this procedure has been transformed from one with a high rate of complications, prolonged recovery, and permanent visual disability to one of the great successes of medical technology and surgical skill, with rapid recovery to a level of function often better than before the development of the cataract, and at a small fraction of the earlier cost.

Our goal is to create a definitive resource for cataract surgeons at all stages of their careers. The text ranges from preoperative fundamentals and operative techniques through avoidance and management of complications and special situations, ending with a glimpse of new technology. We pay tribute to the leaders who have brought us to this level, and we salute all cataract surgeons who are committed to the never-ending pursuit of perfect surgery.

Roger F. Steinert, MD

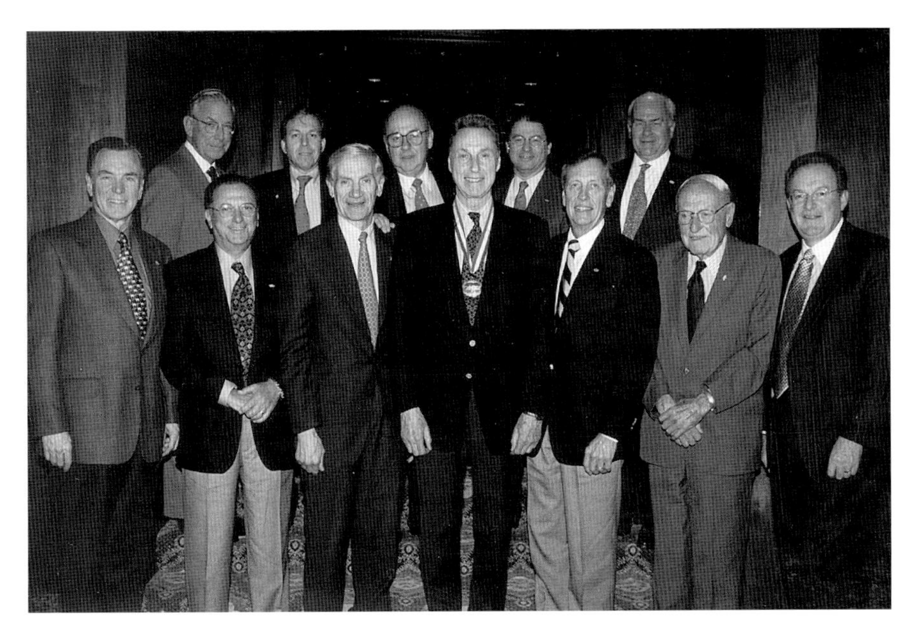

Some of the original leaders of the American Society of Cataract and Refractive Surgery. *Front Row:* Spencer P. Thornton, Charles D. Kelman, Manus C. Kraff, Robert M. Sinskey, Guy E. Knolle, John E. Gilmore, Executive Director David Karcher. *Back Row:* Robert C. Drews, Kenneth J. Hoffer, Jack M. Dodick, Stephen A. Obstbaum, John D. Hunkeler.

ACKNOWLEDGMENTS

The Second Edition represents a doubling of the original text. In the First Edition, we created a teaching textbook that thoroughly covered all the basics of cataract surgery and its complications. In the Second Edition, our goal was not only to update that text, but also to include virtually all the nuances of cataract surgery and its complications in a variety of settings. Our many contributors, worked long hours to produce extraordinary chapters on virtually all of the many ramifications of cataract surgery. This text was only possible because of the time-honored medical ethic of donating one's time and talent freely to educate one's colleagues and to advance the level of care. There is no way to adequately thank all of you, except to gratefully acknowledge your gifts!

At Elsevier, we were supported by a dedicated staff. Four Managing Editors have seen this large project through, beginning with Kim Cox and her successor, Allan Ross, who approved the Second Edition and oversaw its organization, through Natasha Andjelkovic, PhD, who oversaw most of the writing phase, to Paul Fam, who has been in charge of the final production. Agnes Hunt Byrne, Managing Developmental Editor, has been the cornerstone of the text editing and assembly process. Mike McConnell of Graphic World Publishing Services managed the production of the textbook. They have all been highly professional and a pleasure to work with.

The artwork has been created by Laurel Cook Lhowe, the principal artist for both editions. Her ability to grasp the concepts of the authors and translate them into drawings with striking clarity is legendary. I have had the pleasure of working with Laurel for nearly two decades, and I remain awed by her ability to capture the essence of surgical subtleties.

Each of the authors, as well as the editors, sacrificed free time and asked for forbearance from their families and their staff. You are too numerous to name, but each of us thanks you deeply for your support.

Finally, all of us wish to give special acknowledgement to the central role of Charles Kelman, MD, in the innovations that have brought our surgical specialty to its current level. Charlie is generally acknowledged as the most influential cataract surgeon in the twentieth century. The ramifications of his enormous number of insights have yet to be fully appreciated. Every cataract surgeon, and, more importantly, every cataract patient, has directly benefited from Charlie's creativity. Charlie, we thank you every day!

Roger F. Steinert, MD

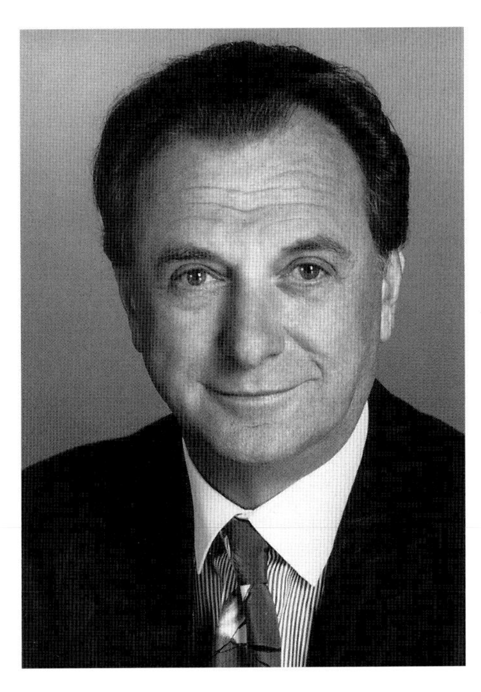

Charles Kelman, MD

CONTENTS

†Deceased.

The Pathology of Cataracts

1

Terrence S. Spencer, MD
Nick Mamalis, MD

Lens Embryology

Knowledge of the embryology of the lens helps one better understand its normal anatomy and the nature of cataracts. Lens cells form early during embryogenesis from surface ectoderm. The optic vesicles (neuroectodermally derived outpouchings of the diencephalon) enlarge to come in contact with the surface ectoderm, which thickens to form the lens plate. At the same time, the optic vesicle begins invaginating, and an indentation called the lens pit forms in the lens plate. The lens pit continues to invaginate as surface ectoderm cells multiply. Eventually, a sphere of cells called the lens vesicle breaks off from the stalk, which kept it connected to the remainder of the surface. The lens vesicle at this point contains a single layer of cuboidal cells within an outer basement membrane. The outer basement membrane forms the lens capsule.

The posterior cells of the lens vesicle begin to elongate anteriorly to become the primary lens fibers (Figure 1-1). These primary lens fibers meet the anterior lens cuboidal cells, obliterating the lumen of the lens vesicle. The primary lens fibers make up the embryonic nucleus, and the anterior lens cuboidal cells are now called the lens epithelial cells. The layer of lens epithelium maintains its presence anteriorly and just posterior to the equator, but no epithelial cells are normally present in the posterior part of the lens.

Secondary lens fibers form from lens epithelial cells near the equator, which begin to multiply and elongate anteriorly under the lens epithelium and posteriorly under the lens capsule. These secondary lens fibers form the fetal nucleus during gestation and continue to grow in this manner, adding new layers. As the lens fibers grow, they extend from the equator to meet anteriorly and posteriorly, forming Y-shaped sutures where they meet during fetal growth. During childhood and adolescence, lens fibers surround the fetal nucleus to become the adult nucleus. Subsequent lens fibers grow to surround the entire nucleus, forming lens cortex.

During fetal development the lens nucleus becomes enveloped within the tunica vasculosa lentis, a nutritive support structure supplied by the hyaloid artery. This structure atrophies and usually disappears by birth.

Normal Anatomy of the Lens

The lens is normally a clear, biconvex structure (Figure 1-2). Viewed from the side, it has an elliptical shape, measuring about 3.5 to 4 mm anterior-posterior by 9 to 10 mm in diameter. It is located posterior to and loosely apposed to the iris. Lens transparency is a function of regular cell shape, regular cell volume, minimal extracellular space, and minimal scatter elements.[1]

The lens is held in place by the zonules, which attach it to the ciliary body. The zonular fibers arise from the basement membrane of the nonpigmented epithelium of the ciliary body and attach just anteriorly and posteriorly to the equator of the lens. Tension on the zonules is reduced by contraction of the ciliary muscle, allowing the lens to become more spherical for accommodation.

The lens is lined on its outer surface by the lens capsule, which is responsible for elasticity, allowing the lens to accommodate. The lens capsule varies in thickness and is thinnest at the posterior pole. Histologically, the lens capsule stains positive with periodic acid–Schiff stain because it is a true basement membrane of the lens epithelial cells.

Lens epithelial cells are arranged in a single row of cuboidal cells along the anterior surface of the lens and end at the lens bow, where new lens fibers are produced. Nutrients and waste products pass through the lens capsule by diffusion and active transport from the anterior epithelium. The equatorial bow region of the lens (Figure 1-3), just posterior to the equator, is where lens epithelial cells elongate to form lens fiber cells. Normally, there are no lens epithelial cells along the posterior pole of the lens capsule.

The cortex and nucleus make up the substance of the lens. The fibers derived earliest lie centrally and form the embryonic, fetal, and, finally, adult nucleus. The lens cortex is formed from the most peripheral fibers found between the nucleus and

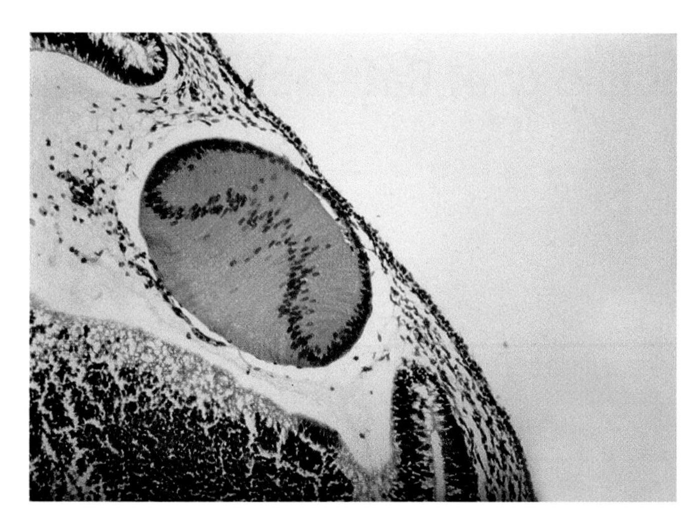

FIGURE 1-1 Embryo lens. Posterior epithelial cells of the lens vesicle elongate to become lens fibers. (Hematoxylin and eosin [H & E] stain; ×10.)

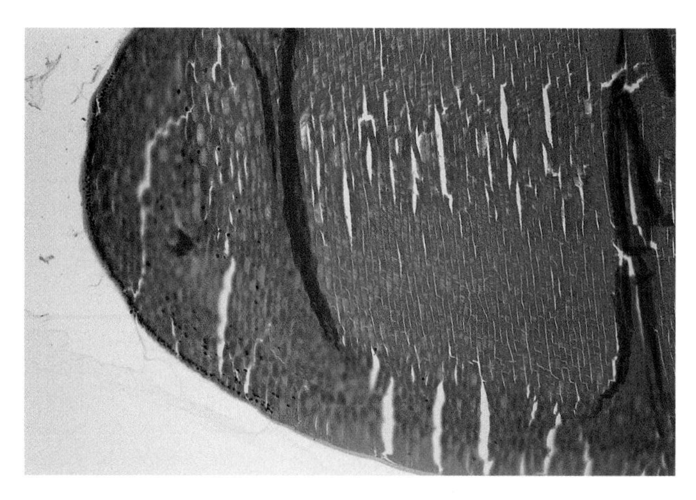

FIGURE 1-3 Lens bow. Lens epithelial cells elongate from the equator to form new lens fibers. The nuclei appear to fan out from the edge of the lens seen in cross section. There are no epithelial cells beneath the posterior surface of the lens capsule. (H & E stain; ×10.)

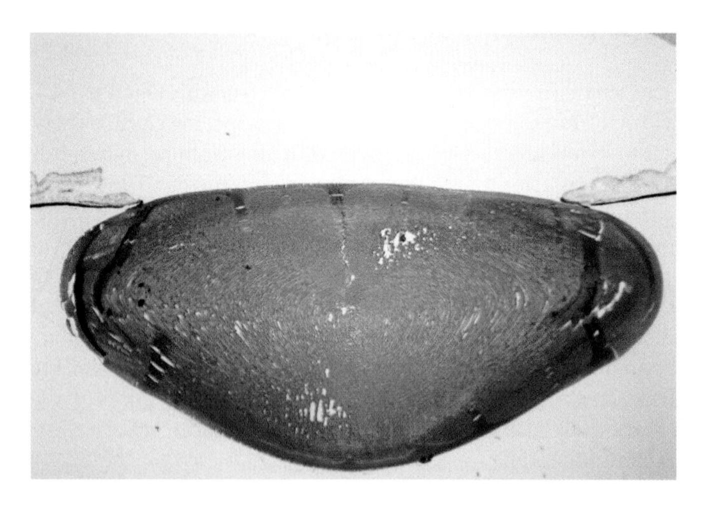

FIGURE 1-2 Normal lens. Histologic section of a normal lens from an enucleated globe showing artifactual clefts and folds. (H & E stain; ×2.)

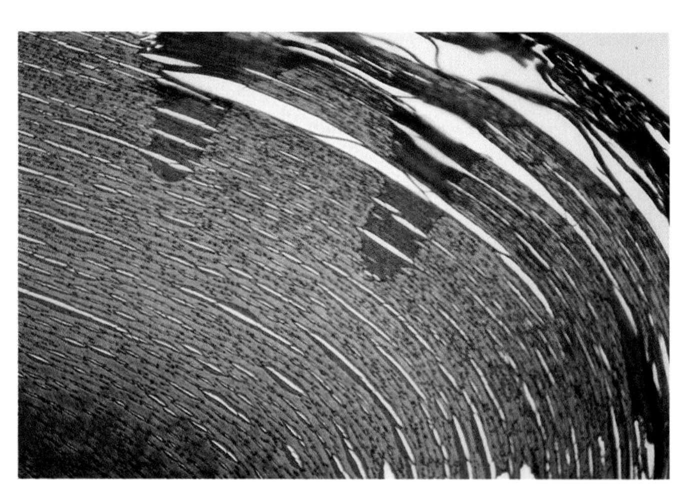

FIGURE 1-4 Lens substance. Normal fibers appear in layers at the periphery of the lens. The clefts are artifacts from histologic sectioning. (Trichrome stain; ×20.)

capsule (Figure 1-4). As more cortical fibers are produced at the periphery, inner fibers are added to the defined adult lens nucleus.

Introduction to Cataract Pathology

The term *cataract* refers to any opacity of various degree of the crystalline lens, which is normally almost completely transparent. A variety of methods can be used to classify cataracts clinically, but pathologic examination of cataracts may be difficult. The lens tends to survive fairly well postmortem because it does not have its own blood supply, but it does not have the same gross appearance as its clinical appearance in vivo. Hardness of the explanted lens correlates highly with clinical grading of nuclear sclerosis, but not with cortical or subcapsular opacities.[2,3] One problem with pathologic examination of a cataract is the alteration in the appearance of the lens when it is placed in fixatives for preservation of tissue. The microscopic alterations that are seen on histologic sections do not necessarily correlate with the severity of cataract and visual dysfunction seen clinically. When the lens is processed and sectioned for histologic examination, numerous artifacts appear in its structure.

With normal aging, the lens increases in overall size and loses its ability to accommodate. Continued growth of lens fibers with aging causes the nucleus to become compressed and less pliable (nuclear sclerosis).[2,4] Nuclear lens proteins aggregate and are chemically modified to produce pigmentation, decreasing transparency. The increase in pigmentation causes the lens nucleus to appear yellow or, with excess pigmentation, brown (brunescent cataract). Proteins within the cytoplasm of lens cells are modified in a manner that scatters visible light, resulting in opacification.[5] A decrease in metabolic transport of antioxidants in an aging lens, as a result, may allow oxidation of nuclear components.[6] Hydrogen peroxide (H_2O_2), one oxidant, is found at elevated concentrations in some patients with maturity-onset cataract. The activities of glutathione peroxidase, the major enzyme that metabolizes H_2O_2, and other antioxidant enzymes may be reduced in older individuals.[7] The oxidative damage is thought to start in the nucleus of the lens where metabolic activities would be lowest and where modified proteins, susceptible to oxidation, would accumulate with age.[8]

Changes within the lens nucleus are usually accompanied by changes in other parts of the lens. Aging causes nuclear, cortical, and posterior subcapsular cataracts, each to varying degrees. When these changes cause a cataract in the lens, the patient may experience visual impairment, loss of contrast, and dulling perception of color and may also become increasingly myopic. In addition to loss of visual acuity, cataract development may be associated with visual aberrations such as monocular double or triple vision.[9] Clinically mature or "ripe" cataracts may result in total opacification and liquefaction. A hypermature or "overripened" cataract sometimes progresses from the stage of morgagnian cataract (discussed under Cortical Cataracts) to a shrunken membranous cataract after spontaneous loss of liquid protein and resorption of liquefied cortex.

Cataracts are clinically classified in different manners according to location, age of onset, appearance, or cause. The other sections of this book thoroughly cover the etiology of cataracts related to disease and medications. This chapter focuses primarily on the histopathologic features of cataracts based mainly on location of the cataract within the lens.

Congenital Cataracts

Congenital cataracts are present at birth or noted shortly afterward. The morphology of congenital cataracts can be helpful in establishing their cause and prognosis.[10] They are usually bilateral and may occur in association with other medical problems. The insult to the developing lens is often mild enough that the resultant opacity does not interfere with vision.

Congenital zonular cataracts are characterized by opacities situated in one layer of the lens and surrounded by clear lens. A central nuclear cataract from an insult early in development of the lens would be displaced deeper into the lens substance as new fibers grow throughout life.[11] An *embryonal nuclear cataract* results from an injury to the lens during the first 2 months of gestation and would be seen as a small central opacification. A *fetal nuclear cataract* (Figure 1-5) results from an insult at about the third month of gestation and would lie between the level of the anterior and posterior Y sutures or at the sutures *(sutural cataract)*. Sutural opacities with secondary arborization or branching signify a teratologic insult later in gestation. A *perinuclear* or *lamellar zone* from a later insult would be arranged concentrically to the lens capsule with the cataractous layer surrounding the nucleus. The lamellar cataract takes its name from the laminar or sheetlike anatomy of the lens and is surrounded by the more peripheral clear cortical layers of the lens.[12,13]

Polar cataracts are opacities located on the anterior or posterior pole. Fibrous metaplasia of the anterior lens epithelium causes an *anterior polar cataract* (Figure 1-6). When caused by hyperplasia of the embryonal pupillary membrane, a conical mass of connective tissue (pyramidal cataract) protrudes into the anterior chamber. Histologically, a localized loss of epithelial cells with an anterior subcapsular plaque is seen (see also Anterior Subcapsular Abnormalities later in this chapter).

A *posterior polar cataract* is a larger disc-shaped opacity resulting from persistent hyperplastic primary vitreous and can result in degeneration of the posterior subcapsular cortex with progressive opacification. A hyaloid vessel remnant, called a *Mittendorf dot,* is a small, dense white spot on the posterior surface of the lens and is clinically insignificant.

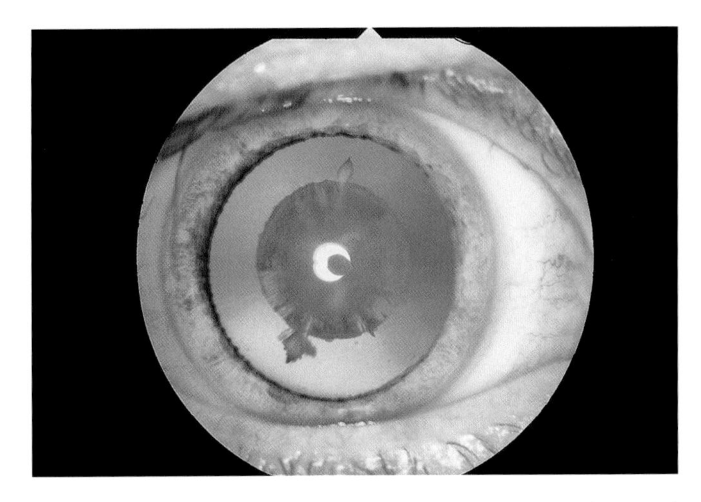

FIGURE 1-5 Fetal nuclear cataract. Clinical appearance of a central cataract surrounded by normal lens tissue.

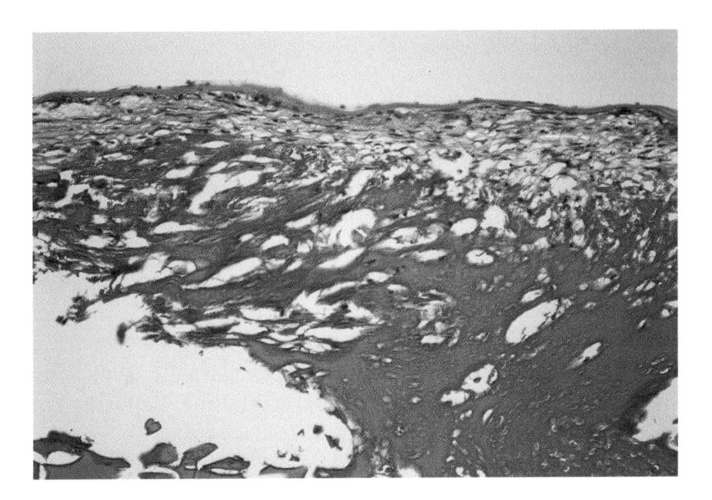

FIGURE 1-6 Anterior polar cataract. The lens epithelium has been replaced by fibrous metaplasia. (H & E stain; ×20.)

Nuclear Cataracts

The most common age-related opacity of the lens is the nuclear sclerotic cataract (Figure 1-7). Increased compaction of nuclear fibers in age-related cataracts may be a contributing factor for excessive scatter in nuclear opacification.[14] Clinically, cataractous lens nuclei have decreased transparency in addition to the increased amount of pigmentation often found in normal

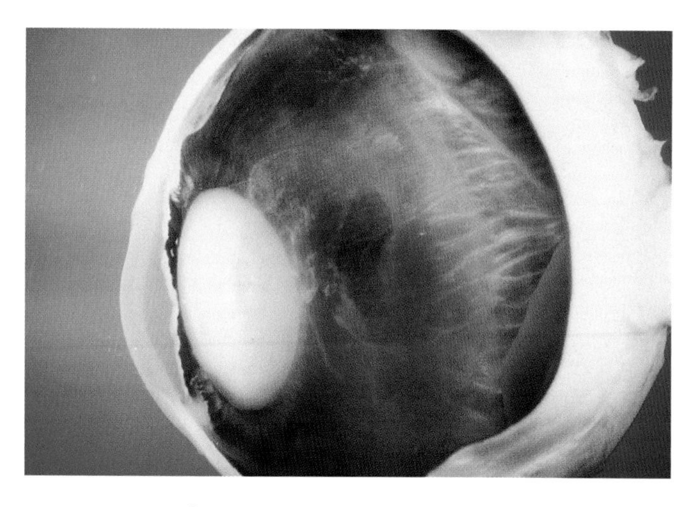

FIGURE 1-7 Cataractous lens. This enucleated globe is sectioned sagitally to show the gross appearance of a cataractous lens.

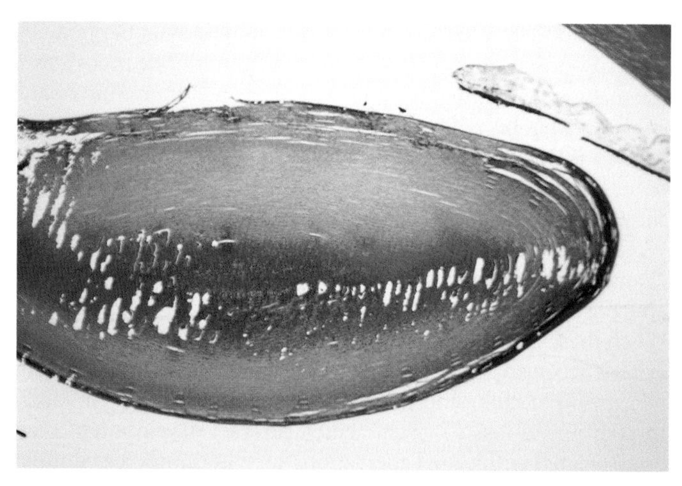

FIGURE 1-8 Nuclear sclerotic cataract. The nucleus from this postmortem globe with a senile cataract takes on a dense homogenous appearance. Changes are often subtle, as in this specimen. (Trichrome stain; ×2.)

aging. The lens nucleus normally appears histologically to have cellular laminations, which become more compact with aging. Lenses with nuclear sclerotic cataracts are characterized histopathologically by subtle changes with a dense homogeneous appearance (Figure 1-8). The laminations fade, and the nucleus becomes amorphous, taking on a more uniform eosinophilic staining characteristic. In an isolated nuclear sclerotic cataract, the surrounding cortical fibers would microscopically retain visible outlines of the cytoplasmic membranes. The increase in lens pigmentation seen clinically is not usually evident by histopathologic examination, but crystalline deposits are sometimes observed.[15]

Cortical Cataracts

Aging changes in the lens cortex result in cortical cataracts. Lens epithelium likely plays a role in the loss of transparency of the cortex.[16] Insoluble proteins are assumed to be characteristic of cortical cataractous epithelium, which is also accompanied by various morphologic abnormalities such as spokes or rosettes[17] (Figure 1-9). Histopathologically, accumulation of eosinophilic fluid between lens cells with displacement and degeneration of bordering cells characterizes cortical cataracts (Figure 1-10). Clefts seen microscopically correspond to visible changes observed clinically by slit lamp examination. Spherical droplets or globules of released protein from breakdown of cortical cell walls are called *morgagnian globules* (Figure 1-11). Encountering these droplets during surgical cataract excision may release milky fluid. These globules may accumulate, and they may eventually replace the entire cortex and result in a mature morgagnian cataract.[18] The central dense nucleus at this point would become gravity dependent, often displaced inferiorly to the lower equatorial region of the lens (Figure 1-12).

The deep cortex of some lenses has been found to have crystalline deposits, which can appear as a "Christmas tree

A

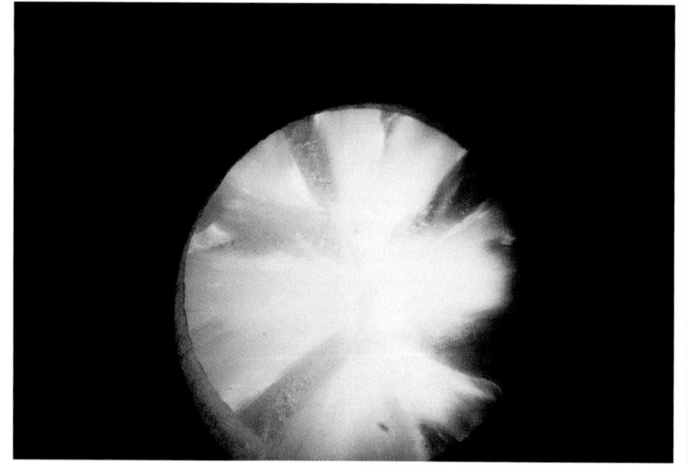

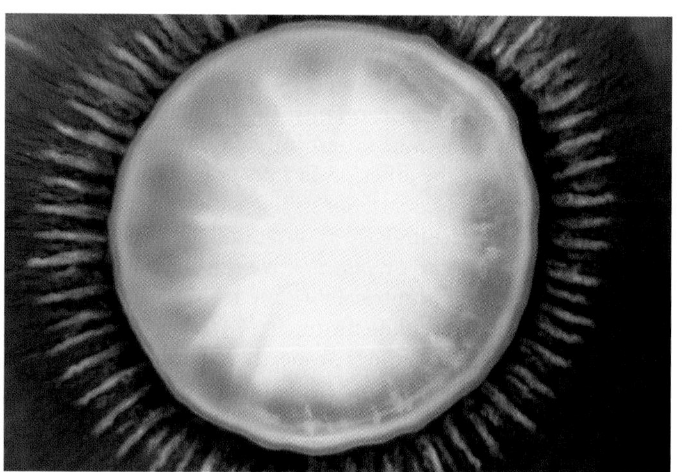

B

FIGURE 1-9 Cortical cataract. **A,** Clinical photograph of a senile cataract with cortical fluid clefts. **B,** Posterior view of an enucleated globe with cortical spokes.

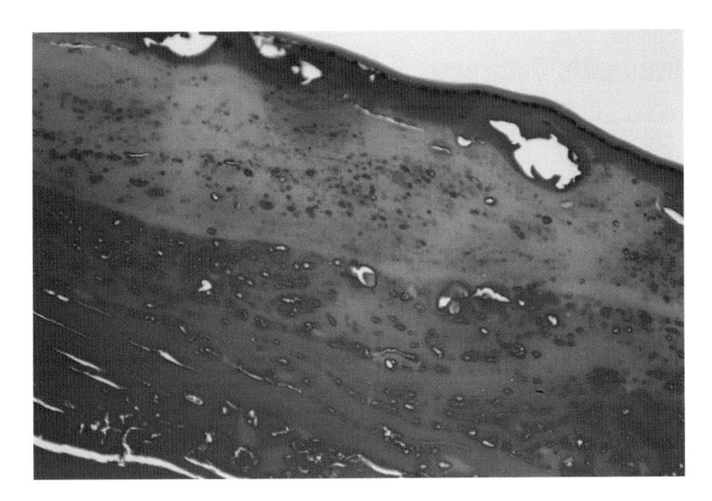

FIGURE 1-10 Cortical cataract. Histologic section of an early cortical cataract with accumulation of eosinophilic fluid between lens fibers. (H & E stain; ×10.)

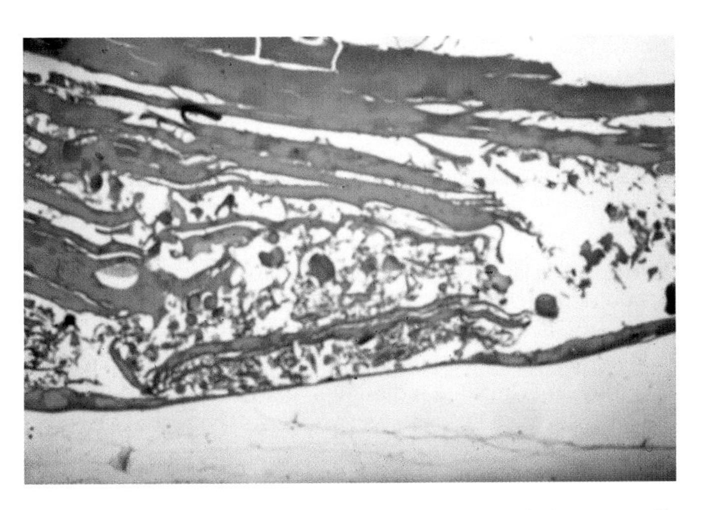

FIGURE 1-11 Morgagnian globules. Advanced cortical cataract with breakdown of lens proteins, histologically appearing as eosinophilic-staining spheres. (H & E stain; ×10.)

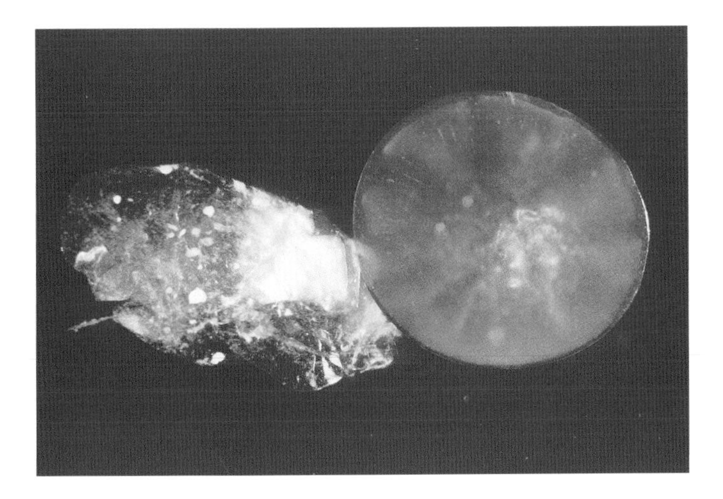

FIGURE 1-12 Morgagnian cataract. Gross appearance of a dense lens nucleus and its associated capsule in a mature morgagnian cataract.

cataract."[19] The crystals may be formed from cholesterol, lipids, calcium, or other compounds and in many cases do not decrease visual acuity unless other forms of cataracts coexist, but these crystals can be associated with phacolytic glaucoma.[20] Some forms of crystals are visible on histologic examination by use of cross-polarized filters.

Posterior Subcapsular Cataracts

Clinically visible opacification located just anterior to the posterior lens capsule may be formed idiopathically or after an injury to the posterior area of the lens. In addition, posterior subcapsular cataracts may form secondary to multiple medications such as corticosteroids and in association with various systemic conditions. These posterior subcapsular cataracts appear as focal, dotlike granular areas or plaques in the posterior subcapsular cortex (Figure 1-13). This type of cataract is associated with degeneration of subcapsular posterior cortical cells followed by proliferation of peripheral lens epithelial cells, which migrate posteriorly beyond the lens bow at which it normally terminates.[21] The posterior migration of lens epithelial cells possibly represents an attempt to replace the degenerate, sometimes liquefied lens substance in the cataractous lens and can be seen in diverse cataract conditions. The abnormally positioned epithelial cells enlarge and are called bladder or Wedl cells.[22] The nuclei of the bloated bladder cells are visible in histologic sections (Figure 1-14).

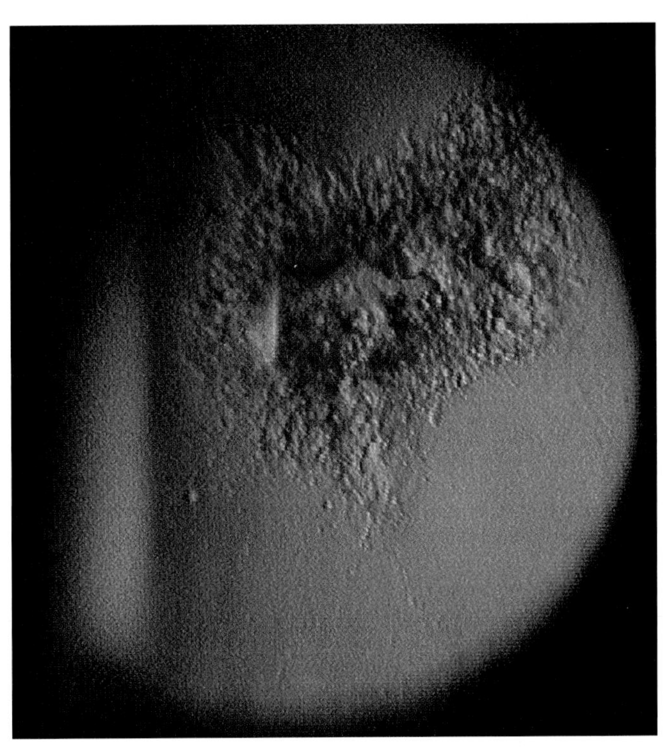

FIGURE 1-13 Posterior subcapsular cataract. Clinical photograph of a focal granular area in the posterior subcapsular cortex.

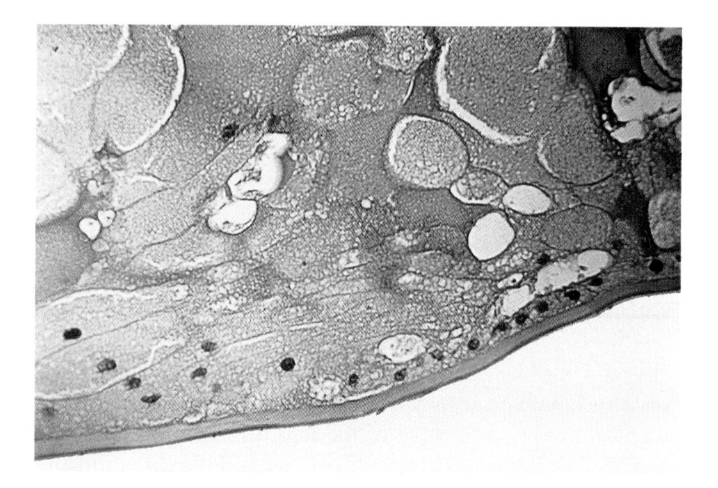

FIGURE 1-14 Bladder cells (Wedl cells). Lens epithelial cells have become swollen after abnormally migrating to the posterior pole of the lens. (H & E stain; ×20.)

Anterior Subcapsular Abnormalities

Subepithelial lens opacities have been observed following an attack of acute glaucoma, and, when such an association exists, are described as *glaukomflecken*. The severe elevation of intra-aocular pressure may form grayish opacities localized beneath the anterior lens capsule, which histologically appear as focal areas of epithelial cell necrosis.[23] Epithelial cell degeneration can be in response to other insults such as radiation and inflammation.

An *anterior subcapsular plaque* can form from proliferation and subsequent degeneration of lens epithelial cells leading to opacities. This type of cataract is usually the result of irritation, from uveitis, or disruption from trauma (discussed later in this chapter). Histologically, the plaque of the anterior or equatorial lens epithelium appears as a thin layer of fibrous tissue (fibrous metaplasia).[24] Multiple layers of such plaques may be laid down with intervening layers of normal cortex to form a reduplication cataract (Figure 1-15).

Traumatic Cataracts

Contusion of the eye may be severe enough to cause deposition of iris pigment on the lens capsule (Vossius ring). A Vossius ring is an imprint of the pupillary margin of the iris, and the pigment may resolve with time. Severe enough blunt force may cause formation of a cataract, which initially appears stellate with opacities lying in the cortex or capsule. Disruption of the lens zonular fibers from injuries can cause the lens to be dislocated or partially dislocated (subluxated). Some blunt traumas cause both cataract formation and dislocation of the lens. The dislocation may be in any direction. Changes leading to lens opacity in traumatic cataracts appear to involve epithelial and subsequent cortical fiber deterioration.[25]

Laceration or perforation of the lens capsule from trauma results in a localized opacity usually progressing to opacification of the entire lens. Histologically, the ruptured capsule typically appears as a wrinkled membrane. Opacities from small capsular injuries may remain stable as a focal cortical cataract, but exposed cortex often swells, expanding through the capsular tear. This process may induce a granulomatous inflammatory response of the remaining lens nucleus. Retained metallic foreign bodies within the lens may cause focal, rusty appearing opacities (siderosis lentis).

The lens is susceptible to damage induced by ionizing radiation, with cataract formation often occurring many years after the initial exposure. Cataracts induced by radiation are usually observed in the posterior region of the lens, often in the form of a posterior subcapsular cataract.[26] Radiation exposure of the lens has a cumulative effect, but large doses can cause sudden injury to lens epithelial cells and subsequent opacity of the entire lens. Infrared radiation and intense heat exposure to the lens, as seen in glass blowers, has caused cobweblike cortical opacities and changes in the lens capsule.

When only a small portion of lens epithelial cells and cortical material remain in the periphery of the capsule after trauma or cataract extraction, a *Soemmering's ring cataract* may form (Figure 1-16). The epithelial remnants undergo proliferation or

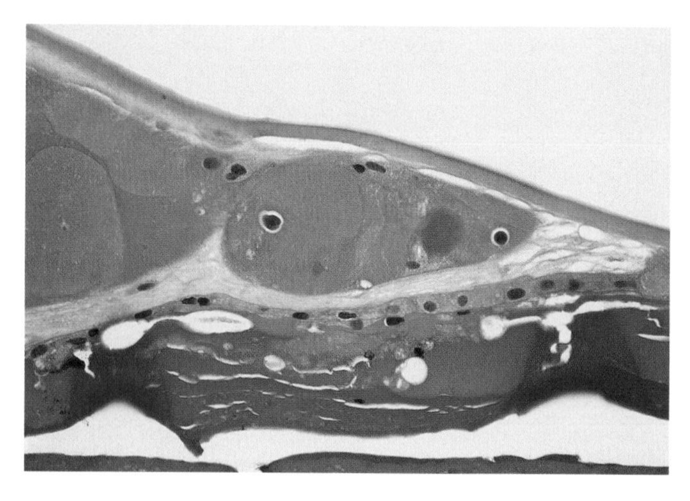

FIGURE 1-15 Anterior subcapsular cataract. Epithelial cells appear posterior to an abnormal fibrous plaque. (H & E stain; ×20.)

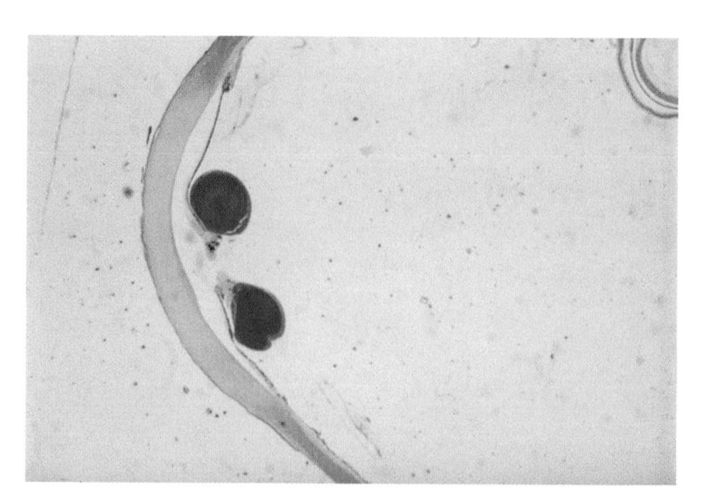

FIGURE 1-16 Soemmering's ring cataract. Soemmering's ring in this eye formed after traumatic rupture of the capsule and loss of most of the lens contents. (H & E stain, ×2.)

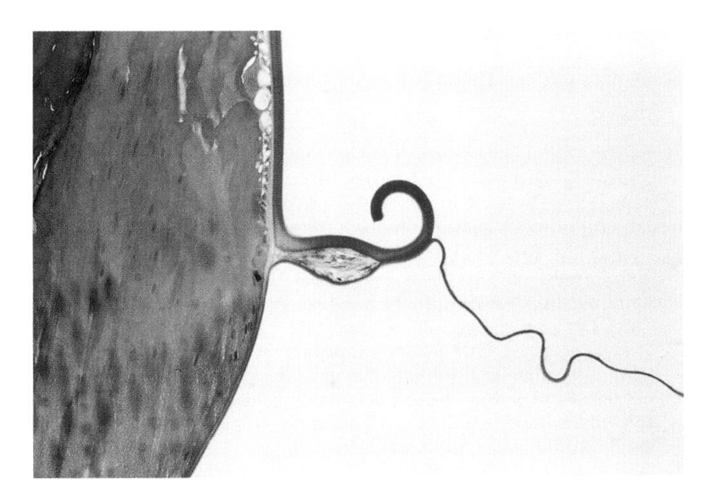

FIGURE 1-17 Soemmering's ring cataract. Lens epithelial cells proliferate in the periphery of the lens capsule. (Trichrome stain; ×40.)

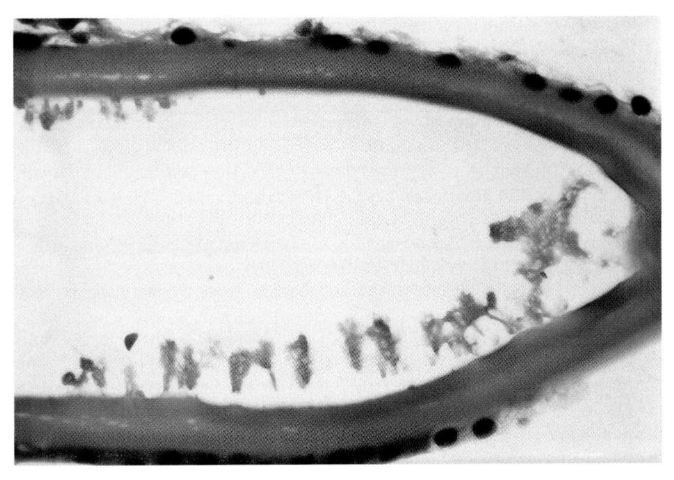

FIGURE 1-18 Pseudoexfoliation. This curled-up piece of anterior lens capsule removed during cataract surgery shows deposits lined up, resembling iron filings on a magnet. The outer surface of the lens capsule is opposite the remaining lens epithelial cells. (H & E stain; ×100.)

fibrous metaplasia to form a doughnut-shaped ring. A histologic examination of the Soemmering's ring would reveal a barbell-shaped cross section with a residual lens capsular membrane forming the shaft that connects a bulbous prominence of retained lens cortex at one or both equators[27] (Figure 1-17).

Lens epithelial cells displaced through the capsule by accidental or surgical trauma can regenerate and proliferate in an abnormal location to form *Elschnig pearls.* Microscopically the pearls resemble clusters of the bladder cells (Wedl cells) found in the posterior aspect of a cataractous lens, except they are found in the anterior chamber on the lens surface or iris stroma.

Pseudoexfoliation and True Exfoliation

Exfoliation syndrome (pseudoexfoliation) is a different entity than *true exfoliation.*[28] True exfoliation is a rare delamination of the lens capsule, which peels off in outward curling scrolls. Most patients with true exfoliation have a history of exposure to intense heat or infrared radiation. Histologically, the lens capsule appears thickened, and the outer portion may peel away from the intact layer closest to the lens epithelium. The peripheral portion of lens capsule often appears normal.[29]

In contrast, the more common pseudoexfoliation material is believed to be basement membrane material arising within the anterior chamber and appearing on the lens, iris, corneal endothelium, and trabecular meshwork. The material, initially believed to be a deposit on the lens,[28] is synthesized from lens epithelial cells and by cells of the iris and ciliary epithelium.[30] Clinically, the deposit appears on the anterior lens capsule as a central disc surrounded by a relatively clear zone, surrounded by peripheral granular area. Pseudoexfoliation can cause secondary open-angle glaucoma called *glaucoma capsulare.* Weakening of the zonular fibers can complicate cataract surgery in these patients. Histopathologically, the lens capsule surface appears to have straight deposits resembling iron filings aligned on a magnet (Figure 1-18). The material may also be found on or within the iris, trabecular meshwork, and the corneal endothelium.

Conclusion

In conclusion, cataracts can present with a large variety of histopathologic changes. These cataractous changes can involve any of the structures of the lens, including the nucleus, cortex, and anterior and posterior subcapsular areas. A thorough understanding of the pathology of various types of cataracts will allow the surgeon to more adequately prepare for the removal of a cataractous lens.

REFERENCES

1. Garner MH, Kuszak JR: Cations, oxidants, light as causative agents in senile cataracts, *P R Health Sci J* 12:115-122, 1993.
2. Heyworth P, Thompson GM, Tabandeh H et al: The relationship between clinical classification of cataract and lens hardness, *Eye* 7:726-730, 1993.
3. Assia EI, Medan I, Rosner M: Correlation between clinical, physical, and histopathological characteristics of the cataractous lens, *Graefes Arch Clin Exp Ophthalmol* 235:745-748, 1997.
4. Duncan G, Wormstone IM, Davies PD: The aging human lens: structure, growth, and physiological behaviour, *Br J Ophthalmol* 81:818-823, 1997.
5. Clark JI, Clark JM: Lens cytoplasmic phase separation, *Int Rev Cytol* 192:171-187, 2000.
6. Truscott RJ: Age-related nuclear cataract: a lens transport problem, *Ophthalmic Res* 32:185-194, 2000.
7. Spector A: Oxidation and aspects of ocular pathology, *CLAO J* 16(1 suppl): S8-10, 1990.
8. Augusteyn RC: Protein modification in cataract: possible oxidative mechanisms. In Duncan G, editor: *Mechanisms of cataract formation in the human lens,* London, 1981, Academic Press, pp 72-111.
9. Campbell C: Observations on the optical effects of a cataract, *J Cataract Refract Surg* 25:995-1003, 1999.
10. Lambert SR, Drack AV: Infantile cataracts, *Surv Ophthalmol* 40:427-458, 1996.
11. Eagle RCJ, Spencer WH: Lens. In Spencer WH, editor: *Ophthalmic pathology: an atlas and textbook,* ed 4, vol 1, Philadelphia, 1996, WB Saunders, pp 372-437.
12. Grottrau PD, Schlotzer-Schrehardt U, Dorfler S et al: Congenital zonular cataract: clinicopathologic correlation with electron microscopy and review of literature, *Arch Ophthalmol* 111:235-239, 1993.

13. Potter WS: Pediatric cataracts, *Pediatr Clin North Am* 40:841-851, 1993.
14. Al-Ghoul KJ, Nordgren RK, Kuszak AJ et al: Structural evidence of human nuclear fiber compaction as a function of aging and cataractogenesis, *Exp Eye Res* 72:199-214, 2001.
15. Zimmerman LE, Johnson FB: Calcium oxalate crystals within ocular tissues, *Arch Ophthalmol* 60:372-383, 1958.
16. Worgul BV, Merriam GRJ, Medvedovsky C: Cortical cataract development: an expression of primary damage to the lens epithelium, *Lens Eye Toxic Res* 6:559-571, 1989.
17. Kalariya N, Rawal UM, Vasavada AR: Human lens epithelial layer in cortical cataract, *Indian J Ophthalmol* 46:159-162, 1998.
18. Bron AJ, Habgood JO: Morgagnian cataract, *Trans Ophthalmol Soc U K* 96:265, 1976.
19. Shun-Shin GA, Vrensen GFJM, Brown NP: Morphologic characteristics and chemical composition of Christmas tree cataract, *Invest Ophthalmol Vision Sci* 34:3489-3496, 1993.
20. Flocks M, Litwin CS, Zimmerman LE: Phacolytic glaucoma: a clinicopathologic study of one hundred thirty-eight cases of glaucoma associated with hypermature cataract, *Arch Ophthalmol* 54:37, 1955.
21. Eshaghian J, Streeten BW: Human posterior subcapsular cataract: an ultrastructural study of the posteriorly migrating cells, *Arch Ophthalmol* 98:134-143, 1980.
22. Wedl C: *Atlas der pathologischen Histologie des Auges*, Leipzig, 1860-1861, Wigand.
23. Anderson DR: Pathology of the glaucomas, *Br J Ophthalmol* 56:146-157, 1972.
24. Font RL, Brownstein S: A light and electron microscope study of anterior subcapsular cataracts, *Am J Ophthalmol* 78:972-984, 1974.
25. Rafferty NS, Goossens W, March WF: Ultrastructure of human traumatic cataract, *Am J Ophthalmol* 78:985-995, 1974.
26. Lipman RM, Tripathi BJ, Tripathi RC: Cataracts induced by microwave and ionizing radiation, *Surv Ophthalmol* 33:200-210, 1988.
27. Apple DJ, Rabb MF: Lens and pathology of intraocular lenses. In Klein EA, editor. *Ocular pathology*, ed 3, St Louis, 1985, Mosby, pp 118-159.
28. Dvorak-Theobald GD: Pseudo-exfoliation of the lens capsule, *Am J Ophthalmol* 37:1-12, 1954.
29. Callahan A, Klien BA: Thermal detachment of the anterior lamella of the anterior lens capsule: a clinical and histopathologic study, *Arch Ophthalmol* 59:73-80, 1958.
30. Eagle RCJ, Font RL, Fine BS: The basement membrane exfoliation syndrome, *Arch Ophthalmol* 97:510-515, 1979.

Surgical Anatomy, Biochemistry, Pathogenesis, and Classification of Cataracts

2

Leo T. Chylack, Jr., MD

In the United States today, surgical extraction of the age-related cataract is the most frequently reimbursed operation in patients older than 65 years of age.[1] More than 1.4 million extractions per year are performed to restore visual function to older Americans. The technology supporting this procedure has evolved rapidly over the past 25 years as ophthalmic surgeons shifted from intracapsular to extracapsular techniques and as intraocular lenses (IOLs) replaced contact and spectacle lenses. The technology continues to evolve today as new techniques and materials reduce costs and surgical complexity and improve the optical quality of IOLs and functional end results. In developing countries, modern techniques are being adapted by surgeons serving huge numbers of patients with cataract-related blindness. Age-related cataract (Figure 2-1) is the leading cause of visual impairment in the world today; more than 50 million individuals have cataract-related visual impairment.[2]

The timely dissemination of up-to-date surgical knowledge is one way in which skilled surgeons can address the worldwide problem of cataract-related visual impairment and blindness. This chapter focuses on the evaluation and surgical care of individual patients and thus may be more useful to the young surgeon beginning his or her training in cataract surgery or the older surgeon contemplating a change in surgical technique than to the public health official charged with organizing the treatment of cataract in millions of indigent patients. However, the most modern surgical techniques are being applied successfully even in the most primitive settings to alleviate visual loss, and we hope that this text facilitates the transfer of surgical knowledge to those areas of the world where it is badly needed.

Surgical Anatomy of the Lens

The crystalline lens grows throughout life, changing its shape from a slightly rounded ovoid in childhood to a more flattened ovoid in old age. After the filling of the lens vesicle with lens fiber cells and the beginning of cortical fiber formation, the lens always contains a capsule, an anterior and equatorial layer of epithelium, a peripheral cortical region, and an inner nuclear core. In children and young adults with visually disabling cataracts, the capsule is strong, the vitreous is firm, and the ease with which the cortex and nucleus are removed is equal. In contrast, for older adults with age-related cataracts the surgeon must deal with an increasingly fragile capsule, a syneretic vitreous body, and a nucleus that may behave more like a piece of stone than a piece of living tissue. Knowledge of the surgical anatomy of the lens and of the changes that each region undergoes with age helps the surgeon plan and execute a successful procedure regardless of the age of the patient.

Capsule

The capsule originates as the basement membrane of the epithelial cells of the embryonic lens vesicle, which it encapsulates in its entirety. As the posterior vesicle cells elongate anteriorly and fill the vesicle, the capsule assumes an anterior and posterior aspect. The anterior capsule remains a basement membrane for the epithelial cells, but the posterior capsule is now a thin membrane that is merely adherent to the fiber cells growing along its inner surface. A twofold increase in anterior capsule thickness occurs with age[3]; the capsule is always thinnest posteriorly.[4]

For more than a century accommodative changes in the lens have been attributed to the intrinsic elasticity of the capsule. It has been assumed that relaxation of lens zonules allowed capsular elasticity to deform (round up) the lens and increase accommodative power. However, more modern techniques have shown that the capsule distributes other forces on the lens (i.e., from the ciliary body) but does not act primarily to deform the shape of the lens. Mathematical modeling[5] of accommodation of the human lens has progressed and now is able to characterize some of the age-associated changes in this process.[6]

The surgeon performing neodymium: yttrium-aluminum-garnet (Nd:YAG) laser capsulotomy knows that the intrinsic elasticity or scrollability of the capsule is responsible for the expansion of the opening made by the laser pulse, and the scrolling usually occurs along the external surface of the capsular bag, suggesting that greater stress acts on the outer rather than the inner filaments of the capsule. The elastic characteristics of the capsule change with secondary cataract formation as a layer of epithelial and fibrous cells are laid down on the inner surface of the capsular scaffold. Less tendency to scroll externally exists; often, cut flaps remain protruding stiffly into the optical zone. The formation of a capsular opacity may simply represent the continuation of the sliding movement of epithelial cells along the capsule that occurs normally in the

A

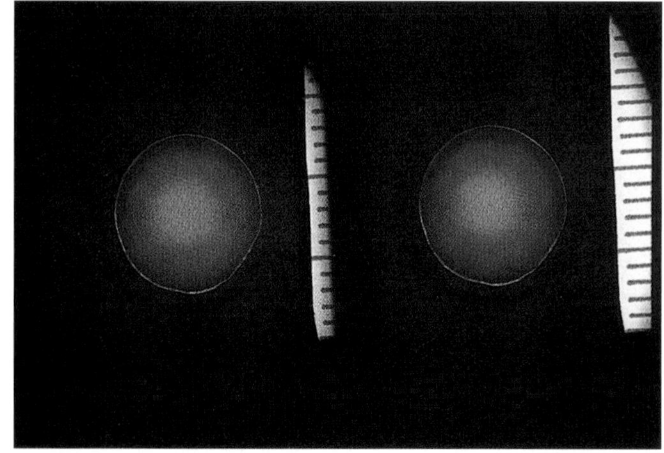

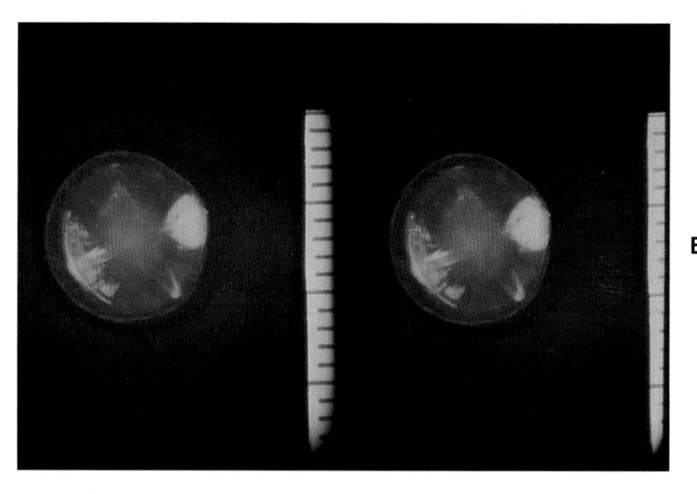

B

C

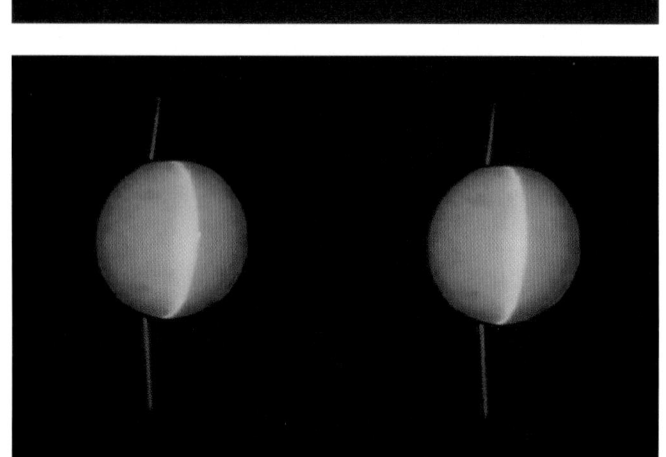

FIGURE 2-1 **A,** Minimal age-related nuclear cataract in an intracapsularly extracted lens. **B,** Moderately advance mixed corticonuclear age-related intracapsularly extracted cataract. **C,** Hypermature age-related cataract.

lens. On the inner surface of the anterior capsule of the intact lens, the anterior epithelial cells move from the midperiphery to the equatorial region, where they differentiate into fiber cells. Lacking a cortical region to join, the cells may continue to move posteriorly along the intact capsule and form balloon cells and fibrous or glassy plaques.

The expenditure of funds to cover the costs of treating posterior capsule opacification (PCO) is exceeded only by the cost of cataract surgery,[7] so there has been considerable interest in understanding the mechanism by which PCO occurs and devising treatments for it. Many articles have emphasized the reduction in incidence of PCO if foldable acrylic IOLs are used.[8,9] It may be possible to reduce (or eliminate) PCO by developing improved IOL design, but a great deal of effort has been invested in studying the cell biology of this process using a variety of experimental systems (cultured human capsular bags obtained postmortem, cell culture systems, in vivo animal model systems, and in situ human observation).[10] Human lens epithelial cells can survive and multiply in serum-free cell culture, so there are intrinsic mechanisms sustaining these cells. If serum is added, however, the replication rate increases dramatically. This has led to the search for paracrine factors (proteins from other cells), and a number of candidates have been found (transferrin, basic fibroblast growth factor, epithelial growth factor, and transforming growth factor beta [TGF-β]) that either accelerate proliferation or stimulate transdifferentiation of epithelial cells into fiber cells. Also, autocrine factors (transferrin) and other cytokines have been found.[11,12] Simply performing a capsulorhexis will stimulate epithelial cell proliferation[13] compared with the rate in the intact lens.

In a recent study of the effects of TGF-β2 on lens epithelial cells in capsular bag cultures, Wormstone et al[14] showed that a human monoclonal antibody CAT-152 (lerdelimumab) completely neutralized the effect of the TGF-β2-induced effects on the lens epithelial cells, leading to PCO. Other approaches to preventing or minimizing PCO involve the addition of cytotoxins to the haptics and/or the IOLs, but in these cases, toxicity to other intraocular cells (particularly the corneal endothelium) is a major concern. These are all well reviewed in Wormstone's article.

A point about the anterior capsule that has surgical relevance is that it is thickest in the midperiphery. More peripherally the capsule thins considerably. This may be part of the reason why a capsulorhexis placed too far peripherally extends into the equatorial region. The capsule tears easily as a circular disc if the tear is kept within the thicker zone.

Epithelium

With age, the height of the epithelial cells decreases and the width increases. Some studies have shown that a decrease in the number of epithelial cells occurs with cataract formation; other studies have been unable to find decreased numbers of cells. No anatomic features of the epithelium exist that influence surgical technique, but all ophthalmic surgeons recognize that the epithelium is exquisitely sensitive to trauma; its key metabolic role makes it the "Achilles' heel" of the lens.

In addition to the accelerated proliferation of lens epithelial cells in response to paracrine, autocrine, and mechanical factors, these same cells may undergo apoptosis (programmed cell death) in response to oxidative stress and TGF-β2. Oxidative stress in a well-known risk factor for age-related cataract, and TGB-β2 is a growth factor associated with the cellular changes underlying PCO. It may be possible, however, to use this growth factor to increase apoptotic death of cells remaining on the posterior capsule after cataract surgery.

An excellent review of aspects of the lens epithelium that make it generally interesting to biologic scientists (no tumors were found in lens epithelium, and it is an excellent model for the effects of age on epithelial cell function) has been published.[15]

Another publication reveals the dramatic changes that occur in the lens epithelium with age.[16] There were many "black holes" representing large areas of severely attenuated epithelial cells. In some areas there was no coverage of the overlying lens capsule. Other features (furrows, and cloudlike stuctures) were found in the aged epithelium, but none of these was associated with the type or severity of age-related cataract. It was hoped that noncontact specular microscopy could be used to identify patients at risk for cataract formation, but the changes noted were more a manifestation of aging than opacification.

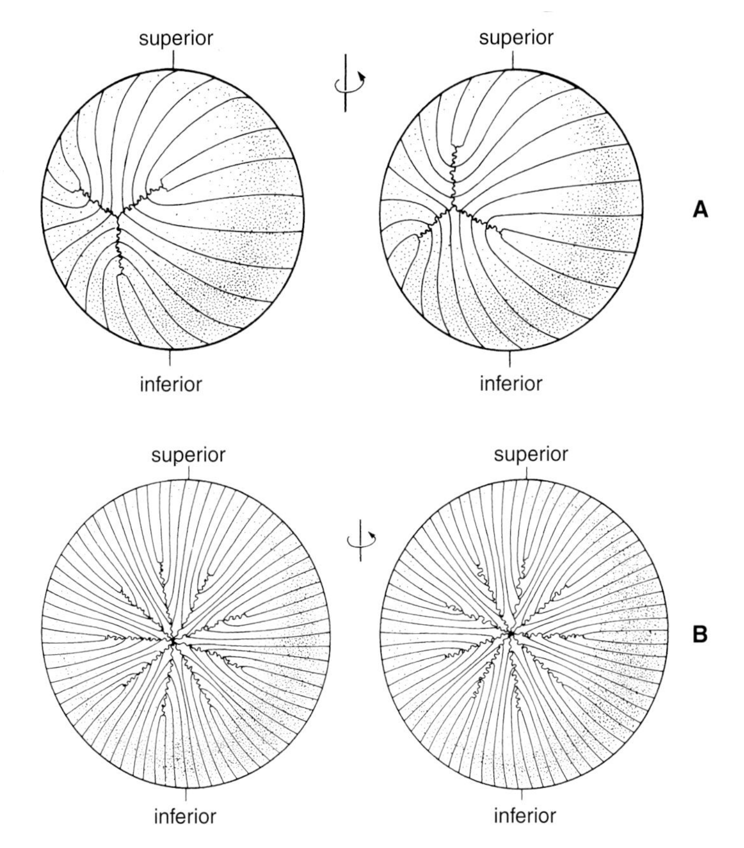

FIGURE 2-2 A, Scale computer-assisted drawings of the Y suture seen in normal human lenses at birth and in the fetal nucleus of senescent lenses. *Left,* Anterior Y suture. *Right,* Posterior inverted Y suture. Compare and contrast the irregular ends of secondary fiber cells overlapping to form suture branches with the regular and orderly juxtaposition of fiber cells along their length. The anterior and posterior suture patterns are directly offset as a result of opposite fiber cell end curvature. **B,** Scale computer-assisted drawings of the star suture seen in the cortex of normal, young adult human lenses and in the adult nucleus of normal, noncataractous, senescent lenses. *Left,* Anterior; *right,* posterior. (From Kuszak JR, Deutsch TA, Brown HG: Biochemistry of the crystalline lens. In Albert DM, Jakobiec FA, editors: *Prinicples and practice of ophthalmology,* vol 1, Philadelphia, 1994, WB Saunders, p 569.)

Cortex

The three-dimensional structure of the fiber cells in the developing lens has been published by Shestopalov and Bassnett.[17] Using expression of green fluorescent protein in cells transfected by two different methods, they were able to show that the formation of the anterior and posterior sutures is asynchronous and that the disorganization of deep nuclear fiber cells seen in the aged lens is actually characteristic of the primary lens fibers in the embryonic lens, not a consequence of aging.

Several anatomic terms are used today to describe the different regions of the adult lens cortex.

- *Peripheral cortex* is just beneath the anterior epithelium or the posterior capsule.
- *Supranuclear cortex* is adjacent to the adult nucleus.
- *Epinucleus* is equivalent to the supranuclear region.
- *Sutures* are the lines formed by abutting ends of lens fibers.

Kuszak et al[18] have demonstrated in several studies the complex anatomy of human lens sutures (Figure 2-2). The dendritic suture structure of the adult cortical cataract often outlines the opaque cortical spoke.

Additional layers of cortical fibers are added throughout life, but the posterior cortex is always thinner than the anterior cortex. What was the subcapsular region in the young child is the supranuclear or epinuclear region in the adult.

An interesting difference exists in the relationships among the capsule, the anterior epithelial cells, and the posterior lens fibers. The posterior fibers peel off easily from the capsule during stripping and aspiration, possibly because a potential space (the embryonic lens vesicle) exists between the posterior fibers and the posterior capsule. The anterior epithelial cells remain adherent to the anterior and equatorial capsule during stripping, perhaps because the capsule is part of the cell itself (its basement membrane) and not just a structure adjacent to it.

One may see the term *followability* in descriptions of the technique of aspirating lens cortex. It refers to the ease with which the cortex follows the aspiration tip as it strips the cortical fibers off the posterior capsule. Also, it means easily "aspiratable." Soft cortex is "followable"; stiff nuclear material is not.

Nucleus

Several anatomic terms refer to different concentric layers of the nucleus (Figure 2-3).

- *Epinucleus* is the outermost nucleus or innermost cortex.
- *Adult nucleus* is the next innermost layer.

- *Fetal nucleus* corresponds to the cotyledonous areas of light scattering in the clear adult lens.
- *Embryonal nucleus* is the innermost core of nucleus.

Surgically, the nucleus is characterized by a densely sclerotic posterior third, a slightly less sclerotic central core, and a softer peripheral shell. Occasionally in older patients, even the outermost nuclear shell is very rigid.

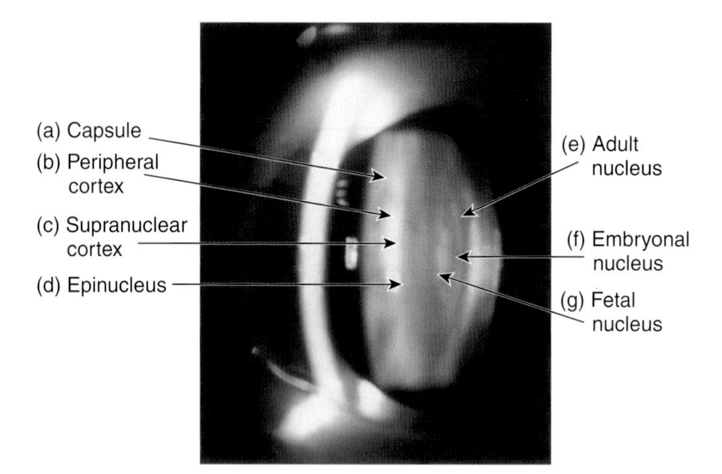

FIGURE 2-3 Color slit lamp photograph of a clear lens showing the different cortical and nuclear layers.

Nuclear sclerosis is an ambiguous misnomer often used inconsistently by clinical ophthalmologists to describe the yellowing and opacification of the nucleus with age. Modern systems of cataract classification identify the features of color change (brunescence) and opacification (opalescence) separately.

The term *sclerosis* is reserved for describing a tactile property of the nucleus—the increasing rigidity of the nucleus with age. This occurs as more cholesterol is incorporated into the phospholipids of the lens membranes. The cholesterol-to-phospholipid ratio is a measure of capsular elasticity; it increases steadily with age and even more sharply after age 60 years.[19] Increasing nuclear sclerosis is responsible in part for the loss of the lens's focusing power at near—a clinical age-related condition called presbyopia. Advanced sclerosis is also a major obstacle to phacosonication of the nucleus. If it is too sclerotic, the nucleus must be removed intact (as in a planned extracapsular extraction).

Opacification (or opalescence) of the nucleus is caused by the formation of light-scattering foci either in the nuclear fiber cytoplasm or on the nuclear plasma membranes. Light is scattered by huge protein aggregates that are formed as sulfhydryl (-SH) groups are oxidized to form protein-protein disulfide (-SS-)

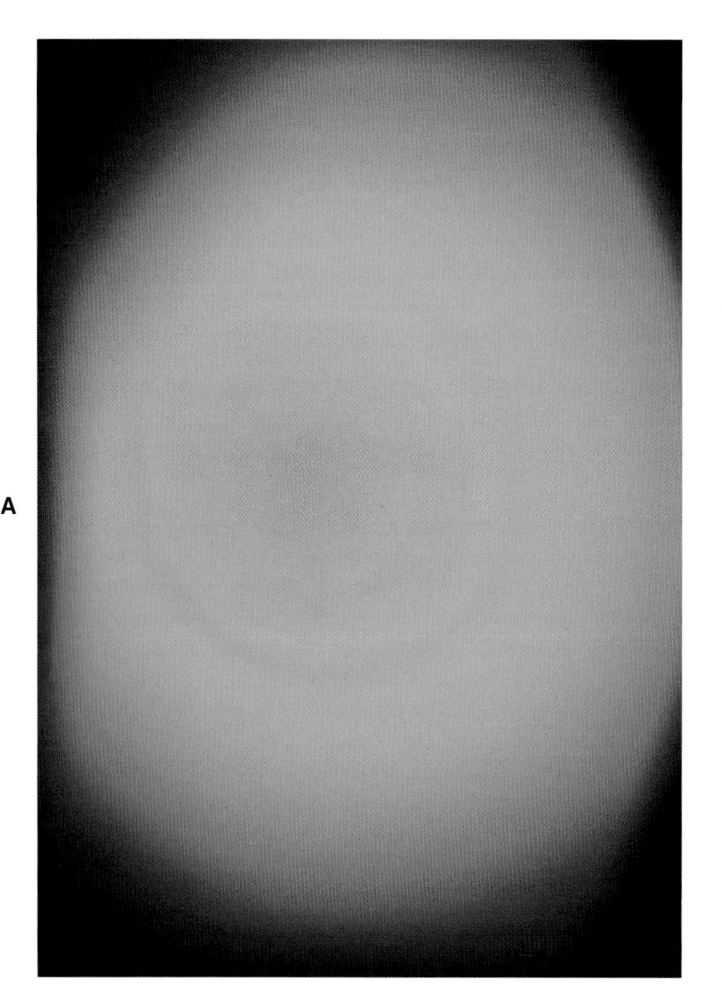
A

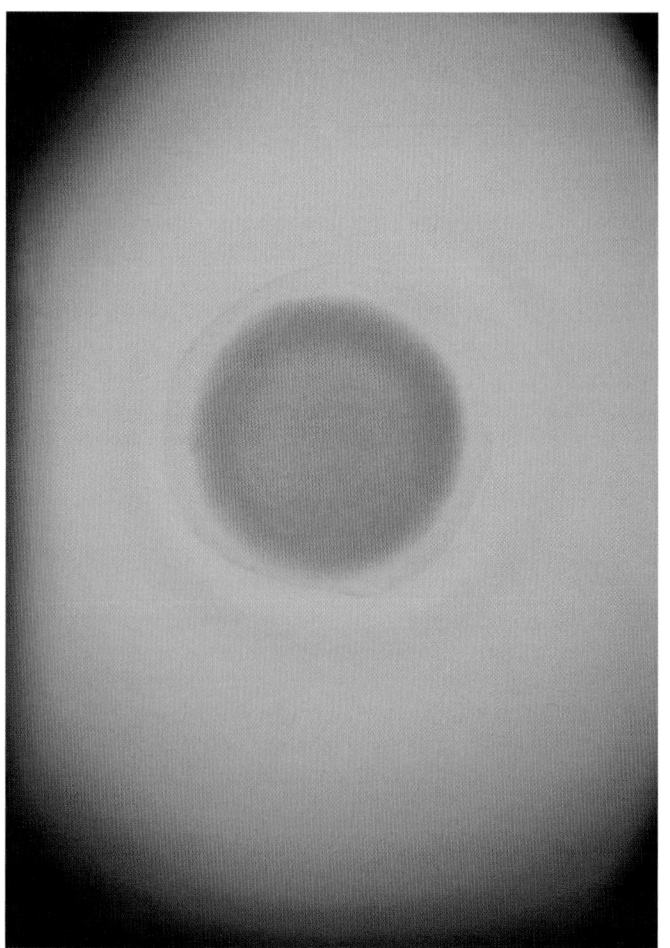
B

FIGURE 2-4 **A,** Minimal nuclear brunescence in an intracapsularly extracted lens photographed against a white background. **B,** Advanced nuclear brunescence in an intracapsularly extracted lens photographed against a white background.

bonds and by larger molecular aggregates that have higher refractive indices than the monomeric proteins.[20]

The nucleus also changes color with age. The fetal lens is just a faintly perceptible yellow color; in the aged lens the nucleus may be golden yellow, orange, reddish brown, or black. This change in color is called *brunescence* (Figure 2-4). The change is distinct from the age-related increase in the light scattering (opalescence) of the nucleus. It is due to the accumulation of oxidized tryptophan (*N*-formylkynurenine), nonenzymatically glycated protein, and other chromophores. Moderate amounts of brunescence may be beneficial because chromophores absorb blue light and reduce glare. However, advanced brunescence causes a reduction in high-contrast acuity and contrast sensitivity independent of the opalescence of the nucleus.[21,22]

Good clinical correlation exists between the intensity of the brunescence and the hardness of the posterior nucleus. The intensity of the light scattering (opalescence) is also well correlated to the hardness of the nucleus.

Optical Basis of Transparency of the Normal Lens and Light Scattering in Cataract

The transparency of the normal lens is derived from its regular fiber arrangement and the minimal spatial variation in the index of refraction relative to the wavelength of incident light.[23,24]

In the cataractous lens, more abrupt changes occur in the index of refraction because of (1) the accumulation of fluid with a low index of refraction between fiber cells in cortical and subcapsular cataracts, (2) the formation of very high-molecular-weight cytoplasmic protein aggregates in nuclear cataracts, and (3) the binding of high-molecular-weight aggregates to cellular membranes in all forms of cataracts.[25-27]

Biochemistry

The structural proteins of the lens are divided into three main groups (alpha, beta, and gamma crystallins) in order of decreasing molecular weight. Most of the enzymes are the size of beta-crystallins. They compose the pathways of aerobic metabolism in the organelle-rich epithelium and most superficial cortical fiber cells and anaerobic metabolism in the organelle-free fiber cell cytoplasm. The main metabolic substrate of lens is glucose derived from the aqueous humor, and the energy derived from glucose is used in protein-lipid synthesis, active transport of ions and amino acids, and maintenance of normal lens hydration. Kador[28] has provided an excellent summary of lens biochemistry and metabolism.

Physiology

Active transport mechanisms are found predominantly in the epithelium, and they are involved in the movement of ions, amino acids, and other metabolites. The movement of water in the lens is governed by the movement of ions or osmotically active substances, and a disruption of the normal movement of water in the lens can lead to acute cataract formation. In patients with insulin-dependent, acidotic diabetes who are brought back to euglycemia too rapidly, a mature or hypermature cataract occasionally forms within a few hours. The cataract is caused by the rapid movement of water into the lens to neutralize the hyperosmolarity in the fiber cytoplasm resulting from the abundant sorbitol (an impermeable sugar alcohol) found there. Sorbitol is the sugar alcohol of glucose; as it accumulates in the cytoplasm, it renders the cytoplasm hypertonic relative to the extracellular space, and water moves rapidly into the fiber cell. The abrupt lowering of the index of refraction of the cytoplasm as water enters the cell results in light scattering. Trauma may disrupt epithelial active transport and water flux and result in rapid loss of lens clarity.

Although it has been known for decades that ascorbic acid is actively transported into the lens, only recently the transport proteins have been identified.[29] The specific ascorbic acid transporter SVCT2 was found in an epithelial cell line, and its gene expression was upregulated by oxidants and other cytokines. This paper suggests that such a transport system and the important antioxidant ascorbic acid may respond to the level of ambient oxidative stress.

Rae[30] provides an excellent review of lens physiology.

Mechanisms of Cataract Formation

The following sections discuss the known mechanisms of cataract formation.

Osmotic Stress

Osmotic stress in the diabetic cataract has been discussed previously. A similar mechanism is believed to apply in the human galactosemic cataract. In both the galactosemic and diabetic cataract, sugars are converted to their respective sugar alcohol by the enzyme aldose reductase in what is called the *sorbitol pathway*. The sorbitol pathway is composed of the enzymes aldose reductase and polyol dehydrogenase (iditol dehydrogenase). Like sorbitol, galactitol (dulcitol) cannot pass through plasma membranes, and once formed, it remains in the cytoplasm. Water enters the cell to neutralize the hyperosmolarity of the cytoplasm, and the epithelial and fiber cells swell. Also, low-index refraction fluid accumulates between fiber cells in sugar cataracts. Both intracellular and intercellular changes combine to create light-scattering foci and lens opacification.

The role of the sorbitol pathway in human diabetic age-related cataract is uncertain; there is very little aldose reductase activity in the human lens epithelium and even less in the fiber cell cytoplasm of the cortex and nucleus.

When performing intraocular surgery, it is important to maintain the proper tonicity (ion concentration) and osmolarity of fluids infused into the eye. Before the introduction of salt solutions with the proper tonicity, osmolarity, and nutrient content, osmotically induced secondary cataracts were a frequent intraoperative or postoperative complication in vitrectomy surgery. In fact, the clear lens was often removed prophylactically during vitrectomy because postoperative osmotic secondary cataract formation was seen so often.

Protein Aggregation

None of the individual crystallin proteins in the clear lens is large enough to scatter light. In the aging lens and in the nuclear cataract, however, the different crystallins combine to form huge aggregates that are large enough to scatter light. The aggregation of millions of light-scattering foci in the lens constitutes a cataract. These aggregates may exist free in the cytoplasm (in nuclear cataracts) or may be bound to cell membranes (in cortical and posterior subcapsular cataracts).

Oxidative Stress

Oxidative stress denotes the adverse effects of oxygen and its various redox forms on the constituents of the lens. Oxygen can exist as hydrogen peroxide, singlet oxygen, hydroxyl radical, and superoxide. There are enzyme systems in the lens that produce and destroy these redox species. The relative balance between systems that produce and systems that destroy these oxidants determines whether or not the lens suffers oxidative damage. If the defense mechanisms are deficient, hydrogen peroxide can accumulate and (1) deactivate sulfhydryl-dependent enzyme systems, (2) aggregate proteins by forming protein-protein disulfide bridges, (3) change lens color by forming chromophores, or (4) disrupt membrane structure.

An excellent brief review of glutathione (GSH), an important antioxidant in the lens, has been published.[31] GSH participates in a redox cycle in the lens and is able to detoxify hydrogen peroxide, hydroxyl radical, and dehydroascorbic acid. Loss of GSH is associated with membrane damage and protein aggregation—factors underlying early opacification.

Posttranslational Protein Changes

In addition to oxidative damage, other changes in lens proteins occur after the protein is formed; these constitute *posttranslational* changes and include nonenzymatic glycosylation, racemization, and aggregation.

Phase Separation

One reversible mechanism of aggregation is phase separation.[32] As temperature drops, certain protein molecules form large groups; although the individual protein molecules are not covalently bound together, the size of the group is large enough to scatter light. This mechanism applies to the cold cataract often seen in cooled calf lenses. Its relevance to human cataract is yet unknown. Whether or not phase-separated proteins are more likely to form covalently bound aggregates remains to be determined.

Metabolism

Aberrant lens metabolism is suspected as a causative mechanism in many cataracts, but there is little evidence supporting this suspicion in humans. When specific abnormalities have been sought in cataractous lens epithelium, surprisingly normal metabolic activity has often been found. In the older human lens, there is little metabolic activity in the cortex and nucleus, even in the clear lens. Except for the declining ability of the lens to metabolically resist oxidative damage, there is little evidence that cataract formation is a metabolic event.

Of particular interest is the ability of the lens to accumulate dietary antioxidants. A recent study of one of the dietary carotenoids, lycopene, showed that this substance reduced the osmotic effects associated with galactose exposure and the extent of oxidative damage.[33] This report suggests that this dietary carotenoid can get into the lens where it does help to offset osmotic and oxidative stress.

Cataract Classification

Rationale

Until recently, there has been little need to accurately classify cataract type or severity. Traditionally, clinicians have used anatomic (cortical, nuclear, etc.) or etiologic (radiation, steroid, etc.) terms to describe the type of cataract. Descriptors of cataract severity have been based on coarse, subjective scales and have included terms such as *immature, advanced immature, and mature*. As basic scientists developed means of identifying and quantitating mechanisms of human cataract formation, it became necessary to more accurately and consistently describe or classify cataracts.[34-37] Also, as pharmaceutical companies encountered drugs with cataractogenic toxicity and as epidemiologists began to study the risk factors of human cataract formation, better systems of cataract classification were needed. Several have been developed, and they include the Lens Opacities Classification System, versions I to III (LOCS I to III)[38-40]; the Oxford Cataract Classification System[41,42]; the Wilmer System[43,44]; and the Wisconsin System.[45] The World Health Organization (WHO) in collaboration with many of the originators of the other cataract classification systems sponsored the development and testing of a "simplified" cataract grading scheme. It was published in 2002.[46] The simplification refers to the ability to use this system in the field and the reduced number of standards needed to grade the severity of cataract. The WHO anticipates using this system to estimate the type and severity of cataracts in patients who are blind from cataract. Such data will help host countries to plan their programs to care for these patients and for patients likely to soon become cataract blind. The reduced number or standard images in the WHO's system may reduce the applicability of this system to studies aimed at detecting the smallest amount of cataractous change in the shortest possible period (e.g., assessing the cataractogenic potential of new system drug candidates or measuring the impact of nonsurgical treatments of age-related cataract in the shortest possible time).

Lens Opacities Classification System

The LOCS III set of standards is reproduced in Figure 2-5.[40] In the LOCS III system, the grader, working at the slit lamp microscope with a set of standards on a nearby light box, estimates separately the extent of cortical and subcapsular cataract, the intensity of light scattering in the nucleus, and the

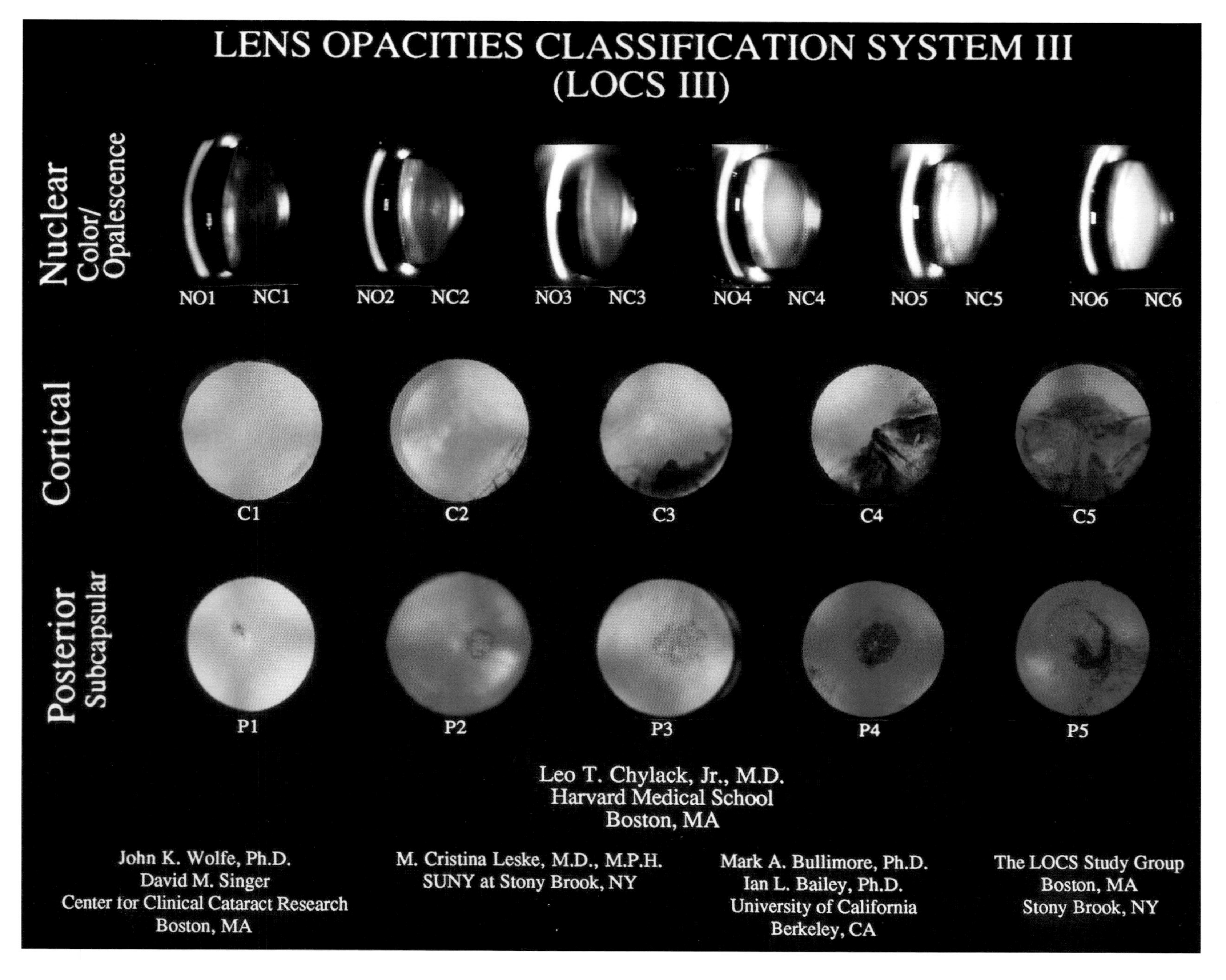

FIGURE 2-5 Lens Opacities Classification System, version III (LOCS III). This set of standards consists of six standards to grade nuclear opalescence *(NO)* and nuclear color *(NC)*, five to grade cortical cataract *(C)*, and five to grade posterior subcapsular cataract *(P)*. (Copyright 1992 by Leo T. Chylack, Jr, MD. Reprinted with permission from *Archives of Ophthalmology*.)

color of the nucleus. Grades are in decimal form; for example, a cortical cataract, the severity of which is judged to be intermediate between cortical standards 2 and 3, would be graded 2.5. Similar grades could be generated for different degrees of nuclear opalescence and nuclear color. The LOCS II and III systems have been validated[47] and used widely in pharmaceutical trials, natural history studies, and other epidemiologic studies.

There has been some interest in using the LOCS II and III systems in clinical practice. It has been considered helpful in following the severity of a cataract and communicating information about cataract type and severity to patients. It has also been used to grade the intensity of nuclear opalescence and color in planning phacoemulsification surgery.[48] The greater the LOCS III grade for nuclear opalescence and nuclear color, the more likely it is that the nucleus will be sclerotic. Little apparent correlation exists between the ease of aspirating an opaque cortex or subcapsular lens fibers and the LOCS III grade. Clear cortex can be aspirated as easily as opaque cortex.

Objective Documentation of Cataract

Even finer grading of cataract severity is possible with standardized lens photography and techniques of image analysis. Such techniques include measurement of nuclear density,[49,50] the area of cortical or subcapsular opacity,[51,52] or the color of the nucleus[53,54] using Scheimpflug slit images, retroillumination images, or color slit images, respectively. These techniques allow measurement of the rates of change in cataract severity in different populations.

Epidemiology, Risk Factors, and Medical Treatment of Cataract

Epidemiology and Risk Factors of Age-Related Cataract

Many risk factors of age-related cataract have been identified during the past 20 years.[55-57] Factors that increase the risk of age-related cataract include female sex, smoking, heavy alcohol intake, limited education, use of corticosteroids, increased sun exposure, black race, dehydrating diarrhea, myopia, protein-deficient and specific amino acid–deficient diets, and diabetes mellitus. Factors that lower the risk of cataract include the use of multivitamin supplements and, possibly, aspirin.[58,59]

Medical Treatment of Cataract

Many surgeons have expressed their conviction that surgery is the only appropriate treatment of cataract-related visual loss or blindness. In many parts of the world, however, there are too few surgeons and too many patients with visually disabling cataract. In these situations, the ability to address the age-related cataract problem with a medical, nutritional, or environmental approach would greatly reduce suffering and the need for medical and surgical care. Viewing cataract-related blindness from a worldwide perspective places the nonsurgical management of cataract in the proper context.

In many parts of the world, drugs with alleged anticataract efficacy are marketed widely and enjoy huge sales. None of these preparations has been shown effective with rigorous clinical investigative methods. Until recently, many countries were allowed to market drugs proved safe even though they were not proved effective. In countries in which medical practitioners are unable to offer cataract surgery to patients with cataract-related visual loss, use of preparations with purported anticataract efficacy and positive placebo effects might be understandable. However, the economic cost of using these nostrums is high, and such economic resources might be better spent on delivering better surgical care to such patients.

A National Eye Institute–sponsored 5-year study of the natural history of age-related cataract formation (the Longitudinal Study of Cataract) has been completed.[60,61] This study measured the rates of cortical, nuclear, and posterior subcapsular cataract formation and rates of nuclear brunescence. It also related personal, environmental, occupational, and nutritional data to these rates and provided insights into nonsurgical methods of intervening to slow the rates of age-related cataract formation (e.g., decrease smoking, use multivitamin antioxidants, avoid high body mass index [obesity]).

Two prospective, randomized, placebo-controlled clinical trials of the effect of antioxidant vitamins on the rate of age-related cataract have been published.[62,63] Interestingly, the Roche European American Cataract Trial (REACT) showed that a micronutrient mixture containing vitamin C, vitamin E, and beta-carotene was able to produce a small deceleration of progression of age-related cataract. The Age-Related Eye Disease Study (AREDS) trial using a similar mixture, but with lower dosages, showed no beneficial effects on cataract progression. Knowing whether or not these vitamins and beta-carotene slow age-related cataract will have to await the completion of a third randomized, placebo-controlled trial.

Unfortunately, at present, few additional medical anticataract agents have potential. In the United States, a phase separation inhibitor was tested as a means of slowing or preventing the nuclear cataract that follows vitrectomy and was found to have no beneficial effect. At present, it is particularly frustrating to have the technology to test anticataract drug efficacy but few anticataract agents to test.

Fortunately, in countries with great shortages of surgical practitioners, there are now low-cost, modern, surgical options for caring for patients with cataract-related blindness. From the cataract camps in India to the technician-staffed operating rooms in Africa, one sees ingenious ways of providing surgical care for patients with cataract where it is most needed.

REFERENCES

1. Stark WJ, Sommer A, Smith RE: Changing trends in intraocular lens implantation, *Arch Ophthalmol* 107:1441, 1989.
2. International Agency for the Prevention of Blindness: *World blindness and its prevention*, New York, 1980, Oxford University Press.
3. Tripathi RC, Tripathi BJ: Lens morphology, aging, and cataract, *J Gerontol* 38:258, 1983.
4. Fincham EF: The mechanism of accommodation, *Br J Ophthalmol* 8(suppl):5, 1937.
5. Koretz JF, Handelman GH: A model for accommodation in the young human eye: the effects of elastic anisotropy on the mechanism, *Vision Res* 23:1679, 1983.
6. Burd HJ, Judge SJ, and Cross JA: Numerical modeling of the accommodating lens, *Vision Res* 42:2235, 2002.

7. Bertelmann E, Kojetinsky C: Posterior capsule opacification and anterior capsule opacification, *Curr Clin Ophthalmol* 12:35, 2001.
8. Apple DJ, Peng Q, Visessook N et al: Eradication of posterior capsule opacification: documentation of a marked decrease in Nd:YAG laser posterior capsulotomy rates noted in an analysis of 5416 pseudophakic human eyes obtained post-mortem, *Ophthalmology* 108:505, 2001.
9. Javdani SM, Huygens MM, Callebaut F: Neodymium:YAG capsulotomy rates after phacoemulsification with hydrophobic and hydrophilic acrylic intraocular lenses, *Bull Soc Belge Ophtalmol* 283:13, 2002.
10. Wormstone M: Posterior capsule opacification: a cell biological perspective, *Exp Eye Res* 74:337, 2002.
11. Majima K: Human lens epithelial cells proliferate in response to exogenous EGF and have EGF and EGF receptor, *Ophthalmic Res* 27:356, 1995.
12. Wormstone IM, Tamiya S, Marcantonio JM et al: Hepatocyte growth factor and c-Met expression in human lens epithelial cells, *Invest Ophthalmol* 41:4216, 2000.
13. Rakic JM, Galand A, Vrensen GF: Separation of fibers from the capsule enhances mitotic activity of human lens epithelium, *Exp Eye Res* 64:67, 1997.
14. Wormstone IM, Tamiya S, Anderson I et al: TGF-beta2-induced matrix modification and cell transdifferentiation in the human lens capsular bag, *Invest Ophthalmol Vis Sci* 43:2301, 2002.
15. Bhat SP: The ocular lens epithelium, *Biosci Rep* 21:537, 2001.
16. Balaram M, Kuszak JR, Ayaki M et al: Noncontact specular microscopy of human lens epithelium, *Invest Ophthalmol Vis Sci* 41:474, 2000.
17. Shestopalov VI, Bassnett S: Three-dimensional organization of primary lens fiber cells, *Invest Ophthalmol Vis Sci* 41:859, 2000.
18. Kuszak JR, Bertram BA, Macsai MS et al: Sutures of the crystalline lens: a review, *Scanning Electron Microsc* 3:1369, 1984.
19. Li LK, So L, Spector A: Age-dependent changes in the distribution and concentration of human lens cholesterol and phospholipids, *Biochim Biophys Acta* 917:112, 1987.
20. Siezen RJ, Owen EA: Physicochemical characterization of high-molecular-weight alpha-crystallin subpopulations from the calf lens nucleus, *Biochim Biophys Acta* 749:227, 1983.
21. Chylack LT Jr, Padhye N, Khu PM et al: Loss of contrast sensitivity in diabetic patients with LOCS II classified cataract, *Br J Ophthalmol* 77:7, 1993.
22. Chylack LT Jr, Jakubicz G, Rosner B et al: Contrast sensitivity and visual acuity, as functions of cataract type and extent, *J Cataract Refract Surg* 19:399, 1993.
23. Benedek GB: Theory of transparency of the eye, *Appl Opt* 10:459, 1971.
24. Trokel S: The physical basis for transparency of the crystalline lens, *Invest Ophthalmol* 1:493, 1962.
25. Tripathi RC, Tripathi BJ: Morphology of the normal, aging, and cataractous human lens. II. Optical zones of discontinuity and senile cataract, *Lens Res* 1:43, 1983.
26. Harding CV, Maisel H, Chylack LT Jr et al: The structure of the human cataractous lens. In Maisel H, editor: *The ocular lens: structure, function and pathology*, New York, 1985, Marcel Dekker.
27. Vrenson G, Willekens B: Biomicroscopy and scanning electron microscopy of early opacities in the aging human lens, *Invest Ophthalmol Vis Sci* 31:1582, 1990.
28. Kador PF: Biochemistry of the lens: intermediary metabolism and sugar cataract formation. In Albert DM, Jakobiec FA, editors: *Principles and practice of ophthalmology (basic sciences)*, Philadelphia, 1994, WB Saunders, p 146.
29. Kannan R, Stolz A, Ji Q et al: Vitamin C transport in human lens epithelial cells: evidence for the presence of SVCT2, *Exp Eye Res* 73:159, 2001.
30. Rae J: Physiology of the lens. In Albert DM, Jakobiec FA, editors: *Principles and practice of ophthalmology (basic sciences)*, Philadelphia, 1994, WB Saunders, p 123.
31. Giblin FJ: Glutathione: a vital lens antioxidant, *J Ocular Pharmacol Ther* 16:121, 2000.
32. Clark JI, Benedek GB: Phase diagram for cell cytoplasm from the calf lens, *Biochem Biophys Res Commun* 95:482, 1980.
33. Mohanty I, Joshi S, Trivedi D et al: Lycopene prevents sugar-induced morphological changes and modulates antioxidant status of human lens epithelial cells, *Br J Nutr* 88:347, 2002.
34. Marcantonio JM, Duncan G, Davies PD et al: Classification of human senile cataracts by nuclear color and sodium content, *Exp Eye Res* 31:227, 1980.
35. Chylack LT Jr, Lee MR, Tung WH et al: Classification of human senile cataractous change by the American Cooperative Cataract Research Group (CCRG) Methods I: instrumentation and technique, *Invest Ophthalmol Vis Sci* 1983;24:424, 1983.
36. Chylack LT Jr, White O, Tung WH: Classification of human senile cataractous change by the American Cooperative Cataract Research Group (CCRG) Methods II: staged simplification of cataract classification, *Invest Ophthalmol Vis Sci* 25:166, 1984.
37. Chylack LT Jr, Ransil BJ, White O: Classification of human senile cataractous change by the American Cooperative Cataract Research Group (CCRG) Methods III: the association of nuclear color (sclerosis) with extent of cataract formation, age and visual acuity, *Invest Ophthalmol Vis Sci* 1984;25:174, 1984.
38. Chylack LT Jr, Leske MC, Sperduto R et al: Lens Opacities Classification System, *Arch Ophthalmol* 106:330, 1988.
39. Chylack LT Jr, Leske MC, McCarthy D et al: Lens Opacities Classification System II (LOCS II), *Arch Ophthalmol* 107:991, 1989.
40. Chylack LT Jr, Wolfe JK, Singer DM et al: The Lens Opacities Classification System, Version III (LOCS III), *Arch Ophthalmol* 111:831, 1993.
41. Sparrow JM, Bron AJ, Brown NAP et al: The Oxford clinical cataract classification and grading system, *Int Ophthalmol* 9:207, 1986.
42 Sparrow JM, Ayliffe W, Bron AJ et al: Inter-observer and intra-observer variability of the Oxford clinical cataract classification and grading system, *Int Ophthalmol* 11:151, 1988.
43. West SK, Taylor HR: The detection and grading of cataract: an epidemiological perspective, *Surv Ophthalmol* 31:175, 1986.
44. Taylor HR, West SK: The grading of lens opacities, *Aust NZ J Ophthalmol* 17:81, 1989.
45. Klein BEK, Magii YL, Neider MW et al: Wisconsin system for classification of cataracts from photographs. NTIS Accession No. PB 90-138306. Available from National Technical Information Service, 5285 Port Royal Rd., Springfield, VA 22161.
46. Thylefors B, Chylack LT Jr, Konyama K et al: A simplified cataract grading system, *Ophthalmic Epidemiol* 9:83, 2002.
47. Maraini G, Pasquini P, Tomba MC, et al, and The Italian-American Cataract Study Group: An independent evaluation of the Lens Opacities Classification System (LOCS II), *Ophthalmology* 96:611, 1989.
48. Davison JA, Chylack LT Jr: Clinical application of the lens opacities classification system III in the performance of phacoemulsification. *J Cataract Refract Surg* 29:138-145, 2003.
49. Chylack LT Jr, Mantel G, Wolfe J et al: Monitoring cataract with LOCS II and counterpart objective measures: lovastatin and the human lens, results of a two year study, *Optom Vis Sci* 70:937, 1993.
50. Chylack LT, McCarthy D, Khu P: Use of Topcon SL-45 Scheimpflug slit photography to measure longitudinal growth of nuclear cataracts in vivo, *Lens Res* 5:83, 1988.
51. Wolfe JK, Chylack LT Jr: Objective measurement of cortical and subcapsular opacification in retroillumination photographs, *Ophthalmic Res* 22(suppl 1): 62, 1990.
52. Wolfe JK, Chylack LT Jr: Differentiation between cortical and posterior subcapsular cataract using pattern matching in computerized image analysis, *Invest Ophthalmol Vis Sci* 31(ARVO suppl):353, 1989.
53. Herzberg S, McCarthy D, Kansupada K et al: Positional dependence of objective measures of nuclear color in the lens: correlation with LOCS II score, *Invest Ophthalmol Vis Sci* 31(ARVO suppl):352, 1989.
54. Chylack LT Jr, Wolfe JK, Friend J et al: Quantitating cataract and nuclear brunescence: the Harvard and LOCS systems, *Optom Vis Sci* 70:886, 1993.
55. Leske MC, Chylack LT, Suh-Wuh W et al: The lens opacities case control study: risk factors for cataract, *Arch Ophthalmol* 109:244, 1991.
56. The Italian-American Study Group: Risk factors for age-related cortical, nuclear, and PSC cataracts, *Am J Epidemiol* 133:541, 1991.
57. Harding JJ, van Heyningen R: Epidemiologv and risk factors for cataract, *Eye* 1:537, 1987.
58. Cotlier E, Sharma YR: Aspirin and senile cataracts in rheumatoid arthritis, *Lancet* 1:338, 1981.
59. Seddon JM, Christen WG, Manson JE et al: Low-dose aspirin and risks of cataract in a randomized trial of US physicians, *Arch Ophthalmol* 109:252, 1991.
60. Leske MC, Chylack LT Jr, Wu SY et al: Incidence and progression of nuclear opacities in the Longitudinal Study of Cataract, *Ophthalmology* 103:705, 1996.
61. Leske MC, Chylack LT Jr, He Q et al: Incidence and progression of cortical and posterior subcapsular opacities: the Longitudinal Study of cataract, *Ophthalmology* 104:1987, 1997.
62. Chylack LT Jr, Brown NP, Bron A et al:. The Roche European American Cataract Trial (REACT): a randomized clinical trial to investigate the efficacy of an oral antioxidant micronutrient mixture to slow the progression of age-related cataract, *Ophthalmic Epidemiol* 9:49, 2002.
63. AREDS Research Group: A randomized, placebo-controlled, clinical trial of high-dose supplementation with vitamins C and E and beta-carotene for age-related cataract and vision loss: AREDS Report No. 9, *Arch Ophthalmol* 119:1439, 2001.

Preoperative Evaluation of the Patient with Visually Significant Cataract

3

Samuel Masket, MD

Advanced cataract formation produces a characteristic symptom, profound visual loss, which may be deduced from the patient's medical history. Likewise, the physical findings of a well-developed cataract can be determined during a basic ocular examination, which includes simple tests of visual function. Cataracts in earlier stages or in eyes with concomitant disease, however, require a greater degree of diagnostic skill and clinical investigation to determine the visual significance of the cataract and how to best advise and treat the patient in question.

Until recently, the only device used to assess the loss of visual function associated with cataract formation was Snellen acuity testing developed by Dr. Hermann Snellen during the middle of the nineteenth century. Snellen testing employs high-contrast familiar letter optotypes. As such, it is a measure of the optical resolving power of the ocular system. Moreover, Snellen testing is performed under the controlled lighting conditions (generally darkened) of the refracting lane and therefore does not simulate the varied visual challenges of daily life. Patients with certain types of cataract in relatively early stages often note diminished visual function although good Snellen acuity may be maintained.[1-4]

Given that "real life" conditions present a far more complex series of visual clues to interpret than does Snellen testing, there has been an interest in and a need for the development of additional methods for testing visual function. Such devices have been referred to as tests of "functional vision," which are designed to simulate the visual disability induced by ocular disease and its impact on the visual tasks presented under conditions of daily life. Two general categories of functional vision testing devices have been developed; one system tests for glare disability, or diminution of vision induced by ambient light, and the other evaluates contrast sensitivity function (CSF), which tests visual recognition of varying target sizes against backgrounds of differing contrasts. Although the two testing systems have significant overlaps and a reduction in one function often leads to a diminution of the other, they are distinctly different, but vital, aspects of functional vision evaluation. They are useful in assessing the visual loss attributed to cataract and other ocular diseases when good Snellen acuity is noted despite significant visual complaints offered by the patient. Tests of visual function are designed to aid in the determination of the visual significance of cataract formation; they are not intended to be used as screening devices or to induce patients without functional complaints to have surgery.

Preoperative evaluation of the patient with cataract additionally requires an appreciation of the visual prognosis for surgery, or potential visual acuity. This is particularly valuable for patients with ocular disease occurring in association with cataract formation. Several methods are available to help determine the potential postoperative vision.

During the last decade, the Agency for Health Care Policy and Research, a previous arm of the Department of Health and Human Services, performed a comprehensive review of cataract care and issued a set of guidelines outlining suggested preoperative, intraoperative, and postoperative management of the adult with cataract.[5] They were a framework on which a paradigm (see further on) was constructed for the evaluation of the adult with cataract. Included in the guidelines, among other material, was a review of the ophthalmic literature regarding preoperative functional vision testing. The guidelines recognized that functional vision loss may be noted with certain cataract types and good Snellen acuity. Yet, on the basis of the rigid criteria for the literature review, there was no recognition of the value of any specific test of glare disability, CSF, or potential visual acuity. Primarily there has been no standardization for ancillary preoperative tests of usual function. Nevertheless, clinicians often find that tests for these parameters are useful in evaluating patients with cataracts that have not reached maturity. A survey of members of the American Society of Cataract and Refractive Surgery indicated that 65% of the respondent members employed either glare disability testing or CSF in evaluating the patient with cataract.[6]

On the other hand, advanced cataracts, those that prohibit adequate ophthalmoscopy, require evaluation for the potential visual benefit of their removal because the integrity of the retina and optic nerve cannot be assessed by routine means.

Glare Disability

Glare may be considered a subjective visual response to light. In the absence of significant ocular disease, bright light may induce *discomfort glare* before retinal photic adaptation; visual function, however, is unimpaired by discomfort glare. Conversely, *disability glare* implies that there is a reduction in visual function caused by the scattering of incoming light by inhomogeneity of the ocular media. As in other ocular diseases that induce partial

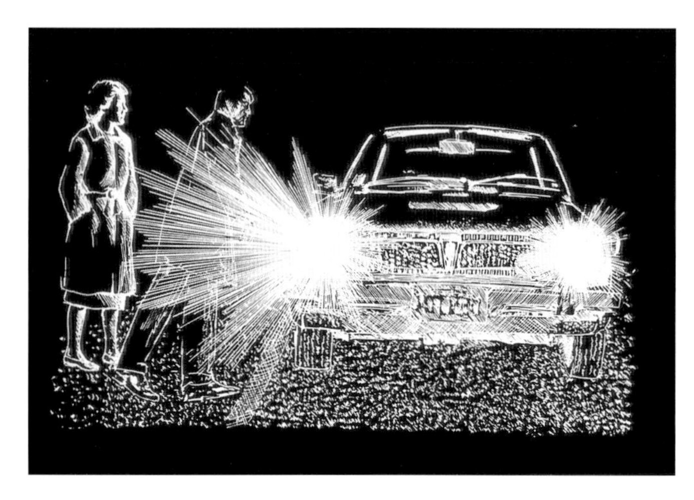

FIGURE 3-1 Glare resulting from oncoming car headlight hinders the ability to view pedestrians, as the dispersed light veils the objects. Glare loss is inversely related to the distance between the glare source and the object of regard. The pedestrian nearer the headlight is obscured more than is the pedestrian farther from the light. (From Koch DD: Glare and contrast sensitivity testing in cataract patients, *J Cataract Refract Surg* 15:158-164, 1989.)

opacification of the ocular media, cataracts disperse incoming light, creating forward light scatter and a "veiling luminance" that interferes with the perception of the visual object of regard. More commonly, this phenomenon is called *glare disability* (Figure 3-1).[3] In general, opacities of the anterior segment (cataract being the most typical) are associated with glare disorders, whereas posterior segment abnormalities are less likely to induce disabling glare. The closer the media opacity is to the retinal image plane, the less the geometric opportunity for light scattering and obscuring of the image. Therefore corneal edema is a more likely source of glare than is macular edema.[7] Cataracts disperse incoming light and are anterior in the path of light. Therefore patients with cataracts may exhibit marked disability glare while retaining good visual acuity under favorable lighting conditions, such as the darkened refracting lane. Cortical and posterior subcapsular cataracts generally cause daytime glare more readily than do nuclear cataracts, which are more prone to cause nighttime glare.[4,8] Glare disability therefore is a common cataract-related symptom, and testing for glare should be sufficiently sensitive to correlate well with patient complaints and adequately specific to avoid confusion with posterior segment disorders.

Several useful devices for determining and measuring glare disability have been employed in clinical practice (Table 3-1.) These devices, which may be in short supply today, are generally designed to test a function of vision with and without the addition of an offending light or glare source. The difference in visual function with and without the glare source is attributed to glare disability. However, each testing system uses a different glare source (central or peripheral point light sources, diffuse background illumination, and so on) and test of visual function (letter optotypes, sine wave gratings, Landolt ring, and so on). The brightness acuity tester (BAT) (Figure 3-2)[9] is in common use because it is readily portable, compact, and relatively inexpensive and may be used in conjunction with the Snellen chart of the refracting lane. The BAT offers three levels of background illumination in a small hemispheric bowl held near the eye. As a result, one possible source of error is pupil constriction by the illuminator; certain patients with cataract will perform better with pupil constriction, thereby giving a false-negative test. Conversely, the third level of brightness is dazzling, inducing false-positive results. Moreover, because no

TABLE 3-1

Automated Instruments for Measuring Glare Disability

Instrument	Manufacturer	Test Format	Glare Light
BAT	Mentor	Letter acuity	Background
Eye Con 5	Eye Con	Letters	Background
IRAS GT	Randwal Instrument Co	Sine wave acuity	4-point
MCT 8000	Vistech	Sine wave contrast	Points or background
Miller-Nadler	Titmus Optical	Landolt C contrast	Background
TVA	Innomed	Letter acuity	Point

From *Ocular surgery news,* Stack, Inc, Thorofare, NJ.

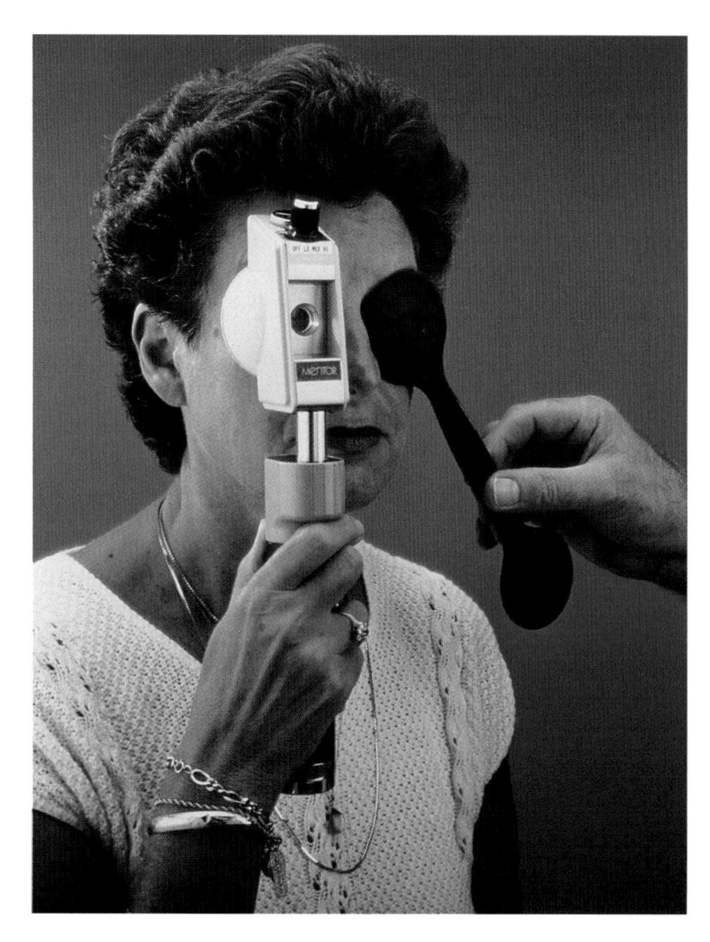

FIGURE 3-2 Brightness acuity tester (BAT). Handheld device allows patient to view distance charts. The bowl presents diffuse background illumination at three levels of light intensity. (Courtesy Mentor O & O, Santa Barbara, Calif.)

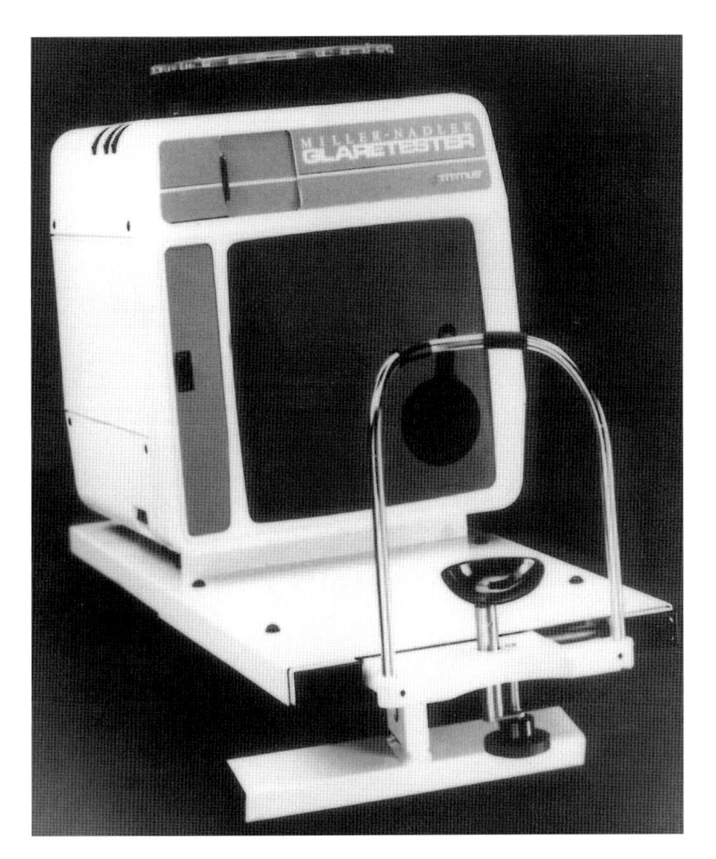

FIGURE 3-3 Clinical model Miller-Nadler glare tester. The unit is a modified tabletop projector. Glare is induced by the background illumination of the projector. The chin rest support system maintains consistent testing distance. (From Masket S: Reversal of glare disability after cataract surgery, *J Cataract Refract Surg* 15:165-168, 1989. Courtesy Titmus Optical, Inc., Petersburg, Va.)

point source of light is used, the BAT does not simulate night driving conditions.

Another popular device is the Miller-Nadler glare testing device (Figure 3-3).[10] This unit relies on a modified tabletop slide projector to provide diffuse background illumination against which the patient views one of a series of 20/400-sized Landolt rings that sit on a constant-contrast background circle. The rings vary in contrast to the background. Because the Miller-Nadler system employs background glare with a contrast test, it may be useful in simulating daytime glare disability but has been faulted for offering only one object size.[11]

As noted in Table 3-1, other automated devices have been developed and marketed. Moreover, simple, albeit noncalibrated, methods may also be used to assess glare disability. One simple means is to measure Snellen acuity indoors and then retest the patient outdoors with the chart positioned in front of the direct sunlight. Another method is to direct a penlight obliquely toward the pupillary margin while Snellen testing is underway; the difference between the Snellen acuity with and without the penlight is attributed to glare disability.[12]

No uniform standards have been established for glare testing devices, a fact that limits their acceptance by rigidly scientific criteria. Nevertheless, it appears that measurement of disabling glare is most useful because it correlates well with cataract symptoms and is reversible with successful cataract surgery.[13-15]

Contrast Sensitivity

Activities of daily living, such as driving an automobile, confront the individual with an ever-changing set of visual targets, luminances, and contrasts that require rapid visual interpretation. CSF evaluates the patient's ability to perceive a variety of coarse, intermediate, or fine details at differing contrasts relative to the background (Figure 3-4). In such fashion, contrast testing seeks to objectively assess the equivalent of the patient's visual function in daily life.

Contrast sensitivity testing is somewhat analogous to audiometry, which measures hearing threshold sensitivity to audible tones of differing intensities and audio frequencies. Snellen testing of visual acuity, which is performed only at high contrast, is similar to audiometry performed at only one volume, or much like listening to music in which all notes are played at maximum loudness. Therefore contrast sensitivity testing is a much more complete form of vision analysis than is Snellen testing.[16] Nevertheless, because different object sizes are tested in both systems, a clear relationship exists between visual acuity and contrast sensitivity. The 20/20 "E" optotype subtends a total of 5′ arc on the retina, with each arm and each space accounting for 1′. As noted in Figure 3-5, a contrast grating pattern correlates to the arm and space of the letter "E." One dark and one light bar together equal one cycle. Thirty cycles

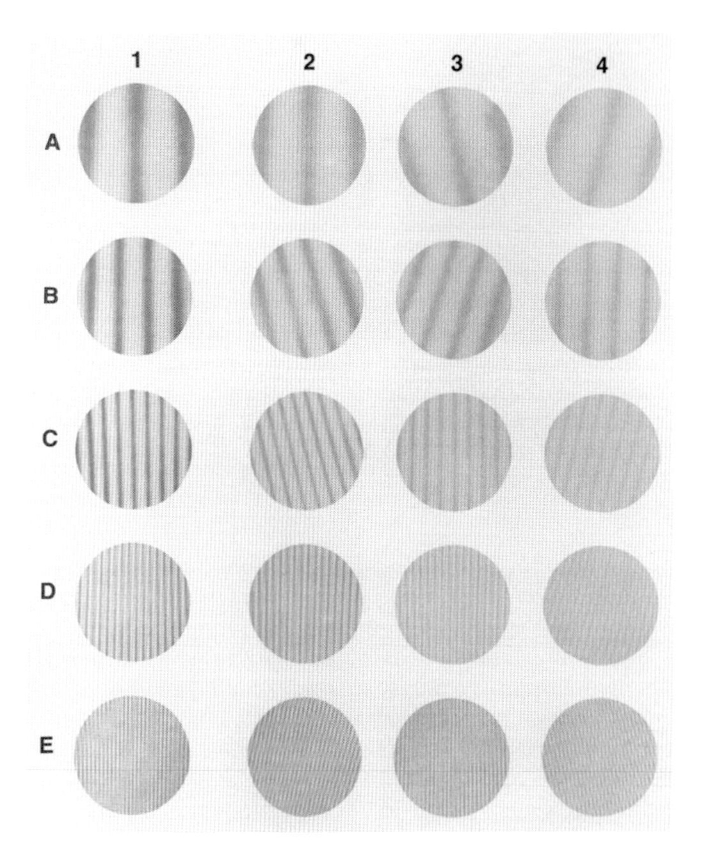

FIGURE 3-4 Representative portion of preprinted contrast sensitivity test plates. Note varied orientation of contrast bars. (Courtesy Vistech, Inc., Dayton, Ohio.)

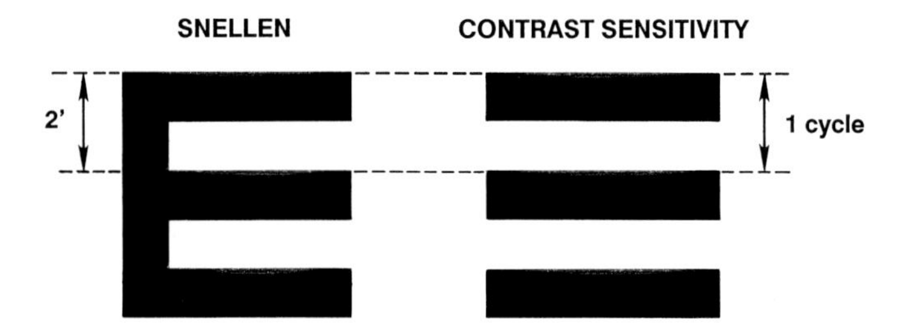

FIGURE 3-5 Comparison between 20/20 letter "E" optotype and contrast sensitivity bars. Note that the arm and space of the letter substend 2′ arc and are equal in size to a contrast bar and space at 30 cycles per degree. Therefore at high contrast the 30 cycles per degree bar is equivalent to 20/20 Snellen acuity. (From Masket S: Glare disability and contrast sensitivity function in the evaluation of symptomatic cataract, *Ophthalmol Clin North Am* 4:365-380, 1991.)

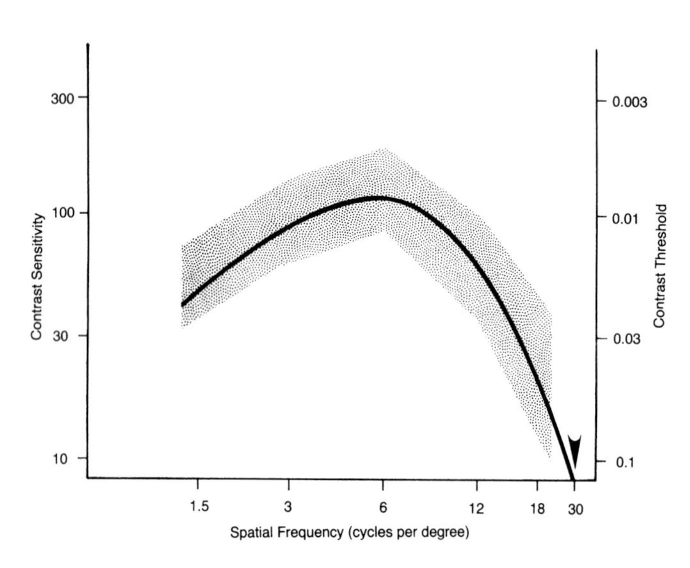

FIGURE 3-6 CSF curve typical for the normal eye depicted as solid line with surrounding gray area that corresponds to 2 standard deviations of the normal mean. Note that peak sensitivity occurs near six cycles per degree of subtended retinal arc. The *arrow* denotes the portion of the curve that corresponds to 20/20 Snellen acuity. (From Masket S: Glare disability and contrast sensitivity function in the evaluation of symptomatic cataract, *Ophthalmol Clin North Am* 4:365-380, 1991.)

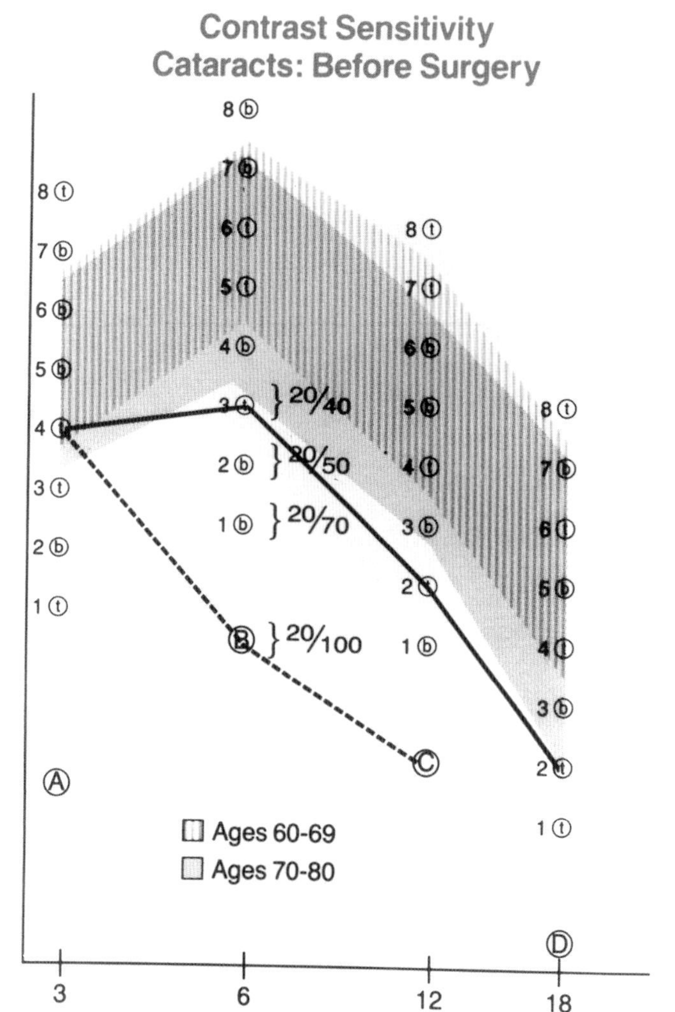

FIGURE 3-7 Typical CSF curve of the presurgical cataract patient. Note that the CSF curve of both eyes falls below the range of the accepted norm (90th percentile). The left eye *(broken line)* has markedly diminished contrast sensitivity yet the same high-contrast Snellen acuity as the right eye. (Courtesy Vector Vision, Inc., Dayton, Ohio.)

per 1 degree (or 60′) of retinal arc therefore correspond to the spacing of a 20/20 optotype. It follows then, that just one point, 30 cycles per degree, on a contrast sensitivity curve (Figure 3-6) at high contrast corresponds to the 20/20 line of Snellen testing. The typical human contrast sensitivity curve, noted in Figure 3-6, reveals that the peak contrast sensitivity of the visual system occurs at image sizes near six cycles per degree as subtended on the retina. An object that subtends six cycles per degree on the retina corresponds in size to a 20/100 optotype. This indicates that the human visual system requires higher contrast for perception at higher spatial frequencies. Therefore it is possible that the eye may perceive small target sizes at high contrast while not recognizing larger objects at reduced contrast levels. This concept offers an explanation for the visual complaints of patients who retain reasonably good Snellen acuity yet express difficulty in "real life" visual function.

Given that CSF is analogous to a greatly expanded form of Snellen testing, it stands to reason that reduced contrast function will occur at high spatial frequencies when visual acuity is reduced for any reason, including uncorrected refractive errors and a number of anterior segment abnormalities, for example, keratoconus and pterygium.[17] CSF therefore is quite sensitive but not as specific as disability glare testing when evaluating symptomatic cataract.[18] It has been reported that early cataracts reduce contrast sensitivity primarily at high and intermediate frequencies (Figure 3-7),[19,20] whereas optic neuropathies are purported to reduce contrast sensitivity at low frequencies. Reduced CSF has also been noted and reported in a host of posterior segment disorders, including macular degeneration and diabetic retinopathy.[17]

In addition, interest has centered on the effect of monocular cataract on binocular visual function. By means of CSF testing, it has been established that at high spatial frequencies, binocular contrast sensitivity decreases to a level below that of the cataractous eye alone. This demonstrates binocular visual inhibition and indicates that a patient with one cataract may suffer significant visual disability, even when the noncataractous eye has normal monocular vision.[21-22] Furthermore, this information suggests that correcting only one eye in a patient with binocular cataracts may not fully improve functional vision; often the second eye will require surgery for the patient to gain the benefits of cataract rehabilitation. Moreover, a patient's perceived visual disability with cataract may correlate better with tests of binocular contrast sensitivity than with any of the monocular tests of visual function.[23]

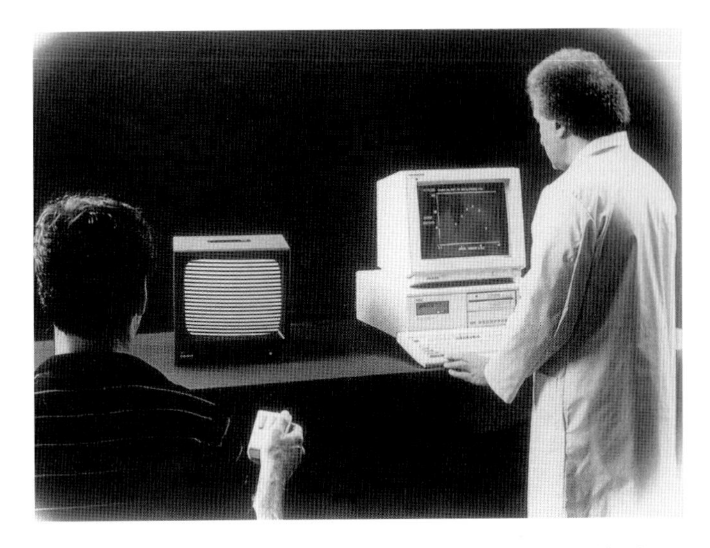

FIGURE 3-9 Computerized contrast sensitivity apparatus used for determining CSF. Contrast patterns are presented on a video display terminal as generated by the computer. (From Jindra LF, Zermon V: Contrast sensitivity testing: a more complete assessment of vision, *J Cataract Refract Surg* 15: 141-148, 1989.)

Measurement of Contrast Sensitivity Function

The determination of a CSF curve for the eye requires measurement of two separate functions: (1) the perceived contrast threshold between the object and the background and (2) the target size of the object subtended on the retina and measured in cycles per degree. Originally used as a research tool in the evaluation of ocular and neural diseases, early contrast testing systems used a series of sinusoidal (sine wave) grating patterns (Figures 3-4, 3-8, and 3-9). Currently, the familiar letter optotype contrast charts (Table 3-2) designed by Terry (Figure 3-10), Pelli-Robson (Figure 3-11), and Regan are used as clinical alternatives to sine wave gratings, and CSF is often measured in a fashion similar to Snellen testing, with the patient reading letter charts of differing contrasts. The Regan charts each employ log MAR optotypes between 20/200 and 20/20 at varying contrasts of 96%, 50%, 25%, 11%, and 4%. The 25% and 11% Regan

A

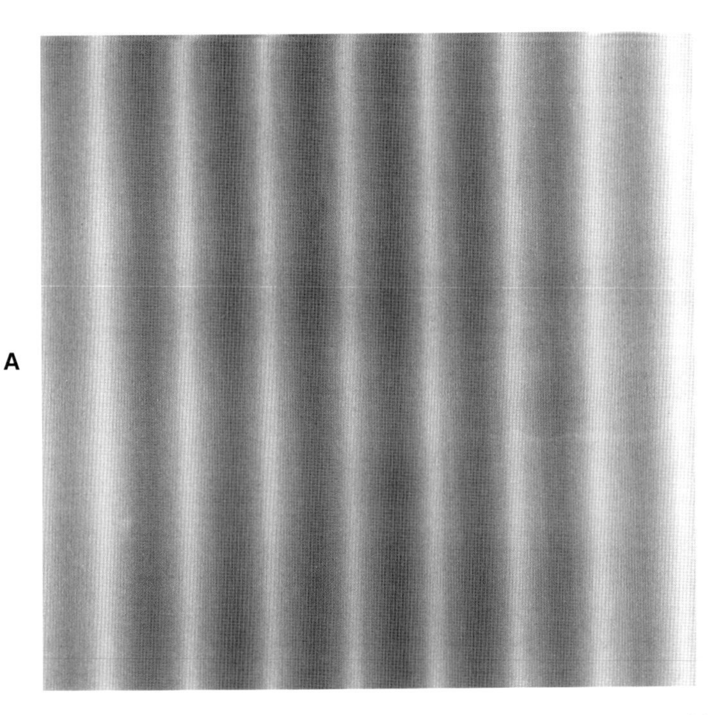

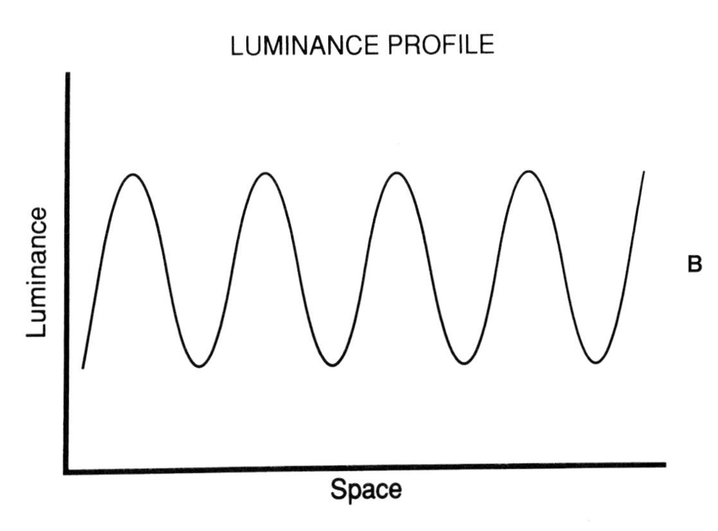

B

FIGURE 3-8 A, Sinusoidal grating pattern used in testing contrast sensitivity. **B,** Luminance versus spatial relationship in sinusoidal grating patterns. (From Jindra LF, Zermon V: Contrast sensitivity testing: a more complete assessment of vision, *J Cataract Refract Surg* 15:141-148, 1989.)

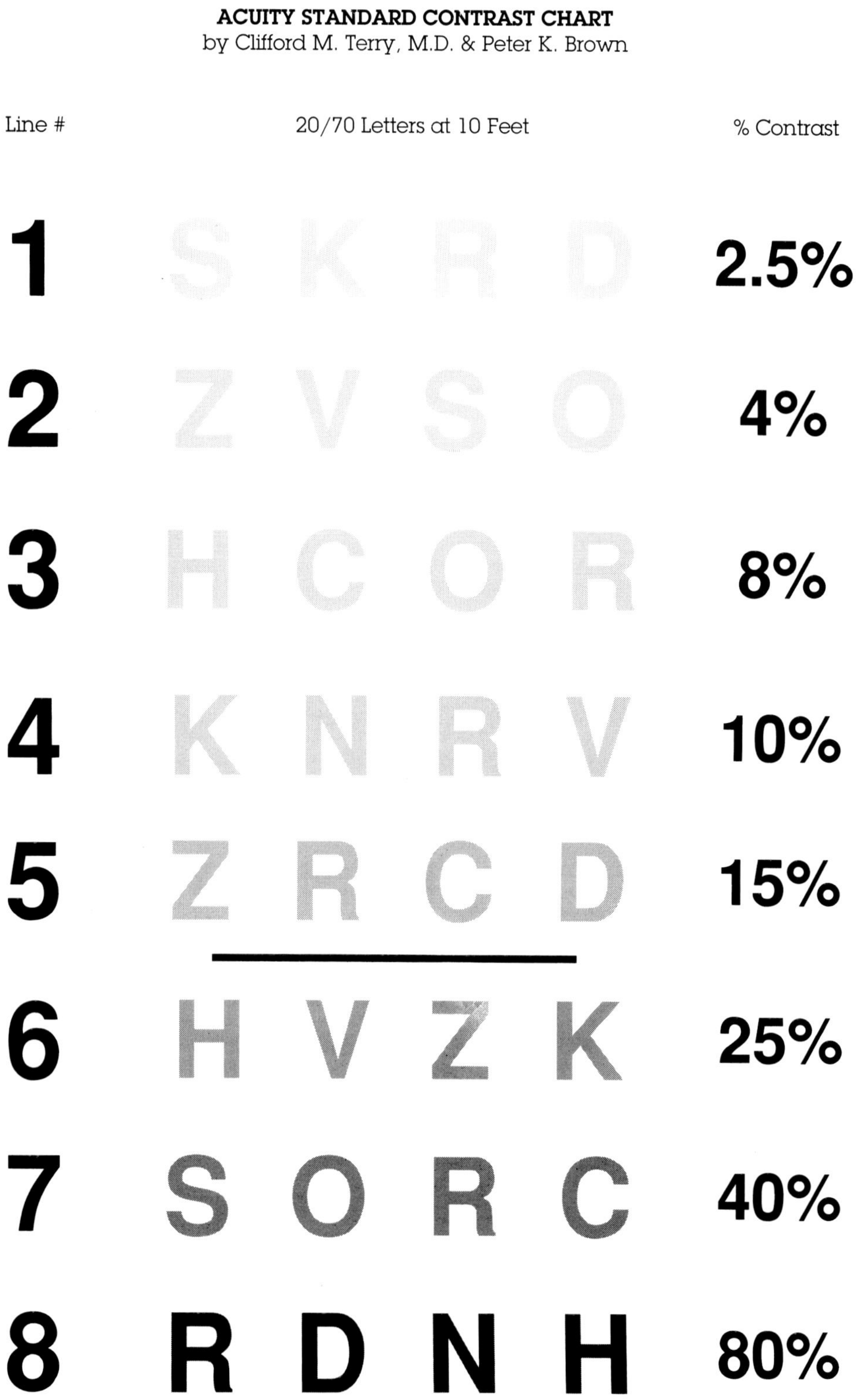

ACUITY STANDARD CONTRAST CHART
by Clifford M. Terry, M.D. & Peter K. Brown

Line #	20/70 Letters at 10 Feet	% Contrast
1	S K R D	2.5%
2	Z V S O	4%
3	H C O R	8%
4	K N R V	10%
5	Z R C D	15%
6	H V Z K	25%
7	S O R C	40%
8	R D N H	80%

FIGURE 3-10 The Terry acuity standard contrast chart. Letter optotype chart with contrast between letters and background varying between 2.5% and 80%. Letter size is equal to 20/70 optotype viewed at 10 ft. Nighttime driving may be hazardous for the patient who cannot read line 5 or above. This chart is for demonstration purposes only. (From Masket S: Glare disability and contrast sensitivity function in the evaluation of symptomatic cataract, *Ophthalmol Clin North Am* 4:365-380, 1991.)

TABLE 3-2
Letter Optotype Charts for Contrast Sensitivity Testing

	Pelli-Robson	Regan	Terry
Contrast range	1%-100%	4%, 11%, 25%, 50%, 96%	2.5%-80%
Letter sizes	20/80	20/20-20/200	20/70
Testing distance	10 ft	10 ft	10 ft

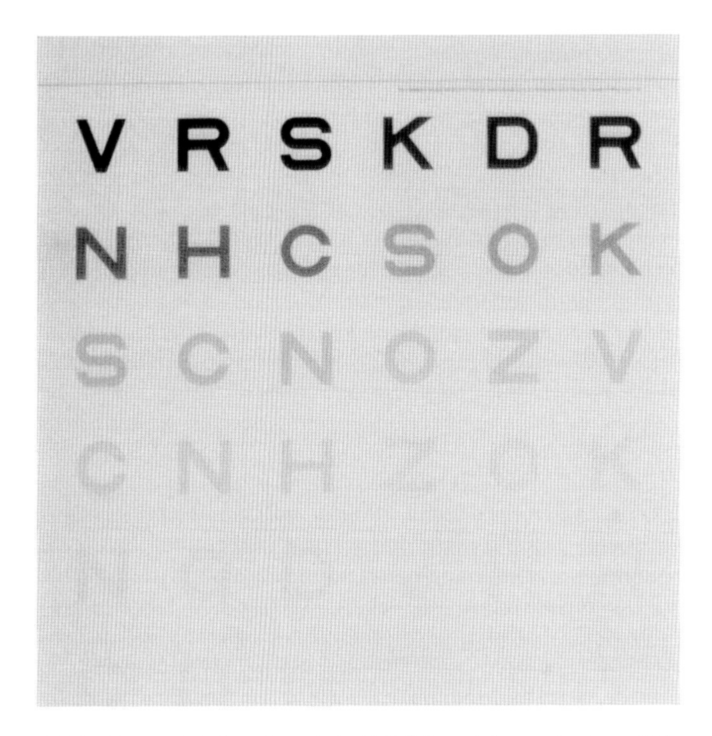

FIGURE 3-11 A portion of the Pelli-Robson letter contrast sensitivity chart. Note that the letters are of equal size but differ in contrast. (From Pelli DG, Robson JG, Wilkins AJ: The design of a new letter chart for measuring contrast sensitivity. In *Clinical vision science*, vol 2, Oxford, 1988, Pergamon Press, Ltd, p 187.)

contrast charts have been found particularly useful in evaluating cataract patients.[24] Because the Regan charts present letter targets of differing sizes at varied contrasts, they can be used to establish a true CSF curve for the eye, whereas the Pelli-Robson and Terry charts offer only one size of letter targets. Both attempt to evaluate the most sensitive part of the contrast sensitivity curve, near six cycles per degree. Without targets of varied sizes, a complete contrast curve for the eye cannot be determined.

When contrast sensitivity is measured with letter charts, the room and chart illumination must be standardized. Self-contained tabletop vision testing devices offer the possible advantage of uniform internal illumination for enhanced reproducibility. Table 3-3 lists the available automated devices for evaluating CSF. Unfortunately, as in the case of glare disability testing, there has been no consensus on the appropriate standards for contrast sensitivity testing, and a number of devices are available to determine CSF, with each of them employing a somewhat different method.

TABLE 3-3
Contrast Sensitivity Testing Devices

Device	Manufacturer	Format	Target Type
B-VAT II	Mentor	Computer screen	Sine wave
CSV 1000	Vector Vision	Illuminated wall chart	Sine wave
Eye Con 5	Eye Con	Computer screen	Letters
MCT 8000	Vistech	Tabletop view box	Sine wave
Optec 1000	Stereo Optical	Tabletop view box	Sine wave
Optec 2000			
TVA	Innomed	Computer screen	Square wave
VCTS	Vistech	Near-far charts	Sine wave

From *Ocular surgery news,* Stack, Inc, Thorofare, NJ.

Combination of Glare and Contrast Sensitivity Testing

It has been well established that glare disability reduces the contrast sensitivity of the visual system.[25] Therefore certain glare testing systems, such as the Miller-Nadler glare tester, evaluate the effect of a glare source on contrast targets to determine glare disability. Testing of CSF or low-contrast visual acuity in the presence of glare is superior to the testing of disability glare with high-contrast targets in assessing cataract patients with essentially normal neuroretinal function.[26] It has become common practice to evaluate visual function when combining the BAT as a glare source with the Regan or Pelli-Robson contrast sensitivity charts.[23] This form of testing has been adopted by the United States Food and Drug Administration as requisite for determining visual function after placement of multifocal lens implants. Conversely, separate glare or contrast tests may have specific value for assessing other neural-visual conditions.[11] Given that high-contrast testing alone is of limited value in simulating the visual complaints of the patient with cataracts, it is likely that clinicians will accept into daily practice the combination of low-contrast visual acuity testing with an added glare source as the most effective means to quantify cataract-induced visual symptoms. A simple and gross system employs a penlight as a glare source in combination with Pelli-Robson contrast charts.[27] Hopefully, standard means for combining glare and contrast testing for the evaluation of patients with symptomatic cataract will be established and widely accepted among academicians, clinical practitioners, and regulating organizations.

Assessment of Potential Visual Function Following Cataract Removal

Patients with symptomatic cataract formation and otherwise normal ocular examinations can anticipate amelioration of their diminished vision with successful cataract removal. However, patients with cataract and concomitant ocular disease, for example, macular degeneration, may present a dilemma in management because ophthalmoscopy may be misleading or particularly difficult with advanced cataracts. Often, the patient and surgeon are reluctant to consider cataract surgery when the prognosis for return of visual function is limited. Nevertheless, in some cases of multiple ocular disease, cataract rehabilitation may prove significantly beneficial to the patient. Determination of the expected visual improvement after surgery may allow the patient to arrive at an appropriate decision for or against surgery. Toward that end, a few devices for the determination of potential retinal function or visual return have been brought to the clinical arena (Tables 3-4 and 3-5).

Testing devices for the determination of potential visual acuity attempt to project visible targets through the cataract to reach the retina for subjective interpretation. One system, the Guyton-Minkowski potential acuity meter (PAM),[28] is temporarily attached to a slit lamp and uses a reduced Snellen chart that is projected through a pinhole aperture onto the macular region; refractive errors may be compensated for by the apparatus. The principle of using a pinhole aperture to assess the potential visual acuity after proposed cataract surgery has been further adapted in the Potential Acuity Pinhole test.[29] In this method, the increased depth of focus afforded by pinhole apertures is combined with bright light from a transilluminator to assess potential vision in the presence of a cataract. It is reported to be more accurate than the PAM.[30] The second type of potential acuity apparatus uses laser-generated interference stripes or fringes that are projected onto the retinal surface through the ocular media; the width of the fringes, corresponding to acuity, is variable.[31-34] Refractive errors need not be corrected with interferometry testing because projection of the laser images on the retina is not affected by ametropia.

The potential acuity devices—whether the Snellen chart, the PAM, or the interferometry fringes—are subjective methods that require an alert and cooperative patient in addition to a skilled and compassionate examiner. Moreover, these tests are of greatest value when the cataract has not advanced past the 20/200 level because very dense lens opacities may yield false-negative results. A clinical rule of thumb indicates that a predicted improvement of four lines of vision by the acuity tester suggests a good prognosis for cataract surgery. Typically, if a patient's best corrected visual acuity is recorded at 20/70, a 20/30 potential acuity response is considered indicative of significant visual improvement with surgery. Caution must be exercised in interpreting the results of potential acuity testing because some cases of maculopathy may yield a false-positive response, whereas extremely dense cataracts may produce false-negative results.

In addition, simple and less expensive clinical tools may be useful in determining the visual prognosis after cataract removal in cases of suspected macular disease. One method is the yellow filter test suggested by Koch.[35] In this system, when a transparent yellow filter is placed over reading material, it is noted to worsen vision in the presence of a significant cataract but might be noted to improve vision if the macular degenerative process is more significant than the cataract.

Occasionally, a cataract or other media opacity may be sufficiently dense to preclude any view of the posterior segment; in such cases, the prognosis for return of vision cannot be assessed by the aforementioned testing devices. A number of alternative means to determine gross potential acuity in patients with markedly advanced cataracts have been developed over time and may be useful. Two-point discrimination, penlight-generated entoptoscopy, gross color perception, blue-field entoptoscopy, and Maddox rod testing are among the available tests of certain value (see Table 3-5). Standard B-scan ultrasonographic imaging and electrophysiologic studies, such as electroretinography and the visual evoked potential, may provide useful information when considering an eye with totally opaque media, but these methods may be too costly for routine use in determining indication for cataract surgery.

In two-point discrimination testing, two light sources of equal intensity are held about 25 inches (or 62 cm) from the patient. If the patient can correctly identify the two lights, retinal function is assumed to be grossly intact. No information is learned about macular potential. This test is most useful in cases of fully mature cataracts or otherwise dense ocular media. Similarly, gross color perception may be useful as a tool to establish general retinal integrity; the cobalt blue light source or the green filter (red-free source) of the slit lamp may be useful for this purpose.

Tests of entoptic phenomena have also been used to assess the function of the retina. A penlight or transilluminator may be placed over the closed lid or directly on the globe to stimulate perception of the Purkinje vascular tree images. Although some patients may observe and describe the retinal vasculature, optic nerve, and macular region accurately, other patients, even with intact retinas, cannot observe the Purkinje images. Therefore the test is most useful in comparing the two eyes of one patient, assuming that one eye is normal and the involved eye has opaque media. In patients with one normal eye and one eye with densely opaque media, testing for an afferent pupillary defect may also be beneficial because at virtually all stages of development, cataracts do not induce abnormal pupillary reactions.

TABLE 3-4

Devices for Determination of Potential Visual Acuity

Device	Method
Guyton-Minkowski Potential Acuity Meter (Mentor)	Reduced Snellen chart
Lotmar Visometer (Haag-Streit)	Laser interferometer
Rodenstock (Rodenstock)	Laser interferometer
IRAS Interferometer (Randwal)	Laser interferometer

TABLE 3-5

Methods for Determination of Retinal Function-Integrity

Method	Function
Blue-field entoptoscopy (Mira)	Foveal capillary net
Visual evoked potential	Evoked cortical responses
Electroretinography	Electroretinography
B-scan ultrasonography	Imaging
Pinhole acuity	Potential acuity
Penlight entoptic phenomena	Purkinje images
Maddox rod	Gross macular function
Two-point discrimination	Gross retinal function
Color perception	Gross macular function

Blue-field entoptoscopy is more specific for macular function and is based on the ability of the patient to observe the flow of white blood cells in the parafoveal capillaries. Blue light is absorbed by the red blood cells but not the white blood cells. As a result, with proper filters and an appropriate bright light source, the patient can observe "flying corpuscles" or white blood cells if the fovea is functionally intact. Unfortunately, the test requires a special apparatus, relies on a carefully discerning patient as observer, and may yield false-negative results with dense cataracts.

A Maddox rod may be used as a simple test of macular function in patients in whom the ocular media is not totally opaque. The Maddox rod is held in front of the eye to be tested, and a light source is held approximately 14 inches (or 35 cm) away. If the patient observes an unbroken red line, one may assume macular integrity. A discontinuity of the red line suggests a macular lesion. A totally opaque cataract or vitreous will not allow perception of the Maddox rod.

Imaging with B-scan ultrasonography may be helpful to determine the presence of vitreous hemorrhage or retinal detachment in cases of mature cataract. However, little to no information about macular function can be learned from imaging, whereas simple clinical testing (light projection, two-point discrimination, etc.) may offer an impression sufficient to determine an indication for surgery.

Electroretinography, which estimates overall rod function, is of little value in determining postoperative vision potential. Although evaluation of visual evoked potential is more specific for macular function than is electroretinography, simpler clinical tests are generally as valuable to establish a surgical indication, given the high success rate and low complication rate associated with modern cataract surgery.

Scanning laser ophthalmoscopy, a relatively new testing tool, is capable of imaging the retina in the presence of a significant cataract.[36] However, the cost of the device makes it impractical to use for the sole purpose of presurgical screening.

A Paradigm for the Clinical Evaluation of the Patient with Cataract

At present, there is no single specific valid objective test of visual function to indicate the presence of an operable cataract. Rather, new testing tools add to the battery of ocular function tests and, when combined with a careful analysis of patient symptoms, physical findings, and assessment of potential visual function, they offer a rational means of determining an indication for cataract surgery.

Above all, and central to the issue of appropriate indications for cataract surgery, is the patient's history of visual disturbance and what impact the visual deficit has on the patient's daily tasks of life. A history of significant functional impairment may make it appropriate to remove a posterior subcapsular cataract despite distance Snellen acuity of 20/25 or better, if near vision is reduced or disabling glare is present. Conversely, an asymptomatic sedentary individual with a dense uniocular brunescent nuclear cataract may not perceive a significant benefit from surgery if visual symptoms are not noted. An old clinical adage suggests that it is impossible to help an asymptomatic patient; that concept remains valid today. Written entries in the patient's medical record should clearly state the patient's symptoms and the effect they have on activities of daily living. An activities-of-life scale, with written record for documentation, has been proposed as a means of evaluating the subjective significance of a patient's cataract.[37] Moreover, the patient's symptoms should correspond to the vision loss associated with cataract formation, whereas the progressive inability to see traffic signs under night lighting or against background glare could certainly be induced by evolving cataracts.

The objective ocular examination of the patient with cataract must be comprehensive to establish the absence or presence of concomitant ocular and systemic disease that might also produce visual symptoms or bear on the prognosis for recovery of vision. In addition, contraindications for surgery, such as untreated active blepharitis or uncontrolled intraocular pressure, should also be ascertained.

Best (spectacle) corrected acuity for distance and near vision should be determined; meaningful refractive changes might be significant because nuclear cataracts often induce a myopic shift.

Given that cataract extraction with lens implantation is the most common procedure performed under Medicare coverage and accounts for $3 billion of health care expenditures, patients, third-party payers, and regulatory agencies have an understandable interest in the appropriateness of cataract surgery. As a result, certain agencies (e.g., State Professional Standard Review Organizations) have set limits of visual acuity (generally 20/50 spectacle corrected distance acuity) as appropriate for cataract surgery. However, it has long been well established that Snellen visual acuity alone is not an adequate means to establish indication for surgery.

Consideration of compromised near vision is often overlooked by review organizations. Posterior subcapsular cataracts are noted for their deleterious effect on reading acuity well in advance of marked reduction in distance acuity. Unfortunately, there are no governmentally ordained minimum requirements for near vision. Conversely, posterior subcapsular (and cortical) cataracts tend to induce symptoms of daytime glare with attendant visual disability. Although no specific glare testing device has received the tacit approval of review organizations, the clinician can employ any of the appropriate methods (see Table 3-1) to measure glare disability to establish documentation for proposed cataract surgery deemed necessary by patient symptoms. Daytime glare disability is best simulated by tests that use a diffuse background glare source.

Nuclear cataracts ordinarily reduce distance vision more than they do near vision. As a result, patients who are visually symptomatic with nuclear cataracts are more likely than patients with posterior subcapsular cataract to fall within review organizations' guidelines for surgical indications. This may be particularly true for some patients with opalescent (oil droplet appearance on retinoscopy) nuclear cataracts who may experience early loss of distance acuity. However, in some cases, advanced nuclear brunescence may be observed without a marked loss in Snellen acuity; the patients, however, are likely to complain about difficulty with nighttime vision, particularly while driving. Moreover, color perception may be significantly hampered by dense brunescent nuclear cataracts. If patients offer significant complaints regarding visual function in the presence of a nuclear cataract yet retain better than 20/50 Snellen acuity, it is likely that CSF will be reduced. In addition, tests of glare disability that simulate nighttime glare (peripheral or paracentral light spots rather than diffuse background illumination) are likely to demonstrate significant abnormality. Combinations of glare and contrast testing are certain to be best in documenting loss of vision function associated with nuclear cataracts.

Assuming that the patient's history suggests a significant visual deficit and that the physical findings support the presence of cataract formation commensurate with the functional vision loss, cataract surgery may be entertained. The patient must be the final arbiter in the decision to have cataract surgery. Moreover, it is essential to determine the prognosis for return of vision with the proposed cataract surgery. Tests of potential visual acuity must be entertained when the ocular findings include other pathologic features, particularly macular degeneration or optic neuropathy. When pupillary reactions are normal (no afferent defect) and the view of the fundus is sufficient to determine the lack of pathologic condition, specific tests of potential acuity are not necessary. However, if optic neuropathy is suspected, visual field studies should be performed. Moreover, in cases of macular degeneration, in which subretinal neovascularization may be considered, fluorescein angiography may be a useful diagnostic adjunct although its quality is limited by media opacification. When employed in cases of questionable prognosis, specific tests of potential visual function may provide important information for clinician and patient. Given that the PAM, laser interferometers, and the potential acuity pinhole test can bypass some corneal disease, irregular astigmatism, and refractive errors, they are otherwise useful guides when the relative visual significance of a cataract is difficult to measure in view of concomitant disease of the posterior pole. In cases of extraordinarily dense or mature cataracts, one might consider the use of B-scan ultrasonography in addition to tests of entopic phenomena and so on.

Once the diagnosis of a visually significant, surgically remediable cataract has been established, the patient (and family members, as appropriate) should be counseled in regard to the findings and prognosis for return of vision. It is almost exclusively a patient-oriented decision whether to have surgery, as is the timing for the procedure. Assuming the patient chooses corrective surgery, it is then incumbent on the practitioner to ascertain the social and supportive needs of the patient during the perioperative period. Can the patient comply with the instructions for postoperative use of eyedrops or other medications? How will the patient be transported for surgery and postsurgical care? What assistance might the patient need for preparing meals early after surgery? These are a few of the pertinent questions.

When planning surgery for any given patient after determining that it is appropriate for and commensurate with the needs of the patient, a careful assessment of the eye to be operated on should be performed and a surgical plan established. The patient may wish to share in deciding the expected postoperative refraction, which is a particularly important consideration in cases of high preoperative ametropia. Presurgical planning should also consider corneal astigmatism and wound placement and construction. Size and type of intraocular lens might also be affected by the desired spherical and astigmatic results of surgery.

The comprehensive examination should also uncover potentially complicating factors, such as medication allergies, uncontrolled intraocular pressure, corneal endothelial compromise, a narrow chamber angle, a poorly dilating pupil, pseudoexfoliation, lens subluxation, posterior capsular defects (as in patients with posterior polar cataracts), a vitreoretinal pathologic condition with lattice peripheral retinal degeneration, and open retinal tears. In the days just before surgery, an external examination is helpful to rule out conjunctivitis or active blepharitis.

Requirements for presurgical medical evaluation may vary from region to region. However, elderly patients with cataract are subject to a range of general medical disorders. It may be beneficial to include the primary care physician in surgical planning, giving careful consideration to certain conditions, including diabetes, systemic hypertension, cardiovascular disease, pulmonary disorders, hyperthyroidism, anticoagulation, and long-term corticosteroid use.

In summary, the presurgical evaluation of the patient with a symptomatic cataract can be a significant and cognitive exercise. Depending on the density of the cataract and the degree of visual symptoms, the clinician must decide what tests are appropriate and necessary to fully evaluate the patient. After a thorough examination process, the patient can be informed of the findings and can make an educated selection from the options for care. If surgery is indicated and entertained, the patient's general medical and social conditions must also be explored before determining the best course of action.

REFERENCES

1. Hess RF, Woo GC: Vision through cataracts, *Invest Ophthalmol Vis Sci* 17:428-435, 1978.
2. Cinotti AA: Evaluation of indications for cataract surgery, *Ophthalmic Surg* 10:25-31, 1979.
3. Jaffe NS: Glare and contrast: Indications for cataract surgery, *J Cataract Refract Surg* 12:372-375, 1986.
4. Koch DD: Glare and contrast sensitivity testing in cataract patients, *J Cataract Refract Surg* 15:158-164, 1989.
5. Cataract Management Guideline Panel: *Cataract in adults: management of functional vision impairment.* Clinical Practice Guideline, Number 4, Rockville, Md, US Department of Health and Human Services, Public Health Service, Agency for Health Care Policy and Research, AHCPR Pub No. 93-0542, February 1993.
6. Koch DD, Liu JF: Survey of the clinical use of glare and contrast sensitivity testing, *J Cataract Refract Surg* 16:707-711, 1990.
7. Carney LG, Jacobs RJ: Mechanisms of visual loss in corneal edema, *Arch Ophthalmol* 102:1068-1071, 1984.
8. Neumann AC, McCarty GR, Steedle TO et al: The relationship between cataract type and glare disability as measured by the Miller-Nadler glare tester, *J Cataract Refract Surg* 14:40-45, 1988.
9. Holladay JT, Prager TC, Trujillo J et al: Brightness acuity test and outdoor visual acuity in cataract patients, *J Cataract Refract Surg* 13:67-70, 1987.
10. Hirsch RP, Nadler PM, Miller D: Clinical performance of a disability glare tester, *Arch Ophthalmol* 102:1633-1636, 1984.
11. Elliot DB, Bullimore MA: Assessing the reliability, discriminative ability, and validity of disability glare tests, *Invest Ophthalmol Vis Sci* 34:108-119, 1993.
12. Maltzman BA, Horan C, Rengel A: Penlight test for glare disability of cataracts, *Ophthalmic Surg* 19:356-358, 1988.
13. Masket S: Reversal of glare disability after cataract surgery, *J Cataract Refract Surg* 15:165-168, 1989.
14. Cink DE, Sutphin JE: Quantification of the reduction of glare disability after standard extracapsular cataract surgery, *J Cataract Refract Surg* 18:385-390, 1992.

15. Rubin GS, Adamsons IA, Stark WJ: Comparison of acuity, contrast sensitivity, and disability glare before and after cataract surgery. *Arch Ophthalmol* 111:56-61, 1993.
16. Jindra LF, Zermon V: Contrast sensitivity testing: a more complete assessment of vision, *J Cataract Refract Surg* 15:141-148, 1989.
17. Masket S: Glare disability and contrast sensitivity function in the evaluation of symptomatic cataract, *Ophthalmol Clin North Am* 4:365-380, 1991.
18. American Academy of Ophthalmology: Contrast sensitivity and glare testing in the evaluation of anterior segment disease (ophthalmic procedures assessment), *Ophthalmology* 97:1233-1237, 1990.
19. Adamsons I, Rubin GS, Vitale S et al: The effect of early cataracts on glare and contrast sensitivity: a pilot study, *Arch Ophthalmol* 110:1081-1086, 1992.
20. Drews-Bankiewicz MA, Caruso RC, Datiles MB et al: Contrast sensitivity in patients with nuclear cataracts, *Arch Ophthalmol* 110:953-959, 1992.
21. Pardhan P, Gilchrist J: The importance of measuring binocular contrast sensitivity in unilateral cataract, *Eye* 5:31-35, 1991.
22. Taylor RH, Mission GP, Moseley MJ: Visual acuity and contrast sensitivity in cataract, *Eye* 5:704-707, 1991.
23. Elliot DB, Hurst MA, Weatherill J: Comparing clinical tests of visual function in cataract with the patient's perceived visual disability, *Eye* 4:712-717, 1990.
24. Regan D: The Charles F. Prentice Award Lecture 1990: specific tests and specific blindnesses: keys, locks, and parallel processing, *Optom Vis Sci* 68:489-512, 1991.
25. Abrahammson M, Sjostrand J: Impairment of contrast sensitivity function (CSF) as a measure of disability glare, *Invest Ophthalmol Vis Sci* 27:1131-1136, 1986.
26. Elliot DB, Hurst MA, Weatherill J: Comparing clinical tests of visual loss in cataract patients using a quantification of forward light scatter, *Eye* 5:601-606, 1991.
27. Williamson TH, Strong NP, Sparrow J et al: Contrast sensitivity and glare in cataract using the Pelli-Robson chart, *Br J Ophthalmol* 76:719-722, 1992.
28. Minkowski JS, Palese M, Guyton DL: Potential acuity meter using a minute serial pinhole aperture, *Ophthalmology* 90:1360-1368, 1983.
29. Hofeldt AJ, Weiss MJ: Illuminated near card assessment of potential acuity in eyes with cataract, *Ophthalmology* 105:1531-1536, 1998.
30. Meliki SA, Safar A, Martin J, Ivanova A et al: Potential acuity pinhole: A simple method of measure potential visual acuity in patients with cataracts: comparison to potential acuity meter, *Ophthalmology* 106:1262-1267, 1999.
31. Faulkner W: Laser interferometric prediction of postoperative visual acuity in patients with cataracts. *Am J Ophthalmol* 95:626-636, 1983.
32. Tabbat SE, Lindstrom RL: Laser retinometry versus clinical estimation of media: a comparison of efficacy in predicting visual acuity of patients with lens opacities, *J Cataract Refract Surg* 12:140-145, 1986.
33. Goldstein J, Hecht SD, Jamara RJ et al: Clinical comparison of the SITE IRAS hand held interferometer and Haag-Streit Lotmar visometer, *J Cataract Refract Surg* 14:208-211, 1988.
34. Bernth-Petersen P, Naeser K: Clinical evaluation of Lotmar visometer for macula testing in cataract patients, *Acta Ophthalmology* 60:525-532, 1982.
35. Koch P: Testing useful for cataract/macular disease patients, *Ophthalmology Times* 17:1, 30, 1992.
36. Kirkpatrick JN, Manivannan A, Gupta AK et al: Fundus imaging in patients with cataract: role for a variable wavelength scanning laser ophthalmoscope, *Br J Ophthalmol* 79:892-899, 1995.
37. Mangione CM, Phillips RS, Seddon JM et al: Development of the "activities of daily vision scale." A measure of visual functional status, *Med Care* 30:1111-1126, 1992.

Intraocular Lens Implant Power Calculation, Selection, and Ocular Biometry

4

Kenneth J. Hoffer, MD, FACS

Since Sir Harold Ridley experienced a 21-diopter "surprise" in lens power calculation in his first two cases in 1949 to 1950, we have been seeking ways to calculate intraocular lens (IOL) power with greater accuracy (Figure 4-1). The science is rather dry and does not stimulate great interest among the majority of cataract surgeons. To make the subject more interesting, we break it down into its component parts.

The three major components of IOL power calculation are (1) biometry, (2) formulas, and (3) clinical variables. *Biometry* can be divided into its components necessary to calculate IOL power: the axial length, the corneal power, and the IOL position. *Formulas* can be divided into their generations, their usage, and their personalization. *Clinical variables* deal with patient needs and desires, special circumstances, and problems and errors.

When the human lens is replaced with an IOL, the optical situation becomes a two-lens system (cornea and IOL) projecting an image onto the macula. The distance between the two lenses (X) affects the refraction, as does the distance between the two-lens system and the macula (Y). X is defined as the distance from the anterior surface of the cornea to the effective principal plane of the IOL in the visual axis. Y is defined as the distance from the principal plane of the IOL to the photoreceptors of the macula in the visual axis. It is easy to see that X + Y is equal to the visual axis axial length of the eye (Z). Therefore knowing X and Z will allow the calculation of Y (Y = Z – X).

To calculate the IOL power, we must know the vergence of the light rays entering the cornea (refractive error [R]). For emmetropia, R is zero. The relationship of the factors (X, Y [Z – X], P, K, R) are such that a formula can be written to describe it. Knowing the values of any four of these allows calculation of the fifth.

Biometry

Axial Length

If the crystalline lens (cataract) is to be removed, obtaining an accurate axial length (AL) is mandatory. If the lens has already been removed (aphakia/pseudophakia) or will not be removed (phakic refractive lens [PRL]), an AL is not always necessary because the correct implant lens power can be calculated using a refraction formula (see Refraction Formula). Because this formula requires an accurate vertex distance, it is not dependable in cases of aphakia where errors in the vertex distance of a high-powered refraction can have a significant effect.

The important considerations for obtaining accurate ultrasound AL are listed in Table 4-1.

AXIAL LENGTH INSTRUMENTS

Until now, all AL measuring instruments have been A-scan ultrasound units. Many A-scan instruments are available, and ensuring that the unit you are using has been calibrated and is capable of accurate measurements is important. The instrument must have an oscilloscope screen such that true echo spikes are observed in determining axiality. Instruments that merely report a numerical reading of the AL ("black box" or spike simulation) do not allow clinical decision making during the examination and are fraught with potential errors. A major step in improving accuracy would be to replace such an instrument with one that has an oscilloscope screen.

A new method for measuring AL was introduced in 1999 by Zeiss Jena/Humphrey (Figure 4-2). It uses laser tomography to measure AL. The instrument, called the IOLMaster, performs four functions; it measures the AL, the corneal power, and the anterior chamber depth (the latter two by optical means) and performs the formula IOL power calculations using modern theoretic formulas. Side-by-side analysis of the accuracy of the instrument compared with standard techniques is now being performed. Initial reports from Germany (Wolfgang Haigis, PhD) conclude that results in 10% of eyes cannot be obtained because of either density of the cataract or the patient's inability to fixate. So far, obtaining an AL measurement in eyes with posterior subcapsular cataracts has been considerably difficult, but overall results have been impressive.

WARNING: *Index of Refraction (IR) User Adjustable. The IOLMaster allows the user to change the IR in the setup program. This is used to convert K readings from radius of curvature (in mm) to diopters (D). It must be set to 1.3375 to obtain the correct results for the Hoffer Q formula.*

IMMERSION TECHNIQUE

The immersion technique of Ossoinig[1] has been shown to be more accurate than the standard applanation technique in

FIGURE 4-1 Uncorrected 20/20 vision in an eye with a Ridley posterior chamber IOL implanted by Harold Ridley in 1951. (Photo taken by author in 1979.)

TABLE 4-1

Considerations for Obtaining Accurate Measurements*

Considerations
A. Ultrasound axial length
1. A-scan ultrasound instrument
2. Real-time oscilloscope screen
3. Immersion technique
4. Experienced technician
5. Appropriate ultrasound velocities
6. B-scan backup
B. Corneal power
1. Instrumentation
2. Contact lens wear
3. Astigmatism
4. Previous refractive surgery
5. Corneal transplant eyes
6. IR of 1.3375 in IOLMaster

*Considerations are listed in order of importance.

A
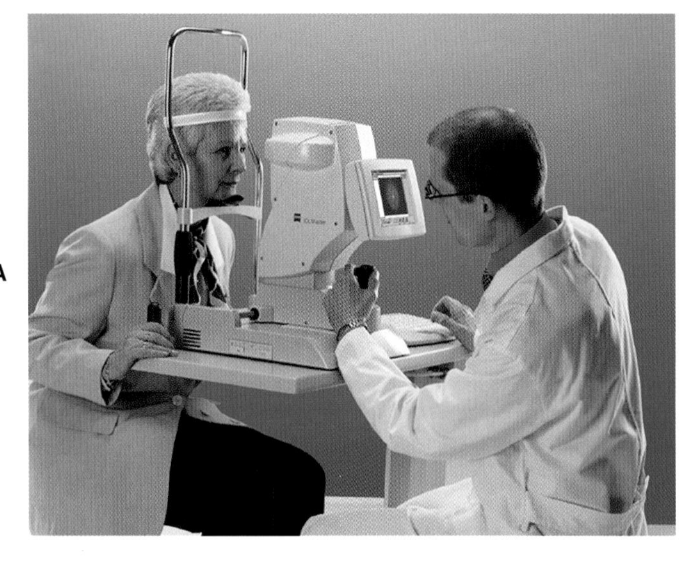

B
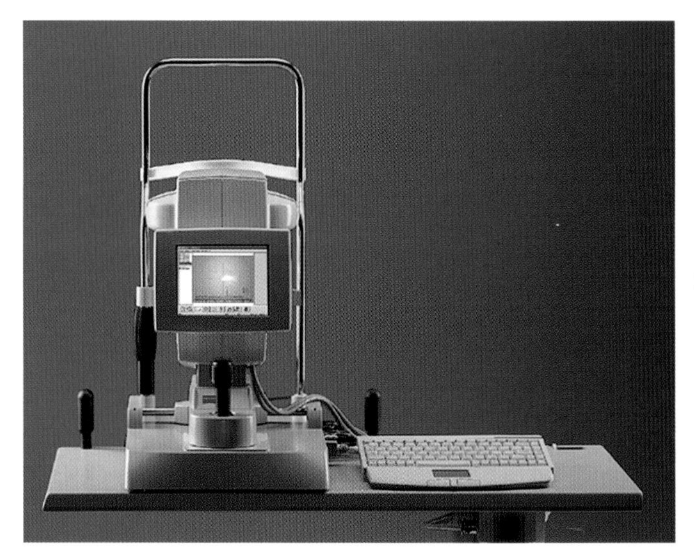

FIGURE 4-2 Zeiss IOLMaster laser tomography axial length measurement instrument. **A,** Side view. **B,** Front view.

several studies[2,3] over the past 15 years. They report a mean average shortening of the AL of 0.25 to 0.33 mm using applanation compared with immersion. A consistent error could be compensated for by the addition of a constant or by formula personalization, but this is not possible because the compression error varies from eye to eye.

Arguments against immersion are that it is time consuming, expensive, and messy and requires the patient to be supine. On the contrary, the examination can be performed in a standard ophthalmic examination chair reclined back at a 45-degree angle with the headrest set back so that the patient's AL is perpendicular to the floor (Figure 4-3). To maintain a non-leaking fluid bath in the Ossoinig scleral shell,* we use a 50/50 dilution of 2.5% hydroxypropyl methylcellulose (Goniosol) in Dacriose solution. Once the eye is anesthetized topically, the scleral shell is gently placed between the lids and filled three-fourths full with the solution. Any air bubbles should be removed with a short silicone tube attached to a syringe. The latter can also be used to remove the solution at the completion of the procedure. The ultrasound probe is placed into the solution and positioned parallel to the axis of the eye (Figure 4-4). Axiality is judged by watching for the correct spike patterns on the oscilloscope screen as the probe position is adjusted.

*Hansen Ophthalmic Development Labs, 2412 Towncrest Dr., Iowa City, IA 52240; 319-338-1285.

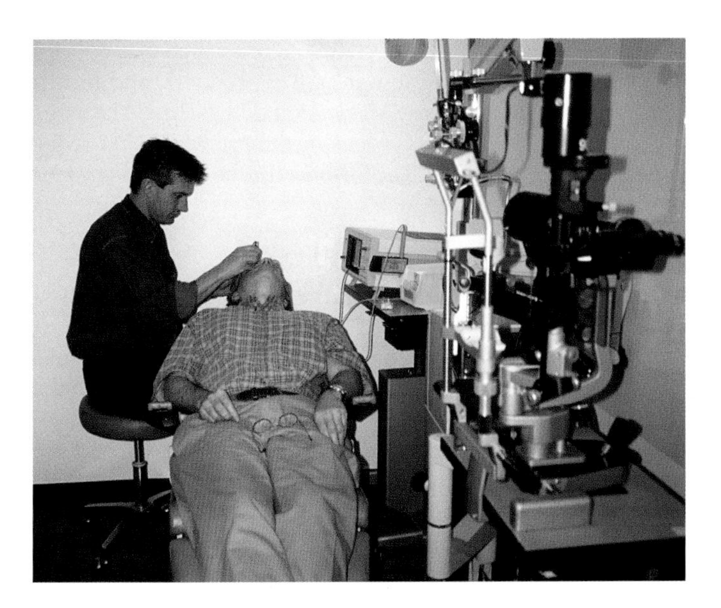

FIGURE 4-3 Immersion technique setup for patient in normal ophthalmic examination chair.

WARNING: *If the AL is very difficult to obtain and the eye appears to have a length greater than 25 mm, suspect a* ***staphyloma.*** *By direct ophthalmoscopy (with patient fixating on cross-hair target), measure the distance from the target (macula) to the edge of the optic nerve (in disc diameters). B-scan exam is then performed to measure the AL at that distance from the edge of the optic nerve shadow (Figure 4-5).*

WARNING: *When measuring an eye containing an IOL, ignore multiple reduplication echoes noted in the vitreous space, which are caused by the IOL.*

WARNING: *If planning silicone oil injection into the vitreous space, perform an accurate AL measurement before doing so and make this information available to the patient. It is practically impossible to measure an eye filled with silicone oil using ultrasound (try using a velocity of 1000 m/sec.). The Zeiss IOLMaster is purported to measure eyes filled with silicone oil and should be used if available. Alternatively, consider performing a secondary IOL after an aphakic refraction is obtained.*

WARNING: *Measuring the AL of both eyes is prudent and customary.*

Always measure AL to the nearest hundredth of a millimeter and record it carefully. Errors in AL are the most significant and amount to ~2.5 D/mm in IOL power; however, be aware that this error drops to ~1.75 D/mm in very long eyes (30 mm) but jumps to ~3.75 D/mm in very short eyes (20 mm). Greater care must be taken in measuring short eyes.

ULTRASOUND VELOCITIES

The ultrasound velocities[4,5] for the various parts of the eye, IOL materials, and average pseudophakic velocities are shown in Table 4-2.

WARNING: *Measuring an eye containing a silicone IOL with standard phakic velocity (1555 m/sec) can amount to an error of 3 to 4 D.*

Because of the inversely proportional change in the axial ratio of solid to liquid as the eye increases in length, the average phakic velocity of a short 20-mm eye is 1560 m/sec, and that of a long 30-mm eye is 1550 m/sec instead of the nominal 1555 m/sec (Figure 4-6). This factor amounts to only a small (0.25 D) error in the extremes of AL, but it can be corrected. This inversely proportional relationship is greater in pseudophakic eyes but is not a factor in aphakic eyes.

If an eye has been measured using the wrong velocity, it can be easily corrected without remeasuring the eye by using the following formula:

$$AL_{CORRECTED} = [(AL_{MEASURED}) \times (V_{CORRECT})] \div V_{MEASURED}$$

where V is the ultrasound velocity.

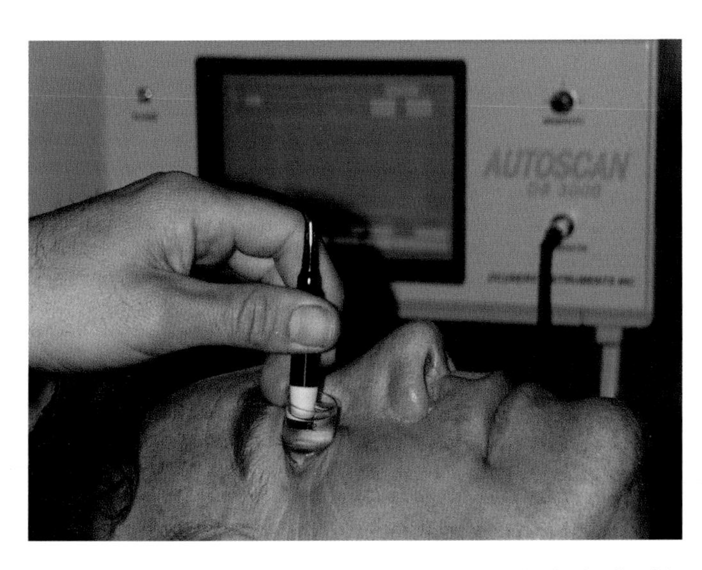

FIGURE 4-4 Immersion technique showing the probe in the Ossoinig shell filled with Goniosol.

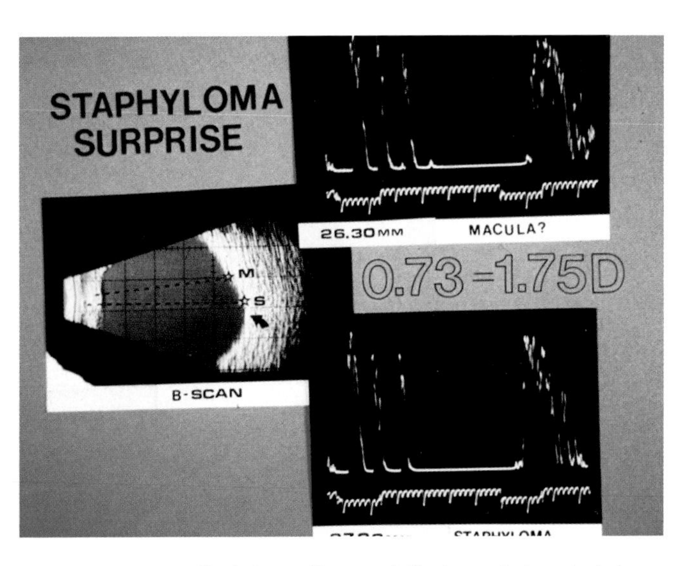

FIGURE 4-5 Staphyloma. B-scan *(left)* demonstrates staphyloma. A-scans show shorter reading at macula *(upper)* than at posterior pole *(lower)*.

TABLE 4-2
Ultrasound Velocities[5] (at Body Temperature)

A. From the following sound velocity values[4,5]:	
• Cornea and lens	1641 m/sec
• Aqueous and vitreous	1532 m/sec
• PMMA IOL	2660 m/sec
• Silicone IOL	980 m/sec
• Acrylic IOL	2026 m/sec
• Glass IOL	6040 m/sec
• Silicone Oil	987 m/sec
B. The average sound speeds[4] for various conditions of a 23.5 mm eye are calculated:	
• Phakic eye	1555 m/sec
• Aphakic eye	1534 m/sec
• PMMA pseudophakic	1556 m/sec
• Silicone pseudophakic	1476 m/sec
• Acrylic pseudophakic	1549 m/sec
• Glass pseudophakic	1549 m/sec
• Phakic silicone oil	1139 m/sec
• Aphakic silicone oil	1052 m/sec

IOL, Intraocular lens.

This is because the instrument does not measure length or distance (d) directly. Instead, it measures the time (T) it takes the sound to traverse the eye and converts it to a linear value using the velocity (V) formula, where d = V × T.

Optional CALF method. Holladay[6] has offered an optional method to measure the AL that attempts to decrease the error inherent in changes in average velocity caused by the length of the eye. All eyes, regardless of status, are measured at a velocity of 1532 m/sec (as if the eye were a bag of water), and to this value is added the corrected AL factor (CALF). The CALF value represents the thickness of a lens in the eye whether it is the crystalline lens or an IOL. The formula for the CALF of any lens (including the cornea) is:

$$\text{CALF} = T_L \times (1 - 1532/V_L),$$

where T_L is the axial thickness of the lens and V_L is the sound velocity through that lens.

Holladay computes the thickness of the human cataractous lens using $T_L = 4 + \text{Age}/100$, and the sound velocity through the cataract using $V_L = 1659 - ([\text{Age} - 10]/2)$. Substituting these two formulas into the previous CALF formula, the CALF formula for the crystalline lens yields:

$$\text{CALF} = \left[4 + \frac{\text{Age}}{100}\right] \times \left[1 - \frac{1532}{\left(1659 - \left(\frac{\text{Age} - 10}{2}\right)\right)}\right]$$

The CALF for the cataractous lens is therefore calculated using only the age of the patient. Holladay recommends using a CALF value of 0.28 (value for a 70-year-old) for all ages because the value for a 1-year-old is 0.306 and that for a 100-year-old is 0.224. The maximum error in CALF for those younger than 70 is 0.026 (0.07 D), and for those older than 70 it is 0.056 (0.14 D).

The reasoning behind this method is that if an "average" eye velocity is incorrect, it affects the entire AL measurement. However, if the estimate of the CALF value is wrong, it only affects a small percentage of the overall AL, that is, only the lens portion. Holladay's formulation, however, ignores the factor of the corneal thickness (0.55 mm). To correct this, I recommend

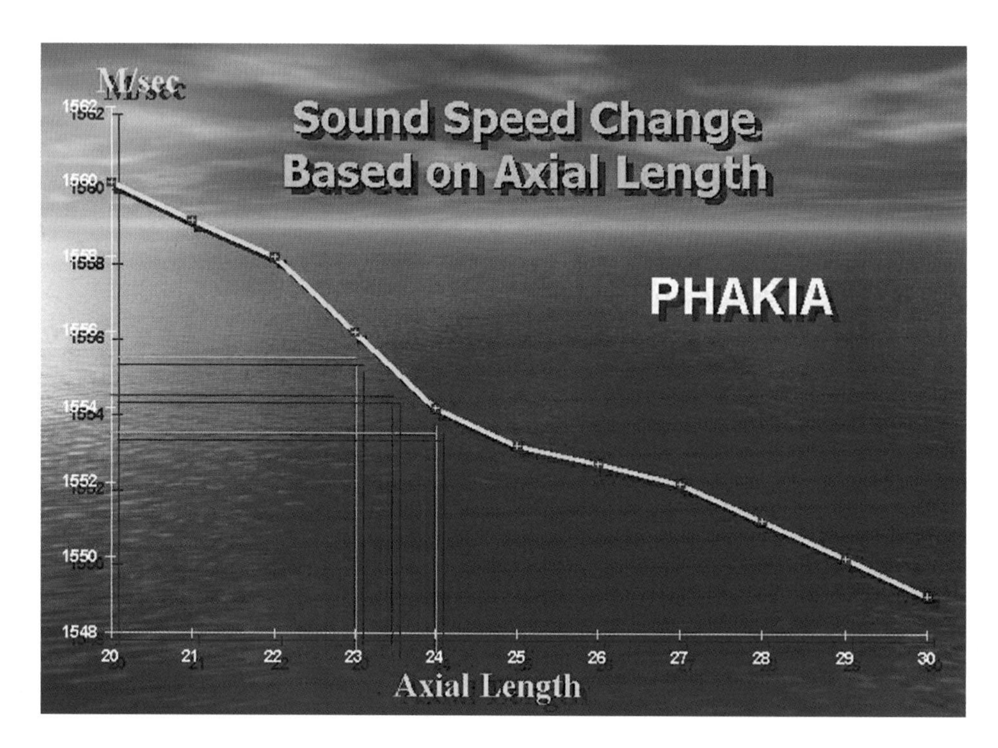

FIGURE 4-6 Phakic velocity. Graph of decline in average sound velocity of a phakic eye as the axial length increases.

TABLE 4-3
Formulas for Calculating Biometric Parameters

A. CALF factors for pseudophakic eyes (using CALF = $T_L \times (1 - 1532/V_L)$, where T_L is the axial thickness of the lens and V_L is the sound velocity for the IOL material in the eye:

- $CALF_{PMMA} = T_L \times (1 - 1532/2660) = +0.424 \times T_L$
- $CALF_{Silicone} = T_L \times (1 - 1532/980) = -0.563 \times T_L$
- $CALF_{Acrylic} = T_L \times (1 - 1532/2026) = +0.243 \times T_L$

B. The correction for the cornea:

- $CALF_{Cornea} = T_C \times (1 - 1532/1641) = 0.55 \times 0.066423 = 0.037$

C. Knowing the thickness of the implanted IOL,* the following formulas can be used:

- PMMA eye $AL = AL_{1532} + 0.424 \times TL + 0.037$
- Silicone eye $AL = AL_{1532} - 0.563 \times TL + 0.037$
- Acrylic eye $AL = AL_{1532} + 0.243 \times TL + 0.037$
- Piggyback IOLs $AL = AL_{1532} + T1 \times (1 - 1532/V_1) + T2 \times (1 - 1532/V_2) + 0.037$, where T_1 and T_2 are the thickness and V_1 and V_2 are the velocity of each IOL

*The IOL thickness can be obtained from the manufacturer.
AL, Axial length; *CALF*, corrected AL factor.

using a CALF of 0.32 (0.28 + 0.037). The correction for the cornea is calculated in Table 4-3.

A similar method can be used for pseudophakic eyes using CALF = $T_L \times (1 - 1532/V_L)$ and the known V_L for each IOL material (see Table 4-3). Knowing the thickness of the implanted IOL, the formulas in Table 4-3 can be used. If the IOL thickness cannot be obtained, the one published by Holladay[7] can be used. The AL of an eye containing two IOLs of different materials can be obtained using the formula in part C of Table 4-3.

Retinal thickness factor. Some formula writers add a value to the ultrasonic AL measurement to take into account the additional distance from the surface of the retina to the level of the receptive end of the cones. This value has been estimated to be 0.20 to 0.25 mm, and it is automatically added to the AL in some formulas (Binkhorst, Holladay) and not used at all in others (Colenbrander, Hoffer Q).

Corneal Power

The first lens in the ocular system is the cornea. The important factors to consider in obtaining accurate corneal power are listed in Table 4-1.

INSTRUMENTATION

Most manual keratometers (Bauch & Lomb, Marco) measure the front surface of the cornea and convert the radius (r) of curvature obtained to diopters (K) using an index of refraction (IR) of 1.3375 (K = 337.5/r).* Many postulate that the 1.3375 index is too high, and Holladay[6] recommends using 4/3 instead. To correct for this, the K reading obtained is multiplied by the factor 0.98765431, which will result in ~0.54-D decrease in corneal power (range 0.43 D for 35-D cornea to 0.62 D for 50-D cornea). If the keratometer uses a different IR, you can change from an IR of 1.332 to 1.3375 by: 1.3375 × K/1.332.

WARNING: *Before using this refractive index correction factor clinically, test it out on a series of previously operated eyes to see what effect it would have had on your accuracy.*

To ensure accuracy, manual keratometers must be calibrated on a regular schedule using the special set of 3 calibration spheres.

Corneal topography units also supply simulated corneal power values. I performed a prospective comparison study of the manual keratometer (B&L) with one such unit (TechnoMed C-Scan, Tubinger, Germany) on 172 cataract eyes. The mean of the central (3-mm zone) readings was 0.24 D flatter with the topography unit (43.55 D vs. 43.79 D), which may be explained by the index of refraction discussed previously. When personalization was performed on both instrument data sets, however, IOL power calculation accuracy was statistically equal.

WARNING: *Hard contact lenses should be removed permanently for at least 2 weeks prior to measuring corneal power for IOL power calculation.*

ASTIGMATISM

Regular astigmatism is not a factor in IOL power calculation because the goal is to predict the postoperative spherical equivalent refractive error. Therefore the average of the two K readings is the only value used and should result in mixed astigmatism. If a myopic cylinder were desired, the flattest K reading could be used instead. If astigmatism is surgically corrected at the time of lens implantation, it would be important to know the effect of this surgery on the final average corneal power and adjust the K reading used to calculate the IOL power accordingly. Because of the coupling ratio, this effect is usually zero, but an analysis of previous cases would be useful.

PREVIOUS REFRACTIVE SURGERY

Previous corneal refractive surgery changes the architecture of the cornea such that standard methods of measuring the corneal power cause it to be underestimated. Radial keratotomy (RK) causes a relatively proportional equal flattening of both the front and back surface of the cornea, leaving the index of refraction relationship the same. On the other hand, photorefractive keratectomy (PRK) and laser-assisted intrastromal keratomileusis (LASIK) flatten only the front surface. This changes the refractive index calculation, creating an underestimation of the corneal power by about 1 diopter for every 7 diopters of refractive surgery correction obtained.

The major cause of error is the fact that most keratometers measure at the 3.2-mm zone of the central cornea, which often misses the central flatter zone of effective corneal power. The following two methods are used to better estimate the corneal power in these refractive surgery eyes.

Clinical History Method.[8-14] This method is based on the fact that the final change in refractive error the eye obtains from surgery was due only to a change in the effective corneal power. If this refractive change is added to the presurgical corneal power, the effective corneal power the eye has now is obtained.

*Other manual keratometers (Jena, Haag-Streit) use different IR values.

WARNING: *All patients having corneal refractive surgery should be given the following data for their personal health records: (1) preoperative corneal power, (2) preoperative refractive error, and (3) postoperative healed refractive error (before lens changes effected it). They should be told to give this data to anyone planning to perform cataract or IOL surgery on them.*

All attempts should be made to obtain the preceding information from the refractive surgeon records. It is not beneficial to vertex-correct the spectacle refraction as was originally recommended.

The estimated effective corneal power (K) can be calculated with the following formula:

$$K = K_{PREOP} + R_{PREOP} - R_{PO}$$

where:
R = Refractive error
PREOP = Preoperative
PO = Postoperative

Contact Lens Method.[8-14] This method is based on the principle that if a hard PMMA contact lens (CL) of plano power (P) and a base curve (B) equal to the effective power of the cornea is placed on the eye, it will not change the refractive error of the eye; that is, the difference between the manifest refraction with the contact lens (R_{CL}) and without it (R_{NoCL}) is zero. The formula to calculate the estimated corneal power is as follows:

$$K = B + P + R_{CL} - R_{NoCL}$$

where:
B = Base curve
P = Power of CL
R = Refractive error
NoCL = Bare refraction

Again, the refractive errors are not vertex-corrected to the corneal plane. Several computer IOL power calculation programs calculate these two methods automatically when needed (Hoffer Programs, Holladay IOL Consultant).

If the results of the previous two methods differ, the lowest estimated corneal power should be used. Rarely are such eyes myopic after IOL surgery. Obviously, the former method cannot be used if the historical data is not available, and the latter method is impossible if the cataract precludes performing a refraction. In such cases, it might be wise to delay the IOL implantation and calculate the secondary implant power using the aphakic refractive error in the refraction formula or use a piggyback lens or phakic refractive lens (PRL) to correct any deficiency.

CORNEAL TRANSPLANT EYES

A problem also arises when attempting to predict what the corneal power will be after a corneal transplant. Some have suggested using the corneal power of the other eye (if available) or using an average of one's posttransplant corneal powers, but published reports show a very large range of prediction and refractive errors with these attempts. In 1986 Hoffer[15,16] suggested performing the IOL implantation after the corneal transplant has settled down, and in 1990 Geggel[17] reported excellent refractive results (Figure 4-7) using this two-stepped approach (66% had 20/40 or better acuity without correction). A secondary piggyback IOL or PRL is another alternative to correct residual ametropia.

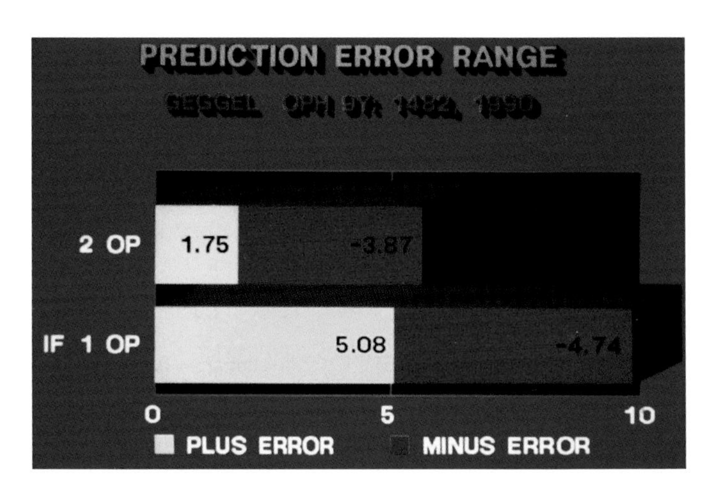

FIGURE 4-7 Corneal transplants. Dramatic decrease in range of IOL prediction error when IOL is implanted secondarily after transplant heals (5.62 D) versus a triple procedure (9.82 D).

IOL Position

This factor was historically referred to as the anterior chamber depth (ACD) because the optic of all IOLs in the early era was positioned in front of the iris in the anterior chamber. Because most IOLs today are positioned behind the iris, new terms have been offered, such as effective lens position (ELP) by Holladay[6] and actual lens position by the Food and Drug Administration.

ACD is defined as the axial distance between the two lenses (cornea and IOL) or, more exactly, the distance from the front surface (anterior vertex) of the cornea to the effective principal plane of the IOL (or front surface of the crystalline lens). This value is required for all formulas, and it is incorporated into the A constant specific to each IOL style for regression formulas or as an ACD, both supplied by the manufacturer. Some have proposed that it would be useful to measure the preoperative anatomic ACD (corneal epithelium to anterior capsule) either with an A-scan unit or by optical pachymetry. I performed such a comparison study on 44 eyes and showed that the optical method resulted in a mean 0.20 (±0.35) mm deeper ACD than obtained by ultrasound using 1548 m/sec (3.14 vs. 2.93 mm).

The IOL position has been considered the least important of the three variables as a cause of IOL power error, but in 1998, I saw an early postoperative IOL patient with a shallowed ACD and myopia of –2.50 change to plano in 3 days, after the chamber deepened by 2 mm. IOL position has received the most attention from formula writers over the past 10 years. The major effort has been directed toward a better prediction of where the IOL will ultimately rest. A recent study on a series of 270 eyes receiving a silicone plate haptic lens showed that the IOL shifted a mean of 0.06 mm posteriorly at 3 months, compared with its position on the first day after surgery. This was commensurate with a mean 0.21-D shift toward hyperopia.

WARNING: *An IOL intended for capsular bag placement should be decreased by 0.75 to 1.00 D (depending on the IOL power) when placed in the ciliary sulcus.*

Formulas

Generations

FIRST GENERATION

The first IOL power formula was published by Fyodorov and Kolonko[18] in 1967. Colenbrander[19] wrote his in 1972, followed by the Hoffer[20] formula in 1974. Binkhorst[21] published his formula in 1975, which became widely used in America. In 1978, first Lloyd and Gills,[22,23] followed by Retzlaff[24] and later Sanders & Kraff,[25] each developed a regression formula based on analysis of their previous IOL cases. This work was amalgamated in 1980 to yield the SRK I formula.[26] All these formulas depended on a single constant for each lens that represented the predicted IOL position (ACD).

SECOND GENERATION

In 1982 at the Welsh Cataract Congress in Houston, Hoffer[27,28] showed a direct relationship between the position of a PMMA posterior chamber IOL and the AL and presented a formula to better predict ACD. Others (Binkhorst,[29] SRK II[30] [1988]) developed different mechanisms to apply this predictive relationship, which Holladay defined as the second generation.

THIRD GENERATION

In 1988 Holladay[31] proposed a direct relationship between the steepness of the cornea and the position of the IOL. He modified the Binkhorst formula to incorporate this, as well as the AL relationship. Instead of ACD input, the formula would calculate the predicted distance from the cornea to the iris plane (using a corneal height formula by Fyodorov) and add to it the distance from the iris plane to the IOL. The latter he called the *surgeon factor* (SF), and it is specific to each lens. Retzlaff[32] followed suit and modified the Holladay I formula to allow use of A constants, calling it the SRK/T theoretic formula in 1990. It was intended to replace the previous SRK regression formulas, but 50% of American surgeons still use them. In 1992 Hoffer[33] developed the Q formula using a tangent function to accomplish the same effect.

FOURTH GENERATION

In 1990 Olsen et al.[34] proposed using the preoperative ACD and other factors to better estimate the postoperative IOL position and published algorithms for this approach. After several studies showed the Holladay I formula was not as accurate as the Hoffer Q in eyes shorter than 22 mm, Holladay used the preoperative ACD measurement, as well as corneal diameter, lens thickness, refractive error and age, to calculate an estimated scaling factor (ESF) that multiplies the IOL-specific ACD. This Holladay II formula has been promulgated since 1996 but has yet to be published.

REFRACTION FORMULA

Holladay[35] published a formula in 1993 to calculate the power of an IOL for an aphakic eye or ametropic pseudophakic eye (piggyback IOL) or a refractive lens (PRL) for a phakic eye. It does not need the AL but requires the corneal power, preoperative refractive error, and desired postoperative refractive error, as well as the vertex distance of both. I do not recommend its use in aphakic eyes because the vertex distance is difficult to measure accurately, and because of the high power of their refractive error, greater errors can result. It is, however, a good check against the AL formula calculation.

Usage

BASED ON AXIAL LENGTH

My study[33] of 450 eyes (by one surgeon using one IOL style [Figure 4-8]) showed that in the normal range (72%) of AL (22 to 24.5 mm) almost all formulas function adequately but that the SRK I formula is the leading cause of poor refractive results in eyes outside this range. It also showed that the Holladay I formula was the most accurate in medium-long eyes (24.5 to 26 mm) (15%) and that the SRK/T was more accurate in very long eyes (>26 mm) (5%). In short eyes (<22 mm) (8%) the Hoffer Q formula was most accurate, and this was confirmed ($p > 0.0001$) in an additional large study of 830 short eyes, as well as in a multiple-surgeon study by Holladay. Holladay has postulated that the other formulas overestimate the shallowing of the ELP in these very short eyes.

A more recent study[36] I performed on 317 eyes showed that the Holladay II formula equaled the Hoffer Q in short eyes but was not as accurate as the Holladay I or Hoffer Q in average and medium-long eyes (Table 4-4). Eyes shorter than 19 mm are extremely rare (0.1%) and may well be benefited by using the Holladay II formula. In attempting to improve the accuracy of the Holladay formula, the addition of more biometric data input has improved the Holladay II formula in the extremes of AL but deteriorated its excellent performance in the normal and medium-long range of eyes (22 to 26 mm), which is 82% of the population.

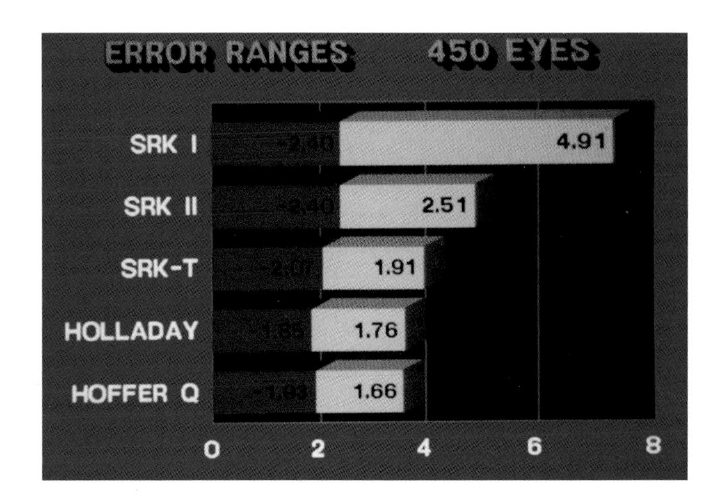

FIGURE 4-8 Error range. Range of IOL power error in study of 450 eyes using regression formulas compared with modern theoretic formulas.

TABLE 4-4

Results of Accuracy of Four Theoretical Formulas on 317 Eyes Using the Holladay IOL Consultant for Analysis*

	Mean Absolute Error						All 317 Eyes	
Formula	**Short Eyes <22 mm**	**Normal Eyes 22-24.5 mm**	**Medium-Long Eyes 24.5-26 mm**	**Very Long >26 mm**	**All Long Eyes <24.5 mm**	**All Eyes**	**Maximum Error**	**>±2D Error**
Holladay II	**0.72**	0.56	0.51	0.49	0.50	0.55	−1.60	0%
Holladay I	0.85	**0.42**	**0.37**	0.56	0.43	**0.43**	−1.44	0%
Hoffer Q	**0.72**	**0.43**	0.47	0.58	0.50	**0.45**	−1.61	0%
SRK/T	0.83	0.46	**0.35**	**0.44**	**0.36**	**0.44**	−1.45	0%
Average	0.78	0.47	0.42	0.52	0.45	0.47		
Best	H-Q H-II	H-Q H-I	SRK/T H-I	SRK/T	SRK/T			

From Hoffer KJ: Clinical results using the Holladay 2 intraocular lens power formula, *J Cataract Refract Surg* 26:1233-1237, 2000.
*Boldface numbers = recommended formulas.

A

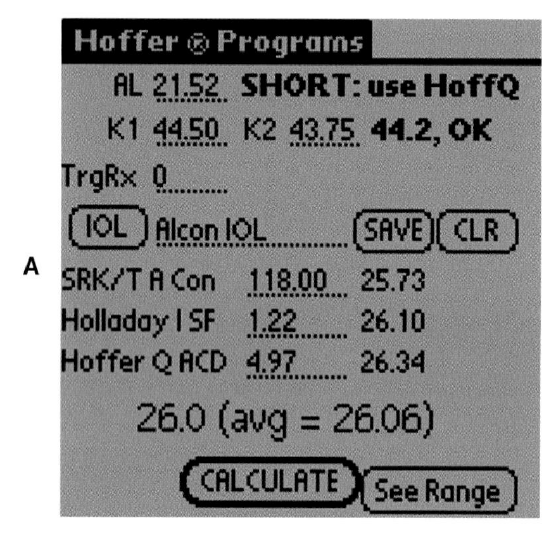

B

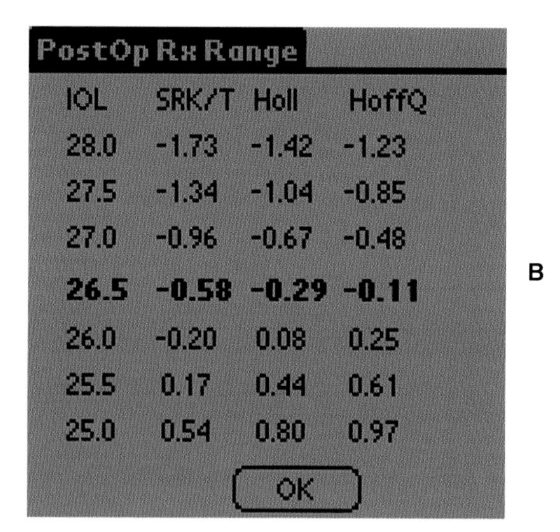

FIGURE 4-9 Hoffer Programs IOL power program on a Palm personal digital assistant. **A,** Main calculation screen using Hoffer Q, Holladay, and SRK/T formulas. **B,** Next screen showing refractive results of different IOL powers.

METHODOLOGY

There are several means by which to use these newer formulas, including A-scan instruments; handheld calculators; computer programs that run on DOS, Windows, and Macintosh systems; and the handheld Palm PDA operating system (Figure 4-9). Also, the published ones can be programmed on a spreadsheet. It is important to check the errata in references 32 (SRK/T) and 33 (Hoffer Q). The most popular commercial programs are the Hoffer Programs System* (1990) and the Holladay IOL Consultant* (1997), which include several formulas and the ability to personalize them, as well as routines to deal with odd clinical situations.

Personalization

The concept of personalizing a formula based on a surgeon's past experience and data was introduced by Retzlaff[37] using the A constant to refine the formula. Holladay incorporated this concept into backsolving for the surgeon factor, and Hoffer backsolved for his personalized ACD. Several studies have proved that formula personalization definitely improves formula accuracy significantly.

The following parameters are required from postoperative eyes for personalization:

1. Axial length (preoperative)
2. Corneal power (preoperative)
3. IOL power
4. Postoperative refractive error (stable)

The eyes should all contain the same lens style by one manufacturer implanted by one surgeon. The same biometry instruments and technician should also have been used. Eyes with postoperative surprises or acuity worse than 20/40 should not be included because of the poor accuracy in obtaining refractive error. Personalization involves backsolving for the exact IOL position that would produce that refractive error with that AL and K. Then all the "ideal" IOL positions are averaged to arrive at the personalized value to use in the future. Personalization can be easily performed using the Hoffer Programs or Holladay IOL Consultant computer programs.

*Available from EyeLab, Inc., 1605 San Vicente Blvd, Santa Monica, CA 90402; 310-451-2020.

Clinical Variables

Patient Needs and Desires

Most surgeons have developed their own plan for deciding on the clinical needs of their patients. A common recommendation is to aim patients for mild postoperative myopia (–0.5 to –1.5 D) so that if the error is on the plus side, they will be emmetropic, and if on the minus side, they will have reading vision. This is necessary because of the larger range of IOL power errors generally experienced. When the bell-shaped curve of prediction error is squeezed down to 67% within ±0.50 D, it is possible to aim most patients for emmetropia. This is even more important when implanting a multifocal IOL. Senior citizens are much more active today then in the past, and in emergency situations it would be a lot safer if they were emmetropic to escape to safety.

There are several exceptions, however. Patients who have been lifelong myopes are never happy being hyperopes postoperatively. Patients that would wind up with a large anisometropia should be stimulated to be fit with a contact lens in the other eye before deciding on an emmetropic IOL. Monocular contact lens wearers are more successful than binocular. It is wise to document all discussions in unusual situations.

Special Circumstances

MONOCULAR CATARACT IN BILATERAL HIGH AMETROPIA

The dilemma is whether to make the surgical eye emmetropic or match the large ametropia of the other eye, which may never need surgery. Until now, I have convinced most patients to accept a contact lens or ignore the other eye and go for the "brass ring" of emmetropia. In the future, those who can't tolerate contact lenses could have a PRL either placed in the other eye or placed over the IOL to eliminate aniseikonia and have it removed if the other eye ultimately has surgery.

PEDIATRIC EYES

Children have always posed a dilemma[38] in IOL power selection in that the eye will grow in length and become more myopic if a fixed emmetropic power is implanted. The study of pediatric eyes by Gordon and Donzis[39] shows a steep AL growth rate from premature babies to age 2, increasing by 6 mm (~20 D), whereas corneal power drops from 54 D to 44 D, offsetting 10 D. If IOLs are used in this age-group, it might be best to place piggyback lenses with the more posterior IOL having the average adult emmetropic power and the anterior IOL being the added power needed to reach emmetropia now. As the child grows, the vision can be corrected with myopic glasses until he or she is old enough to have the anterior IOL removed.

Between the ages of 2 to 5 years, growth slows to about 0.4 mm per year and only increases another 1 mm from age 5 to 10 while corneal power remains stable. From age 2 to 10, it might be wise to aim for 1.5 to 2 D of hyperopia postoperatively, which allows for reasonable uncorrected vision and light spectacle correction in amblyopia treatment. When the child matures, he or she will become emmetropic or mildly myopic, depending on age at implantation. Growth slows after age 10 to 15, and emmetropia can be the aim. Future use of implantable PRLs over the top of IOLs may be very helpful in these kids because they can easily be exchanged as the eye grows, keeping them emmetropic throughout life.

BIFOCAL IOL

In 1991 the author[40] reported that to obtain –2.75 D myopia (reading at 14 to 16 inches), the IOL power in the near vision region must be about 3.75 to 4.00 D stronger than the emmetropic power. Also, the amount of this additional power in a bifocal IOL is not affected at all by the AL and is affected very little by the corneal power. However, it is affected by the IOL position, and an AC lens would need less add power than a PC lens. In multifocal IOL implantation, to negate the need for any glasses, it is important to aim for emmetropia, but mild postoperative hyperopia is far better than even the mildest myopia. The distance vision will be reasonable in the former (they can easily obtain readers if necessary); whereas in the latter it will not. Bifocal IOL patients with myopia are not happy, and everything should be done to avoid this situation because minus power "readers" are not readily available. In the future, a PRL could be implanted over the top of the bifocal to make the eye emmetropic.

SILICONE OIL REFRACTIVE EFFECT

The second problem that arises when the vitreous is replaced with silicone oil is that the refractive index of the oil is much less than that of vitreous, and it acts as a negative lens in the eye, which must be offset with more power in the IOL. This effect depends on the shape factor of the back surface of the IOL in that a biconvex IOL creates the worst problem and a concave posterior lens (no longer commercially available) causes practically none. In between the two is the plano-posterior lens, which is recommended in these cases. With a plano-convex lens, 2 to 3 D must be added to the IOL power to compensate for this silicone effect, and 5 to 6 D for a biconvex lens.

PIGGYBACK LENSES

Either piggyback lenses can be placed primarily or the second lens placed secondarily over a previously healed IOL. In the former, the anterior IOL forces the posterior IOL more posteriorly a distance equal to the central thickness of the anterior lens. This causes the posterior lens (whose focal point is moved farther behind the retina) to require more power to maintain the same focus. This effect diminishes the thinner (lower power) the anterior lens is, and a thinner lens is easier to remove if necessary. Primary piggyback lenses necessitate special calculations to adjust for the posterior lens shift.

Secondary piggyback lenses can be calculated with the refraction formula or by a more simple formula based on the fact that the healed primary IOL is more stable. Because of the different effect on vertex power changes between plus and minus lenses, the following formulation works well.

$$\text{Hyperopic: Piggyback IOL} = 1.5 \times Rx_{\text{ERROR}}$$
$$\text{Myopic error: Piggyback IOL} = 1.0 \times Rx_{\text{ERROR}}$$

where *Rx* is postoperative spherical equivalent refractive error.

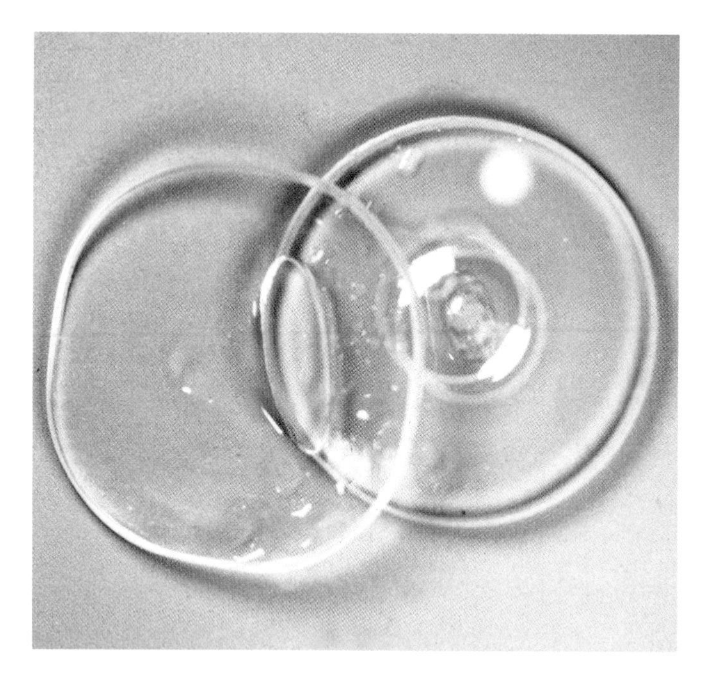

FIGURE 4-10 McReynolds IOL lens power analyzer.

Problems and Errors

The major problem is an unacceptable postoperative refractive error. The sooner it is discovered, the sooner it can be corrected. Therefore it is wise to perform K readings and a manifest refraction on the first postoperative day. Immediate surgical correction[41] (24 to 48 hours) allows easy access to the incision and the capsular bag, one postoperative period, and excellent uncorrected vision. The majority of medicolegal cases today are due to a delay in diagnosis and treatment of this iatrogenic problem. Until now, this problem could only be corrected by lens exchange, which creates the dilemma of determining which factor created the IOL power error: AL, corneal power, mislabeled IOL, or a combination. Today, with the advent of low-powered IOLs, the best remedy may be a piggyback IOL. With a piggyback IOL, it is not necessary to determine what caused the error or to remeasure the AL of the freshly operated pseudophakic eye. The power of an explanted IOL can be confirmed by using the McReynolds lens analyzer* (Figure 4-10).

A shallow AC can lead to as much as 3 D of myopia (depending on the power of the IOL), which will disappear when the AC reforms. An RK eye has a propensity for the cornea to flatten postoperatively, causing large hyperopic surprises. It may take up to 3 to 4 months for the cornea to resteepen; therefore surgical correction should not be attempted until then.

Conclusion

Simple steps and attention to detail can be very useful in preventing IOL power errors, and recent advances in IOL power range availability have made this problem more easily corrected. Since the first American ultrasound IOL power calculation[42] in 1974, the past quarter century has seen great improvement in the accuracy of postoperative refractive prediction. Future improvements may someday eliminate the problems that remain.

*William McReynolds, MD, 1111 Main St., Quincy, IL 62301; 217-222-6656.

REFERENCES

1. Ossoinig KC: Standardized echography: basic principles, clinical applications, and results, *Int Ophthalmol Clin* 19:127, 1979.
2. Shammas HJF: A comparison of immersion and contact techniques for axial length measurements, *J Am Intraocul Implant Soc* 10:444-447, 1984.
3. Schelenz J, Kammann J: Comparison of contact and immersion techniques for axial measurement and implant power calculation, *J Cataract Refract Surg* 15:425-428, 1989.
4. Hoffer KJ: Ultrasound speeds for axial length measurement, *J Cataract Refract Surg* 20:554-562, 1994.
5. Mark HF, Bikales N, Overberger CG et al, editors: *Encyclopedia of Polymer Science & Engineering*, vol 1, New York, 1989, Wiley and Sons, pp 147-149.
6. Holladay JT: Standardizing constants for ultrasonic biometry, keratometry, and intraocular lens power calculation, *J Cataract Refract Surg* 23:1356-1370, 1997.
7. Holladay JT, Prager TC: Accurate ultrasonic biometry in pseudophakia, *Am J Ophthalmol* 107:189-190, 1989.
8. Holladay JT: IOL calculations following radial keratotomy surgery, *Refract Corneal Surg* 5:36A, 1989.
9. Hoffer KJ: IOL power calculation in RK eyes, *Phaco Foldables* 7:6, 1994.
10. Hoffer KJ: Calculation of intraocular lens power in post-radial keratotomy eyes, *Ophthalmic Practice (Canada)* 12:242-243, 1994.
11. Hoffer KJ: Ways to calculate IOL power in RK eyes. Refractive surgery update (Thornton), *Ocular Surg News* 13:86, 1995.
12. Hoffer KJ: Intraocular lens power calculation for eyes after refractive keratotomy, *J Refract Surg* 11:490-493, 1995.
13. Hoffer KJ: How to do cataract surgery after RK, *Review Ophthalmol* 20: 117-120, 1996.
14. Hoffer KJ: Intraocular lens power calculation for eyes after refractive keratotomy, consultation section, *Ann Ophthalmol* 28:67-68, 1996.
15. Hoffer KJ: The triple procedure: a plea for three, *Geriatric Ophthalmol* 2:7, 1986.
16. Hoffer KJ: Triple procedure for intraocular lens exchange, *Arch Ophthalmol* 105:609, 1987.
17. Geggel HS: Intraocular lens implantation after penetrating keratoplasty: improved unaided visual acuity, astigmatism, and safety in patients with combined corneal disease and cataract, *Ophthalmology* 97:1460-1467, 1990.
18. Fyodorov SN, Kolonko AI: Estimation of optical power of the intraocular lens, *Vestnik Oftalmologic (Moscow)* 4:27, 1967.
19. Colenbrander MC: Calculation of the power of an iris-clip lens for distance vision, *Br J Ophthalmol* 57:735-740, 1973.
20. Hoffer KJ: Intraocular lens calculation: the problem of the short eye, *Ophthalmic Surg* 12:269-272, 1981.
21. Binkhorst RD: The optical design of intraocular lens implants, *Ophthalmic Surg* 6:17-31, 1975.
22. Gills JP: Regression formula, *J Am Intraocul Implant Soc* 4:163, 1978 (editorial).
23. Gills JP: Minimizing postoperative refractive error, *Contact Intraocular Lens Med J* 6:56-59, 1980.
24. Retzlaff J: A new intraocular lens calculation formula, *J Am Intraocul Implant Soc* 6:148, 1980.
25. Sanders DR, Kraff MC: Improvement of intraocular lens power calculation: regression formula, *J Am Intraocul Implant Soc* 6:263, 1980.
26. Sanders DR, Retzlaff J, Kraff MC et al: Comparison of the accuracy of the Binkhorst, Colenbrander and SRK implant power prediction formulas, *J Am Intraocul Implant Soc* 7:337-340, 1981.
27. Hoffer KJ: Biometry of the posterior capsule: a new formula for anterior chamber depth of posterior chamber lenses. In Emery JC, Jacobson AC, editors: *Current concepts in cataract surgery (Eighth Congress)*, New York, 1983, Appleton-Century Crofts, pp 56-62.
28. Hoffer KJ: The effect of axial length on posterior chamber lenses and posterior capsule position, *Curr Concepts Ophthalmic Surg* 1:20-22, 1984.
29. Binkhorst RD: Biometric A-scan ultrasonography and intraocular lens power calculation. In Emery JE, editor: *Current concepts in cataract surgery: selected proceedings of the Fifth Biennial Cataract Surgical Congress*, St Louis, 1987, Mosby, pp 175-182.

30. Sanders DR, Retzlaff J, Kraff MC: Comparison of the SRK II formula and the other second generation formulas, *J Cataract Refract Surg* 14:136-141, 1988.
31. Holladay JT, Prager TC, Chandler TY et al: A three-part system for refining intraocular lens power calculations. *J Cataract Refract Surg* 14:17-24, 1988.
32. Retzlaff J, Sanders DR, Kraff MC: Development of the SRK/T intraocular lens implant power calculation formula, *J Cataract Refract Surg* 16:333-340, 1990; Errata: 16:528, 1990.
33. Hoffer KJ: The Hoffer Q formula: a comparison of theoretic and regression formulas, *J Cataract Refract Surg* 19:700-712, 1993; Errata: 20:677, 1994.
34. Olsen T, Oleson H, Thim K et al: Prediction of postoperative intraocular lens chamber depth, *J Cataract Refract Surg* 16:587-590, 1990.
35. Holladay JT: Refractive power calculation for intraocular lenses in the phakic eye, *Am J Ophthalmol* 116:63-66, 1993.
36. Hoffer KJ: Clinical results using the Holladay 2 intraocular lens power formula, *J Cataract Refract Surg* 26:1233-1237, 2000.
37. Retzlaff J: Calculating the surgeon's personal A-constant. In Retzlaff J, Sanders DR, Kraff MC, editors: *Lens implant power calculation manual*, ed 3, Thorofare, NJ, 1990, Slack Inc, pp 12-13.
38. Hoffer KJ: Selection of lens power for implantation in infants and children, *J Am Intraocul Implant Soc* 1:49, 1975.
39. Gordon RA, Donzis PB: Refractive development of the human eye, *Arch Ophthalmol* 103:785-789, 1985.
40. Hoffer KJ: Lens power calculation for multifocal IOLs. In Maxwell A, Nordan LT, editors: *Current concepts of multifocal intraocular lenses*, Thorofare, NJ, 1991, Slack Inc, pp 193-208.
41. Hoffer KJ: Early lens exchange for power calculation error, *J Cataract Refract Surg* 21:486-487, 1995.
42. Hoffer KJ: The history of IOL power calculation in North America. In Kwitko ML, Kelman CD, editors: *The history of modern cataract surgery*, The Hague, Netherlands, 1998, Kuglen Publications, pp 193-208.

Ophthalmic Viscosurgical Devices: Physical Characteristics, Clinical Applications, and Complications

5

Stephen S. Lane, MD

The introduction of viscoelastic agents (now termed *ophthalmic viscosurgical devices* [OVDs] by the International Standards Organization) for use in ophthalmic intraocular procedures has had a significant impact on the practice of ophthalmology. OVDs possess a unique set of properties, based on their chemical structure, that enable them to protect the corneal endothelium from mechanical trauma and to maintain an intraocular space, even with an open incision. Viscosurgery,[1] a term used to designate the procedures and manipulations performed with OVDs, has been used in a broad spectrum of ophthalmic procedures. The use of OVDs has become commonplace in anterior segment surgery, and the widespread use and availability of these materials most likely have facilitated and helped ease the transition in the conversion first from intracapsular to planned extracapsular surgery and then to phacoemulsification.

The physical properties of OVDs are the result of chain length and intrachain and interchain molecular interactions. The diverse rheologic properties of any given OVD directly affect the clinical characteristics of that particular material. A thorough understanding of these properties allows ophthalmic surgeons to choose an OVD that is task specific. For example, a specific substance may be selected because of its space maintenance qualities, its corneal endothelial protection qualities, or its coating qualities.

Rheologic and Physical Properties

The rheologic characteristics of OVDs that are most relevant when considering their usefulness in ophthalmic surgery are viscoelasticity, viscosity, pseudoplasticity, and surface tension (Tables 5-1 and 5-2).

Viscoelasticity

Elasticity refers to the ability of a solution to return to its original shape after being stressed. The rheologic property of viscoelasticity is the essence of the usefulness of these materials as surgical tools in ophthalmology. Elasticity allows the anterior chamber to reform after deformation by depression on the cornea when external forces are released. A nonelastic solution such as balanced salt solution (BSS) will show no such reformation after release of forces.

The terms *viscosity* and *viscoelasticity* are not synonymous. Viscosity, viscoelasticity, and pseudoplasticity, however, are interrelated. The amount of elasticity of an elastic compound increases with increasing molecular weight and greater chain length of the molecules. Unfortunately, comparison of the different OVDs with regard to elasticity is not easily made because of the different ways and nonuniform expression of values by the various manufacturers.

Viscosity

Viscosity (see Table 5-1) reflects a solution's resistance to flow, which is in part a function of the molecular weight of the substance. Viscosity of viscoelastics is measured in centipoise (cP) or centistokes (cSt), which are measures of the resistance to flow relative to a given shear force. Liquid solutions are generally considered to have viscosities of less than 10,000 cSt at rest, whereas solutions with resting viscosities greater than 100,000 cSt are gel-like. The higher the solution's molecular weight, the more it resists flow. Molecular weight, on the other hand, reflects the size of the solution's molecules. Viscosity depends on the degree of movement of a solution, which is also known as the shear rate, and varies inversely with temperature. The viscosity of a solution can be increased by increasing either the concentration or the molecular weight of the solution.

To facilitate optimal intraocular manipulation, an OVD should maintain space and protect tissues (possess a high viscosity at low shear rates), allow movement of instruments, aid in intraocular lens (IOL) implantation (possess a moderate viscosity at medium shear rates), and allow easy introduction into the eye through a small cannula (possess a low viscosity at high shear rates).[2] At the present time, no OVD fulfills all of these requirements.

Pseudoplasticity

Pseudoplasticity refers to a solution's ability to transform when under pressure, from a gel-like substance to a more liquid substance. The more pseudoplastic a material is, the more rapidly it changes from being highly viscous at rest to a thin,

Dr. Lane has no commercial or proprietary interest in the products discussed and will not receive any remuneration resulting from their use.

TABLE 5-1

Physical Properties of OVD Substances

	Resting Viscosity (cP)*	Dynamic Viscosity (cP)‡	Color	Pseudoplasticity	Contact Angle
Healon	>200,000	40,000-64,000	Clear	+++	60 degrees
Healon GV	2,000,000	80,000	Clear	++++	†
Amvisc	100,000	40,000	Clear	+++	60 degrees
Amvisc Plus	102,000	55,000	Clear	+++	†
Chondroitin sulfate	17,000 at 50%	30 at 20%	Yellow	No	†
Viscoat	41,000	40,000	Clear	++	52 degrees
Ocucoat	†	4000	Clear	+	52 degrees
Vitrax	40,000	30,000	Clear	+++	†
ProVisc	†	39,000	Clear	+++	†
Healon 5	7 million	60,000-80,000	Clear	++++	†
Cellugel	**40,000**	30,000	Clear	++	†

Modified from Liesegang TJ: Viscoelastic substances in ophthalmology, *Surv Opththalmol* 34:268-293, 1990.
*At shear rate of zero; data from Arshinoff S, personal communication.
†Not available.
‡At shear rate of 2/s, 25 °C. Pseudoplasticity key: + = slight; ++ = fair; +++ = good; ++++ = excellent.

TABLE 5-2

Physical Properties of Various OVD Materials

	Source	Manufacturer Molecular Mass (daltons)	Content	pH Buffer Solvent	Osmolality (mOsm/kg H_2O)	Concentration (mg/ml)
Healon 5	Rooster combs	Pharmacia Pfizer	2.3% sodium hyaluronate	7.0-7.5 phosphate-buffered saline	320	23
Healon GV	Rooster combs	Pharmacia Pfizer 5×10^6	1.4% sodium hyaluronate	7.0-7.5 phosphate-buffered saline	302	14
Healon	Rooster combs	Pharmacia Pfizer $2.5\text{-}3.8 \times 10^6$	1% sodium hyaluronate	7.0-7.5 phosphate-buffered saline	309	10
Vitrax	Rooster combs	Advanced Medical Optics 5×10^5	3% sodium hyaluronate	7.0-7.5 physiologic BSS	310	30
Amvisc	Rooster combs	Bausch & Lomb 2×10^6	1% sodium hyaluronate	6.5-7.2 physiologic saline	318	10
Amvisc Plus	Rooster combs	Bausch & Lomb 2×10^6	1.6% sodium hyaluronate	7.2 physiologic saline	340	16
Viscoat	Bacterial fermentation (sodium hyaluronate): shark fin cartilage (sodium chondroitin sulfate)	Alcon 500×10^3; 25×10^3	3% sodium hyaluronate; 4% sodium chondroitin sulfate	7.0-7.5 physiologic phosphate buffer	360	Sodium hyaluronate 30; chondroitin sulfate 40
Ocucoat	Wood pulp	Bausch & Lomb 86×10^3	2% HPMC	7.2 BSS and variable buffers	319	20
ProVisc	Bacterial fermentation	Alcon 1.9×10^6	1% sodium hyaluronate	7.25 physiologic sodium chloride phosphate buffer	310	10
Cellugel	Wood pulp	Alcon 3×10^5	2% HPMC	N/A	315	N/A

BSS, Balanced salt solution; *HPMC,* hydroxypropyl methylcellulose.

watery solution at high shear rates. A change in molecular structure accompanies this pseudoplastic behavior. In clinical terms, a high-molecular-weight, high-viscosity OVD at rest (zero shear force) acts as an excellent lubricant, coats tissues, and maintains space very well. When under the influence of stress (i.e., a high shear rate), however, the OVD will become an elastic molecular system behaving as an excellent shock-absorbing gel. The highest shear rates occur when a solution is passed through a cannula, and viscosity becomes independent of molecular weight. When the molecules align themselves in the direction of flow, the viscosity is determined solely by the concentration. Pseudoplastic solutions therefore have a low

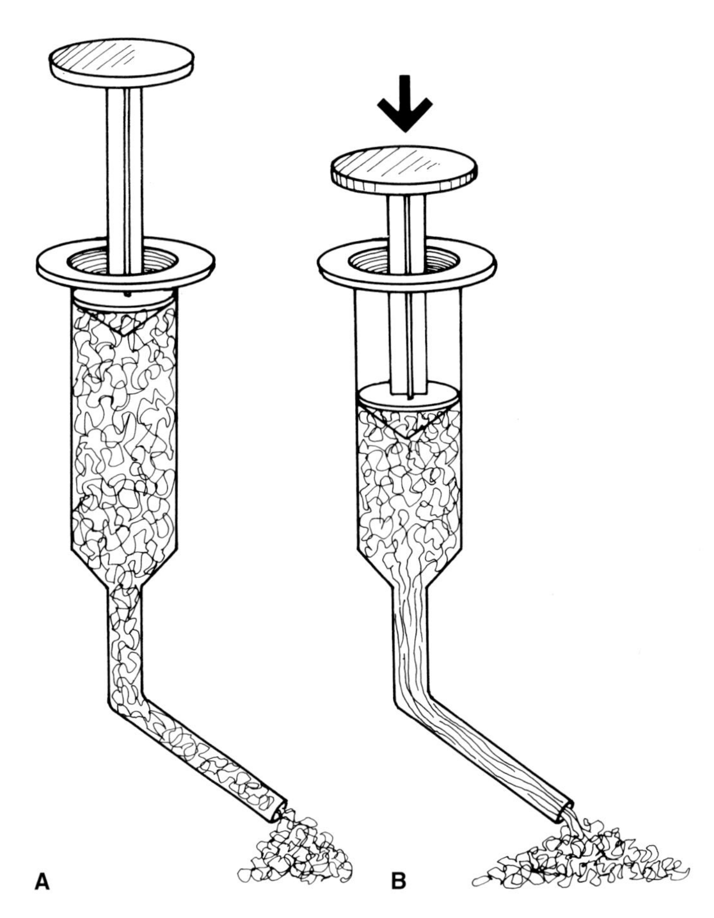

FIGURE 5-1 **A,** When shear is applied (flow through a cannula), the large, randomly entangled coils begin to uncoil, allowing flow. **B,** With increasing shear (more pressure on the syringe plunger), unfolding increases, entanglement drops, and the viscous solution flows easily through the cannula.

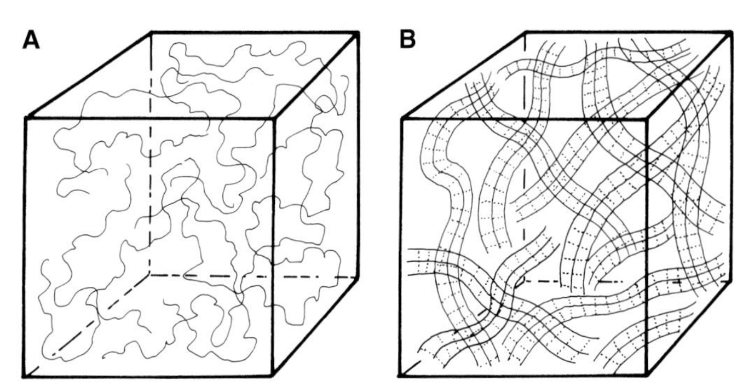

FIGURE 5-2 **A,** Sodium hyaluronate (NaHA) molecules in low concentration at rest (zero shear rate). In solution the NaHA chain folds on itself and forms a long, loose, randomly arranged coil. **B,** As the concentration of these large NaHA molecules is increased, the individual molecular coils start to overlap and become compressed. This crowding of the chains increases the chances for various noncovalent chain-chain interactions. This in turn increases the viscosity of the solution and also increases the elasticity of the solution.

viscosity at high shear rates and can be extruded easily through a small-diameter cannula (27 or 30 gauge) (Figure 5-1). The viscosity of a viscoelastic substance at rest (zero shear rate) is a function of concentration, molecular weight, and the size of the flexible molecular coils of the material (Figure 5-2). At high shear rates, the viscosity is independent of molecular weight and is determined mainly by the concentration.[3]

Surface Tension

The coating ability of an OVD is determined not only by the surface tension of the material itself but also by the surface tension of the contact tissue, surgical instrument, or IOL. By measuring the angle formed by a drop of the OVD on a flat surface (the contact angle), the coating ability of a substance can be estimated. Lower surface tension and lower contact angle indicate a better ability to coat. In this respect a solution of sodium hyaluronate has a significantly higher surface tension and contact angle than does a solution of chondroitin sulfate, sodium hyaluronate–chondroitin sulfate in combination, or hydroxypropyl methylcellulose (HPMC), thus indicating these latter solutions provide superior coating.[3]

A comparison of the various physical properties of OVDs is summarized in Tables 5-1 and 5-2.

Cohesion and Dispersion

In an attempt to help us better understand the interaction among these various rheologic properties and their clinical usefulness, Arshinoff[4] has divided OVDs into two categories:

- *Viscocohesive* OVDs are characterized by high-viscosity material, which adheres to itself through intramolecular bonds or intermolecular entanglement and resists breaking apart. In general, OVDs with long molecular chains will be more cohesive because the molecules become entangled. Cohesive OVDs possess a high molecular weight, a high degree of pseudoplasticity, and high surface tension.
- *Viscodispersive* OVDs exhibit opposite characteristics. They possess lower viscosity and adhere well to external surfaces, such as tissues and instruments. These materials tend to break apart easily compared with cohesive materials and exhibit lower molecular weight, lower surface tension, and lower pseudoplasticity.

Although cohesiveness and dispersiveness are not measurable rheologic properties in themselves, they are useful constructs when considering the clinical behavior of OVDs.

Recently, a new descriptive term, *viscoadaptive,* has been introduced. This term refers to the ability of an OVD to adapt its behavior to the intended surgical task without the surgeon having to do anything except perform the task at hand. Unlike devices that fit one of the two aforementioned categories, the viscoadaptive agent ideally functions as both, *adapting* its behavior to a changing parameter in its environment. That changing parameter under most circumstances is the degree of turbulence present.

Desired Properties of OVDs

As mentioned earlier, the interplay among the various rheologic properties is responsible for the clinical characteristics desired in performing ophthalmic surgery. As a corollary, the degree to

TABLE 5-3
Desired Properties of an Ideal OVD

Desired Properties of an Ideal OVD
Ease of infusion
Retention under positive pressure in the eye
Retention during phacoemulsification
Easy removal or no removal required
Does not interfere with instruments or IOL placement
Protects the endothelium
Nontoxic
Does not obstruct aqueous outflow
Clear

IOL, Intraocular lens; *OVD,* ophthalmic viscosurgical device.

which we can maximize these desirable clinical characteristics is, for the most part, based on our ability to optimize the unique rheologic and physical properties that each OVD possesses. The desired properties of an ideal OVD are listed in Table 5-3.

Viscoelastic Compounds, the Building Blocks of Commercially Available Viscoelastic Materials

Sodium Hyaluronate

Sodium hyaluronate (NaHA) is a biopolymer occurring in many connective tissues throughout the body, including both the aqueous and vitreous humors. Its basic structural unit is a disaccharide, joined by a beta-1,4-glucosidic bond, which is linked in a repeating fashion with beta-glucosidic bonds to form a long unbranched chain. This mucopolysaccharide chain subsequently forms a random coil when placed in a solution such as physiologic saline. As the concentration of large sodium hyaluronate molecules is increased (>0.5 mg/ml), individual molecular coils start to overlap and are compressed (see Figure 5-2). This crowding of the chains increases the chances for various noncovalent chain-chain interactions. This, in turn, causes a considerable increase in the viscosity of the solution. For example, the kinematic viscosity of a 2 mg/ml concentration of sodium hyaluronate in physiologic buffer is only in the 100-cSt range: at 10 mg/ml, it is in the 100,000-cSt range. Therefore a fivefold increase in the concentration causes a 1000-fold increase in the viscosity of the solution. With this increase in viscosity, the elastic properties of the solution also increase. This forms the rationalization of Amvisc Plus and Healon GV. The elastic behavior of a concentrated (>0.5 mg/ml) sodium hyaluronate solution depends greatly on the mechanical energy (shear force) applied to the solution. On a molecular level, this means that under the imposed strain, the polysaccharide coils slip between each other, and conformational and configurational rearrangements occur while the solution exhibits viscous flow (see Figure 5-2). The noninflammatory fraction of sodium hyaluronate (NIF-NaHA)[5] used for ophthalmic procedures has a high molecular weight (2 to 5 million daltons [d]) and a low protein content (<0.5%) and carries a single negative charge per disaccharide unit.

This fraction is highly purified and has been shown to be sterile, nontoxic, nonantigenic,[6] noninflammatory,[7] and pyrogen free. In primate vitreous humors, sodium hyaluronate has a half-life of approximately 72 days.[8] In primate aqueous humors the half-life is 2 to 7 days depending on the viscosity.[9] Clinical observations in humans have supported this result.

Chondroitin Sulfate

Chondroitin sulfate is another viscoelastic biopolymer that is found as one of the three major mucopolysaccharides in the cornea. Its structure is similar to hyaluronic acid, consisting of the same repeating disaccharide unit. Chondroitin sulfate is of medium molecular weight in the range of 50,000 d.

Chondroitin sulfate, like sodium hyaluronate, does not appear to be metabolized but is eliminated from the anterior chamber in approximately 24 to 30 hours.

Hydroxypropyl Methylcellulose

HPMC is yet another viscoelastic material used for intraocular procedures.[10] Unlike the previous two compounds, it does not occur naturally in animals but is distributed widely as a structural substance in plant fibers such as cotton and wood. It is a cellulose polymer composed of D-glucose molecules linked together by beta-glycosidic bonds.

Special care must be taken in the filtration of this material to ensure a highly purified preparation, as Rosen, Gregory, and Barnett[11] noted the presence of vegetable fibers and other contaminates in samples they examined. Methylcellulose is a nonphysiologic compound; as such, it does not appear to be metabolized intraocularly but is eliminated from rabbit anterior chambers in approximately 3 days. It is also quite hydrophilic and hence can be irrigated from the eye.

Commercial OVD Preparations

Healon, Healon GV, Healon 5

The first commercially available sodium hyaluronate, Healon, was developed by Balazs,[12] who sold the rights to Pharmacia. In 1958 Balazs suggested the use of hyaluronic acid as a vitreous substitute, and, subsequently, two different ophthalmic preparations were developed. Etamucaine (Laboratories Chibert, Clermount-Ferrand, France), a bovine hyaluronic acid preparation of low viscosity and concentration, was found to be well tolerated as a vitreous replacement despite a mild intravitreal inflammatory response.[13]

The second preparation, Healon, truly initiated the age of viscosurgery. This high-viscosity, high-molecular-weight sodium hyaluronate derived primarily from rooster combs was developed and purified by Balazs and associates to produce a specific non-inflammatory fraction.[7,8,12,14] In 1972 the first human intraocular injections of Healon into the vitreous and anterior chambers were reported, and its use in surgical procedures, varying from vitreoretinal diseases to cataract extraction and keratoplasty, was suggested. These suggestions have been pursued actively, and, subsequently, OVDs have become an invaluable tool in a broad array of applications.

By increasing both the molecular weight and concentration, Pharmacia introduced Healon GV (greater viscosity) in 1992.

With a resting viscosity of 2 million cSt (at least 10 times more viscous than most other viscoelastics), Healon GV provides superior viscosity for particularly demanding surgery.[15] Despite positive vitreous pressure, Healon GV is able to create and maintain a deep anterior chamber where other OVDs may fail. (It has 3 times the resistance to pressure as Healon in the presence of high positive vitreous pressure.) Procedures dealing with small pupils, pediatric cataract extraction, and capsulorhexis during positive vitreous pressure are facilitated with the use of Healon GV. However, because of its highly cohesive nature, Healon GV leaves the anterior chamber very quickly during irrigation and aspiration or phacoemulsification, leaving the corneal endothelium susceptible to compromise.

Pharmacia and Pfizer have developed a new OVD, which they believe possesses all of the best properties of Healon GV and yet is retained in the anterior chamber throughout the phacoemulsification procedure. Healon 5 is the result of this effort and has been hailed as the first viscoadaptive OVD by the manufacturer. When exposed to low flow rates, it behaves as a superviscous cohesive device like an enhanced Healon GV. However, as flow rates increase, Healon 5 begins to fracture into smaller pieces, making its behavior mimic some of the properties of dispersive OVDs. It was released for sale in the United States in early 2001.

Amvisc, Amvisc Plus

Amvisc is another sodium hyaluronate product extracted from rooster combs. It was first distributed by Precision-Cosmet and now is distributed by Bausch & Lomb Surgical. Released in 1983, Amvisc is slightly less viscous than Healon. Amvisc Plus, a 1.6% sodium hyaluronate product with a higher viscosity than Amvisc, is also available. The viscosity of Amvisc Plus is 55,000 cP compared with Amvisc (40,000 cP). This higher viscosity obtained by increasing the total concentration (16 mg/ml) and using a sodium hyaluronate molecule of lower molecular weight allows improved space maintenance, tissue manipulation, and tissue immobilization when compared with Amvisc.[16]

AMO Vitrax

AMO Vitrax (Advanced Medical Optics) is a low-molecular-weight viscoelastic preparation of a highly purified NIF-NaHA dissolved in BSS. Despite the relatively low molecular weight, AMO Vitrax is highly concentrated, which provides a significantly viscous material. Unlike other sodium hyaluronic compounds, AMO Vitrax requires no refrigeration and has a shelf life of 18 months. AMO Vitrax (like Viscoat) possesses a lower viscosity than Healon at rest (zero shear) but maintains its viscosity under medium shear, whereas Healon decreases sharply in a linear fashion.

ProVisc

ProVisc (Alcon Surgical, Inc.) is a sterile, nonpyrogenic, high-molecular-weight, highly purified NIF-NaHA dissolved in physiologic sodium chloride phosphate buffer. ProVisc material is obtained from microbial fermentation by a purified proprietary process. In this respect, it is similar to the process involved in the sodium hyaluronate fraction of Viscoat. Clinical testing demonstrates that ProVisc is equal to Healon in its efficacy for protecting the corneal endothelium and in its level of safety.[17] Like Viscoat, ProVisc requires refrigeration.[14]

Viscoat

Viscoat (Alcon Surgical, Inc.) is a 1:3 mixture of 4% chondroitin sulfate and 3% sodium hyaluronate manufactured by Alcon Surgical, Inc. The sodium hyaluronate fraction, like ProVisc, is produced by bacterial fermentation through genetic engineering techniques. The chondroitin sulfate is obtained from shark fin cartilage. This combination of the compounds combines the higher viscosity and chamber-maintaining properties of sodium hyaluronate with the coating and cell protection properties of chondroitin sulfate. Koch et al.,[18] in a prospective randomized study, compared the endothelial protective effect of Healon and Viscoat during iris-plane phacoemulsification and posterior chamber phacoemulsification. In the iris-plane phacoemulsification group, Viscoat provided greater corneal endothelial cell protection than Healon. In the posterior chamber phacoemulsification group, however, no significant differences in cell protection were noted, with both materials exhibiting excellent endothelial cell protection.

Ocucoat

Ocucoat (Bausch &Lomb Surgical) is a highly purified synthetic, nonprotein, nontoxic preparation of 2% HPMC. Ocucoat has been marketed as a viscoadherent rather than a viscoelastic because of its significant coating ability and its relative lack of elastic properties. The reader must be aware that formulations produced by individual hospital pharmacies are not consistent proprietary products and can contain various solid particles, mainly vegetable matter remaining from the raw material.[11] Ocucoat is manufactured from the highest pharmaceutical-grade HPMC and is subjected to a special dual-filtration process. A study presented in 1988 verified that Ocucoat is as free of particulate debris as Healon (Smith SG, European Intraocular Implant Council Meeting, 1988). Because of its poor elastic properties, a larger-bore cannula and increased infusion pressure are necessary for injection. Unlike other OVDs, Ocucoat can be sterilized by autoclaving and stored at room temperature. Because the raw materials are ubiquitous, there is potential for decreased cost. The complex biotechnical processes required to ensure purity, however, may limit this.

Cellugel

Cellugel (Alcon Surgical, Inc) is a sterile, nonpyrogenic, non-inflammatory, single-use OVD of highly purified 2% HPMC. It is supplied in a disposable syringe delivering 1 ml, packaged in a sterile peel pouch, and terminally sterilized by autoclaving. Like Ocucoat, Cellugel can be stored at room temperature. Unlike Ocucoat, Cellugel has a tenfold greater viscosity and fourfold higher molecular weight. As a result, the ability to maintain space is greater with Cellugel than with Ocucoat despite both being 2% HPMC.

Clinical Uses of OVDs

Anterior segment surgery by its very nature induces corneal damage, as documented by specular microscopy and pachymetry studies. Endothelial damage may occur at any stage in even routine procedures, from the opening of the anterior chamber with manipulation of the cornea to insertion of an IOL after cataract extraction. Hence the introduction of OVDs to anterior segment surgery can be easily appreciated from the perspective of corneal endothelial protection alone. Additional applications of these materials, however, have quickly become manifest, and the field of viscosurgery has broadened rapidly. Alpar[19] outlined some of the applications that have been used in anterior segment surgery, many of which were developed specifically for cataract surgery. OVDs can be applied externally to provide corneal and conjunctival epithelial protection throughout the procedure without impairing visibility.[20] Both intraocularly and extraocularly, OVDs can be used to form a mechanical barrier to control hemorrhage. Maintenance of the anterior chamber while fashioning the surgical wound and during intraocular manipulations can be accomplished with the injection of an OVD through a small incision. The iris and other intraocular tissues can be manipulated with the "soft instrument" effect of OVDs even in the face of increased vitreous or orbital pressure, and they may contribute to greater surgical control in the case of an expulsive hemorrhage. Finally, the use of OVDs may help to decrease the incidence of postoperative cystoid macular edema by appropriate maintenance of intraocular pressure and alteration of the refraction of the operating microscope light (Table 5-4).

A review of each of the OVD's attributes should make it apparent that the use of a single agent during most ophthalmic intraocular procedures is accompanied by compromises in surgical suitability. In phacoemulsification, for example, the ideal single OVD would offer a combination of cohesive and dispersive characteristics that would fulfill the range of needs through the course of the phacoemulsification procedure (Table 5-5).

TABLE 5-4
Clinical Uses of OVDs

Cataract surgery
Corneal surgery and penetrating keratoplasty
Glaucoma surgery
Anterior segment reconstruction as a result of trauma
Posterior segment surgery

OVDs, Ophthalmic viscosurgical devices.

Although a combination of agents can fulfill both cohesive and dispersive needs, the use of multiple agents may be cost prohibitive. Therefore, by employing a needs-specific approach that takes into account the surgical needs (requirements), surgeons can more astutely match agent with task to improve clinical outcomes. The viscoadaptive agent Healon 5 is an attempt to provide both cohesive and dispersive properties in a single agent. Continued experience with this agent will determine if this claim holds true.

Complications of OVD Use

Despite the many positive attributes of OVDs, their drawbacks and complications also must be given careful consideration. Most important is the elevation of intraocular pressure noted postoperatively after use in cataract surgery. First noted with the use of Healon,[21] the elevation is especially severe and prolonged if the material is not thoroughly removed at the conclusion of surgery,[22] giving rise to what has been termed *Healon-block glaucoma*. This increase in intraocular pressure is dose related and of a transient nature, occurring in the first 6 to 24 hours and typically resolving spontaneously within 72 hours postoperatively. This ocular hypertensive effect is presumed to be the result of large molecules of the OVD creating mechanical resistance in the trabecular meshwork and hence decreasing outflow facility.

The clearance of an OVD through the trabecular meshwork is believed to depend on a combination of the material's viscosity and molecular weight.[22] Theoretically, materials possessing lower viscosities and lower molecular weights clear the eye faster, thereby creating less intraocular pressure elevation.

Recently, attention has been directed at the importance of early (1 to 8 hours) postoperative intraocular pressure measurements when evaluating the effects of Healon[23] and other OVDS[21,24] on postoperative intraocular pressure. Significant intraocular pressure spikes can be missed if only 24-hour postoperative measurements are taken.

Lane et al.[25] compared the early postoperative intraocular pressures after the use of Healon, Viscoat, and Ocucoat in ECCE and IOL implantation. In this study, the Viscoat and Ocucoat groups were further randomized into subgroups in

TABLE 5-5
OVD Requirements During Phacoemulsification

Surgical Task	Primary Viscoelastic Function	Required Properties	Agent Category
Capsulorhexis	Maintain deep anterior chamber	High viscosity at low shear rates; elasticity	Cohesive
Emulsify nucleus	Stay in eye to cushion and coat tissues, provides endothelial coating	Low molecular weight; low surface tension; high viscosity at high shear rates	Dispersive
Remove cortex	Endothelial coating	Low surface tension	Dispersive
Open bag, insert IOL	Maintain deep anterior chamber and capsular bag	High viscosity at low shear rates; elasticity	Cohesive
Remove OVD at conclusion of surgery	Remove quickly and completely	High molecular weight; high surface tension	Cohesive

which the material was either retained at the conclusion of surgery or removed with irrigation and aspiration. The results of this study showed significant increases in intraocular pressure in all groups at the 4 ± 1 hour postoperative period. At 24 hours all groups except for the Viscoat-removed group showed significant elevations in intraocular pressures from baseline values. More recently, Rainer et al.[26] confirmed this, noting a significant intraocular pressure (IOP) rise over baseline for both Healon 5 and Viscoat in the early postoperative period.

To blunt the postoperative intraocular pressure rise, diluting, removing, or aspirating the OVD from the eyes at the conclusion of cataract surgery has been advocated by many.[13,21,27-31] However, this procedure has been shown only to shorten or reduce the incidence rather than eliminate the elevation of intraocular pressure.[29,30,32] Others recommend the use of pharmacologic prophylactic treatment in minimizing postoperative intraocular pressure rises. Acetazolamide,[33] intracameral miotics, beta-blockers such as timolol[24,34] or levobunolol,[35] and pilocarpine 4% gel[36] have all been shown to be effective in reducing postoperative intraocular pressure.

All OVDs, as well as the surgical procedure alone, are capable of increasing the intraocular pressure in the early postoperative period. Removal of the viscoelastic substance and use of acetazolamide, as well as other glaucoma medications, blunt intraocular pressure elevations but not in a predictable fashion. The intraocular pressure response in any given individual after cataract surgery is only in part caused by which OVD is used.

Several other disadvantages of viscosurgery deserve brief mention. Because of the viscous nature and electrostatic charge of these materials, inflammatory and red blood cells may remain suspended in the anterior chamber after surgery, giving the appearance of a plastic anterior uveitis. Intraocular hemorrhage also may be trapped between the vitreous space and the OVD within the anterior chamber and hence mimic the appearance of a vitreous hemorrhage.[37]

Calcific band keratopathy has occurred as a complication peculiar to the initial formulation of chondroitin sulfate–containing OVDs. Several investigators noted that postoperative subepithelial corneal deposits identified histochemically as calcium phosphate precipitates were associated with the use of the intracameral Viscoat.[29,38-40] Since the reformulation of Viscoat, this complication has not recurred.

Summary

OVDs have found applications within ophthalmology and have become indispensable tools in a variety of ophthalmic surgical procedures. The viscoelastic properties of these materials enable them to protect the corneal endothelium and epithelium effectively, maintain intraocular spaces, manipulate intraocular tissues, and control intraocular hemorrhage. Viscosurgery has helped to decrease the amount of corneal damage sustained during surgery and to facilitate difficult and delicate intraocular manipulations. At present, we have a choice of 10 commercially available substances; 7 sodium hyaluronate materials (Healon, Healon GV, Healon 5, Amvisc, Amvisc Plus, AMO Vitrax, and ProVisc), a combination of sodium hyaluronate and chondroitin sulfate (Viscoat), and 2 HPMC products (Ocucoat and Cellugel).

Widespread success in clinical situations has been achieved with the pure hyaluronate and combination hyaluronate–sodium chondroitin sulfate material. Ocucoat and Cellugel possess the potential advantages of lower cost, no requirement of refrigeration, and a larger quantity of the material per unit (1 mL) while maintaining absolute purity because of the extensive refinement and filtration process. Because of the success of all these products, a great deal of interest has been stimulated to develop other OVDs, and a number of new materials may become available in the coming years.

Currently, no single OVD is ideal under all circumstances. For any particular surgical task, the surgeon should consider the multiple physiochemical characteristics of each OVD available, as well as their desirable and undesirable clinic effects, and then choose the most appropriate substance. With the current armamentarium of OVDs, the ophthalmic surgeon can now optimize the surgical result by selecting the OVD most appropriate for the procedure. As new materials are developed and as our knowledge of the physical properties, clinical effects, and surgical indications are better defined, the selection process for choosing the best product should improve.

REFERENCES

1. Balazs EA, Miller D, Stegmann R: Viscosurgery and the use of Na hyaluronate in intraocular lens implantation. Presented at the International Congress and First Film Festival on Intraocular Implantation, Cannes, France, 1979.
2. Bothner H, Wik O: Rheology of intraocular solutions, *Viscoelastic Mater* 2:53-70, 1986.
3. Bothner H, Wik O: Rheology of hyaluronate, *Acta Otolaryngol (Stockh) Suppl* 442:25-30, 1987.
4. Arshinoff S: The safety and performance of ophthalmic viscoelastics in cataract surgery and its complications. In Arshinoff S, editor: *Proceedings of the Sixth Annual National Ophthalmic Speakers Program 1993,* Montreal, 1994, Medicopea International, pp 21-28.
5. Balazs EA: Sodium hyaluronate and viscosurgery. In Miller D, Stegman R, editors: *Healon: a guide to its use in ophthalmic surgery,* New York, 1983, John Wiley, pp 5-28.
6. Richter AW, Ryde EM, Zetterstrom EO: Non-immunogenicity of a purified sodium hyaluronate preparation in man, *Int Arch Allergy Appl Immunol* 59:45-48, 1979.
7. Denlinger JL, Eisner G, Balazs EA: Age-related changes in the vitreous and lens of rhesus monkeys *(Macaca mulatta).* I. Initial biomicroscopic and biochemical survey of free-ranging animals, *Exp Eye Res* 31:67-69, 1980.
8. Denlinger JL, Balazs EA: Replacement of the liquid vitreous with sodium hyaluronate in monkeys. I. Short-term evaluation, *Exp Eye Res* 31:81-99, 1980.
9. Schubert H, Denlinger JL, Galzs EA: Na-hyaluronate injected into the anterior chamber of the owl monkey: effect on IOP and range of disappearance, *ARVO Abstr* 9:118, 1981.
10. Fechner PU, Rechner MU: Methylcellulose and lens implantation, *Br J Ophthalmol* 67:259-263, 1983.
11. Rosen ES, Gregory RPF, Barnett F: Is 2% hydroxy propylmethylcellulose a safe solution for intraoperative clinical applications? *J Cataract Refract Surg* 12:679-684, 1986.
12. Balazs EA: Physiology of the vitreous body. In Schepens CL, editor: *Importance of the vitreous body in retina surgery with special emphasis on reoperations,* St Louis, 1960, Mosby, pp 29-48, 144-146.
13. Girod P, Rouchy JP: L'acide hyaluronique dans la chirurgie du corps vitre: reflexions a propos de 24 cas, *Annals Oculist* 203:25-40, 1970.
14. Denlinger JL, El-Mofty AAM, Balazs EA: Replacement of the liquid vitreous with sodium hyaluronate in monkeys. II. Long-term evaluation, *Exp Eye Res* 30:101-117, 1980.
15. Hutz WW, Exkhardt B, Kohnen T: Comparison of viscoelastic substances used in phacoemulsification, *J Cataract Refract Surg* 22:955-959, 1996.
16. Probst L, Nichols B: Endothelial and intraocular pressure changes after phacoemulsification with AmVisc Plus and Viscoat, *J Cataract Refract Surg* 19:725-730, 1993.

17. Lehman R, Brint S, Stewart R et al: Clinical comparison of ProVisc and Healon in cataract surgery, *J Cataract Refract Surg* 21:543-547, 1995.
18. Koch DD, Liu JF, Glasser DB et al: A comparison of corneal endothelial changes after use of Healon or Viscoat during phacoemulsification, *Am J Ophthalm*ol 115:188-201, 1993.
19. Alpar JJ: Viscoelastic surgery, *Ann Ophthamol* 19:350-353, 1987.
20. Norn MS: Preoperative protection of cornea and conjunctiva, *Acta Ophthalmol* 59:587-594, 1981.
21. Barron BA, Busin M, Page C et al: Comparison of the effects of Viscoat and Healon on postoperative intraocular pressure, *Am J Ophthalmol* 100: 377-384, 1985.
22. Pape LG: Intracapsular and extracapsular technique of lens implantation with Healon, *J Am Intraocul Implant Soc* 6:342-343, 1980.
23. Henry JC, Olander K: Comparison of the effect of four viscoelastic agents on early postoperative intraocular pressure, *J Cataract Refract Surg* 22:960-966, 1996.
24. Cherfan GM, Rich WJ, Wright G: Raised intraocular pressure and other problems with sodium hyaluronate and cataract surgery, *Trans Ophthalmol Soc U K* 103:227-279, 1983.
25. Lane SS, Naylor DW, Kullerstrand LJ et al: Prospective comparison of the effects of Occucoat, Viscoat, and Healon on intraocular pressure and endothelial cell loss, *J Cataract Refract Surg* 17:21-26, 1991.
26. Rainer G, Menapace R, Findl O et al: Intraocular pressure after small incision cataract surgery with Healon 5 and Viscoat, *J Cataract Refract Surg* 26:271-276, 2000.
27. Choyce DP: Healon in anterior chamber lens implantation, *J Am Intraocul Implant Soc* 7:138-139, 1981.
28. Miller D, Stegmann R: The use of Healon in intraocular lens implantation, *Int Ophthalmol Clin* 22:177, 1982.
29. Nevyas AS, Raber IM, Eagle RC et al: Acute band keratopathy following intracameral Viscoat, *Arch Ophthalmol* 105:958-964, 1987.
30. Olivius E, Thorburn W: Intraocular pressure after cataract surgery with Healon, *J Am Intraocul Implant Soc* 11:480-482, 1985.
31. Kohnen T, vonEhr M, Schutte E et al: Evaluation of intraocular pressure with Healon and Healon GV in sutureless cataract surgery with foldable lens implantation, *J Cataract Refract Surg* 22:227-237, 1996.
32. Glasser DB, Matsuda M, Edelhauser HF: A comparison of the efficacy and toxicity of and intraocular pressure response to viscous solutions in the anterior chamber, *Arch Ophthalmol* 104:1819-1824, 1986.
33. Lewen R, Insler MS: the effect of prophylactic acetazolamide on the intraocular pressure rise associated with Healon-aided intraocular lens surgery, *Ann Ophthalmol* 17:315-318, 1985.
34. Percival P: Complications from use of sodium hyaluronate (Healonid) in anterior segment surgery, *Br J Ophthalmol* 66:714-716, 1982.
35. Weidle EG, Lisch W, Thiel HJ: Excision of the posterior lens capsule without damaging the anterior vitreous face, *Fortschr Ophthalmol* 82:256-258, 1985.
36. Ruiz RS, Wilson CA, Musgrove KH: Management increased intraocular pressure after cataract extraction, *Am J Ophthalmol* 103:487, 1987.
37. Nirankari VS, Karesh J, Lakhanpal V: Pseudo vitreous hemorrhage: a new intraoperative complication of sodium hyaluronate, *Ophthalmic Surg* 12:503-504, 1981.
38. Binder PS, Deg JK, Kohl S: Calcific band keratopathy after intraocular chondroitin sulfate, *Arch Ophthalmol* 105:1243-1247, 1987.
39. Coffman MR, Mann PM: Corneal subepithelial deposits after use of sodium chondroitin, *Am J Ophthalmol* 102:279-280, 1986.
40. Ullman S, Lichtenstein SB, Heerlein K: Corneal opacities secondary to Viscoat, *J Cataract Refract Surg* 12:489-492, 1986.

Biomechanical Characteristics of Suture Materials and Needles in Cataract Surgery

6

Carl B. Tubbs, MD
Robert C. Allen, MD

Although the perfect needle-suture combination (see further on) might be modified by many contemporary ophthalmic surgeons to include the "invisible" suture (as in sutureless surgery), there will always be a need for suture use in the management of some primary cataract surgeries, as well as in most secondary surgical interventions. In addition, eye surgeons have always strived for precise instrumentation, and suture materials are no exception. The demands placed on the surgeon arise in part from the enhanced visibility of the operative field provided by the development of the surgical loop and, especially, by the introduction of the coaxial ophthalmic operating microscope. Minute ocular tissues that are manipulated and reapposed are generally more rigid and have a higher collagen content than do other tissues in the body; transincisional pressure gradient and fluid barrier stability requirements are similar to those needed in vascular surgery. The ultimate goal of ophthalmic surgery is improved visual outcome, which is directly related to the construction and closure of the ocular incision. These factors, coupled with the microsurgical techniques required to manipulate thin and often friable tissues, form the basis for the production of highly developed needles and suture materials.

The ideal needle-suture combination would be easy to manipulate in the operative field, be strong enough to withstand instrument manipulation and several atraumatic passages through fairly dense tissue, and allow satisfactory tissue support for good incisional apposition during the healing process. Ideally, it would provide watertight closure by using a sharp needle with a front-cutting surface and a small enough tract so that the suture that follows would plug the needle incision but also allow tissue support without "cheese-wiring" through tissue. The suture material itself would be inert and noninflammatory and have a tensile strength sufficient to last through the healing process. Because small changes in incisional construction and closure strongly influence visual outcome by affecting astigmatism, the demands for the manufacture of appropriate needle and suture materials are quite high.

We hope to elucidate the background of the development of needles and sutures for ophthalmic use and apply this knowledge to form a rational basis for the selection of needle and suture materials for specific ophthalmic procedures, concentrating on cataract surgery. Although this chapter is not intended to be a comprehensive review of all current ophthalmic products, it should provide, for both the beginning and the experienced surgeon, a basis for selecting surgical materials that would enhance the performance of the surgery, as well as postoperative patient comfort and ultimately good visual outcome.

Needles

Before 1959 in the United States, eyed needles were commonly used for ocular procedures.[1,2] Such needles worked much as standard cloth sewing needles used today. The major drawback to such a design was that each needle passage drew through the incision two pieces of suture, and only one suture piece would be used for closure, so the needle tract was necessarily large compared with that of the suture diameter. The development of the needle swage (permanent attachment of the suture to the needle at the time of manufacture), introduced in 1914,[3] overcame this design flaw and allowed less traumatic suturing techniques to be applied to ocular surgery.

Needle Swages

Three basic models of needle swage have been developed. For relatively large (>0.36-mm diameter) wire gauges (such as the Alcon P-5 needle with a wire diameter of 0.4 mm and the Ethicon G2 with a wire diameter of 0.423 mm), a mechanical drill has historically been used to bore a hole in the trailing end of the needle. The suture is then fixed into the hole. Mechanical drilling techniques are not reliable for smaller needle wire sizes; therefore either a channel-style fixation technique or a laser drilling technique has been used for small needles. The channel-style needle swage involves the use of a tool that forms a planed cut (approximately 4 times as long as a laser-bored hole) half the thickness of the needle wire along the trailing end of the needle with a depression to which the suture is fixed. This is an advantage over the eyed needles, but the process leaves a groove and an unevenly rounded surface at the needle end. Grasping the needle with a needle holder in the relatively large swage area can loosen the attachment of the suture or deform the needle itself by deforming the swage. Laser-drilled swages, however, allow a continued smooth needle trailing end with less wire bulk removal during manufacture. This process provides more local wire strength and thus more posterior allowance in grasping the needle for use.

The biomechanical performance of laser-drilled and channel-style needles has been investigated by comparing similar Ethicon needles in a standardized, reproducible grading system.[4] Both channel-style and laser-drilled needles had comparable suture attachment strengths, but the force required to draw the channel-style needle through a test membrane was significantly greater (nearly threefold) than that required with the laser-drilled needle. When needle strength performance studies were performed 3 mm from the needle end (1.5 mm distant to the 1.5-mm laser-drilled hole but inside the 6-mm channel swage), the forces required to reversibly deform, irreversibly deform, and fracture the needle in this area were all much less in the channel-style needle. Both needle types, however, performed similarly with forces applied to the body of the needle (where it is usually grasped with an instrument), away from the swage site. These authors recommended that laser drilling be used for all needle types, a processing technique that has continued to be advanced.

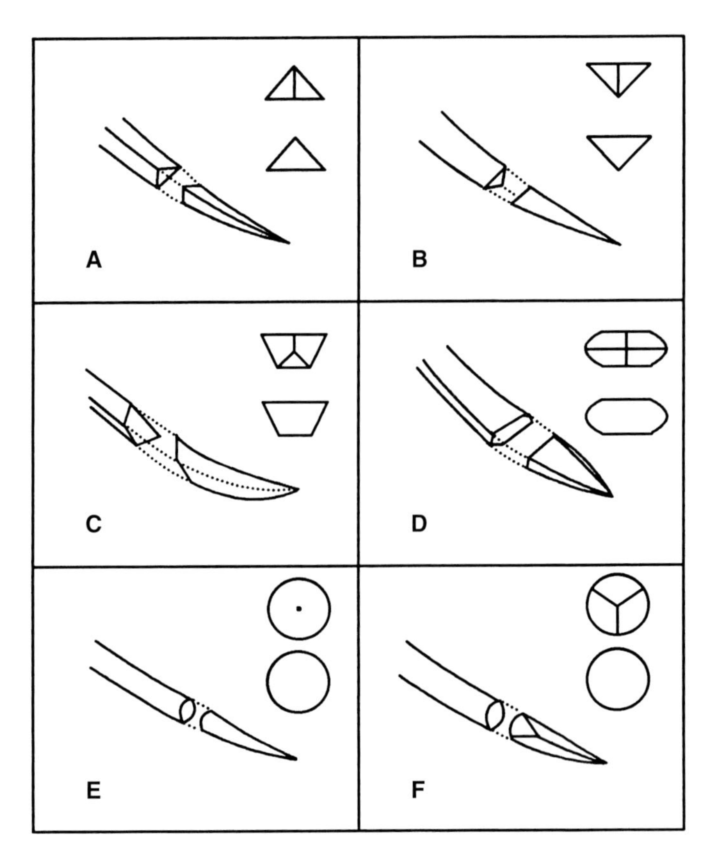

FIGURE 6-1 Schematic drawings of selected needles. **A,** Conventional needle (cutting concave: sharper than reverse cutting). **B,** Reverse cutting (cutting convex). **C** and **D,** Spatula design (best for lamellar work). **E,** Taper-point (best for watertight closure but requires force for passage). **F,** Tapercut (watertight closure with less passage force).

Properties of the Surgical Needle

The surgical needle should have inherent properties that allow the gentle but secure reapposition of tissues by the administration of the general surgical techniques so elegantly described by Halsted.[5] The ideal needle has been lauded as one with the following characteristics: (1) sufficiently rigid so that it does not bend; (2) long enough so that it can be grasped by the needle holder for passage and then be retrieved without damage to its point; (3) of sufficient diameter to permit a slim-point geometry and a sharp cutting edge, resulting in a tract large enough to allow the knot to be buried; and (4) as nontraumatic as possible.[6] Theoretically, the needle composition should provide enough strength to withstand mechanical forces so that the needle may be passed through tissue without becoming dull and grasped with a clamp without becoming permanently deformed. It should also be able to yield enough (not be brittle) so that it does not fracture easily if unduly stressed. The size and style of the needle obviously depend on the intended use.

Standard architectural characteristics define the type or style of needle, and these are typically included with the cataloged needle description. It is more rare to find the metallurgical composition or brand of wire used to fashion the needle, although this may be obtained from the manufacturer. Typical characteristics required to define a needle style include point cutting edge (Figure 6-1), curvature (circle fraction or degrees) (Figure 6-2), chord length and radius (Figure 6-3), wire diameter, and needle length. In general, the half-circle (higher degree) needles are appropriate for deep and shorter bites, and larger bites are better obtained with the flatter one-quarter to three-eighths circle (lower degree) needles.[7] Spatula-style needles tend to work well for intralamellar work, such as lamellar keratoplasty, standard cataract incision closure, deep corneal incision closure, and strabismus surgery, whereas the standard and reverse cutting needles better traverse tougher tissue, such as full-thickness scleral grafts and through-and-through corneal bites. The tapered-point needle has the advantage of causing a

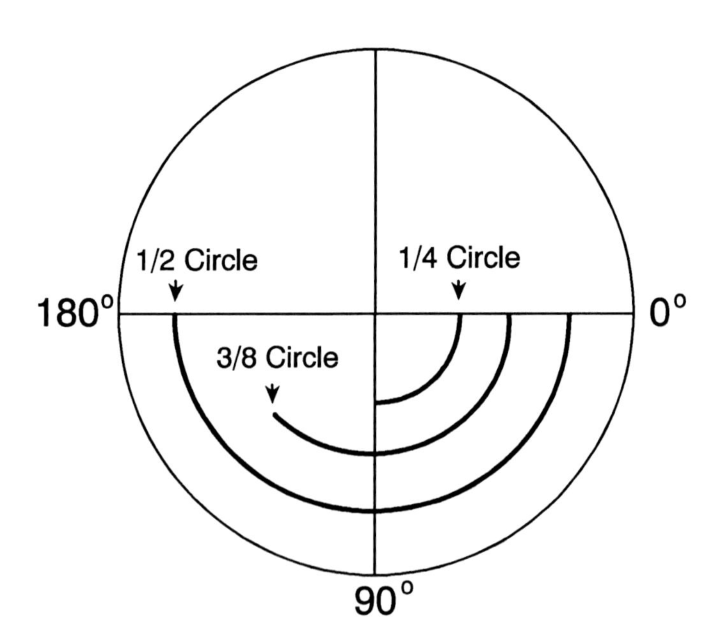

FIGURE 6-2 Needle circle and degrees. Needle curvature and length are defined in terms of circle arc and circle degrees. The less curved, lower-arc needles are better suited for more shallow tissue penetration and thus larger "bites" of tissue.

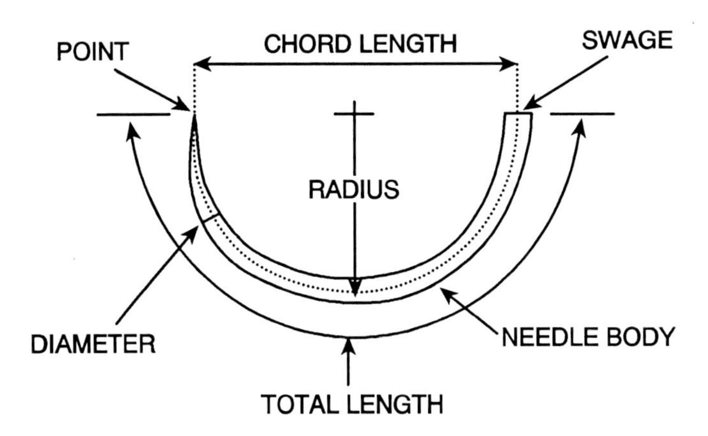

FIGURE 6-3 Schematic terminology of a surgical needle. The needle body is usually grasped with the needle driver away from the swage because the swage is usually round and also relatively weak when compared with the body. The wire diameter can be small enough so that the trailing suture fills the needle tract.

smaller tract in soft tissue such as conjunctiva, but its relative lack of cutting surface causes it to be more difficult to pass through tissue; it is especially difficult to penetrate the more collagenous cornea and sclera with this needle.

Ophthalmic surgeons generally develop familiarity with and a preference for a particular needle based on clinical performance. Although clinical testing and assessment are the ultimate measure of needle performance, standardized biomechanical testing has been developed for in vitro use. Parameters of performance, such as sharpness, cutting edge design, resistance to bending, resistance to breakage, and metallurgical analysis, allow the evaluation of needles before clinical use and can serve as an objective measure of a needle's predicted clinical utility.

NEEDLE SHARPNESS

Needle sharpness is a measure of the needle's ability to be passed through tissue; sharper needles require less force for initial tissue penetration and for the passage of the needle along its length of curvature. Sharper needles therefore require less applied force and thus induce less trauma to the surrounding tissues. The overall clinical needle performance in regard to sharpness in vivo depends on the particular surgeon and the use of appropriate techniques, such as tissue countertraction and following the needle curvature during needle passage.

The in vitro assessment of needle sharpness has been reported using a standardized technique and has been correlated to scanning electron micrographs of the tested surgical needles. In one study,[8] the force required to pass curved, reverse cutting needles through a thin, laminated synthetic membrane was measured. Comparable needles from three different manufacturers were used. Increased sharpness was correlated with smaller wire diameter. Extra finishing techniques such as electrohoning and hand-honing produced sharper needles than did simple machine grinding. Scanning electron micrographs and elemental analysis of the needles also correlated with sharpness; sharper needles had a longer, more narrow cutting edge and were fabricated from an American Society for Testing and Materials (ASTM) 45500 alloy that had better performance than did ASTM alloys 42000 or 42020. The authors concluded that Ethicon manufactured the sharpest needles tested, followed by Davis & Geck, and then Deknatel. These relationships are further supported by more recent investigations.[9]

CUTTING EDGE DESIGN

The cutting edge configuration might also be expected to influence surgical needle sharpness.[10] Both the conventional and the reverse cutting needles have a triangular configuration with two sharpened lateral edges. The conventional needle has the third cutting edge on the concave surface, whereas the reverse cutting needle has the third edge on the convex, or outer, surface (see Figure 6-1). Standardized in vitro measurement of sharpness comparing the Ethicon PC-1 and P-1 needles showed that the conventional cutting needle required significantly lower forces to penetrate a test membrane. The increased sharpness appeared to be related to the thinner cutting edge geometry as determined by scanning electron micrograph analysis.

An additional modification of the conventional cutting edge needle (Ethicon PC Prime), manufactured from the ASTM 44500 alloy (Figure 6-4), combined with a slightly different heat treatment process during manufacturing, has been shown to further enhance sharpness as measured in vitro, as well as in clinical use in the emergency room for suturing skin lacerations.[12] Heat treatment after the modified conventional needle is bent to its final curvature serves to enhance the biomechanical properties by relieving stress, reviving elastic properties, and enhancing the resistance to bending.[13] The increased cutting angle along the concave surface enhances tissue penetration.

Cardiovascular needles (taper point) are often used in conjunctival closure, in which a watertight closure of the incision is desired. Such a needle has been recommended for closure of oral mucous membranes by Thoma.[14] The biomechanical performance of several taper-point needle types from different

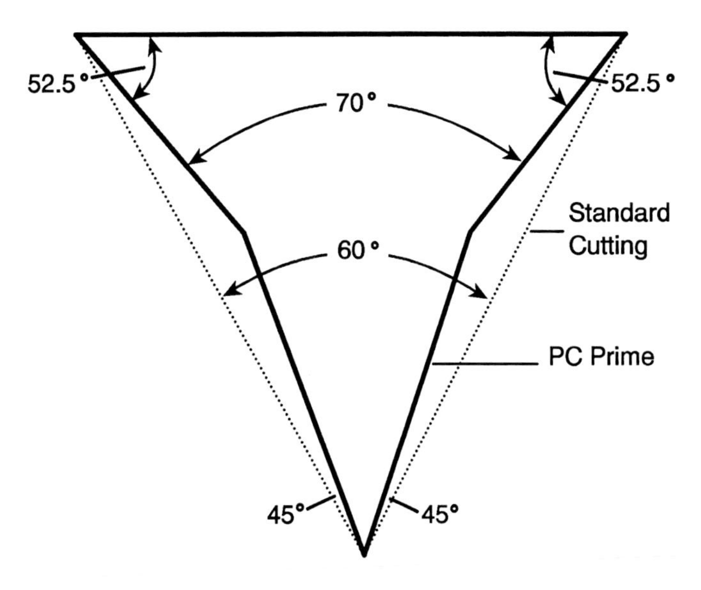

FIGURE 6-4 Standard cutting and PC Prime needle. Modification of the cutting point edges by steepening the angulation of each of the cutting surfaces *(solid lines)* allows increased sharpness as measured in vitro and in vivo, when compared with a conventional cutting needle *(dashed lines)*. Tissue penetration is enhanced with the same driving force.

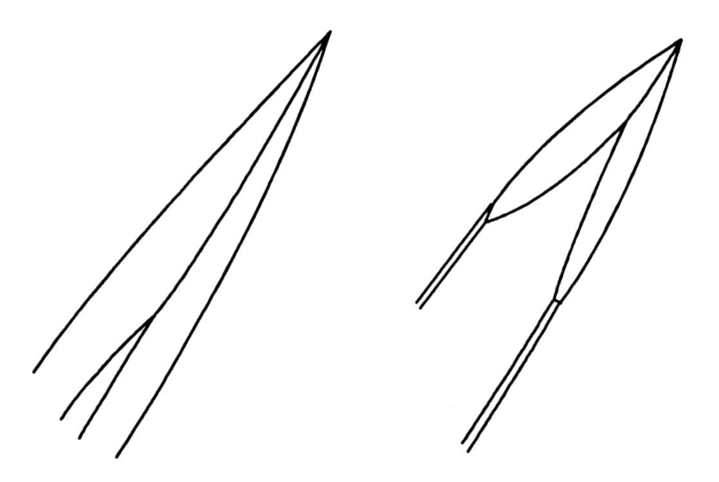

FIGURE 6-5 Schematic drawing of reverse cutting and Tapercut needles. The Tapercut needle combines characteristics of the reverse cutting and the taper-point needles. Note the shorter cutting surfaces of the Tapercut; penetration force is less than with the taper-point needle, and less tissue trauma occurs than with the standard reverse cutting needle.

manufacturers has been studied using standardized testing and scanning electron micrographic analysis.[15] For the smallest wire size (0.2 mm), there does not appear to be significant differences among required needle penetration forces, but this does not hold true for the other sizes tested (0.25 mm and 0.36 mm). Again, the manufacturer, finishing procedure, and alloy composition have significant effects on needle sharpness. Scanning electron micrographs show the Ethicon taper point to be the least affected by geometric irregularity, which is thought to account, in part, for its increased sharpness.

A modification of the taper-point needle is the Tapercut needle,[16] which is a modified taper-point needle with a short reverse cutting point that quickly blends into a taper-point body (Figure 6-5). Although the initial penetration forces of this needle are essentially the same as for a similar standard reverse cutting needle, the Tapercut needle requires more force for full needle passage in vitro because of the more limited cutting surface. Clinically, this means that the Tapercut needle should penetrate virgin tissue more easily than a standard taper point would, and if passed in the curve of the needle without bending, the Tapercut needle would cause less overall tissue cutting and provide a more watertight closure than would the reverse cutting needle.

RESISTANCE TO BENDING, DUCTILITY, AND CLAMPING MOMENT

Although needle sharpness is a key aspect of overall needle performance, it is also important to discuss other needle characteristics to form a rational basis for needle selection. These other factors include needle resistance to bending, needle ductility, and clamping moment. The mechanical resistance to bending allows the needle to be grasped and passed less traumatically through tissues.[17] A needle that bends easily can cause tissue injury via the application of cutting forces by the needle point or edge; it can also cause unwanted tissue trauma resulting from passing a deformed needle body. Needle ductility, strictly speaking, would be a measurement of the needle's ability to be "fashioned into a new form" (plasticity) and has been quantified mechanically as the amount of deformation that a needle can withstand without breakage.[18]

With respect to needle bending, a standardized procedure has been developed that allows the generation of a bending force–angular deformation curve[9,17] and the determination of the forces required to reversibly and irreversibly deform a needle. A typical graph for a curved needle shows an initial elastic region followed by an irregular nonlinear plastic region of deformation. The determinants of needle-bending response to applied stress relate to needle diameter, needle material, and the manufacturer.

Similarly, needle ductility can be quantitatively assessed[9,18] by determining the work required to completely fracture a surgical needle by repeatedly bending it back and forth through a 90-degree arc. Superior ductility grading was seen in needles manufactured with the ASTM 45500 alloy, with additional improvement provided by the electrohoning process.

The definition of *clamping moment* is more complex and deals with the interplay of forces that develop when a particular needle holder (with flat clamping jaws) grasps a particular needle.[9] Because the needle holder acts as a lever, the clamping force of the needle holder is directly related to the length of the handles and inversely related to the length of the jaws, with the surgeon having ultimate control of the force applied to the handles. This force from the handles to the jaws is transmitted to the curved needle, which lies within the flat clamping area of the needle holder. For the needle holder jaws to close completely, the needle segment that lies within the jaws of the needle holder must of necessity flatten, deforming the needle. The maximum clamping moment of a needle holder is defined as the product of the clamping force at one end of the needle (applied by the jaws of the holder at one of the two concave contact areas of the needle and the holder) and the length of the moment arm (one half of the jaw width of the needle holder in which the needle lies). For assessment of needle performance with a specific needle holder, a needle "yield moment" can be defined, which is the maximal force that can be applied to a needle without permanent deformation. If the clamping moment of the needle holder exceeds the yield moment of the needle, permanent needle deformation will occur, resulting in a less curved needle with increased chord length.

Clamping moment has been investigated using the Halsey, Mayo-Hegar, Crile-Wood, and DeBakey needle holders with larger needles than usually used in ophthalmic surgery.[9] All the listed needle holders had clamping moments that were sufficient to overcome the yield moments of the 0.43-mm-diameter needles tested (i.e., the needles would irreversibly deform with clamping). Although the clamping moments and yield moments of instruments specific to ophthalmic surgery have not been tested to date, the common use of narrow-tipped nonlocking needle holders, coupled with microscopic visualization of the needle–needle holder interface and tissue response, makes the clamping moment theoretically a less important issue in overall ophthalmic needle performance.

The performance of specific ophthalmic surgical needles has been studied, with attention to sharpness, resistance to

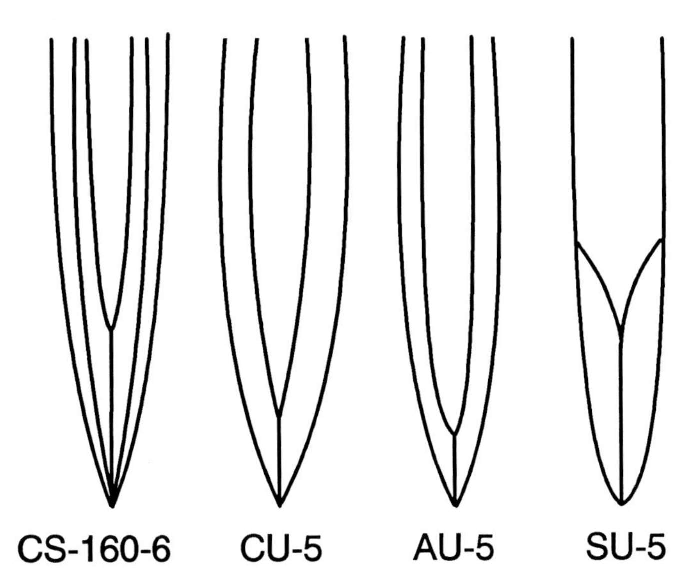

FIGURE 6-6 Schematic drawings of selected ophthalmic needle points. The cutting surface geometry has a strong influence on biomechanical needle performance. When tested in vitro, the CS-160-6 design provides easier tissue penetration than the other designs shown. New designs might be tested in vitro to predict clinical performance.

ductility, and bending.[19] Specifically, similar-sized needles were evaluated and included the CS-160-6 needle (Ethicon, Inc.) and the AU-5, CU-5, and SU-5 needles (Alcon, Inc.). The CS-160-6 needle (Figure 6-6) had superior biomechanical performance in standardized testing, which appeared to be related to the needle geometry, as well as to the needle alloy composition. Clearly, additional biomechanical investigation of ophthalmic needles may be accomplished in the future, with objective in vitro performance used as a guide to estimate clinical utility.

We can thus summarize the general characteristics of high-performance ophthalmic surgical needles. The needles would be sharp (with the smallest possible wire size and would be electrohoned or hand honed in addition to mechanical grinding), strong (resist bending, deformation, and breakage), and as free as possible of mechanical defects. The ASTM alloy 45500 appears to be the most appropriate steel for needle manufacture, and heat treating after needle bending appears to provide additional needle strength. The intended surgical use defines the necessary cutting edge style and overall needle dimensions, so a variety of surgical needle types should remain available to the surgeon.

Sutures

Myriad materials for general surgical suturing have been used historically, including linen, twine, horsehair, and silver wire, among others. The two earliest advances in modern suture technologies came with the development of catgut and silk suture materials. Catgut, actually prepared from the intestinal intima of sheep and cattle, was studied in the late 1800s by Lister and Macewen.[20,21] It was Lister who first presented observations on catgut treated with chromic acid and carbolic acid, a process that extended the strength of the material for much more than the few days that untreated catgut could hold. Lister had some initial success with investigations on sterilizing silk, and Halsted noted the advantages of silk over catgut in the early 1900s.[22] Synthetic materials became available in the 1940s, with nylon and polyester (Dacron) finding application in the operating room shortly thereafter. More recently, additional synthetic materials such as polyglycolic acid, polyglactin 910, polydioxanone, and polybutester have been manufactured for use as suture material.

Suture Characteristics

The search for the ideal suture material continues, and great advances have been made within the past century. Because a typical tissue incision has little inherent strength for at least the first week, the appropriate apposition of the edges of the incision is important in closure to minimize the amount of healing required by relieving local stresses and assisting in the promotion of hemostasis. Once granulation tissue and fibroblastic activity have increased the incisional strength, suture strength itself becomes less important; however, scar modulation continues for several months,[23,24] and incised skin, for example, is never as strong as the original tissue. The eye presents a particular problem in this respect. Healing requires an active cellular response and thus a blood supply, and ocular tissue such as the sclera, although juxtaposed to vascular tissue, is in itself avascular. The iris, although vascular, typically does not respond to surgical manipulation with a scarring response, and long-term suture strength for iridotomy closure is required. The cornea is the ultimate example of avascular tissue in which long-term suture strength is required; incisional dehiscence might cause endophthalmitis, and suture slippage may cause significant visual loss because of an astigmatic refractive error. Animal studies have documented the rate of corneal healing, with approximately 50% of the inherent corneal strength regained between 6 months and 1 year.[25,26]

The ideal suture would be strong, yet easily manipulated in the surgical field. Knots in the material should be easily tied and have minimal bulk and lasting strength without slippage. The inflammatory reaction provoked by the material should be minimal, unless used in a situation in which this would be warranted. The suture material should allow suture positioning so that the material would not provide a route of entry of foreign material or infective organisms or an egress of body fluids.

Obviously, no one suture type is appropriate for all types of ocular surgery, and several different types of surgical material may work equally well for a particular procedure. In the next section, a description of suture materials is presented with an overview of suture biomechanical characteristics. This should allow the ophthalmic surgeon to review the available materials and make a selection for a particular procedure using a scientific basis. The ultimate test of the chosen suture material will then depend on the clinical performance of that surgeon.[27]

In general terms, a suture may be described as being "*adsorbable*" or *nonabsorbable*, but this is relative terminology. Typically, adsorbable refers to a suture that loses most of its tensile strength within 2 months; catgut is an example of readily proteolized material, whereas nylon is degraded over many months, and polypropylene is relatively inert. There is an official organization that provides the classification of additional properties of suture materials, the United States Pharmacopeia. Such defined properties include the suture configuration (monofilament or multifilament), tensile strength (resistance to breakage with respect to suture diameter), elasticity and plasticity, memory, and knot strength. In addition, tissue reactivity with respect to inflammation and fluid adsorption and suture capillarity are other notable considerations.[28-30]

Specific Suture Materials

The classic adsorbable material is surgical gut, which retains tensile strength for only 4 or 5 days.[24] Gut treated with chromic acid (chromic gut) retains tensile strength for 14 to 21 days. The brief strength afforded by gut, coupled with its relative stiffness and inflammatory response, limits its use mainly to conjunctival closure when lasting tensile strength is not needed; however, hydrated gut is relatively easy to handle and tie.

Polyglycolic acid (Dexon) maintains strength longer, with 60% remaining at 7 days,[31] about 20% remaining at 14 days,[32,33] and 5% remaining at 1 month.[34] The longer tensile strength and less inflammatory response when compared with surgical gut offer advantages, but polyglycolic acid is stiff and so is generally braided for ease of use. Coated polyglycolic acid allows additional utility in terms of suture passage and knot tying.

Polyglactic acid (Vicryl), another braided polymer, is very similar to polyglycolic acid but has somewhat less overall tensile strength.[35] The adsorption curve is similar to that of polyglycolic acid for up to 1 month, but complete adsorption occurs much more quickly than that of polyglycolic acid after that.[34] Like polyglycolic acid, polyglactic acid induces less inflammatory response during adsorption than does surgical gut. Polyglactic acid is commonly used for cases of necessary cunjunctival closure such as cataract surgery combined with a filtration procedure.

Polydioxanone (PDS) is a monofilament polyester with longer lasting tensile strength than either polyglycolic acid or polyglactic acid, retaining about 75% of its original strength at 14 days and 40% at 6 weeks.[36] It is stiffer than the other polyesters and more difficult to manipulate, but it affords minimal tissue reaction after placement.

Polytrimethylene carbonate (Maxon), a newer monofilament, has improved strength and handling characteristics when compared with polydioxanone and retains its characteristic of low inflammation induction. The general strength retention is about 80% at 2 weeks and 30% at 6 weeks.[37] It has a better first-throw holding capacity than does polyglactic acid, making knot positioning easier.[38]

Nylon is a very slowly hydrolyzed polyamide material that is generally used as a monofilament. There are two types of nylon used as surgical material, nylon 6 and nylon 6/6.[39] The maximal tensile strengths of three brands of ophthalmic 10-0 nylon have been measured in vitro and were found to be markedly different. Polyamide 6/6 manufactured by SSC had the greatest maximal tensile strength, followed by Ethicon's nylon 6 and Alcon sutures (nylon formulation unknown). The tensile strength of a single knot, however, was the same for all three.[40] All three types of sutures that were intentionally "bruised" with the tying forceps or injured by submaximal stretching mechanically lost only about 10% of the original tensile strength despite morphologic changes as seen by electron microscopy.

With respect to degradation, in the rabbit model approximately 90% of the original tensile strength remains at 1 year, and 70% remains at 2 years,[41] with an estimated hydrolysis rate of 15% to 20% per year.[42,43] Nylon 6 material used for some two-loop iris fixation lenses shows complete breakdown by electron microscopy after 4 years.[44] A handling problem arises with the use of nylon because of its inherent memory, so additional throws are needed to maintain satisfactory knot security.[28,45]

Monofilament nylon induces less inflammation than does polyglycolic acid,[46] but toxic ocular effects do occur. A series of patients have experienced inflammation thought to be related to nylon suture after uneventful cataract surgery,[47] and there has been a case report of toxicity after vitrectomy closure with nylon.[48] In one study,[49] patients who had incisional closure with 10-0 nylon sutures for cataract surgery were examined over a period of 3 years, and nearly 90% of these patients had broken sutures at 2 and 3 years. Although this is not surprising considering the biodegradation curve of nylon, more than half of these patients were symptomatic because of exposed suture end irritation. A second study[50] found giant papillary conjunctivitis, mucus, epithelial filaments, limbitis, keratoconjuntivitis, and iritis as potential problems related to late nylon suture behavior, with initial loosening within 3 months and later breakage and inflammation as likely causes.

Surgical silk is a processed protein that is treated with silicone or wax to enhance handling. Like nylon, silk is a hydrolyzed material that more rapidly loses its tensile strength within 3 to 4 months and is generally entirely degraded well within 2 years.[43,51] A soft, workable material with little memory and low tensile strength,[52] it typically causes minimal irritation when used on oral mucous membranes[53] but may elicit more inflammation elsewhere.[54] In a rabbit study, corneal inflammation was least apparent with 10-0 nylon and 9-0 silk but was more marked with 7-0 collagen and 8-0 virgin silk. The greatest reaction seen by histopathologic and clinical examination was with 7-0 braided silk.[55] Interestingly, severe reactions have been reported in response to silk in the human eye,[56] and it is postulated that braided silk is a less offensive material because of the removal of sericin (a natural silkworm polymer) during the processing of braided silk, which is not performed during the production of virgin silk.

Polypropylene (Prolene) is a smooth, inert material with low tissue adherence. Its strength is comparable to that of nylon, but the smooth slippery surface makes knot security less dependable unless additional throws are used. Polypropylene has plastic qualities,[57] so once stretched, it tends to remain somewhat elongated. Even though polypropylene tends to become encapsulated in fibrous tissues and is therefore thought to have long-lasting tensile strength,[42,58,59] electron microscopic studies of polypropylene haptics show substantial degradation when examined at 1 and 6.5 years.[60]

Braided polyester (Mersilene, Dacron) sutures have improved handling qualities because of their multifilamentous structure and are comparable to monofilament polyesters in terms of strength and low tissue reactivity. Coated polyester sutures, such as Ethibond, produce less tissue drag than do the uncoated materials, but the coating tends to crack after knots are tied.[61]

Polybutester (Novafil) is an elastic monofilament suture that will stretch twice as much as similar-gauge nylon under low applied tension.[62] An advantage of polybutester over nylon and polypropylene is that the increased elasticity allows a stretching response to tissue edema, with return to a less stretched configuration as edema decreases, thereby maintaining incisional closure without undue tension on edematous tissue or slack once edema subsides. An additional advantage over nylon for corneoscleral section closure is the minimal degradation of polybutester, as evidenced by scanning electron microscopy, compared with the almost total degradation of nylon at 23 months in the rabbit model.[63]

The viscoelastic properties of several suture types have been investigated,[64] including polypropylene, polytrimethylene carbonate, polyglactic acid, and silk. When 4-0 gauge monofilament or multifilament sutures are tested for relaxation properties, it has been shown that both polypropylene and polytrimethylene carbonate relax at 25° C, whereas silk and polyglactic acid remain relatively stiff, further supporting the use of silk or polyglactic acid when the objective is to maintain a temporarily secure incisional closure without elasticity.

Surgical Forceps and Knots

Regardless of the type of suture material used, the suture must be force-loaded to complete a ring closure and to form a knot in one area. Tying forceps or small needle holders with flat, smooth surfaces are generally used. It would be wise to avoid toothed needle holder jaws, because these cause suture damage and a reduction in suture tensile strength.[65] Even the flat tying forceps can cause suture damage as discussed previously, and if the instrument platform forms an acute angle with the stressed suture, the sharp platform edge may weaken or even break the suture before tying is completed. This obviously would become more important if a running suture were used. Good surgical technique involves not only avoiding the suture or knot breaking tension but also grasping the suture with the tying instruments to maintain a parallel configuration with respect to the angle of pull and the angle of the forcep jaws (Figure 6-7).

The surgical knot in an otherwise intact suture is a potential weak area. There has been considerable variation in the style of knot used to secure a suture. An in vitro system has been developed that allows the discrimination between knot slippage and breakage, two common causes of knot failure. When monofilament polypropylene, polydioxanone, and polytrimethylene carbonate, and multifilament braided polyester, polyglycolic acid, and polyglactic acid were tested in vitro with a number of distinct slip and nonslip knot styles, it was found that the standard three-throw square knots provided optimal results for all materials.[66] However, sliding knots with one extra throw, when limited to small monofilament or coated multifilament material, achieved results that would be clinically acceptable.[67] Instrument tying, in general, produces knots (both granny and square) that tend to break before slipping, as compared with the insecure granny knots achieved by hand tying.[68] The use of the granny knot with interrupted 10-0 nylon suture in cataract closure has been recently advocated.[69]

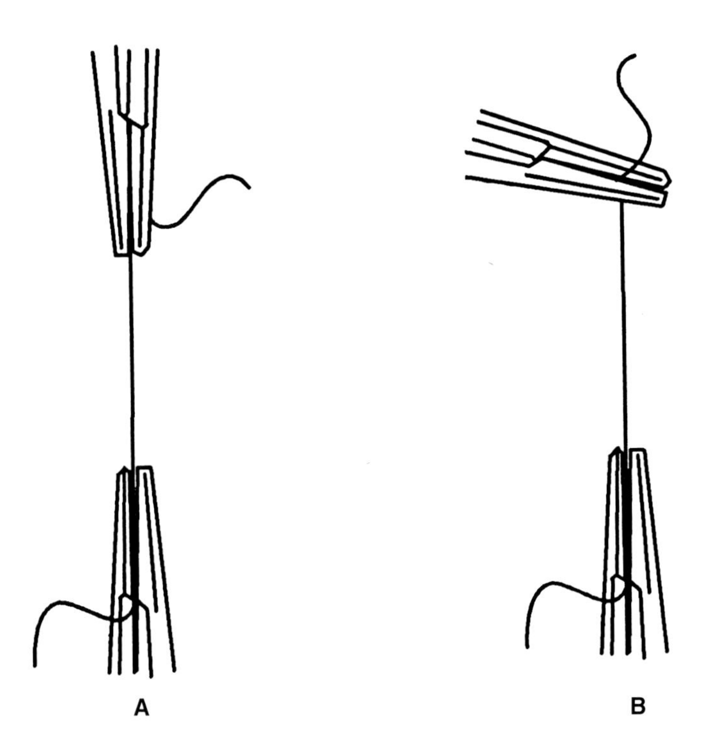

FIGURE 6-7 Suture typing technique to minimize stress. Sutures react to mechanical stress in elastic (forgiving) and inelastic (forgetting) ways. When tying, the reduction of shear forces by maintaining a parallel forceps position **(A)** minimizes suture trauma, as opposed to an angled forceps position **(B)**. This becomes particularly important when using a running suture closure.

The type of knot and suture material used are considerations that affect local wound healing, because the bulk of the surgical knot can promote incisional distortion and local foreign body reaction. Ideally, one would wish to have a continuous suture with no knot, and it is best to attempt to minimize the number of throws to minimize knot bulk while maintaining knot security. Monofilament nylon produces less knot bulk than does coated polyglactic acid, and although a surgeon's knot (two initial loops followed by a single counterthrow) minimizes knot bulk for both materials, the difference in volume is not much greater than a three-throw square knot, which is a more reliable closure.[70] Larger gauge suture materials appear to be a more significant factor in the induction of local inflammation than are extra knot throws. For example, adding two extra throws to a given gauge suture knot increases the knot mass by a factor of 1.5, whereas increasing the suture gauge by a factor of 2 increases the knot volume by a factor of 4 to 6.[71] Besides increasing inflammation, the increased knot bulk from the larger sutures probably also increases the difficulty in burying the knots, an important consideration in cataract surgery in which lid friction causes local irritation.

Suture Material and Outcome

The final astigmatic outcome following cataract surgery is related to incisional construction, incisional closure, steroid use, suture material, personal patient healing characteristics, and preoperative corneal geometry. Incisional construction and closure and suture material are probably the most important considerations for most patients; the former two are difficult to isolate from the latter, but estimations of the effect may be made. The effect of suture material on final astigmatic outcome has been investigated by several authors, both for extracapsular and phacoemulsification techniques. There seem to be distinct differences in the final astigmatic outcome based on the type of suture used for incisional closure. In addition, survey data show that ophthalmic surgeons have fairly consistent preferences.[72] Eighty-seven percent of responding surgeons used nylon sutures, 4% used polyester, and 5% used polypropylene. With respect to nylon sutures, 91% of surgeons favored 10-0 gauge, with 6% using 9-0, and 1% using 11-0 nylon for incisional closure.

It has been well established that the use of adsorbable suture materials in extracapsular cataract surgery, such as polyglactin[73,74] and silk,[75] allows against-the-rule astigmatic shift. In extracapsular surgery, prospective comparisons among closure of a standard incision with virgin 8-0 silk, interrupted 9-0 nylon, and double running 10-0 nylon have supported the finding that virgin silk generally causes an against-the-rule shift, whereas both running and interrupted nylon tended to better maintain with-the-rule astigmatism. The authors concluded that the type of suture material is a more important factor than the use of continuous or interrupted suturing closure.[76] A combination of 9-0 preplaced silk and 10-0 nylon closure in 137 eyes confirms the tendency toward long-term astigmatic drift, with most of the operatively produced with-the-rule cylinder declining in power over the first 2 months.[77]

Although nylon allows less cylindric drift than do adsorbable sutures for extracapsular closure, the biodegradation of nylon certainly allows some astigmatic shift. A prospective study comparing incisional closure with 11-0 braided polyester and 10-0 nylon in 25 patients found no significant difference in astigmatic shift at 6 months.[78,79] When 10-0 nylon was compared with 10-0 polybutester in 60 patients, no significant surgically induced astigmatic shift was noted between the two patient groups, although the polybutesters tended to maintain somewhat greater with-the-rule astigmatism, and the nylon sutures showed more significant degradation by electron microscopic analysis after an average of 18 months.[80] In a large prospective review, postoperative astigmatism was investigated with incisional closure using 10-0 and 9-0 nylon, 10-0 polypropylene, and 10-0 polyester.[81] Significant hydrolysis of nylon was seen at 5 months (10-0) and 12 months (9-0), with late astigmatic drift seen with 9-0 nylon when incisions did not heal normally. When compared with nylon, polypropylene and braided polyester did not show hydrolysis, but the elasticity of polypropylene allowed more against-the-rule shift than did polyester. The author recommended the use of 10-0 braided polyester for incisional closure.

The small "tunnel" incision for phacoemulsification provides earlier incisional stabilization without the large postoperative astigmatic drift generally seen in extracapsular surgery.[75,82-85] Practically speaking, a smaller chord length incisional entry into the anterior chamber should cause less astigmatic drift, although this will still depend on the location and type of incision used. Theoretically speaking, the importance of the suture should diminish with increased tunnel strength and diminished tunnel width.

Using a specific "shoelace" suturing technique with a scleral pocket chord length of 5.5 to 6.5 mm, the postoperative astigmatic response was assessed in 85 eyes while comparing 10-0 and 9-0 nylon with 10-0 polyester for watertight closure.[86] The smaller 10-0 nylon caused less early with-the-rule astigmatic shift, thought to be related to increased elasticity of the suture; late postoperative astigmatic change was not statistically different among the three suture types, but there was a tendency for polyester to be associated with giant papillary conjunctivitis. Long-term follow-up is available for patients with scleral tunnels of 6.5- and 7.5-mm chord length with the scleral groove 1.5 mm posterior to the limbus. With approximately 50 patients randomized to shoelace closure with 10-0 nylon, 10-0 polypropylene, 11-0 polyester, and 10-0 polyethylene, operatively induced astigmatism was followed for a period for more than 2 years. Over the first 3 months, with-the-rule astigmatism was greatest in the polyester group, with comparably less in the polyethylene and nylon groups. The polypropylene group had the least early astigmatic shift but the most rapid decay to against-the-rule astigmatism. At 2 years, against-the-rule cylinder was generally seen in all suture closures, with polyester having the least cylindric decay, followed by polypropylene at 0.5 diopter (D) and nylon at 1.0 D of against-the-rule decay.[87] A short-term comparison of astigmatism in a group of patients who had scleral tunnels closed with horizontally single-stitched 5-, 6-, and 6.5-mm chord length incisions and a group of patients with 5-mm unsutured incisions found no significant differences between the groups at an average of 7 weeks.[88] In general, elastic suture materials such as nylon and polypropylene tend to induce less early surgical astigmatism when compared with polybutester and braided polyester. When only suture material is considered, the late against-the-rule drifts clinically observed are likely caused by suture plasticity, elasticity, and biodegradation.

The advent of smaller tunnel incisions for phacoemulsification (and the introduction of the foldable lens) has provided the ophthalmic surgeon with the opportunity to create an incision that holds itself apposed and prevents fluid flow despite a pressure gradient. Although it is beyond the scope of this chapter to discuss the distinctive styles of such incisional construction, sutures are often thought to be unnecessary in these "watertight" cases. If the incision can gain tensile strength without the induction of hypotony or infection, a sutureless closure should decrease early astigmatic shift from local edema by avoiding the placement of foreign material. It should also allow minimal long-term against-the-rule decay while increasing patient comfort and avoiding the need to remove broken or loose sutures postoperatively. If early additional incisional strength is thought to be of benefit, closure with 10-0 polyglactic acid may allow short-term strength with little induced tissue reaction and reasonable adsorption within 3 months.

REFERENCES

1. Rizutti AB: *Clinical evaluation of suture material and needles in surgery of the cornea and lens,* Somerville, NJ, 1968, Ethicon, Inc.
2. Trier WC: Considerations in the choice of surgical needles, *Surg Gynecol Obstet* 149:84-94, 1979.
3. Minahan PR: Eyeless needle. US Patent Office, No. 1,106,667, Aug 11, 1914.

4. Ahn LC, Towler MA, McGregor W et al: Biomechanical performance of laser-drilled and channel taper point needles, *J Emerg Med* 10:601-606, 1992.
5. Heuer GW: Dr. Halsted, *Bull Johns Hopkins Hosp* 90(suppl):1, 1952.
6. Polack FM, Sanchez J, Eve FR: Microsurgical sutures. I. Evaluation of various types of needles and sutures for anterior segment surgery, *Can J Ophthalmol* 9:42-47, 1974.
7. Polack FM: Microsurgical instrumentation and sutures. In *Corneal transplantation,* New York, 1977, Grune & Stratton, pp 114-121.
8. Thacker JG, Rodeheaver GT, Towler MA et al: Surgical needle sharpness, *Am J Surg* 157:334-339, 1989.
9. Edlich RF, Towler MA, Rodeheaver GT et al: Scientific basis for selecting surgical needels and needle holders for wound closure, *Clin Plast Surg* 17:583-602, 1990.
10. Bernstein G: Needle basics, *J Dermatol Surg Oncol* 11:1177-1178, 1985.
11. Towler MA, McGregor W, Rodeheaver GT et al: Influence of cutting edge configuration on surgical needle penetration forces, *J Emerg Med* 6:475-481, 1988.
12. Kaulbach HC, Towler MA, McClelland WA et al: A bevelled, conventional cutting edge surgical needle: a new innovation in wound closure, *J Emerg Med* 8:253-263, 1990.
13. Masseria V: Heat treating. In *Metals handbook,* vol 4, ed 9, Metals Park, Ohio, 1981, American Society for Metals, pp 621-649.
14. Thoma KH: General surgical procedures. In *Oral Surgery,* vol 1, ed 4, St. Louis, 1963, Mosby.
15. McClelland WA, Towler MA, Kaulbach HC et al: Biomechanical performance of cardiovascular needles, *Am Surg* 56:632-638, 1990.
16. Hoard MA, Bellian KT, Powell DM et al: Biomechanical performance of tapercut needles for oral surgery, *J Oral Maxillofac Surg* 49:1198-1203, 1991.
17. Abidin MR, Towler MA, Rodeheaver JG et al: Biomechanics of curved surgical needle bending, *J Biomed Mater Res* 23:129-143, 1989.
18. Abidin MR, Towler MA, Nochimson GD et al: A new quantitative measurement for surgical needle ductility, *Ann Emerg Med* 18:64-68, 1989.
19. McClung WL, Thacker JG, Edlich RF et al: Biomechanical performance of ophthalmic surgical needles, *Ophthalmology* 99:232-237, 1992.
20. Gibson T: Evolution of catgut ligatures: the endeavors and successes of Joseph Lister and William Macewen, *Br J Surg* 77:824-825, 1990.
21. Goldenberg I: Catgut, silk and silver: the story of surgical sutures, *Surgery* 46:908-912, 1959.
22. Halsted W: Ligature and suture material, *JAMA* 60:1119-1126, 1913.
23. Lober C, Fenske N: Suture materials for closing the skin and subcutaneous tissues, *Aesthetic Plastic Surg* 10:245-247, 1986.
24. Swanson N, Tromovitch T: Suture materials, 1980s: properties, uses and abuses, *Int J Dermatol* 21:373-378, 1982.
25. Gosset AR, Dohlman CH: The tensile strength of corneal wounds, *Arch Ophthalmol* 79:595-602, 1968.
26. Yanoff M, Fine BS: Surgical and non-surgical trauma. In *Ocular pathology,* ed 2, Philadelphia, 1982, Harper and Row, pp 132-138.
27. Lavrich JB, Goldberg DS, Nelson LB: Suture use in pediatric cataract surgery: a survey. *Ophthalmic Surg* 24:554-555, 1993.
28. Forrester JC: Suture materials and their use, *Br J Hosp Med* 578-592, 1972.
29. Moy RL, Waldman B, Hein DW: A review of sutures and suturing techniques, *J Dermatol Surg Oncol* 18:785-795, 1992.
30. Moy RL, Lee A, Zalka A: Commonly used suture materials in skin surgery, *Am Fam Physician* 44:2123-2128, 1991.
31. Morgan MN: New synthetic adsorbable suture material, *Br J Med* 2:308-313, 1969.
32. Herman JB, Kelly RJ, Higgins GA: Polyglycolic acid sutures, *Arch Surg* 100:486-490, 1970.
33. Postlethwaite RW: Polyglycolic acid suture, *Arch Surg* 101:489-499, 1970.
34. Craig PH, Williams JA, Davis KW et al: A biologic comparison of polyglactin 910 and polyglycolic acid synthetic adsorbable sutures, *Surg Gynecol Obstet* 141:1-10, 1975.
35. Blomstedt B, Jacobson S: Experiences with polyglactin 910 in general surgery, *Acta Chir Scand* 143:259-263, 1977.
36. Ray JA, Doddi N, Regula D et al: Polydioxanone (PDS), a novel monofilament synthetic adsorbable suture, *Surg Gynecol Obstet* 153:497-503, 1981.
37. Katz AR, Mukherjee DP, Kaganou AL et al: A new synthetic monofilament adsorbable suture made from polytrimethylene carbonate, *Surg Gynecol Obstet* 161:213-222, 1985.
38. Moy RL, Kaufman AJ: Clinical comparison of polyglactic acid (Vicryl) and polytrimethylene carbonate (Maxon) suture material, *J Dermatol Surg Oncol* 17:667-669, 1991.
39. Weast RC, editor: *Handbook of chemistry and physics 1984,* ed 55, Cleveland, 1984, CRC Press.
40. Kappelhof JP, Swart W, Willekens BLJC: A comparison between three brands of 10-0 nylon sutures, *Doc Ophthalmol* 72:209-213, 1989.
41. Postlethwaite RW: Long term comparison study of nonabsorbable sutures, *Ann Surg* 271:892-898, 1970.
42. Ethicon, Inc: *Wound closure manual,* Somerville, NJ, 1985, Ethicon, Inc, pp 1-101.
43. *The United States pharmacopeia,* ed 20, Washington DC, Official for July 1, 1980.
44. Yamanaka A, Nakamae K, Takeuchi M et al: Scanning electron microscope study on the biodegradation of IOL and suturing materials, *Trans Ophthalmol Soc UK* 104:517-521, 1985.
45. Holmlund DEW: Knot properties of surgical suture materials, *Acta Chir Scand* 140:355-362, 1974.
46. Hartman LA: Intradermal sutures in facial lacerations: comparative study of clear monofilament nylon and polyglycolic acid, *Arch Otolaryngol Head Neck Surg* 103:542-543, 1977.
47. Balyeat HD, Davis RM, Rowsey JJ: Nylon suture toxicity after cataract surgery, *Ophthalmology* 95:1509-1514, 1988.
48. Schechter RJ: Nylon suture toxicity after vitrectomy surgery, *Ann Ophthalmol* 22:352-353, 1990.
49. Jackson H, Bosanquet R: Should nylon corneal sutures be routinely removed? *Br J Ophthalmol* 75:663-664, 1991.
50. Acheson JF, Lyons CJ: Ocular morbidity due to monofilament nylon corneal sutures, *Eye* 5:106-112, 1991.
51. Yu GV, Cavaliere R: Suture materials properties and uses, *Am J Podiatr Med Assoc* 73:57-64, 1983.
52. Herman JB: Tensile strength and knot security of surgical suture materials, *Am Surg* 37:209-217, 1971.
53. Meyer RD, Antonini CJ: A review of suture materials. I. *Compendium* 10:260-265, 1989.
54. Postlethwait RW, Willigan DA, Ulin AW: Human tissue reaction to sutures, *Ann Surg* 181:144-150, 1975.
55. Aronson SB, Moore TE: Suture reaction in the rabbit cornea, *Arch Ophthalmol* 82:531-536, 1969.
56. Soong HK, Kenyon KR: Adverse reactions to virgin silk sutures, *Ophthalmology* 91:479, 1984.
57. Bennett R: Selection of wound closure materials, *J Am Acad Dermatol* 18:619-637, 1988.
58. Stroumtsos D: *Perspectives on sutures,* Pearl River, NY, 1978, Davis and Geck, pp 1-90.
59. Jongebloed WL, Figueras MJ, Humalda D et al: Mechanical and biochemical effects of man made fibres and metals in the human eye: SEM-study, *Doc Ophthalmol* 61:303-312, 1986.
60. Jongebloed WL, Worst JGF: Degradation of polypropylene in the human eye: a SEM-study, *Doc Ophthalmol* 64:143-152, 1986.
61. Macht SD, Krizek TJ: Sutures and suturing: current concepts, *J Oral Maxillofacial Surg* 36:710-712, 1978.
62. Rodeheaver GT, Nesbit WS, Edlich RF: Novafil: a dynamic suture for wound closure, *Am Surg* 204:193-199, 1986.
63. McClellan KA, Billson FA: Long-term comparison of Novafil and nylon in corneoscleral sections, *Ophthalmol Surg* 22:74-77, 1991.
64. von Fraunhofer JA, Sichina WJ: Characterization of surgical suture materials using dynamic mechanical analysis, *Biomaterials* 13:715-720, 1992.
65. Stamp CV, McGregor W, Rodeheaver GT et al: Surgical needle holder damage to sutures, *Am Surg* 54:300-306, 1988.
66. Brouwers JE, Oosting H, deHaas D et al: Dynamic loading of surgical knots, *Surg Gynecol Obstet* 173:443-448, 1991.
67. Van Rijssel EJC, Trimbos JB, Booster MH: Mechanical performance of square knots and sliding knots in surgery: a comparative study, *Am J Obstet Gynecol* 162:93-97, 1990.
68. James JD, Wa MW, Bastra EK et al: Technical considerations in manual and instrument tying techniques, *J Emerg Med* 10:469-480, 1992.
69. Phillips CI: Granny knot for interrupted 10-0 nylon sutures in cataract sections, *Ophthalmol Surg* 24:109-112, 1993.
70. Trimbos JB, Brohim R, vanRijssel EJC: Factors relating to the volume of surgical knots, *Int J Gynecol Obstet* 30:355-359, 1989.
71. van Rijssel EJC, Brand R, Admiraal C et al: Tissue reaction and surgical knots: the effect of suture size, knot configuration, and knot volume, *Obstet Gynecol* 74:64-68, 1989.
72. Leaming DV: Practice styles and preferences of ASCRS members: 1991 survey, *J Cataract Refract Surg* 18:460-469, 1992.
73. Stainer GA, Binder PS, Parker WT et al: The natural and modified course of post-cataract astigmatism, *Ophthalmic Surg* 13:822, 1982.
74. Wishart MS, Wishart PK, Gregor ZJ: Corneal astigmatism following cataract surgery, *Br J Ophthalmol* 70:825, 1986.

75. Reading VM: Astigmatism following cataract surgery, *Br J Ophthalmol* 68:97, 1984.
76. Dekkers NWHM, Buijs J: Corneal astigmatism after cataract surgery, *Doc Ophthalmol* 72:323-327, 1989.
77. Talamo JH, Stark WJ, Gottsch JD et al: Natural history of corneal astigmatism after cataract surgery, *J Cataract Refract Surg* 17:313-318, 1991.
78. Drews RC: Astigmatism shift after extracapsular surgery: Mersilene versus nylon, *Int Ophthalmol* 13:209-210, 1989.
79. Drews RC: Astigmatism shift after cataract surgery: nylon versus Mersilene, *Ophthalmol Surg* 20:695-696, 1989.
80. Seeto R, Ng S, McClellan KA, Billson FA: Nonabsorbable suture material in cataract surgery: a comparison of Novafil and nylon, *Ophthalmol Surg* 23:538-544, 1992.
81. Cravy TV: Long-term corneal astigmatism related to selected elastic, monofilament, nonadsorbable sutures, *J Cataract Refract Surg* 15:61-69, 1989.
82. Lindstrom RL, Destro MA: Effect of incision size and Terry keratometer usage on postoperative astigmatism, *Am Intraocular Implant Soc J* 11:469-473, 1985.
83. Swinger CA: Postoperative astigmatism, *Surv Ophthalmol* 31:219-248, 1987.
84. Masket S: One year postoperative astigmatic comparison of sutured and unsutured 4.0 mm scleral pocket incisions, *J Cataract Refract Surg* 19:453, 1993.
85. Steinert RF, Brint SF, White SM et al: Astigmatism after small incision cataract surgery: a prospective, randomized, multicenter comparison of 4- and 6.5 mm incisions, *Ophthalmology* 98:417, 1991.
86. Masket S: Comparison of suture materials for closure of the scleral pocket incision, *J Cataract Refract Surg* 14:548-551, 1988.
87. Gimbel HV, Raanan MG, DeLuca M: Effect of suture material on postoperative astigmatism, *J Cataract Refract Surg* 18:42-50, 1992.
88. Buzard KA, Shearing SP: Comparison of postoperative astigmatism. with incisions of varying length closed with horizontal sutures and with no sutures, *J Cataract Refract Surg* 17(suppl):734-739, 1991.

The Phaco Machine: The Physical Principles Guiding Its Operation

7

William J. Fishkind, MD, FACS
Thomas F. Neuhann, MD
Roger F. Steinert, MD

Although the surgical techniques of phacoemulsification are often described, there is a tendency to overlook a basic aspect of this type of surgery: the physics of closed-system surgery and how it translates into clinical performance.

In addition, a basic knowledge of the principles of the physics and engineering of the machines, the power generators, and fluidics not only can assist in making a rational decision as to what kind of equipment to use but also can promote the performance of a surgical procedure that is more gentle and efficient, thus improving outcomes and minimizing complications.

All phaco machines consist of a computer to generate ultrasonic impulses and a transducer, usually piezoelectric crystals, to turn these electronic signals into mechanical energy. The energy thus created is harnessed, within the eye, to overcome the inertia of the lens and emulsify it. Once turned into emulsate, the fluidic systems remove the emulsate and replace it with balanced salt solution (BSS) in a closed, steady-state environment.

Basic Principles of Power Generation

The prerequisite for the removal of a cataract through a small incision is a technique to break up the hard nucleus into emulsate for aspiration. Inspired by the technique of dentistry to remove tarter with a metal tip that oscillates longitudinally at frequencies in the ultrasonic range, Kelman[1-3] adopted this principle, combining the oscillating tip and the evacuation tube into a hollow needle.[4] Titanium is the material of choice for such applications because it resists the fragmentation that occurs with more brittle metals. The mechanisms by which such an oscillating tip fragments the nucleus are examined in the following text.

Types of Transducers

MAGNETOSTRICTIVE TRANSDUCERS

Magnetostrictive transducers are based on packs of ferromagnetic lamellae surrounded by an electric coil. The magnetic field induced by the high-frequency electric current flowing through the coil excites the oscillation.

The advantages of magnetostrictive transducers include contact-free excitation, thus avoiding deterioration at the junction of the current and the transducer. These transducers, coupling elements, and the entire handpiece are rugged. They can withstand mechanical injury and have a long life span. Their primary disadvantage is a relative low grade of efficiency. Only a small part of the energy input is transformed into mechanical action; the majority becomes heat. Heating not only carries the risk of tissue burn but also makes the transducer lose efficiency with rising temperatures. Also, in the original design, the concentric aspiration line had to be brought out before the lamellar stack, necessitating two sharp bends that frequently clogged.

Recent improvements include considerably increased efficiency through sophisticated ferromagnetic metal alloys with rare earth elements and engineering modifications that allow both the irrigation and aspiration lines to be concentrically brought straight all the way through the tack to the tip. This not only avoids the clog-prone bends but also provides a double stream of constantly flowing cooling fluid through all the elements of the vibrating system, thus obviating the need for a separate cooling system as was found on the older handpiece.

PIEZOELECTRIC TRANSDUCERS

These transducers are based on the reversal of the piezoelectric phenomenon. Certain crystals, on compression, produce electric current. In reverse, electric current causes the crystal to contract. Applying current to a crystal at high frequency causes it to oscillate at that frequency.

The crystal is mounted on the "horn." This is a piece of tubing of narrowing diameter eventually ending with the attachment of the phaco needle. The decreasing diameter tube acts as an amplifier to generate adequate power for emulsification.

The advantages of piezoelectric crystals include a high grade of efficiency and therefore little inherent heat generation, with no need for extra cooling. Their low mass allows rapid movement and precise control. Some of the newer machines use digital inputs to generate power. Digital control is more precise and instantaneous. Many new handpieces use multiple crystals (usually two to four sets) to maximize responsiveness and provide adequate power to emulsify the mature hard nucleus.

TABLE 7-1
Phaco Machines

Company	Model	Frequency kHz	Pump Type	Pump Comment	Vacuum Range mm Hg	Flow Range ml/min	Comments
Alcon	Legacy Series 20000	40	Turbostatic Peristaltic	High vacuum pack	0-500	0-60	Flared ABS tip; new software: burst and pulse mode
Allergan	Diplomax	40	Peristaltic	Microprocessor control of pump	0-500	0-44	Pulse and burst mode
Allergan	Prestige	47.5	Peristaltic	Microprocessor control of pump	0-500	0-40	Pulse and burst mode
Allergan	Sovereign	38	Peristaltic	Microprocessor control of pump; Shield–fluid coupled Pressure sensor	0-500	0-40	ProSync-onboard computer control; power matrix and digital control allow power down to 5%
Bausch & Lomb	Millennium	28	Venturi or Concentrix	Venturi Hybrid: programmable to emulate Venturi or Peristaltic	0-550	0-60	Dual linear foot pedal; modular upgrades
Paradigm	SIStem	40	Peristaltic	Microprocessor control of pump; variable rise time (VRT)	0-500	0-50	Automatic surge suppression; variable rise time (pump accelerator)
Staar	The Wave	42	Peristaltic	Fluid-coupled aspiration system	0-500	0-50	Surge suppression system; coiled tubing; CD Rom printout of events

ABS, Aspiration bypass system.

Disadvantages include the connection points between crystal and electric current, the connections among the multiple layers of crystals that are necessary to provide adequate stroke amplitudes, and the structural brittleness of the crystal itself. These properties limit the longevity of such transducers. They are delicate and deteriorate both by accidental mechanical injury and by the oscillation they produce.

Tuning

Every material has an inherent frequency at which it vibrates naturally. This is called its resonant frequency. If excited to vibrate at this frequency, the transformation into mechanical amplitude will be optimal, and the creation of other forms of energy, principally heat, will be minimized. The creation of balanced crystals, their attachment to the horn, and the weight of the titanium phaco needle are therefore carefully controlled during manufacturing.

The phaco procedure is performed in a less rigidly controlled environment. In the course of phacoemulsification, the needle is passed through and inside material of inconsistent resistance. The aqueous humor is less resistant than a soft nucleus, and a soft nucleus less resistant than a mature one. Thus, for example, as the phaco needle travels through BSS into a hard nucleus, the resonant frequency must be adjusted, to prevent inefficient emulsification. The result of inefficient emulsification is prolonged phaco time, higher powers, and ensuing increased heat generation.

Therefore all modern phaco systems now have a built-in feedback loop constantly adjusting, or tuning, the oscillating frequency to an optimal resonance. This is a function of the central processing unit of the machine. It reads the change in resistance of the phaco needle and makes minute adjustments in the stroke length or frequency, thus maximizing effectiveness. The rate of repetition with which the machine makes these adjustments is machine dependent. In the AMO Sovereign system, the tuning rate is 20 microseconds. It is intuitive, however, that the greater the frequency of these corrections, the more effective the emulsification.

Power Generation

Power is created by the interaction of frequency and stroke length. *Frequency* is defined as the speed of the needle movement. It is determined by the manufacturer of the machine. Presently, most machines operate at a frequency of between 35,000 cycles per second (c/s; or hertz [Hz]) to 45,000 c/s (Table 7-1). This frequency range is the most efficient for nuclear emulsification. Lower frequencies appear to be less efficient, and higher frequencies create excess heat.[5]

Frequency is maintained constant by tuning circuitry designed into the machine computer. As noted earlier, tuning is vital because the phaco tip is required to operate in varied media. The computer recognizes the change in resistance by sensing a change in load. The appropriate response is then delivered to the phaco tip by a minute change of frequency or stroke length depending on the machine algorithm. The surgeon will subjectively appreciate good tuning circuitry by a sense of smoothness and power.

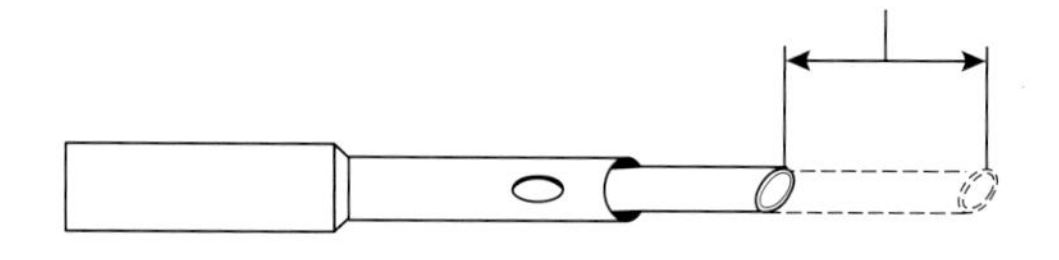

FIGURE 7-1 Stroke length.

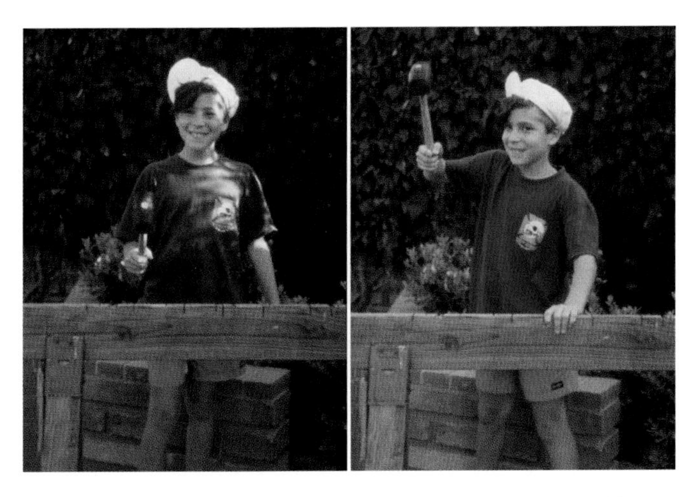

FIGURE 7-2 According to the formula F = MA (Force = Mass × Accleration), as distance to the point of impact is increased, acceleration is increased, resulting in increased force.

Stroke length is defined as the length of the needle movement (Figure 7-1). This length is generally 2 to 6 mils (thousandths of an inch). Most machines operate in the 2- to 4-mil range. Longer stroke lengths are prone to generate excess heat. The longer the stroke length, the greater the physical impact on the nucleus and, in addition, the greater the generation of cavitational forces (Figure 7-2).

Stroke length is determined by foot pedal excursion in position 3 during linear control of phaco power. Although the frequency is unchanged, the amplitude of the sine wave is increased in direct proportion to the depression of the foot pedal (Figure 7-3).

Energy at the Phaco Tip

The actual tangible forces, which emulsify the nucleus, are a blend of the "jackhammer" effect and cavitation energy.[1]

The jackhammer effect is the direct mechanical impact of the physical striking of the needle against the nucleus. The efficiency of this mechanism depends on two main prerequisites:

1. *Rapid forward acceleration of the phaco tip.* This overcomes the inertia of the nucleus penetrating it rather than driving it away.
2. *Close mechanical contact between the tip and the nucleus.* Engineers call this *force coupling*. It is accomplished by pressing the tip against the nucleus or by pressing the nucleus to the tip.

The jackhammer effect can be maximized or minimized depending on the tip selection as discussed in the text that follows.

The cavitation effect is more complex. The phaco needle, moving through the liquid medium of the aqueous humor at ultrasonic speeds, creates intense zones of high and low pressure. Low pressure, created with backward movement of the tip, literally pulls dissolved gases out of solution, thus giving rise to microbubbles (25.4^{-5} mm) in size. Forward tip movement creates an equally intense zone of high pressure. This produces compression of the microbubbles until they implode. At the

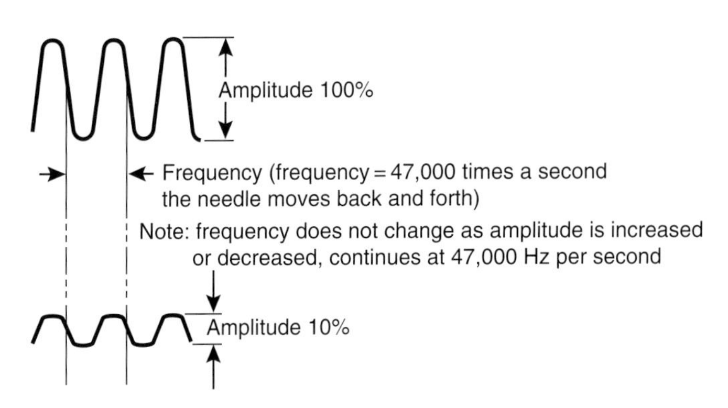

FIGURE 7-3 Frequency remains constant. The amplitude of the sine wave increases. This increases stroke length and resultant jackhammer and cavitational forces.

moment of implosion, the bubbles create a temperature of 7204° C and a shock wave of 75,000 PSI. Of the microbubbles created, 75% implode, amassing to create a powerful shock wave radiating from the phaco tip in the direction of the bevel with annular spread. However, 25% of the bubbles are too large to implode. These microbubbles are swept up in the shock wave and radiate with it.

The cavitation energy thus created can be directed in any desired direction as the angle of the bevel of the phaco needle governs the direction of the generation of the shock wave and microbubbles.

A method of visualizing these forces, called *enhanced cavitation,* has been developed. Using this process, with a 45-degree tip, the cavitation wave is generated at 45 degrees from the tip and comes to a focus 1 mm from it. Similarly a 30-degree tip generates cavitation at a 30-degree angle from the bevel, and a 15-degree tip, 15 degrees from the bevel (Figure 7-4). A 0-degree tip creates the cavitation wave directly in front of the tip, and the focal point is 0.5 mm from the tip (Figure 7-5). The Kelman tip has a broad band of powerful cavitation, which radiates from the area of the angle in the shaft. A weak area of cavitation is developed from the bevel but is inconsequential (Figure 7-6).[6]

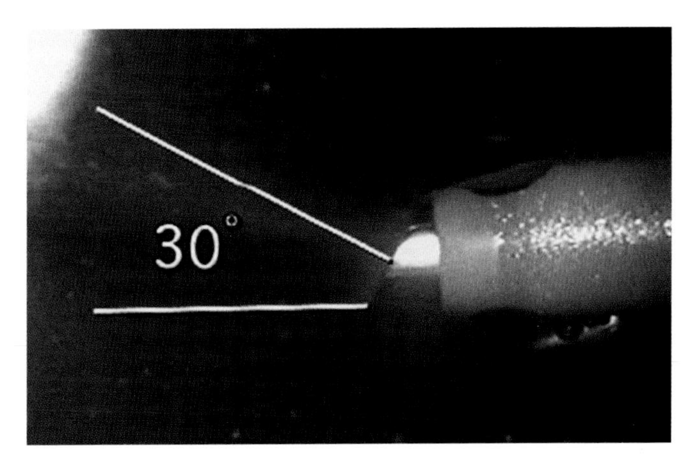

FIGURE 7-4 A 30-degree tip. Enhanced cavitation shows ultrasonic wave focused 1 mm from the tip, spreading at an angle of 30 degrees.

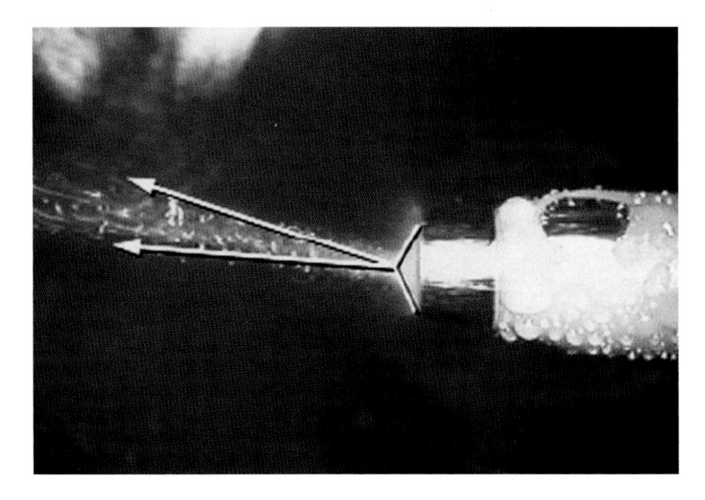

FIGURE 7-5 A 0-degree tip. Enhanced cavitation shows ultrasonic wave focused 0.5 mm in front of the tip, spreading directly in front of it.

Taking into consideration analysis of enhanced cavitation, it can be concluded that emulsification is most efficient when both the jackhammer effect and cavitation energy are integrated. To accomplish this, a 0-degree tip, or when using an angled tip, the bevel of the needle, should be turned toward the nucleus, or nuclear fragment. This simple maneuver causes the broad bevel of the needle to strike the nucleus. This enhances the physical force of the needle striking the nucleus. In addition, the cavitational force is concentrated into the nucleus rather than away from it (Figure 7-7). This causes the energy to emulsify the nucleus and be absorbed by it. When the bevel is turned away from the nucleus, the cavitational energy is directed up and away from the nucleus toward the iris and endothelium (Figure 7-8). Finally, in this configuration, the vacuum force (discussed later in this chapter) can be maximally exploited as occlusion is encouraged.

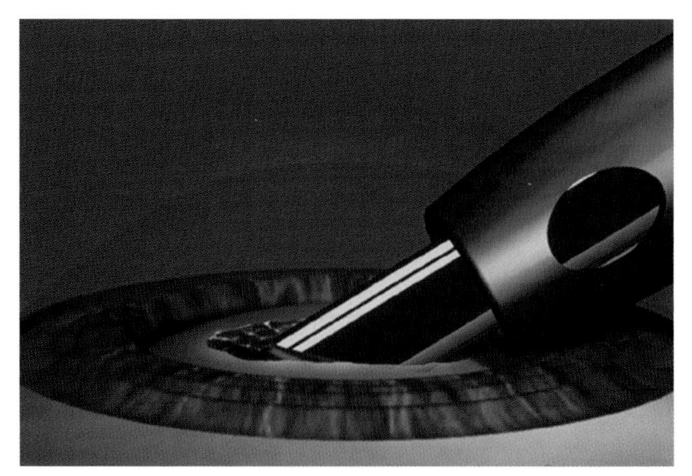

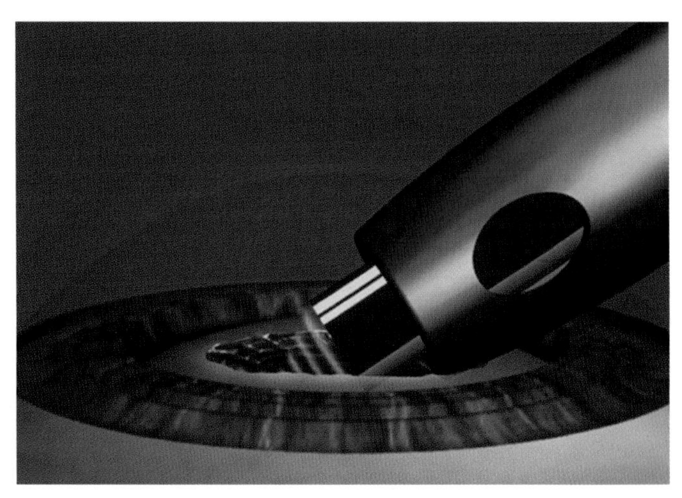

FIGURE 7-7 Turning the bevel of the phaco tip toward the nucleus focuses cavitation and jackhammer energy into the nucleus.

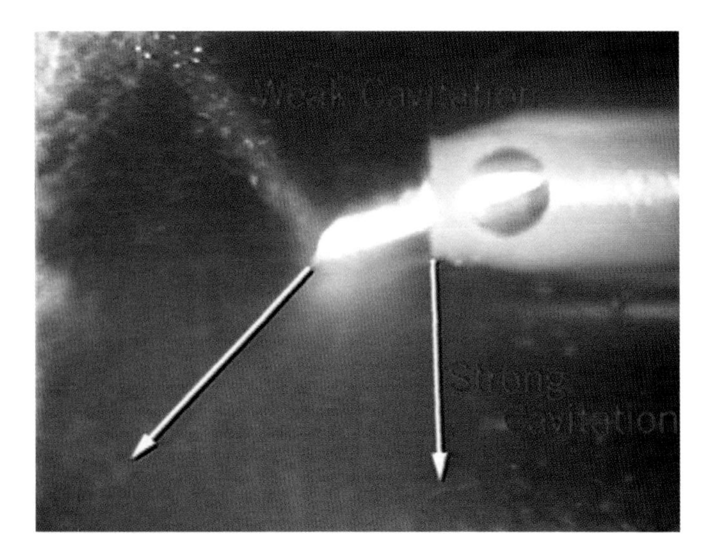

FIGURE 7-6 Kelman tip. Enhanced cavitation shows broad band of enhanced cavitation spreading inferiorly from the angle of the tip. A weak band of cavitation spreads from the tip.

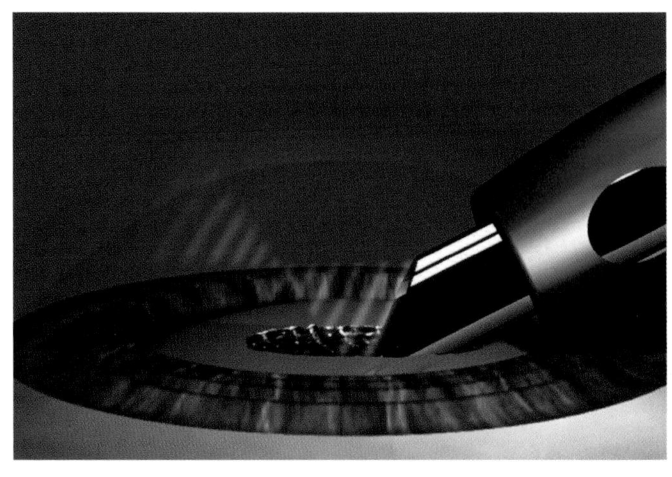

FIGURE 7-8 Bevel is turned away from the nucleus. Jackhammer is the only effect. Cavitation energy is wasted and may damage the iris and endothelium.

Modification of Phaco Power

Modification of phaco power must be accomplished to harness these powerful forces for a controlled phaco surgical procedure.

Application of the minimal amount of phaco power intensity necessary for emulsification of the nucleus is desirable. Unnecessary power intensity is a source of heat with subsequent wound damage. Moreover, excessive cavitational energy is a cause of endothelial cell damage and iris damage with resultant alteration of the blood-aqueous barrier. Phaco power intensity can be modified by altering phaco power amplitude, phaco power duration, and phaco power delivery.

Alteration of Phaco Power Amplitude

Stroke length is determined by foot pedal excursion and therefore foot pedal adjustment. When set for linear phaco, depression of the foot pedal increases stroke length and, consequently, power.

New foot pedals, such as those found in the Allergan Sovereign and the Alcon Legacy machines, permit surgeon adjustment of the throw length of the pedal in position 3. This can refine power application. The Bausch & Lomb Millennium dual linear foot pedal permits the separation of the fluidic aspects of the foot pedal from the power elements.

Alteration of Phaco Power Duration

The duration of application of phaco power has a dramatic effect on overall power delivered to the anterior segment. This is the use of power modulations. Power modulations include the use of burst, multiburst, and pulsed phaco. For example, if continuous power is employed for 1 minute, the effective phaco time is 1 minute. If the power is pulsed at 10 pulses per second, the effective phaco time is 30 seconds. The effective power delivered to the anterior segment is half of the continuous amount. Burst mode in the Allergan Sovereign (parameter is machine dependent) is characterized by 80 or 120 millisecond periods of power combined with fixed short periods of aspiration only. Pulse mode uses fixed pulses of power of 50 or 150 ms with variable short periods of aspiration only (Figure 7-9). Phaco techniques such as choo-choo chop and phaco chop use minimal periods of power in pulse mode to reduce power delivery to the anterior chamber. In addition, the use of pulse mode to remove the epinucleus provides an added margin of safety. When the epinucleus is emulsified, the posterior capsule is exposed to the phaco tip and may move forward toward it because of surge. Activation of pulse phaco mode creates a deeper anterior chamber to work within. This occurs because each period of phaco energy is followed by an interval of no energy. During the interval of absence of energy the epinucleus is drawn toward the phaco tip, producing occlusion, interrupting outflow. This allows inflow to deepen the anterior chamber immediately before onset of another pulse of phaco energy. The surgeon will recognize the outcome as operating in a deeper, more stable anterior chamber.

Recent innovations by Alcon, AMO, and Staar have resulted in new forms of power modulation.

"Jackhammer" Modifications of Software

A recent development in phaco machine technology has been the use of sonic energy. Rather than using ultrasonic frequencies (25,000 to 50,000 c/s), these machines operate below 20,000 Hz (c/s). The Staar Sonic Wave system operates in the 40 to 400 c/s range.

The Alcon NeoSoniX operates in the 100 to 120 Hz range. The Alcon modification also includes the addition of a 2-degree maximum variable oscillatory movement to the phaco tip. These modifications use only the jackhammer energy to emulsify the nucleus. Their subultrasonic frequency generates no cavitational energy or turbulence. This system is claimed achieve emulsification with decreased energy delivered to the anterior segment and decreased heat production.[7]

These modifications are so new that it remains to be seen how successful they will be.

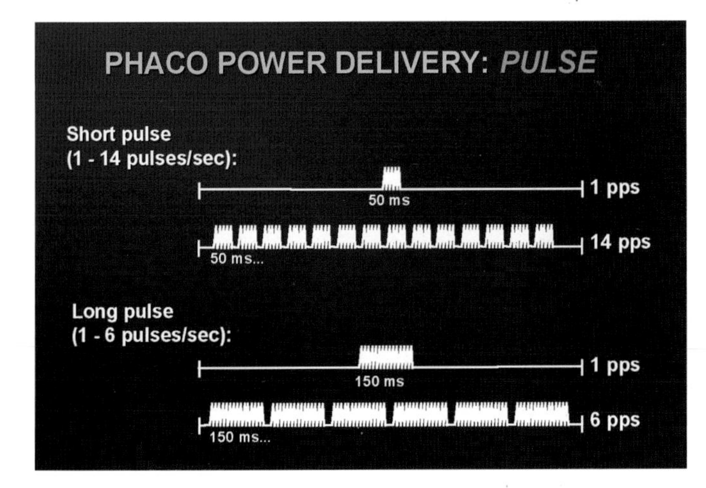

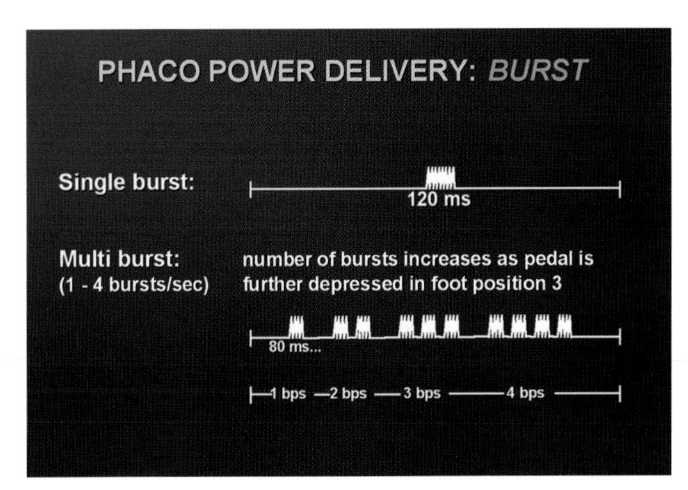

FIGURE 7-9 Graphic representation of pulse mode and burst mode in the AMO Sovereign machine. (Courtesy AMO.)

Cavitational Modifications of Software

Advanced Medical Optics (AMO) has introduced the WhiteStar system. In this modification, extremely short bursts of power are interspersed with similar, extremely short periods of aspiration. The on-off cycle is regulated by the surgeon and may be as short as 2 ms on or off. It can be adjusted with more on time than off time (e.g., 2 ms on 4 ms off) for surgeons who prefer chopping techniques, or more on time than off time (e.g., 4 ms on and 2 ms off) for surgeons who sculpt during divide-and-conquer techniques. The change in phaco duty cycles leads to enhanced followability. The end result is shorter phaco power on times and less delivery of total phaco energy to the anterior segment. In addition, the off time allows effective cooling of the phaco tip.

This is an important characteristic of this software modification. Recent studies have shown that the wound will show the first signs of a wound burn at 45° C and frank signs of burn at 50° C. With WhiteStar, the maximal wound temperature at 100% power was measured at 28° C.[8] Therefore the phaco tip can be placed though the wound without the cooling sleeve. This change allows for the performance of a bimanual phacoemulsification procedure, in which the irrigation is provided by a 20-gauge irrigating chopping instrument inserted through a 1.4-mm clear cornea incision. The 20-gauge, 15-degree or 30-degree phaco tip without the irrigation sleeve is inserted through a 20-gauge clear cornea incision 90 degrees to 100 degrees away. The nucleus is emulsified by either a vertical or horizontal chopping procedure. The wound remains cool and the efficiency of the procedure is enhanced as the separate irrigation tends to wash fragments into the phaco tip.

Alteration of Phaco Power Delivery

The amplitude of phaco energy is modified by tip selection. Phaco tips can be modified to accentuate (1) power intensity, (2) flow, or (3) a combination of both.

Power intensity is modified by altering bevel tip angle. As noted previously, the bevel of the phaco tip focuses power in the direction of the bevel. The 0-degree tip focuses both jackhammer and cavitational force directly in front of it. The 30-degree tip focuses these forces at a 30-degree angle from the phaco tip (see Figures 7-4, 7-5, 7-7, and 7-8). The Kelman tip produces broad powerful cavitation directed away from the angle in the shaft (see Figure 7-6). This tip is excellent for the hardest of nuclei.

Power intensity and flow are modified by using a 0-degree tip. This tip focuses power directly ahead of the tip and enhances occlusion caused by the smaller surface area of its orifice.

New flare and cobra tips direct cavitation into the opening of the bevel of the tip. Thus random emission of phaco energy is minimized. The narrow "neck" of the tip functions as a flow restrictor, increasing resistance to flow and reducing the tendency to create surge (Figure 7-10). Designer tips such as the "flathead" designed by Barry Seibel and power wedges designed by Douglas Mastel offer the ability to fine tune the focus of phaco energy as well as modify the aspiration flow dependent upon the configuration and diameter of the phaco tip.

Small-diameter tips, such as 21-gauge tips, change fluid flow rates. Although they do not actually change power intensity, they appear to have this effect, as the nucleus must be emulsified into smaller pieces for removal through the smaller diameter tip.

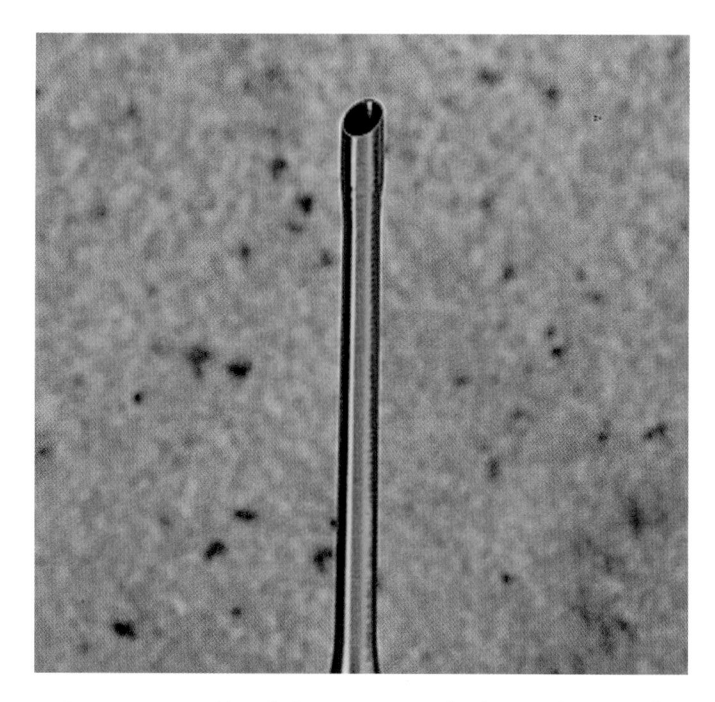

FIGURE 7-10 Flare tip focuses power at the tip secondary to the flare and acts as a flow restrictor secondary to the narrowing at the "neck." (Courtesy Micro Technology Inc.)

The Alcon aspiration bypass system (ABS) tip modification is available with a 0-degree tip, a Kelman tip, or a flare tip. The tip type is a modification of power intensity, and the ABS is a flow modification. In the ABS system a 0.175-mm hole in the needle shaft permits a variable flow of fluid into the needle, even during occlusion (Figure 7-11). The amount of flow through the shaft hole is variable and depends on the vacuum

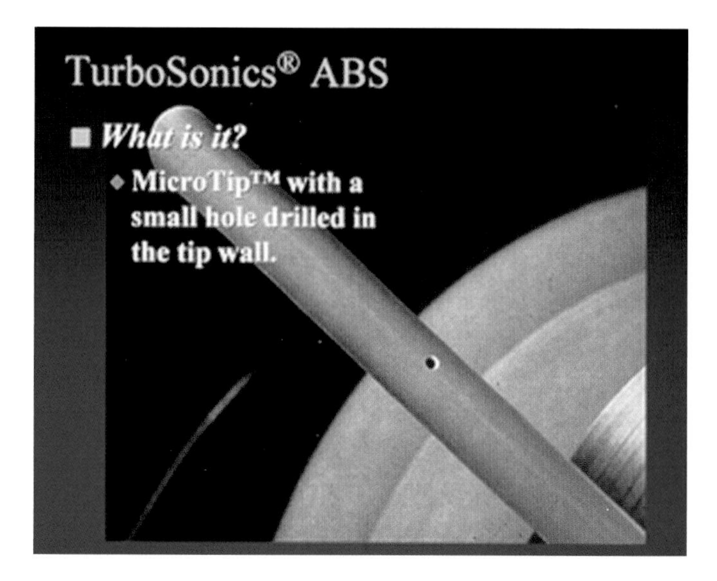

FIGURE 7-11 A 0.175-mm hole drilled in the shaft of the ABS tip provides an alternate path for fluid to flow into the needle when an occlusion occurs at the phaco tip.

level. The higher the vacuum level, the greater the flow. This flow adjustment serves to reduce postocclusion surge.

Flow is modified by using one of the varieties of Microseal tips. These tips have a flexible outer sleeve to seal the phaco incision. They also have a rigid inner sleeve or a ribbed shaft configuration to protect cooling irrigant inflow. Thus a tight seal allows low-flow phacoemulsification without danger of wound burns.

Phaco power intensity is the energy that emulsifies the lens nucleus. The phaco tip must operate in a cool environment and with adequate space to isolate its actions from delicate intraocular structures. This portion of the action of the machine is dependent on its fluidics.

Fluidics

The fluidics aspect of all machines is fundamentally a balance of fluid inflow and fluid outflow. The resultant balance of these two influences will be the maintenance of a constant intraocular volume and therefore a stable and deep anterior chamber. In addition, the intraocular pressure must be maintained within physiologically compatible limits.

Infusion

Inflow (infusion) is the pressure gradient, which drives the infusion flow. In a gravity feed system, the bottle height above the eye of the patient creates an infusion pressure. When infusion pumps are employed, the amount of infusion pressure programmed into the pump will be responsible for the generation of infusion pressure. With recent acceptance of temporal surgical approaches, the eye of the patient may be physically higher than in the past. This requires that the irrigation bottle be adequately elevated. In addition, when the machine flow rate is increased, increased fluid evacuation from the anterior chamber requires increased inflow to maintain the steady-state system. Therefore, when the machine flow rate is increased, the bottle height should also be increased. A shallow, unstable anterior chamber results otherwise.

Infusion tubing diameter and elasticity do not play a significant role in infusion volume control because high pressures and rapid pressure fluxes rarely occur on the irrigation bottle side of the system.

Outflow

Control of outflow is notably more complex because many factors influence both volume and speed of fluid outflow during the phaco procedure. Among these variables are incision size, phaco tip diameter and sleeve diameter, pump type and settings, and tubing diameter and compliance. In addition, computer software design plays a significant role in regulating both outflow volume and speed.

INCISION

The *incision size* is an important variable in the determination of fluid outflow. This is actually a controlled leak determined by the sleeve-incision relationship. The incision length selected should create a snug fit with the phaco tip and sleeve selected. This results in minimal controlled wound fluid outflow with resultant increased anterior chamber stability.

If the incision is too large for the selected phaco tip and sleeve combination, the excessive fluid outflow will necessitate increased fluid inflow to maintain a deep anterior chamber. The increased infusion volume not only is deleterious to the health of the endothelium but usually cannot sustain the sudden changes in volume that occur during the procedure. This leads to considerable chamber instability with increased risk of rupturing the posterior capsule.

If the incision is too small, crimping of the sleeve will lead to decreased inflow with resultant chamber shallowing. In addition, decreased inflow is the origin of decreased cooling and may produce wound burns.

ASPIRATION SETTINGS

Aspiration rate, or flow, is defined as the flow of fluid, in cubic centimeters per minute, through the aspiration tubing. With a peristaltic pump this rate is determined by the speed of the pump. Flow is the fluidic force that determines how well particulate material is attracted to the phaco tip. Flow adjustments act to speed up or slow down events in the anterior chamber. Therefore, if events appear to be occurring too rapidly, the flow rate is slowed. Alternatively, if events are occurring too slowly, the flow rate is increased.

Aspiration level, or vacuum, is a level and measured in millimeters of mercury (mm Hg). It is defined as the magnitude of negative pressure created in the tubing. Vacuum is the fluidic force determinant of how well, once occluded on the phaco tip, particulate material will be held to the tip.

Flow therefore is the setting that controls how well material is attracted to the phaco tip. Vacuum is the setting that determines how well material is held against the tip once occlusion occurs.

Vacuum Sources

The origin for the development of vacuum is the vacuum pump. The three categories of vacuum sources or pumps are (1) flow pumps, (2) vacuum pumps,[3] and (3) hybrid pumps.

The prototype example of the *flow pump* is the peristaltic pump (Figure 7-12). This pump consists of a series of rotating rollers that successively compress the aspiration tubing, moving fluid within the tubing and creating vacuum. The speed of rotation of the pump head governs the flow rate. One important advantage of this class of pumps is the ability to allow *independent control of both aspiration rate and aspiration level.*

The primary example of the vacuum pump is the Venturi pump (Figure 7-13). In the Venturi pump, compressed gas is passed through a Venturi, which creates a vacuum. The Venturi is attached to a rigid reservoir that is attached to the aspiration tubing. The velocity of the compressed gas passage through the Venturi creates greater or lesser vacuum that is then transferred through the reservoir to the aspiration line. This results in varying amounts of vacuum.

Additional examples of this pump type are the rotary vane and diaphragmatic pumps.

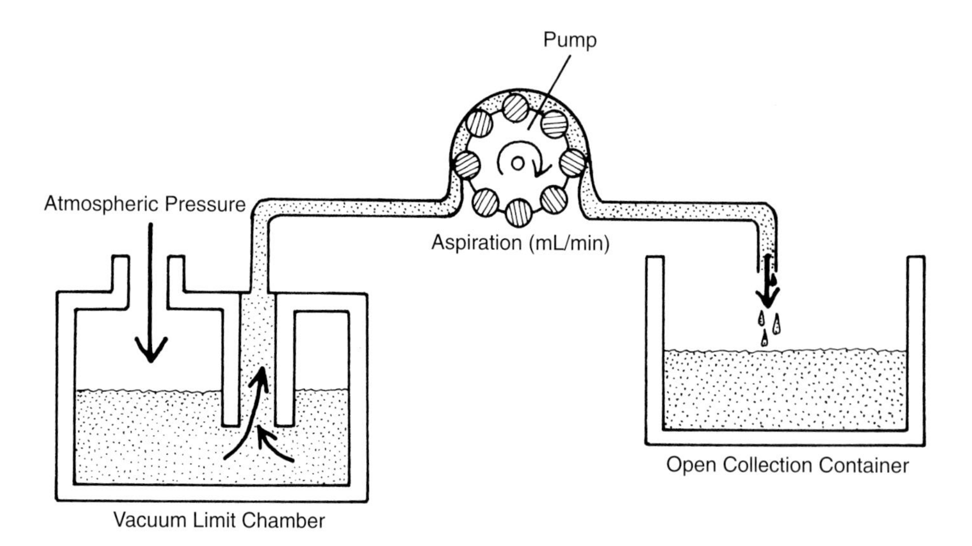

FIGURE 7-12 Peristaltic pump uses a rotating wheel with rollers to pinch off segments of the aspiration tubing, thereby moving separate columns of fluid through the tubing at a controlled rate of aspiration or flow. The vacuum limit is set separately and independently, limiting the maximal vacuum that is tolerated in the condition of complete occlusion of the aspiration line. The collection chamber, located after the vacuum limit chamber and the aspiration pump, is open to atmosphere.

Vacuum pumps allow direct control of only vacuum level. Flow control is dependent on the vacuum level setting. *There is no independent setting of aspiration flow.*

Modern modifications of the basic pump types have prompted the creation of a new pump category, the *hybrid pump.* These pumps are interesting in that they can act like either a vacuum or flow pump, independent of their original design, depending on their programming. They are the most recent supplement to pump types. They are universally controlled by digital inputs, producing extraordinary flexibility and responsiveness.

The primary example of the hybrid pump is the Allergan Sovereign peristaltic pump (Figure 7-14) or the Bausch & Lomb Concentrix pump (Figure 7-15).[9]

The challenge to the surgeon is to balance the effect of phaco power intensity, which tends to push nuclear fragments away from the phaco tip, with the effect of flow, which attracts fragments toward the phaco tip, and vacuum, which holds the fragments on the phaco tip. Generally, low flow slows down intraocular events, and high flow or vacuum speeds them up. Low or zero vacuum is helpful during sculpting of a hard or a

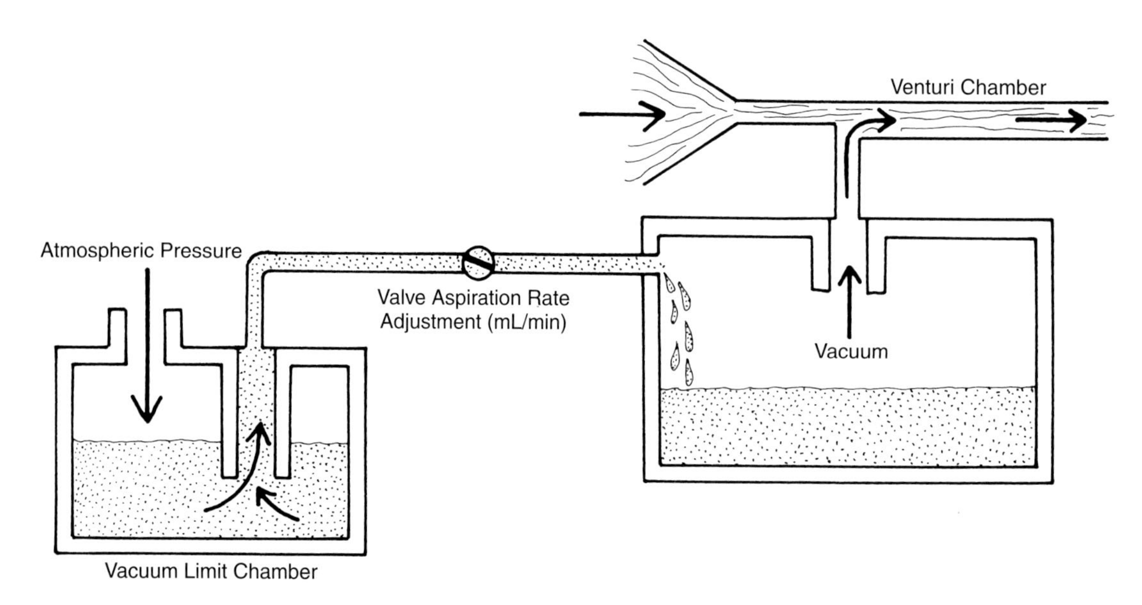

FIGURE 7-13 In a Venturi pump system, the flow of gas passed through tubing with increasing diameter creates a vacuum. The collection chamber is therefore a closed system. A separate valve can control the aspiration rate. A separate vacuum limit can be set, but a continuous internal vacuum is necessary to drive the aspiration of the fluid.

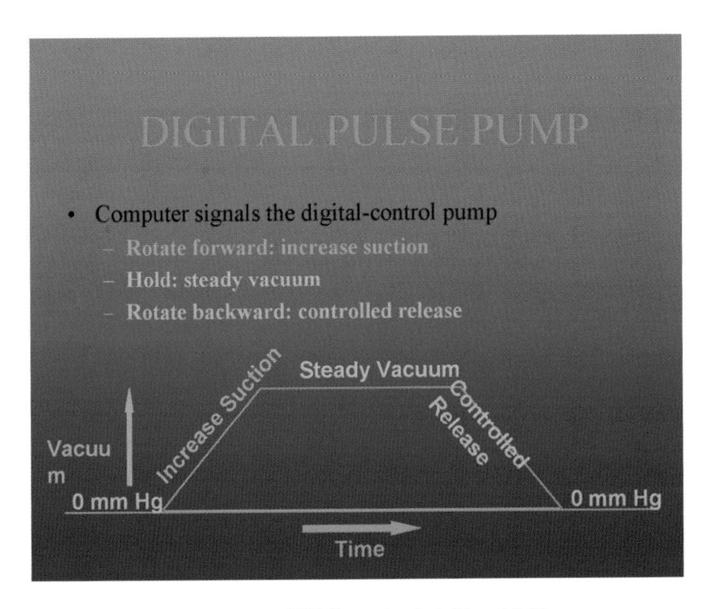

FIGURE 7-14 AMO Sovereign hybrid peristaltic pump.

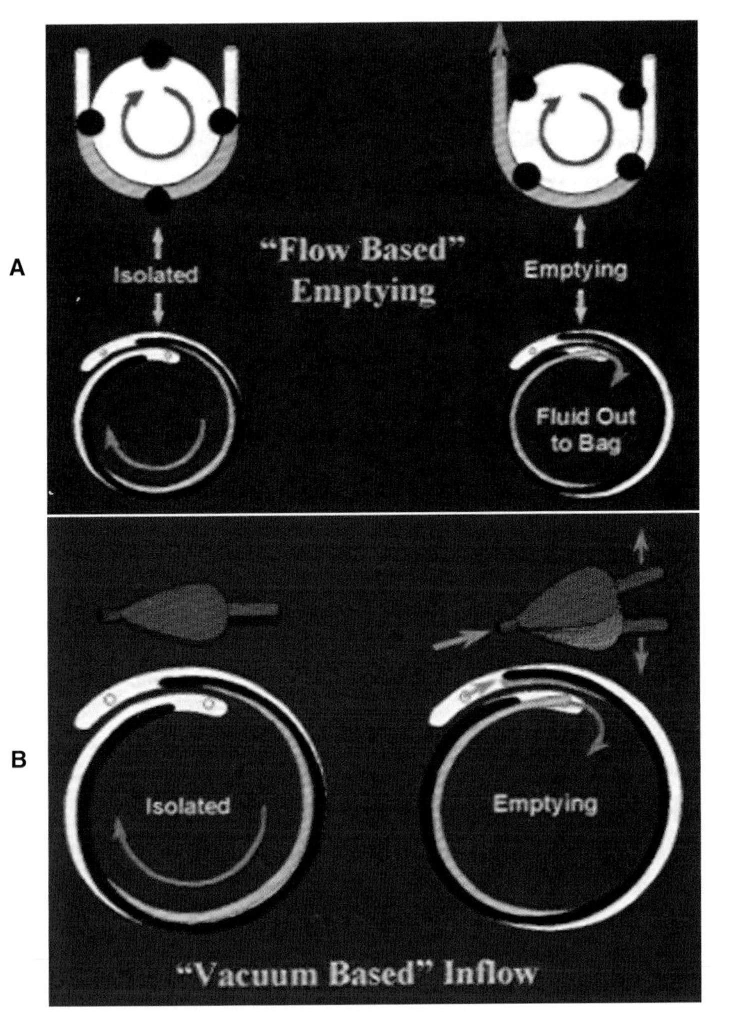

FIGURE 7-15 A, The scroll pumps' emptying phase is flow based, analogous to a peristaltic system. **B,** During the inflow phase, the male scroll opens like a bellows, creating vacuum response similar to a Venturi system.

large nucleus. In this circumstance, the large, hard endonucleus may cause the surgeon to phacoemulsify near or under the iris, or anterior capsule, with a high-power intensity. With normal aspiration the phaco tip may aspirate the iris. The high power will cause immediate, severe damage to the iris. Therefore zero (or very low) vacuum will prevent inadvertent aspiration of the iris or capsule, preventing significant morbidity.

Surge

A principal limiting factor in the selection of high levels of vacuum or flow is the development of surge. When the phaco tip is occluded, flow is instantly interrupted, and vacuum rapidly builds to its preset maximum level (Figure 7-16). Emulsification of the occluding fragment then clears the occlusion. Flow instantaneously begins at the preset level in the presence of the high vacuum level. In addition, if the aspiration line tubing is not reinforced to prevent collapse (tubing compliance), the tubing will have constricted during the occlusion. It then expands on occlusion break. The expansion is an additional source of brisk vacuum production. These factors cause a rush of fluid from the anterior segment into the phaco tip (Figure 7-17). The fluid in the anterior chamber may not be replaced by infusion rapidly enough to prevent its shallowing. Therefore subsequent, rapid anterior movement of the posterior capsule occurs. Often the cornea collapses. The violent snapping of the posterior capsule, or abrupt forceful stretching of the bag around nuclear fragments, may be a cause of capsular tears (Figure 7-18). In addition, the posterior capsule can be literally sucked into the phaco tip, tearing it. The magnitude of the surge is contingent on the presurge settings of flow and vacuum.

The phaco machine manufacturers help to decrease surge by providing noncompliant aspiration tubing. This does not constrict in the presence of high levels of vacuum.

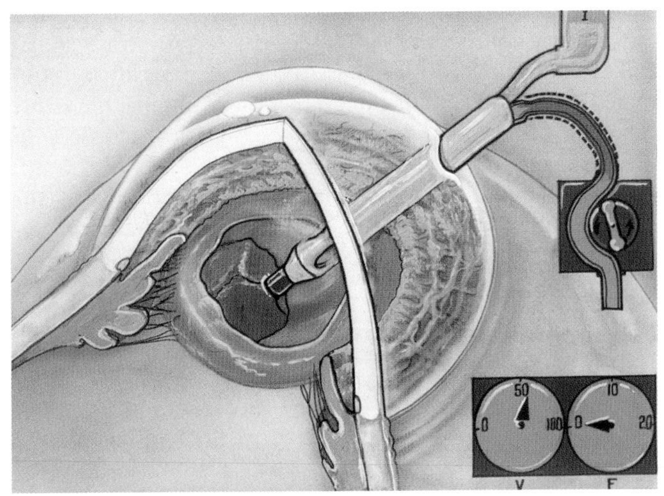

FIGURE 7-16 Immediate presurge. The nuclear fragment has occluded the phaco tip. Flow instantaneously drops to zero. Vacuum begins to rise toward the maximum preset. The aspiration tubing begins to collapse. The chamber is deep. (Courtesy Thieme Publications, New York.)

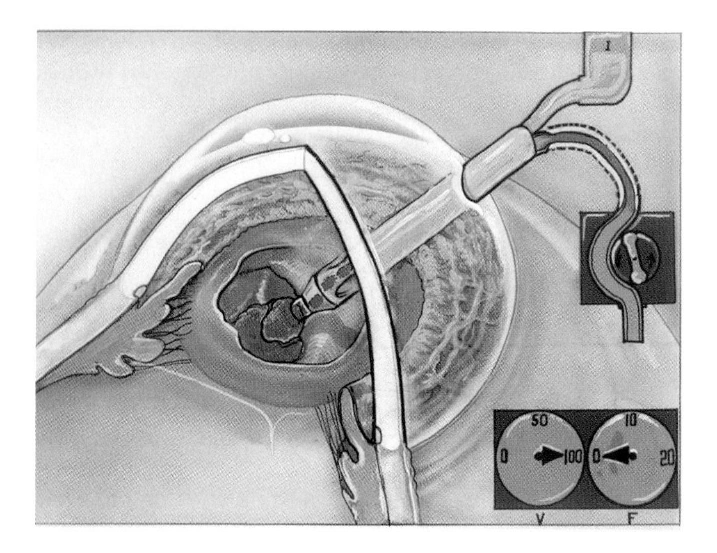

FIGURE 7-17 Early surge. Phaco power has partially emulsified the fragment. Flow is about to resume and instantaneously rise to the preset maximum. Vacuum, at maximum, is about to precipitously drop. The tubing is expanding. Outflow is exceeding inflow. The chamber is beginning to collapse. The posterior capsule is beginning to bulge around the remaining heminucleus. (Courtesy Thieme Publications, New York.)

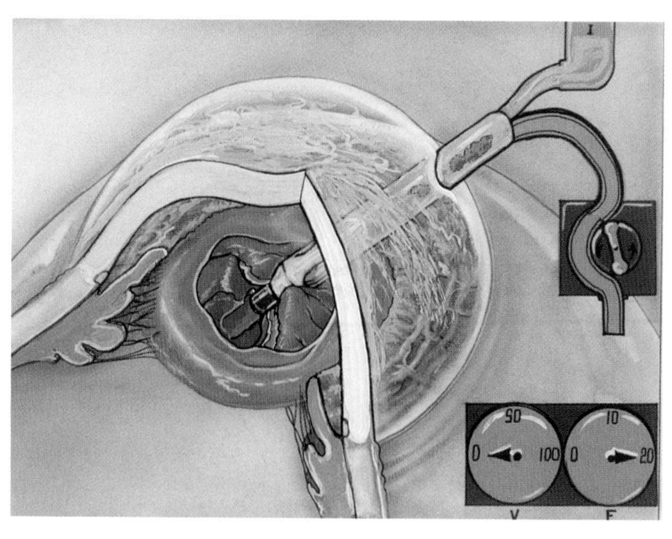

FIGURE 7-18 Midsurge. Flow is now at preset maximum. Vacuum is zero. The anterior chamber is markedly shallowed. The posterior capsule has snapped around the heminucleus, causing a tear. The cornea has collapsed. (Courtesy Thieme Publications, New York.)

Most manufacturers have created algorithms in their software that emulate the anterior chamber moment to moment during the phaco procedure. These algorithms can anticipate microsecond changes in the real anterior chamber and make appropriate pump adjustments to minimize surge.

Surge Modification

Surge is undoubtedly an unwanted event. The trampolining of the posterior capsule caused by surge has the effect of creating dismay among surgeons. In an effort to prevent capsular tears, they move the nucleus is anteriorly, closer to iris and endothelium. To promote a more safe procedure and to spare the iris and endothelium unnecessary trauma, the astute surgeon will consider the changes in fluidics necessary to prevent surge.

If the defining instant in the generation of surge is the occlusion break, the entire episode can be divided into preocclusive, occlusive, and postocclusive segments.

Preocclusion

Historically, the only way to modify surge was to select lower levels of flow and vacuum. This category would be a modification in preocclusion (Figure 7-19). At present, many other methods exist to decrease surge. Another approach to surge management, in all phases of occlusion, is the use of an anterior chamber maintainer. The constant flow of this device acts to deepen the chamber in all phases of phacoemulsification. Constant infusion, when available, is another preocclusion modification, although its benefits are not significant.

OCCLUSION

Only a few modifications take place at the moment of occlusion. The first is the use of the Alcon ABS tip. This tip, discussed earlier, has a 0.175-mm hole drilled in the shaft of the phaco needle. When occlusion occurs at the tip, fluid flows into this hole. The amount of flow depends on the vacuum and flow settings. For example, the flow through this hole is 4 cc/min at a vacuum of 50 mm Hg and 11 cc/min at a vacuum of 400 mm Hg. Because some flow always exists, in reality there is never complete occlusion. This prevents the rise of high vacuum levels and thus diminishes postocclusion surge. This modification must be used with the high vacuum tubing or it does not function properly.

The second, as employed by the Paradigm unit, is a variable rise time. By slowing the pump speed during occlusion, the generation of high vacuum levels is decelerated, and surge is diminished.

POSTOCCLUSION

Once occlusion has occurred, decreasing the vacuum or flow instantaneously to dramatically decrease flow into the phaco tip is a powerful method of diminishing surge.

The model for this type of surge modification is found in the AMO Sovereign unit. In this machine, microprocessors sample vacuum and flow parameters 50 times a second, creating a "virtual" anterior chamber model. At the moment of surge, the machine computer senses the increase in flow and instantaneously slows or reverses the pump to stop surge production. Pump management, rather than venting, is the mechanism to control surge.

In addition, this device has a programmable occlusion threshold setting. When the vacuum reaches this threshold, a new flow, as well as a new power modulation, can be programmed. Therefore, if a hard nucleus is being emulsified, when the

A

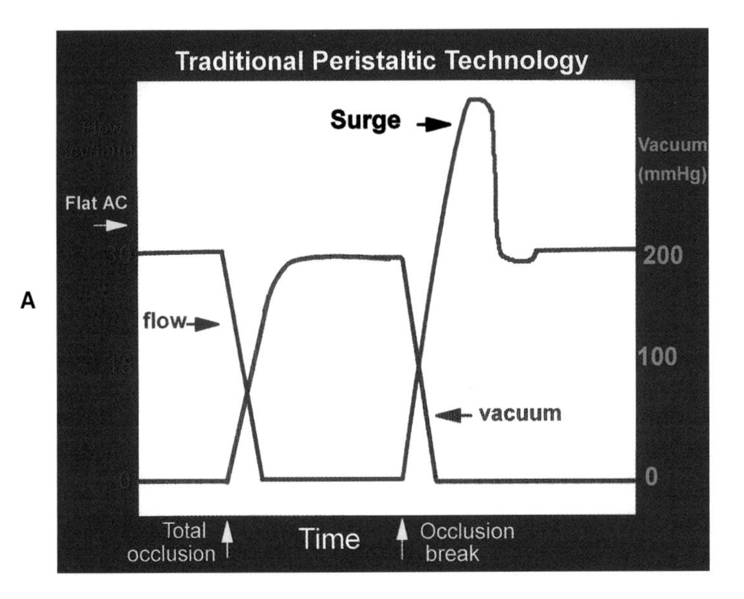

B

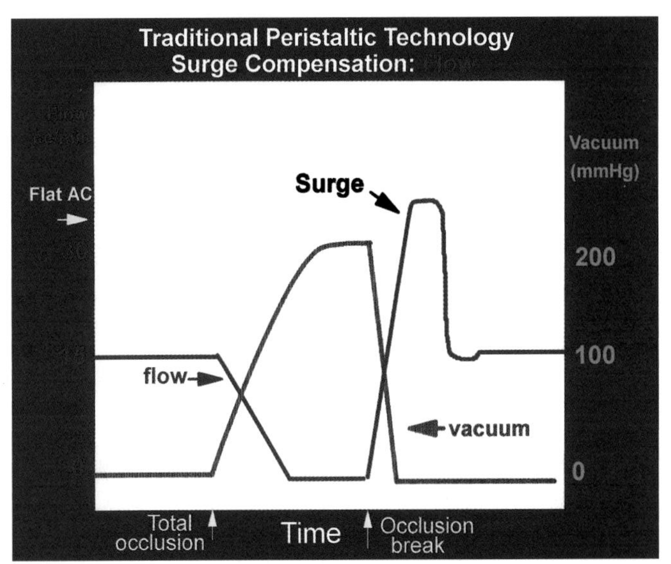

C

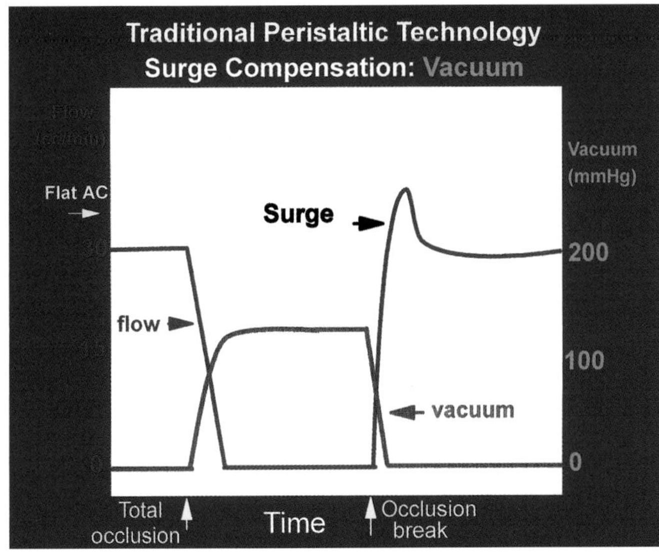

D

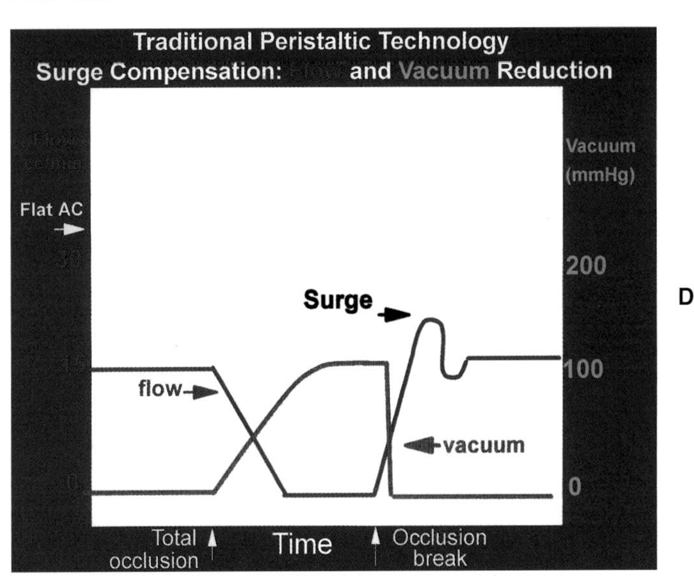

FIGURE 7-19 The dynamics of vacuum and flow, with particular emphasis on the phenomenon of surge. The values shown are illustrative and not necessarily those of any particular commercial system or surgical technique. **A,** In traditional peristaltic technology, flow ideally can be set at a relatively high rate just below that which would flatten the anterior chamber. In a nonoccluded system, the flow can be high, and the vacuum level at the phaco tip is nearly zero. When the tip is occluded, the aspiration rate rapidly falls to zero. The vacuum level rises correspondingly. The more rapid the flow rate, the more quickly the vacuum level rises. The vacuum level continues to build up to the preset limit, after which fluid is bled into the aspiration line, limiting the maximum vacuum. When occlusion is relieved, the vacuum then rapidly falls back to a near zero level at the tip. The stored potential energy in the aspiration line causes a momentary "surge" in the fluid flow before the flow stabilizes at the original level determined by the rotation of the peristaltic pump. If the potential energy causes a surge of fluid flow greater than the combined rate of irrigation fluid inflow and wound leak, flattening of the anterior chamber results. **B,** One mechanism for compensating for surge is to reduce flow. When flow or aspiration rate is reduced, two effects are seen. First, after occlusion is obtained, the rate at which the vacuum rises is slower. Ultimately, however, the vacuum still builds to the preset level. Second, after occlusion break, the height of the fluid surge is the same as in panel **A.** However, the surge is relative to the baseline level of nonoccluded flow. Because the flow has been reduced, the overall surge level may be at or below the level of a momentary flattening of the anterior chamber. **C,** An alternative compensation for surge is to reduce the vacuum level. Because the flow rate is unchanged, the speed at which the maximum vacuum is achieved is unchanged compared with the buildup of vacuum seen in panel **A.** After the occlusion is relieved, the amount of surge is reduced because the stored potential energy is reduced through the lower vacuum level. Because of the high flow rate, however, even this reduced amount of surge may exceed the level at which flattening of the anterior chamber is seen. **D,** In common clinical practice, both the flow and vacuum levels are reduced below the theoretical maximum to guard against surge. As illustrated, the reduction in flow rate and maximal vacuum level reduced the surge below the level at which the anterior chamber flattens. Through these compromises, safe phacoemulsification can be clinically performed. *(Continued)*

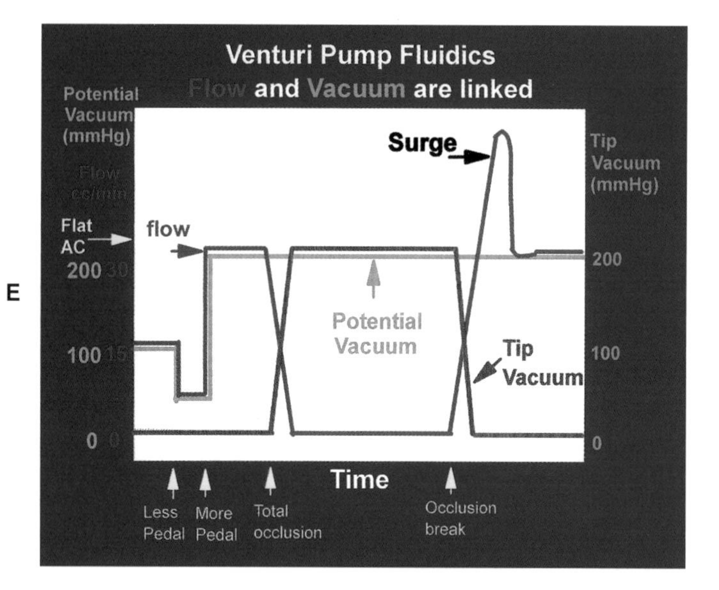

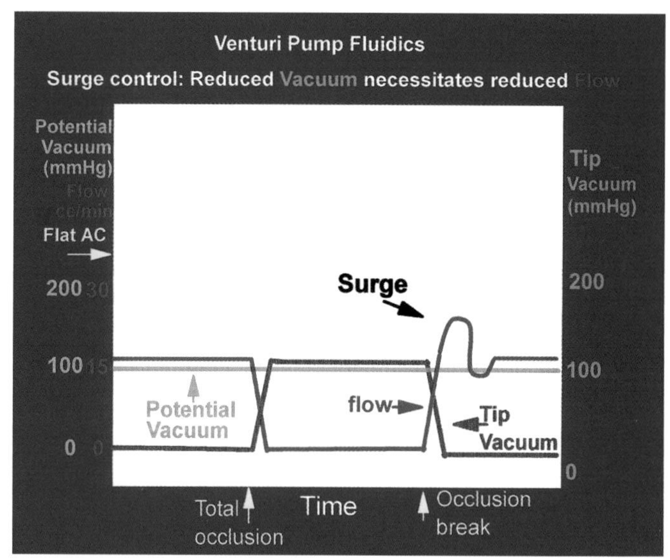

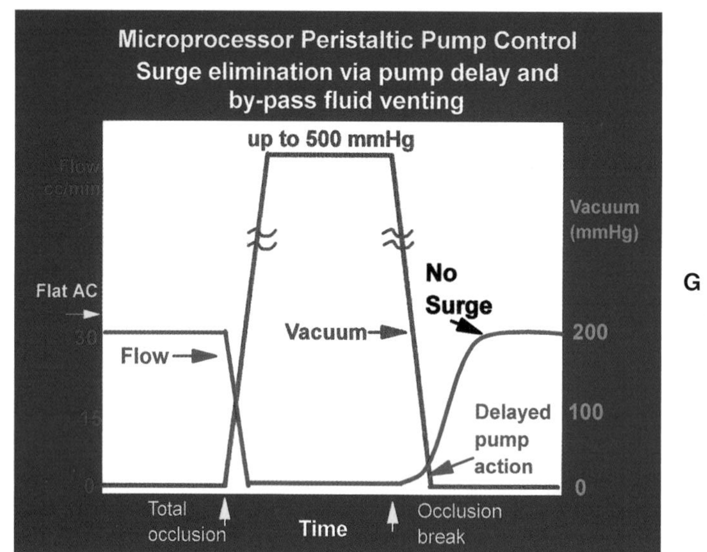

FIGURE 7-19, cont'd The dynamics of vacuum and flow, with particular emphasis on the phenomenon of surge. The values shown are illustrative and not necessarily those of any particular commercial system or surgical technique. **E,** In a Venturi or diaphragm pump, flow and vacuum are intrinsically linked. The potential vacuum within the system caused by the Venturi and diaphragm pump is the principal determinant of the flow level. As illustrated in the left side of the figure, one attribute of the Venturi system is the rapid response time of the flow rate achieved by varying the potential vacuum within the system. After total occlusion occurs clinically, however, the performance at the phaco tip is similar to that of the peristaltic pump. The vacuum level at the tip rises to the preset level of the internal pump while the flow rate drops to zero. When occlusion is relieved, the vacuum at the tip once again drops to nearly zero. The stored potential energy in the system is translated into the clinical phenomenon of surge, just as in a peristaltic system. After the surge phenomenon, the flow rate stabilizes at the level determined by the internal vacuum of the Venturi pump. **F,** To compensate for surge and to maintain the anterior chamber, typically maximum potential vacuum and flow rate are reduced. Because of the intrinsic linkage of flow and vacuum in a Venturi or diaphragm pump system, reduction of the internal potential vacuum necessitates a reduced flow rate. By reducing both the flow and maximum vacuum, the surge level can be reduced below the level of flattening of the anterior chamber. **G,** New technology offers enhanced control over the surge phenomenon. As a result, phacoemulsification can be performed at vacuum levels that were previously highly unsafe. As illustrated, a microprocessor peristaltic pump control system may allow vacuum levels to build up to 500 mm Hg or more. After a break in the occlusion, the microprocessor delays the action of the pump by delaying its onset. In this manner, combined with other steps, such as reducing the compliance of the vacuum tubing, the phenomenon of surge is reduced to clinically tolerable levels, and high vacuum can be employed as a clinical tool without danger of collapse of the anterior chamber.

vacuum reaches 80 mm Hg, for example, the flow, which might have been set at 350 ml/min, can now be automatically decreased to 100 ml/min. The result will be a noteworthy decrease in surge. Moreover, the pulse rate can be simultaneously slowed to further stabilize the anterior chamber.

Another solution to this problem is demonstrated in the Bausch & Lomb Millennium machine. The dual linear foot pedal can be programmed to separate both the flow and vacuum from power. In this way, flow or vacuum can be lowered before beginning the emulsification of an occluding fragment. The emulsification therefore occurs in the presence of a lower vacuum or flow so that surge is minimized.

Finally, the Starr Wave machine solves this problem in another manner. The patented coiled aspiration tubing acts as a flow resistor. At low flow settings, up to 50 ml/min, the tubing acts like normal tubing. When flow exceeds this level, turbulence in the tubing inhibits further increases in flow. This dampens the fluid outflow, and subsequent vacuum rise. The result is decreased surge.

Venting

Often during the performance of phacoemulsification, or irrigation and aspiration (I&A), undesirable material is aspirated on the phaco tip. This could be posterior capsule or a piece of nucleus that is too large for efficient emulsification. Often the aspiration of these structures requires hasty release. Venting is the mechanism for this release by neutralizing vacuum in the aspiration line.

When the surgeon lifts the foot pedal from position 2 or 3, the venting mechanism is engaged. This allows air or fluid to flow into the aspiration line. Generally, venting to air has been abandoned by most manufacturers. When the aspiration line is vented to air, bubbles form in the aspiration tubing. When the foot pedal is again depressed, the development of vacuum is slowed because the air in the line must first be aspirated before vacuum can once more rise.

The preferred venting material is therefore fluid. Most machines use fluid from the infusion bottle for this purpose. The fluid flows into the aspiration tubing, neutralizing vacuum and permitting the release of unwanted material. Because no air has been introduced into the system, when the foot pedal is again engaged, there is brisk redevelopment of flow and vacuum. This technique produces a more responsive system.

In some machines, venting also occurs when the selected vacuum level is attained. Controlled venting stops further generation of vacuum and maintains the commanded vacuum level.

Irrigation and Aspiration

Fluidic management techniques used in the phaco mode are now applied to the I&A segment. Therefore surge management systems function to prevent surge when a large or "sticky" piece of cortex is aspirated.

Most I&A tips use a 0.3-mm orifice. They are now available in straight and angled configurations. Soft or hard metal sleeves are also offered to provide coaxial fluid inflow. Soft sleeves are now preferred to provide a tighter uniform seal within the surgical wound. This lessens superfluous outflow and leads to a more stable anterior chamber.

Alcon has recently introduced a clever steerable I&A tip. It is an articulated silicone tip with angulation that is controlled by the foot pedal. The advantage is that it can be twisted into any desired angulation to remove hard to reach cortex. In addition, the silicone aspiration port is reported to be "capsular friendly," in that it can aspirate the posterior capsule with 450 mm Hg vacuum without tearing it.[4]

Bimanual Irrigation and Aspiration

Introduced in Europe by Dr. Peter Brauweiler, the use of separate cannulas for I&A has been widely accepted. In this technique, small paracentesis-like incisions are made for placement of the cannulas. The small incisions and smaller cannulas offer controlled inflow and outflow, which promotes anterior chamber stability. The ability to more easily reach recalcitrant cortex provides surgeons with a technique that simplifies I&A. The relative positions of the cannulas are simply exchanged to reach new areas of cortex.

Bimanual techniques are especially suited to removal of cortex in difficult situations. When the posterior capsule is torn, the additional control of aspiration cannula placement, as well as the decreased anterior chamber fluid fluctuations, minimizes the risk of rupturing the vitreous face with subsequent necessity for vitrectomy. In addition, in cases of zonular dehiscence, the added flexible placement and maneuverability of the aspiration cannula provide a margin of safety removing cortex without further disruption of zonules.

Vitrectomy

All current machines have vitrectomy capability. Generally the same I&A tubing are used. They are attached to the vitrectomy handpiece. In the vitrectomy mode the foot pedal controls irrigation and aspiration and activates the vitrectomy handpiece cutter. If the cutter is actuated by compressed air, it must be connected with the dedicated compressed air tubing to the machine attachment port.

Vitrectomy Instruments

The three types of vitrectomy handpieces are rotary, oscillatory, and guillotine cutters.

Rotary cutters have a sharp blade, or blades, which rotate perpendicular to the long axis of the aspiration tube. They have the advantage of being self-sharpening and therefore perform excellent cutting when in proper working order. They are often actuated electrically. The potential problem with these cutters occurs when the blades are dull from extensive usage or are out of alignment. The rotatory movement of the blades then has the capability of pulling the vitreous into the instrument without cutting it. The result is "spooling" of the vitreous, which is often the cause of postoperative vitreous traction with subsequent cystoid macular edema or retinal detachment.

Oscillatory cutters function similarly to rotary cutters, but rather than spinning in 360-degree circles, they rotate 180 degrees and then reverse direction. They can be self-sharpening. They are electrically driven. Because they do not completely spin, they cannot spool the vitreous and are therefore safer to use. They require periodic maintenance because they are usually reusable.

Guillotine cutters are presently the most popular form of vitrectomy handpiece. The blade moves up and down in the long axis of the aspiration tube. These blades cannot be self-sharpening because of their design. Therefore these instruments are usually disposable rather than reusable. This feature offers the benefit of well-lubricated, sharp blades each time they are used. They are actuated by compressed air. They remove vitreous cleanly, without spooling.

Vitrectomy Technique

When vitrectomy is necessary it can be performed from the limbus or pars plana. In either case a bimanual vitrectomy technique is preferred. The irrigation sleeve is removed from the vitrectomy handpiece and discarded. The main incision is closed. If not self-sealing, it should be sutured. The paracentesis incision is used for infusion. A 23-gauge cannula attached to the infusion bottle is inserted through the paracentesis. The infusion bottle is lowered to an adequate height to maintain the anterior chamber without excessive outflow. A new 2-mm paracentesis is created in a comfortable position. The vitrectomy handpiece, without the infusion sleeve, is placed through this incision. The machine is set to low vacuum (50 to 100 mm Hg). If a peristaltic pump is used, a flow of 18 to 22 ml/min will provide adequate generation of vacuum without excessive turbulence. The cutting speed should be high (300 to 400 cuts/min) so that the aspirated vitreous is cut before the vitreous strands are allowed to place traction on the vitreous base.

The tip of the cutter is placed into the anterior vitreous, and the vitrectomy is performed until vitreous is removed to the level of the posterior capsule (Figure 7-20). In this way the vitreous is literally shelled out of the posterior segment without disturbing the vitreous base at the pars plana or the vitreous connections to the macula or optic nerve. This approach minimizes the risk of postoperative cystoid macular edema and retinal detachment.

If performed from the pars plana, similar settings and techniques are used. The vitrectomy instrument is introduced through an incision created precisely 3.0 to 3.5 mm posterior to the limbus with a microvitreoretinal (MVR) blade. Under direct visualization the vitrector is placed into the anterior vitreous with the aspiration port up, and vitrectomy is performed as noted previously (Figure 7-21).[10]

Phaco Technique and Machine Technology

The patient will have the best visual result when total phaco energy delivered to the anterior segment is minimized. In addition, phaco energy should be focused into the nucleus. This step will prevent damage to iris blood vessels and endothelium. Finally, proficient emulsification will lead to shorter overall surgical time. Therefore a lesser amount of irrigation fluid will pass through the anterior segment.

The general principles of power management are to focus phaco energy into the nucleus, vary fluid parameters for efficient sculpting and fragment removal, and minimize surge.

All phaco techniques require three phases: removal of the endonucleus, removal of the epinucleus with or without attached cortex, and I&A of cortex.

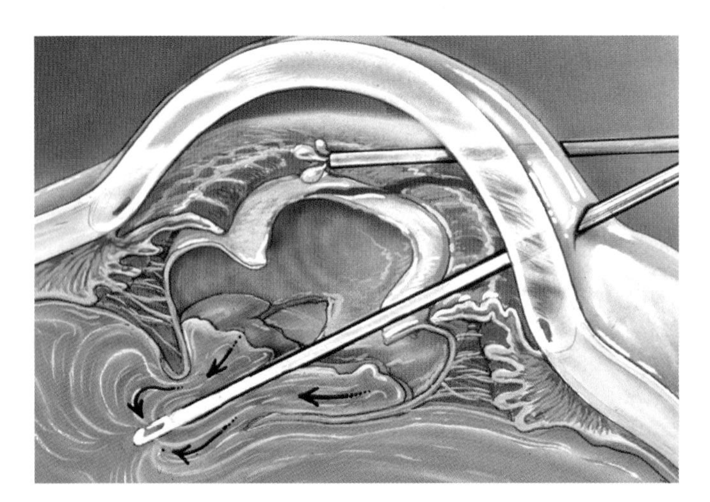

FIGURE 7-20 The vitrector, with the Charles Sleeve removed is placed through a paracentesis into the vitreous. Irrigation is provided by a 23-gauge cannula placed through another paracentesis. The vitreous is drawn back into the posterior segment and removed to the level of the posterior capsule. (Courtesy Thieme Publications, New York.)

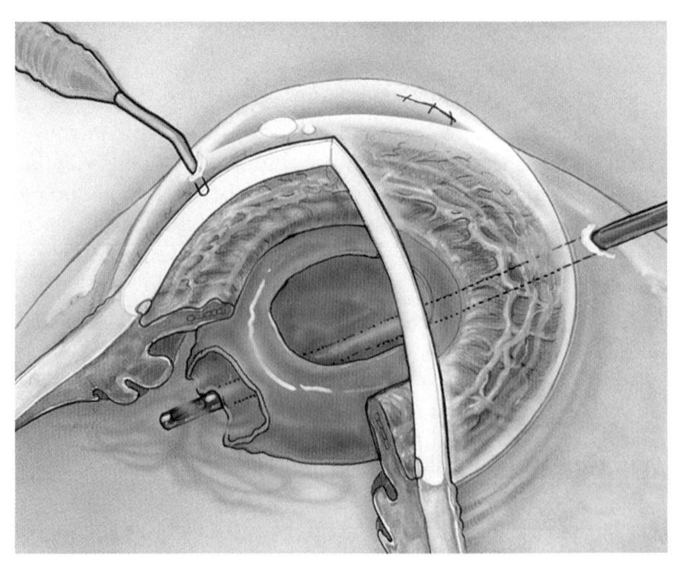

FIGURE 7-21 Vitrectomy through the pars plana. After an incision is made 3.5 mm posterior to the limbus with an MVR blade, the vitrectomy instrument is placed into the anterior vitreous under direct observation. (Courtesy Thieme Publications, New York.)

The endonucleus can be emulsified in situ as seen with divide and conquer techniques. Alternatively, it can be manipulated within the capsular bag and iris plane as seen with phaco chop or supracapsular techniques.

Divide and Conquer Phaco

SCULPTING

To focus cavitation energy into the nucleus a 0-degree tip or a 15-degree or 30-degree tip turned bevel down should be used. Zero or low vacuum (depending on the manufacturer's recommendation) is mandatory for bevel-down phaco to prevent occlusion. Occlusion during sculpting is undesirable. At best, it causes excessive movement of the nucleus during sculpting. At worst, occlusion occurring near the equator is the cause of tears in the equatorial bag early in the phaco procedure, and occlusion at the bottom of a grove cause phaco through the posterior capsule. Once the grove is judged to be adequately deep, the bevel of the tip should be rotated to the bevel-up position to improve visibility and prevent the possibility of phaco through the posterior nucleus and posterior capsule.

QUADRANT AND FRAGMENT REMOVAL

The tip selected, as noted previously, is retained. Vacuum and flow are increased to reasonable limits subject to the machine being used. The limiting factor to these levels is the development of surge. The bevel of the tip is turned toward the quadrant or fragment. Low pulsed or burst power is applied at a level high enough to emulsify the fragment without driving it from the phaco tip. Chatter is defined as a fragment bouncing from the phaco tip as a result of aggressive application of phaco energy.

EPINUCLEUS AND CORTEX REMOVAL

For removal of epinucleus and cortex the vacuum is decreased while flow is maintained. This allows grasping of the epinucleus just deep to the anterior capsule. The low vacuum helps the tip hold the epinucleus on the phaco tip without breaking off chunks. This will occur in the presence of high vacuum. Once the epinucleus is occluded on the phaco tip, it will rotate around the equator and can then be pulled to the level of the iris. There, low-power pulsed phaco is employed for emulsification. If cortical cleaving hydrodissection has been performed, the cortex will be removed concurrently.

Stop and Chop Phaco

Groove creation is performed as noted earlier in the discussion of divide and conquer sculpting techniques.

Once the grove is adequate, vacuum and flow are increased to improve holding ability of the phaco tip. The tip is then burrowed into the mass of one heminucleus using pulsed linear phacoemulsification. The sleeve should be 1 mm from the base of the bevel of the phaco tip to created adequately exposed needle length for sufficient holding power. Excessive phaco energy application is to be avoided because it will cause nucleus immediately adjacent to the tip to be emulsified. The space thus created in the vicinity of the tip is responsible for interfering with the seal around the tip and therefore the capability of vacuum to hold the nucleus. The nucleus will then pop off the phaco tip, making chopping more difficult. With a good seal the heminucleus can be drawn toward the incision, and the chopper can be inserted at the endonucleus-epinucleus junction. After the first chop a second similar chop is performed. The pie-shaped piece of nucleus thus created is removed with low-power pulsed phacoemulsification, as discussed in the divide and conquer section.

Epinucleus and cortex removal is also performed as noted previously.

Phaco Chop

Phaco chop requires no sculpting. Therefore the procedure is initiated with high vacuum and flow and linear pulsed phaco power. For a 0-degree tip, when emulsifying a hard nucleus, a small trough may be required to create adequate room for the phaco tip to borrow deep into the nucleus. For a 15-degree or a 30-degree tip, the tip should be rotated bevel down to engage the nucleus. A few bursts or pulses of phaco energy allow the tip to be buried within the nucleus. It then can be drawn toward the incision to allow the chopper access to the epinucleus-endonucleus junction. If the nucleus comes off the phaco tip, excessive power has produced a space around the tip, reducing vacuum holding power as noted previously. The first chop is then produced by sliding the chopper over the nucleus with its tip in contact with the nucleus to prevent inadvertent damage to the anterior capsular rim. The chopper is dropped into the separation between endonucleus and epinucleus. The chopper is drawn down and left while simultaneously the phaco tip is lifted up and pushed to the right. This maneuver creates the first chop. Minimal rotation of the nucleus allows creation of the second chop in like manner. The first pie-shaped segment of nucleus is mobilized with high vacuum and elevated to the iris plane. There it is emulsified with low linear power, high vacuum, and moderate flow. The remaining first heminucleus is chopped in turn. The second heminucleus is then rotated to a position opposite the wound and is chopped and emulsified in a similar manner.

Supracapsular Phaco

After creation of a capsulorhexis large enough to allow prolapse of the entire lens nucleus, hydrodissection only is performed. With the anterior chamber fully filled with viscoelastic, the nucleus is gently flipped into a supracapsular position. It is then emulsified with a carouselling technique, working at the edge with moderate vacuum and flow settings.

Phaco Machine Settings

Currently, many new-generation sophisticated machines (see Table 7-1) are available. Each of these controls the balance of power generation and fluidic features by different methods. In addition, surgeons now can tailor the machine parameters not only to their style of surgery but also to each individual segment of the phaco procedure. Therefore a listing of different settings for each procedure is beyond the scope of this chapter. However,

TABLE 7-2

Allergan Sovereign Settings for Phaco Chop* for William J. Fishkind, MD, FACS

	Phaco 1	Phaco 2	Phaco 3	Phaco 4	I/A 1	I/A 2	I/A 3
Segment description	Hard nucleus Chopping	Hard nucleus Chopping and segment removal	Moderate nucleus	Epinucleus and cortex	I&A	Caps vac	VE removal
Aspiration: linear or panel (ml)	Panel	Panel	Panel	Panel	Panel	Panel	Panel
Unoccluded	26	22	11	20	26	6	36
Occluded		24	12	12			
Vacuum (mm Hg)	Linear	Linear	Linear	Linear	Linear	Linear	Linear
Occlusion threshold		150	80	100			
Maximum vacuum	330	330	300	200	500	10	500
Phaco power							
Unoccluded % power	20	25	15	10			
Unoccluded attributes	LP/2 pps	SP/4 pps	LP/3 pps	SP/6 pps			
Occluded % power		25	10	10			
Occluded attributes		LP/3 pps	SP/6 pps	LP/3 pps			
Bottle height (inches)	28	30	28	28	28	12	26

*With 2.8-mm temporal clear corneal incision, 20-gauge 0-degree tip.
I&A, Irrigation and aspiration; *LP,* long pulse; *SP,* short pulse; *VE,* viscoelastic.

a representative listing of different parameters for three surgeons using the same machine is illustrated in Tables 7-2 to 7-4. These tables show how power, flow, and vacuum vary from surgeon to surgeon and for each phase of phacoemulsification.

Conclusion

It has been said that the phaco procedure is blend of technology and technique. Awareness of the principles that influence phaco machine settings is required to perform a proficient and safe operation. In addition, often during the procedure, the initial parameters must be modified. A thorough understanding of fundamental principles will enhance the surgeon's capability to respond appropriately to this requirement.

It is a fundamental principle that through relentless evaluation of the interaction of the machine and the phaco technique, the skillful surgeon will find innovative methods to enhance technique. "The road to success is always under construction."

TABLE 7-3

Allergan Sovereign Settings for Nonstop Phaco Chop* for David Chang, MD

	Phaco 1	Phaco 2	Phaco 3	Phaco 4	I/A 1	I/A 2	I/A 3
Segment description	Burst for dense nuclei	Nuclear fragments	Epinucleus and soft nuclei	Sculpting	Cortex removal	Cap vac and epinucleus	VE removal
Aspiration: linear or panel (ml)	Panel	Panel	Panel	Panel	Panel	Linear	Panel
Unoccluded	18	20	26	14	26	40	40
Occluded	16	16	22				
Vacuum (mm Hg)	Linear	Linear	Linear	Linear	Linear	Panel	Linear
Occlusion threshold	90	90	125	30			
Maximum vacuum	400	400	200		500	350	500
Phaco power							
Unoccluded % power	35	30	25	50			
Unoccluded attributes	Multiburst	Continuous	Continuous	Continuous			
Occluded % power	20	30	25				
Occluded attributes	LP/4 pps	SP/8 pps	SP/8 pps				
Bottle height (cm)	71	71	71	71	71	71	71

*With 2.5-mm clear corneal incision, 20-gauge 15-degree tip.
LP, Long pulse; *SP,* short pulse; *VE,* viscoelastic.

TABLE 7-4

Allergan Sovereign Settings for Choo-choo Chop and Flip* Phaco for I. Howard Fine, MD

	Phaco 1	Phaco 2	Phaco 3	I/A 1	I/A 2	I/A 3
Segment description	Chop	Trim	Flip	Cortex	VE	Cap. vac. removal
Aspiration: linear or panel (ml)	Panel	Panel	Panel	Panel	Linear	Panel
Unoccluded	30	30	28	30	40	6
Occluded	34	26	22			
Vacuum (mm Hg)	Linear	Linear	Linear	Linear		Linear
Occlusion threshold	190	20	80			
Maximum vacuum	375	150	150	500	300	10
Phaco power						
Unoccluded % power	40	20	20			
Unoccluded attributes	LP/2 pps	LP/2 pps	LP/2 pps			
Occluded % power	40	20	20			
Occluded attributes	LP/2 pps	LP/2 pps	LP/2 pps			
Other modes	Continuous irrigation	Continuous irrigation	Continuous irrigation	Continuous irrigation	Continuous irrigation	Continuous irrigation
Bottle height (inches)	30	30	30	30	30	22

*With 2.5-mm clear corneal incision, 20-gauge 30-degree tip.
LP, Long pulse; *SP,* short pulse; *VE,* viscoelastic.

REFERENCES

1. Kelman CD: Phaco-emulsification and aspiration, *Am J Ophthalmol* 64: 23-35, 1967.
2. Kelman CD: History of emulsification and aspiration of senile cataracts, *Trans Am Acad Ophthalmol Otolaryngol* 78:35-38, 1974.
3. Kelman CD: Phacoemulsification in the anterior chamber, *Ophthalmology* 86:1980-1982, 1979.
4. Kratz RP, Colvard DM: Kelman phacoemulsification in the posterior chamber, *Ophthalmology* 86:1983-1984, 1979.
5. Cimino WW, Bond LJ: Physics of ultrasonic surgery using tissue fragmentation. II. *Ultrasound Med Biol* 22:101-117, 1996.
6. Fishkind WJ: *Pop goes the microbubbles,* Video Film Festival ASCRS 1998, Grand Prize winner ESCRS, 1998.
7. Serafano D: Upgrades to phaco system give surgeons more options, *Ophthalmol Times* 26:16-17, 2001.
8. Soscia W, Howard JG, Olson, RJ: Microphacoemulsification with WhiteStar. A wound-temperature study. *J Cataract Refract Surg* 28:1044-1046, 2002.
9. Seibel BS: Section 1. In *Phacodynamics, mastering the tools and techniques of phacoemulsification surgery,* ed 3, Thoroughfare, NJ, 1999, Slack Inc, pp 14-85.
10. Nichamin LD: Prevention pearls. In Fishkind WJ, editor: *Complications in phacoemulsification,* New York, 2001, Thieme, pp 260-270.

BIBLIOGRAPHY

Fishkind, WJ, editor: *Complications in phacoemulsification, avoidance, recognition and management,* New York, 2001, Thieme.

Seibel BS: *Phacodynamics, mastering the tools and techniques of phacoemulsification surgery,* ed 3, Thoroughfare, NJ, Slack Inc.

Retrobulbar and Peribulbar Anesthesia for Cataract Surgery

8

Robert C. (Roy) Hamilton, MB, BCh, FRCPC

Advances in surgical techniques, especially small-incision phacoemulsification, have lessened the universal demand for akinetic anesthesia using regional blocks. Other methods, including sub-Tenon's, subconjunctival, and solely topical corneoconjunctival anesthesia, have been introduced. However, solid regional block anesthesia including muscle akinesia is still the preferred choice of anesthesia for many cataract surgeons. Although peribulbar blocks were popularized in 1986, claiming to avoid serious complications of the retrobulbar method,[1] a recent survey of the annual American Society of Cataract and Refractive Surgeons with input from 1342 members indicates 30% using retrobulbar and 24% using peribulbar blocks.[2]

Desirable Prerequisites

Knowledge of the basic science disciplines (pharmacology of ocular and local anesthetic drugs, physiology of the eye, anatomy of the orbit and its contents) is essential to safe practice of orbital regional anesthesia, including retrobulbar block.[3] Observation of and subsequent initial supervision by personnel with wide clinical experience and knowledge are recommended. The goal for each practitioner is to build up an experiential database from which increasingly good judgment can result. Even when the blocking practitioner is an ophthalmologist, a strong argument can be made for the routine presence of an anesthesiologist.[4,5] Noninvasive blood pressure, electrocardiographic, and oxygen saturation monitoring should be routinely used before and during the induction of anesthesia and intraoperatively.

Anatomy and Applied Anatomy

In this chapter the adjective *retrobulbar* refers to the conical compartment within the confines of the four rectus muscles and their intermuscular septa. Compared with the peripheral orbit where fat is more dense, the retrobulbar cone contains fat that is arranged in large globules, which permit free movement of the intraorbital portion of the optic nerve in the various duction positions of the globe. A matrix of connective tissues, which support and allow dynamic function of the orbit contents, controls the spread of local anesthetic solutions.[6]

Motor nerves enter the muscle bellies of the four rectus muscles from their conal surface, 1 to 1.5 cm from the apex of the orbit. Local anesthetics in blocking concentration have to reach and diffuse to the core of an exposed 5- to 10-mm segment of each of these motor nerves in the posterior retrobulbar space for conduction block of those nerves, and resulting akinesia of their supplied muscles, to occur. Retained activity of the superior oblique muscle is often seen after retrobulbar local anesthetic injection because its motor nerve, the trochlear, runs outside the muscle cone. Total blockade of the smaller-diameter sensory and autonomic nerves including the ciliary ganglion, on the other hand, is more easily achieved. Corneal and perilimbal conjunctival sensory innervation, along with the superior-nasal quadrant of the peripheral conjunctival sensation, are mediated through the nasociliary nerve, which lies within the retrobulbar space. The remainder of the peripheral conjunctival sensation, however, is supplied through the lacrimal, frontal, and infraorbital nerves coursing outside the muscle cone.[7] Because of this, intraoperative pain may be experienced in the peripheral orbit following a solely retrobulbar block.[8]

Ophthalmic Regional Block Anesthesia

Traditional Retrobulbar Block and Its Inherent Problems

In 1934 Atkinson[9] described a technique that evolved into the traditional method of retrobulbar blockade. In his article:

> [With the patient's gaze directed] upward and inward, [a 35-mm needle entered percutaneously] a short distance below the inferior-temporal margin of the orbit ... the skin is moved upward with the needle so that the point just clears the inferior orbital margin. The needle is then directed upward and inward, midway between the external and inferior recti muscles, and advanced toward the apex of the orbit for a distance of from 2.5 to 3.5 cm.

Although Atkinson did not use such a directive in his text (however, illustrations in his article may have led to the interpretation), traditional teaching regarding the inferior-temporal needle entry point has been to locate it at the junction of the medial two thirds and lateral third of the inferior orbital rim. Generations of ophthalmology residents were trained in this way as a result; in fact, the technique continues to be reproduced in ophthalmology and anesthesiology texts even though "there is now no doubt that [it] is unsafe and there are medicolegal implications."[10] Unsöld, Stanley, and DeGroot[11] demonstrated conclusively in a cadaver model that the Atkinson "up-and-in" globe position places a stretched and taut optic nerve and the posterior pole of the globe in line for potential damage from the tip of the needle approaching from the inferior-temporal quadrant. In addition, tangential puncture of the optic nerve sheath can occur, leading to injection of anesthetic agent into the subarachnoid space resulting in brainstem anesthesia.[12] Pautler et al. [13] reported two cases of optic nerve trauma with resultant catastrophic loss of vision from long and sharp needles injected toward the orbital apex with the globe in the up-and-in position. Using information gained from the Unsöld paper, they recommended that for retrobulbar blocks patients should fixate in primary gaze and that needle length be reduced to 32 mm ($1\frac{1}{4}$ inch) and directed toward an imaginary point behind the macula rather than aiming for the orbital apex. They reported that in the primary gaze globe position the optic nerve lies in a nontaut manner on the nasal side of the sagittal plane passing through the visual axis, in which location and state the risk of nerve damage is much reduced (Figure 8-1).

Katsev et al.[14] analyzed the dimensions of 120 orbits from 60 human skulls related to the length of needles used for retrobulbar anesthesia. The distance from the inferior orbital rim to the optic foramen ranged from a maximum of 58 mm to a minimum of 42 mm. Because a 38-mm ($1\frac{1}{2}$-inch) needle fully inserted toward the posterior orbit had the potential of damaging vital structures in fully one fifth of the orbits examined (i.e., those of smaller dimension), they recommended that depth of needle penetration into the orbit be limited to a maximum of 31.5 mm ($1\frac{1}{4}$ inch) from the inferior orbital rim to avoid damage to the tightly packed important structures (nerves, blood vessels, muscles) at the orbital apex.

Liu, Youl B, Moseley[10] repeated Unsöld's cadaver experiment in vivo using magnetic resonance imaging and confirmed the findings of a taut optic nerve in up-and-in position and of a sinuous loose nerve in the primary gaze position.

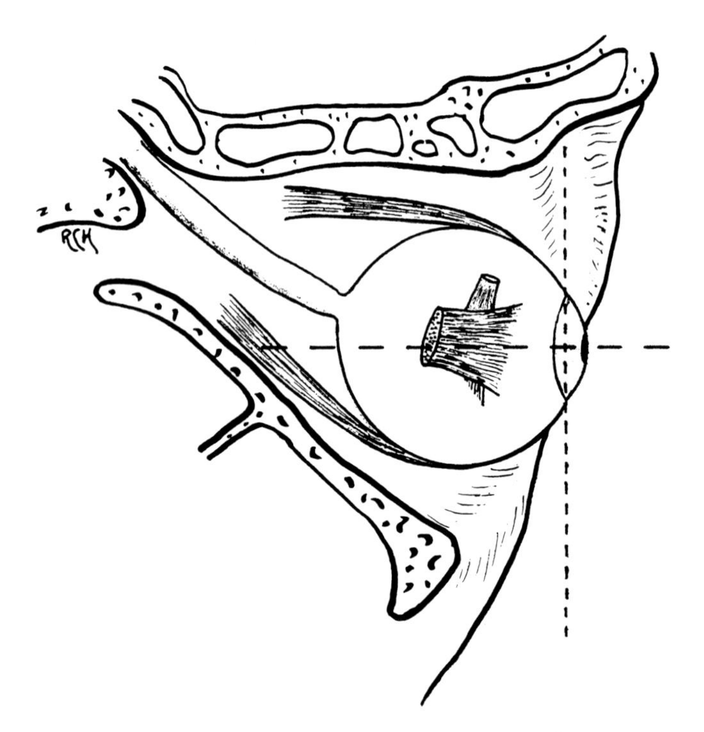

FIGURE 8-1 Plane of the iris and midsagittal plane of the globe in primary gaze; view from above. *Fine dashed line* indicates the plane of the iris (useful in gauging depth of needle advancement); *coarse dashed line* indicates the midsagittal plane of the eye and the visual axis through the center of the pupil. The optic nerve lies on the nasal side of the midsagittal plane of the eye. Note how the temporal orbital rim is set back from the rest of the orbital rim at or about the globe equator, making for easy needle access to the retrobulbar compartment. (Courtesy Gimbel Educational Services.)

Complications of Ophthalmic Regional Block Anesthesia

OPTIC NERVE INJURY

Injection at the orbital apex, as was advocated in the distant past[15] and is now outmoded, has the potential of frank optic nerve injury. Katsev et al.[14] recommended that needle length introduced beyond the orbital rim for both intraconal and periconal injections should not exceed 31 mm ($1\frac{1}{4}$ inches) to avoid damage to the optic nerve in all patients. In the execution of orbital blocks, it is possible for the needle tip to enter the optic nerve sheath and produce not only brainstem anesthesia, as described below, but also tamponade of the retinal vessels within the nerve and/or the small vessels supplying the nerve itself either by the volume of drug injected or by provoking intrasheath hemorrhage.[13,16-19]

BRAINSTEM ANESTHESIA

Brainstem anesthesia is caused by direct spread of local anesthetic to the brain from the orbit along submeningeal pathways. It is the eyeblock complication most likely to warrant cardiopulmonary resuscitation. An essential prerequisite in all locations where regional ocular anesthesia is performed is the provision of oxygen saturation monitoring in the room where the block is done and in the operating room,[12] along with equipment to provide respiratory support and cardiopulmonary resuscitation.[5] The incidence has been reported as 1 in 350 to 500 retrobulbar injections.[12]

GLOBE PENETRATION AND PERFORATION

The incidence range of globe penetration (solely entrance wound) and perforation (entrance and exit wounds) has been reported as low as 0 in a series of 2000 peribulbar blocks[1] to 1 in a series of 1000 retrobulbar blocks.[20] In myopic patients the incidence may be as high as 1 in 140 blocks.[21] The true incidence is not known because many cases are not reported[22]; more than 50% of cases go unrecognized at the time of their occurrence.[23] A rare and devastating complication, ocular explosion, has been reported several times[24,25]; it results from excessively high pressure being applied to the injecting syringe following unrecognized ocular penetration by the needle. Ultimate visual outcome is very poor.

EXTRAOCULAR MUSCLE MALFUNCTION

Because extraocular muscle malfunction can result from local anesthesia agent myotoxicity or needle trauma,[26,27] it is important to choose a block technique in which the needle placement avoids needle contact with muscle. The most common muscles affected, in order of frequency, are the inferior rectus muscle (Figure 8-2),[28-31] the inferior oblique muscle (including injury and trauma to its motor nerve) (Figure 8-3),[28] the superior rectus muscle (Figure 8-4),[32] and the medial rectus muscle (Figure 8-5).[33]

HEMORRHAGE

Retrobulbar hemorrhages vary in severity. Some are of venous origin and spread slowly. Signs of severe arterial hemorrhage are rapid and taut orbital swelling, marked proptosis with immobility of the globe, and massive blood staining of the lids and conjunctiva.[34] Serious impairment of the vascular supply to the globe may result.[35,36] By constant vigilance and keen observation of the signs immediately following needle withdrawal, bleeding may be minimized and confined by rapid application of digital pressure over a gauze pad placed on the closed lids. The incidence of serious retrobulbar bleeding was reported to be 1% to 3% in one paper[16] and as 0.44% in a series of 12,500 cases.[37] A strong argument can be made in favor of fine disposable needles over those of larger gauge,[8,13,38] on the

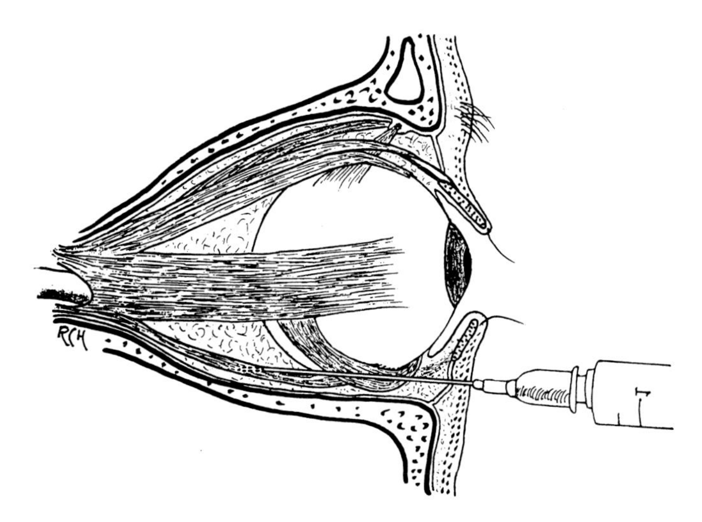

FIGURE 8-2 Inferior rectus muscle trauma, lateral view. A straight 31-mm (1¼-inch) needle being advanced from the inferior-temporal quadrant in an attempt to enter the retrobulbar compartment has failed to adequately rise from the orbit floor. The needle tip has entered the belly of the inferior rectus muscle. Hemorrhage into the muscle with subsequent fibrosis, or intramuscular injection of local anesthetic with subsequent myotoxicity, may result in prolonged or permanent imbalance between the superior and inferior rectus muscles and vertical diplopia.[31] (Courtesy Gimbel Educational Services.)

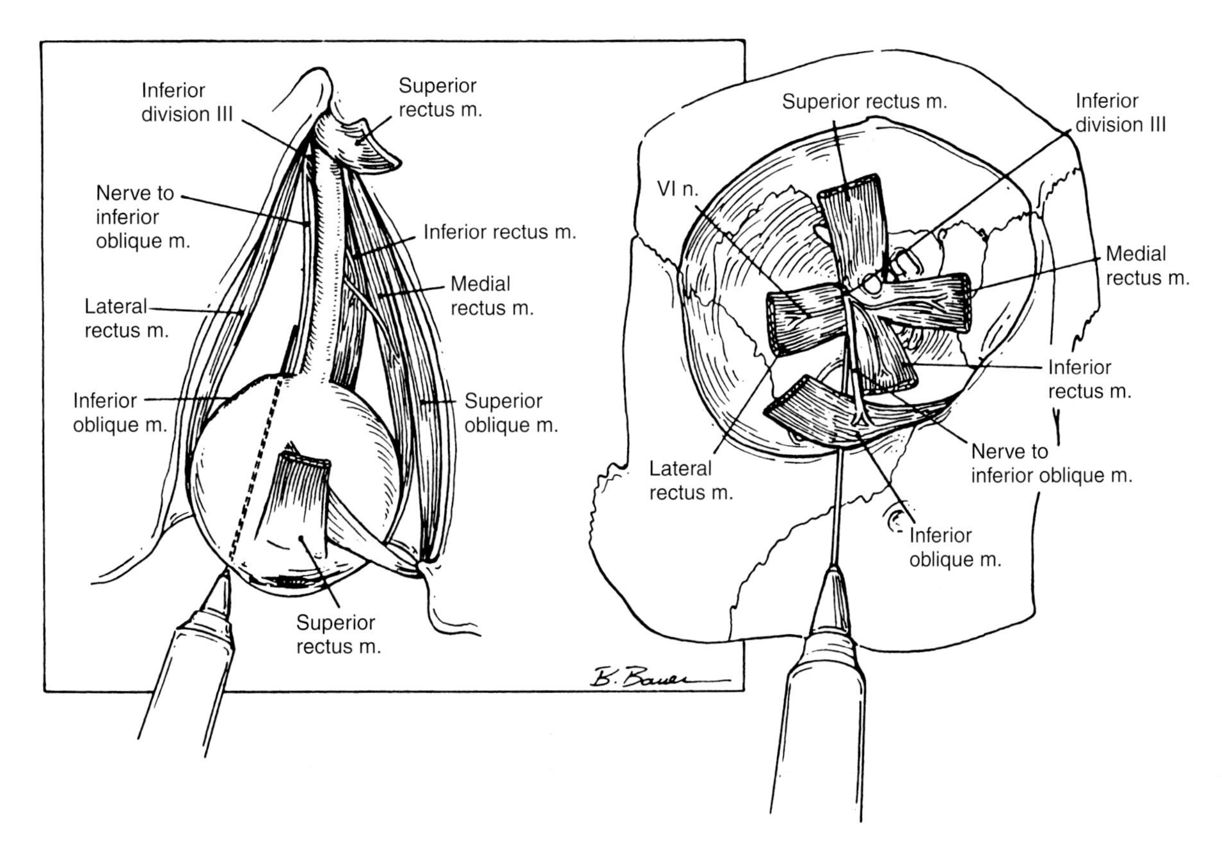

FIGURE 8-3 Risks of injection from the traditional entry point. Right orbit: **A,** view from above; **B,** view from in front with the globe removed. Observe the proximity of the needle path to the inferior oblique muscle belly, its motor nerve, and the lateral border of the inferior rectus muscle. One or more of these three structures can easily be damaged by a traditionally placed retrobulbar needle. (From Hunter DG, Lam GC, Guyton DL: Inferior oblique muscle injury from local anesthesia for cataract surgery, *Ophthalmology* 102:508, 1995.)

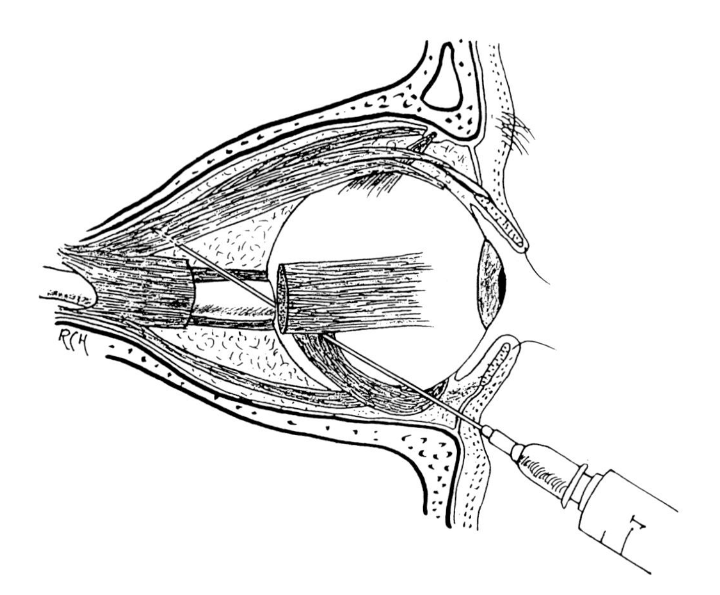

FIGURE 8-4 Superior rectus muscle trauma, lateral view. A straight 38-mm ($1\frac{1}{2}$-inch) needle being advanced from the inferior-temporal quadrant through the retrobulbar compartment too deeply has entered the belly of the superior rectus muscle. Hemorrhage into the muscle with subsequent fibrosis, or intramuscular injection of local anesthetic with subsequent myotoxicity, may result in prolonged or permanent imbalance between the superior and inferior rectus muscles and vertical diplopia.[32] (Courtesy of Gimbel Educational Services.)

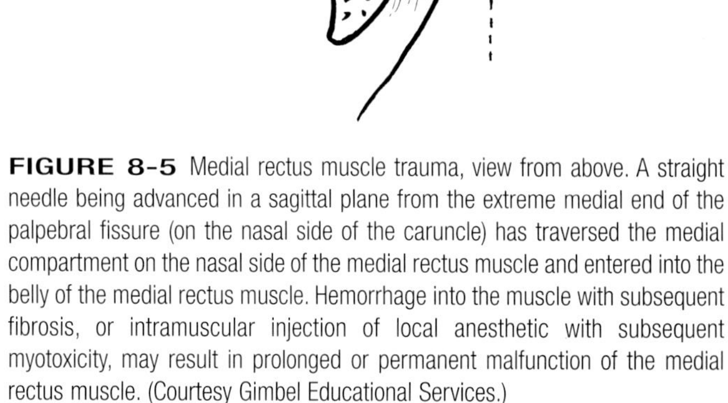

FIGURE 8-5 Medial rectus muscle trauma, view from above. A straight needle being advanced in a sagittal plane from the extreme medial end of the palpebral fissure (on the nasal side of the caruncle) has traversed the medial compartment on the nasal side of the medial rectus muscle and entered into the belly of the medial rectus muscle. Hemorrhage into the muscle with subsequent fibrosis, or intramuscular injection of local anesthetic with subsequent myotoxicity, may result in prolonged or permanent malfunction of the medial rectus muscle. (Courtesy Gimbel Educational Services.)

grounds that if a vessel is perforated, less bleeding occurs through a small rent and the bleeding is less precipitous. Because the orbital apex contains the largest vessels entering and exiting the orbit, the depth to which needles are inserted should be strictly limited. When serious bleeding occurs in this area, there is not only the problem of general increase in orbital pressure, making surgery difficult, but also the potential for obstruction to the blood supply to and from the globe.

The anterior orbit generally has smaller vessels than exist posteriorly. Two anterior orbital locations, which are relatively avascular and frequently used sites for needle placement, are the inferior-temporal quadrant and the compartment directly on the nasal side of the medial rectus muscle. Needle placement into the superior nasal compartment should be avoided because the end vessels of the ophthalmic artery system are located there, as are some large veins and the complex trochlear mechanism of the superior oblique muscle.

In intraocular surgery it is considered advantageous if the intraocular pressure is low and pressure fluctuations are kept to a minimum.[39] The attainment of a "soft eye" in the avoidance of complications, particularly suprachoroidal hemorrhage,[40,41] was more important in a former era. Phacoemulsification techniques, which require a smaller surgical incision, are associated with smaller swings in intraocular pressure than the older intracapsular or extracapsular methods. At the completion of retrobulbar and peribulbar injections, mechanical orbital decompression devices[42-45] are commonly used to promote ocular hypotony and a reduction in vitreous volume,[46] especially when larger volumes of orbital injectate have been used (as in peribulbar blockade).

GENERAL COMMENT ON COMPLICATIONS

The occurrence or avoidance of the complications mentioned previously is directly influenced by block technique. Elimination of known hazards (e.g., inappropriate globe position during block, inappropriate choice of needle path, inappropriate depth of needle placement) is the key to successfully avoid complications.

Comparison of Retrobulbar with Peribulbar Blockade

As discussed earlier, the peribulbar technique was introduced in 1986 as a less hazardous alternative to retrobulbar anesthesia in response to a concern about complications of the latter.[1] The rationale was that peribulbar technique, by avoiding needle placement within the rectus muscle cone, would avoid optic nerve damage and globe perforation. However, after initial enthusiasm a significant number of globe perforations were reported.[47-49] Higher volumes of injectate were required to achieve akinesia, onset time of blockade was much slower than with retrobulbar, and repeat injections (each with inherent risk of complication) were more frequently required. Although there are proponents of both retrobulbar and peribulbar techniques, safe anesthesia can be accomplished by both methods; likewise, serious complications can arise with both if carried out incorrectly. Two published large series preferred the more dependable outcome of retrobulbar needle placement.[8,50] Therefore, rather than condemn the retrobulbar technique outright, it merits revisitation and revision in the light of better understanding of the cause of various complications.[51]

Revised retrobulbar block

SITE AND DEPTH OF INJECTION

The inferior-temporal orbital quadrant is the preferred location for retrobulbar needle placement because it provides easy access to the retrobulbar cone compartment (see Figure 8-1). To avoid complications (hemorrhages, optic nerve trauma, brainstem anesthesia, muscle damage), needles must never be inserted deeply to the orbital apex.[14] Injectate placement in the anterior retrobulbar compartment is much safer; from there, posterior spread occurs to achieve motor nerve blocking concentration at the apex of the cone.[52]

NEEDLE TYPE AND SYRINGE SIZE

Traditional teaching favored dull-tipped, intermediate-gauge needles with the supposed advantages that blood vessels were pushed aside rather than traumatized and that tissue planes could be more accurately defined. Although a commonly held belief among ophthalmologists,[47] it is not true that it is more difficult to penetrate the globe, the optic nerve sheath, or blood vessels with a blunt needle.[3] Larger dull needles, compared with fine disposable ones, cause more serious damage if the globe is penetrated.[3] Because disposable cutting needles produce minimal tissue distortion, little or no pain results. Tactile discrimination is progressively reduced with increasing needle size.[38] The use of blunt-tipped, wider-gauge needles should be abandoned.[53] Special attention should be paid to the length of needle entering beyond the orbital rim; 31 mm as measured from the orbital rim should never be exceeded to rule out optic nerve impalement.[14] In regional block techniques (both retrobulbar and peribulbar), all needles should be orientated tangentially to the globe with the bevel opening faced toward the globe.[8] Because less force has to be exerted, a change in resistance to injectate flow is more easily detected by the injecting hand when using a needle mounted on a smaller syringe as compared with a larger size. This ability to more easily detect change in resistance to injection is important in avoiding complications, as is the regular use by all practitioners of standard sets of needles and syringes so that they become familiar with the normal flow resistance characteristics of their equipment. In addition, an "inject-as-you-advance" technique provides added safety.[54]

ADVANTAGE OF MINIMAL OR NO SEDATION

Fully conscious or minimally sedated patients on whom regional ophthalmic blocks are done painlessly can accurately report symptoms or demonstrate signs that may indicate onset of undesirable block complications. Thus, by being conscious, they act as their own monitors. For example, the devastating complication of ocular explosion described previously[24,25] is not likely to occur in a conscious patient because the pain experienced by the patient would be so great. Elderly patients require less pharmacologic support for anxiety at the time of surgery than do young patients and take the discomforts of life more easily "in their stride." For a small percentage of elderly patients who benefit from preoperative sedation, fine judgment is required to select the correct drug dosage to produce a calm patient who remains alert and cooperative. The advantages of regional anesthesia can be negated rapidly with excessive use of sedation.[55] A recent multicenter study confirmed that intravenous anesthetic agents administered to reduce pain and anxiety are associated with an increased incidence of side effects and adverse medical events.[56] Incomplete regional anesthesia is best managed with block supplementation until complete; operating in the presence of obvious block failure subjects the patient to an unpleasant and stressful experience; and use of intravenous sedation to cover gross block inadequacy is hazardous and inappropriate.

Painless block techniques are achievable through the use of fine, sharp disposable needles and precision placement methods. The author strongly recommends a preblock transconjunctival injection of local anesthetic diluted 10 times with sterile balanced salt solution, which renders the percutaneous injection to follow totally painless (Figure 8-6).[57] This transconjunctival injection is carried out through conjunctiva previously rendered anesthetic with topical local anesthetic eye drops.

PREBLOCK ASSESSMENT

A safe prerequisite to regional anesthesia of the orbit is to know the axial length measurement of the eye before the block to warn of the higher risk in longer-than-average eyes.[58] In cataract surgery a precise axial length measurement is usually available because it is required for intraocular lens diopter power calculation. In the presence of high myopia, peribulbar block or even general anesthesia, as opposed to retrobulbar block, may be more prudent. Similar caution would apply when a preexisting scleral buckle exists from an earlier retinal operative procedure.

The axial length of the globe to be blocked is noted, as is the position of the globe in the orbit (enophthalmos versus exophthalmos), by observing the plane of the iris and the location of the globe equator relative to the temporal orbital rim.

RECOMMENDED BLOCK TECHNIQUE

The author, with an experience of 27,500 retrobulbar blocks and 5,700 peribulbar blocks over the past 18 years, has adopted a rational approach to safe retrobulbar blocking that stresses the importance of aiming the retrobulbar needle (27-gauge sharp disposable, 31-mm length) "midway between the inferior and lateral rectus muscles"[30] from an inferior-temporal entry point at the junction of the temporal and inferior orbital rims (Figure 8-7). This modified entry point allows easy and safe access to the retrobulbar space because the temporal orbital rim is set back from the rest of the orbital rim (see Figure 8-1).

The inferior-temporal rim of the orbit is palpated and the desired entry point chosen just inside the orbital rim at the 7:30 position for the right eye (Figure 8-8, *A*) or the 4:30 position for the left eye. With the patient's eyes in primary gaze, the needle is advanced in a sagittal plane with 10-degree upward inflection from the transverse plane, at first invaginating the skin while being directed safely between the globe and temporal orbit wall. It very soon penetrates the skin and can then be advanced to the depth of the globe equator before being redirected upward and

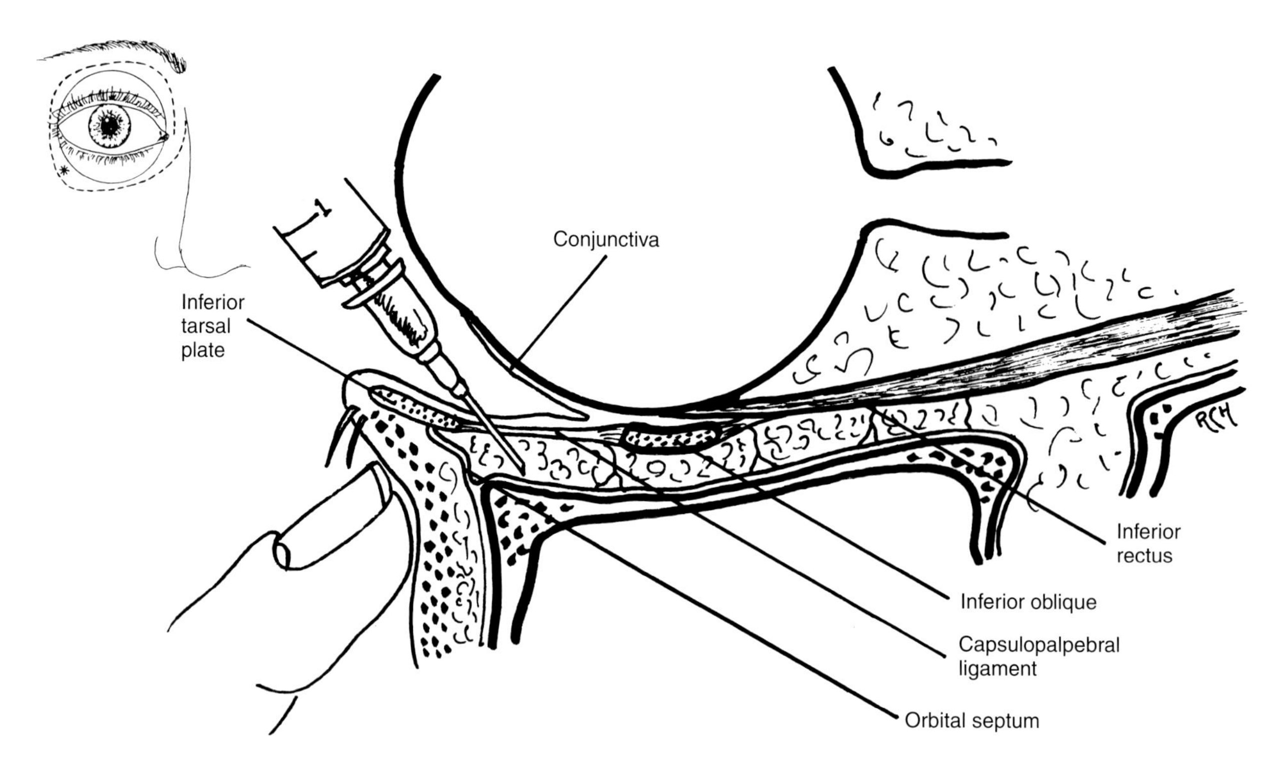

FIGURE 8-6 Injection of "painless local" in inferior-temporal quadrant, lateral view. After instillation of topical anesthesia drops in the inferior conjunctival fornix, the lower eyelid is gently retracted with a finger. A 30-gauge 12-mm needle enters transconjunctivally in the inferior-temporal area just posterior to the inferior tarsal plate with the shaft of the needle arranged tangentially to the globe. Following test aspiration, the initial injection is of 1 ml painless local* to a depth of 1 cm from the conjunctiva. The needle has easily and painlessly penetrated the conjunctiva, and deep to it the capsulopalpebral fascia. The needle entry point is at the lower end of the lateral orbital rim *(small insert)*. After an interval of 3 to 4 minutes, the skin overlying the site of injection (lateral third of lower lid) will be anesthetic. (Courtesy Gimbel Educational Services.)

*Painless local made up from 1 part full-strength local anesthetic injectate and 10 parts balanced salt solution.[57]

inward toward an imaginary point behind the pupil, approaching but not passing the midsagittal plane (see Figures 8-1, 8-8, and 8-9). The globe is continuously observed during needle placement to detect globe rotation that would indicate engagement of the sclera by the needle tip. During this latter action the circumference of the globe can be "palpated" with the shaft of the needle as it passes around it (Martin Livingston, MD, personal communication). The modified entry position provides safer access to the orbit because there is more physical space here compared with the traditional entry point (see Figure 8-7). In addition, the modified technique avoids possible needle damage to the inferior rectus and inferior oblique muscles and to the motor nerve supply to the inferior oblique (see Figure 8-3).[28] A percutaneous as opposed to a transconjunctival needle entry point is used because it avoids having to combat the orbicularis tone often present in the inferior eyelid or the problems created when there is a narrow palpebral fissure and wide lateral canthal fold. Slow needle advancement following first penetration of the skin is ideal, with injections of minidoses of anesthetic solution at multiple intervals. Having reached the desired final needle-tip location, and after checking by aspiration for inadvertent intravascular placement, a slow injection of the desired volume of anesthetic solution is made. This interval method of needle advancement provides not only patient comfort but also constantly updated information about tissue resistances along the needle path. Should the needle tip penetrate the globe, the next minidose injection will announce itself loud and clear as severe pain (provided, of course, there has not been use of excessive sedation to render the patient beyond being able to act as his or her own monitor). A globe penetration picked up accurately and early in this fashion is far better than rapid needle placement to full depth in one swift motion with the possibility of globe perforation and its late diagnosis. Final depth of needle penetration of the orbit is gauged by observing the hub-shaft junction of the 31-mm needle in relation to the plane of the iris (Figures 8-1 and 8-8), instead of measuring from the inferior orbital rim as in the traditional technique; thus, in dealing with enophthalmic and exophthalmic globes, there is automatic correction for the anomaly. In dealing with a globe of average axial length (23.5 mm), when the midpoint of the 31-mm needle is at the plane of the iris, the point of the needle will already have passed the globe equator. In like manner, ovoid globes in myopic patients (greater axial length measurement) will require a longer section of the advancing needle to guarantee passage beyond the globe equator before redirection into the retrobulbar compartment. The final desired

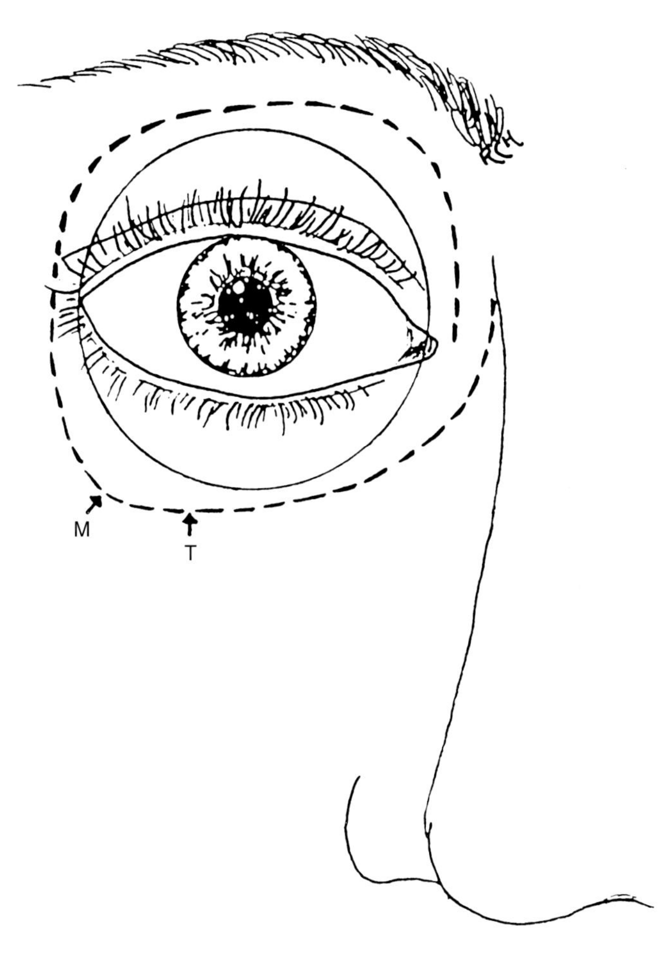

FIGURE 8-7 Traditional and modified needle entry positions. The outline of the globe is superimposed on a template of the orbital rim. Traditional inferior block injection site is just inside the orbital rim at *T.* The author's modified injection site is inferior-temporal, just inside the orbital rim at *M.* (Courtesy Gimbel Educational Services.)

needle-tip position lies between the lateral rectus muscle and the optic nerve, as depicted in the cadaver dissection (see Figure 8-9).

INJECTATE MIXTURE AND VOLUME

The selection of anesthetic agent with additives depends mainly on the desired duration of effect. Concentrations up to but not exceeding 2% lidocaine (or agent of equivalent potency) are appropriate. Admixture with epinephrine is commonly used to prolong block duration and to increase block solidity, but it may be contraindicated if orbital vascular pathology is present; a concentration of 1:200,000, given the volume of injectate used in ophthalmic regional anesthesia, is devoid of systemic effects.[59] Hyaluronidase, a highly purified bovine testicular enzyme that hydrolyzes extracellular hyaluronic acid,[60] is a desirable component for promotion of spread within the orbit and for hypotony.[61,62] Recently the product has been in short supply and, in fact, is no longer being produced.[60] Anecdotal reports have linked its absence from local anesthetic mixtures with a higher rate of complications, notably diplopias resulting from toxic levels of anesthetic in the extraocular muscles.[63] Having attained the desired safe depth of placement in the anterior retrobulbar compartment, and following a negative test aspiration for possible intravascular penetration, a volume of up to 4 ml of the chosen mixture is slowly injected. Younger adults present more of a challenge in achieving akinesia than the elderly because of more dense connective tissues hindering the access of anesthetics to the motor nerves to the extraocular muscles.[64]

Complementary Medial Block

Because peripheral orbit sensation may be retained following retrobulbar block, as mentioned earlier (anatomy paragraph), a small-volume peribulbar local anesthetic injection provides an

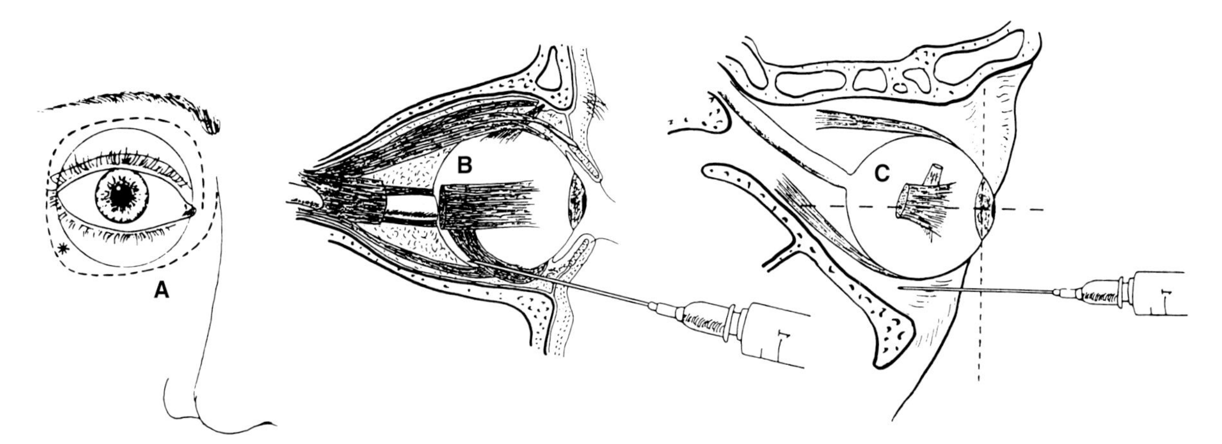

FIGURE 8-8 Revised inferior-temporal retrobulbar block. **A** and **D,** Frontal views; **B** and **E,** lateral views; **C** and **F,** views from above. The inferior-temporal rim of the orbit is palpated and the desired entry point (*) chosen just inside the orbital rim at the 7:30 position for the right eye **(A)** or the 4:30 position for the left eye. With the patient's eyes in primary gaze, the 27-gauge 31-mm (1¼-inch) sharp disposable needle is advanced in a sagittal plane **(C)** with 10-degree upward inflection from the transverse plane **(B)**, at first invaginating the skin while being directed safely between the globe and temporal orbit wall **(C)**. It very soon penetrates the skin and can then be advanced to the depth of the globe equator (**B** and **C**). (If the needle were further advanced in the sagittal plane, contact with the lateral wall of the orbit would occur.)

Continued

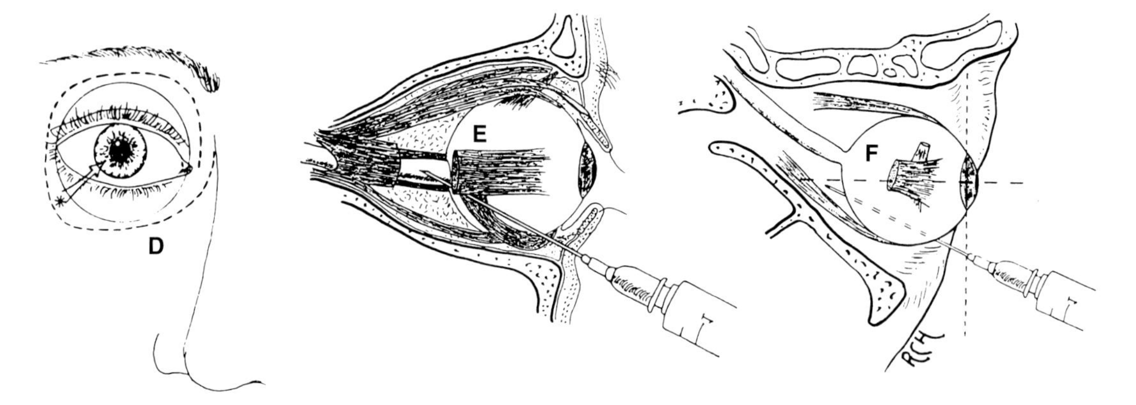

FIGURE 8-8, cont'd Revised inferior-temporal retrobulbar block. The needle is then redirected with medial and upward components (**D** and **E**) toward an imaginary point behind the pupil, approaching but not passing the midsagittal plane **(F).** The needle enters the retrobulbar space by passing through the intermuscular septum between the lateral and inferior rectus muscles **(E).** The globe is continuously observed during needle placement to detect globe rotation that would indicate engagement of the sclera by the needle tip. During needle placement, continuing observation of the relationship between the needle-hub junction and the plane of the iris establishes an appropriate depth of orbit insertion (**E** and **F**). In a globe with normal axial length as illustrated here, when the needle-hub junction has reached the plane of the iris, the tip of the needle lies 5 to 7 mm beyond the hind surface of the globe (**E** and **F**). Following test aspiration, up to 4 ml of anesthetic solution is *slowly* injected. (Courtesy Gimbel Educational Services.)

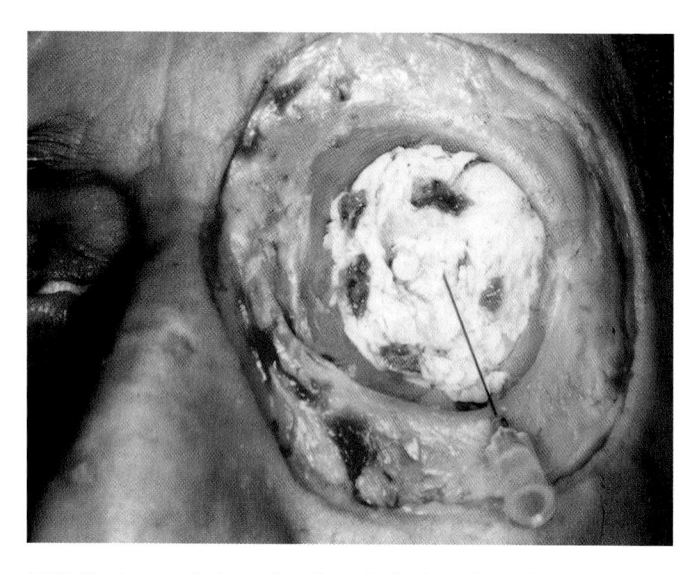

FIGURE 8-9 Cadaver dissection with final needle position in retrobulbar compartment; photograph of the left orbit. The anterior orbital contents have been removed as far back as 5 mm behind the posterior pole of the globe. Note the optic nerve stump and the amputated bellies of the four rectus muscles and the superior oblique muscle. The inferior oblique muscle has been removed along with the globe itself. A 27-gauge sharp disposable needle of 31 mm length has entered the retrobulbar compartment. It has passed between the lateral and inferior rectus muscles. Its tip lies between the lateral rectus muscle and the optic nerve. Note the medial and upward angling of the needle required for it to access its final desired location. (Courtesy Gimbel Educational Services.)

excellent complement. The site of choice is injection into the peribulbar fat compartment on the nasal side of the medial rectus muscle (Figure 8-10).[33] In addition to peripheral orbital anesthesia, this complemental injection provides effective blockade of the central fibers of orbicularis oculi, thus avoiding the need for van Lint or other type of facial nerve blockade. Injection into this compartment at a depth of 25 mm will contribute useful extraocular motor-nerve blockade, whereas more superficial placement (for which a 12-mm needle may be chosen) will provide excellent central orbicularis muscle blockade. The patient's eyes are directed in primary gaze. With the bevel facing the medial orbital wall, the needle is directed toward the interaural line and toward the midline of the skull at the occiput[65] and inserted to the desired depth. The volume injected can be within the range of 1 to 5 ml of local anesthetic solution, depending on the desired effect.

Peribulbar Block

The adjective *peribulbar* refers to that location external to the confines of the four rectus muscles and their intermuscular septa. In the technique known as peribulbar block, local anesthetic agents or mixtures are deposited within the orbit but do not enter within the geometric confines of the cone of rectus muscles. The mechanism whereby it works was elucidated by Koornneef,[6] who demonstrated that the intermuscular septum between the rectus muscles was incomplete and permitted anesthetic deposited outside the cone of rectus muscles to spread centrally. Introduced as a safer method than intraconal blocking to avoid serious complications,[1] these nevertheless have been reported.[47-49] Knowledge of orbital anatomy is just as important as with the older method, and there are disadvantages to using periconal blocking. Davis and Mandel[1] in 1986 were first to publish a paper on the peribulbar block method. Calling their block technique *posterior peribulbar,* they used two intraorbital needle placements outside the muscle cone, one above and one below the cone, each to a depth of 3.5 cm with a total of up to 10 ml of solution injected.[1] Bloomberg[66] championed the cause of shorter needle peribulbar regional anesthesia and

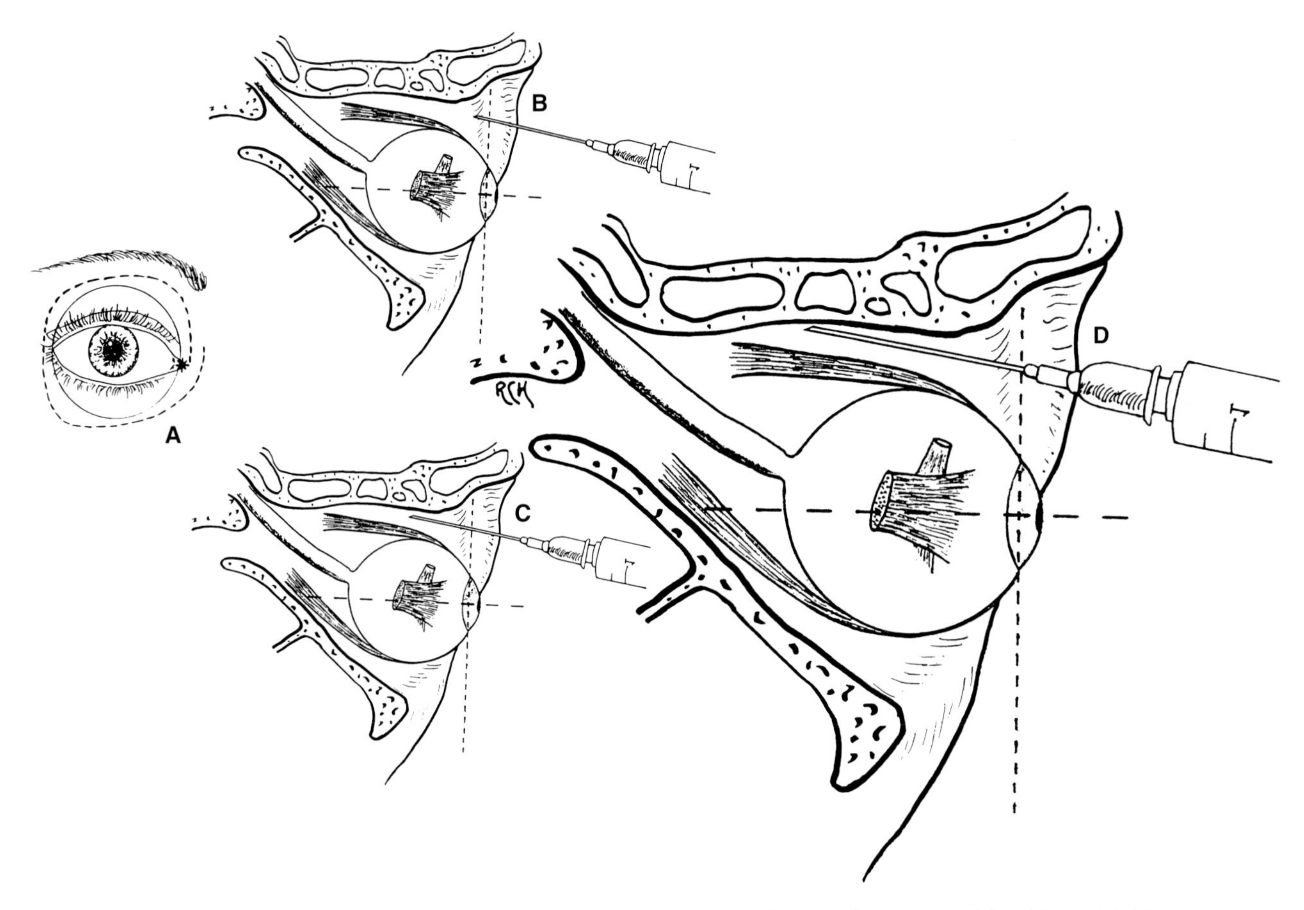

FIGURE 8-10 Complementary peribulbar block. Medial pericone block: needle entry point (*) is on the medial side of the caruncle at the extreme medial angle of the palpebral fissure (**A** and **B**). The patient's eyes are directed in primary gaze. With the bevel facing the medial orbit wall, the needle is directed toward the interaural line and toward the midline of the skull at the occiput[65]; that is, at about 5 degrees toward the medial orbit wall (**B** to **D**). Continuing observation of the relationship between the needle-hub junction and the plane of the iris controls appropriate depth of insertion **(D).** In a globe of normal axial length, the 25-mm needle tip will be at the depth of the hind surface of the eye. The eye in the drawing is 23.5 mm in diameter, and the needle is 25 mm long. Injection at a depth of 25 mm will contribute useful extraocular motor-nerve blockade, whereas more superficial placement will favor blockade of the central fibers of the orbicularis muscle. Volume injected can be within the range of 1 to 5 ml of local anesthetic solution, depending on the desired effect. (Courtesy Gimbel Educational Services.)

called his technique *periocular block*. In Bloomberg's method a 2.5-cm, 25- or 27-gauge needle entered the inferior-temporal orbital quadrant and was directed "deliberately toward the orbit floor" to a depth of 2 cm; a single 8- to 10-ml injection was given. He stated that only 5% of patients required supplemental blocking. Other authors report up to 50% failure to achieve akinesia with periconal blocking.[5,67] Onset of akinesia is considerably slower than with intraconal block,[5,68-70] volume requirement is greater,[71] postinjection orbital pressure is greater,[72] and the supplementation rate to achieve total akinesia is higher.[5,73,74] The incidence of periorbital ecchymoses[68] and conjunctival chemosis is also greater.[67,69,75] Of the many variations of the peribulbar technique, a common one is placement in two locations, one inferior-temporal and the other in the superior nasal orbit (a site that is vascular and therefore prone to hematoma formation). For those who wish to practice peribulbar blocking, the author suggests a two-needle technique: the first being an injection in the inferior-temporal quadrant, as described in Figure 8-11, and the second an injection into the medial fat compartment on the nasal side of the medial rectus muscle (complementary block as described in the previous section). Up to 5 ml of local anesthetic solution is injected at each site. Because there is insufficient space between the lateral rectus and inferior rectus muscles and the lateral and inferior walls of the orbit, respectively, these areas cannot be used without risking extraocular muscle injury.

Parabulbar (Sub-Tenon's) Block

Anesthesia for cataract surgery produced by injection beneath Tenon's capsule of small volumes of local anesthetic were first described by Swan[52] in 1956. He indicated that the sub-Tenon's method produced better iris and anterior segment anesthesia than did subconjunctival injection. Since 1990 the sub-Tenon's

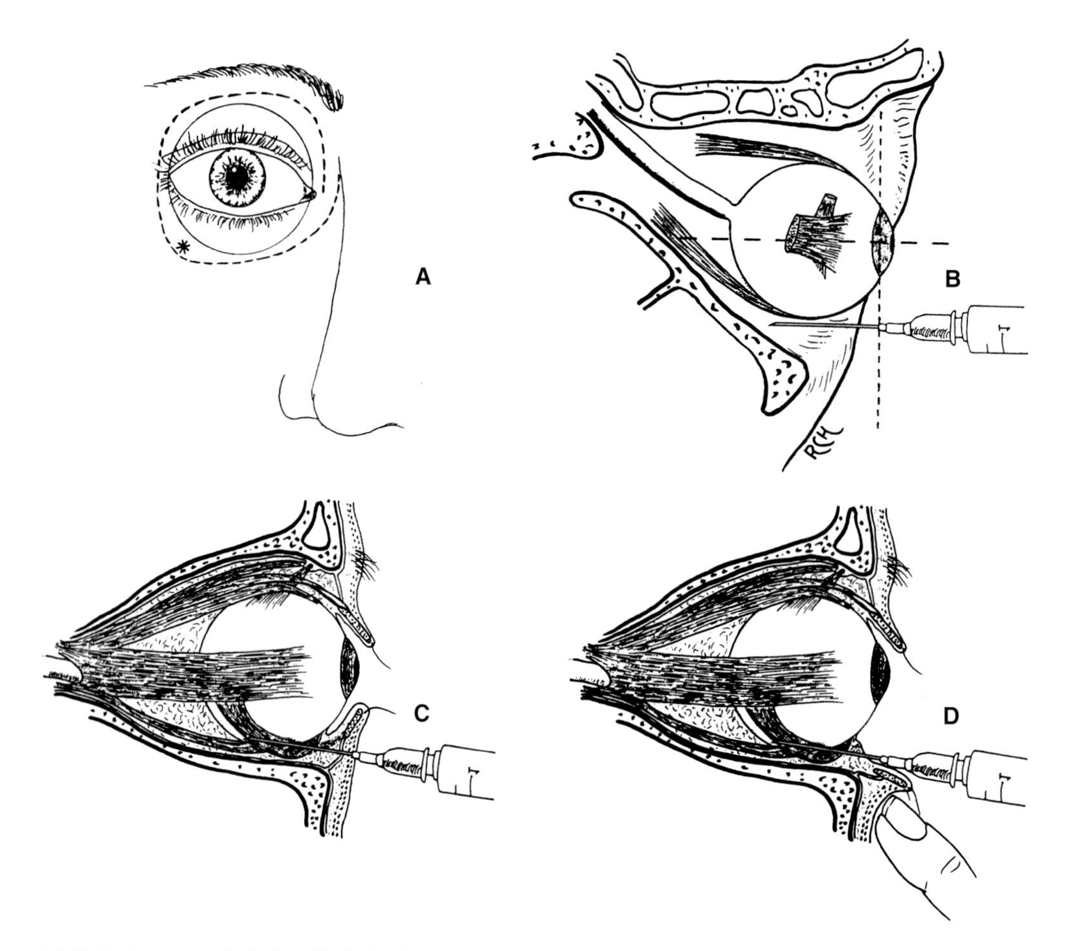

FIGURE 8-11 Peribulbar block, inferior-temporal injection. **A,** Frontal view; **B,** view from above; **C** and **D,** lateral views. The inferior-temporal rim of the orbit is palpated and the desired entry point (*) chosen just inside the orbital rim at the 7:30 position for the right eye **(A)** or the 4:30 position for the left eye. With the patient's eyes in primary gaze, the 27-gauge 25-mm sharp disposable needle is advanced in a sagittal plane **(B)** with 10-degree upward inflection from the transverse plane (**C** and **D**), and passes the globe equator to a depth controlled by observing the needle-hub junction reach the plane of the iris **(B).** Percutaneous needle entry is the preferred technique **(C);** however, the transconjunctival route is also possible **(D).** (Courtesy Gimbel Educational Services.)

injection technique has been extensively used.[76] This injection technique evolved into anesthesia produced by blunt cannula insertion[77] after surgical dissection into the sub-Tenon's space.[77-79] Onset of anesthesia is rapid.[80,81] The degree of abolition of extraocular muscle movement is proportional to the volume of injectate. Following placement of local anesthetic by cannula beneath Tenon's capsule, spread occurs into the anterior retrobulbar space.[82] Disadvantages of the method are an increased incidence of conjunctival chemosis and hemorrhage and the potential of damaging one of the vortex veins.[77] Conjunctival hemorrhage is common if diathermy is not used.[82] Peripheral orbital anesthesia may be incomplete; supplemental local anesthetic injections may be necessary to achieve patient comfort.[83] Repeat sub-Tenon's injections can be performed simply in the presence of incomplete anesthesia.[53] Unlike topical corneoconjunctival anesthesia, sub-Tenon's, retrobulbar, and peribulbar techniques easily abolish iris and ciliary body sensation and can be used to produce globe akinesia.[83]

REFERENCES

1. Davis DB, Mandel MR: Posterior peribulbar anesthesia: an alternative to retrobulbar anesthesia, *J Cataract Refract Surg* 12:182-184, 1986.
2. Leaming DV: Practice styles and preferences of ASCRS members: 1999 survey, *J Cataract Refract Surg* 26:913-921, 2000.
3. Grizzard WS, Kirk NM, Pavan PR et al: Perforating ocular injuries caused by anesthesia personnel, *Ophthalmology* 98:1011-1016, 1991.
4. Javitt JC, Addiego R, Friedberg HL et al: Brain stem anesthesia after retrobulbar block, *Ophthalmology* 94:718-724, 1987.
5. Morgan GE: Retrobulbar apnea syndrome: a case for the routine presence of an anesthesiologist, *Reg Anesth* 15:106-107, 1990 (letter).
6. Koornneef L: Orbital septa: anatomy and function, *Ophthalmology* 86: 876-880, 1979.
7. Atkinson WS: Local anesthesia in ophthalmology, *Am J Ophthalmol* 31:1607-1618, 1948.
8. Hamilton RC, Gimbel HV, Strunin L: Regional anaesthesia for 12,000 cataract extraction and intraocular lens implantation procedures, *Can J Anaesth* 35:615-623, 1988.
9. Atkinson WS: Local anesthesia in ophthalmology, *Trans Am Ophthalmol Soc* 32:399-451, 1934.
10. Liu C, Youl B, Moseley I: Magnetic resonance imaging of the optic nerve in

extremes of gaze: implications for the positioning of the globe for retrobulbar anaesthesia, *Br J Ophthalmol* 76:728-733, 1992.
11. Unsöld R, Stanley JA, DeGroot J: The CT-topography of retrobulbar anesthesia, *Albrecht Von Graefes Arch Klin Exp Ophthalmol* 217:125-136, 1981.
12. Hamilton RC: Brain-stem anesthesia as a complication of regional anesthesia for ophthalmic surgery, *Can J Ophthalmol* 27:323-325, 1992.
13. Pautler SE, Grizzard WS, Thompson LN et al: Blindness from retrobulbar injection into the optic nerve, *Ophthalmic Surg* 17:334-337, 1986.
14. Katsev DA, Drews RC, Rose BT: An anatomic study of retrobulbar needle path length, *Ophthalmology* 96:1221-1224, 1989.
15. Gifford H: Motor block of extraocular muscles by deep orbital injection, *Arch Ophthalmol* 41:5-19, 1949.
16. Morgan CM, Schatz H, Vine AK et al: Ocular complications associated with retrobulbar injections, *Ophthalmology* 95:660-665, 1988.
17. Brod RD: Transient central retinal occlusion and contralateral amaurosis after retrobulbar anesthetic injection, *Ophthalmic Surg* 20:643-646, 1989.
18. Giuffrè G, Vadala M, Manfrè L: Retrobulbar anesthesia complicated by combined central retinal vein and artery occlusion and massive vitreoretinal fibrosis, *Retina* 15:439-441, 1995.
19. Sullivan KL, Brown GC, Forman AR et al: Retrobulbar anesthesia and retinal vascular obstruction, *Ophthalmology* 90:373-377, 1983.
20. Cibis PA. Discussion. In Schepens CL, Regan CDJ, editors: *Controversial aspects of the management of retinal detachments*, Boston, 1965, Little, Brown, p 251.
21. Duker JS, Belmont JB, Benson WE et al: Inadvertent globe perforation during retrobulbar and peribulbar anesthesia, *Ophthalmology* 98:519-526, 1991.
22. Schepens CL: A comparison of peribulbar and retrobulbar anesthesia for vitreoretinal surgical procedures, *Arch Ophthalmol* 114:502, 1996 (letter).
23. Ginsburg RN, Duker JS: Globe perforation associated with retrobulbar and peribulbar anesthesia, *Semin Ophthalmol* 8:87-95, 1993.
24. Magnante DO, Bullock JD, Green WR: Ocular explosion after peribulbar anesthesia, *Ophthalmology* 104:608-615, 1997.
25. Bullock JD, Warwar RE, Green WR: Ocular explosions from periocular anesthetic injections, *Ophthalmology* 106:2341-2353, 1999.
26. Carlson BM, Emerick S, Komorowski TE et al: Extraocular muscle regeneration in primates, *Ophthalmology* 99:582-589, 1992.
27. Rainin EA, Carlson BM: Postoperative diplopia and ptosis: a clinical hypothesis on the myotoxicity of local anesthetics, *Arch Ophthalmol* 103:1337-1339, 1985.
28. Hunter DG, Lam GC, Guyton DL: Inferior oblique muscle injury from local anesthesia for cataract surgery, *Ophthalmology* 102:501-509, 1995.
29. Ong-Tone L, Pearce WG: Inferior rectus muscle restriction after retrobulbar anesthesia for cataract extraction, *Can J Ophthalmol* 24:162-165, 1989.
30. Hamed LM: Strabismus presenting after cataract surgery, *Ophthalmology* 98:247-252, 1991.
31. Hamed LM, Mancuso A: Inferior rectus muscle contracture syndrome after retrobulbar anesthesia, *Ophthalmology* 98:1506-1512, 1991.
32. Capó H, Roth E, Johnson T et al: Vertical strabismus after cataract surgery, *Ophthalmology* 103:918-921, 1996.
33. Hustead RF, Hamilton RC, Loken RG: Periocular local anesthesia: medial orbital as an alternative to superior nasal injection, *J Cataract Refract Surg* 20:197-201, 1994.
34. Feibel RM: Current concepts in retrobulbar anesthesia, *Surv Ophthalmol* 30:102-110, 1985.
35. Goldsmith MO: Occlusion of the central retinal artery following retrobulbar hemorrhage, *Ophthalmologica* 153:191-196, 1967.
36. Kraushar MF, Seelenfreund MH, Freilich DB: Central retinal artery closure during orbital hemorrhage from retrobulbar injection, *Trans Am Acad Ophthalmol Otolaryngol* 78:65-70, 1974.
37. Edge KR, Nicoll JMV: Retrobulbar hemorrhage after 12,500 retrobulbar blocks, *Anesth Analg* 76:1019-1022, 1993.
38. Grizzard WS: Ophthalmic anesthesia. In Reinecke RD, editor: *Ophthalmology annual*, New York, 1989, Raven Press, pp 265-294.
39. Mackool RJ: Intraocular pressure fluctuations, *J Cataract Refract Surg* 19:563-564, 1993 (letter, comment).
40. Atkinson WS: Akinesia of the orbicularis, Am J Ophthalmol 36:1255-1258, 1953.
41. Atkinson WS: Observations on anesthesia for ocular surgery, *Trans Am Acad Ophthalmol Otolaryngol* 60:376-380, 1956.
42. Buys NS: Mercury balloon reducer for vitreous and orbital volume control. In Emery J, editor: *Current concepts in cataract surgery*, St Louis, 1980, Mosby, p 258.
43. Davidson B, Kratz R, Mazzocco T et al: An evaluation of the Honan intraocular pressure reducer, *J Am Intraocul Implant Soc* 5:237, 1979.
44. Drews RC: The Nerf ball for preoperative reduction of intraocular pressure, *Ophthalmic Surg* 13:761, 1982.
45. Gills JP: Constant mild compression of the eye to produce hypotension, *J Am Intraocul Implant Soc* 5:52-53, 1979.
46. Palay DA, Stulting RD: The effect of external ocular compression on intraocular pressure following retrobulbar anesthesia, *Ophthalmic Surg* 21: 503-507, 1990.
47. Kimble JA, Morris RE, Witherspoon CD et al: Globe perforation from peribulbar injection, *Arch Ophthalmol* 105:749, 1987 (letter).
48. Mount AM, Seward HC: Scleral perforations during peribulbar anaesthesia, *Eye* 7:766-767, 1993.
49. Gillow JT, Aggarwal RK, Kirby GR: A survey of ocular perforation during ophthalmic local anaesthesia in the United Kingdom, *Eye* 10:537-538, 1996.
50. Loots JH, Koorts AS, Venter JA: Peribulbar anesthesia: a prospective statistical analysis of the efficacy and predictability of bupivacaine and a lignocaine/bupivacaine mixture, *J Cataract Refract Surg* 19:72-76, 1993.
51. Hamilton RC: Retrobulbar block revisited and revised, *J Cataract Refract Surg* 22:1147-1150, 1996.
52. Swan KC: New drugs and techniques for ocular anesthesia, *Trans Am Acad Ophthalmol Otolaryngol* 60:368-375, 1956.
53. Gardner S, Ryall D: Local anaesthesia within the orbit, *Curr Anaesth Crit Care* 11:299-305, 2000.
54. Kuhn F, Mester V, Berta A: The continuous-injection technique to reduce complications during retrobulbar anesthesia, *Ophthalmic Surg Lasers* 30: 67-68, 1999.
55. Smith DC, Crul JF: Oxygen desaturation following sedation for regional analgesia, *Br J Anaesth* 62:206-209, 1989.
56. Katz J, Feldman MA, Bass EB et al: Adverse intraoperative medical events and their association with anesthesia management strategies in cataract surgery, *Ophthalmology* 108:1721-1726, 2001.
57. Farley JS, Hustead RF, Becker KE: Diluting lidocaine and mepivacaine in balanced salt solution reduces the pain of intradermal injection, *Reg Anesth* 19:48-51, 1994.
58. Hamilton RC, Grizzard WS: Complications. In Gills JP, Hustead RF, Sanders DR, editors: *Ophthalmic anesthesia*, Thorofare, NJ, 1993, Slack Inc, pp 187-202.
59. Sarvela J, Nikki P, Paloheimo M: Orbicular muscle akinesia in regional ophthalmic anaesthesia with pH-adjusted bupivacaine: effects of hyaluronidase and epinephrine, *Can J Anaesth* 40:1028-1033, 1993.
60. American Academy of Ophthalmology Wydase Task Force Report, 2001.
61. Nicoll JMV, Treuren B, Acharya PA et al: Retrobulbar anesthesia: the role of hyaluronidase, *Anesth Analg* 65:1324-1328, 1986.
62. Dempsey GA, Barrett PJ, Kirby IJ: Hyaluronidase and peribulbar block, *Br J Anaesth* 78:671-674, 1997.
63. Brown SM, Brooks SE, Mazow ML et al: Cluster of diplopia cases after periocular anesthesia without hyaluronidase, *J Cataract Refract Surg* 25:1245-1249, 1999.
64. Morsman CD, Holden R: The effects of adrenaline, hyaluronidase and age on peribulbar anaesthesia, *Eye* 6:290-292, 1992.
65. Sarvela J, Nikki P: Comparison of two needle lengths in regional ophthalmic anesthesia with etidocaine and hyaluronidase, *Ophthalmic Surg* 23:742-745, 1992.
66. Bloomberg LB: Anterior periocular anesthesia: five years experience, *J Cataract Refract Surg* 17:508-511, 1991.
67. Wang HS: Peribulbar anesthesia for ophthalmic procedures, *J Cataract Refract Surg* 14:441-443, 1988.
68. Drews RC, Malbran ES: Anesthesia, speculum free eye surgery, intraoperative fundus observation with the surgical microscope. In Boyd BF, editor: *Highlights of ophthalmology*, vol 1, Cali, Colombia, 1993, Carvajal, 1993, pp 1-26.
69. Arora R, Verma L, Kumar A et al: Peribulbar anesthesia in retinal reattachment surgery, *Ophthalmic Surg* 23:499-501, 1992.
70. Khalil SN: Local anaesthesia for eye surgery, *Anaesthesia* 46:232, 1991 (letter, comment).
71. Straus JG: A new retrobulbar needle and injection technique, *Ophthalmic Surg* 19:134-139, 1988.
72. Stevens J, Giubilei M, Lanigan L et al: Sub-Tenon, retrobulbar and peribulbar local anaesthesia: the effect upon intraocular pressure, *Eur J Implant Ref Surg* 5:25-28, 1993.
73. Ali-Melkkilä TM, Virkkilä M, Jyrkkiö H: Regional anesthesia for cataract surgery: comparison of retrobulbar and peribulbar techniques, *Reg Anesth* 17:219-222, 1992.
74. Lebuisson DA: Simplified and safer peribulbar anaesthesia, *Eur J Implant Ref Surg* 2:123-124, 1990.
75. Weiss JL, Deichman CB: A comparison of retrobulbar and periocular anesthesia for cataract surgery, *Arch Ophthalmol* 107:96-98, 1989.

76. Tsuneoka H, Ohki K, Taniuchi O et al: Tenon's capsule anaesthesia for cataract surgery with IOL implantation, *Eur J Implant Ref Surg* 5:29-34, 1993.
77. Stevens JD: A new local anaesthesia technique for cataract extraction by one quadrant sub-Tenon's infiltration, *Br J Ophthalmol* 76:670-674, 1992.
78. Mein CE, Woodcock MG: Local anesthesia for vitreoretinal surgery, *Retina* 10:47-49, 1990.
79. Greenbaum S: Parabulbar anesthesia, *Am J Ophthalmol* 114:776, 1992.
80. Greenbaum S: Anesthesia for cataract surgery. In Greenbaum S, editor: *Ocular anesthesia*, Philadelphia, 1997, WB Saunders, pp 1-55.
81. Markoff DD: Sub-Tenon's anesthesia, *Operative Techniques Cataract Refractive Surg* 3:127-131, 2000.
82. Stevens JD, Restori M: Ultrasound imaging of no-needle 1-quadrant sub-Tenon local anaesthesia for cataract surgery, *Eur J Implant Ref Surg* 5:35-38, 1993.
83. Simcock PR, Raymond GL, Lavin MJ: Peribulbar injection and direct infiltration for vitreoretinal surgery, *Arch Ophthalmol* 110:1357-1358, 1992 (letter, comment).

Topical Intracameral Anesthesia

9

Alan S. Crandall, MD

Anesthesia

Modern intraocular surgery involves many new technologies. These include phacoemulsification, foldable intraocular lenses, clear corneal incisions, and capsular tension rings (and Cionni variations), among many others. This infusion of new techniques has forced a reevaluation of the anesthetic needs for anterior segment surgery.

In the 1985 survey of members of the American Society of Cataract and Refractive Surgeons (ASCRS),[1] 76% of the responding ophthalmologists used a retrobulbar injection with a facial block; 4% used a periocular block, and 4% used general anesthesia. Thus, in 1985, 92% of the ophthalmologists who returned their survey used a retrobulbar anesthetic for cataract surgery. A similar survey conducted among members of the American Academy of Ophthalmology[2] showed that in 1992, 71% of those responding used retrobulbar anesthesia for cataract surgery, whereas 28% used a peribulbar technique. Subsequent ASCRS surveys showed a steady decline in the number of respondents using retrobulbar anesthesia.[3-11] By the 1998 survey, anesthesia preferences for cataract surgery had changed dramatically, with 32% of respondents using retrobulbar anesthesia; 27% using a periocular block; and 37% of respondents using topical anesthesia for cataract surgery, an anesthetic technique not even listed in the 1985 survey.

One might conclude from this data that topical anesthesia for cataract surgery is an entirely new notion. However, more correctly, one would say that topical anesthesia has been rediscovered. In 1884 Karl Koller first described the topical use of cocaine as an anesthetic agent for ocular surgery.[12] Later that same year, Knapp[13] described a method for enucleation using a retrobulbar injection of cocaine.[12] Widespread acceptance of injected cocaine anesthesia for cataract surgery was limited, however, by the toxicity of the drug. Thus, at the turn of the century, topical instillation of cocaine was the standard for cataract surgery. Topical cocaine, however, was not without local toxicity. Tetracaine later became available and was less locally toxic than cocaine; therefore it was commonly substituted for cocaine as a topical agent for cataract surgery. Tetracaine, however, did not provide the same depth of anesthesia for intraocular structures as did cocaine. This fact, along with the more complicated surgical techniques developed in the 1920s and 1930s, pushed many ophthalmologists away from topical anesthesia to rely more on retrobulbar procaine injections for adequate surgical anesthesia for cataract surgery.[14] Infiltration of retrobulbar anesthetic was really the standard cataract surgery technique for decades thereafter. Ironically, it has been the complications associated with these infiltration anesthetic techniques that have led the ophthalmic community full circle, back to topical anesthesia for cataract surgery.

Topical Anesthesia

Topical anesthesia is not new. In fact, it was considered an important discovery when Karl Koller observed that a solution of cocaine applied to the eye could prevent pain during eye surgery. (Koller likely also introduced Sigmund Freud[15] to cocaine). With further advances in anesthesia and changes in ocular surgery, general anesthesia and injection techniques became the standard of care. The use of topical anesthesia was reintroduced by Fichman[16] in the early 1990s. This technique used topical 0.5% tetracaine. Soon other agents also became acceptable because other drops (such as 0.75% Marcaine [Sanofi Winthrop Pharmaceuticals, New York] and 1% to 2% lidocaine) were less toxic to the corneal epithelium.

Initially, some patients were not completely comfortable with the use of topical anesthesia only, so some surgeons used intravenous sedation and analgesics to give further comfort. However, in 1995 Gills, Cherchio, and Raanan[17] introduced the use of nonpreserved lidocaine (1%) given intracamerally, which would provide further anesthesia. In an attempt to evaluate the new procedures, Patel et al.[18] randomized patients to receive a retrobulbar block versus topical anesthesia. A visual pain analogue scale was used to assess pain during surgery. They concluded that topical anesthesia can be used safely and that patient discomfort was only marginally higher postoperatively. Furthermore, the same group then randomly allocated patients to receive topical plus balanced salt solution, versus topical plus intracameral lidocaine, and found very slight differences between the two groups. They also found slightly better patient

Supported in part by a grant from Research to Prevent Blindness, Inc., New York, NY, to the Department of Ophthalmology and Visual Sciences, University of Utah.

TABLE 9-1
Techniques of Anesthesia for Cataract Surgery

General anesthesia
Retrobulbar
Peribulbar
Parabulbar
Topical

TABLE 9-2
Contraindications to Topical Anesthesia

RELATIVE
Language barrier
Deafness
Uncooperative patients
Difficult surgery
Extended time for surgery
Nystagmus
ABSOLUTE
Allergy to the anesthetic
Coarse nystagmus

cooperation in the group that received the intracameral lidocaine.[19]

In routine small-incision cataract surgery, ocular anesthesia with topical anesthetics will usually suffice (Table 9-1). However, depending on the surgeon's experience,[20] there may contraindications (relative and absolute) to the use of topical anesthesia (Table 9-2).

Currently, this author uses topical anesthesia for cataract surgery, combined cataract and glaucoma surgery, trabeculectomy, viscocanalostomy, secondary lens implants, sutured posterior chamber intraocular lens, and sutured Cionni rings.

Parabulbar (Sub-Tenon's) Anesthesia

Tenon's capsule is, of course, an anterior extension of dura. It fuses with conjunctiva near the surgical limbus. Therefore it can provide access to the retrobulbar space. Hansen, Mein, and Mazzoli[21] reported the use of sub-Tenon's surgery in 1990. Greenbaum[22] designed a specific flexible cannula to deliver the anesthesia. In this procedure, a dissection is made through conjunctiva and Tenon's capsule down to bare sclera; the Greenbaum cannula (or other blunt cannula) is used; and, by making the incision small enough, the fluid can be forced to dissect posteriorly, and, usually, only a few milliliters of anesthesia are required. The anesthesia is of rapid onset, but the globe akinesia takes a few minutes to occur. A similar technique was described by Stevens[23]; however, he used a blunt, curved, metal cannula and started his incision 5 mm posterior to the limbus.

Techniques for Topical Anesthesia

1. In outpatients, drops with 0.5% proparacaine are initiated. Dilating drops and antibiotic plus Voltaren (Novartis Pharmaceutical Corp., East Hanover, NJ) are administered twice. Beginning with the third set and approximately 15 minutes before surgery, one more set of dilating drops and two sets of 0.75% bupivacaine drops are instilled (Figure 9-1). Next, two to three drops of half-strength Betadine (Purdue Frederick Co., Norwalk, Conn.) are instilled into the cul-de-sac (Figure 9-2).

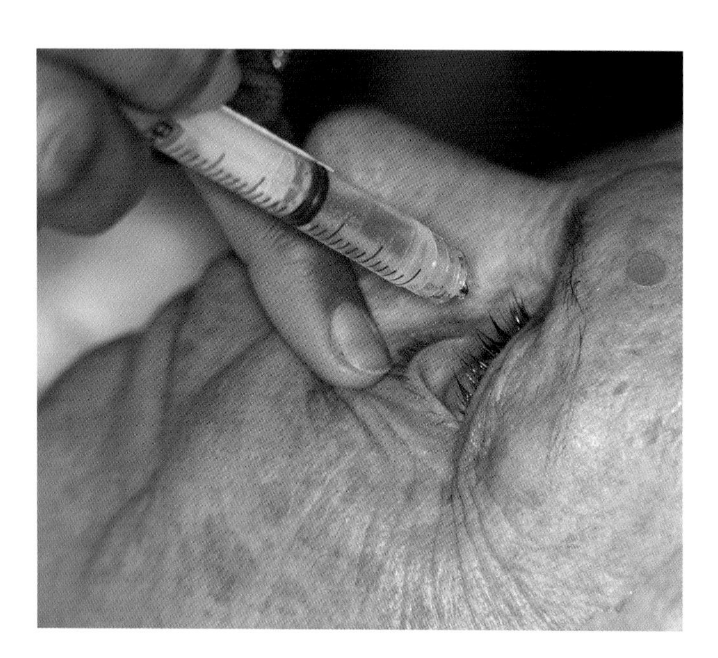

FIGURE 9-1 Bupivacaine 0.75% drops administered initially every 10 minutes ×3.

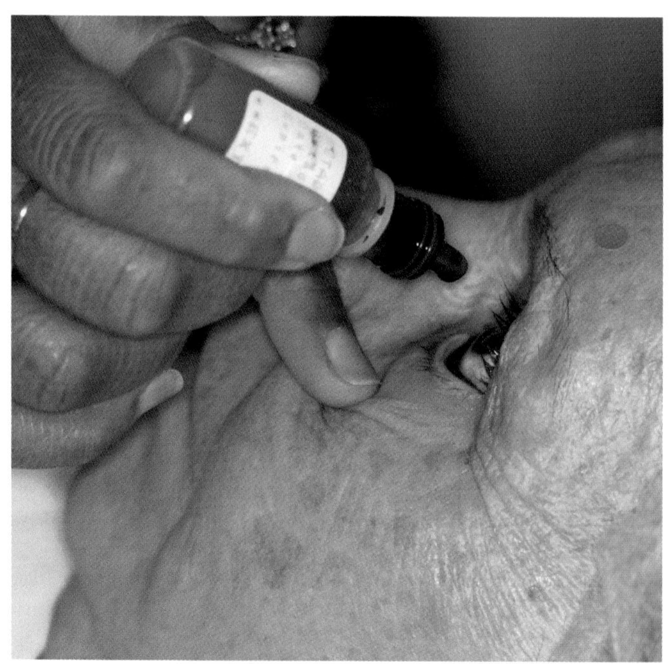

FIGURE 9-2 Betadine 5% drops administered before lidocaine gel.

2. Just before entering the operating room, viscous lidocaine is instilled into the cul-de-sac (Figure 9-3).
3. Once in the operating theater, one more drop is instilled and the patient has the sterile skin preparation administered. Another drop of anesthetic can be administered.
4. During draping, the patient's upper lid is held with a sterile 4 × 4 gauze bandage, and the patient is asked to look down. This usually allows application of the drape without difficulty (Figure 9-4). The patient can be told that there is an odd feeling during the process, especially when placing the lid speculum (Figure 9-5, *A* and *B*). Most patients are quite comfortable once the speculum is in place. It is important that the lashes are covered with the drape to reduce the stimulus. The light source is very low and slowly raised as the patient becomes comfortable.
5. A stab incision is made, and 0.3 ml of 1% unpreserved lidocaine is slowly injected. Patients can be warned that they may feel a slight sting although most do not (Figures 9-6 and 9-7).
6. Versed (Roche Laboratories, Nutley, NJ), 0.5 to 1 mg, usually will be administered, although many patients require none.

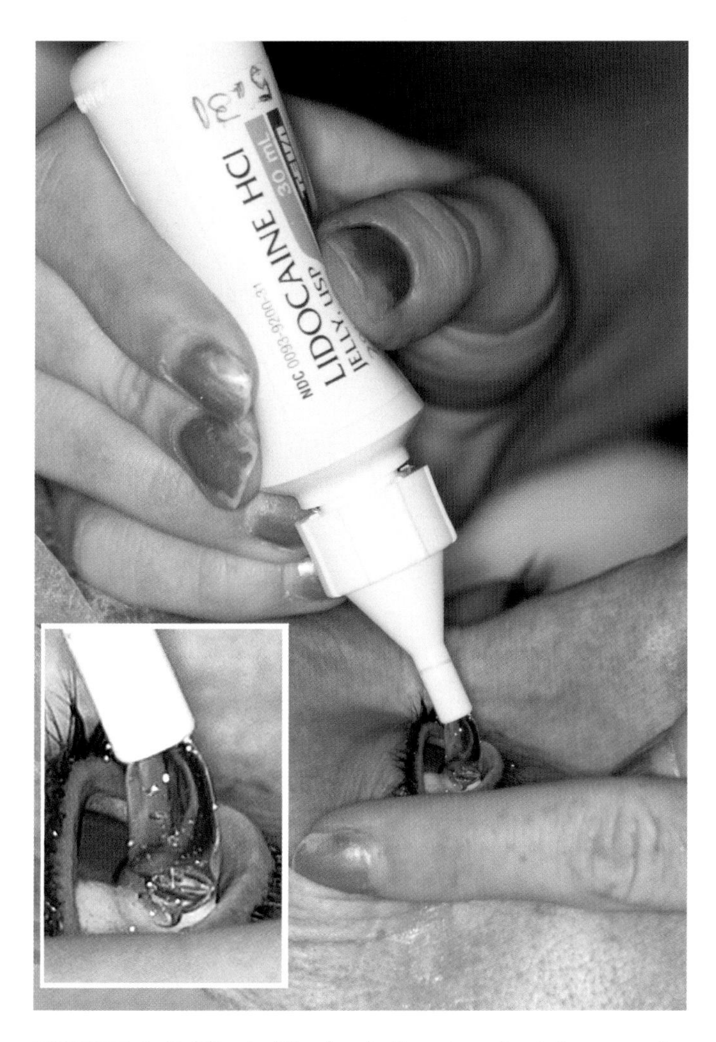

FIGURE 9-3 Lidocaine 2% gel applied to ocular surface before preparation and draping of patient.

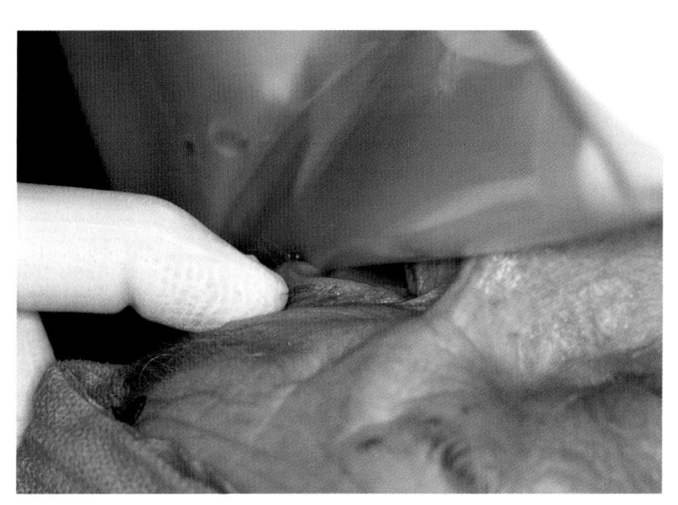

FIGURE 9-4 Drape applied after sterile prep as lids are retreated and patient looks down.

A

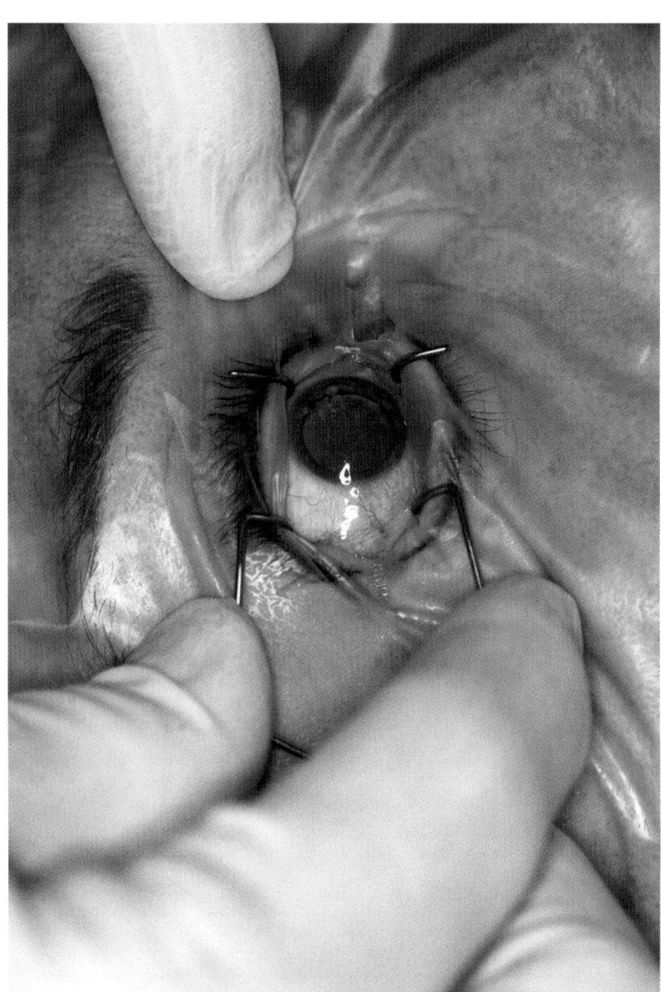

B

FIGURE 9-5 **A** and **B,** Lid speculum placed after incision of drape, ensuring adequate coverage of lid margin and lashes.

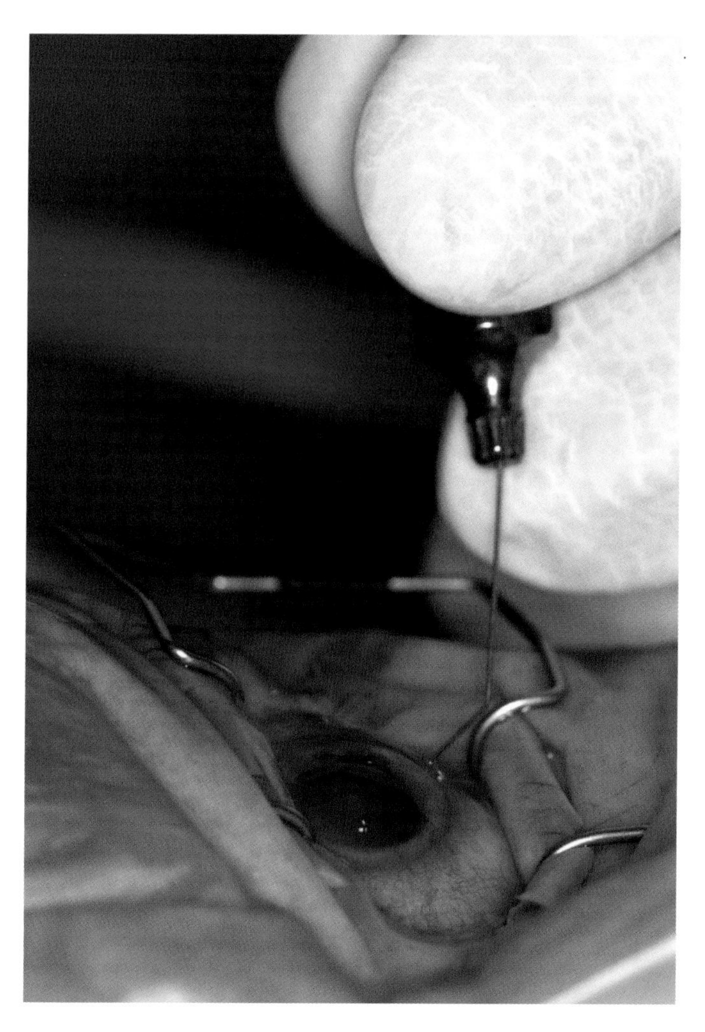

FIGURE 9-6 Nonpreserved lidocaine 1% injected into anterior chamber.

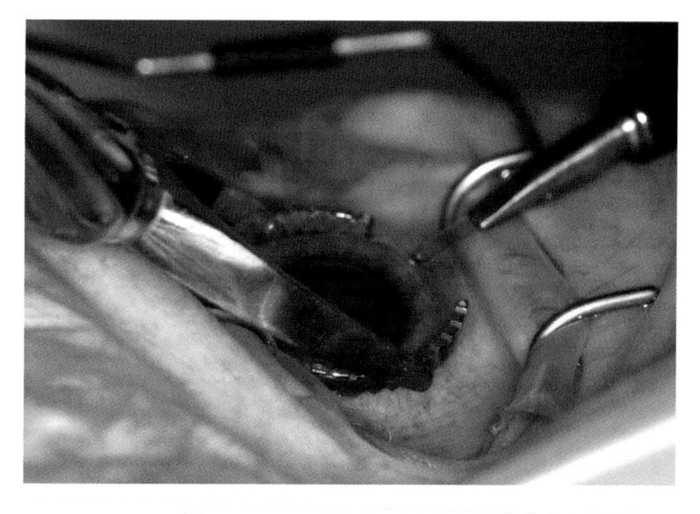

FIGURE 9-7 Thornton fixation ring used to stabilize globe for paracentesis.

REFERENCES

1. Leaming DV. Practice styles and preferences of ASCRS members—1985 survey, *J Cataract Refract Surg* 12:380-384, 1968.
2. Schein OD, Bass EB, Sharkey P et al: Cataract surgical techniques: preferences and underlying beliefs, *Arch Ophthalmol* 113:1108-1112, 1995.
3. Leaming DV: Practice styles and preferences of ASCRS members—1987 survey, *J Cataract Refract Surg* 14:552-559, 1988.
4. Leaming DV: Practice styles and preferences of ASCRS members—1988 survey, *J Cataract Refract Surg* 15:689-697, 1989.
5. Leaming DV: Practice styles and preferences of ASCRS members—1989 survey, *J Cataract Refract Surg* 16:624-632, 1990.
6. Leaming DV: Practice styles and preferences of ASCRS members—1991 survey, *J Cataract Refract Surg* 18:460-469, 1992.
7. Leaming DV: Practice styles and preferences of ASCRS members—1983 survey, *J Cataract Refract Surg* 20:459-467, 1994.
8. Leaming DV: Practice styles and preferences of ASCRS members—1994 survey, *J Cataract Refract Surg* 21:378-385, 1995.
9. Leaming DV: Practice styles and preferences of ASCRS members—1995 survey, *J Cataract Refract Surg* 22:931-939, 1996.
10. Leaming DV: Practice styles and preferences of ASCRS members—1996 survey. *J Cataract Refract Surg* 23:527-535, 1997.
11. Leaming DV: Practice styles and preferences of ASCRS members—1997 survey, *J Cataract Refract Surg* 24:552-561, 1998.
12. Altman AJ, Albert DM, Fournier GA: Cocaine's use in ophthalmology: our 100-year heritage, *Surv Ophthalmol* 29:300-306, 1985.
13. Knapp H: On cocaine and its use in ophthalmic and general surgery, *Arch Ophthalmol* 13:402-448, 1884.
14. Russell DA, Guyton JS: Retrobulbar injection of lidocaine (Xylocaine) for anesthesia and akinesia, *Am J Ophthalmol* 38:78-84, 1954.
15. Karch SB: Coca java and the Southeast Asia coca industry. In Karch SB, editor: *A brief history of cocaine*, Boca Raton, 1997, CRC Press, pp 71-81.
16. Fichman RA: Use of topical anesthesia alone in cataract surgery, *J Cataract Refract Surg* 22:612-614, 1996.
17. Gills JP, Cherchio M, Raanan M: Unpreserved lidocaine to control discomfort during cataract surgery using topical anesthesia, *J Cataract Refract Surg* 23:545-550, 1997.
18. Patel BCK, Burns TA, Crandall A et al: A comparison of topical and retrobulbar anesthesia for cataract surgery, *Ophthalmology* 103:1196-1203, 1996.
19. Crandall AS, Zabriskie NA, Patel BCK et al: A comparison of patient comfort during cataract surgery with topical anesthesia versus topical anesthesia and intracameral lidocaine, *Ophthalmology* 1006:60-66, 1999.
20. Patel BCK, Clinch TE, Burns TA et al: Prospective evaluation of topical versus retrobulbar anesthesia: a converting surgeon's experience, *J Cataract Refract Surg* 24:853-860, 1998.
21. Hansen EA, Mein CE, Mazzoli R: Ocular anesthesia for cataract surgery: a direct sub-Tenon's approach, *Ophthalmic Surg* 21:696-699, 1990.
22. Greenbaum S: Anesthesia in cataract surgery. In Greenbaum S, editor: *Ocular anesthesia*, Philadelphia, 1997, WB Saunders, pp. 1-55.
23. Stevens JD: A new local anesthesia technique for cataract extraction by one quadrant sub-Tenon's infiltrations, *Br J Ophthalmol* 76:670-674, 1992.

Extracapsular Cataract Surgery: Indications and Techniques

10

Jared Emery, MD
Roger F. Steinert, MD

Extracapsular cataract surgery, strictly speaking, includes both phacoemulsification and planned extracapsular cataract extraction. By convention, the terms *extracapsular* and *planned extracapsular* refer to an operation in which the lens nucleus is delivered intact through a limbal incision of about 10 mm.

Since 1970, phacoemulsification and extracapsular cataract surgery have replaced intracapsular cataract extraction, except for rare instances such as subluxated lenses or eyes in which a question of patient sensitivity to lens material exists. Phacoemulsification was used in about 15% to 20% of cataract cases in the United States from the mid-1970s through 1987. Phacoemulsification then rapidly gained in popularity, becoming the procedure of choice for about 50% of surgeons by 1990, for 70% of surgeons by 1992,[1] and nearly 100% of responding surgeon members of the American Society of Cataract and Refractive Surgery in a survey in 2000.[2] However, the extracapsular cataract operation is still used by many surgeons in specific situations. In some cases, it is the procedure of choice. Every cataract surgeon should be skilled in extracapsular cataract surgery.

Indications

The extracapsular operation can be used successfully for almost any cataract. The method is not appropriate for luxated or subluxated lenses. Its main disadvantages compared with phacoemulsification include greater induced astigmatism,[3-7] less stability of the postoperative refraction,[3,8,9] more early postoperative inflammation,[10,11] and a higher rate of posterior capsular opacification.[12] Its main advantage is that in some cases it can provide a greater margin of safety. In cases in which the nucleus is very dense, the pupil dilates poorly, posterior synechiae are present, or zonular integrity is in question (as in pseudoexfoliation syndrome or after pars plana vitrectomy), some surgeons have a greater margin of safety with the extracapsular procedure.

The surgeon should use the procedure that is likely to give the most successful result. For example, if the surgeon perseveres with phacoemulsification made difficult by poor exposure, he or she might face a higher likelihood of capsular rupture with vitreous loss than might have been the case had the surgery been converted to large-incision extracapsular extraction. The careful surgeon judges each case in advance and chooses phacoemulsification or planned extracapsular surgery based on his or her expectation that this will produce the best result for the patient. In the majority of cases, this decision can be made before surgery. For some cases, however, one might choose during surgery to switch from phacoemulsification to a planned extracapsular technique. The extracapsular technique of Emery (discussion to follow) allows the surgeon to switch readily from phacoemulsification to large-incision planned extracapsular surgery at any stage of the operation.

Techniques

The best cataract surgical techniques give consistently reproducible results. The surgeon remains in control. The operation accomplishes removal of the nucleus with minimal stress on the zonules, secure placement of an intraocular lens (IOL) with an intact capsular bag, and closure with a watertight incision that gives minimal astigmatism. The procedure should be as simple as possible to promote success and should apply with minimal variations to all types of cases.

Preparation

After aseptic preparation of the operative site, dry the lid margins using cellulose sponges. Apply a large unperforated plastic drape (3M) to the open lids and incise (Figure 10-1).

Retract the upper and lower lids using the Jaffe wire lid speculum. Attach a rubber band to each speculum and use a hemostat to clip the rubber band to the drapes, applying the minimum amount of tension that will give adequate exposure of the globe. Place 4-0 black silk sutures beneath the insertions of the superior and inferior rectus muscles. Tuck in the flaps of the drape and attach the sutures to the rubber bands (Figure 10-2). Use only the necessary tension to produce adequate exposure above the superior limbus and maintain visibility of the inferior limbus.

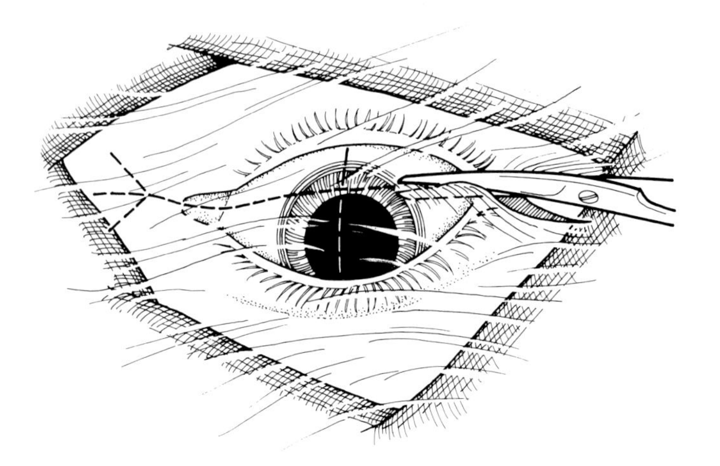

FIGURE 10-1 Technique for incision of plastic drape.

Conjunctival Incision

Make a fornix-based flap to expose the limbus using a 7-mm peritomy with oblique relaxing incisions extending from the limbus about 3 mm posteriorly, as illustrated (Figure 10-3).

Apply light wet-field cautery to obliterate all visible surface vessels posterior to the intended incision site, which will be approximately 3 mm posterior to the anterior limbus (Figure 10-4). Clean the limbus with a Tooke knife to "squeeze" residual blood from vessels near the limbus. Avoid fraying the scleral surface with excessive scraping.

Scleral Incision

Using calipers, measure a 10-mm chord length on the sclera, with the points positioned 3 mm posterior to the limbus (Figure 10-5). Make a 10-mm partially penetrating incision using a 30-degree disposable steel microsurgical blade. The incision groove will run parallel with the limbus and 3 mm posterior to the anterior limbal margin (Figure 10-6). The groove should be perpendicular to the scleral surface and to a depth of 50% to 75% of the scleral wall thickness.

Make a lamellar scleral dissection using a disposable crescent blade. Begin this dissection at the base of the preplaced groove. Dissect the flap anteriorly, beginning at the apex of the groove. Continue tangential to the globe for about 1 mm along the entire length of the groove. Then extend the tunnel in one direction, wherever access is easiest (Figure 10-7). Gradually come anterior, being careful to depress the heel of the crescent blade to avoid premature penetration at the site where the corneoscleral curvature steepens. Bring the incision anterior into clear cornea just beyond (central) to the limbal arcade (Figures 10-7 and 10-8). About 4 mm of scleral-corneal dissection should extend to the point of anterior chamber entry. Keeping the blade fully inserted as in Figure 10-7, gently extend the plane of dissection right and left to the full 10-mm width; stabilize the globe by grasping the sclera posterior to the groove. Avoid grasping the scleral flap because it might tear. Judge the depth of the scleral-corneal dissection by viewing the blade through the translucent sclera. Keep the sclera moist to give greater visibility of the blade (see Figures 10-7 and 10-8).

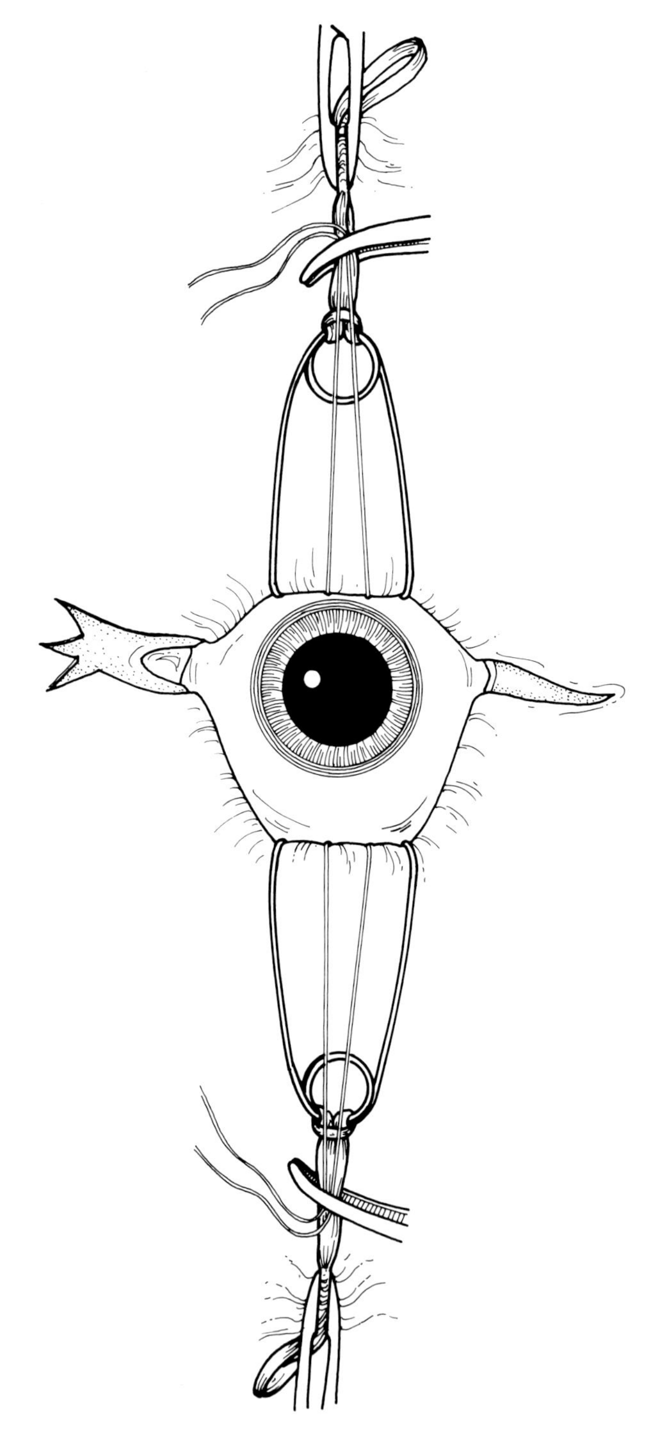

FIGURE 10-2 Surgeon's view of placement of Jaffe wire lid specula and rectus sutures. Note that good exposure of the operative site is achieved while still allowing visibility of the inferior limbus.

Use a disposable phaco keratome to penetrate the anterior chamber, making an incision parallel to the iris plane. It helps to aim the point of the blade somewhat posteriorly until initial penetration is achieved to avoid sliding up along corneal lamellae and entering the anterior chamber more centrally than desired. After penetration of the blade point, level out the blade

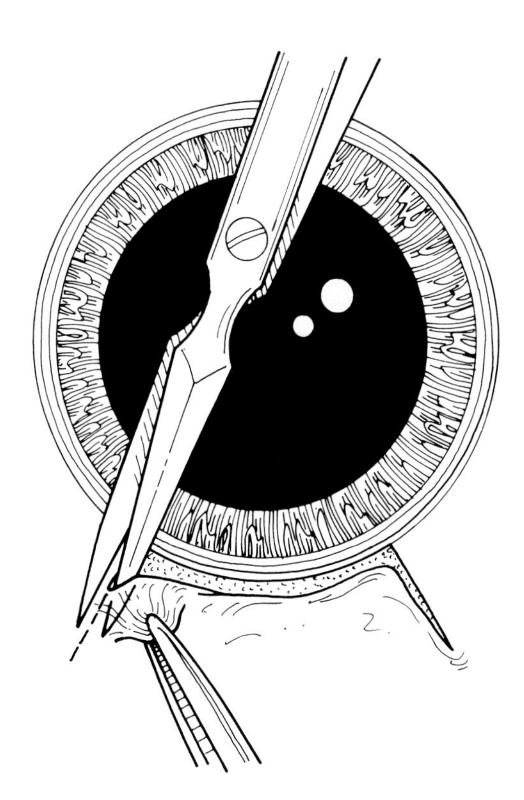

FIGURE 10-3 Expose the superior limbus with a 7-mm peritomy and oblique relaxing incisions.

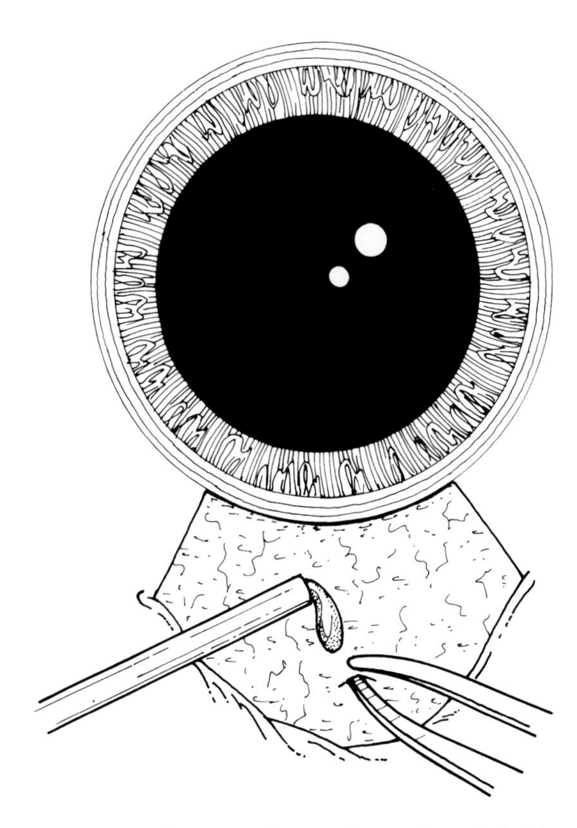

FIGURE 10-4 Cauterize surface vessels posterior to the incision site.

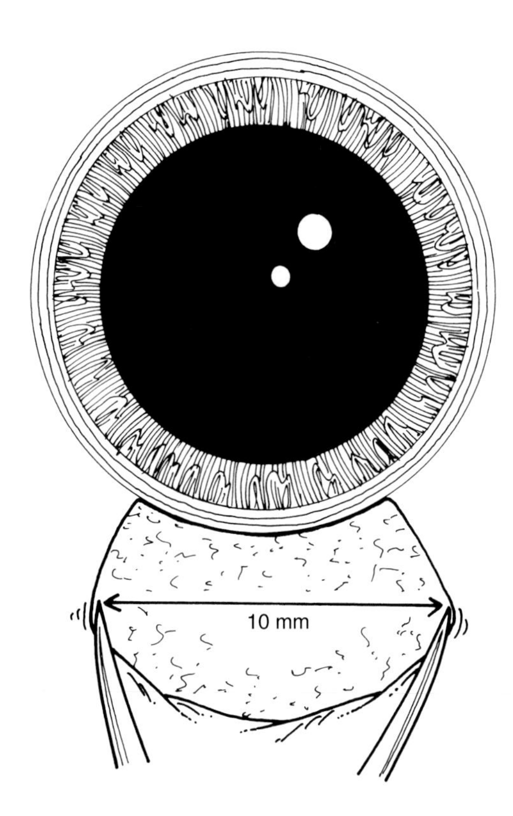

FIGURE 10-5 Incision site: a 10-mm chord length 3 mm posterior to the limbus.

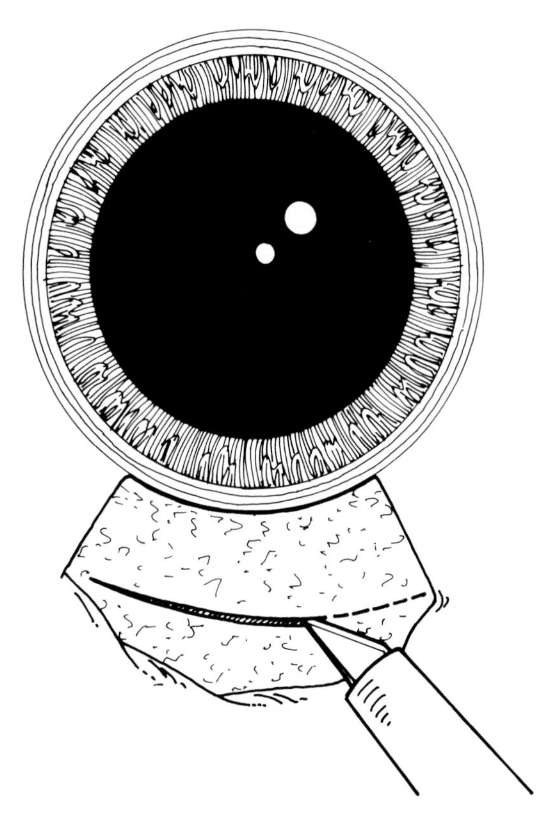

FIGURE 10-6 Place incision groove parallel with the limbus 3 mm posterior to the anterior limbal margin.

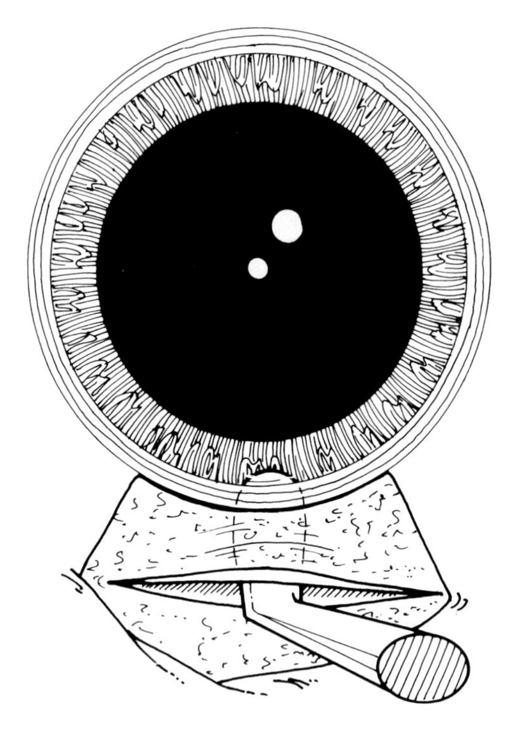

FIGURE 10-7 Dissection of scleral tunnel using crescent blade.

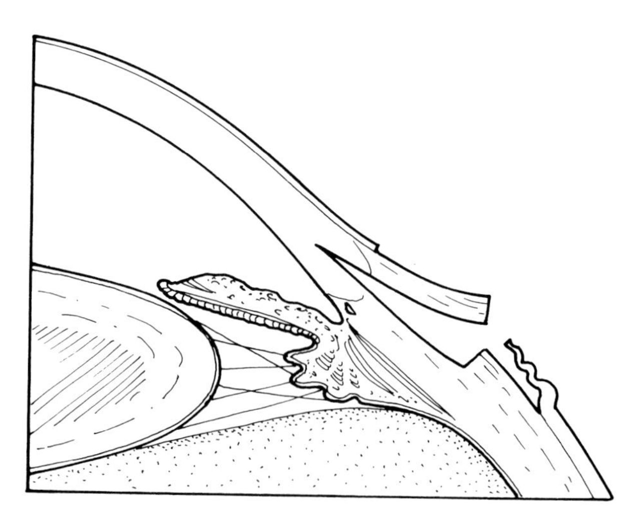

FIGURE 10-8 Cross-sectional view of cornea and sclera showing depth and extent of scleral tunnel.

so that it remains parallel to the plane of the iris and then push in to make a 1.5-mm opening. You will extend this incision later after the anterior capsulectomy (Figure 10-9).

Anterior Capsulectomy

Fully inflate the anterior chamber with a viscoelastic such as sodium hyaluronate. Use a 27-gauge disposable needle with a small microhook at its tip to create a 6- or 7-mm circular anterior capsulectomy. Make very small bites directed parallel with the pupillary margin. Each bite after the first should begin on top of the anterior capsule about 1 mm from the adjacent capsular incision (Figure 10-10). A fluid movement of the microhook should first puncture the capsule with slight posterior pressure and then sweep parallel with the pupillary margin until the tear joins the adjacent incision.

The capsulectomy should be at least 6 mm in diameter. Smaller-diameter openings lead to rather large tears of the peripheral capsule that tend to destabilize the lens implant. An opening of 6 to 7 mm gives a reasonable margin of peripheral anterior capsule, while allowing the nucleus to prolapse with less pronounced radial tearing.

After completion of the circular anterior capsulectomy, reinsert the blade that was used to make the original entry into the anterior chamber and extend the entry site to about 3 mm. Inject additional viscoelastic before this step as needed. (The surgeon may make the initial entry 3 mm wide to skip this step. The 1.5-mm initial entry was suggested to help retain the viscoelastic and to maintain the depth of the anterior chamber throughout the capsulectomy.) Remove the fragment of anterior capsule using toothless forceps. Insert the crescent blade and extend the third plane of the incision parallel to the iris plane to the full 10-mm width of the previous flap dissection (Figure 10-11). Use pushing strokes of the crescent blade to cut the third plane; this helps make a watertight valve incision.

Removal of the Nucleus

Put three interrupted 8-0 Vicryl or 9-0 black silk sutures across the lips of the scleral groove, taking about a 1-mm bite on each side. Place them so that when they are tied they will be equally spaced across the wound, giving four 2.5-mm openings for passage of the irrigation-aspiration instrument (Figure 10-12). Loop the sutures around the margins of the groove, as shown in Figure 10-12.

Using the McIntyre 26-gauge cannula attached to an irrigating cystotome handpiece, prolapse the superior lens nucleus into the anterior chamber. Pass the McIntyre 26-gauge cannula into the anterior chamber at the 12 o'clock position. Move the tip over to the 2 o'clock position and slide it beneath the margin of the anterior capsular leaflet. Retract the leaflet toward the lens equator rather firmly to allow the cannula to pass beyond the equator. Then, press slightly posterior with the whole shaft (not just the tip) of the cannula while gently irrigating with gravity flow through the handpiece. Maintain posterior pressure against the scleral wound while holding the shaft of the instrument parallel to the plane of the iris to help bring the nucleus forward. The lens nucleus begins to cleave from the posterior capsule, allowing the tip of the cannula to pass beneath the equator of the nucleus. After cleavage begins and irrigation forms a space between the edge of the nucleus and the posterior capsule, lift slightly on the edge of the nucleus to enhance the cleavage, slide the cannula slightly to the right in the cleavage, lift on the edge of the nucleus again, depress slightly and slide into the cleavage to the right again, lift again on the nucleus, and so on, repeating this movement slowly to allow the nucleus to cleave and lift away from the posterior capsule. The movement should be slow and deliberate to give the nucleus time to separate gently from the posterior capsule. Continue this movement until the superior quarter to half of

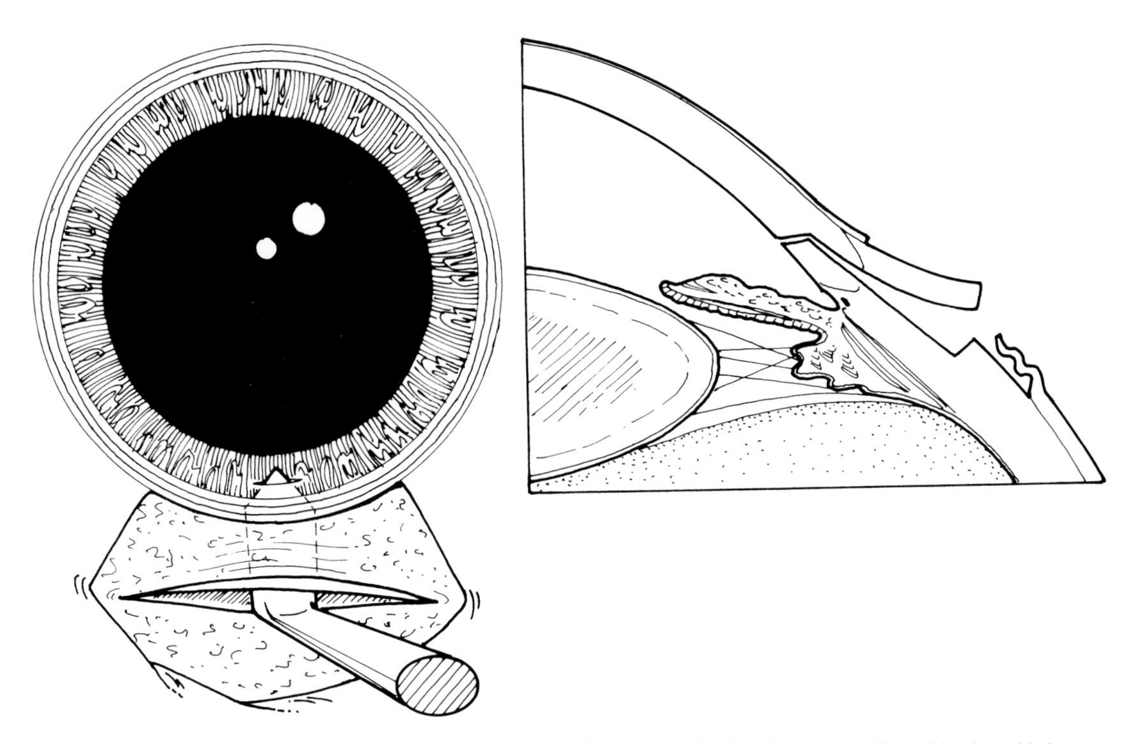

FIGURE 10-9 Plane three of the incision: penetration into the anterior chamber using a disposable phaco blade. Inset shows cross-sectional view of incisional planes.

the nucleus emerges through the pupil into the anterior chamber (Figures 10-13 and 10-14).

Attach a Knolle-Pearce irrigating lens loop (Storz E0631) in the irrigating handpiece and adjust the bottle height to get a rapid drip of fluid. Pass the lens loop through the incision and then gently beneath the nucleus, allowing time for the fluid to dissect ample space between the nucleus and the posterior capsule. Lift slightly on the nucleus, slide into the cleavage plane, lift slightly again, slide further into the cleavage plane, and so on. Repeat this sequence until the nucleus floats up away from the posterior capsule and toward the wound. The lens loop should now be positioned beneath the central nucleus.

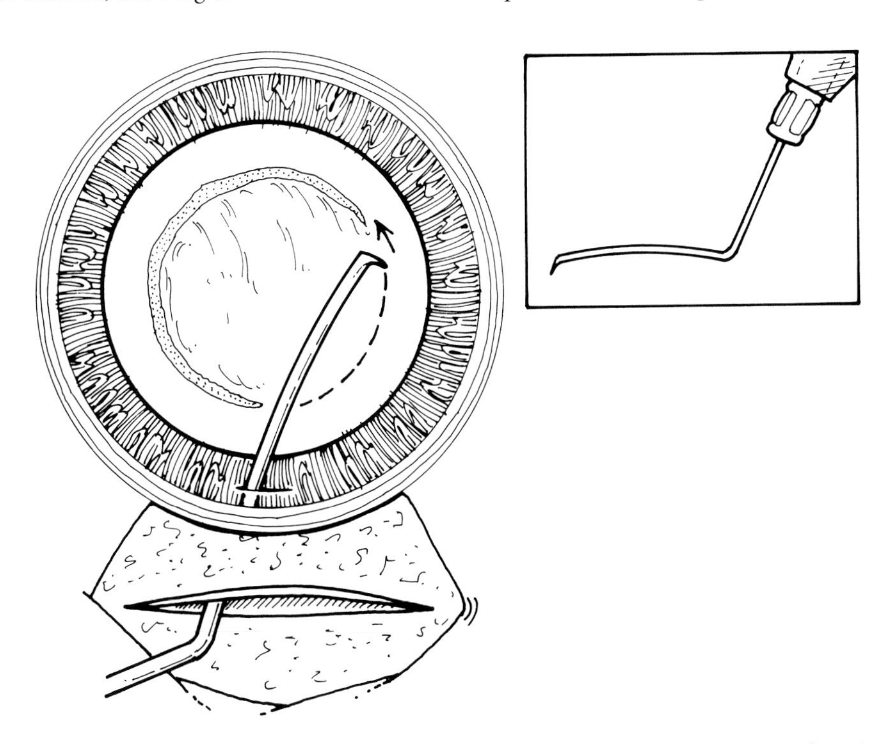

FIGURE 10-10 Anterior capsulectomy. For this, bend a 27-gauge disposable needle into the configuration shown in the inset. Attach the needle to a small syringe, which serves as a handle.

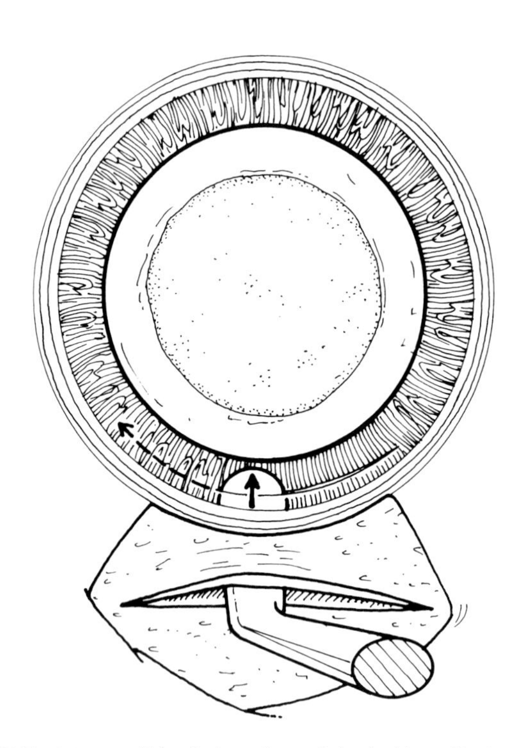

FIGURE 10-11 Extend plane three of the incision with the crescent blade.

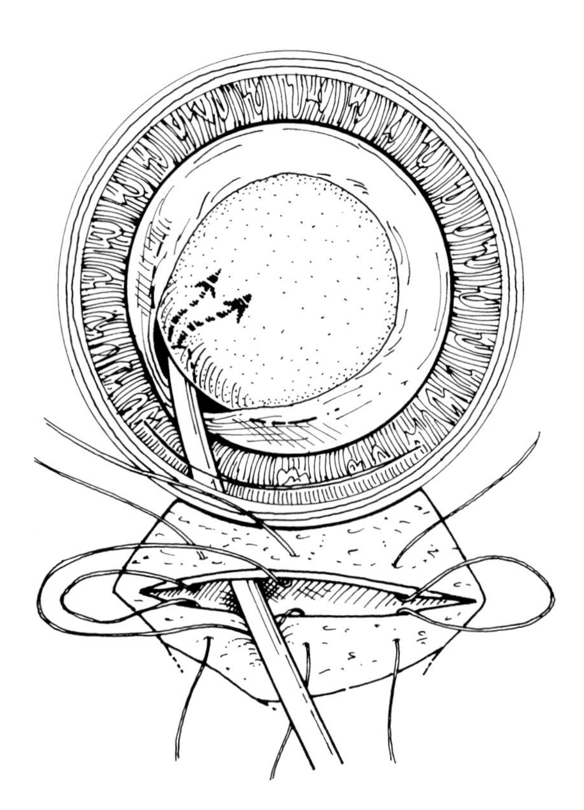

FIGURE 10-13 Technique for prolapse of superior nucleus into the anterior chamber using the McIntyre 26-gauge cannula with irrigation.

Hesitate until fluid builds up and pushes the nucleus against the internal lip of the wound. Then withdraw the loop while applying slight posterior pressure at the same time, lift slightly on the anterior scleral lip with forceps held in the free hand. Most nuclei come readily through a 10-mm incision, but an occasional large hard compact nucleus comes out more readily after extending the scleral incision to a width of 11 mm (Figures 10-15 and 10-16).

Commonly, a rumpled shell of epinuclear cortex strips away from the nucleus as it passes out of the eye and remains

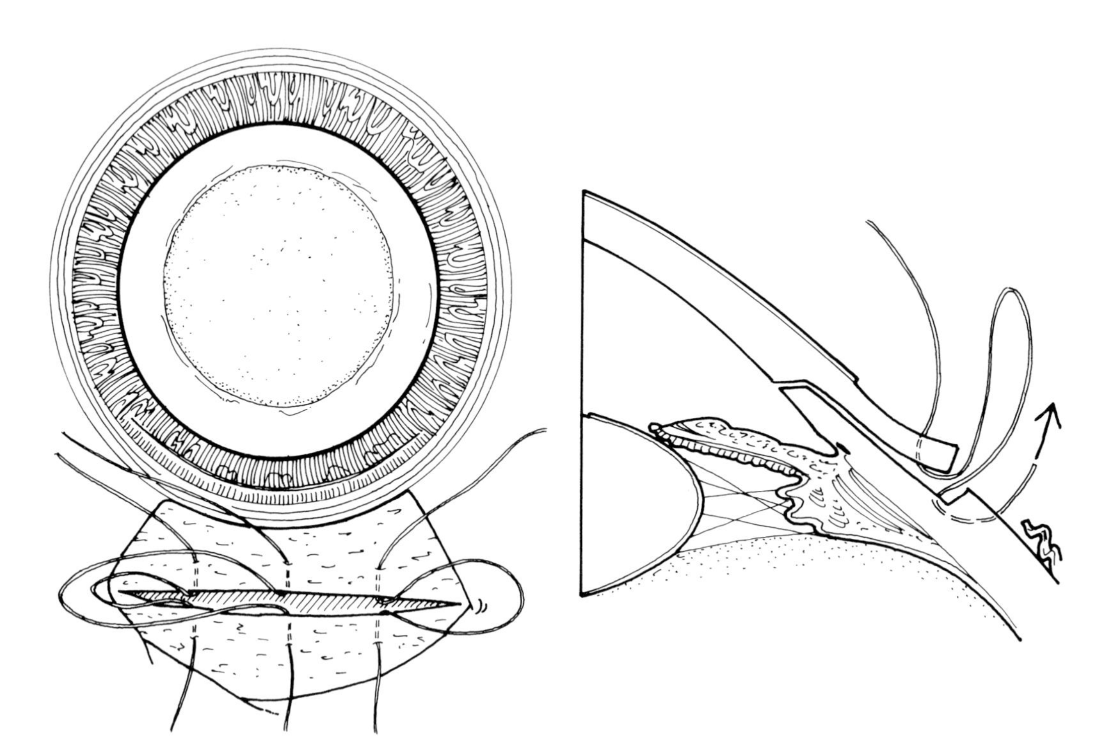

FIGURE 10-12 Technique for placement of three interrupted 9-0 black silk sutures.

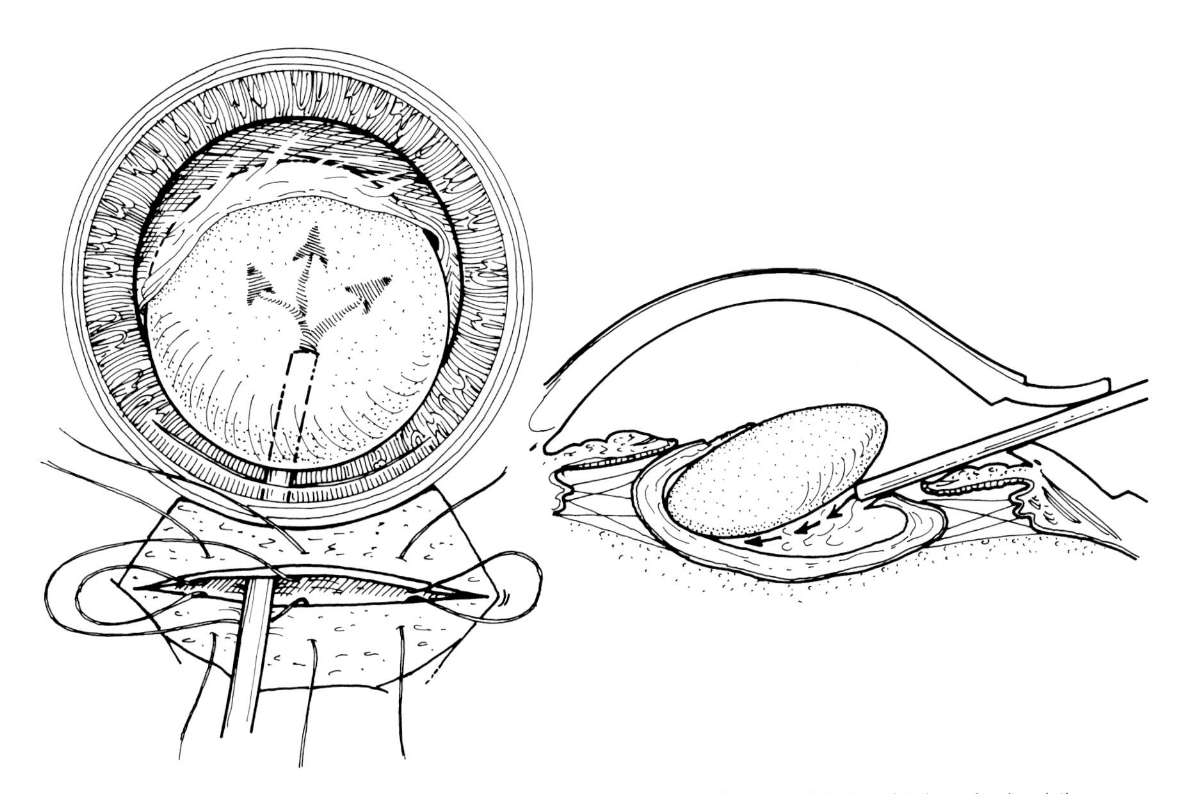

FIGURE 10-14 Prolapse of nucleus into anterior chamber is facilitated by infusion of balanced salt solution posterior to nucleus.

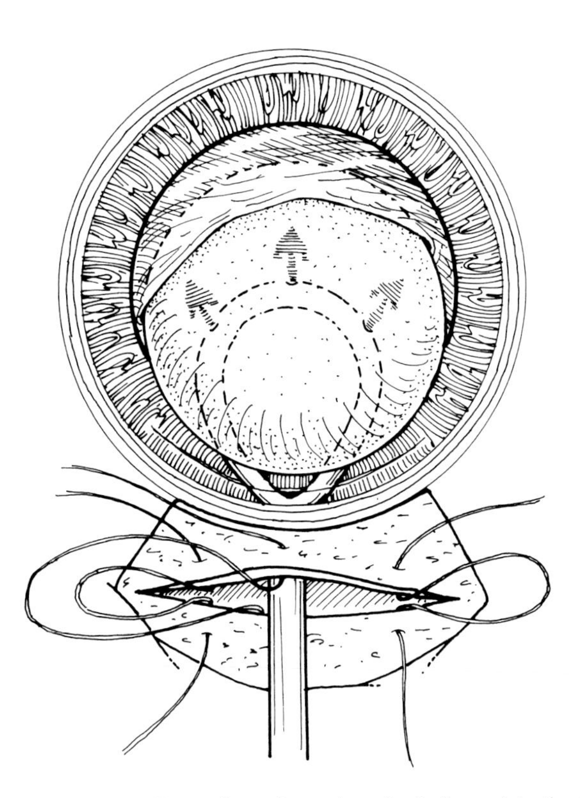

FIGURE 10-15 Extract the nucleus using a Knolle-Pearce irrigating lens loop.

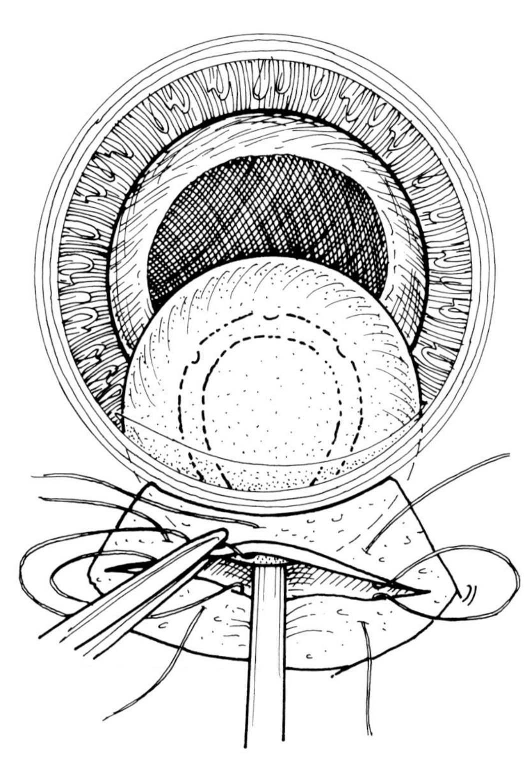

FIGURE 10-16 The lens loop draws the nucleus through the wound.

adjacent to the internal lip of the wound. Irrigate this loose cortex from the anterior chamber using a Randolph cannula attached to a squeeze bottle of balanced solution.

Removal of the Cortex

Tie the three preplaced sutures. Use either an automated irrigation-aspiration device, such as that found with equipment supplied for phacoemulsification or extracapsular surgery, or a manual irrigation-aspiration instrument. Insert the tip of the irrigation-aspiration device through any of the 2.5-mm wound segments between the sutures as needed for easy access. Insert the instrument with the aspiration hole aimed anteriorly.

Place the tip of the instrument gently into the capsular fornix while keeping close to the posterior capsule to avoid aspirating the free anterior capsular flap. This allows the cortex in the capsular fornix to occlude the opening as aspiration begins, helping prevent aspiration of the anterior capsular leaflet. About 1 second after initiating gentle aspiration, withdraw the tip of the aspiration device into the pupillary space to verify that cortex is attached to it. Once the surgeon confirms that the irrigation port is aspirating cortex and is free of other unwanted attachments, the aspiration vacuum can be increased to complete aspiration of the attached cortical fragment. Remove the cortex sequentially from adjacent sites until all has been removed. As each fragment is aspirated, slowly bring the tip of the instrument into the center of the pupil to strip cortex away from the posterior capsule and simultaneously to aspirate it.

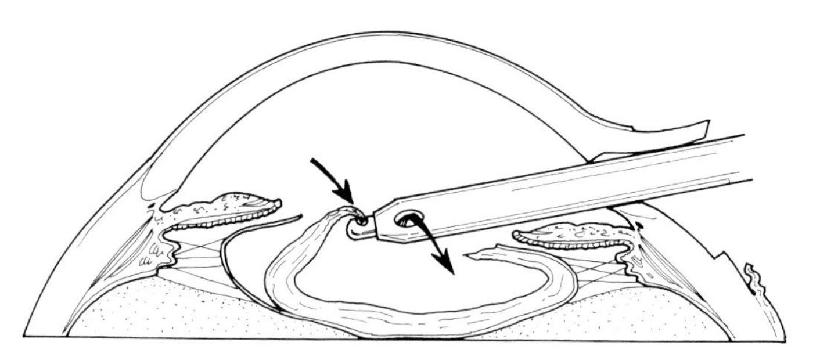

FIGURE 10-18 Cross-sectional view of cortical aspiration.

Begin aspirating cortex at the 6 o'clock position and then remove it gradually as illustrated until cortex remains only adjacent to the wound. Usually cortex adjacent to the wound can be removed by inserting the aspiration tip at the far right side of the incision to remove cortex next to the left part of the incision, and vice versa. If cortex near the wound is adherent, irrigate it using a curved Binkhorst aspiration cannula attached to a syringe. This usually loosens it so that it can be more easily removed by the aspiration tip (Figures 10-17 to 10-20). If these maneuvers do not remove the cortex, aspirate it carefully using a curved Binkhorst cannula attached to a syringe containing balanced salt solution after inflating the capsular bag with a viscoelastic agent.

Polish the posterior capsule with a capsule polishing instrument (Figure 10-21). Any cortex that can be readily removed will

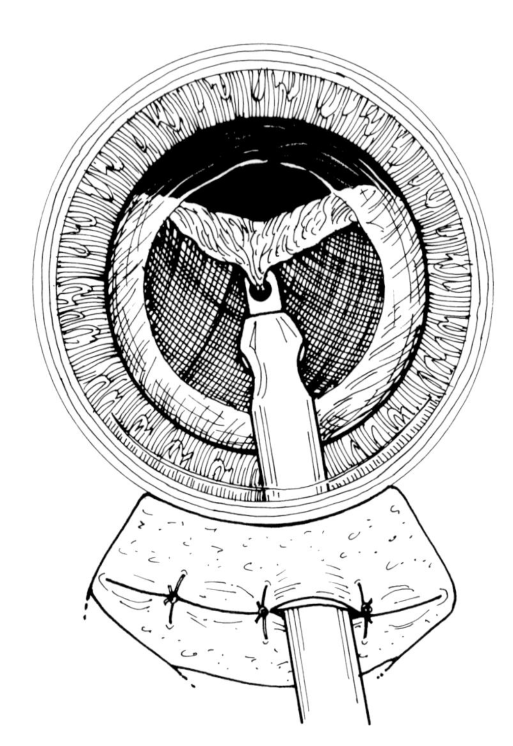

FIGURE 10-17 Remove residual cortex from posterior capsule using irrigation-aspiration instrument beginning at the 6 o'clock position (surgeon's view).

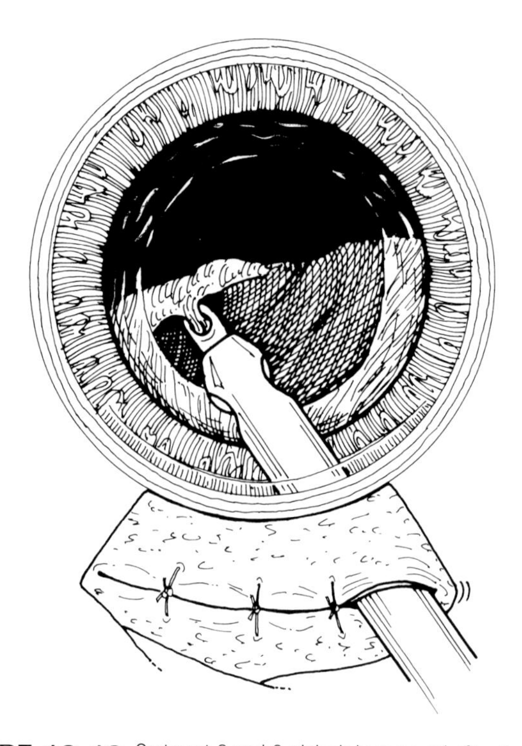

FIGURE 10-19 Cortex at 3 and 9 o'clock is removed after the inferior cortex.

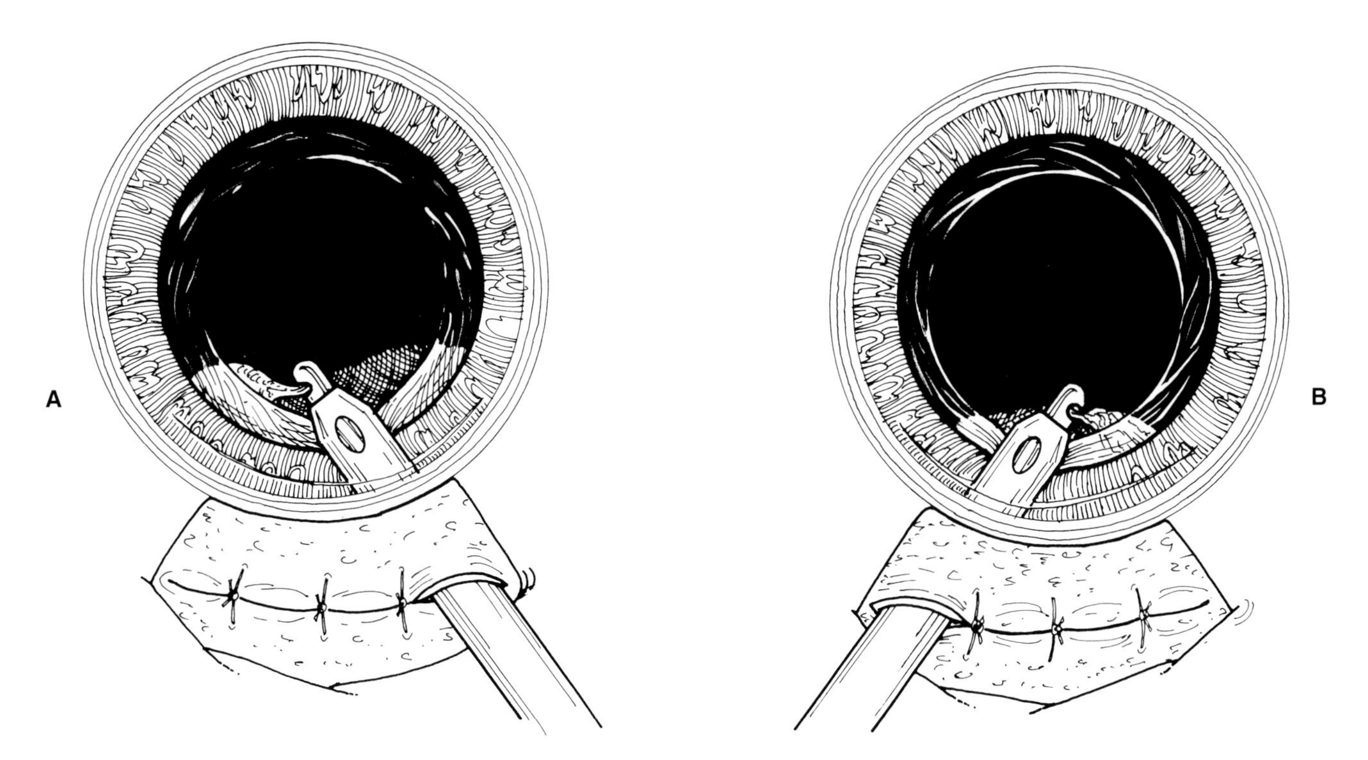

FIGURE 10-20 Aspiration of cortex at 12 o'clock position is made easier by inserting the irrigation-aspiration instrument through the far right side of the incision to remove cortex at the 12 to 1 o'clock position **(A)** and through the far left of the incision to remove cortex at the 11 to 12 o'clock position **(B).**

be rubbed off the capsule. If residual fibrotic material does not readily come off, this may be left for later neodymium:yttrium-aluminum-garnet laser capsulotomy. With an appropriate aspiration device that includes a "capsule vacuuming" mode, residual cortical material can be vacuumed away from the posterior capsule with reasonable safety (Figure 10-22).

Implantation of the Intraocular Lens

With a viscoelastic agent, fill the central anterior chamber and place additional viscoelastic beneath the anterior capsular flaps to inflate the capsule for in-the-bag IOL insertion. If the surgeon desires to place the lens implant into the ciliary sulcus, such as in a situation when the posterior lens capsule has ruptured, use viscoelastic beneath the iris to flatten the residual anterior capsule flap against the posterior capsule to inflate the space of the ciliary sulcus rather than inflating the lens capsule as described previously.

Remove the 11 o'clock and 12 o'clock temporary sutures in preparation for the lens insertion. Holding the lens with lens-insertion forceps (such as Bechert forceps), slide it into the anterior chamber. As the optic passes through the wound, tilt it to position the haptic to pass into the capsular bag (or sulcus, if desired). The inferior haptic should slide close to the posterior capsule and into the bag (or sulcus) as the optic passes through the wound incision (Figure 10-23). As the right hand releases the optic, the left hand, holding the superior haptic, pushes it in and to the left, thereby rotating the inferior haptic of the lens somewhat toward the 7 or 8 o'clock position.

After releasing the optic, grasp the superior haptic of the lens at its midpoint. In the left hand, use a blunt iris hook (Katena K3-5422) (Figure 10-24). Grasp the residual margin of the anterior capsule along with the margin of the iris and retract slightly toward the wound, using the blunt iris hook in the left

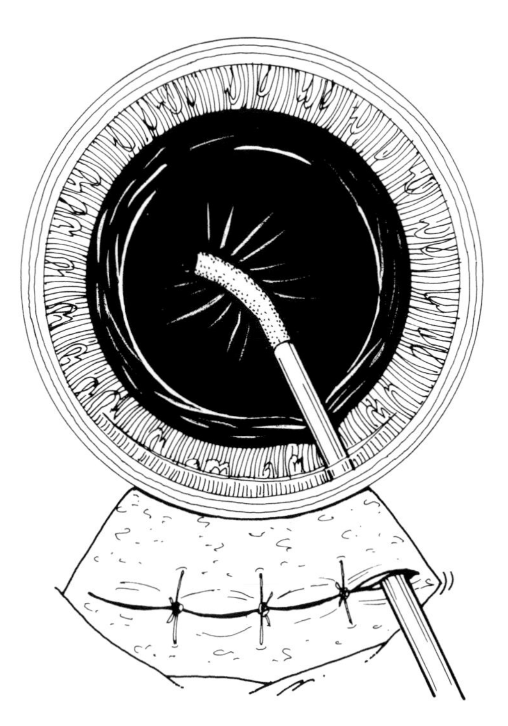

FIGURE 10-21 Polish the posterior capsule with a Kratz scratcher.

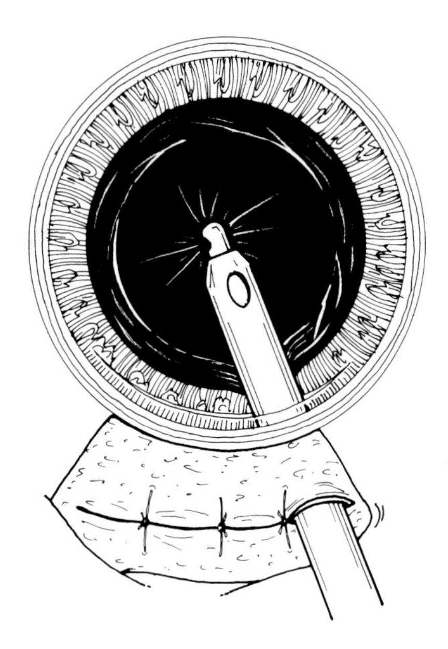

FIGURE 10-22 Aspiration of residual cortical material using irrigation-aspiration instrument and "capsule vacuuming" mode.

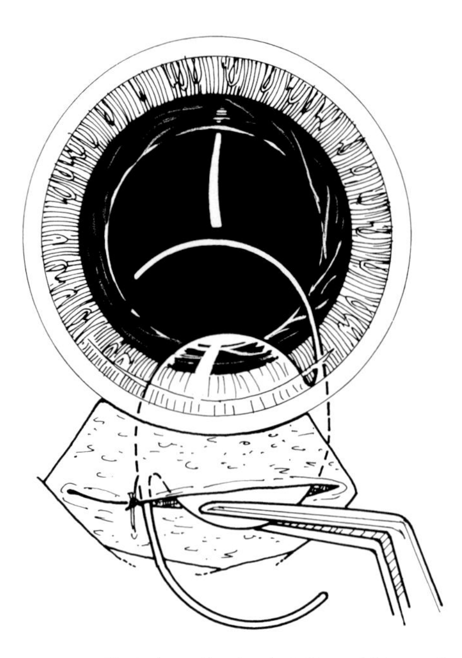

FIGURE 10-23 Technique for implantation of intraocular lens using viscoelastic.

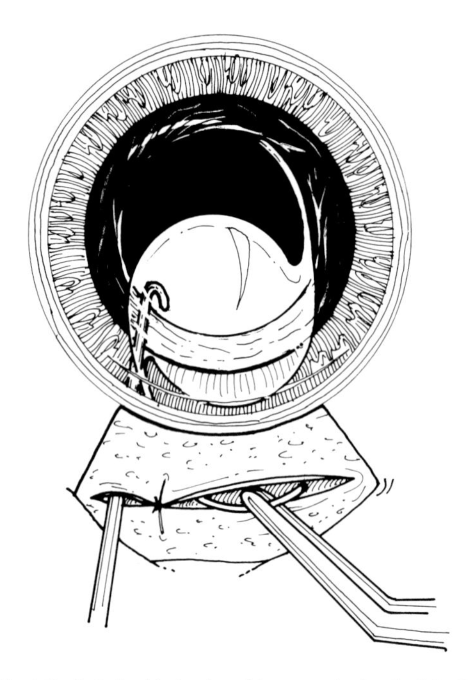

FIGURE 10-24 An iris hook guides superior haptic into the capsular bag.

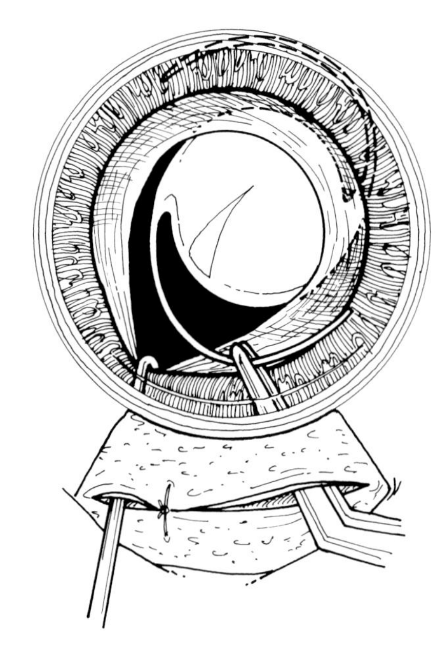

FIGURE 10-25 The iris hook can retract the anterior capsule and iris if necessary to allow accurate placement of the superior haptic into the capsular bag.

hand while passing the superior haptic into the anterior chamber and using the right hand with a vector of movement toward the position of the iris hook (Figure 10-25). This causes the lens to rotate into a horizontal position. The superior haptic is flexed sufficiently to clear the margin of the iris and the anterior capsule and to pass beneath the edge of the iris hook, which can in effect "shoe-horn" the superior haptic into the capsular bag by gliding the haptic beneath the hook. Once the superior haptic has been released into the capsule bag, a Sinskey hook may be used to rotate the lens slightly clockwise to settle it into a central position. Minimize manipulation of the lens to avoid dislocating a haptic from the bag into the ciliary sulcus.

Wound Closure

Place a corneal cover over the central cornea to block light from the microscope. Leave the temporary suture in place at the

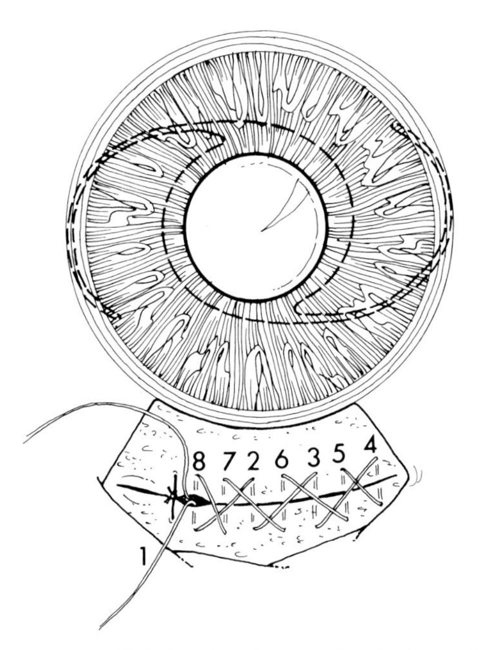

FIGURE 10-26 Technique for placement for shoelace suture—each bite is numbered in order. Suture is tied with knot in wound.

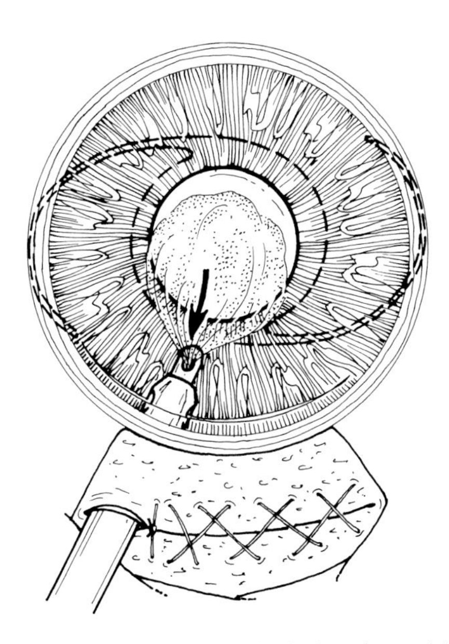

FIGURE 10-27 Removal of viscoelastic through remaining unsutured part of wound. Inject intraocular carbachol 0.01% to constrict pupil after removal of viscoelastic.

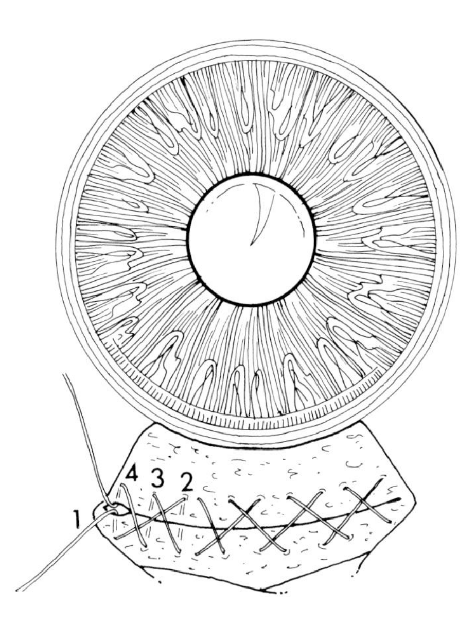

FIGURE 10-28 Remove remaining 9-0 silk suture and place 10-0 nylon shoelace suture as indicated, with each bite numbered in order of placement.

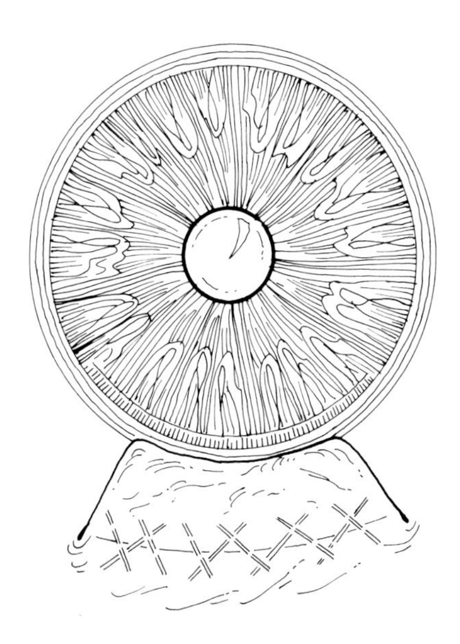

FIGURE 10-29 Appearance showing constricted pupil (carbachol) and conjunctival flap in place.

1 o'clock position; close the incision to the right of that suture with a running 10-0 nylon suture placed in a shoelace fashion as illustrated. In Figure 10-26, the initial penetration point of each bite of the suture is labeled sequentially to demonstrate how the suture is placed. The first bite starts within the lips of the wound and passes through only the posterior lip; the final bite passes only through the anterior lip, thereby allowing the two suture ends to come together and to be tied within the wound. Begin each suture bite after the first, about 1 mm from the anterior lip of the incision.

Pass the needle though the flap, then intralamellarly along the bed of the scleral dissection and finally through intact sclera. Exit 1 mm posterior to the scleral groove. Bury the knot within the lips of the wound next to the remaining temporary suture.

Aspirate residual viscoelastic material by passing the irrigation-aspiration instrument through the incision remaining open to the left of the temporary suture (Figure 10-27). Inject an intraocular miotic agent to constrict the pupil. Close the remainder of the wound with a 10-0 nylon suture using a modified shoelace configuration, as indicated (Figure 10-28). Close the conjunctival flap by applying wet-field coaptation forceps in the usual fashion along the oblique cuts nasally and temporally (Figure 10-29).

REFERENCES

1. Leaming DV: Practice styles and preferences of ASCRS members—1992 survey, *J Cataract Refract Surg* 19:603, 1993.
2. Leaming DV: Practice styles and preferences of ASCRS members—2000 survey, *J Cataract Refract Surg* 27:948-955, 2001.
3. Steinert RF, Brint SF, White SM et al: Astigmatism after small incision cataract surgery: a prospective, randomized, multicenter comparison of 4- and 6.5-mm incisions, *Ophthalmology* 98:417-423, 1991.
4. Hayashi K, Hayashi H, Nakao F, et al: The correlation between incision size and corneal shape change in sutureless cataract surgery, *Ophthalmology* 102:550-556, 1995.
5. Kohnen T, Dick B, Jacobi KW: Comparison of induced astigmatism after temporal clear corneal tunnel incisions of different sizes, *J Cataract Refract Surg* 21:417-424, 1995.
6. Oshika T, Nagahara K, Yaguchi S et al: Three year prospective, randomized evaluation of intraocular lens implantation through 3.2 and 5.5 mm incisions, *J Cataract Refract Surg* 24:509-514, 1998.
7. Olson RJ, Crandall AS: Prospective randomized comparison of phacoemulsification cataract surgery with a 3.2-mm vs a 5.5-mm sutureless incision, *Am J Ophthalmol* 125:612-620, 1990.
8. Werblin TP: Astigmatism after cataract extraction: 6-year follow-up of 6.5- and 12-millimeter incisions, *Refract Corneal Surg* 8:448, 1992.
9. Watson A, Sunderraj P: Comparison of small-incision phacoemulsification with standard extracapsular cataract surgery: postoperative astigmatism and visual recovery, *Eye* 6(part 6):626, 1992.
10. Laurell CG, Zetterstrom C, Phillipson B et al: Randomized study of the blood-aqueous barrier reaction after phacoemulsification and extracapsular cataract extraction, *Acta Ophthalmol Scand* 76:573-578, 1998.
11. Pande MV, Spalton DJ, Kerr-Muir MG et al: Postoperative inflammatory response to phacoemulsification and extracapsular cataract surgery: aqueous flare and cells, *J Cataract Refract Surg* 22(suppl 1):770-774, 1996.
12. Minassian DC, Rosen P, Dart JK et al: Extracapsular cataract extraction compared with small incision surgery by phacoemulsification: a randomized trial, *Br J Ophthalmol* 85:822-829, 2001.

Phacosection Cataract Surgery

11

David J. McIntyre, MD

This chapter describes my current choices for the various details, stages, techniques, and instrumentation used during routine cataract surgery. Personal reasons and justifications are briefly stated.

Anesthesia and Oculopression

We have returned to the use of topical anesthesia in routine cataract surgery based on the effectiveness of nonpreserved 2% lidocaine gel. Premedication is usually Versed 2.5 mg, sublingual, on a sponge spear, 20 minutes preoperatively. The dose is varied according to age, health, and weight. The gel is applied in the conjunctival sac before dilation and again as the patient is taken into the OR.

In order to achieve a consistent vitreous "softness," we apply 20 minutes of oculopression during the dilation and prep. The Oculopressor (Microsurgical Technology, Inc.) produces the equivalent of 30 mm Hg pressure (Figure 11-1). During the dilation and topical 50% iodophor solution is instilled. The same solution is used as a skin prep immediately before surgery. With this protocol patients are comfortable and cooperative, and intracameral lidocaine is seldom needed.

Limbus-Based Conjunctival Flap

A limbus-based conjunctival flap is an additional barrier to possible postoperative infection. Only time and sufficient experience will prove the necessity for this otherwise inconvenient and occasionally unsightly step in the procedure. Bipolar cautery is used sparingly, only for significant feeder vessels.

Location of Incision

There is no need for a bridal suture when a temporal incision is used. It also provides more direct access to the anterior chamber and cataract. There may be less astigmatic effect from the surgical procedure, although I doubt the significance of incision location. The traditional superior location is used when the procedure is combined with trabeculectomy.

The Anterior Chamber Maintainer

Pressurization of the anterior chamber (anterior chamber maintainer) is a distinct surgical aid during dissection of the tunnel incision, debulking of the lens, extraction of nucleus fragments, extraction of the epinucleus, aspiration of the cortex, and insertion of the intraocular lens (IOL) (Figure 11-2). Balanced salt solution (BSS) is supplied by gravity infusion to the chamber maintainer. I use an electric IV pole (with foot switch for the surgical assistant) to provide quick and convenient raising and lowering of the BSS bottle (Figure 11-3). Antibiotics are added to the BSS: gentamicin 4 mg/500 ml and vancomycin 10 mg/500 ml.

Self-Sealing Tunnel Incision

The self-sealing (frown) tunnel incision is made in stages (Figures 11-4 and 11-5). The incision is sized for the intended IOL. I use a 6-mm incision and a 5.5-mm one-piece IOL. The self-sealing incision has minimal effect on astigmatism. The patient has a safer, more durable postoperative course, and the surgical procedure is slightly faster. In addition, there is no requirement for expensive corneoscleral sutures and needles. The technique is as follows:

1. The superficial incision is marked and outlined on the surface of the sclera; I use a trifaceted diamond knife (Figures 11-6 and 11-7).
2. A thin or superficial tunnel dissection is made with a crescent knife. The tunnel is less than half the scleral thickness (Figure 11-8). The anterior chamber is not entered at this stage of the procedure.
3. A separate peripheral clear corneal stab puncture is made at a convenient location (Figure 11-9). I make this puncture near the end of the tunnel to my right-hand side.

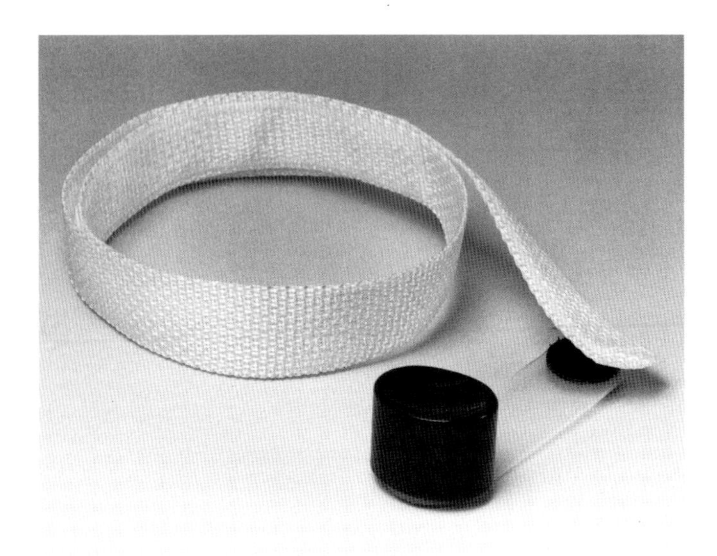

FIGURE 11-1 The Oculopressor conveniently provides an equivalent of 30 mm Hg pressure.

A

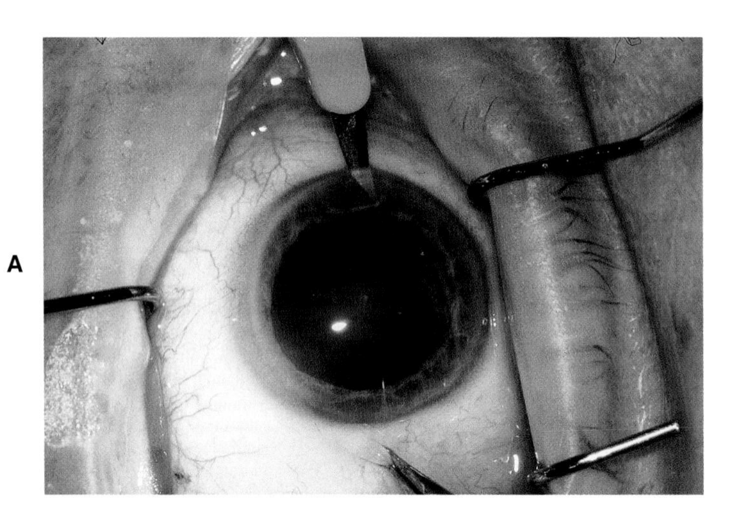

B

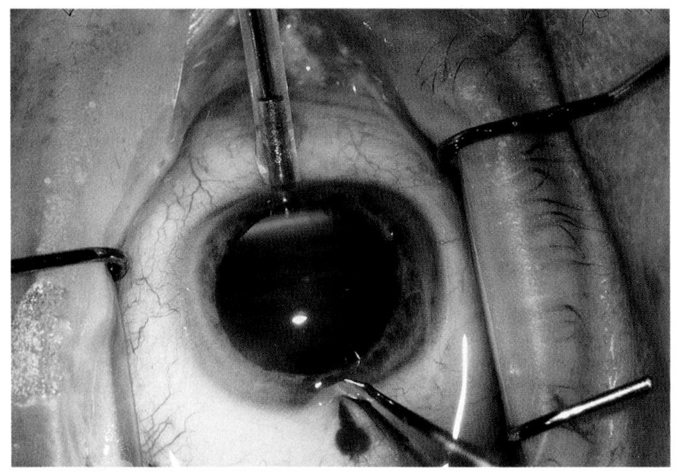

FIGURE 11-2 A and **B,** A 1-mm peripheral corneal puncture is made to allow insertion of a chamber maintainer with 0.6-mm inside diameter.

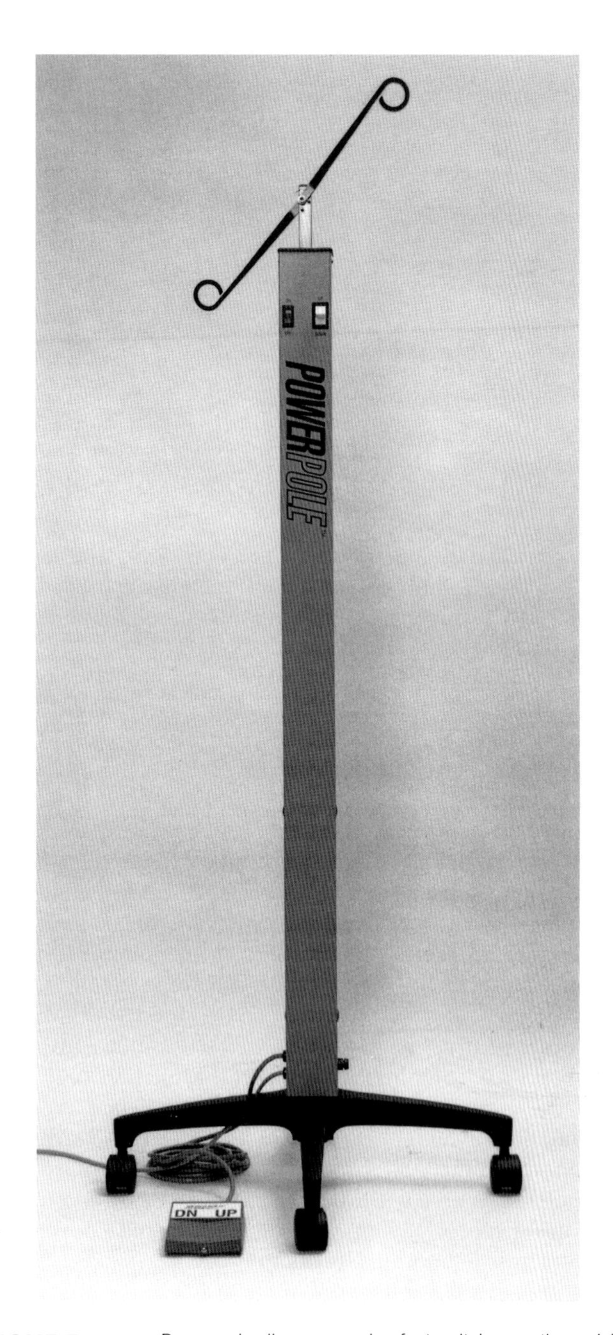

FIGURE 11-3 Power pole allows manual or foot switch operation, raising and lowering the infusion bottle as desired.

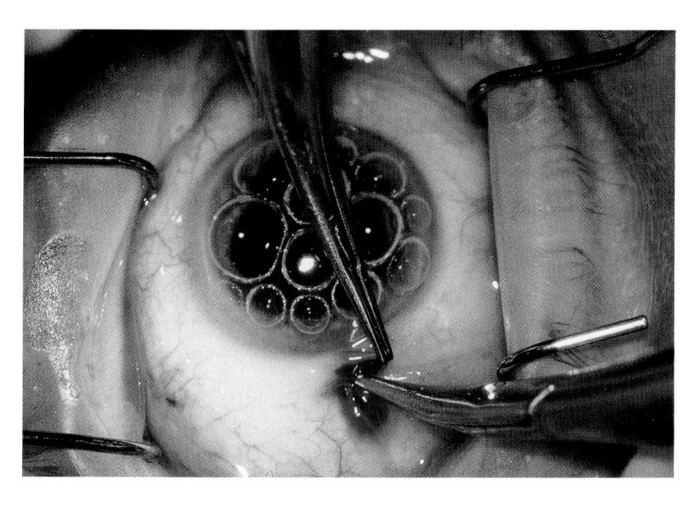

FIGURE 11-4 Limbus-based conjunctival flap is raised.

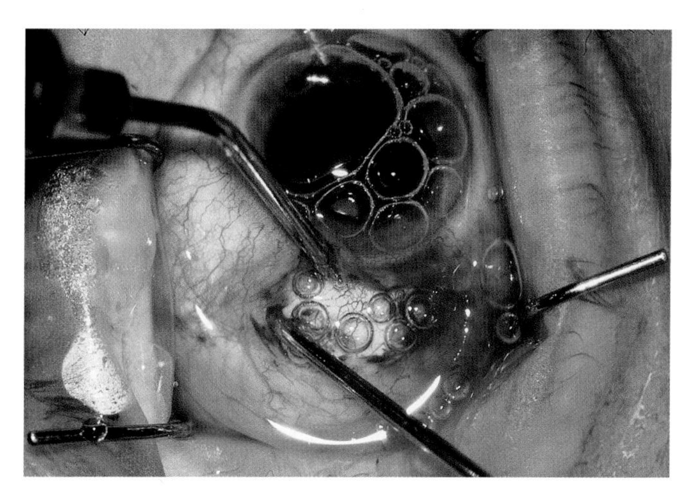

FIGURE 11-5 Episcleral feeder vessels are cauterized with bipolar.

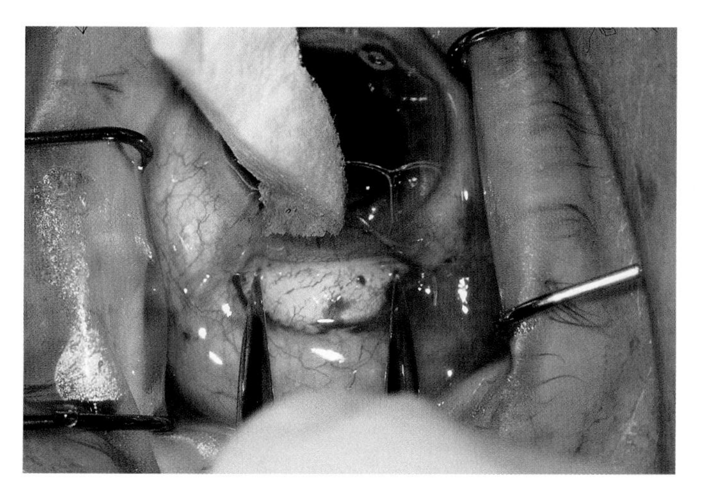

FIGURE 11-6 A 6-mm tunnel incision is marked in anticipation of the insertion of a 5.5-mm one-piece IOL.

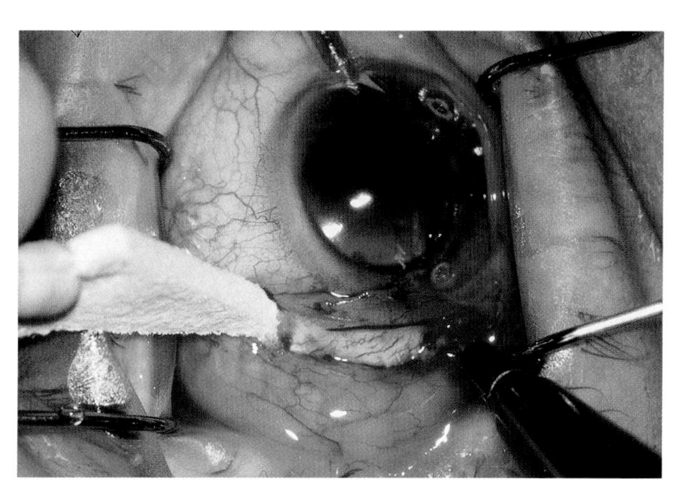

FIGURE 11-7 Initial scleral incision has a radius equal but opposite to the limbus.

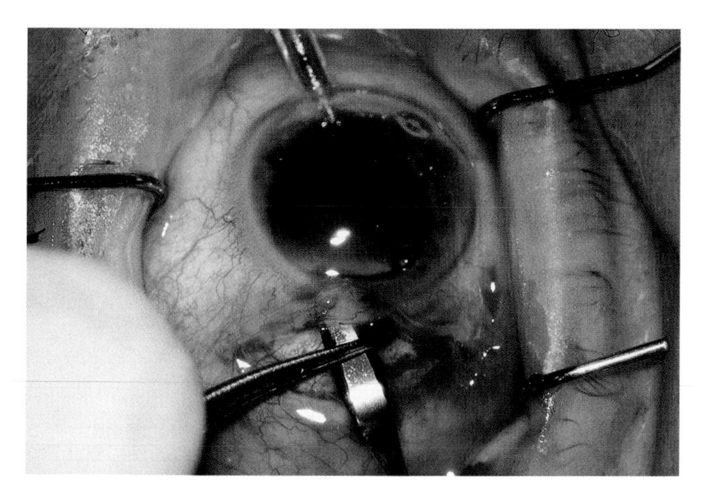

FIGURE 11-8 Tunnel is dissected at one-third scleral thickness without entering the anterior chamber.

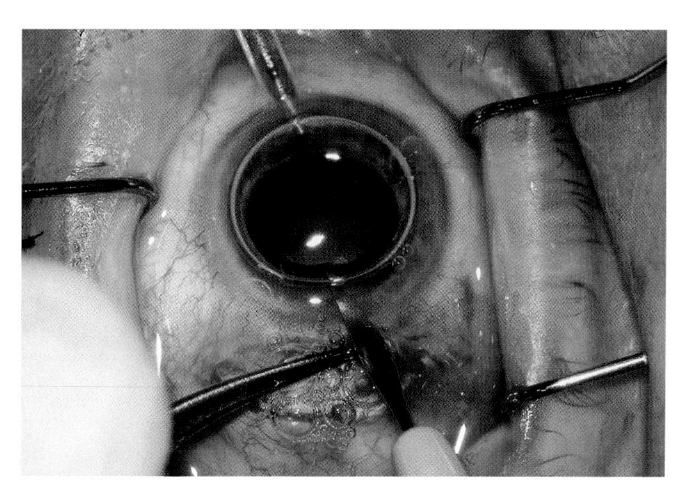

FIGURE 11-9 Separate peripheral clear corneal puncture allows manipulations in the anterior chamber while the tunnel remains sealed.

A

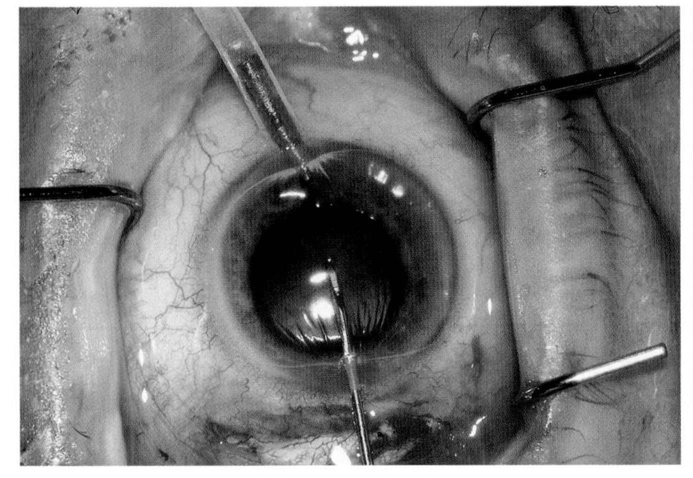

B

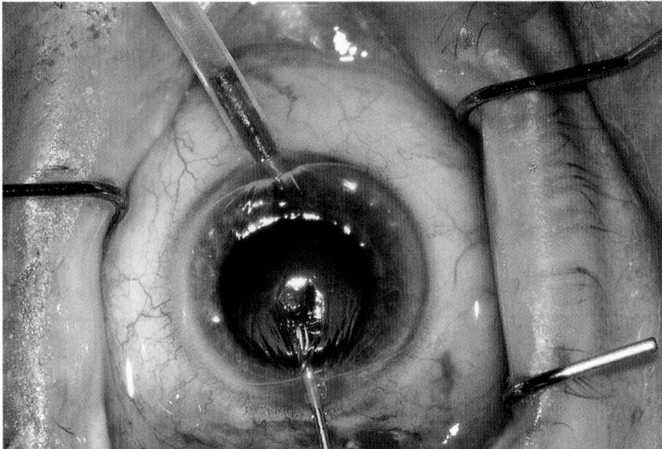

C

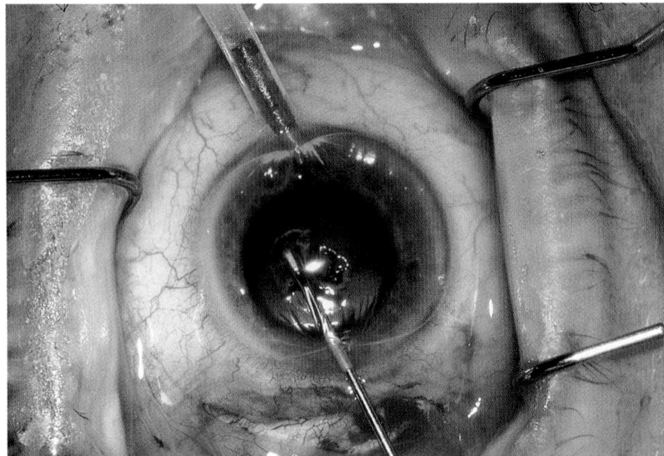

FIGURE 11-10 A, Chamber maintainer is shut off while a hooked cystotome introduces additional air and begins the capsulorhexis. **B,** Capsule is torn clockwise beginning in the subincisional area. **C,** Large air bubble enhances the visualization of the tear, controls the position of the torn fragment, and eliminates the magnification effect of the cornea.

Continuous Circular Capsulorhexis

With a continuous circular capsulorhexis there is less chance for extension of a capsular tear into the posterior capsule (Figure 11-10). The size of the continuous circular capsulorhexis must be adequate for the nucleus technique and for the size of the nucleus in the individual patient. The technique for a continuous circular capsulorhexis is as follows:

1. I prefer to use a hooked needle, entering through the stab puncture. The needle is attached to a small handpiece, and the extension tubing is attached to an air-filled syringe managed by the surgical assistant.
2. The anterior chamber maintainer is turned off.
3. As the anterior chamber is entered, a large air bubble is injected. In my opinion, this improves visualization during the capsulectomy and helps to press the flap of capsule against the surface of the cataract. The air bubble neutralizes the magnification effect of the cornea, which is normally 10% to 15%. Consequently, under an air bubble an apparent 6.5-mm capsulectomy circle is in fact 6.5 mm.
4. I begin with a small puncture at the center of the anterior capsule and then generate a tear that begins toward the incision and extends in clockwise fashion. In most cases, the phacosection technique is safely completed through a 6.5-mm capsulectomy.

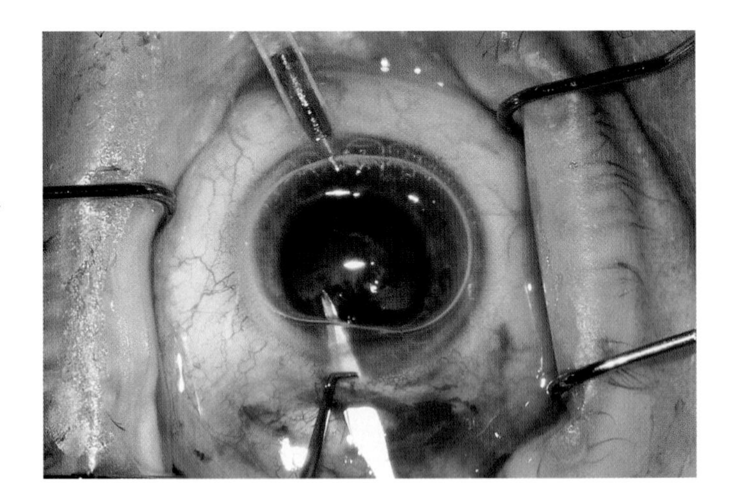

FIGURE 11-11 Chamber maintainer is turned on, and the anterior chamber is entered through the center of the tunnel dissection.

Following the anterior capsulectomy, the anterior chamber maintainer is turned on again. I use the 15-degree supersharp to enter the anterior chamber through the center of the dissected tunnel (Figure 11-11). The incision is then extended to its full length with the crescent blade (Figure 11-12).

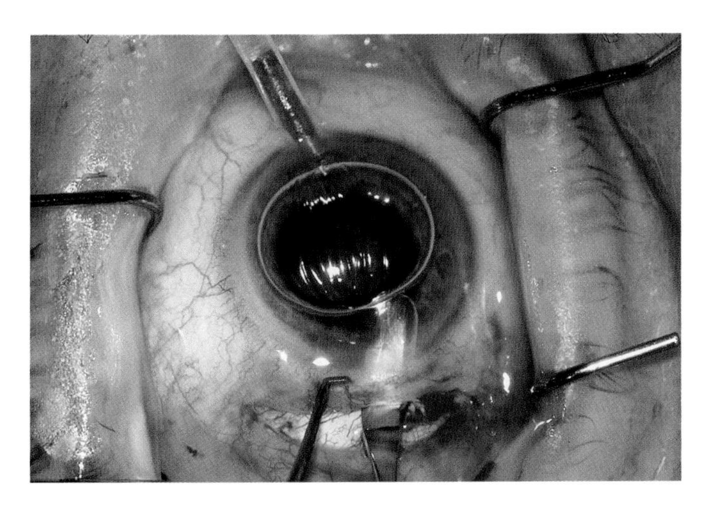

FIGURE 11-12 Tunnel opening into the anterior chamber is completed with the dissecting blade.

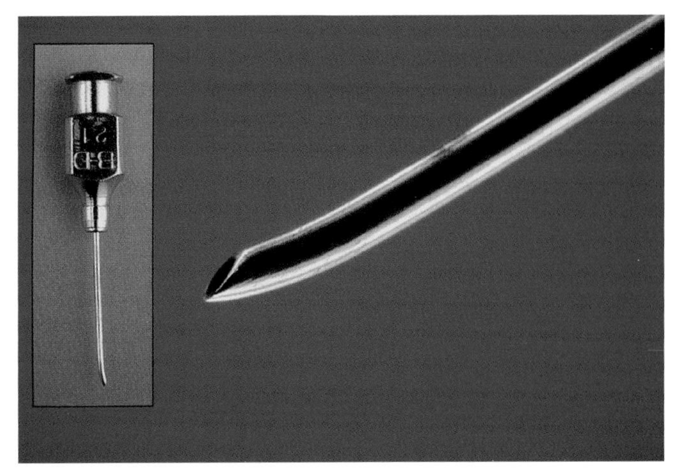

FIGURE 11-13 Oblique pointed 21-gauge aspirating cannula provides for large-bore aspiration.

Debulking the Cataract

To facilitate dissection and removal of the compact central nucleus when debulking the cataract, the cortex and epinuclear tissue lying over the nucleus are aspirated. When a youthful, soft nucleus is present in patients up to the age of 55 or 60 years, the entire lens content may often be aspirated. This then becomes a phacoaspiration cataract procedure rather than a phacosection procedure. The technique is as follows:

1. The anterior chamber maintainer bottle is raised.
2. The special 21-gauge aspirating needle (Figure 11-13), which is attached to a 5- to 6-ml syringe, enters through the peripheral corneal stab puncture.
3. The residual air bubble and fragment of anterior capsule are aspirated.
4. The cortex and epinucleus are aspirated (Figure 11-14), with special attention to removing the epinucleus toward the equator of the nucleus.

Removal of the Nucleus

The nucleus is removed by the phacosection technique. I emphasize that this is dependent on the use of a viscoelastic agent. The technique is as follows:

1. With the anterior chamber maintainer running on a low pressure, the anterior chamber is entered through the stab wound with a special 27-gauge cannula (Figure 11-15) on a 2- to 3-ml syringe.
2. The point of the cannula is introduced at the expected equator of the nucleus and is moved gently along the

A

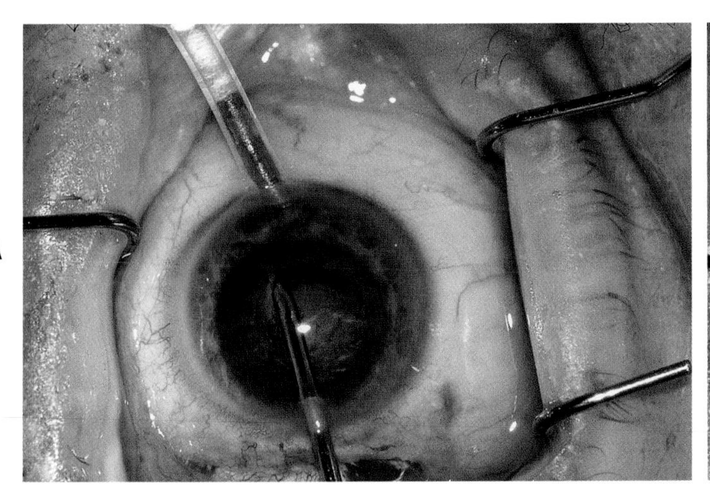

B

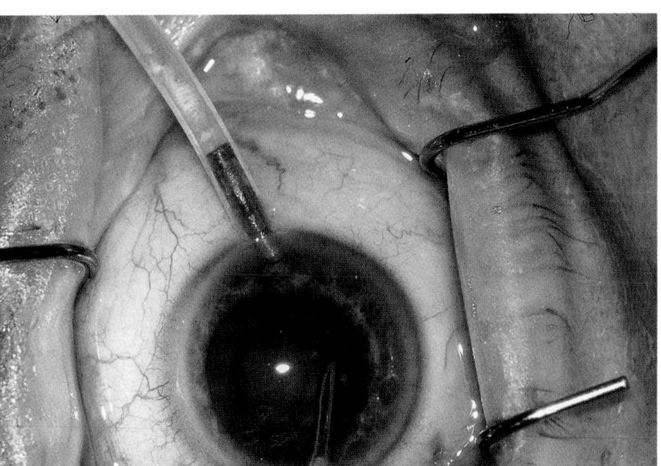

FIGURE 11-14 **A,** The 21-gauge aspirating cannula removes air and the capsulorhexis fragment and begins aspirating the anterior cortex and epinucleus. **B,** Debulking is carried to the surface of the compact nucleus, creating a furrow at its equator.

circumference of the equator while making minimal injections of BSS.
3. I customarily begin this dissection on the margin of the equator to my right.

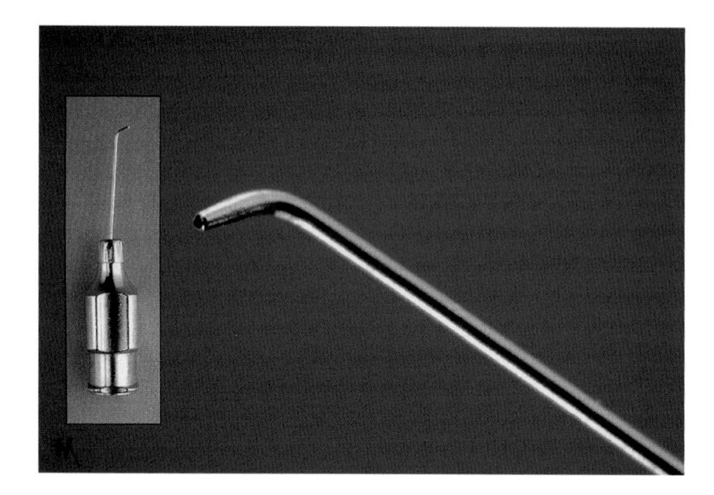

FIGURE 11-15 Semicurved 27-gauge cannula is used for hydrodissection.

4. The dissection is carried clockwise toward the incision and across my left.
5. When one third to one half of the equator has been dissected, the nucleus can often be tilted forward out of its nuclear sheath (Figure 11-16).
6. When the nucleus has been defined and loosened, the 27-gauge cannula is removed, the chamber maintainer is turned off, and viscoelastic material is injected through its cannula through the main tunnel incision. The viscoelastic material is used to provide a cushion in front of the nucleus and to ensure that the nucleus is free from its epinuclear sheath (Figure 11-17).
7. The nucleus cutters are then inserted over and under the nucleus (Figure 11-18). If the nucleus is quite small, the maintainer is again turned on and the nucleus is simply extracted. If the nucleus is larger than the tunnel incision, it is cut into three segments and the center portion is removed with the cutters, again with the anterior chamber maintainer running.
8. If the nucleus has been cut, two fragments will remain in the anterior chamber. The anterior chamber maintainer is turned off, and additional viscoelastic

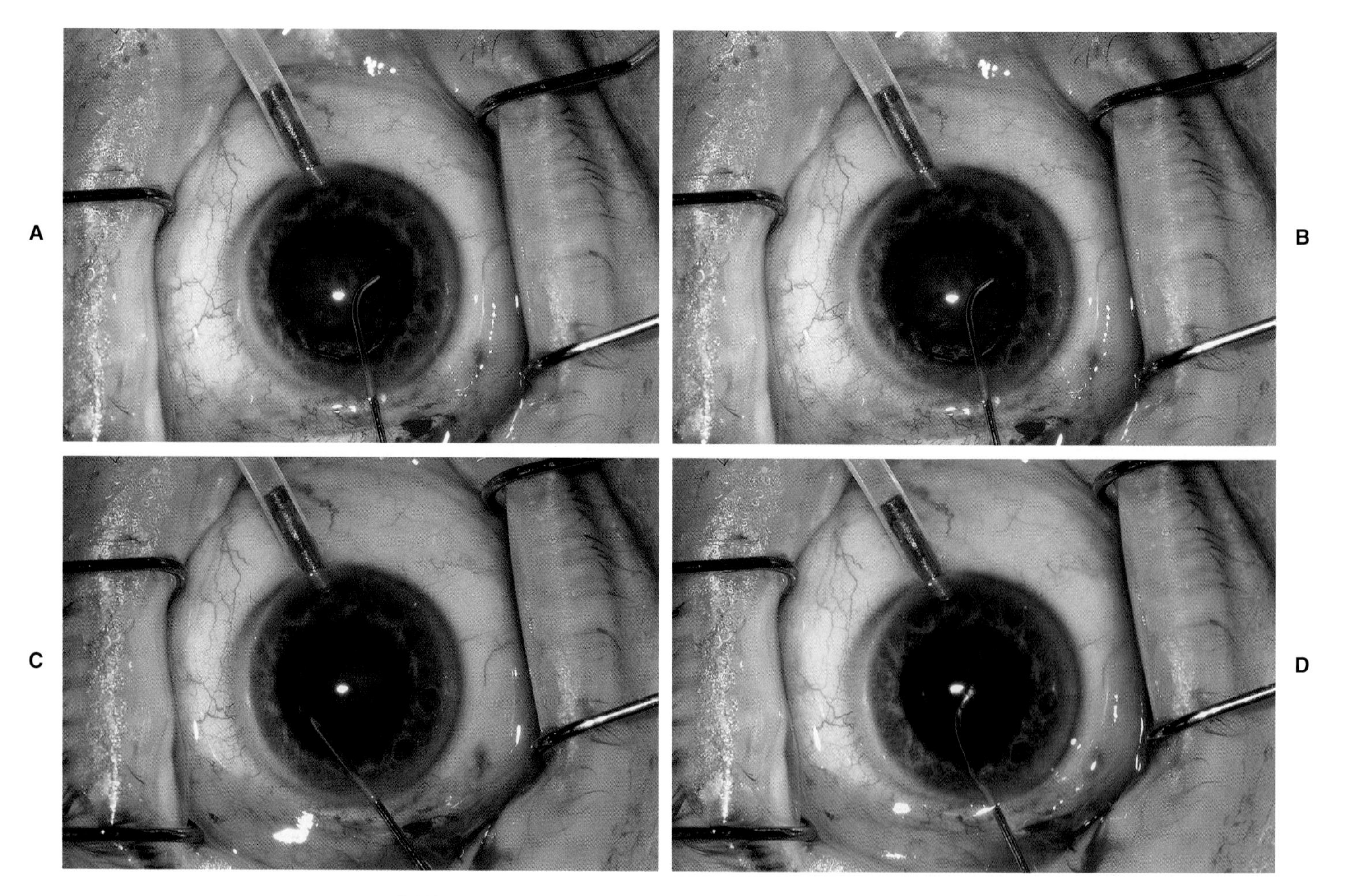

FIGURE 11-16 **A,** With balanced salt solution and the 27-gauge semicurved cannula, the equator of the nucleus is dissected. **B** to **D,** Sequentially, when one third to one half of its circumference is dissected, the nucleus can be elevated from the epinucleus by rotation of the semicurved cannula.

material is used to deepen the chamber over the second fragment and to stabilize its position (Figure 11-19, *A*).

9. The cutters are then used to grasp the second fragment, which is extracted with the anterior chamber maintainer turned on (see Figure 11-19, *B*).

10. If a third fragment remains, the anterior chamber maintainer is again turned off, additional viscoelastic agent is injected, and the fragment is extracted with the cutters while the anterior chamber maintainer is once again turned on.

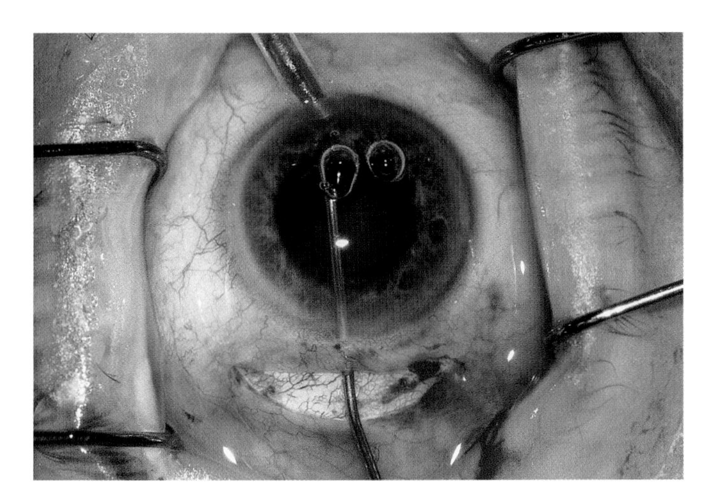

FIGURE 11-17 Anterior chamber maintainer is shut off while viscoelastic is placed over the compact nucleus.

The Epinucleus

Although it is possible to aspirate the epinucleus, particularly with the special 21-gauge cannula, this can be a somewhat dangerous procedure. It is often facilitated by removing the epinucleus in a single mass (Figure 11-20).

With the anterior chamber maintainer running, the 27-gauge cannula and BSS are used to hydrodissect extensively under the margins of the capsulectomy. Normally, the epinucleus will be extruded from the capsular bag as a solid mass and will come to be center of the pupillary space. In this position, the irrigating spoon is inserted under a portion of the epinucleus, and with the pressure of the chamber maintainer and intermittent additional injection of fluid through the irrigating spoon, the epinucleus is expulsed from the anterior chamber.

If the epinucleus is aspirated with a 21-gauge cannula, very gentle forces must be applied to the syringe to avoid grasping and possibly damaging the posterior capsule.

A

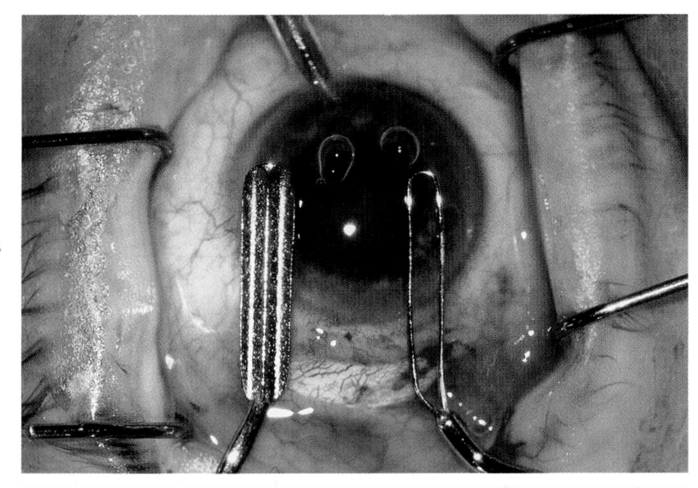

B

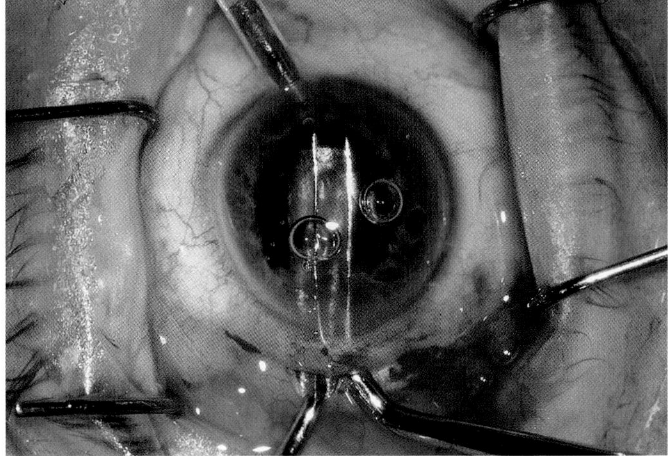

C

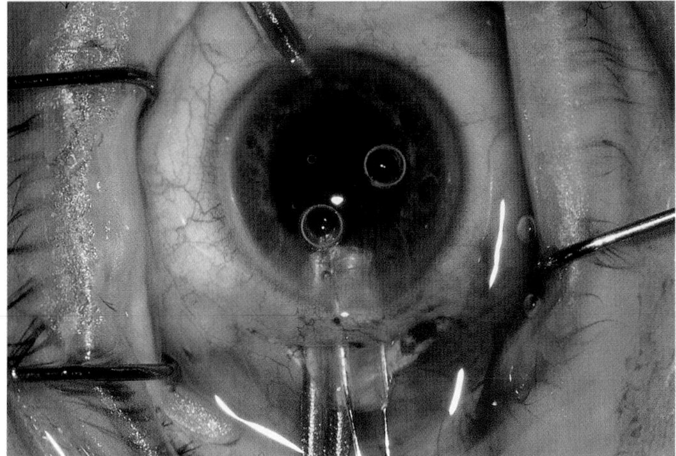

FIGURE 11-18 **A,** Majority of nuclei are sectioned with the double cutter and spatula. **B,** Spatula and double cutter are inserted into the anterior chamber to surround the compact nucleus. **C,** Cutter is pressed against the spatula, and as the contained fragment is extracted, the chamber maintainer is turned on.

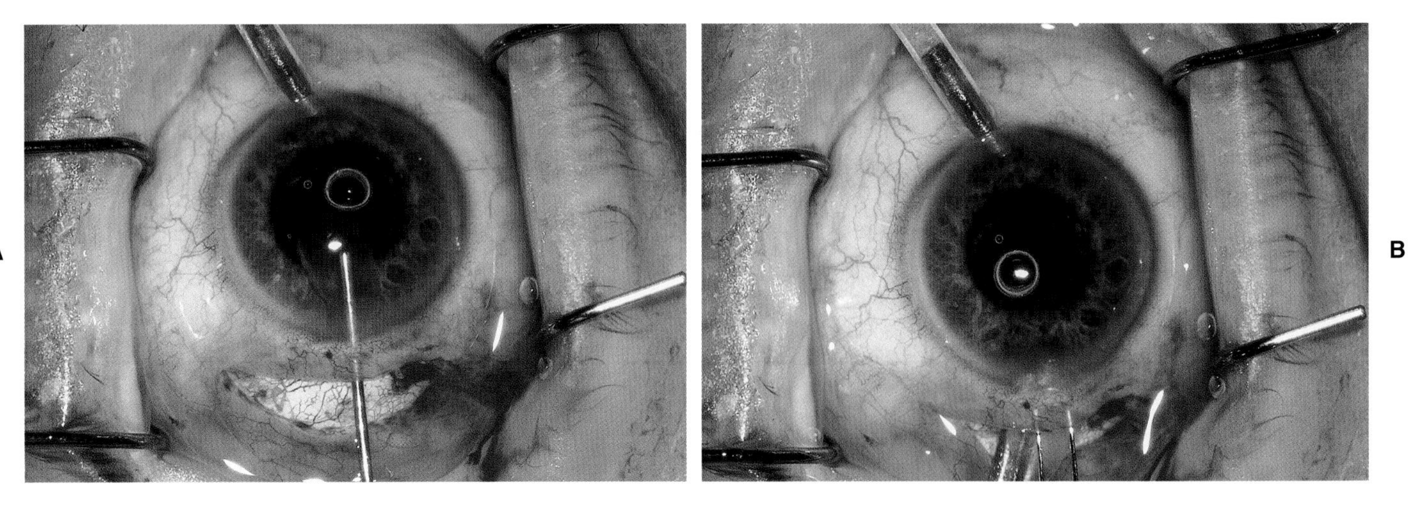

FIGURE 11-19 A, Before extraction of each nuclear fragment, the fragment is repositioned and surrounded with viscoelastic while the maintainer is shut off. **B,** Chamber maintainer is turned on again during extraction of each fragment.

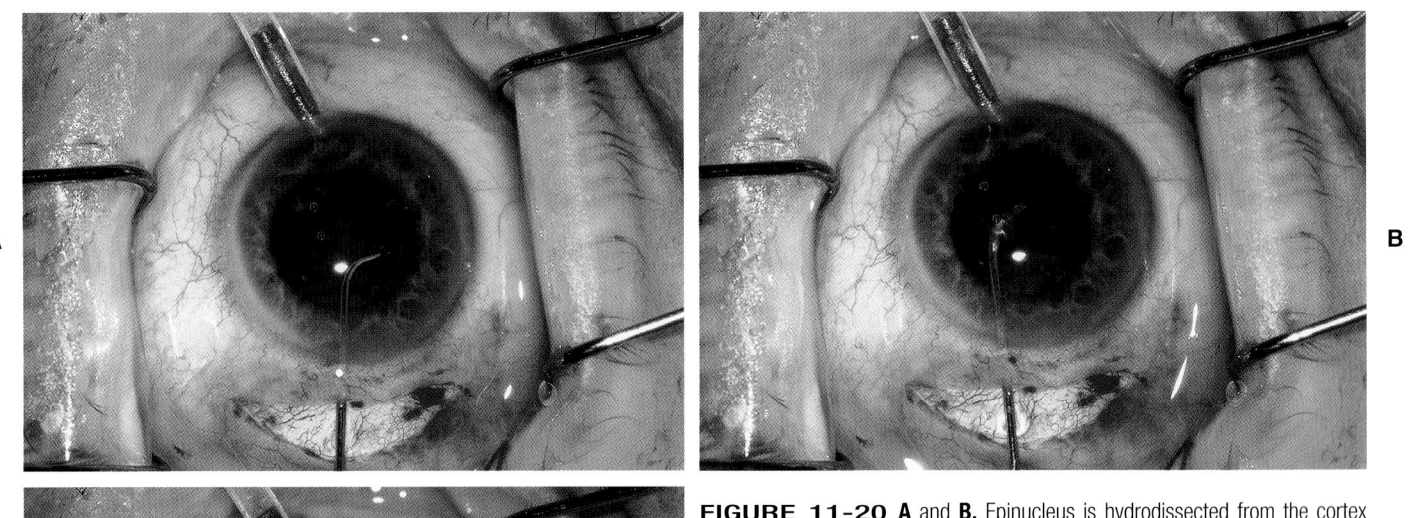

FIGURE 11-20 A and **B,** Epinucleus is hydrodissected from the cortex with the semicurved 27-gauge cannula and balanced salt solution. **C,** Entire epinucleus is extracted with the irrigating spoon and the chamber maintainer.

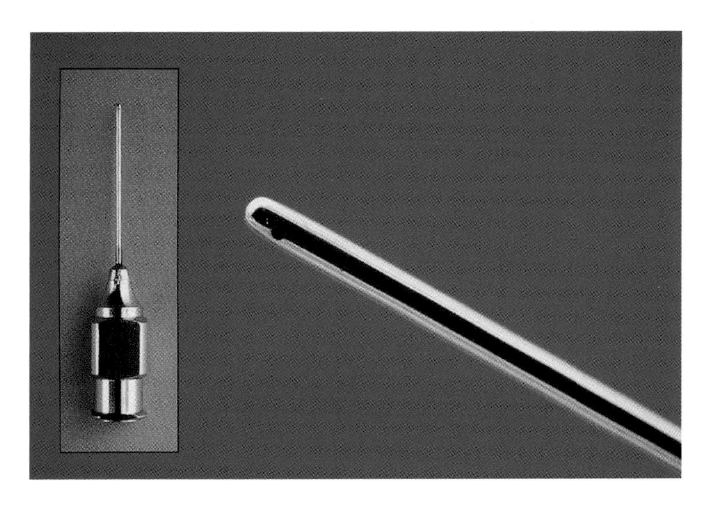

FIGURE 11-21 Straight 23-gauge side-ported aspiration cannula safely facilitates aspiration of residual cortex.

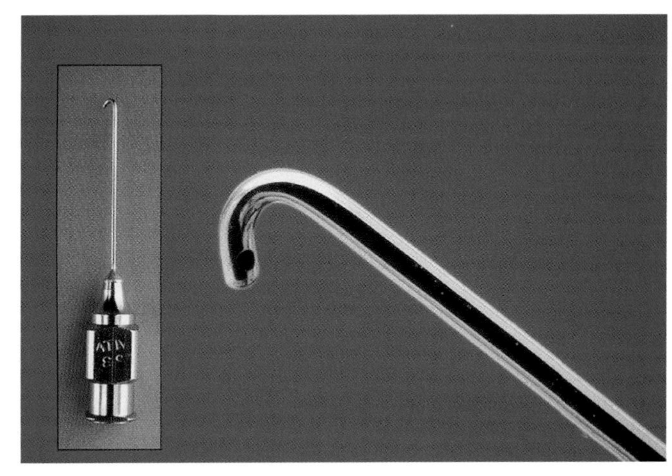

FIGURE 11-23 Binkhorst curved, side-ported cannulas provide ready access to the subincisional capsular bag.

Cortex

The cortex can be aspirated with the 21-gauge cannula; however, maximal control is obtained with the side-port 23-gauge cannula on the 5- to 6-ml syringe (Figure 11-21).

With the anterior chamber maintainer running and the bottle elevated slightly, the straight, side-ported aspirating cannula is inserted through the stab puncture. The tip reaches into the capsular bag, coming into contact with the fibrous residual cortex, which is pulled from the peripheral capsular bag into the pupillary aperture and aspirated (Figure 11-22, *A*). Aspiration forces are intermittent; they are supplied with the fingertips on the syringe, and each fragment is stripped from the periphery toward the center.

A major benefit of the side-ported 23-gauge cannula is the restriction of flow of aqueous after each cortical fragment is aspirated. This restriction is sufficient to allow the surgeon time to release the aspirating force and protect the posterior capsule from damage. Areas of the peripheral capsular bag under the tunnel incision are easily reached for stripping of the cortex (see Figure 11-22, *B*) with the side-ported aspirating hook cannula (Figure 11-23).

Polishing the posterior capsule is completed with the straight, side-ported 23-gauge aspirating cannula (Figure 11-24). The anterior chamber maintainer is of course continuing to run at medium flow.

Lens Implantation

My current preference for lens implantation is a 5.5-mm round, one-piece IOL placed in the capsular bag. I prefer a 2:1 posterior convexity ratio to maximize the pressure against the posterior capsule, hoping to minimize the clouding that may later require a posterior capsulotomy. To minimize the adhesion of the lens

A

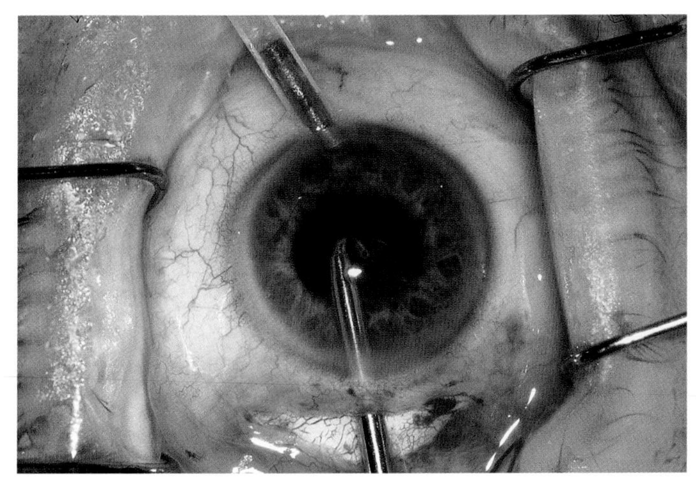

B

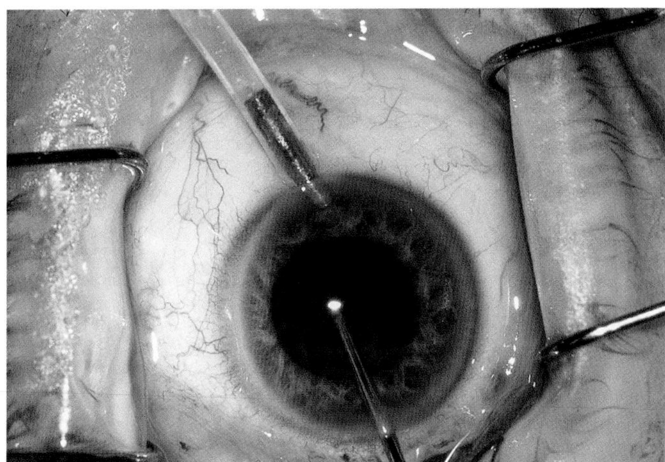

FIGURE 11-22 A, Residual cortex is aspirated with the side-ported 23-gauge aspirating cannula, entering through the side puncture. **B,** Subincisional residual cortex is extracted with the side-ported Binkhorst curved cannula.

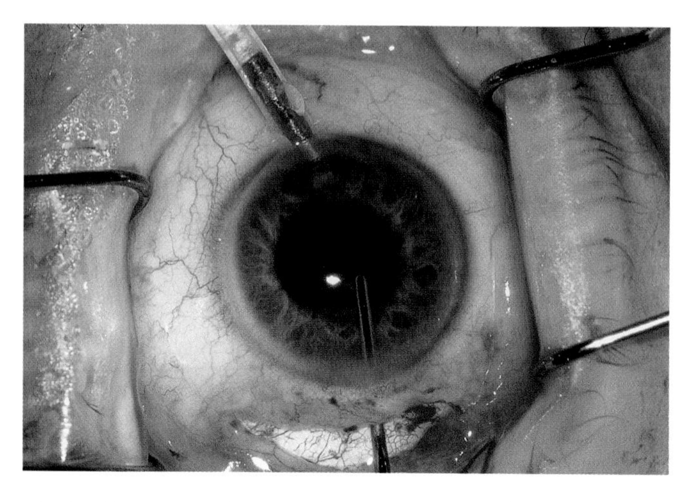

FIGURE 11-24 Central posterior capsule is polished with the side-ported 23-gauge aspirating cannula turned posteriorward.

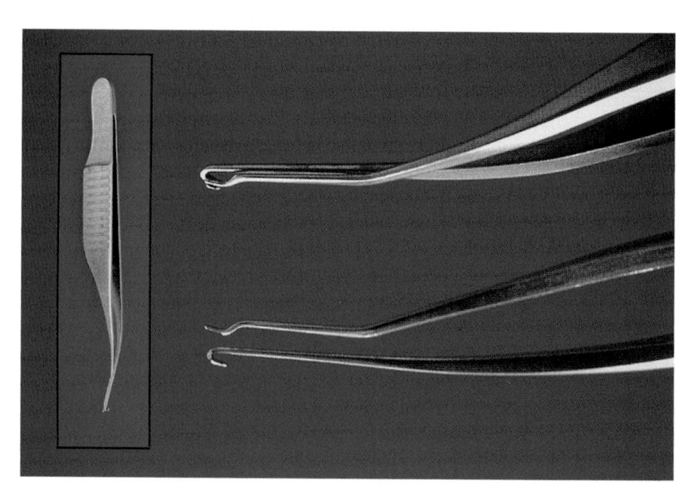

FIGURE 11-26 Ducek forceps facilitate placement in the bag of the trailing haptic loop.

A

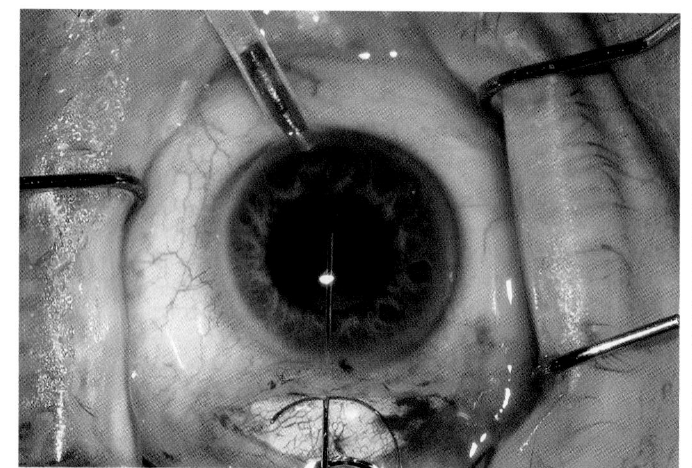

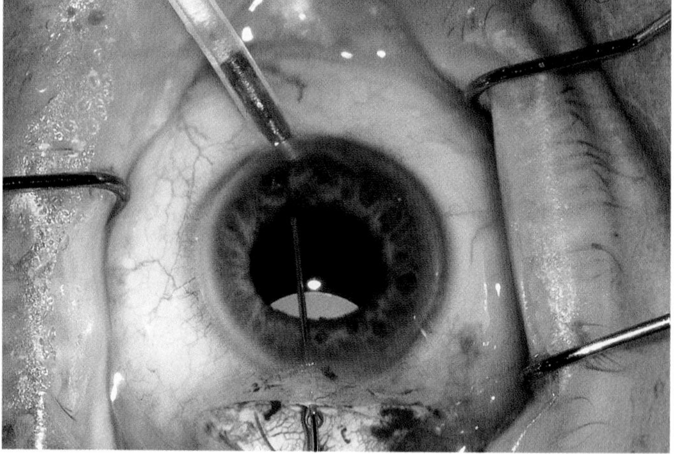

B

C

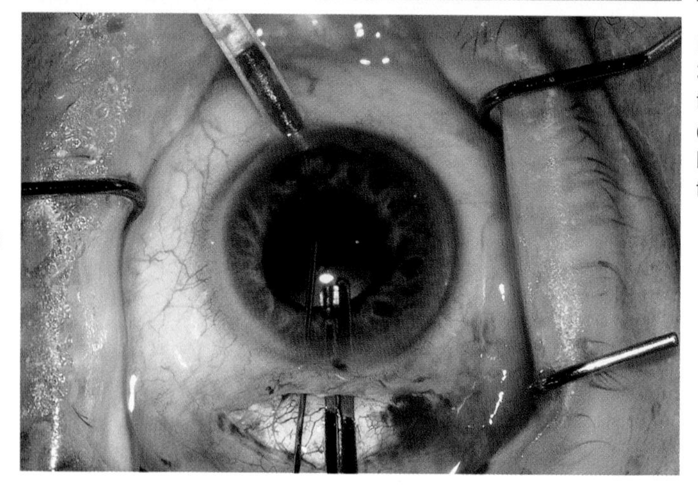

FIGURE 11-25 **A,** With the maintainer running on low flow, the assisting 30-gauge cannula enters the anterior chamber with its tip under the margin of the capsulorhexis. **B,** IOL is inserted under the 30-gauge cannula directly into the capsular bag opposite the tunnel incision. **C,** The 30-gauge cannula stabilizes the IOL while the insertion forceps are removed and the trailing haptic is inserted into the bag with Ducek forceps.

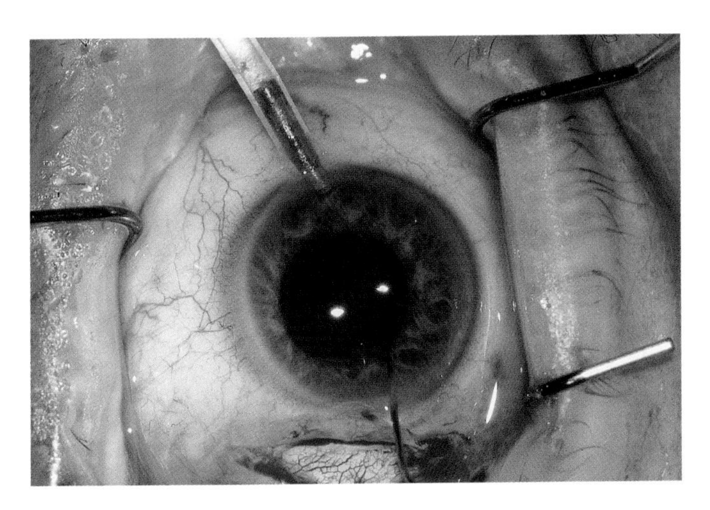

FIGURE 11-27 Through the side puncture with the maintainer running, the lens position may be verified and rotated as necessary.

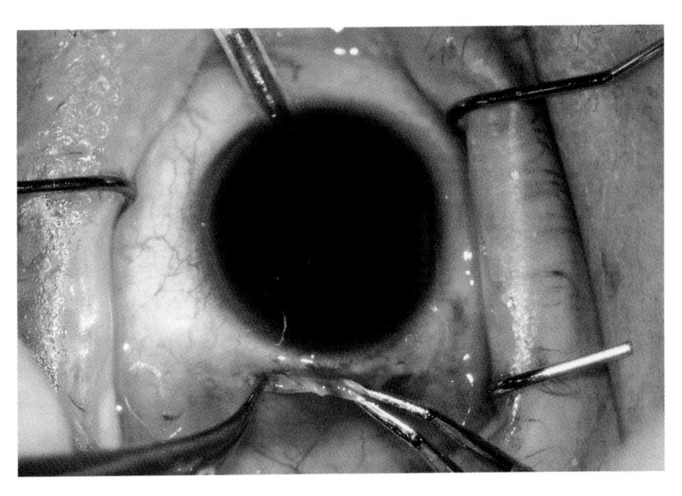

FIGURE 11-28 Conjunctiva is closed with coaptation cautery while unneeded light is eliminated by the eclipse filter.

optic to the posterior capsule during insertion, resulting in possible damage to the capsule, a minimal amount of viscoelastic agent is placed on the posterior lens surface and margin. The lens is inserted with a Kelman-MacPherson forceps assisted by a 30-gauge cannula and the chamber maintainer with the bottle in a low position (Figure 11-25). The trailing loop of the implant is inserted directly into the capsular bag using a Ducek forceps (Figure 11-26). The 30-gauge cannula is used to rotate the IOL into a horizontal position and confirm its positioning within the capsular bag (Figure 11-27).

The conjunctiva is then closed with coaptation cautery (Figure 11-28). The anterior chamber maintainer is turned off and removed and, finally, the anterior chamber is inflated with BSS through the stab puncture (Figure 11-29). However, I emphasize once again that the phacosection technique depends on the use of a viscoelastic agent during management of the nucleus. This is extremely important for protection of the corneal endothelium; with the chamber maintainer, methylcellulose appears to be an entirely adequate agent.

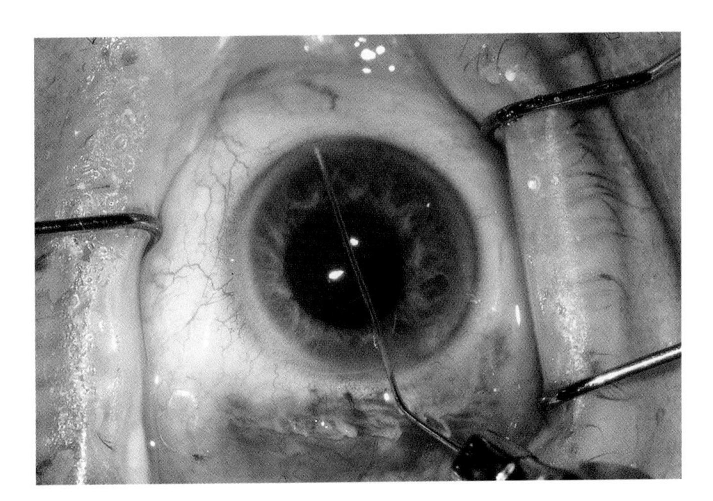

FIGURE 11-29 After maintainer removal, the 30-gauge cannula ensures the absence of iris entrapment and further deepens the anterior chamber.

Incision Construction

12

I. Howard Fine, MD
Richard S. Hoffman, MD
Mark Packer, MD

During the 1960s and in the early 1970s, most cataract surgeries in the United States and Europe were performed by the intracapsular cataract extraction technique using a limbal incision under a conjunctival flap. With few exceptions, there was little interest in reducing, minimizing, or altering surgically induced astigmatism.[1,2] The last 25 years have produced a rapid advancement in cataract surgery wound architecture. As the technology for removing cataracts has advanced, there has been a gradual trend toward smaller incisions, moving from the superior scleral to the temporal clear corneal location, in an attempt to reduce intraoperative complications and postoperative astigmatism.

Evolution of Small Incisions

With the advent of phacoemulsification, Kelman[3] predicted that incisions 3 mm wide would be astigmatism neutral because of their reduced size. However, within a very short time after the introduction of phacoemulsification, intraocular lens (IOL) implants became more commonplace. This necessitated enlargement of the phacoemulsification incision to 6.5 to 7 mm for lens implantation.

Kratz is generally credited as the first surgeon to move from the limbus posteriorly to the sclera to increase appositional surfaces, thus enhancing wound healing and reducing surgically induced astigmatism (Figure 12-1).[4,5] Girard and Hoffman[6] were first to call the posterior incision a *scleral tunnel incision* and were, along with Kratz, the first to make a point of actually entering the anterior chamber through the cornea, creating a corneal shelf. This corneal shelf was designed to prevent iris prolapse. Maloney, who was a fellow of Kratz, advocated a corneal shelf to his incisions, which he described as strong and waterproof.[7]

With the availability of small-incision lenses that could be introduced through incisions of 4 mm or less, the stage was set for the development of techniques that resulted in the achievement of both relative astigmatism-neutral and self-sealing incisions. In 1989, Shepherd[8] introduced the *single horizontal suture*, which was actually a vertical mattress suture, for the closure of 4-mm scleral tunnel incisions in phacoemulsification and foldable lens implantation (Figure 12-2). The achievement of astigmatism neutrality was impressive. Others rapidly recognized that the compressive force of the single horizontal suture was tangential to the limbus and therefore exerted no force on the cornea, which would alter its curvature. As a result, variations of the Shepherd single stitch were soon developed for closure of incisions 5 to 7 mm wide, including the Fine infinity suture (Figure 12-3),[9] Masket's horizontal anchor suture (Figure 12-4),[10] and Fishkind's horizontal overlap suture (Figure 12-5).[11]

In 1989, McFarland[12] used the corneal shelf incision architecture and recognized that these incisions sized for foldable IOLs allowed for the phacoemulsification and implantation of lenses without the need for suturing. This involved lengthening the scleral tunnel and, in his early attempts, creating partial-thickness grooves in the floor of the scleral tunnel parallel to the long axis of the tunnel so that the incision could be reversibly stretched to admit a foldable lens.

Ernest[13] observed McFarland's surgery and recognized that McFarland's long scleral tunnel incision terminated in a decidedly corneal entrance and that the posterior lip of the incision, the so-called corneal lip, acted as a one-way valve imparting to this incision its self-sealing characteristics (Figure 12-6). Koch[14] described what he called the *incisional funnel* (Figure 12-7), indicating that there were certain characteristics of self-sealing incisions with respect to length and configuration that imparted not only self-sealability but also astigmatism neutrality to these incisions.

Self-sealing scleral tunnel incisions have varied with respect to width and the configuration of the groove (which represents the external or scleral incision as opposed to the internal or corneal portion of the incision). The groove has varied from circumlimbal to straight (Figure 12-8) to frown (Figure 12-9) or chevron shaped.[15-18]

Surgical Techniques for Scleral Tunnel Incisions

In the following passage, we describe in detail the construction of a self-sealing scleral tunnel incision using a straight external scleral groove and a tunnel width of 4 mm, recognizing that the same tunnel can be made 7 mm wide with enlargement of

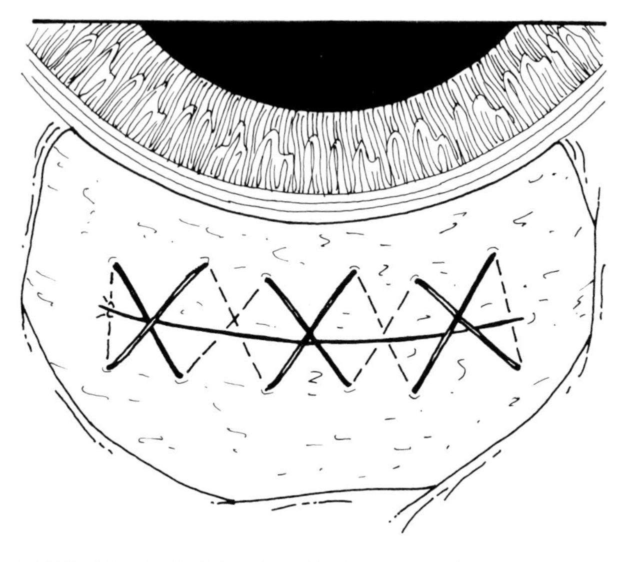

FIGURE 12-1 Scleral tunnel incision and running suture closure.

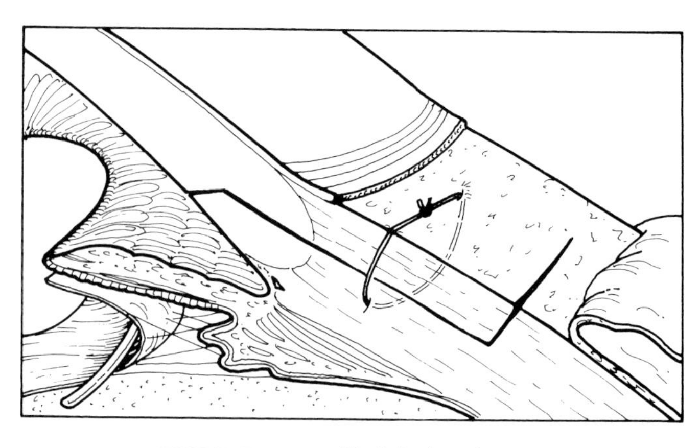

FIGURE 12-2 Single horizontal suture.

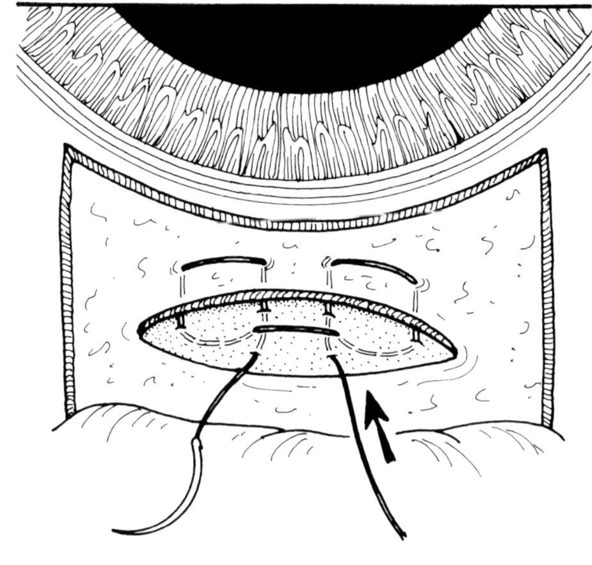

FIGURE 12-4 Horizontal anchor suture.

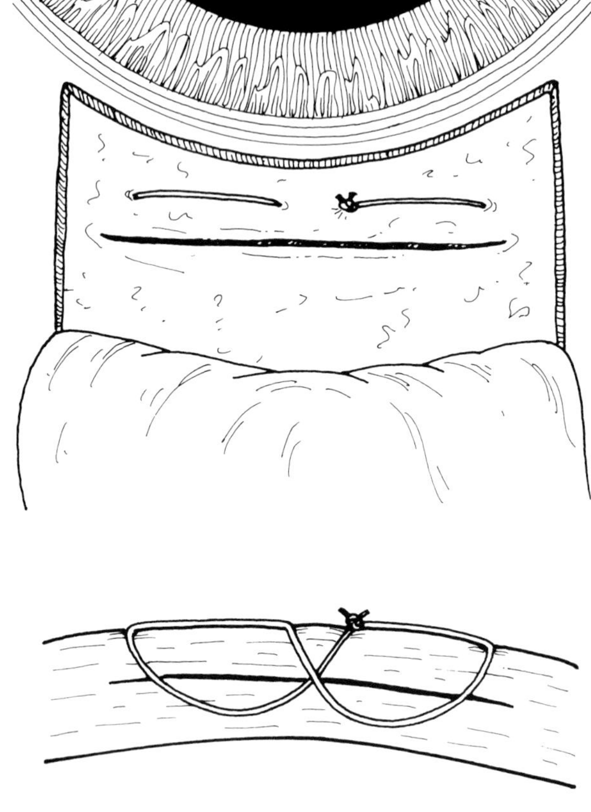

FIGURE 12-3 Infinity suture.

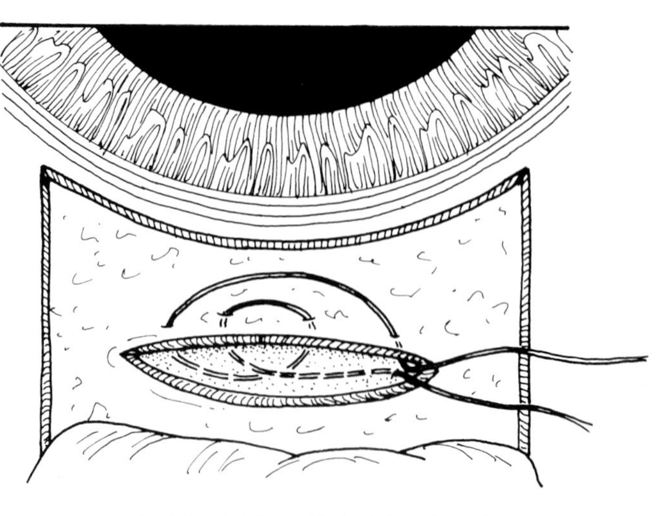

FIGURE 12-5 Horizontal overlap suture.

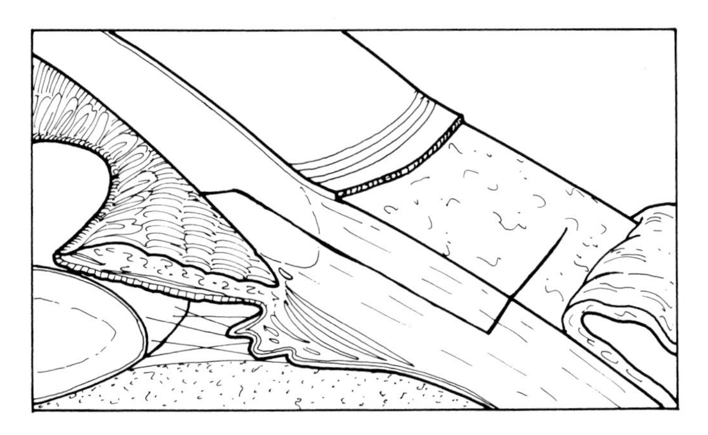

FIGURE 12-6 Self-sealing "corneal lip" scleral tunnel incision.

the internal opening from 3 to 7 mm following completion of phacoemulsification and cortical cleanup and just before lens implantation.

A conjunctival flap is made precisely by marking the width of the scleral tunnel at the limbus (Figure 12-10) and making vertical releasing incisions in the conjunctiva and Tenon's at exactly that width. These vertical releasing incisions extend back approximately 5 mm. The sub-Tenon's space is bluntly dissected with a scissors (Figure 12-11) before a peritomy (Figure 12-12). After the peritomy, the conjunctiva-Tenon's flap is folded at its base upside down on top of the posterior conjunctiva. The peritomy leaves approximately 0.5- to 1-mm lip of conjunctiva attached to the limbus. This acts as a buttress postoperatively to prevent anterior migration of the conjunctiva so that the flap never overhangs the limbus.

Mild cautery is performed near the limbus. Posteriorly, however, heavier cautery is used. The large vessels emanating from the rectus muscle and perforating the sclera between the muscle and the beginning of the tunnel are cauterized directly and adequately. (If these perforating vessels are

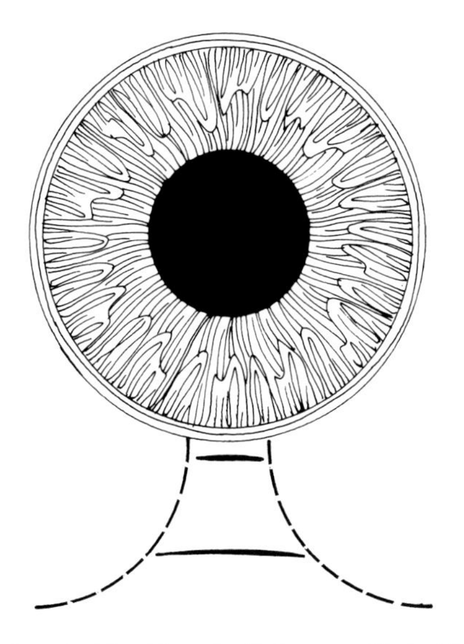

FIGURE 12-7 Incisional funnel with two possible incisions illustrated, both astigmatism neutral.

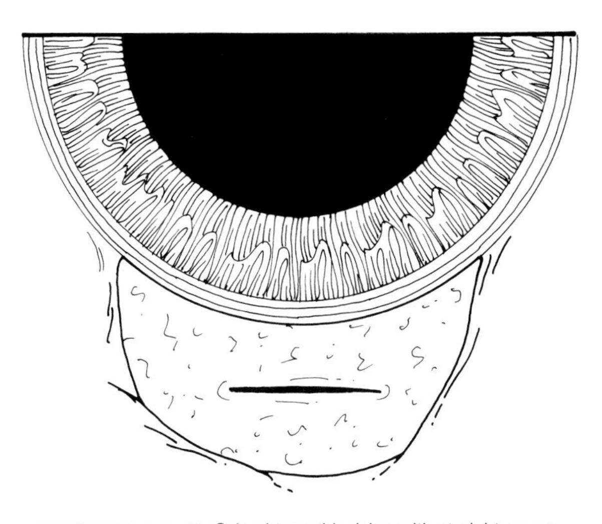

FIGURE 12-8 Scleral tunnel incision with straight groove.

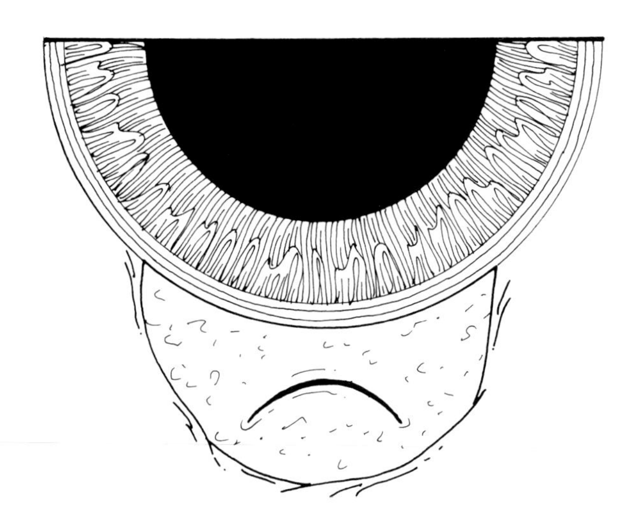

FIGURE 12-9 Frown incision.

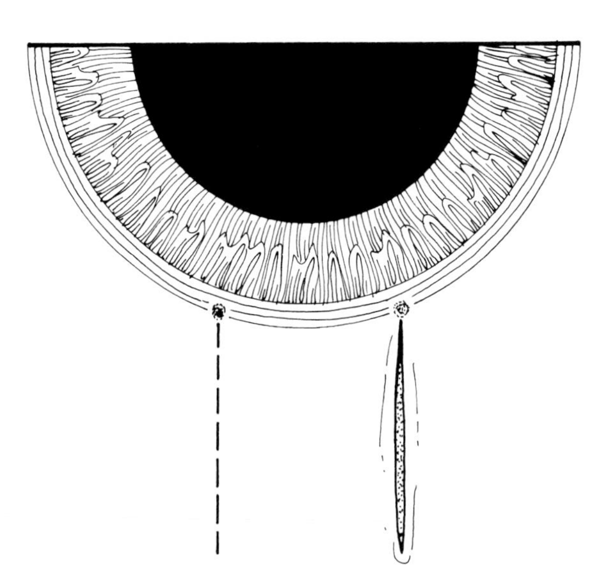

FIGURE 12-10 Blunt dissection of sub-Tenon's space with closed scissors.

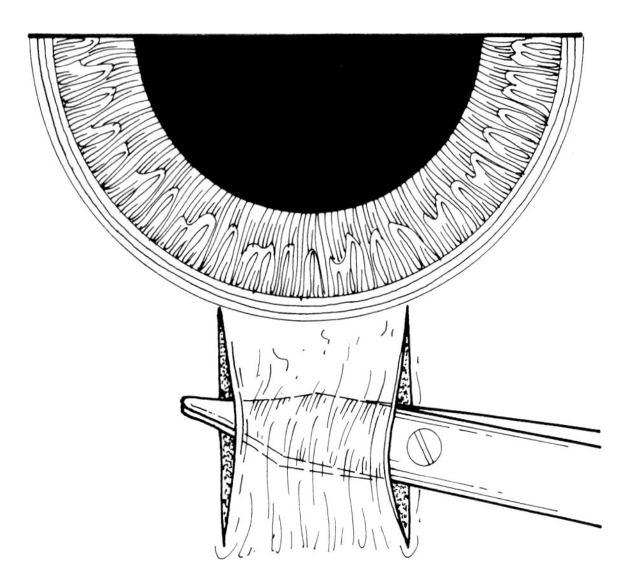

FIGURE 12-11 Peritomizing the conjunctival flap.

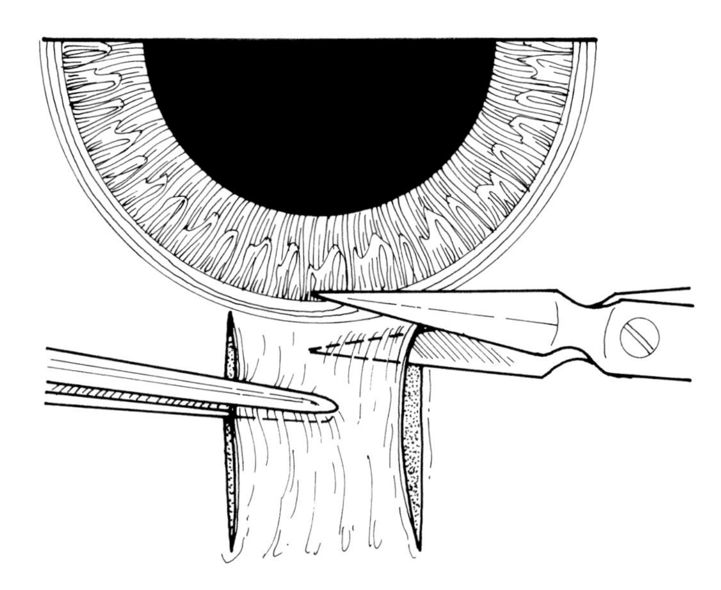

FIGURE 12-12 Millimeter grid on bare scleral bed.

cauterized before they enter the sclera, the tunnel should be dry during the entire procedure and there should be no bleeding either intraoperatively or postoperatively resulting in hyphema.)

Following cautery, a Fine millimeter marker (Rhein Medical No. 8-12106) is stamped in methylene blue and then pressed to the scleral bed, creating a 5 × 8 mm grid of dots 1 mm apart starting 1 mm posterior to the anterior edge of the corneal vascular arcade (Figure 12-13). This allows selection of an incision length and location with great precision and reproducibility. The globe is fixated with a twist grip (Weck No. 7640) posteriorly in the area of bared sclera, and the sclera is cut perpendicularly to make a groove by incising the appropriate dots (Figure 12-14). The groove is sufficiently deep that the surgeon can look down the groove and pick the depth within the sclera at which he or she will dissect the scleral tunnel. A slight anterior edge is elevated with the No. 64 Beaver blade that is used to make the groove, and from that point on an Alcon bevel-up crescent knife (Figure 12-15) (Alcon 8065-940002) is used to dissect the scleral tunnel. (It is important to keep the leading edge of the knife down, whether cutting anteriorly or to either side, as one moves the knife. This is a sharp knife that makes a very clean dissection in the scleral plane.) The dissection is carried forward to the Descemet's membrane at the anterior edge of the vascular arcade (Figure 12-16).

At this point, a side port is made with a trifacet freehand diamond knife (No. KOI KM218R). Viscoelastic is exchanged for aqueous humor through the side port by injecting the viscoelastic into the distal angle. As the expanding wave of viscoelastic moves toward the paracentesis, aqueous humor is expressed. This results in a very stiff and stable anterior chamber. A 3.5-mm keratome blade (Beaver No. 5530) is lubricated with viscoelastic and brought into the tunnel. The blade is advanced so that its point is just at the anterior edge of the vascular arcade. The point is tipped slightly posteriorly, resulting in a dimple on the anterior surface of the cornea

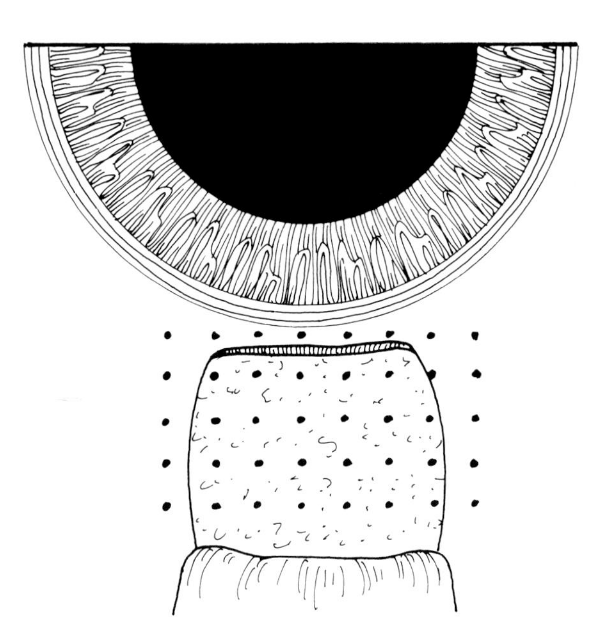

FIGURE 12-13 Initiation of the groove or external incision.

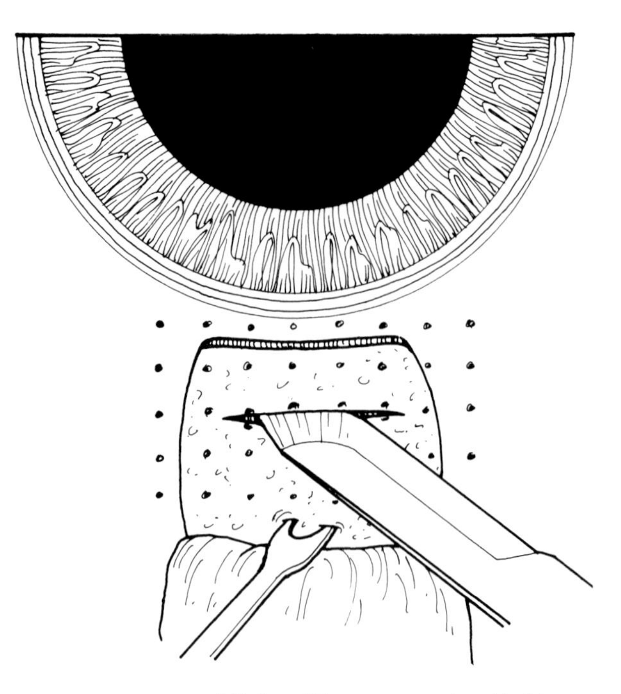

FIGURE 12-14 Initiation of the groove or external incision.

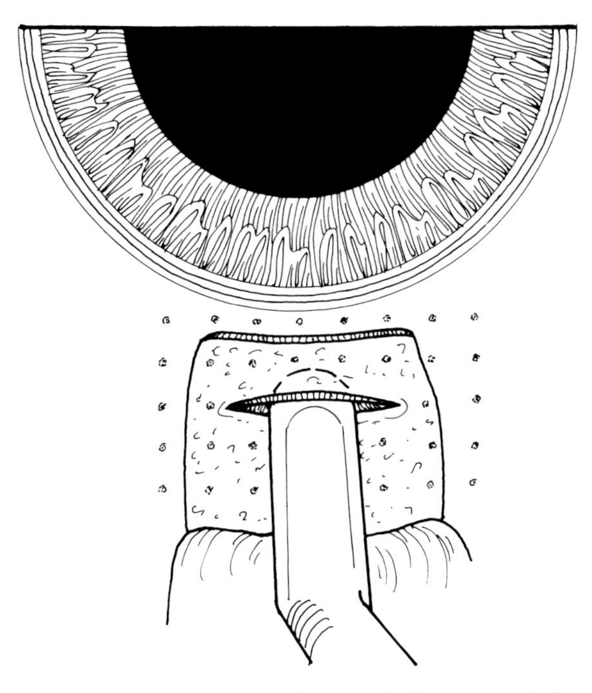

FIGURE 12-15 Initiation of the tunnel with a crescent knife.

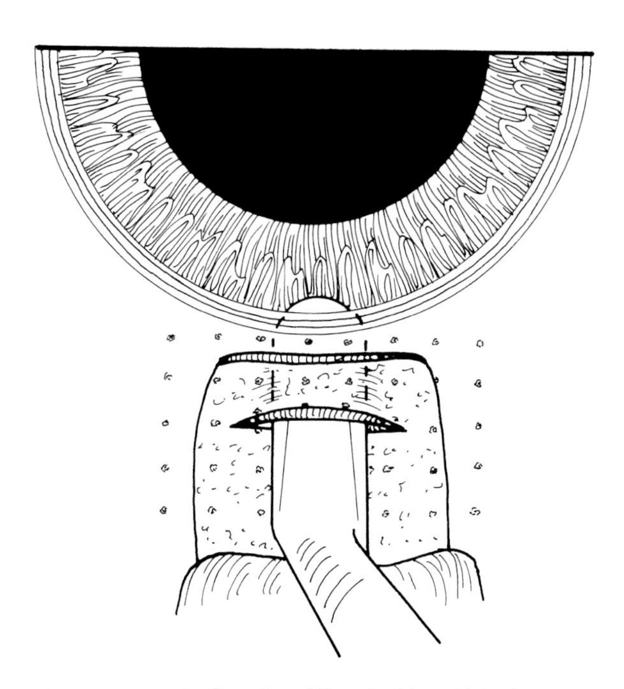

FIGURE 12-16 Dissection of the scleral tunnel into clear cornea.

whose center is directly on the anterior edge of the arcade. The dimple is frequently outlined by a semicircular light reflex (Figure 12-17) with the tip of the keratome at the center. The keratome is then advanced horizontally, parallel to the iris. This results in a linear horizontal cut through Descemet's membrane into the anterior chamber, 0.5 mm anterior to the edge of the vascular arcade (Figure 12-18).

The surgeon must continuously guide the tip of the keratome as it is brought into the anterior chamber. If it is pointed too posteriorly, the cut in Descemet's membrane will start to curve posteriorly at the ends in a "frown" configuration. On the other hand, if the tip of the keratome is elevated too much, the cut in Descemet's membrane will start to curve forward in a "smile" configuration rather than proceed straight across and parallel to the groove. If the keratome is tilted to one side or the other, an S-shaped configuration may result. In all instances, observation of the cut as it proceeds in Descemet's membrane by advancing the keratome can allow for correction of the orientation of the keratome. A straight cut in Descemet's membrane is necessary for the correct architecture of the incision.

The incision is complete when the parallel shoulders of the keratome enter the anterior chamber. The incision can be characterized by the presence of a short posterior lip of clear cornea that acts as a one-way valve.[19] Following the completion of the procedure, this valve is held closed by intraocular pressure, which also acts to collapse the scleral tunnel.

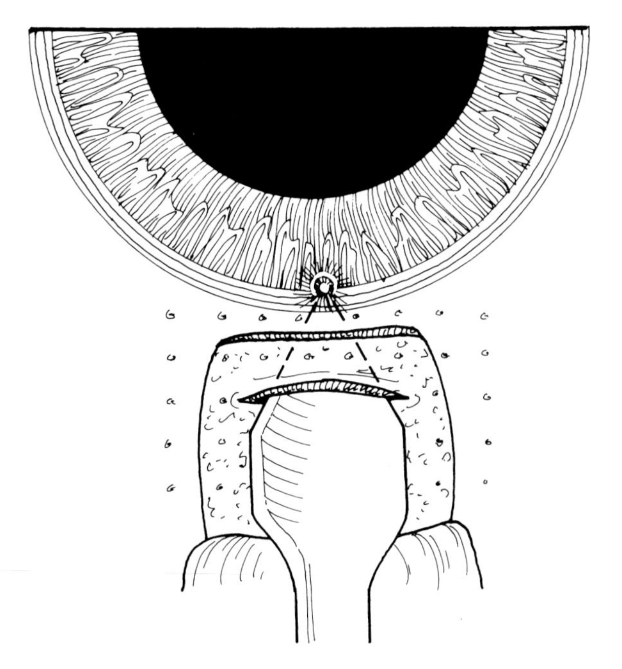

FIGURE 12-17 Dimpling of the cornea by depressing the point of the keratome.

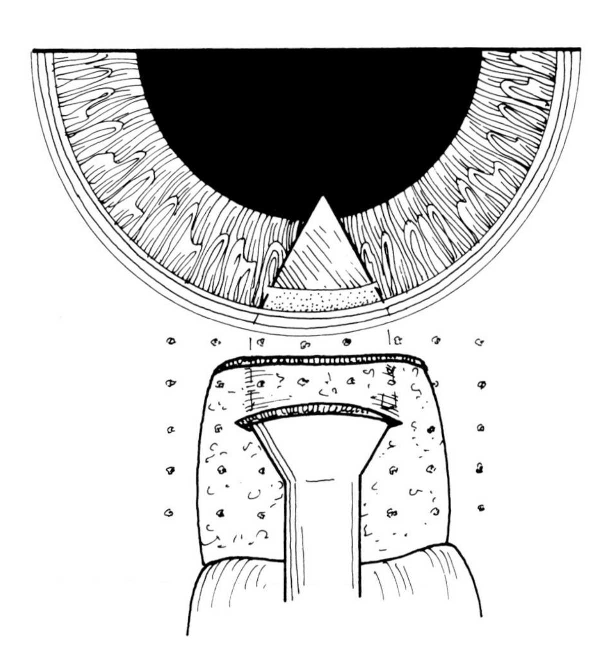

FIGURE 12-18 Straight-line incision in Descemet's membrane 0.5 mm anterior to the vascular arcade.

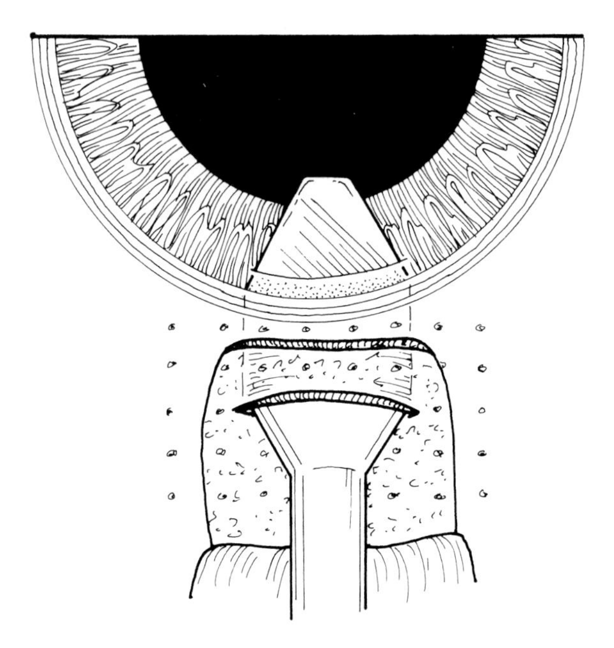

FIGURE 12-19 Enlargement of the 3.5-mm incision to 4.0 mm with a blunt-tipped keratome.

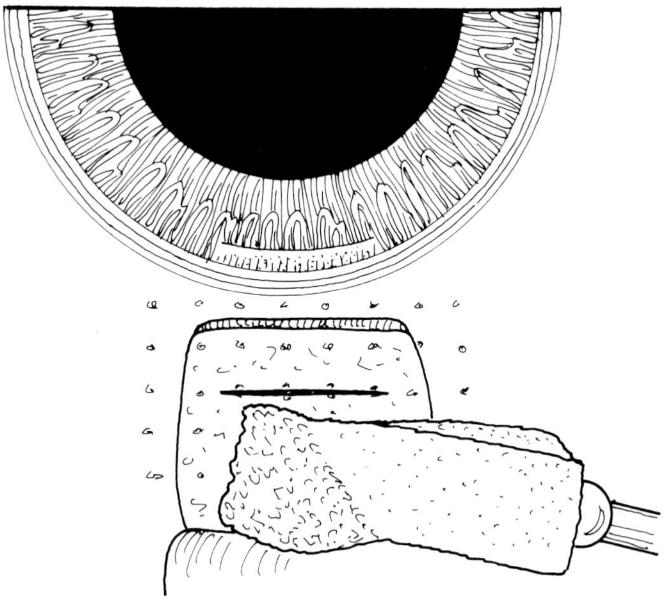

FIGURE 12-20 Testing the scleral incision for watertightness.

If one goes more anteriorly into clear cornea before incising Descemet's membrane, the visualization during phacoemulsification is markedly impaired because of the striae that occur as the phaco tip is tilted down for endolenticular phacoemulsification.

It is important to avoid putting traction on the roof of the scleral tunnel with a forceps. A bridle suture is used during incision construction, and the twist grip is placed posterior to the dot grid to stabilize the globe during construction of the scleral tunnel. The forceps is used to elevate the tunnel roof in placing the keratome inside the tunnel, but countertraction is placed on the posterior lip of the groove rather than the anterior lip during the cutting of Descemet's membrane with the keratome.

Phacoemulsification and later evacuation of viscoelastic take place with the bridle suture unattached to minimize stretching of the tunnel roof. The use of chilled balanced salt solution (BSS) maximizes cooling of the phaco tip, thus minimizing shrinkage of the tunnel. (BSS is kept at approximately 4° C overnight in a refrigerator). After cortical cleanup and expansion of the bag with viscoelastic, the incision in Descemet's membrane is widened with a 4-mm blunt-tip keratome (Figure 12-19) (Beaver No. 374732) for folded silicone lenses. For 6-mm lenses, the initial keratome incision is enlarged with a supersharp knife (15-degree Alcon ophthalmic knife No. 8065-921502) taking care to incise Descemet's membrane as a continuation of the straight-line cut made by the 3.5-mm keratome.

Following IOL implantation and evacuation of residual viscoelastic, the anterior chamber is fully repressurized with BSS through the side port. The lips of the wound are tested by applying pressure with a Weck cell sponge against the posterior lip of the wound (Figure 12-20) in an effort to make the incision leak. If it does leak, which happens less than 5% of the time, a single horizontal suture is placed (in the case of incisions 5 mm or larger, an infinity suture is placed). If no leakage is observed, the conjunctival flap is unfolded back over the incision and smoothed in place. Its corners are returned to the corners of the bed from which they were derived, up against the remaining lip of conjunctiva attached to the limbus (Figure 12-21). The flap is frequently adherent within 1 hour, as observed in one-eyed patients who are not patched at the conclusion of surgery. A Maloney keratometer is used to estimate astigmatism at the conclusion of the surgery (Figure 12-22).[15]

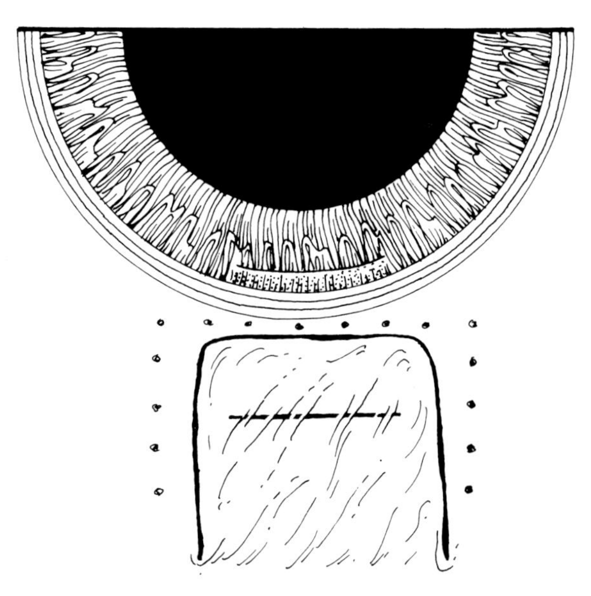

FIGURE 12-21 Conjunctival flap repositioned in its bed.

Development of Clear Corneal Incisions

There have been many surgeons who have favored corneal incisions for cataract surgery before their recent popularization. In 1968, Kelman[3] stated that the best approach for performing cataract surgery was with phacoemulsification through a clear corneal incision using a triangular-tear capsulotomy and a grooving and cracking technique in the posterior chamber. Harms and Mackenson[20] in Germany published an intracapsular technique using a corneal incision in 1967 in an atlas, called *Ocular Surgery Under the Microscope.* Troutman was an early

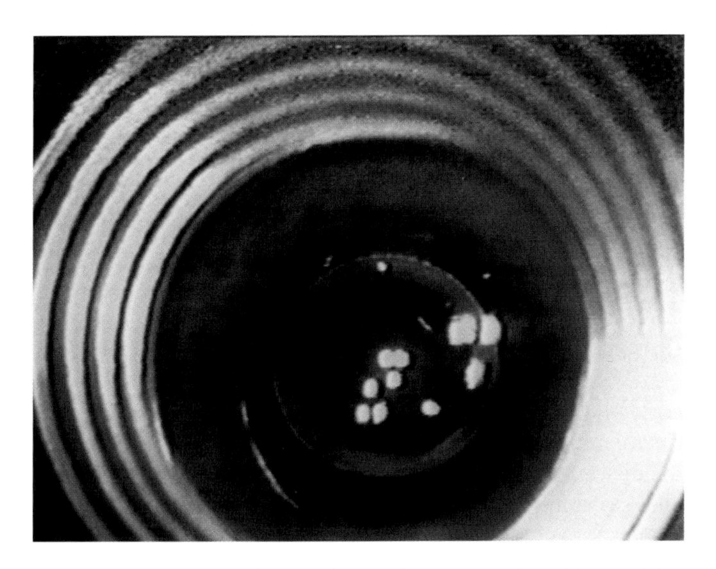

FIGURE 12-22 Estimation of corneal curvature using a Maloney intraoperative qualitative keratometer.

advocate of controlling surgically induced astigmatism at the time of cataract surgery by means of the corneal-incision approach.[21] Arnott[22] in England used clear corneal incisions and a diamond keratome for phacoemulsification although he had to enlarge the incision for introducing an IOL. Galand[23] in Belgium used clear corneal incisions for extracapsular cataract extraction in his envelope technique, and Stegman of South Africa has a long history of having used the cornea as the site for incisions for extracapsular cataract extraction (Stegmann R. Personal communication, December 3, 1992). In April of 1992, Fine presented his self-sealing temporal clear corneal incision at the annual meeting of the American Society of Cataract and Refractive Surgery.[24] In May of 1992, at the Island Ophthalmology Seminar, Kellan demonstrated on video a technique that he referred to as the scleral-less incision. It was essentially a corneal limbal stab incision through conjunctiva and the limbus, entering the anterior chamber through clear cornea, leaving a corneal shelf or lip (Figure 12-23). Finally, perhaps the leading proponent of clear corneal incisions for modern era phacoemulsification was Kimiya Shimizu of Japan.[25]

Fine's personal experience with corneal incisions began in 1979 when the temporal clear cornea was used as the site for secondary anterior chamber IOL implantation. The temporal approach was preferred because of the unpredictable nature of the disturbed anatomy present at the superior limbus in eyes that had previous intracapsular cataract extraction. As soon as foldable lenses were available in 1986, he used sutured clear corneal incisions for phacoemulsification and foldable IOL implantation in patients who had preexisting filtering blebs. After these procedures, a marked reduction in surgically induced astigmatism was noted despite the fact that these incisions were corneal rather than scleral. In 1992, Fine began routinely using clear corneal cataract incisions for phacoemulsification and foldable IOL implantation with incision closure using a tangential suture modeled after Shepherd's technique.[8] Within a very short period, the suture was abandoned in favor of self-sealing corneal incisions.[26]

Indications for Clear Corneal Incisions

Initially, the use of clear corneal incisions was limited to those patients with preexisting filtering blebs, patients taking anticoagulants or with blood dyscrasias, or patients with cicatrizing disease such as ocular cicatricial pemphigoid or Stevens-Johnson syndrome. Subsequently, because of the natural fit of clear corneal cataract incisions with topical anesthesia, the indications for clear corneal cataract surgery expanded. With the ability to avoid any injections into the orbit and use of intravenous medications, those patients who had cardiovascular, pulmonary, and other systemic diseases that might have contraindicated cataract surgery became surgical candidates. Subsequently, through the safety and increasing use of these incisions by some pioneers in the United States, including Williamson, Shepherd,

A

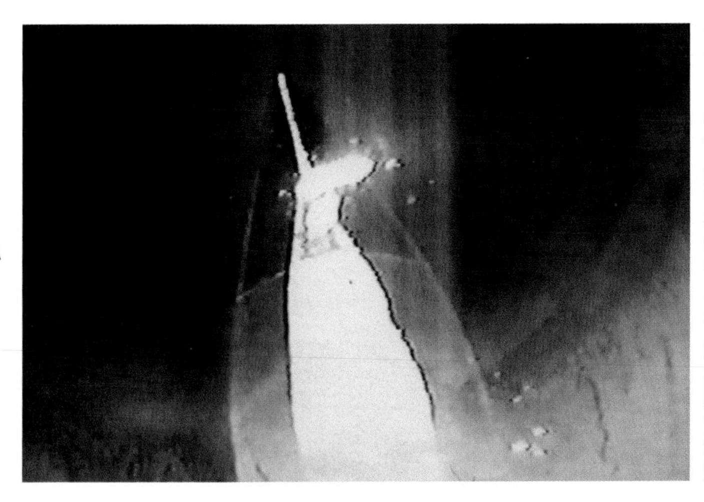

B

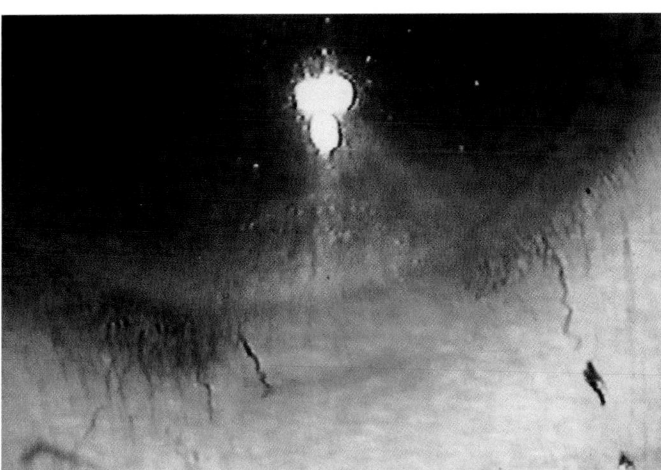

FIGURE 12-23 A, Kellan's corneal limbal stab incision through conjunctiva and the limbus. **B,** Corneal limbal incision following removal of the steel keratome.

Martin, and Grabow,[27] these incisions became increasingly popular and were used on an international basis.

Studies by Rosen[28] using topographic analyses of these incisions demonstrated that clear corneal incisions sized 3 mm in width or less were topographically astigmatism neutral. This led to an increasing interest in these incisions because of an increasing use of techniques including T-cuts, arcuate cuts, and limbal relaxing incisions for managing preexisting astigmatism at the time of cataract surgery. Without astigmatism neutrality in the cataract incision, the predictability of adjunctive astigmatism-reducing procedures would be decreased, making it more difficult to achieve the desired result. In the initial studies and ultimate use of multifocal IOLs, the need for astigmatism neutrality was again a factor for stimulating interest in clear corneal incisions. Finally, the availability of phakic IOLs and the need for control of astigmatism at the time of implantation of these lenses have driven many surgeons to consider clear corneal incisions as the route for phakic IOL implantation.

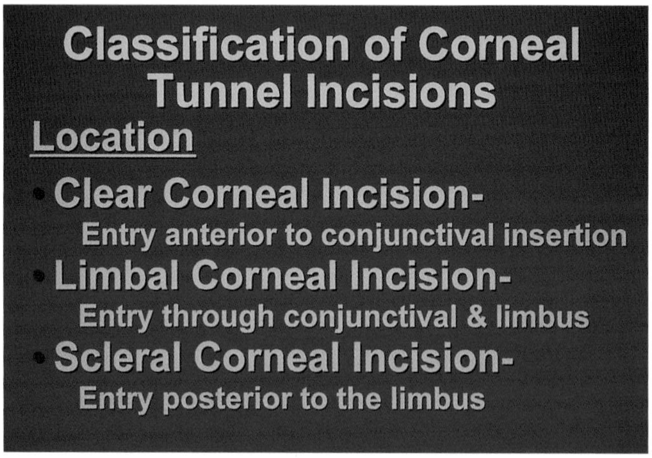

Classification of Corneal Tunnel Incisions
Location
- Clear Corneal Incision- Entry anterior to conjunctival insertion
- Limbal Corneal Incision- Entry through conjunctival & limbus
- Scleral Corneal Incision- Entry posterior to the limbus

FIGURE 12-24 Classification of corneal tunnel incisions by external incision location.

Other advantages of the temporal clear corneal incision include better preservation of preexisting filtering blebs,[29] preservation of options for future filtering surgery, increased stability in the refractive results because of the neutralization of the forces from lid blink and gravity, the ease of approach to the incision site, the lack of need for bridle sutures and resultant iatrogenic ptosis, and, finally, the location of the lateral canthal angle under the incision, which facilitates drainage.

Classification of Clear Corneal Incisions

Early on there was criticism surrounding the use of self-sealing clear corneal incisions because of a fear of a possible increased incidence of endophthalmitis secondary to poor wound healing and sealability. This potential controversy stimulated many studies into the strength and safety of clear corneal incisions compared with limbal and scleral tunnel incisions. Unfortunately, because of a lack of standardization in the definition of what constitutes a limbal versus clear corneal incision, considerable confusion has been generated in this area, making it difficult for surgeons to communicate and compare the relative claims of their individual techniques. Based on Hogan's *Histology of the Human Eye* ("The conjunctival vessels are seen with the slit lamp as fine arcades that extend into clear cornea for about 0.5 mm beyond the limbal edge")[30] and topographic studies of incisions done by Menapace[31] in Vienna, Fine[32] has categorized these incisions using the parameters of location and architecture. An incision is termed *clear corneal* when the external edge is anterior to the conjunctival insertion, *limbal corneal* when the external edge is through conjunctiva and limbus, and *scleral corneal* when it is posterior to the limbus (Figure 12-24). In addition to the anatomic designation of the external incision, these incisions are also classified by their architecture as being *single plane* when there is no groove at the external edge of the incision, *shallow groove* when the initial groove is less than 400 μm, and *deeply grooved* when it is deeper than 400 μm (Figures 12-25 and 12-26). To reduce the confusion and facilitate communication regarding these incisions, we

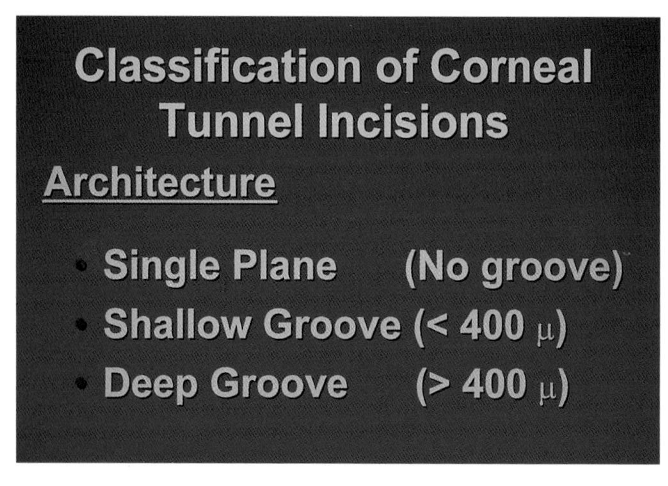

FIGURE 12-25 Classification of corneal tunnel incisions by wound architecture.

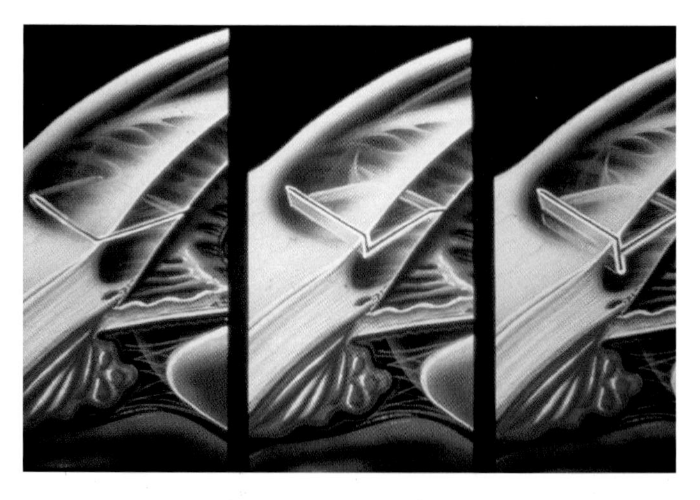

FIGURE 12-26 Cross-sectional view of single-plane, shallow-groove, and deep-groove (hinged) clear corneal incisions.

believe they should be classified as clear corneal, limbal corneal, or scleral corneal incisions and as single planed, shallow grooved, or deep grooved.

Controversies Surrounding Clear Corneal Incisions

One of the most controversial criticisms of clear corneal incisions has been their relative strength compared with limbal or scleral incisions. Ernest et al.[33,34] demonstrated that rectangular clear corneal incisions in cadaver eye models were less resistant to external deformation using pinpoint pressure than were square limbal or scleral tunnel incisions. Subsequently, Mackool and Russell[35] demonstrated that once the incision width was 3.5 mm or less and the length 2 mm or greater, there was an equal resistance to external deformation in clear cornea incisions compared with scleral tunnel incisions. In Ernest's work as well, as incision sizes became increasingly small, the force required to cause failure of these incisions became very similar for limbal and clear corneal incisions, and thus this could be used to further document the safety of incisions sized 3 mm or less.

A major criticism of these cadaver studies is the lack of functioning endothelium contributing to wound sealing. Others have also indicated that cadaver eye incision strength cannot be compared with incisions in vivo.[28] Ernest and Neuhann[36] have compared in vivo posterior limbal incisions with clear corneal incisions and found that deep grooved incisions performed better than shallow-grooved or single-plane incisions in addition to finding that posterior limbal incisions performed better than clear corneal incisions when challenged by pinpoint pressure.

Many surgeons have called into question the validity of pinpoint pressure as a clinically relevant test for cataract wound strength because the probability that anyone would challenge their own incision by pressing on it with something as fine as the instruments used to apply pinpoint pressure in these studies is highly unlikely. Regardless of whether more posteriorly placed incisions demonstrate increased strength compared with clear corneal incisions, the real question is whether that added strength is clinically significant or relevant. Fine[37] and others have demonstrated the stability of clear corneal incisions when a knuckle or a fingertip, the most likely way patients would challenge these incisions, was used. In addition, it is well known that a 1-mm "hypersquare" paracentesis will leak the day after surgery if pinpoint pressure is applied to its posterior lip; however, the likelihood of any paracentesis incision leaking spontaneously or with blunt pressure the day following surgery is extremely low.

One final point of controversy regards the studies in cat eyes performed by Ernest et al.[38] These studies revealed a fibrovascular response in incisions placed in the limbus with extensive wound healing in 7 days compared with a lack of fibrovascular healing in clear corneal incisions. This study has been used to propose an increased safety for limbal incisions as compared with clear corneal incisions. Unfortunately, the real issue for these various incisions is not healing but sealing. We believe that as long as an incision is sealed at the conclusion of surgery and remains sealed, the time before complete healing of the incision is accomplished is almost irrelevant, especially because there is still a 7-day period in which limbal incisions are not truly "healed." An analogy can be drawn to the sealing that takes place during lasik refractive surgery in which there is no fibrovascular healing of the clear corneal interface, which has little effect on the strength, effectiveness, or safety of the wound and, in fact, is an advantage by limiting scarring and an inflammatory healing response. Ultimately, the relative safety of one incision over another in the clinical setting will only be determined with the findings of a difference in the rate of incision-related complications, which to date have not been demonstrated.

One of the clear disadvantages of limbal corneal incisions is the greater likelihood of ballooning of conjunctiva, which can make visualization of anterior chamber structures during the surgical procedure more difficult. In addition, studies by Park et al.[29] demonstrated that violation of the conjunctiva threatens the integrity not only of preexisting filtering blebs but also of the conjunctiva that would participate in filtering surgery at some future date. Finally, the presence of subconjunctival hemorrhage, although not important with respect to the ultimate function of the eye, may be of importance from a cosmetic perspective to the patient, as well as to the survival of filtering blebs.

Contraindications for clear corneal incisions include the presence of radial keratotomy incisions that extend to the limbus that might be challenged by clear corneal incisions,[39] marginal degenerations associated with thinning of the peripheral cornea, and perhaps advanced corneal endothelial dystrophy.

Preoperative Evaluation

Certain studies that may be of value as part of a preoperative workup include endothelial cell counts in patients with endothelial dystrophies and perhaps computerized corneal topography when refractive surgical procedures are going to be combined with cataract surgery in the management of pre-existing astigmatism. This is especially true when refractive and keratometric measurements do not coincide. There has been a recent trend for surgeons to use fluoroquinolone drops four times per day for 3 days prior to the day of surgery.

Techniques

Single-plane incisions, as first described by Fine,[40] used a 3-mm diamond knife.

A Fine-Thornton 13-mm fixation ring (Mastel Instruments, Rapid City, SD) (Figure 12-27) stabilizes the globe and allows manipulation without creating conjunctival tears, subconjunctival hemorrhages, or corneal abrasions (Figure 12-28). Aqueous humor is replaced by viscoelastic material through the side-port incision (Figure 12-29). After pressurization of the eye with viscoelastic, a 300-μm groove may be placed at the anterior edge of the vascular arcade (Figure 12-30); however, this is optional. If the groove has been placed, an incision is made by depressing the posterior edge of the groove with the diamond blade, flattening the blade against the surface of the eye. The knife is moved in the plane of the cornea until the shoulders, which are 2 mm posterior to the point of the knife, touch the external edge of the incision and then a dimple down technique is used to

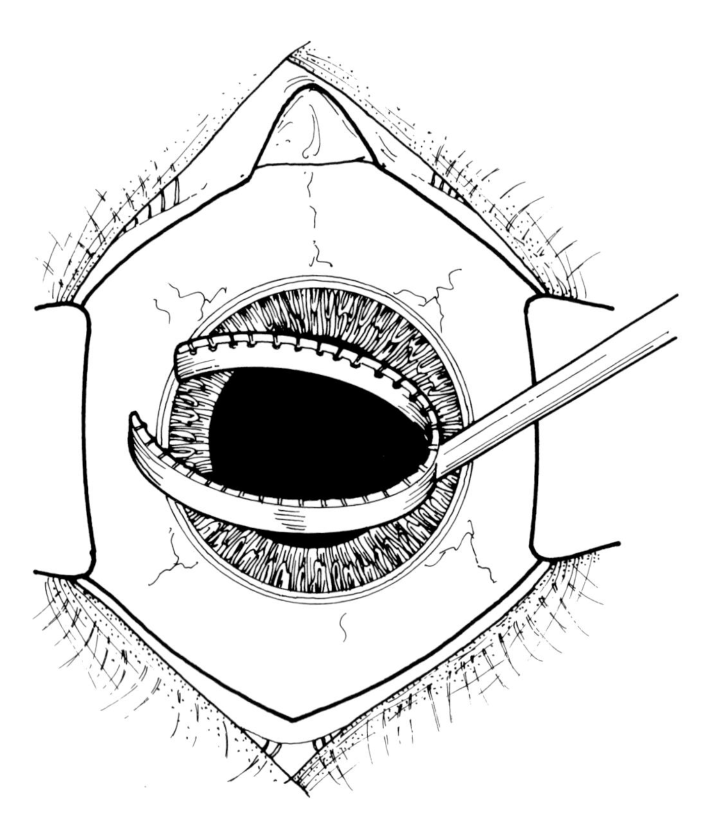

FIGURE 12-27 Fine-Thornton ring, shown in partial profile. Temporal limbus is seen inferiorly.

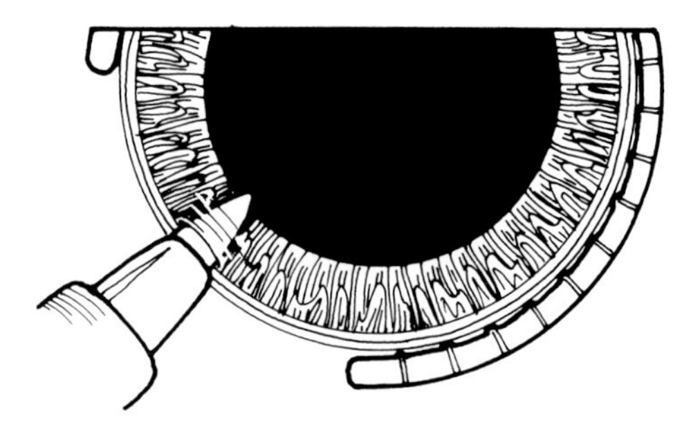

FIGURE 12-29 Paracentesis being made.

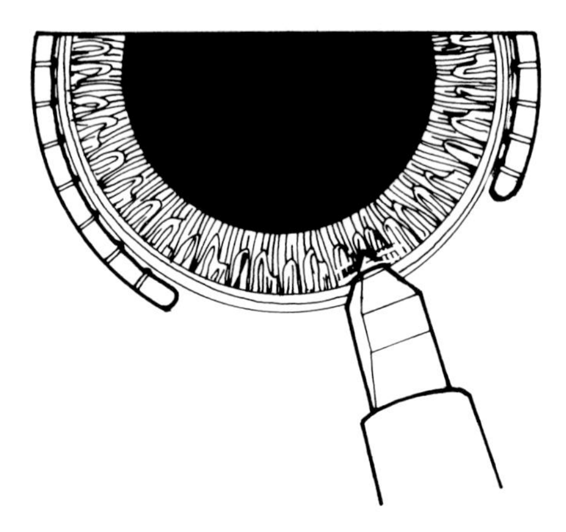

FIGURE 12-30 Grooving of the peripheral cornea.

initiate the cut through Descemet's membrane. After the tip enters the anterior chamber, the initial plane of the knife is reestablished to cut through Descemet's membrane in a straight line configuration (Figure 12-31). Following phacoemulsification, lens implantation, and removal of residual viscoelastic, stromal hydration of the clear corneal incision can be performed to help seal the incision.[26] This is performed by placing the tip of a 26- or 27-gauge cannula in the side walls of the incision and gently irrigating BSS into the stroma (Figure 12-32). This is performed at both edges of the incision to help appose the roof and floor of the incision. Once apposition takes place, the hydrostatic forces of the endothelial pump will help seal the incision. In those rare instances of questionable wound integrity, a single radial 10-0 nylon suture is placed to ensure a tight seal.

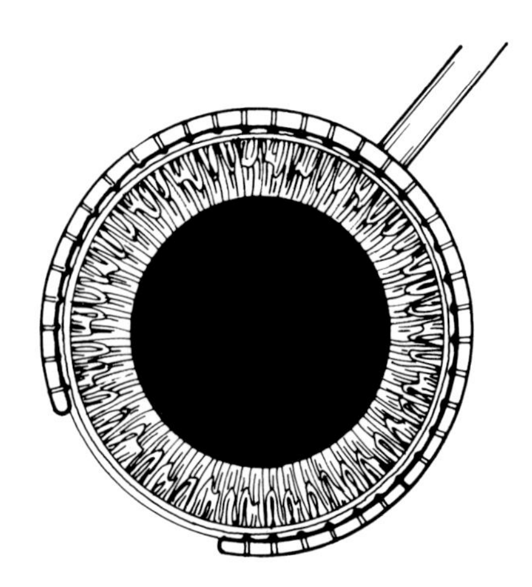

FIGURE 12-28 Purchase of the globe by the Fine-Thornton ring.

Williamson[41] was the first to use a shallow 300- to 400-μm grooved clear corneal incision. The rationale for the Williamson incision was that it led to a thicker external edge to the roof of the tunnel and less likelihood of tearing. Langerman[42] later described the single hinge incision in which requirements for the initial groove were 90% of the depth of the cornea anterior to the edge of the conjunctiva. Initially he used a depth of 600 μm and subsequently made the tunnel itself superficially in that groove, believing that this led to enhanced resistance of the incision to external deformation. Minimal differences in surgically induced astigmatism have been demonstrated between beveled and hinged clear corneal incisions.[43]

Adjunctive techniques were used to combine refractive surgery incisions with clear corneal cataract incisions. Until

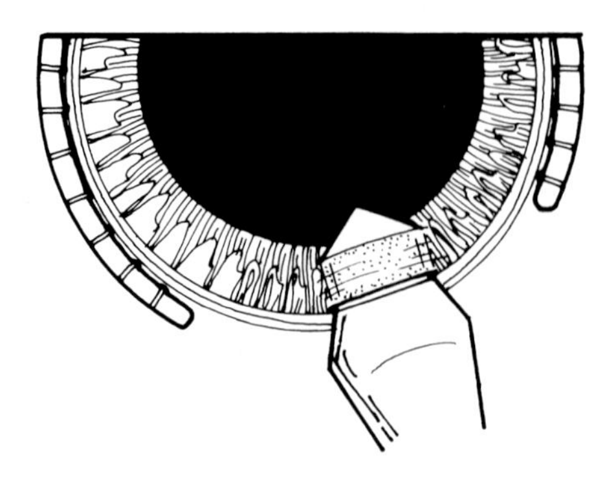

FIGURE 12-31 Construction of the corneal tunnel.

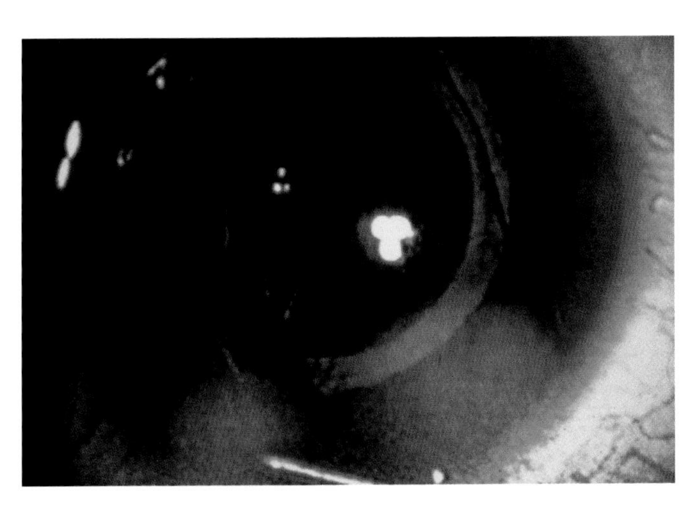

FIGURE 12-32 Stromal hydration of the incision.

recently, Fine used the temporal location for the cataract incisions and added one or two T-cuts made by the Feaster knife (Rhein Medical No. 05-8200) with a 7-mm ocular zone for the management of preexisting astigmatism. Others, including Lindstrom and Rosen, rotated the location of the incision to the steep axis to achieve some increased flattening at the steepest axis to address preexisting astigmatism. Kershner[44] used the corneal incision in the temporal half of the eye by starting with a nearly full-thickness T-cut through which he then made his corneal tunnel incision. For large amounts of astigmatism he used a paired T-cut in the opposite side of the same meridian. Finally, the popularization of limbal relaxing incisions by Gills[45] and Nichamin[46] added an additional means of reducing preexisting astigmatism by using the groove for the limbal relaxing incision as the site of entry for the clear corneal cataract incision. This has been found to be a simple and practical approach for reducing preexisting astigmatism at the time of cataract surgery.[47] At this time Fine places all of his incisions at the temporal periphery and addresses preexisting with limbal relaxing incisions at the steep axis and/or toric IOLs.

New technology blades have been developed that have helped perfect incision architecture. The Fine Triamond knife (Mastel No. 0851913191) was developed in conjunction with Mastel Precision Instruments (Rapid City, SD) so that the incision could be made with an extremely sharp, thin, and narrow knife without a necessity for dimpling down, which resulted in some tendency for tearing of tissue or scrolling of Descemet's membrane. Subsequently, in conjunction with Rhein Medical (Tampa, Fla.), the 3-D blade (No. 05-5083) was developed, which had differential slope angles to the bevels on the anterior versus the posterior surface (Figure 12-33), resulting in an ability to just touch the eye at the site of the external incision location and advance the blade in the plane of the cornea. The differential slopes on the anterior versus posterior aspects of the blade allowed the forces of tissue resistance to create an incision that was characterized by a linear external incision, a 2-mm tunnel, and a linear internal incision without the need to dimple down or distort tissues to create the proper incision architecture.[48] The trapezoidal 3-D blade

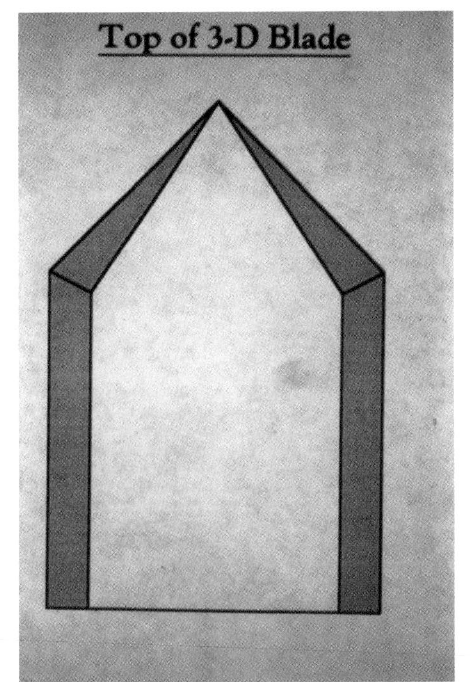

A

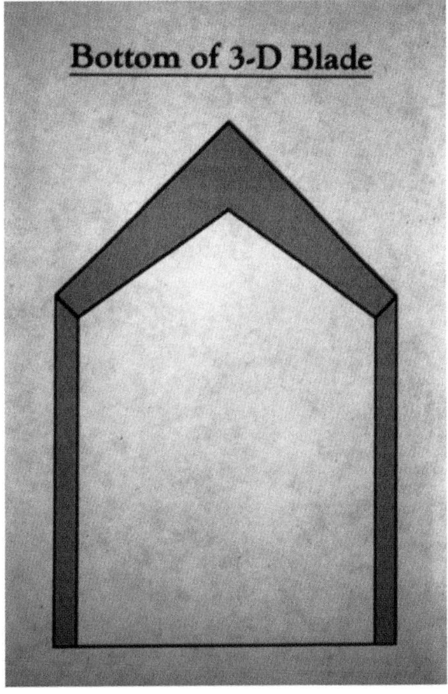

B

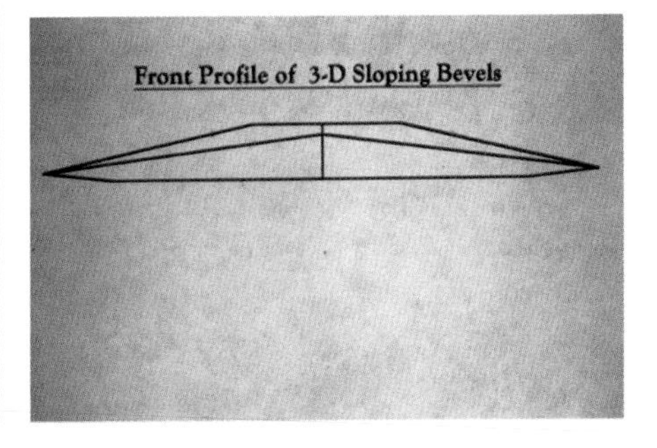

C

FIGURE 12-33 Schematic representation of top view **(A)** and bottom view **(B)** of the 3-mm Rhein 3-D diamond keratome. The front profile of the keratome **(C)** demonstrates the differential slopes on the anterior versus posterior aspects of the blade, which allow the forces of tissue resistance to create the proper incision architecture.

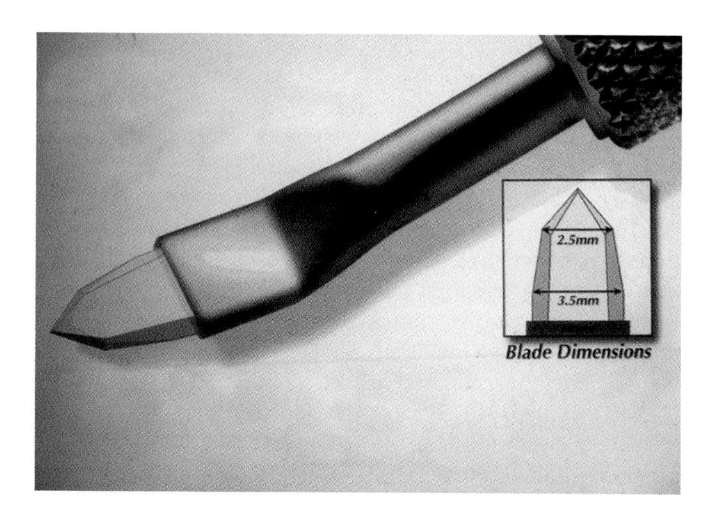

FIGURE 12-34 Rhein 3-D trapezoidal blade with 2.5- to 3.5-mm blade dimensions.

(Rhein No. 05-5086) also allows enlargement of the incision to 3.5 mm for IOL insertion without altering incision architecture (Figure 12-34). Histologic studies of clear corneal incisions performed with steel keratomes and diamond keratomes have shown more disruption of corneal stromal tissue with steel keratomes and more likelihood of severe stromal damage after insertion of foldable IOLs, suggesting that diamond keratomes may have a beneficial effect on incision healing.[49,50]

Many companies, in addition to Rhein Medical, are designing diamond knives for clear corneal incisions. Mastel Precision Surgical Instruments have designed a sleek trapezoidal blade that they have named the Super Stealth (Figure 12-35). The Stealth blade is an ultrathin diamond with asymmetric facets that result in a self-directing bevel similar to the Rhein 3-D blade. American Surgical Instruments Company (ASICO, Westmont, Ill.) has designed two new diamond knives for clear corneal incisions: the Pathfinder (Figure 12-36) and the Clearpath (Figure 12-37). Both blades contain a shelf on the surface of the blade that creates an inner corneal valve of consistent length by forcing the leading edge of the blade into the anterior chamber when the shelf reaches the external incision. Stromal hydration

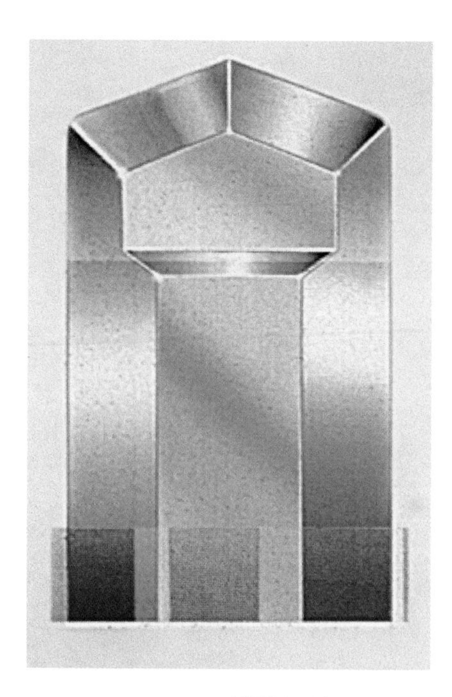

FIGURE 12-36 ASICO Pathfinder Blade.

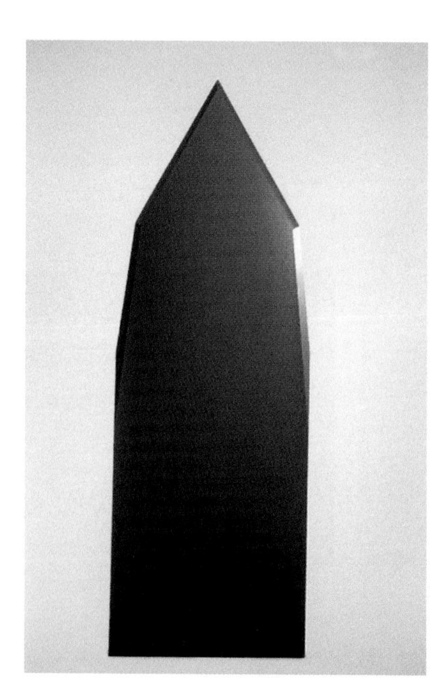

FIGURE 12-35 Mastel Trapezoidal Diamond Stealth blade.

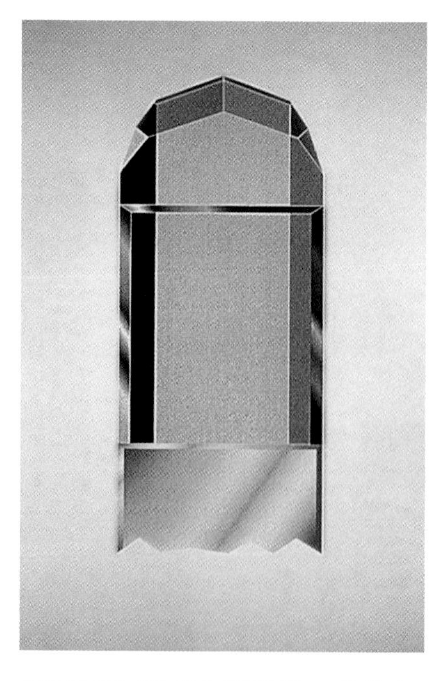

FIGURE 12-37 ASICO Clearpath Blade.

of the wound is claimed to be unnecessary with the Clearpath blade because of the facet design.

A recent study by Mamalis[51] has revealed small predictable enlargements of clear corneal incisions after insertion of foldable IOLs with both forceps and injectors. The degree of wound enlargement increased with higher IOL powers when lenses were inserted with forceps but did not increase with increasing IOL powers when injectors were used. In general, injectors were associated with a smaller percentage increase in wound stretching than forceps, making them a preferable choice for foldable lens insertion through clear corneal incisions.

Intraoperative and Postoperative Complications

Although clear corneal and scleral incision cataract surgery share many of the same intraoperative and postoperative complications, clear corneal incisions by nature of their architecture and location have some unique complications associated with them. If one accidentally incises the conjunctiva at the time of the clear corneal incision, ballooning of the conjunctiva can develop, which may compromise visualization of anterior structures. When this develops, a suction catheter is usually required by the assistant to aid in visualization. Early entry into the cornea might result in an incision of insufficient length to be self-sealing, and thus a single suture may be required to ensure a secure wound at the conclusion of the procedure. A late entry may result in a corneal tunnel incision sufficiently long that the phacoemulsification tip would create striae in the cornea and compromise visualization of the anterior chamber. In addition, incisions that are too short or improperly constructed can result in an increased tendency for iris prolapse.

Manipulation of the phacoemulsification handpiece intraoperatively may result in tearing of the roof of the tunnel, especially at the edges, potentially compromising the ability for the incision to self-seal. Tearing of the internal lip can also occur, resulting in compromised self-sealability or, in rare instances, small detachments or scrolling of Descemet's membrane in the anterior edge of the incision. Of greater concern has been the potential for incisional burns.[52,53] When incisional burns develop in clear corneal incisions, there may be a loss of self-sealability, corneal edema, and severe induced astigmatism.[54] In addition, manipulation of the incision can result in an epithelial abrasion, which can compromise self-sealability because of the lack of a fluid barrier by an intact epithelium. Without an intact epithelial layer, the corneal endothelium does not have the ability to help appose the roof and floor of the incision through hydrostatic forces.

Postoperatively, hypotony might result in some compromised ability for these incisions to seal. Wound leaks and iris prolapse have been very infrequent postoperative complications[55] and are usually present in incisions greater than 3.5 mm in width. In a large survey performed for the American Society of Cataract and Refractive Surgery by Masket and Tennen,[56] there was a slightly increased incidence of endophthalmitis in clear corneal cataract surgery compared with scleral tunnel surgery. However, the survey failed to note the incision sizes in those cases in which endophthalmitis in clear corneal incisions had occurred, and thus it is possible that any increase in the incidence of endophthalmitis was associated with unsutured clear corneal incisions greater than 4 mm in width.

Postoperative Clinical Course and Outcomes

The usual postoperative regimen involves examination on the first postoperative day and a second examination at 10 to 14 days at which time spectacle correction is prescribed. Use of drops postoperatively includes instillation 2 to 3 times a day of a fluoroquinolone, prednisolone acetate, and topical nonsteroidal antiinflammatory. The antibiotic and steroid are discontinued at 10 to 14 days, and the nonsteroidal antiinflammatory agent is continued for an additional 10 days.[57]

Numerous studies have been performed documenting the safety and low magnitudes of astigmatism induced by these incisions, depending on their size. Masket and Tennen[58] have documented by vector analysis 0.50 diopter (D) of induced cylinder and less than 0.25 D of cylinder change in the surgical meridian using 3 × 2.5 mm self-sealing temporal clear corneal incisions. They were also able to demonstrate the refractive stability of these incisions 2 weeks following surgery. Kohnen, Dick, and Jacobi[59] compared the surgically induced astigmatism of 3.5-, 4-, and 5-mm grooved temporal clear corneal incisions and found a mean induced astigmatism of 0.37 D, 0.56 D, and 0.70 D, respectively, after 6 months. A similar study by Pfleger et al.[60] revealed even smaller amounts of induced astigmatism from 3.2-, 4-, and 5.2-mm temporal clear corneal incisions, with the 3.2-mm incision demonstrating astigmatic neutrality with only 0.09 D of induced cylinder.

In addition to comparing the effects of different-sized temporal clear corneal incisions on induced astigmatism, numerous studies have evaluated the relative astigmatic effects of incision location in regard to clear corneal incisions versus corneoscleral incisions, and the temporal versus superior meridian. Nielsen[61] evaluated surgically induced astigmatism from 3.5- and 5.2-mm temporal and superior clear corneal incisions and compared them with 3.5- and 5.2-mm corneoscleral incisions at the superior location. The 3.5-mm clear corneal incisions induced roughly 0.5 D of with-the-rule or against-the-rule drift, depending on temporal or superior location. Larger amounts of astigmatism were induced with the larger clear corneal incisions. He found that the refractive effect of clear corneal incisions was stable between postoperative day 1 and postoperative week 6, making their astigmatic keratotomy effect more useful and predictable if one wished to consider preoperative cylinder when selecting incision type or location.

Cillino et al.[62] compared the astigmatic effects of unsutured 5.2-mm temporal clear corneal incisions with 5.2-mm superior corneoscleral incisions and found comparable amounts of induced astigmatism. Rainer et al.,[63] however, has found a small but significant amount of surgically induced astigmatism continuing up to 5 years postoperatively with 5-mm superior scleral incisions. Although the use of unsutured 5.2-mm clear corneal incisions is considered unsafe because of a possible increase in rates of wound complications and endophthalmitis, Holweger and Marefat[64] have demonstrated that absorbable sutured 5-mm clear corneal incisions were topographically comparable to 3.5-mm sutureless clear corneal incisions, 6 to 8 months postoperatively, making this incision and closure technique a viable option for surgeons.[64]

When temporal clear corneal incisions of 3.2 mm or less have been compared with superiorly placed scleral tunnel incisions of the same size, similar amounts of low induced astigmatism have been documented for the two incision locations.[65,66] In contrast, similarly sized incisions when compared in regard to temporal versus superior clear corneal location have demonstrated more meridional flattening in the superior axis than the temporal axis.[67-69] This has also been demonstrated in the oblique superolateral clear corneal incision compared with a temporal incision, confirming the bias for the temporal location for clear cornea incisions when astigmatic neutrality is desired.[70]

Although small clear corneal incisions appear to have similar astigmatic effects as superior corneoscleral incisions, recent concern has surrounded the possibility of increased endothelial cell loss with these incisions. Grabow[71] reported an increased incidence of endothelial cell loss for superior clear corneal incisions, which increased linearly with increasing ultrasound times. Amon et al.[72] discovered a significant increase in endothelial cell loss in 3.5-mm temporal clear corneal incisions when compared with 3.5-mm superior scleral tunnel incisions. However, a recent study by Dick et al.[73] found that the total endothelial cell loss at 1 year with clear corneal incisions compared favorably with endothelial cell loss rates of other cataract extraction techniques. As ultrasound times decrease in the future with advancing technologies and techniques such as lens chopping and the use of power modulations,[74] endothelial cell loss rates should become insignificant.

Dick et al.[75] have also recently demonstrated that cataract extraction through a clear corneal incision results in less inflammation in the immediate postoperative period when compared with surgery through a sclerocorneal incision. This may ultimately have a beneficial effect in reducing posterior capsule opacification, cystoid macular edema, and keratopathy.

Conclusion

Clear corneal cataract incisions are becoming a more popular option for cataract extraction and IOL implantation throughout the world. Through the use of clear corneal incisions and topical and intracameral anesthesia, we have achieved surgery that is the least invasive of any time in the history of cataract surgery with visual rehabilitation that is almost immediate. Clear corneal incisions with appropriate architecture have had a proven record of safety with relative astigmatic neutrality using the smaller incision sizes. Just 25 years ago, inpatient intracapsular cataract surgery, often performed with general anesthesia, followed by aphakic spectacles was the standard of care. It is striking to realize how far we have come in such a short time.

REFERENCES

1. Paton D, Troutman R, Ryan S: Present trends in incision and closure of the cataract wound, *Highlights Ophthalmol* 14:3, 176, 1973.
2. Jaffe NS, Clayman HM: The pathophysiology of corneal astigmatism after cataract extraction, *Trans Am Acad Ophthalmol Otolaryngol* 79:OP615-630, 1975.
3. Kelman CD: Phacoemulsification and aspiration: a new technique of cataract removal—a preliminary report, *Am J Ophthalmol* 64:23, 1967.
4. Colvard DM, Kratz RP, Mazzocco TR et al: Clinical evaluation of the Terry surgical keratometer, *J Am Intraocul Implant Soc* 6:249-251, 1980.
5. Masket S: Origin of scleral tunnel methods, *J Cataract Refract Surg* 19: 812-813, 1993 (letter).
6. Girard LJ, Hoffman RF: Scleral tunnel to prevent induced astigmatism, *Am J Ophthalmol* 97:450-456, 1984.
7. Maloney WF, Grindle L: *Textbook of phacoemulsification*, Fallbrook, Calif, 1988, Lasenda Publishers.
8. Shephard JR: Induced astigmatism in small incision cataract surgery, *J Cataract Refract Surg* 15:85-88, 1989.
9. Fine IH: Infinity suture: modified horizontal suture for 6.5 mm incisions. In Gills JP, Sanders DR, editors: *Small-incision cataract surgery: foldable lenses, one-stitch surgery, sutureless surgery, astigmatic keratotomy*, Thorofare, NJ, 1990, Slack, Inc, pp 191-196.
10. Masket S: Horizontal anchor suture closure method for small incision cataract surgery, *J Cataract Refract Surg* 17(suppl):689-695, 1991.
11. Fishkind WJ: Horizontal overlap suture: a new astigmatism-free closure, focus on phaco, *Ocular Surg News* 8, Nov. 15, 1990.
12. McFarland MS: Surgeon undertakes phaco, foldable IOL series sans sutures, *Ocular Surg News* 8(5):1, 15, March 1, 1990.
13. Ernest PH: Presentation at the Department of Ophthalmology, Wayne State University School of Medicine, Detroit, Mich, Feb 28, 1990.
14. Koch PS: Structural analysis of cataract incision construction, *J Cataract Refract Surg* 17(suppl):661-667, 1991.
15. Kershner RM: Sutureless one-handed intercapsular phacoemulsification: the keyhole technique, *J Cataract Refract Surg* 17(suppl):719-725, 1991.
16. Fine IH: Architecture and construction of a self-sealing incision for cataract surgery, *J Cataract Refract Surg* 17:672-676, 1991.
17. Singer JA: Frown incision for minimizing induced astigmatism after small incision cataract surgery with rigid optic intraocular lens implantation, *J Cataract Refract Surg* 17(suppl):677-688, 1991.
18. Pallin SL: Chevron sutureless closure: a preliminary report, *J Cataract Refract Surg* 17(suppl):706-709, 1991.
19. Ernest PH: Introduction to sutureless surgery. In Gills JP, Sanders DR, editors: *Small incision cataract surgery: foldable lenses, one-stitch surgery, sutureless surgery, astigmatic keratotomy*, Thorofare, NJ, 1990, Slack, Inc pp 103-105.
20. Harms H, Mackensen G: Intracapsular extraction with a corneal incision using the Graefe knife. In *Ocular surgery under the microscope*, Stuttgart, Germany, 1967, Georg Thieme Verlag, pp 144-153.
21. Paton D, Troutman R, Ryan S: Present trends in incision and closure of the cataract wound, *Highlights Ophthalmol* 14:3, 176, 1973.
22. Arnott EJ: Intraocular implants. *Trans Ophthalmol Soc U K* 101:58-60, 1981.
23. Galand A: *La technique de l'enveloppe*, Liege, Belgium, 1988, Pierre Mardaga publisher.
24. Brown DC, Fine IH, Gills JP et al: The future of foldables. Panel discussion held at the 1992 annual meeting of the American Society of Cataract and Refractive Surgery. *Ocular Surg News*, Aug 15 1992 (supplement).
25. Shimizu K: Pure corneal incision, *Phaco Foldables* 5:5, 6-8, 1992.
26. Fine IH: Corneal tunnel incision with a temporal approach. In Fine IH, Fichman RA, Grabow HB, editors: *Clear-corneal cataract surgery & topical anesthesia*, Thorofare, NJ, 1993, Slack, Inc, pp 5-26.
27. Fine IH, Fichman RA, Grabow HB: *Clear-corneal cataract surgery & topical anesthesia*, Thorofare, NJ, 1993, Slack, Inc.
28. Rosen ES: Clear corneal incisions: a good option for cataract patients: a Roundtable Discussion, *Ocular Surg News*, Feb 1, 1998.
29. Park HJ, Kwon YH, Weitzman M et al: Temporal corneal phacoemulsification in patients with filtered glaucoma, *Arch Ophthalmol* 115:1375-1380, 1997.
30. Hogan MJ, Alvarado JA, Weddell JE, editors: *Histology of the human eye: an atlas and textbook*, Philadelphia, 1971, WB Saunders Company, pp 118-119.
31. Menapace RM: Preferred incisions for current foldable lenses and their impact on corneal topography: Cataract Workshop on the Nile, Luxor-Aswan, Egypt, Nov 20, 1996 (abstract).
32. Fine IH: Descriptions can improve communication, *Ophthalmol Times* 21:30, 1996.
33. Ernest PH, Lavery KT, Kiessling LA: Relative strength of scleral corneal and clear corneal incisions constructed in cadaver eyes, *J Cataract Refract Surg* 20:626-629, 1994.
34. Ernest PH, Fenzl R, Lavery KT et al: Relative stability of clear corneal incisions in a cadaver eye model, *J Cataract Refract Surg* 21:39-42, 1995.

35. Mackool RJ, Russell RS: Strength of clear corneal incisions in cadaver eyes, *J Cataract Refract Surg* 22:721-725, 1996.
36. Ernest PH, Neuhann T: Posterior limbal incision, *J Cataract Refract Surg* 22:78-84, 1996.
37. Fine IH: New thoughts on self-sealing clear corneal cataract incisions. Presented at Hawaii '96, Maui, Hawaii, January 22, 1996.
38. Ernest P, Tipperman R, Eagle R et al: Is there a difference in incision healing based on location? *J Cataract Refract Surg* 24:482-486, 1998.
39. Budak K, Friedman NJ, Koch DD: Dehiscence of a radial keratotomy incision during clear corneal cataract surgery, *J Cataract Refract Surg* 24:278-280, 1998.
40. Fine IH: Self-sealing corneal tunnel incision for small-incision cataract surgery, *Ocular Surg News*, May 1, 1992.
41. Williamson CH: Cataract keratotomy surgery. In Fine IH, Fichman RA, Grabow HB, editors: *Clear-corneal cataract surgery & topical anesthesia*, Thorofare, NJ, 1993, Slack, Inc, pp 87-93.
42. Langerman DW: Architectural design of a self-sealing corneal tunnel, single-hinge incision, *J Cataract Refract Surg* 20:84-88, 1994.
43. Vass C, Menapace R, Rainer G et al: Comparative study of corneal topographic changes after 3.0 mm beveled and hinged clear corneal incisions, *J Cataract Refract Surg* 24:1498-1504, 1998.
44. Kershner RM: Clear corneal cataract surgery and the correction of myopia, hyperopia, and astigmatism, *Ophthalmology* 104:381-389, 1997.
45. Gills JP, Gayton JL: Reducing pre-existing astigmatism. In Gills JP, editor: *Cataract surgery: the state of the art*, Thorofare, NJ, 1998, Slack, Inc, pp 53-66.
46. Nichamin L: Refining astigmatic keratotomy during cataract surgery, *Ocular Surg News*, April 15, 1993.
47. Budak K, Friedman NJ, Koch DD: Limbal relaxing incisions with cataract surgery, *J Cataract Refract Surg* 24:503-508, 1998.
48. Fine IH: New blade enhances cataract surgery, techniques spotlight, *Ophthalmol Times*, Sept 1, 1996.
49. Jacobi FK, Dick B, Bohle R: Histological and ultrastructural study of corneal tunnel incisions using diamond and steel keratomes, *J Cataract Refract Surg* 24:498-502, 1998.
50. Radner W, Menapace R, Zehetmayer M et al: Ultrastructure of clear corneal incisions. I. Effect of keratomes and incision width on corneal trauma after lens implantation, *J Cataract Refract Surg* 24:487-492, 1998.
51. Mamalis N: Incision width after phacoemulsification with foldable intraocular lens implantation, *J Cataract Refract Surg* 26:237-241, 2000.
52. Fine IH: Special Report to ASCRS Members: phacoemulsification incision burns. Letter to American Society of Cataract and Refractive Surgery members, 1997.
53. Majid MA, Sharma MK, Harding SP: Corneoscleral burn during phacoemulsification surgery, *J Cataract Refract Surg* 24:1413-1415, 1998.
54. Sugar A, Schertzer RM: Clinical course of phacoemulsification wound burns, *J Cataract Refract Surg* 25:688-692, 1999.
55. Menapace R: Delayed iris prolapse with unsutured 5.1 mm clear corneal incisions, *J Cataract Refract Surg* 21:353-357, 1995.
56. Endophthalmitis: State of the prophylactic art, *Eyeworld News*, August 1997, pp 42-43.
57. Nishi O, Nishi K, Fujiwara T et al: Effects of diclofenac sodium and indomethacin on proliferation and collagen synthesis of lens epithelial cells in vitro, *J Cataract Refract Surg* 21:461-465, 1995.
58. Masket S, Tennen DG: Astigmatic stabilization of 3.0 mm temporal clear corneal cataract incisions, *J Cataract Refract Surg* 22:1451-1455, 1996.
59. Kohnen T, Dick B, Jacobi KW: Comparison of the induced astigmatism after temporal clear corneal tunnel incisions of different sizes, *J Cataract Refract Surg* 21:417-424, 1995.
60. Pfleger T, Skorpik C, Menapace R et al: Long-term course of induced astigmatism after clear corneal incision cataract surgery, *J Cataract Refract Surg* 22:72-77, 1996.
61. Nielsen PJ: Prospective evaluation of surgically induced astigmatism and astigmatic keratotomy effects of various self-sealing small incisions, *J Cataract Refract Surg* 21:43-48, 1995.
62. Cillino S, Morreale D, Maurceri A et al: Temporal versus superior approach phacoemulsification: short-term postoperative astigmatism, *J Cataract Refract Surg* 23:267-271, 1997.
63. Rainer G, Vass C, Menapace R et al: Long-term course of surgically induced astigmatism after 5.0 mm sclerocorneal valve incision, *J Cataract Refract Surg* 24:1642-1646, 1998.
64. Holweger R, Marefat B: Corneal changes after cataract surgery with 5.0 mm sutured and 3.5 mm sutureless clear corneal incisions, *J Cataract Refract Surg* 23:342-346, 1997.
65. Oshima Y, Tsujikawa K, Oh A et al: Comparative study of intraocular lens implantation through 3.0 mm temporal clear corneal and superior scleral tunnel self-sealing incisions, *J Cataract Refract Surg* 23:347-353, 1997.
66. Poort-van Nouhuijs HM, Hendrickx KHM, van Marle WF et al: Corneal astigmatism after clear corneal and corneoscleral incisions for cataract surgery, *J Cataract Refract Surg* 23:758-760, 1997.
67. Long DA, Monica ML: A prospective evaluation of corneal curvature changes with 3.0 to 3.5 mm corneal tunnel phacoemulsification, *Ophthalmology* 103:226-232, 1996.
68. Simsek S, Yasar T, Demirok A et al: Effect of superior and temporal clear corneal incisions on astigmatism after sutureless phacoemulsification, *J Cataract Refract Surg* 24:515-518, 1998.
69. Roman SJ, Auclin F, Chong-Sit DA et al: Surgically induced astigmatism with superior and temporal incisions in cases of with-the-rule preoperative astigmatism, *J Cataract Refract Surg* 24:1636-1641, 1998.
70. Rainer G, Menapace R, Vass C et al: Corneal shape changes after temporal and superolateral 3.0 mm clear corneal incisions, *J Cataract Refract Surg* 25:1121-1126, 1999.
71. Grabow HB: The clear-corneal incision. In Fine IH, Fichman RA, Grabow HB, editors: *Clear-corneal cataract surgery & topical anesthesia*, Thorofare, NJ, 1993, Slack Inc, pp 29-62.
72. Amon M, Menapace R, Vass C et al: Endothelial cell loss after 3.5 mm temporal clear corneal incision and 3.5 mm superior scleral tunnel incision, *Eur J Implant Refract Surg* 7:229-232, 1995.
73. Dick HB, Kohnen T, Jacobi FK et al: Long-term endothelial cell loss following phacoemulsification through a temporal clear corneal incision, *J Cataract Refract Surg* 22:63-71, 1996.
74. Fine IH: Ongoing research in uses of power modulations to achieve low-energy phacoemulsification of cataracts. Presentation at the ASCRS Innovators' Session, Seattle, April 12, 1999.
75. Dick HB, Schwenn O, Krummenauer F et al: Inflammation after sclerocorneal versus clear corneal tunnel phacoemulsification, *Ophthalmology* 107:241-247, 2000.

Capsulorhexis

13

Thomas Neuhann, MD

History

The rebirth of extracapsular cataract extraction in its modern, refined, microsurgical version has brought with it the need for an adequate technique for anterior capsulectomy. Vogt's technique, using toothed forceps to grasp and rip out a part of the anterior capsule, was definitely thought to be too traumatic, to both the endothelium and the zonular apparatus, as well as too uncontrollable. Kelman's "Christmas tree" technique was a considerable improvement in terms of both better control and less trauma. Soon, however, interconnected perforations of the anterior capsule with a cystotome in a circular pattern, the "can-opener" technique, became the most popular and almost universally used approach worldwide. It allowed relatively precise control of the diameter and shape of the excised anterior capsular flap and, by using a cannula infusion cystotome, allowed the anterior chamber to be maintained throughout the procedure. Later, in an attempt to use the anterior capsule for additional endothelial protection during the surgical procedure, the "letterbox" technique was developed and gained considerable popularity, especially among surgeons preferring planned extracapsular cataract extraction. This two-stage technique also offered considerable advantages for controlled lens implantation into the capsular bag because the anterior capsular window was not completed until after implantation of the intraocular lens (IOL).

Although these techniques and their modifications adequately fulfilled the aim of removing the central part of the anterior capsule, they proved to have one major disadvantage. The necessary manipulations during either phacoemulsification or extraction of the entire nucleus were almost invariably associated with the creation of one or more tears of the remaining peripheral anterior capsular rim, extending at least into the capsular equator. This has a number of undesirable side effects. Not infrequently, the tears extended beyond the capsular equator and into the posterior capsule, accompanied by the associated complications of vitreous loss and loss of the nucleus into the vitreous, especially when occurring early in the course of the operation. In addition, these tears divided the peripheral anterior capsule into a number of separate flaps, which could then interfere with the surgical procedure, especially the aspiration of peripheral cortical remnants. Finally, accumulating clinical evidence led an increasing number of surgeons to prefer IOL implantation into the capsular bag over sulcus implantation; however, it became evident after a while that at least 50% of the IOLs thought to be securely implanted with both loops in the capsular bag had, in reality, only one fixation loop in the bag or none at all. Anterior capsule tears were frequently the source of IOL loops escaping from the capsular bag.

Development of Capsulorhexis

From what may later be called a general surgical "instinct" (which was later fully substantiated by the clinical experience), a number of surgeons had realized for some time that the ideal anterior capsulectomy would be one with a smooth, continuous, ideally circular margin, but the technique to achieve this ideal remained elusive. In 1984, Howard Gimbel in Calgary, Alberta, Canada, and Thomas Neuhann in Munich simultaneously and independently developed a technique that essentially consisted of tearing rather than cutting out a central anterior capsular window. What was so decisively new about this technique was not the tearing itself but the fact that it had been used for part of the anterior capsulotomy before. The difference was that the tear was brought around the entire circumference, resulting in a circular opening with no beginning or end, nor an outward-pointing edge from which a radial tear could originate. Gimbel and Neuhann used different technical approaches, yet with the same underlying basic principle, benefiting from the specific tearing properties of the lens capsule. Much like cellophane, the lens capsule splits easily from a sharp-edged point of departure, whereas it is extremely resistant to tears into a smooth margin. Both surgeons showed their first video film in 1985—Gimbel at the annual meeting of the American Society of Cataract and Refractive Surgery in Boston and Neuhann at the meeting of the German Ophthalmological Society in Heidelberg. In his film, Neuhann also proposed the term *capsulorhexis*. The first formal publication in a scientific journal appeared in 1987[1]; in 1990 Gimbel and Neuhann published a joint article in the *Journal of Cataract and Refractive Surgery*.[2]

Both Gimbel and Neuhann have always regarded capsulorhexis as being developed by both of them equally and independently, respectfully acknowledging the work of others on which it is based.[3]

Terminology

The term *kapsulorhexis* was proposed by Neuhann to make clear that it was a truly new surgical technique, a new surgical principle (namely tearing instead of cutting) and not just another modification of previous techniques. Gimbel originally called his technique "continuous tear capsulotomy." Bringing both their terms together yielded "continuous curvilinear (more general than circular) capsulorhexis" (CCC).

Principles and Advantages of Capsulorhexis

Capsulorhexis leaves a capsular bag with mechanical and structural integrity, despite an opening large enough to deliver the lens through. This is due to the lens capsule's shearing property, which resembles cellophane. Although the capsule tears easily when departing from a sharply pointed defect in an edge, requiring a minimal amount of force, much greater force is required to rupture a straight, smooth margin.[4-6] This property is commonly experienced when opening the cellophane wrapper of a package. Tearing open a cellophane-wrapped package is greatly facilitated when the manufacturer provides a linear break in the wrapper and an arrow to that point with the instructions "Start here." If an opening in the lens capsule has a continuous smooth margin, the remaining capsule stays on stretch like a trampoline, as if no hole were present. The obvious advantages of this are as follows:

1. No tags or flaps of anterior capsule remnants interfere with surgery, especially the aspiration of the peripheral cortex.
2. The mechanical forces exerted onto the capsule and thereby onto the zonules are minimized.
3. The capsular bag is deeply open during surgery with a closed system approach: The posterior capsule is ballooned posteriorly and thus held on stretch, reducing the danger of it getting caught and broken, while the anterior capsule remains on stretch horizontally, maintaining intracapsular space for surgical maneuvers.
4. With an intact capsulorhexis, manipulations within the capsular bag (which are always in some way associated with distention), such as tilting or cracking the nucleus or implanting an IOL, no longer entail the risk of extending radial tears in the anterior capsule into the posterior capsule.
5. Capsulorhexis is the prerequisite for a reproducibly secure, verifiable, and permanent capsular bag fixation of IOL implant haptics.[7]
6. Even in the case of a posterior capsule defect, regardless of its size, an intact anterior capsulorhexis provides the possibility of implanting an IOL safely into the ciliary sulcus. If the capsulorhexis opening is well centered and smaller than the optic, it may be used additionally to fixate the implant by capturing the optic ("rhexis fixation") posteriorly while the haptics remain anterior in the ciliary sulcus.
7. It can be learned "by doing" without exposing the patient or the physician to any risk.
8. Capsulorhexis is the prerequisite for all attempts to minimize or control posterior capsule opacification after cataract formation by the principle of a sharp posterior edge of the IOL.

Current Standard Techniques of Capsulorhexis

There are three basic choices that a surgeon must make for establishing his or her standard technique:

1. The instrument: a cystotome or a forceps
2. The access: via the main incision or via a side-port paracentesis
3. The medium: irrigation with fluid or viscoelastic

Although all three options may theoretically be freely combined, in practice there are two main options:

1. A bent needle or cystotome through a side-port paracentesis under fluid irrigation (or viscoelastic)
2. A forceps through the main incision (or a side-port paracentesis) under viscoelastic

For the **needle technique,** a 23-gauge needle is bent to about a one-quarter circle and with the tip 45 degrees away from the bevel. The needle is mounted on an infusion handpiece, connected to the gravity-fed infusion at maximum height. With the infusion continuously running, the anterior chamber is entered through the side port, the size of which should just be large enough to permit passage of the needle. The chamber will thus be formed as deep as possible. The anterior capsule is perforated near the center with the needle tip and then slitted in a curvilinear manner with the cutting side edge of the needle in such a way that the desired radius of the capsulorhexis is reached in a blend-in manner (Figure 13-1). When about to reach the desired circumference, the capsule is lifted from underneath, close to the leading tear edge, and pushed upward and forward to propagate the tear. Soon, enough of a flap will be created to permit flipping it over and engaging it from its backside, its epithelial side, now facing up toward the cornea.

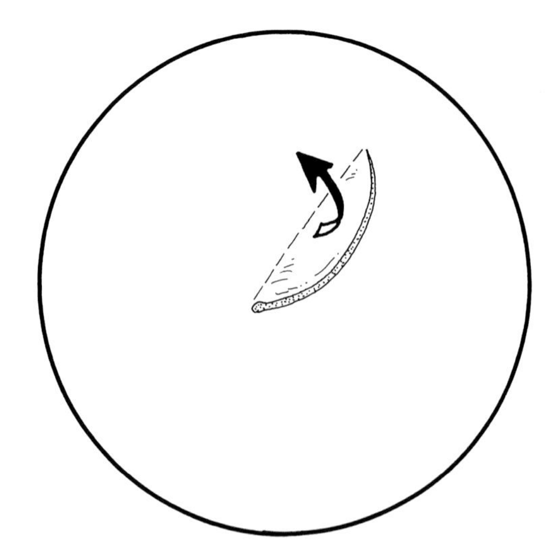

FIGURE 13-1 In the standard technique for capsulorhexis, a central puncture with a cystotome followed by an arched curve creates a slit. The capsular flap is pulled and lifted at its edge.

The needle engages the flap by exerting just enough pressure to create the friction necessary for engagement, but not enough pressure for the needle tip to perforate. Having the capsular flap thus engaged, it is torn in a circular fashion (Figure 13-2, *A*) by appropriately influencing the tear vectors. The more distant the point of engagement is from the leading edge of the tear, the more centripetally one must tear; the closer the point of engagement is to the leading edge, the more directly the tear will follow the direction of traction. It is therefore most advisable to refixate the tear with the cystotome point frequently close to the leading edge—a basic principle that governs the entire technique and its variations. When brought around full circle, the tear is blended into itself, automatically coming from outside in, which is a basic prerequisite to avoid a discontinuity.

The same technique can also be performed with the anterior chamber filled with a viscoelastic substance. One would basically follow the same guidelines, with the exception of the continuously running infusion.

The **forceps technique** makes the use of a viscoelastic substance mandatory to maintain the anterior chamber. When using a Utrata-type forceps, access through the main incision, which for that purpose must be fully widened to at least 3 mm, must be chosen. When using a coaxial forceps of a pars plana–type construction, such as the Koch forceps, a paracentesis opening of appropriate size is sufficient. Otherwise, the forceps technique follows the same principles and guidelines as outlined earlier for the needle technique (see Figure 13-2, *B*).

A

B

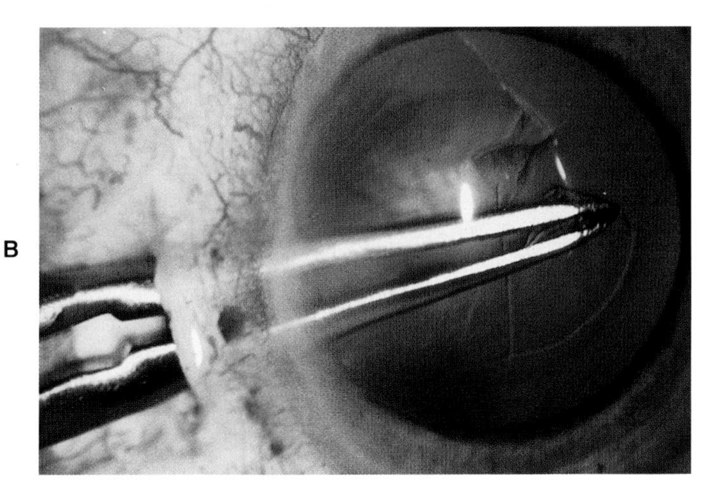

C

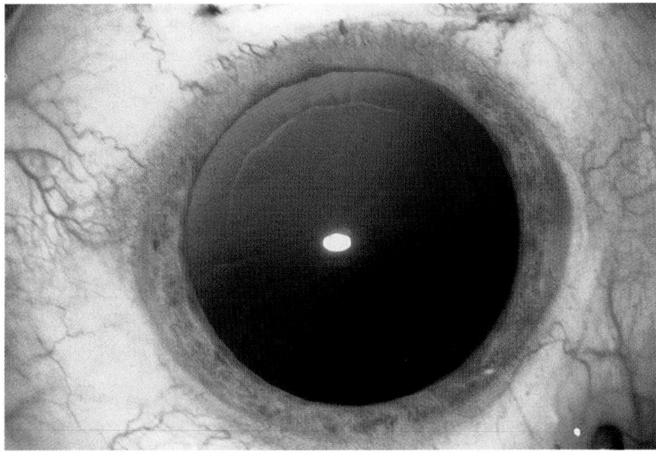

FIGURE 13-2 A, Flap is inverted, and the underside of the capsule edge, now anterior, is engaged with the needle tip or forceps and pulled circularly. **B,** Circular tear capsulorhexis is illustrated using a capsulorhexis forceps. **C,** Perfect large circular capsulorhexis is seen on red reflex through the operating microscope.

TECHNICAL TIPS

Starting the tear somewhere in the center in the capsule has the advantage of virtually eliminating the possibility of creating a discontinuity, which would be caused by finishing the tear from inside out; this becomes especially valuable in cases with reduced visibility (e.g., small pupils, no red reflex). The tear must be performed over the full 360 degrees in the direction in which it was started.

Puncturing the capsule within the contour of the capsulorhexis has the disadvantage that it may cause a stellate burst (with extensions to the capsular periphery) if the needle is not perfectly sharp. If such a burst goes unnoticed (e.g., for visibility reasons) or if its extensions reach too far peripherally to be recovered, a peripheral tear will result at this location (Figure 13-3). In addition, with this technique the risk of inadvertently completing the capsulorhexis from inside out is slightly higher. On the other hand, by beginning with a puncture, the surgeon has two options about where to proceed with the tear, developing it and bringing both ends together at the point of maximal control (Figures 13-2, *C*, and 13-4). Today, most surgeons probably start somewhere in the capsular center.

TECHNICAL TIPS

With irrigation, the capsular flap floats freely in the anterior chamber, improving visualization, maneuverability, and control. Conversely, the incision must be tight, necessitating a very accurate and meticulous fulcrum technique. A viscoelastic substance is more forgiving with a leaking incision. However, visualization, especially of the leading tear edge, may be impaired as the torn-out portion of the capsule gets larger, crimps, and is "frozen" in the viscoelastic, possibly mixed with anterior cortex, and may lead to loss of control over the flap. Therefore the flap should always be well spread out over the undersurface.

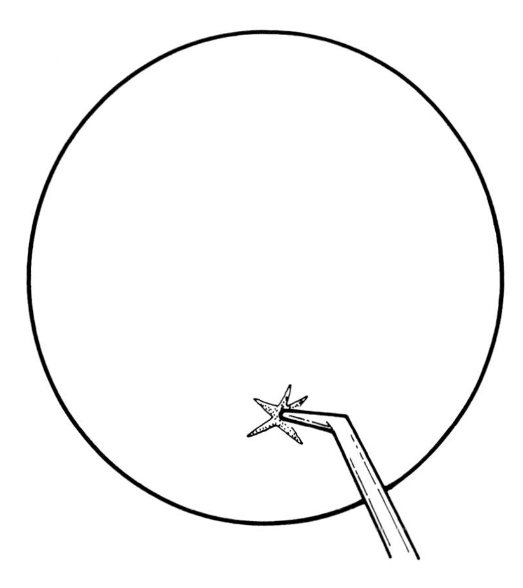

FIGURE 13-3 Use of a blunt needle to puncture the capsule in the periphery may create a stellate burst with outward pointing edges from which peripheral tears may originate.

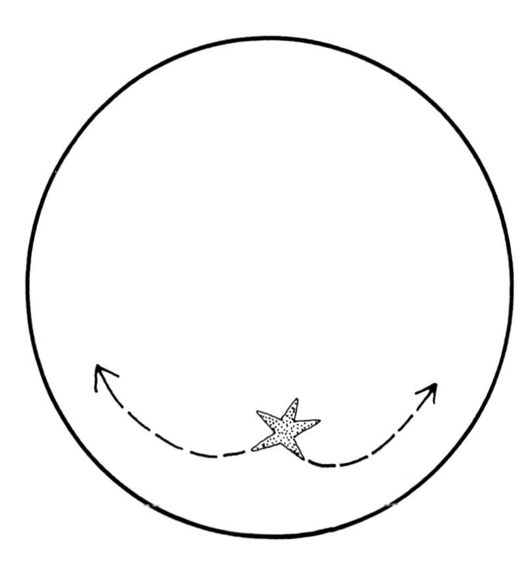

FIGURE 13-4 After a stellate opening, a continuous curve capsulorhexis can be achieved by tearing in both directions from the most peripheral edges of the stellate opening.

TECHNICAL TIPS

A drawback of the forceps technique is that it necessitates a larger incision and therefore can be safely performed only with a viscoelastic agent. Conversely, grasping with a forceps is somewhat more secure than grasping with a needle and is independent of the solidity of the underlying cortical material (which, with the needle technique, really constitutes the "second hand"). This latter aspect also makes it the technique of choice in some special situations (see further on).

Two additional aspects regarding capsulorhexis techniques merit discussion:

The question of the ideal size of the anterior capsule opening. Ideally, the size should be:

- As large as possible. The larger the opening, the easier the manipulation of the nucleus.
- Small enough to allow the anterior capsular margin to just cover the optical part of the IOL, completely sealing it into the capsular bag. This "sealing-in" effect appears to be a prerequisite for the inhibitory effect of sharp IOL edges on the formation of secondary cataract.

Limitations to obtain the ideal size include the following:

- The size of the pupil
- The central insertion of the zonular fibers

The surgeon must recognize that corneal magnification will make the initial capsulorhexis appear larger than its true size; once the IOL is inserted, the capsulorhexis will appear to have shrunken in comparison with the IOL optic.[8]

An asymmetric opening, that is, partly covering and partly not covering the optic margin, is to be avoided because of its potential of causing IOL optic decentration.

Learning capsulorhexis. One of its major advantages is that capsulorhexis can be learned "by doing" without exposing the patient to any additional risk. Coming from whatever prior

TECHNICAL TIPS

When using a Utrata-type forceps through the main incision, insidious loss of viscoelastic is very likely to occur. This leads to a flattening of the anterior chamber and consequently a forward movement of the lens. This, in turn, leads to an increase of the outward vector forces inherent in the lens capsule, making it increasingly more difficult to keep the tear from running outward. Knowing the danger means banning it: refilling the chamber with viscoelastic patiently as losses occur can prevent this most frequent source of losing control over the capsular tear. Instruments that open only at the tip (coaxial vitrectomy type) introduced through a paracentesis reduce viscoelastic loss. Use of a low-molecular-weight, retentive viscoelastic agent also reduces the amount of viscoelastic lost through the main incision.

technique of anterior capsulotomy, the surgeon may begin along the given guidelines. If the tear starts moving into an unwanted direction, the surgeon can revert to the previous technique.

To practice, good surrogates for the lens capsule are cellophane, as used in shrink-wrap packages, or tomato skin. Pigs' eyes, with thicker and more elastic anterior capsules, can serve as excellent models for learning to master the difficulties in infantile and juvenile capsules.

Difficult Situations

Capsulorhexis is best learned under ideal conditions: good to adequate pupillary dilation, good red reflex, deep anterior chamber, and no positive pressure.

The following four basic types of difficulties present challenges for capsulorhexis:

1. No red reflex
2. Small pupil

3. Positive back pressure
4. Extreme elasticity: the infantile/juvenile capsule

Although they often occur in various combinations, each of these situations is discussed separately to clarify the basic principles of management.

No Red Reflex

When there is no adequate reflex from the fundus to retroilluminate the surgical site for visualization, other clues must be used to "detect" the capsular margin in order to control the tear in every moment. The introduction of capsular dyeing, usually with trypan blue, is certainly the most notable progress in solving problems of visualization of the anterior capsule (for details, see Chapter 25, Intumescent Cataract). Additional help can be contributed by other technical details; for instance, inclining the eye slightly with regard to the observation and illumination paths can sometimes produce enough of a red reflex to safely proceed. Also, side illumination, in addition to or instead of coaxial illumination, can be helpful. Often, one can benefit from the orange skin–like specular reflex of the coaxial light source on the capsule. Constant manipulation of the eye position in such a way that the progressing tear edge remains in that reflex zone outlines the tear very clearly. Also, one should always choose as high a magnification as does not interfere with the necessary overview. Finally, proceeding slowly in small steps and with frequent regrasping will help not to lose control of the flap.

The Small Pupil

In addition to precluding visualization of the capsular area where one wishes to place the tear, the small pupil in most instances also causes reduction of the red reflex. Therefore all of the previous measures are advisable as needed. (For an extensive discussion of small-pupil techniques, see Chapter 19.) When the pupil is smaller than the desired capsulorhexis diameter, one may combine different principles. With experience, the surgeon will be able to tear a capsular flap "blindly," larger than the pupil diameter. Starting from the capsular center within the visible pupillary area will ensure completion from "outside in." If one chooses to start the capsulorhexis from the peripheral circumference, the needle may be used to retract the pupillary margin to the desired eccentricity, sliding along it while creating the initial slit and developing the flap away from the site of entry. Previous dyeing of the capsule with trypan blue can be helpful in judging the flap diameter. Measures to increase the pupillary diameter may include injection of atropine and/or epinephrine into the anterior chamber; filling the chamber with viscoelastic; peeling off the fibrous lining of the posterior aspect of the pupil, which so often limits its dilation; dilation of the pupil with self-retaining hooks; or only local dilation of the pupil with a second instrument through a second paracentesis, sliding along the pupillary edge with the progression of the tear. Multiple snip-sphincterotomies or sphincter stretching has been advocated. When in doubt, I prefer a keyhole iridotomy, which is later resutured, because it restores the iris diaphragm and thereby helps prevent later broad adhesions between an atonic, flaccid iris and the anterior capsule or even the posterior capsule from migrating behind the implant. Finally, another possibility is performing phacoemulsification through an initially smaller capsulorhexis and enlarging it later in a two-step-technique.

Positive Pressure

Positive pressure tends to force the tear outward. Therefore these cases require an intentionally small diameter to begin with—which can be widened as soon as the pressure is relieved—and continuous, pronounced centripetal traction in small steps, regrasping frequently close to the tear edge. Also, exerting counterpressure by pushing the lens back with viscoelastic is very helpful.

Infantile/Juvenile Capsule

The special challenge in infantile and juvenile capsulotomy is the increased elasticity of the lens capsule. When placing tension on an anterior capsule flap, it will first distend considerably before propagating the tear; once the tear starts, it has a great propensity to get lost outward because of the tractional "preload" and the elasticity, creating a pronounced outward pulling vector force. It is therefore advisable to intend the tear to be smaller than one really wishes it to be because it will become wider by itself. The capsulorhexis tear should progress slowly, in small steps, and with frequent regrasping and directing the tearing more centripetally than for a typical adult cataract. The disadvantage of the extreme elasticity, however, has a positive side also. Should a discontinuity in the capsulorhexis margin occur, it is for the same reason less likely to progress peripherally when due caution during surgery is maintained.

The only situation in which capsulorhexis is impossible in principle is the totally fibrosed capsule. Cases of heavy fibrosis or fibrous plaques extending so far peripherally that one cannot tear around them without hitting zonules mandate the use of scissors to cut through the fibrosis. The scissor cut should end just barely at the margin of the fibrosis, and from there on into regular capsule the opening should be continued as a tear.

TECHNICAL TIPS

The *intumescent lens* combines the difficulties of positive pressure with those of a lack of red reflex. Filling the anterior chamber with a thick viscoelastic is advisable to block opaque liquefied cortex from leaking into the aqueous humor and compromising visibility. Usually a forceps technique is preferable because the cortex is liquefied and therefore presents no resistance to a needle tip. The second major problem is the increased pressure within the capsule as a result of the swollen lens, which increases the risk of uncontrollable extension of the partially completed capsular opening to the periphery. The surgeon must try to counteract this tendency by filling the anterior chamber with a high-viscosity viscoelastic, to the extent of indenting the anterior lens pole. Sometimes one can decompress the lens by making a small puncture in the central anterior lens and aspirating some of the liquid content.

Special Surgical Techniques

Applying the same basic principles as described earlier has led to the development of maneuvers that may prove helpful in certain situations.

Bimanual Forceps

In certain situations, it may become difficult to grasp and manipulate the capsular flap with just the needle tip. The surgeon may, in these situations, prefer to change to a forceps technique. However, when removing the irrigating cystotome, the lens diaphragm may come forward, causing the tear to divert outward. To avoid this, a bifurcated spatula of the Bechert type (or similar modification) is introduced into the chamber through an opposite paracentesis. The capsular flap is pinched between the needle tip and spatula tip. The capsule flap can then be manipulated as with a forceps.

An alternative is to introduce viscoelastic through the second paracentesis before withdrawing an irrigating cystotome needle. The anterior chamber will remained formed while the surgeon changes to a forceps.

Bimanual/Bi-instrumental Capsulorhexis

When the zonules are very weak, pulling centripetally on the flap may risk disinsertion of the capsule. Holding the flap with capsular forceps with one hand and gently pushing the peripheral margin outward (centrifugally) with a blunt instrument can propagate the tear with less stress on the zonules. The surgeon should strongly consider placing a capsule tension ring as soon as the capsulorhexis is completed in these very tenuous cases.

Posterior Capsulorhexis

Leaving the posterior capsule intact is one of the major objectives of extracapsular surgery. Nevertheless, this goal cannot always be attained. Examples are a dense, nonremovable posterior capsular opacification that will doubtlessly interfere significantly with vision; an infantile cataract in which rapid opacification of the posterior capsule is inevitable and neodymium: yttrium-aluminum-garnet (Nd:YAG) laser capsulotomy is impractical (see Chapter 24, Pediatric Cataracts); or, most frequently, accidental posterior capsular rupture. In all of these cases, the opening in the posterior capsule should have the same quality, if possible, as that of the anterior capsulorhexis, namely being not further extendable because of a continuous smooth margin. This can be obtained by applying the same technique of capsulorhexis to the posterior capsule. In cases of intentional posterior capsule opening, the posterior capsule should be nicked centrally with a needle tip, viscoelastic is injected through the first tiny triangular defect to separate and posteriorly displace the anterior vitreous face, and the posterior capsular triangle is grasped by capsular forceps and torn out as a curvilinear posterior capsulorhexis.

When an unintended capsular defect occurs, extension can be limited by the same technique, as long as the original posterior capsule rent is limited enough to permit this. This technique will then preserve a capsular bag into which an IOL can be implanted securely, maintaining all the advantages of intracapsular implantation.

"Rhexis-Fixation"

In the case of a posterior capsular rupture that cannot be limited by posterior capsulorhexis, another maneuver may maintain most of the advantages of capsular implant fixation. If the anterior capsulorhexis margin is intact and smaller than the IOL optic, the IOL can be implanted into the ciliary sulcus and the optic captured, that is, "buttoned in" backward through the capsulorhexis in the technique first described by Tobias Neuhann. This provides secure mechanical fixation of the lens by the capsule and centration in relation to the capsular opening, with the lens haptics only acting as secondary support. The IOL in this position will have the same optical power as though intracapsularly implanted.

Complications and Pitfalls

The following are three classic intraoperative complications that can occur with capsulorhexis:

1. Discontinuity of the anterior capsular margin
2. Tear into the zonules
3. Diameter too small

The following are two classic postoperative complications:

1. Purse-string contraction
2. Incarceration of viscoelastic

Discontinuity of the Anterior Capsular Margin

The major causative factors are completing the capsulorhexis "from inside outward" (Figure 13-5), nicking an originally intact margin with the second instrument during lens extraction, or breaking the rim with the activated phaco tip. A discontinuity

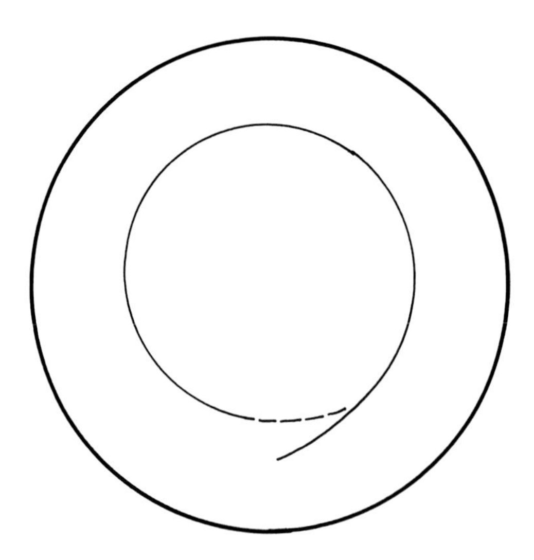

FIGURE 13-5 Illustration of a capsulorhexis that is progressively enlarging so that it finishes from the inside toward the outside.

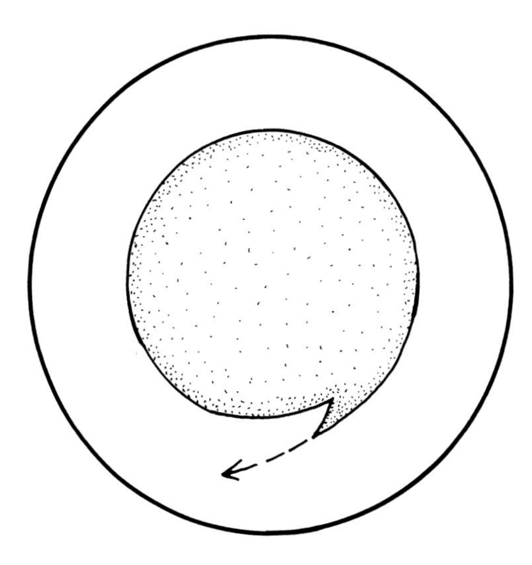

FIGURE 13-6 Discontinuity in the capsule is created by an inside-to-outside finish. From that point, a peripheral tear may originate. The same situation results when a previously intact capsulorhexis margin is cut with an instrument or with the phacoemulsification tip.

in an otherwise intact CCC margin will in most cases extend into a radial tear into the capsular fornix; it will do so very readily because the distensive forces will concentrate on this single point of weakness (Figure 13-6). The risk of this radial tear extending around the capsular fornix into the posterior capsule increases with sparse and friable zonules and with all maneuvers that distend the anterior capsular opening, such as hydrodissection, expression of the nucleus, nuclear fracturing techniques that rely on pushing the nuclear sections widely apart, and IOL implantation maneuvers.

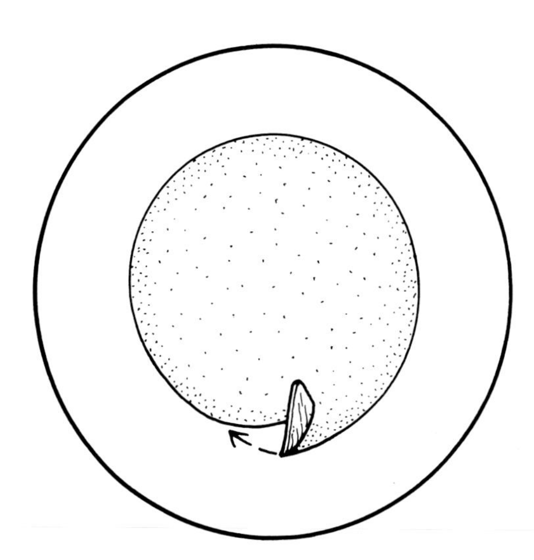

FIGURE 13-7 When an inside-outside discontinuity occurs, it can be repaired by picking up the resulting triangle, inverting it, and tearing centripetally to bring the tear edge back toward the capsulorhexis margin, ultimately blending it in.

TECHNICAL TIPS

The most important rule is to *always close the circle from outside inward.* This will automatically occur when starting the tear somewhere in the center of the capsule, as described earlier (Figure 13-7). If the flap beaks off during the course of the tear, the surgeon must be sure to grasp the remaining flap and continue the outward pointing tear edge. When a discontinuity happens, timely recognition is of key importance. Its edge must instantly be grasped with forceps and blunted off by blending into the main contour (Figure 13-8). When a tear has occurred into the capsular fornix, utmost caution is warranted not to extend the tear further by avoiding the previous risk factors. A relaxing counterincision opposite the first tear may be considered. A radial tear does not preclude capsular bag implantation if manipulations are appropriately gentle. The lens haptics should be placed at 90 degrees from the radial tear. Such a tear is a relative contraindication for implantation of plate haptic IOLs.

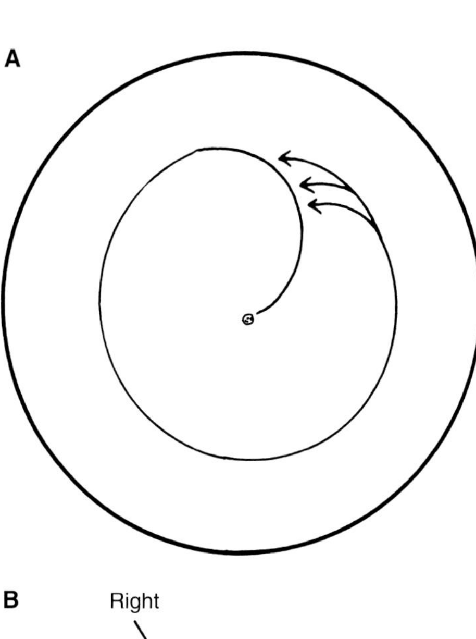

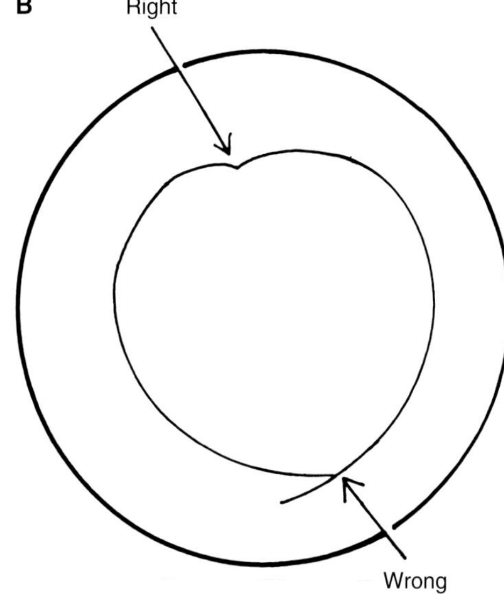

FIGURE 13-8 A, Starting the capsulorhexis from the center makes it virtually impossible to end in an inside-out fashion. Creating a continuous margin is much more likely. **B,** When a capsulorhexis is completed correctly, a small centrally pointing tag is created. When the capsulorhexis is incorrectly finished, a discontinuity occurs.

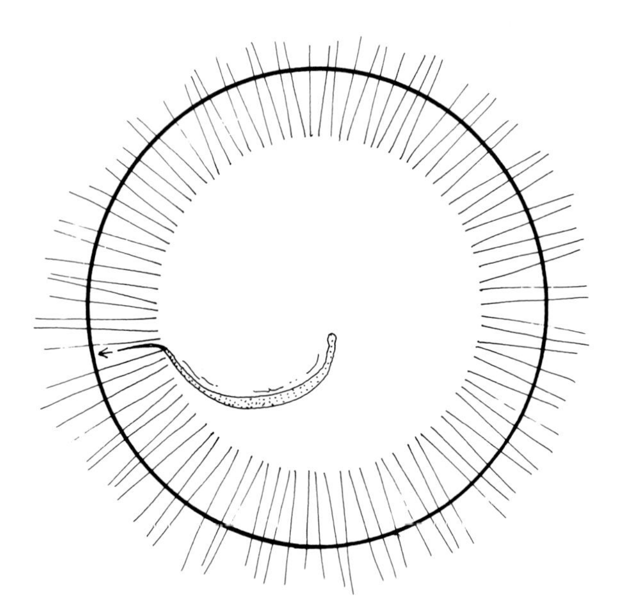

FIGURE 13-9 When a capsular tear encounters a zonular fiber, the resulting zonular forces direct the tear peripherally toward the equator.

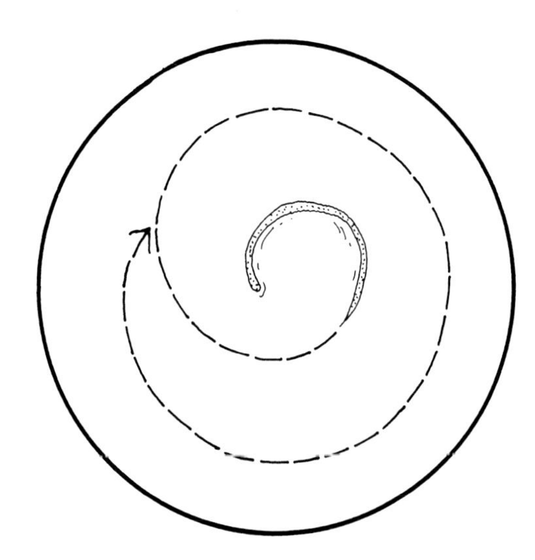

FIGURE 13-10 In performing the capsulorhexis, the surgeon may realize that the original arc is too small. The capsulorhexis can be expanded by "spiraling" outward to the desired diameter and then "closing the circle."

Tear into the Zonules

If the tear encounters zonular fibers, either because it is too peripheral or because zonules are inserting abnormally centrally, it cannot readily be continued. Further tearing will risk deviation of the tear to the periphery, like tearing paper alongside a ruler (Figure 13-9). With the help of high microscope magnification, an optimized red reflex or specular reflex, and optimal focusing, the responsible zonules can be identified and their insertions removed from the capsule with the needle or forceps tip. Then the surgeon brings the tear more centrally and continues. Sometimes this situation can also be managed by grasping the flap close to its edge and briskly pulling it centrally. This maneuver, however, carries a higher risk and is only advised when the more controlled approach does not seem possible.

Healon 5 (Pharmacia), with its exceptionally high density, can also help redirect an extending capsulorhexis tear. A relatively small amount of Healon 5 is injected into the angle, with the expanding bolus reaching the edge of the tear. The dense Healon 5 will help redirect the tear back centrally.

Capsulorhexis with Too Small a Diameter

If the surgeon realizes that the diameter of the CCC is becoming smaller than desired, he or she may just continue the tear in a spiral manner until the desired diameter is reached (Figure 13-10).

When a large and hard nucleus coincides with a very small diameter of the anterior capsular opening, hydrodissection may lead to a pressure-induced rupture of the posterior capsule. The nucleus blocks the capsular opening, and the injected fluid has only one way to escape: posteriorly. An initial bulging forward of the lens followed by a sudden, snaplike drop backward indicates the occurrence. In such an event, conversion to planned extracapsular cataract extraction is indicated. A lens loop behind the nucleus is necessary. Consideration should be given to "posterior assisted levitation" with either an instrument or injection of viscoelastic through a pars plana sclerotomy to support the nucleus from behind.[9]

Purse-String Contraction

The remaining lens epithelial cells on the back surface of the anterior capsule postoperatively undergo fibrous metaplasia. The contraction of this fibrous layer is normally counteracted by the centrifugal forces of the zonular apparatus. However, when either the zonules are weak (e.g., in pseudoexfoliation, trauma, and retinitis pigmentosa) or the fibrosis is excessive (e.g., after increased postoperative inflammation, with some silicone lenses and other factors) or in combinations of both, the anterior capsular opening may contract ("capsular phimosis") (Figure 13-11). The contracture may block the visual axis

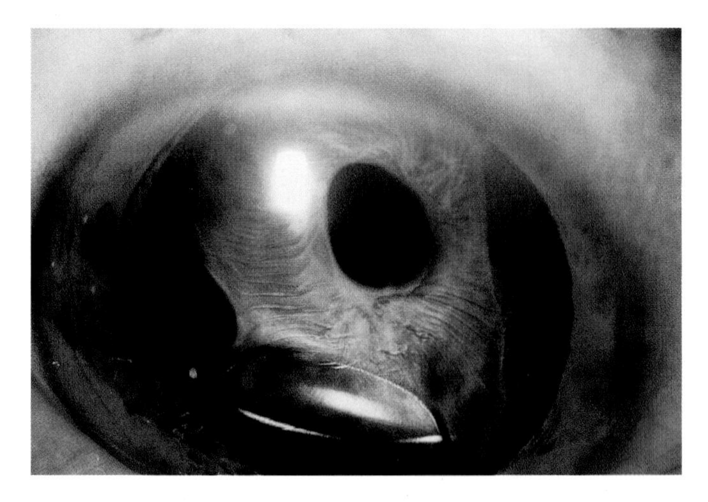

FIGURE 13-11 Postoperative photograph illustrating contracture of the capsulorhexis. This situation is more common when the original capsulorhexis is 4 mm or smaller.

TECHNICAL TIPS

In cases identified at risk for excessive contraction, the surgeon should aim for a relatively large opening, implant lenses with stiff haptics with an overall diameter of about 13 mm, consider implantation of a capsular tension ring (or even two), and perhaps avoid silicone as a lens material. Postoperatively, these cases should be monitored closely. At the first sign of contraction, the anterior capsular margin should be incised with an Nd:YAG laser at three or four equidistant locations. Extension of these discontinuities need not be feared at this stage, owing to the fibrous lining itself and the already secure sealing in of the IOL.

or exert excessive contracture on the ciliary body, leading to hypotony.[10]

Incarceration of Viscoelastic ("Capsular Block Syndrome")

Residual viscoelastic may be trapped behind an implant when the IOL optic margin is completely covered by the capsulorhexis. The retained viscoelastic attracts water osmotically and swells. The implant acts as a valve, permitting the influx of aqueous behind the lens, but not the efflux of the thick viscoelastic-aqueous mixture. This phenomenon is more pronounced with plate haptic lenses but may happen with all types of implants. The consequence may be gross inflation of the capsular bag with posterior ballooning of the posterior capsule and anterior displacement of the IOL, heralded by a shallow anterior chamber and a myopic shift in the refraction.[11]

This complication can best be avoided by complete removal of the viscoelastic material, actively aspirating it from behind the lens. Once capsular block has occurred, the retained material can be released into the anterior chamber by puncturing the anterior capsule beyond the optical margin with Nd:YAG laser pulses. If the pupil cannot be dilated adequately to expose the anterior capsule peripheral to the IOL optic, a laser peripheral iridectomy can be made, followed by further laser pulses deeper through the iridectomy to open the anterior capsule. If this cannot be achieved, the posterior capsule must be punctured, releasing the material into the vitreous. Prophylactic treatment with topical steroids, nonsteroidal antiinflammatory agents, and glaucoma medications is given because of expected transient inflammation and elevated intraocular pressure from the abruptly released viscoelastic agent.

REFERENCES

1. Neuhann T: Theorie und operationstechnik der kapsulorhexis, *Klin Monatsbl Augenheilkd* 190:542-545, 1987.
2. Gimbel HV, Neuhann T: Development, advantages, and methods of the continuous curvilinear capsulorrhexis, *J Cataract Refract Surg* 17:110-111, 1991.
3. Assia EI, Apple DJ, Barden A et al: An experimental study comparing various anterior capsulectomy techniques, *Arch Ophthalmol* 109:642-647, 1991.
4. Thim K, Krag S, Corydon L: Stretching capacity of capsulorhexis and nucleus delivery, *J Cataract Refract Surg* 17:27-31, 1991.
5. Krag S, Thim K, Corydon L: Stretching capacity of capsulorhexis: an experimental study on animal cadaver eyes, *Eur J Implant Refract Surg* 2:43-45, 1990.
6. Assia EI, Apple DJ, Tsai JC et al: The elastic properties of the lens capsule in capsulorhexis, *Am J Ophthalmol* 111:628-632, 1991.
7. Colvard DM, Dunn SA: Intraocular lens centration with continuous tear capsulotomy, *J Cataract Refract Surg* 16:312-304, 1990.
8. Waltz KL, Rubin ML: Capsulorhexis and corneal magnification, *Arch Ophthalmol* 110:170, 1992 (letter).
9. Harris DJ, Specht CS: Intracapsular lens delivery during attempted extracapsular cataract extraction: association with capsulorhexis, *Ophthalmology* 98:623-627, 1991.
10. Fritsch E, Bopp S, Lucke K et al: Pars-plana-kapselresektion zur therapie des okulären hypotoniesyndroms durch kapselschrumpfung mit ziliarkörpertraktion, *Fortschr Ophthalmol* 88:802-805, 1991.
11. Davison JA: Capsular bag distension after endophacoemulsification and posterior chamber intraocular lens implantation, *J Cataract Refract Surg* 16:99-108, 1990.

Hydrodissection and Hydrodelineation

14

I. Howard Fine, MD
Mark Packer, MD
Richard S. Hoffman, MD

Hydrodissection

Hydrodissection of the nucleus in cataract surgery has traditionally been perceived as the injection of fluid into the cortical layer of the lens under the lens capsule to separate the lens nucleus from the cortex and capsule.[1] With increased use of continuous curvilinear capsulorhexis[2,3] and phacoemulsification in cataract surgery, hydrodissection became a very important step to mobilize the nucleus within the capsule for disassembly and removal.[4-8] Following nuclear removal, cortical cleanup proceeded as a separate step, using irrigation and aspiration handpieces.

Fine[9] has previously described cortical cleaving hydrodissection, which is a hydrodissection technique designed to cleave the cortex from the lens capsule and thus leave the cortex attached to the epinucleus. Cortical cleaving hydrodissection usually eliminates the need for cortical cleanup as a separate step in cataract surgery by phacoemulsification, thereby eliminating the risk of capsular rupture during cortical cleanup.

Technique

A small capsulorhexis, 5 to 5.5 mm, optimizes the procedure. The large anterior capsular flap makes this type of hydrodissection easier to perform. The anterior capsular flap is elevated away from the cortical material with a 26-gauge blunt cannula (e.g., Katena Instruments No. K7-5150) before hydrodissection (Figures 14-1 to 14-3). The cannula maintains the anterior capsule in a tented-up position at the injection site near the lens equator. Irrigation before elevation of the anterior capsule should be avoided because it will result in transmission of a fluid wave circumferentially within the cortical layer, hydrating the cortex and creating a path of least resistance that will allow later cortical cleaving hydrodissection (Figure 14-4). Once the cannula is properly placed and the anterior capsule is elevated, gentle continuous irrigation results in a fluid wave that passes circumferentially in the zone just under the capsule, cleaving the cortex from the posterior capsule in most locations. When the fluid wave has passed around the posterior aspect of the lens, the entire lens bulges forward because the fluid is trapped by the firm equatorial cortical-capsular connections (Figures 14-5 and 14-6). The procedure creates, in effect, a temporary intraoperative version of capsular block syndrome as seen by enlargement of the diameter of the capsulorhexis. At this point, if fluid injection is continued, a portion of the lens prolapses through the capsulorhexis. However, if before prolapse the capsule is decompressed by depressing the central portion of the lens with the side of the cannula in a way that forces fluid to come around the lens equator from behind (Figures 14-7 and 14-8), the cortical-capsular connections in the capsular fornix and under the anterior capsular flap are cleaved. The cleavage of cortex from the capsule equatorially and anteriorly allows fluid to exit from the capsular bag via the capsulorhexis, which constricts to its original size, and mobilizes the lens in such a way that it can spin freely within the capsular bag. Repeating the hydrodissection and capsular decompression starting in the opposite distal quadrant may be helpful. Adequate hydrodissection at this point can be demonstrated by the ease with which the nuclear-cortical complex can be rotated by the cannula.

Hydrodelineation

Hydrodelineation is a term first used by Anis[10] to describe the act of separating an outer epinuclear shell or multiple shells from the central compact mass of inner nuclear material, the endonucleus, by the forceful irrigation of fluids (balanced salt solution) into the mass of the nucleus.

Our technique uses the same hydrodissection cannula as previously described. The cannula is placed in the nucleus, off center to either side, and directed at an angle downward and forward toward the central plane of the nucleus. When the nucleus starts to move, the endonucleus has been reached; it is not penetrated by the cannula. At this point, the cannula is directed tangentially to the endonucleus, and a to-and-fro movement of the cannula is used to create a tract within the nucleus. The cannula is backed out of the tract approximately halfway (Figure 14-9), and a gentle but steady pressure on the syringe allows fluid to enter the "empty" distal tract without resistance. Driven by the hydraulic force of the syringe, the fluid will find

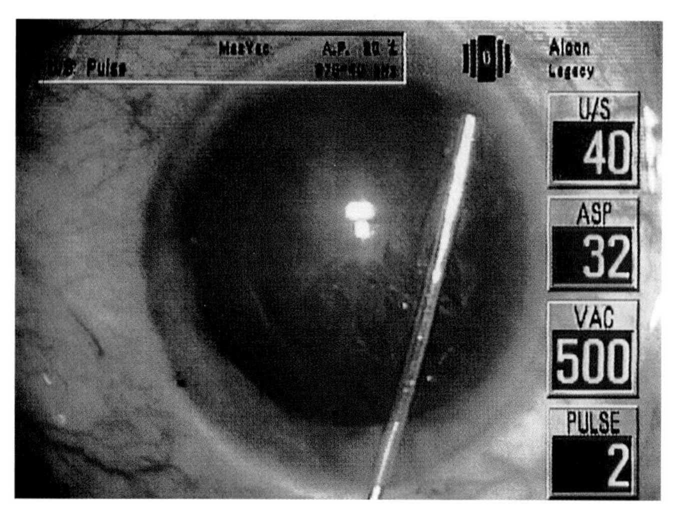

FIGURE 14-1 Placement of the cannula under the anterior capsulorhexis in one of quadrants, elevating the capsule.

A

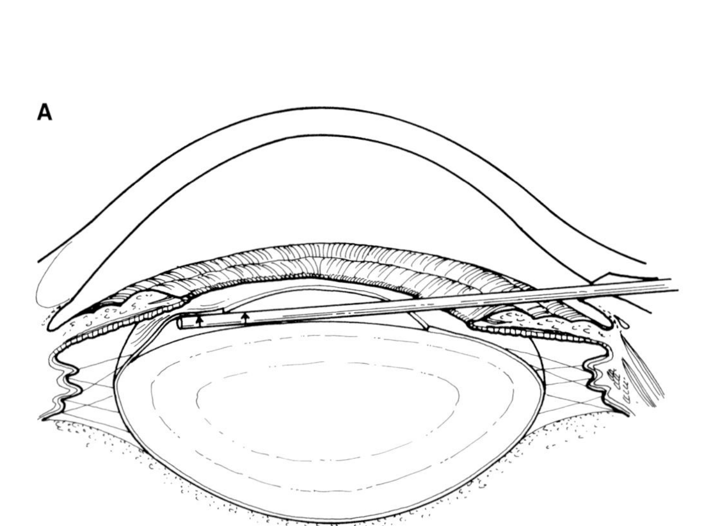

B

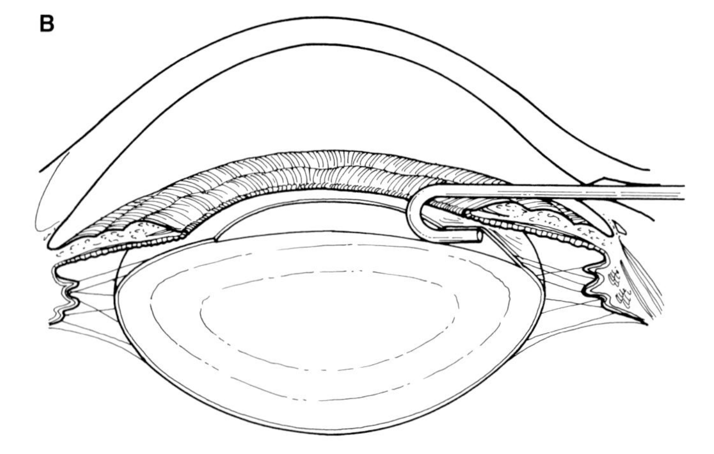

FIGURE 14-2 Cortical cleaving hydrodissection. **A,** In the original technique, the cannula is passed inferiorly, with tenting up of the anterior capsule before injection of fluid. **B,** Alternative technique described by Steinert uses a 180-degree Binkhorst cannula to direct the initial fluid wave superiorly. The cannula is rotated to elevate the anterior capsule and to direct the fluid wave between the capsule and the cortex.

A

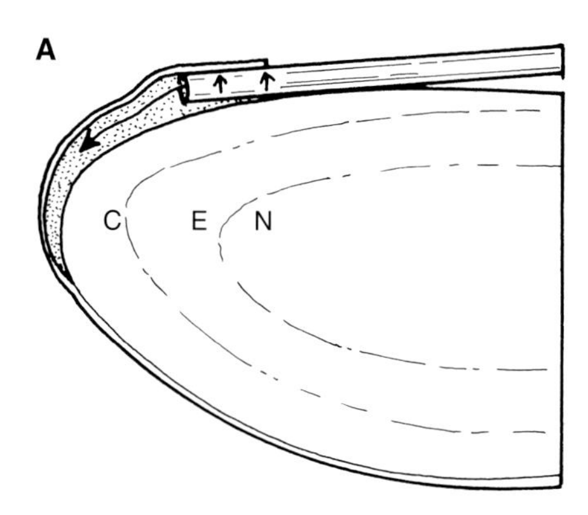

B

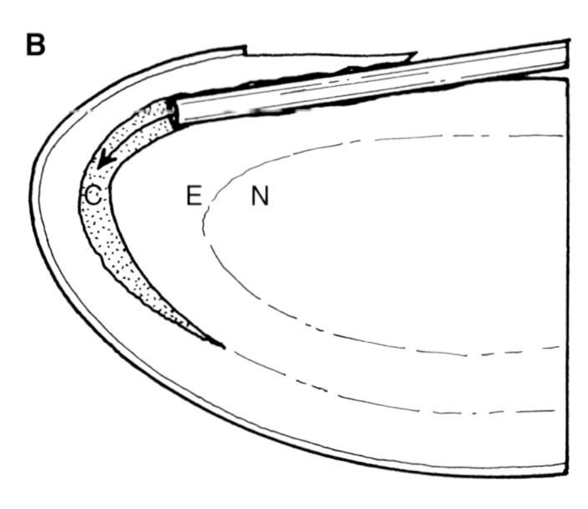

FIGURE 14-3 **A,** In cortical cleaving hydrodissection, the fluid wave passes between the capsule and cortex. **B,** In conventional hydrodissection, the natural fluid cleavage plane is between the cortex and epinucleus. *C,* Cortex; *E,* epinucleus; *N,* nucleus.

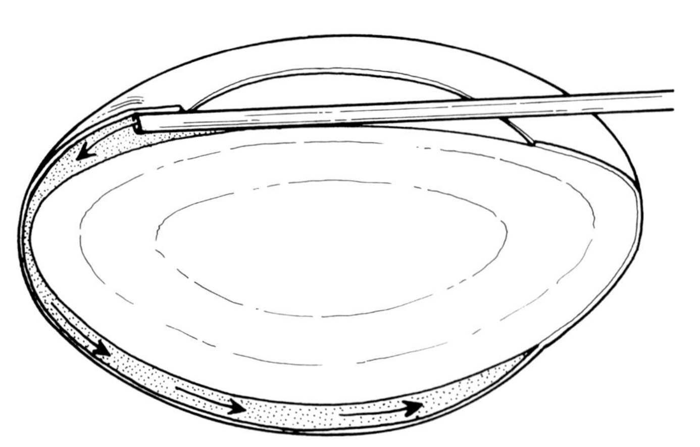

FIGURE 14-4 As the fluid is injected, a posterior fluid wave is created.

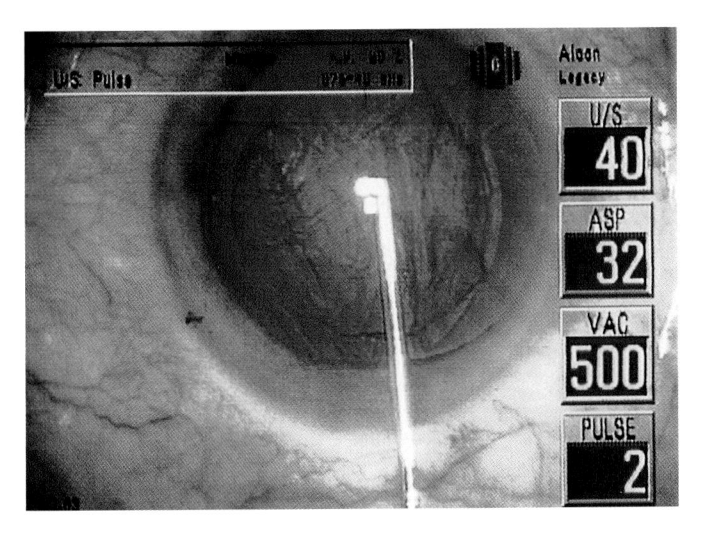

FIGURE 14-5 Enlargement of capsulorhexis as seen following second cortical cleaving hydrodissection fluid wave placed in the opposite distal quadrant just before decompression of the capsular bag.

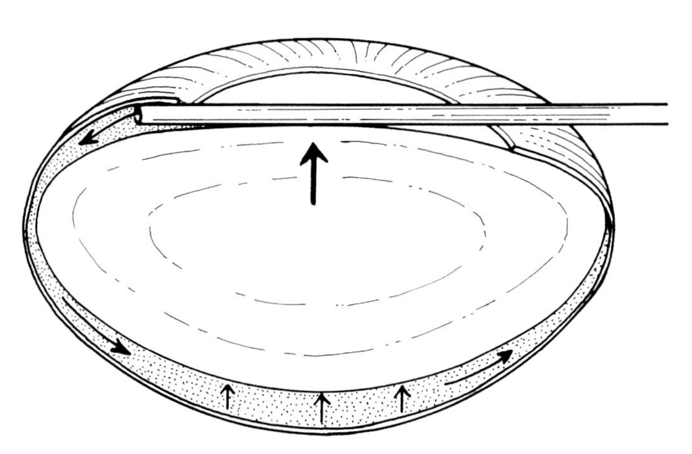

FIGURE 14-6 As cortical cleaving hydrodissection proceeds, fluid is trapped posteriorly, with anterior displacement of the lens in the capsular bag.

the path of least resistance, which is the junction between the endonucleus and the epinucleus, and flow circumferentially in this contour (Figure 14-10). Most often, a circumferential golden ring will be seen outlining the cleavage between the epinucleus and the endonucleus. Sometimes the ring will appear as a dark circle rather than a golden ring.

Occasionally, an arc will result and surround approximately one quadrant of the endonucleus. In this instance, creating another tract the same depth as the first but ending at one end of the arc, and injecting into the middle of the second tract, will extend that arc (usually another full quadrant). This can be repeated until a golden or dark ring verifies circumferential division of the nucleus.

For very soft nuclei, the placement of the cannula allows creation of an epinuclear shell of variable thickness. The cannula may pass through the entire nucleus if it is soft enough, so the placement of the tract and the location of the injection allow an epinuclear shell to be fashioned as desired. In very firm nuclei, one appears to be injecting into the cortex on the anterior surface of the nucleus, and the golden ring will not be seen. However, a thin, hard epinuclear shell is achieved even in the most brunescent nuclei. That shell will offer the same protection as a thicker epinucleus in a softer cataract.

Hydrodelineation circumferentially divides the nucleus and has many advantages. Circumferential division reduces the volume of the central portion of nucleus removed by phacoemulsification by up to 50%. This allows less deep and less peripheral grooving and smaller, more easily mobilized quadrants after cracking or chopping. The epinucleus acts as a protective cushion within which all of the chopping, cracking, and phacoemulsification forces can be confined. In addition, the epinucleus keeps the bag on stretch throughout the procedure, making it unlikely that a knuckle of capsule will come forward, occlude the phaco tip, and rupture.

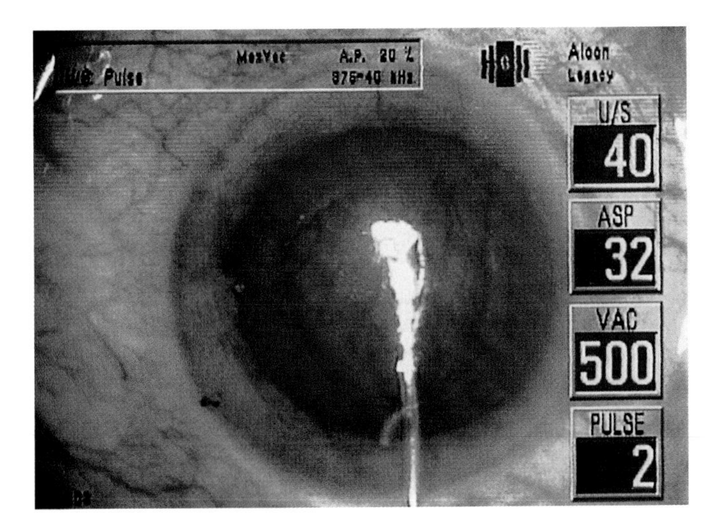

FIGURE 14-7 Return of capsulorhexis to its original size following decompression of the bag.

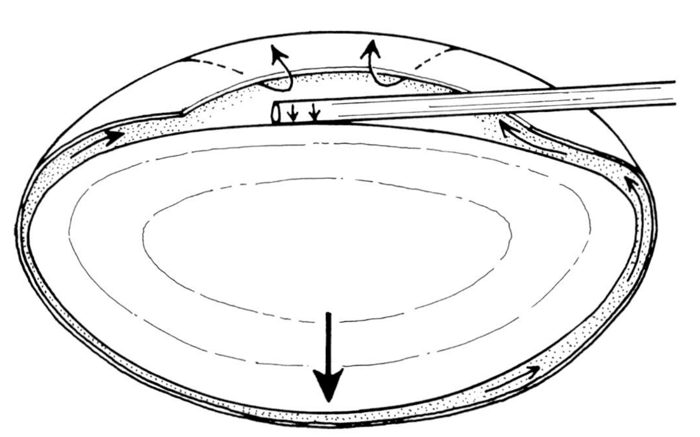

FIGURE 14-8 Posteriorly loculated fluid is decompressed by downward pressure on the lens with the cannula. Trapped fluid then advances around the equator, releasing equatorial cortical-capsular adhesions.

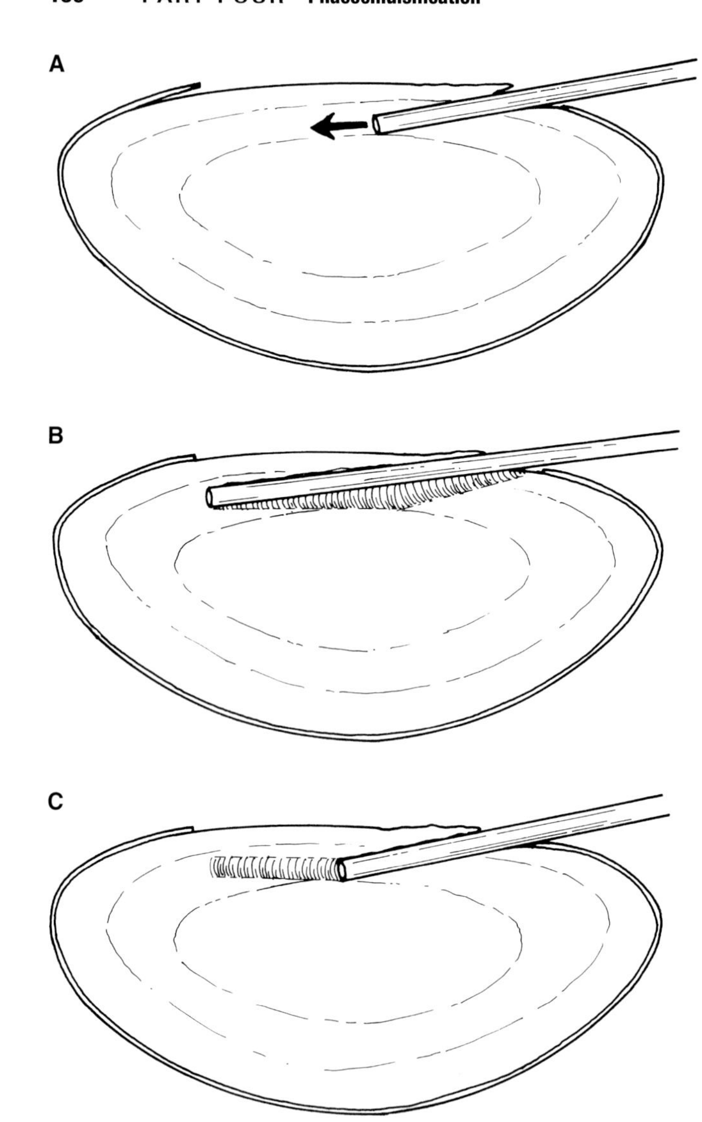

FIGURE 14-9 Hydrodelineation is performed by determining the natural cleavage plane between the nucleus and epinucleus. **A,** Blunt-tipped cannula is advanced as deeply as possible, thereby riding across the tops of the firm nucleus. **B,** Cannula is advanced inferiorly. **C,** Cannula is then partially withdrawn within the tract. Sufficient cannula length is embedded in the lens material to trap the fluid to be injected, but the open tract created allows the fluid pressure to seek out the natural cleavage plane between the inner nucleus and the middle epinuclear layer.

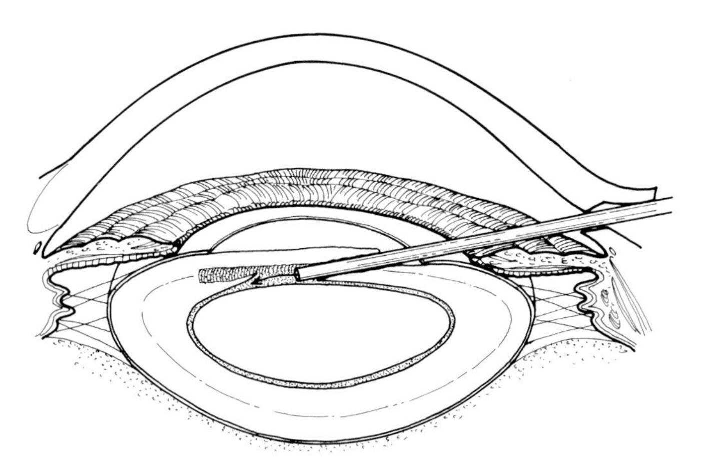

FIGURE 14-10 Complete hydrodelineation is obtained. If the pupil is widely dilated relative to the size of the nucleus, a "golden ring" is seen because of the microscope light reflex.

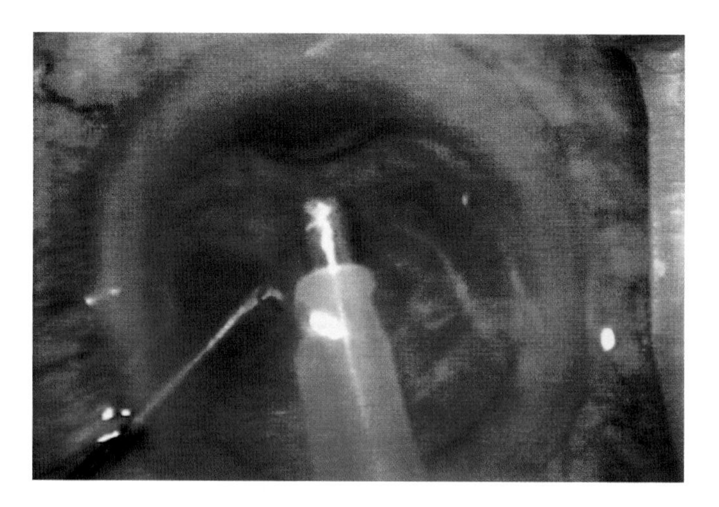

FIGURE 14-11 Purchase of the epinuclear rim and roof in foot position 2, being pulled central to the capsulorhexis. The cortical layer is seen superior to the rim and roof of the epinuclear shell.

Completion of the Procedure

After evacuation of all endonuclear material, the epinuclear rim is trimmed in each of the three quadrants (Figure 14-11), mobilizing cortex as well in the following way. As each quadrant of the epinuclear rim is rotated to the distal position in the capsule and trimmed, the cortex in the adjacent capsular fornix flows over the floor of the epinucleus and into the phaco tip (Figure 14-12). Then the floor is pushed back to keep the bag on stretch until three of the four quadrants of the epinuclear rim and forniceal cortex have been evacuated (Figure 14-13). It is important not to allow the epinucleus to flip too early, thus

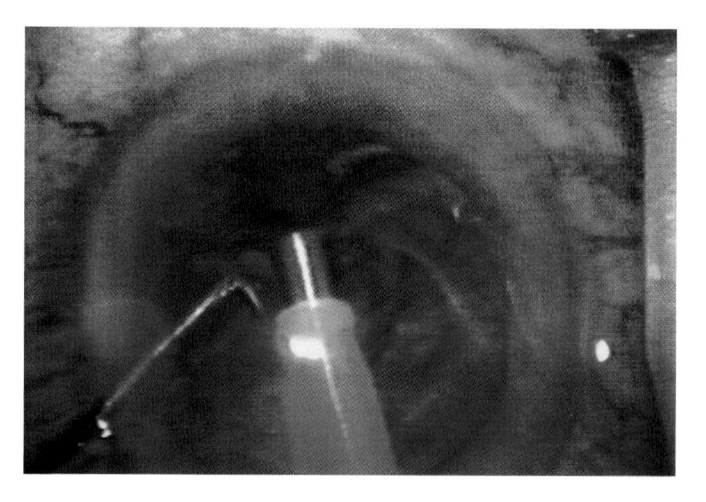

FIGURE 14-12 Following trimming of the initial purchase of the rim and roof in foot position 3, one can see the cortex flow over the floor and into the tip, removing it from that same quadrant.

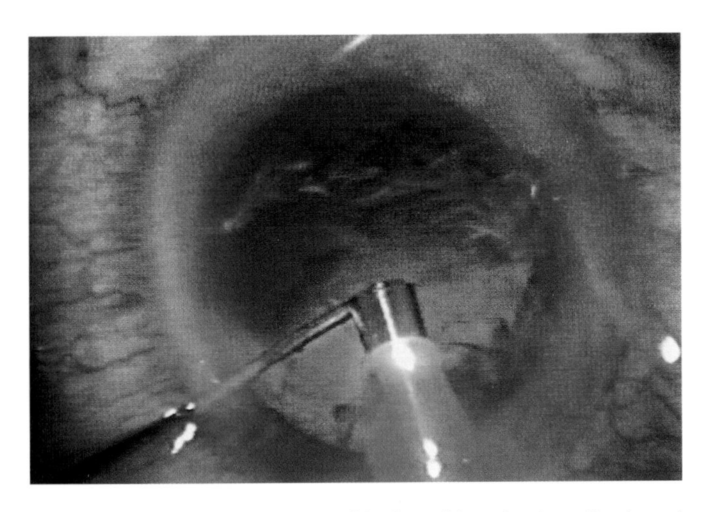

FIGURE 14-13 Repositioning of the floor of the epinucleus after rim and roof of the epinuclear shell have been trimmed and the cortex has been evacuated from the third epinuclear quadrant.

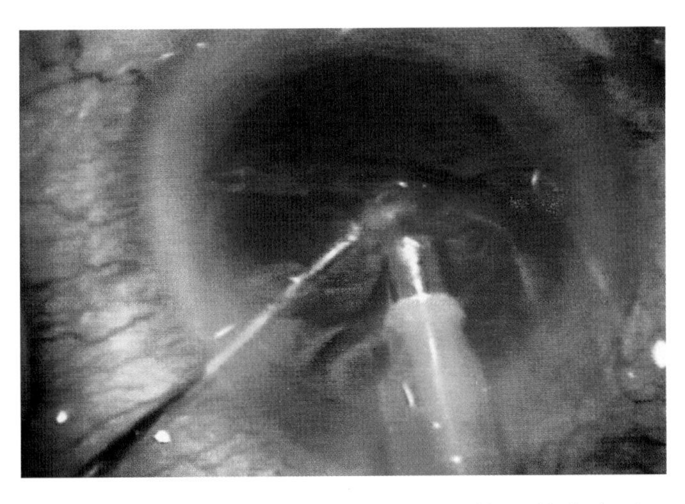

FIGURE 14-14 Initiating the flipping maneuver of the residual epinucleus using the fourth quadrant of epinuclear rim and shell.

avoiding a large amount of residual cortex remaining after evacuation of the epinucleus.

The epinuclear rim of the fourth quadrant is then used as a handle to flip the epinucleus (Figures 14-14 and 14-15). As the remaining portion of the epinuclear floor and rim is evacuated from the eye, 70% of the time the entire cortex is evacuated with it (Figure 14-16).[11] Downsized phaco tips with their increased resistance to flow are less capable of mobilizing the cortex because of the decreased minisurge accompanying the clearance of the tip when going from foot position 2 to foot position 3 in trimming of the epinucleus.

After the intraocular lens is inserted, these strands and any residual viscoelastic material are removed using the irrigation-aspiration tip, leaving a clean capsular bag.

If cortex is still remaining after removal of all the nucleus and epinucleus, there are three options. The phacoemulsification handpiece can be left high in the anterior chamber while the second handpiece strokes the cortex-filled capsular fornices. Often this results in floating up of the cortical shell as a single piece and its exit through the phacoemulsification tip (in foot position 2) because cortical cleaving hydrodissection has cleaved most of the cortical capsular adhesions.

Alternatively, if the surgeon wishes to complete cortical cleanup with the irrigation-aspiration handpiece before lens implantation, the residual cortex can almost always be mobilized as a separate and discrete shell (reminiscent of the epinucleus) and removed without ever turning the aspiration port down to face the posterior capsule (see Figure 14-15).

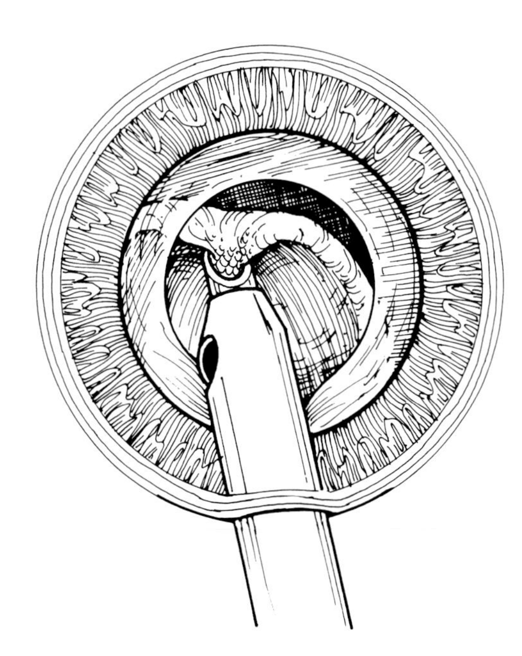

FIGURE 14-15 Aspiration of residual epinuclear and cortical envelope.

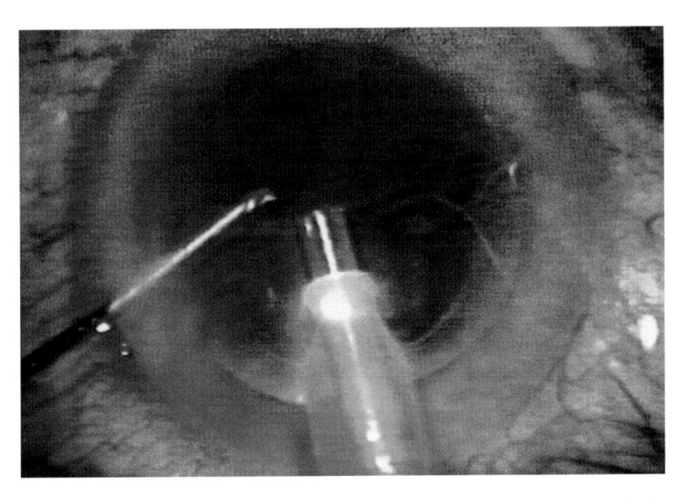

FIGURE 14-16 Capsular bag is clear of cortex, except for a single strand to the right following flipping and evacuation of the residual epinucleus.

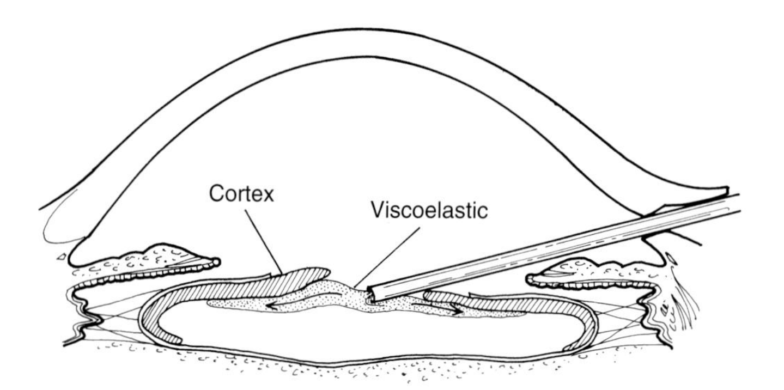

FIGURE 14-17 Residual cortex can be aspirated after IOL insertion. The first step is to carefully instill a viscoelastic agent under the residual cortex.

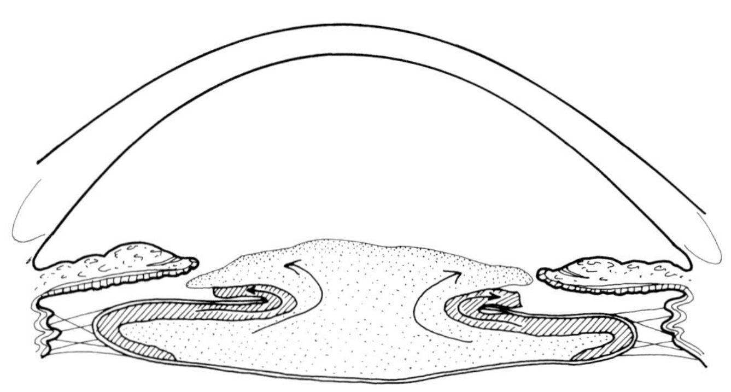

FIGURE 14-18 As the viscoelastic agent fills the capsular bag, tags of remaining cortex are brought anteriorly, draping over the anterior capsule.

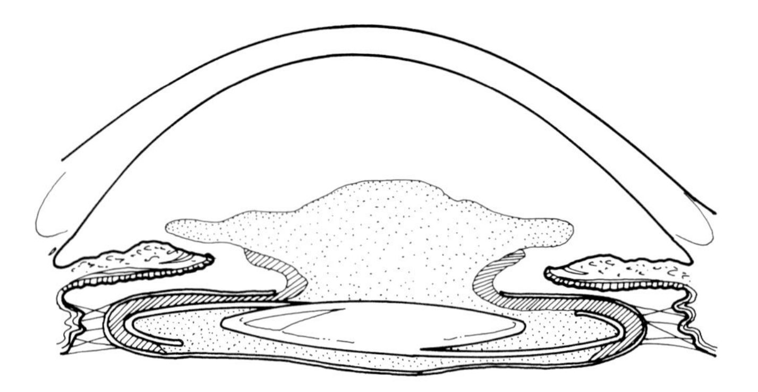

FIGURE 14-19 After the IOL is placed in the capsular bag, residual cortex is then anterior to the IOL optic.

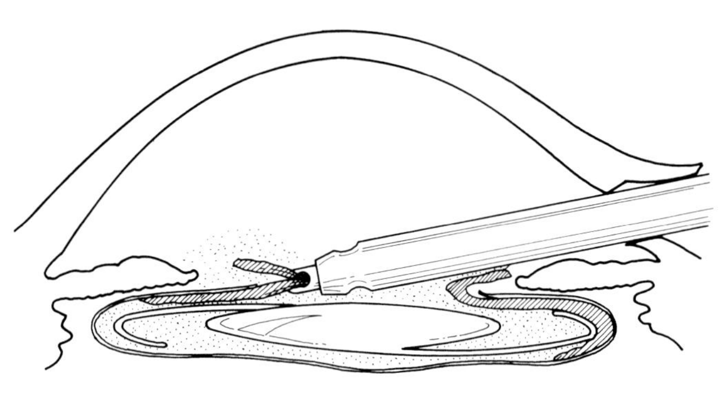

FIGURE 14-20 Irrigation-aspiration tip can now access the remaining cortex and successfully aspirate the cortex while the IOL remains within the capsular bag.

The third option is to viscodissect the residual cortex by injecting the viscoelastic through the posterior cortex onto the posterior capsule. We prefer the dispersive viscoelastic device chondroitin sulfate–hyaluronate (Viscoat). The viscoelastic material spreads horizontally, elevating the posterior cortex and draping it over the anterior capsular flap (Figure 14-17). At the same time, the peripheral cortex is forced into the capsular fornix (Figure 14-18). The posterior capsule is then deepened with a cohesive viscoelastic device (e.g., ProVisc), and the IOL is implanted through the capsulorhexis, leaving the anterior extension of the residual cortex anterior to the IOL (Figure 14-19).

Removal of residual viscoelastic material accompanies mobilization and aspiration of residual cortex anterior to the IOL (Figure 14-20), which protects the posterior capsule, leaving a clean capsular bag.

Conclusions

In summary, the lens can be divided into an epinuclear zone with most of the cortex attached and a more compact central nuclear mass. The central portion of the cataract can be removed by any endolenticular technique, after which the protective epinucleus is removed with all or most of the cortex attached. In most cases, irrigation and aspiration of the cortex as a separate step are not required, thereby eliminating that portion of the surgical procedure and its attendant risk of capsular disruption. Residual cortical cleanup may be accomplished in the presence of a posterior chamber IOL, which protects the posterior capsule by holding it remote from the aspiration port.

REFERENCES

1. Faust KJ: Hydrodissection of soft nuclei, *J Am Intraocular Implant Soc* 10:75-77, 1984.
2. Neuhann T: Theorie und Operationstechnik der Kapsulorhexis, Klin Monatsbl Augenheilkd 190: 542-545, 1987.
3. Gimbel HV, Heuhann T: Development, advantages, and methods of the continuous circular capsulorhexis technique, *J Cataract Refract Surg* 16: 31-37, 1990.
4. Davison JA: Bimodal capsular bag phacoemulsification: a serial cutting and suction ultrasonic nuclear dissection technique, *J Cataract Refract Surg* 15:272-282, 1989.
5. Shepherd JR: In situ fractures, *J Cataract Refract Surg* 16:436-440, 1990.
6. Gimble HV: Divide and conquer nucleofractis phacoemulsification: development and variations, *J Cataract Refract Surg* 17:281-291, 1991.
7. Fine IH: The chip and flip phacoemulsification technique, *J Cataract Refract Surg* 17:366-371, 1991.
8. Fine IH, Moloney WF, Dillman DM: Crack and flip phacoemulsification, *J Cataract Refract Surg* 19:797-802, 1993.
9. Fine IH: Cortical cleaving hydrodissection, *J Cataract Refract Surg* 18: 508-512, 1992.
10. Anis A: Understanding hydrodelineation: the term and related procedures, *Ocular Surg News* 9:134-137, 1991.
11. Fine IH: The choo-choo chop and flip phacoemulsification technique, *Operative Techniques Cataract Refractive Surg* 1:61-65, 1998.

Principles of Nuclear Phacoemulsification

15

Howard V. Gimbel, MD, MPH

Phacoemulsification Today

Cataract surgery using phacoemulsification techniques and instrumentation offers a number of attractive benefits to both the surgeon and patient. The principal advantage is a smaller incision size, which decreases the amount of tissue injury, reduces the amount of postoperative pain and inflammation, and provides a more rapid refractive stabilization[1,2] with less astigmatism induced by the procedure.[1-4] The smaller incision also allows minimal restrictions on the patient's physical activities, even in the early postoperative period.

Although early phacoemulsification techniques performed in the anterior chamber were associated with a high loss of endothelial cells,[5 12] the corneal problems have been significantly minimized by the advent of in situ, or what has become known as posterior chamber, phacoemulsification[13-18] and the protective properties of viscoelastic substances.[19-26] These have in turn enhanced intraoperative safety and surgeon control, while minimizing iris trauma,[27] capsule tears, and the possibility of intraoperative suprachoroidal hemorrhage by maintaining a pressurized surgical environment.

Other advantages of phacoemulsification that are difficult to quantify include a more efficient use of operating room time by the surgeon and staff, highly satisfied patients, and a quicker return to personal independence and to the workforce by many patients, which has tremendous potential economic repercussions.

These benefits and favorable outcomes continue to drive a growing interest in and an acceptance and application of phacoemulsification. In the Leaming studies,[28] phacoemulsification as the surgical procedure of choice increased from 12% in 1985 to 79% in 1992, and it increased further to 97% in 2000. It is worth noting that this survey only reflects the opinion of a portion of the American Society of Cataract and Refractive Surgery membership and may not precisely indicate the trend among American cataract surgeons in general.[29,30] Nonetheless, the upswing in usage of the technique is undeniable. In other countries, such as Australia,[31] the United Kingdom,[32] and Canada, the conversion has probably not been as remarkable, but the momentum for change seems to be building. Similar trends have also been reported in Asia[33-36] and in other parts of Europe.[32,37-40]

The tremendous 15-year growth reflected in the Leaming studies can be directly correlated with the introduction of continuous curvilinear capsulorhexis (CCC) in 1985.[41-43] In concert with the majority of today's in situ phacoemulsification techniques, CCC preserves the anterior capsule rim and helps to ensure in-the-bag placement and long-lasting centration of an intraocular lens (IOL).[44]

The Evolution of Phacoemulsification

The origins of phacoemulsification can be traced to the pioneering efforts of Kelman. In 1967, Kelman described a single-instrument technique for cataract extraction using ultrasound vibration to remove lens material through a 3-mm corneoscleral incision.[45] To minimize posterior capsule tears and dropped nuclei, the nucleus was prolapsed into the anterior chamber and subsequently emulsified. Over the course of the next several years, Kelman shared his experiences with the technique[46-50]; this included publication of results using this new procedure that compared favorably with the results of intracapsular cataract extraction,[51,52] the method of cataract extraction most commonly used at that time. Kelman's enthusiasm for a procedure that reduced astigmatism and provided early rehabilitation was shared by many surgeons. Between 1973 and 1979, the results of thousands of Kelman phacoemulsification cases performed by numerous surgeons were reported.[53-75] However, several factors limited the universal application of Kelman phacoemulsification as the procedure of choice for cataract extraction.

First, a number of reports were published citing damage to the corneal endothelium using the technique. Second was the realization that the very dense, brunescent nucleus resisted ultrasonic fragmentation, making many cases difficult, dangerous, or impossible to accomplish with the techniques and instruments then available. Finally, the shape of intraocular implants of the day required an incision substantially larger than 3 mm, potentially discounting any advantage of a smaller wound to remove the cataract. Nonetheless, Kelman had set the stage for further refinement of his ingenious invention.

In the early 1970s, Sinskey, because of the difficulty of delivering softer nuclei into the anterior chamber, used a

15-degree phacoemulsification tip to sculpt the central nucleus down almost to the posterior capsule before removing the peripheral nuclear shell.[76] By performing the phacoemulsification posteriorly in the capsular bag and thus deep in the anterior chamber, damage to the corneal endothelial cells was significantly reduced.

During this same period, Little[77] and Kratz[78-80] popularized two-handed emulsification of the nucleus using a spatula as a second instrument. Little passed the spatula into the anterior chamber directly alongside the ultrasound tip through the 12 o'clock incision. He sculpted the anterior nucleus centrally with a 45-degree tip, then tilted and prolapsed the remaining nucleus out of the superior equator of the capsular bag for further emulsification. Kratz chose to use a side-port second incision at 3 o'clock for this purpose. The goal of his iris plane–tilt technique was to increase the efficiency of Sinskey's method, especially for lenses with a hard epinucleus, as well as a hard nucleus, while reducing contact with the endothelium and still protecting the posterior capsule. Maloney adopted this technique and taught this to many surgeons.[81]

I was originally trained as an intracapsular surgeon but attended Kelman's New York phacoemulsification course in January 1974. With modifications learned from Kratz, Sinskey, and Little, combined with my own experience and innovation, my technique soon evolved from a one-handed anterior chamber technique to a two-handed posterior chamber technique for soft nuclei with Kratz's tipping technique for hard lenses. I developed the CCC technique in 1984, and by 1985 I had developed the "divide and conquer nucleofractis" method of in situ phacoemulsification.[82,83] This approach evolved because hard, large nuclei could not be tipped out of a 5- to 6-mm CCC and could not be safely emulsified in situ. I found it necessary to emulsify these lenses by systematically dividing and fragmenting the dense nuclear rim after sculpting all that could be safely sculpted. The fracturing technique was then applied to less dense cataracts before extensive sculpting was done. The maneuver of fracturing the nucleus, which I have termed *nucleofractis*[83] can be used in many different ways. It has added efficiency and safety during the emulsification of moderately dense lenses and has allowed all but rock-hard cataracts to be easily conquered by phacoemulsification. The techniques make use of several aspects of lens anatomy.

The Principle of Nucleofractis

Clinical Anatomy of the Lens

The cataractous lens consists primarily of three structures: the capsule, the cortex, and the nucleus (Figure 15-1). The lens capsule is the outermost layer of the lens and consists of the anterior capsule transitioning to the posterior capsule at the equator of the lens.[84-86] Surrounding the central nucleus and epinucleus is the lens cortex. The germinal epithelium of the lens is the source of the lens fibers.[87,88] The nucleus is the central core of the lens and varies in hardness from the center to the periphery in most cataracts, depending on the progression of the cataract. As the typical age-related cataract progresses, the central and then the peripheral nucleus tend to become more brunescent, changing from clear to yellow to dark brown.

A number of lamellar zones are present in the lens, starting with the fetal nucleus, which becomes the hard central nucleus as new fibers are laid down through life.[89,90] These fibers join in a Y-shaped suture anteriorly and posteriorly. The lens thus develops in layers, but orientation of the lens fibers creates radial cleavage planes through which cracks can be made (Figure 15-2). It is my clinical observation that although the Y sutures are the zones most susceptible to fracturing, "fault lines" that may be used for cracking are present to a lesser degree throughout the lens. In a very soft lens such as in a younger person, it may be difficult to identify these fault lines because of decreased fiber density within the nucleus and because interdigitating portions of the lens fibers still hold the nucleus together.

The radial and lamellar zones are analogous to those seen in a tree. If a cross section of a tree is examined, just inside the outer bark, an actively replicating living tissue lays down concentric

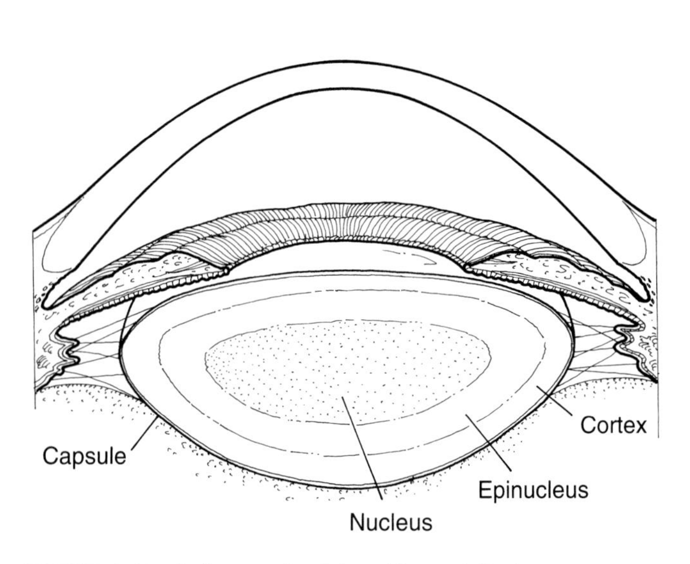

FIGURE 15-1 Cross-sectional view of the crystalline lens.

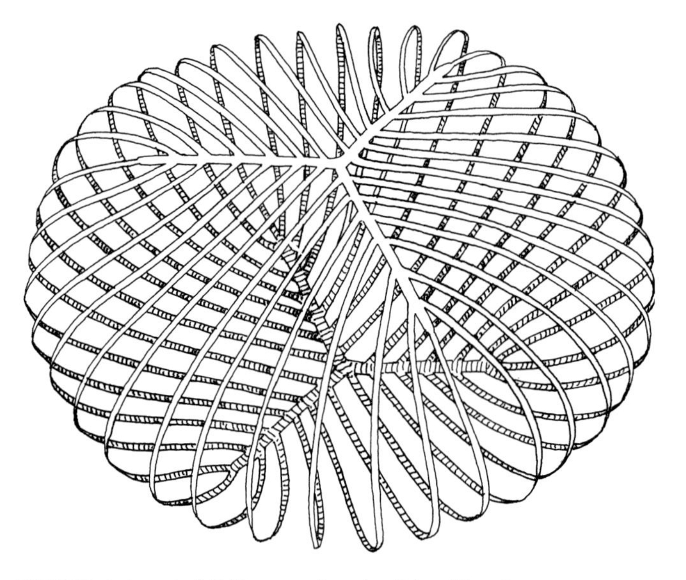

FIGURE 15-2 Artist's conception of radial and lamellar zones.

lamellae of tree fiber. The existence of these lamellae is confirmed by the annular rings of the cut tree trunk. These are less densely packed in the periphery and much more dense and closer together in the center of the tree core. The cataract's outer capsule simulates the tree bark. Just inside the capsule are lens epithelial cells, which lay down concentric lamellae of nuclear tissue that are looser in the periphery and much more dense in the center. A log for use in a fireplace has lamellar separations of bark and annular rings corresponding to the cortex being separated by lamellar hydrodissection. However, for efficient burning, the core of the log is also split with radial fractures, many of which are seen as natural cleavage planes as the wood dries. Another analogy is the watermelon, which has radial, as well as circumferential, cleavage planes. When sculpting down through the nucleus of the cataract, one can often see the natural radial cleavage planes in the nucleus of the lens corresponding to the aforementioned Y sutures seen on slit lamp examination. Although the radial fractures often follow these primary cleavage planes, the instruments can easily create other radial cleavage planes.

Drews[91,92] has used neodymium: yttrium-aluminum-garnet (Nd:YAG) laser energy to demonstrate the position of the core of the lens nucleus, to confirm the existence of these radial fracture lines within the nuclear core, and to provide an anatomic basis for the formation of grooves across the nucleus during phacoemulsification. Hydrodissection of the epinuclear layers from the nuclear core occasionally fractures the nucleus radially, demonstrating the existence of these anatomic divisions. Mechanical fracturing of the nucleus can make very effective use of these anatomic features to achieve safer and more efficient phacoemulsification.

Origins of Nucleofractis

The concept of fracturing or cracking the nucleus is not new. As far back as 1967, Kelman used Ringberg forceps to crack the nucleus (Kelman C, personal communication, 1985). For safety reasons, this technique was abandoned in favor of the nuclear prolapse method. My introduction of a bimanual nucleofractis technique resulted from a combination of a number of factors. In the late 1970s I was using the spatula instrument for rotation of the lens, thereby facilitating sculpting. The spatula was also used as needed during phacoemulsification to stabilize and position the nucleus. By 1984 I was using a technique to subdivide chunks of the nucleus before breaking them up and suctioning them out. In 1985 I also found that rotation of the lens could result in an inadvertent fracture of the nucleus. This discovery led me to devise a technique to purposefully fracture the nuclear rim.

In 1986 I applied the term *divide and conquer* to my in situ phacoemulsification technique, which is derived from the Latin *divide et impera*. I first introduced the divide and conquer technique by way of a videotape at the 1987 European Intraocular Implantlens Council (now called the European Society of Cataract and Refractive Surgery) meeting in Jerusalem. The technique was subsequently presented at numerous courses and was demonstrated by live surgery at the 1988 Canadian Rockies Symposium on Cataract and Refractive Surgery in Calgary, Alberta, Canada.

The fracturing maneuver of divide and conquer can be accomplished once the instruments can be positioned sufficiently deep in the lens, which is achieved after the sculpting of a trough, trench, groove, or crater in the lens nucleus. The goal is then to split the nucleus where it is intact posteriorly and equatorially by a rim of peripheral nucleus. The ideal place to apply the splitting force is at the bottom of the groove first and then at the rim. The reverse can also be used and is the order followed for chopping techniques.

In my experience, this is best accomplished using a bimanual, direct, or at times a cross-fracturing technique in which the phaco probe is moved to the opposite side of the rim and the second instrument is moved to the other. Although I prefer the use of a 0.25-mm cyclodialysis spatula for these purposes, a number of customized instruments, including chopping instruments, have been designed to facilitate this maneuver.[93-95] The nucleus is thus bisected with a minimum of instrument and nuclear movement, so the force is effectively applied at the parallel faces of the groove, splitting the rim directly apart (Figure 15-3). If the instruments are placed too anteriorly in the trench, the bottom of the rim is not split because the inappropriate placement of the instruments has created a torque in this area rather than a splitting force (Figure 15-4).[96] The capsule may redirect the horizontal vector forces and actually compress the deeper nuclear layers.

In addition to the direct and cross-action fracturing techniques, several other methods of cracking are available. Parallel cracking[97] is accomplished by lining up the groove with the point midway between the main incision and the side-port opening. The second instrument is laid deep within the trench while the phaco handpiece rests on top of it. The instruments are then moved away from each other in a parallel position, resulting in easy cracking. The nucleus can be rotated to make additional grooves, and then each groove can be aligned and cracked in exactly the same manner.

Nonrotational cracking is either parallel, direct, or cross handed and takes place within the nucleus without rotation. Learning this technique is advantageous, as it may facilitate nuclear fracturing in the presence of a rent in the CCC opening

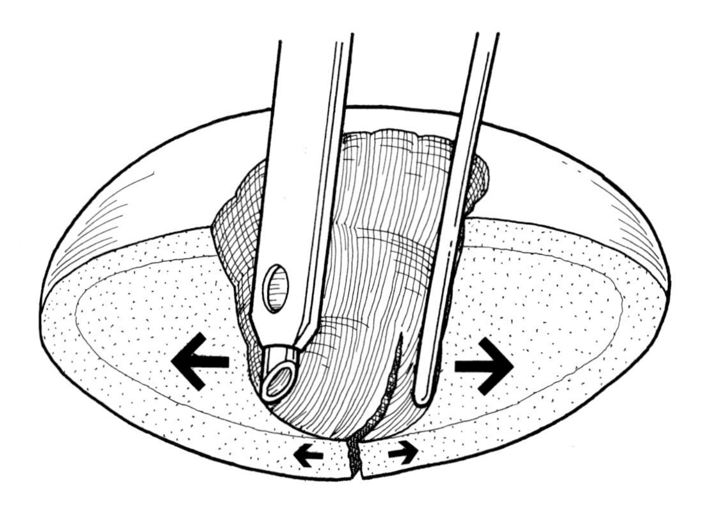

FIGURE 15-3 Posterior placement of the two instruments for bidirectional fracturing or nucleofractis.

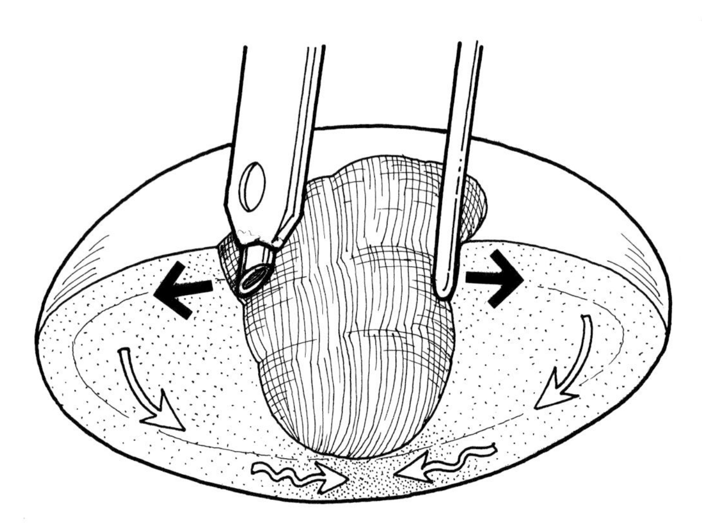

FIGURE 15-4 Inappropriate anterior placement of the instruments, resulting in misapplication of vector forces and ineffective fracturing.

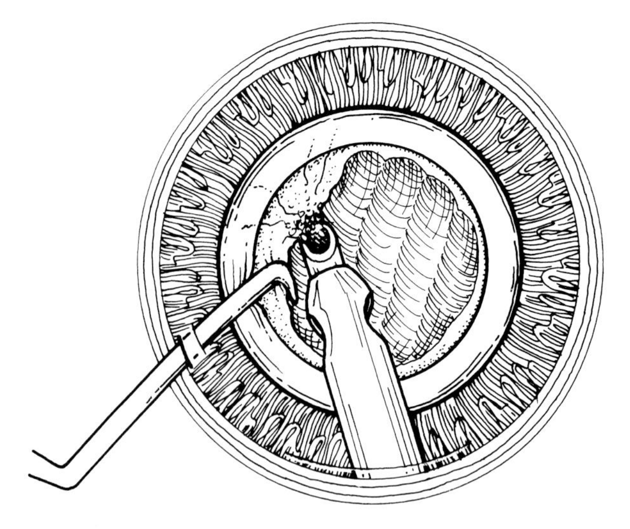

FIGURE 15-5 Crater "divide and conquer" technique. In dense and brunescent cataracts, nucleofractis is facilitated by emulsification of a deep and wide central crater of nucleus.

with less risk of extending the tear. This usually can be safely accomplished by cracking 90 degrees away from the rent to minimize stress to this area. Chopping rather than splitting is the safest method of nucleus disassembly in the presence of an anterior or posterior capsule tear.

Divide and conquer nucleofractis demands a slight stretch or distortion of the lens capsule, and subsequent tears are resisted only by the strong tear-resistant border of the CCC. Conversely, the integrity of the capsule border cannot always be preserved in planned extracapsular extraction or in anterior chamber phacoemulsification, particularly when attempted in large, dense, brunescent nuclei. Hence a clear interdependence has been recognized between the two techniques. Thus the technique of in situ phacoemulsification is uniquely suited to the technique of CCC. The demand for the coexistence of the two techniques is furthered by the great resilience and strength of the smooth-edged border of the CCC, which has been demonstrated experimentally,[98-100] and by protection of the corneal endothelium by a larger rim of anterior capsule during in situ or in-the-bag phacoemulsification.[101]

Because of the mechanics and complexities of nucleofractis, the advent of divide and conquer rendered sculpting no longer a random process but a defined means of achieving nuclear cracking. In fact, two broad variations of divide and conquer nucleofractis[83,102-104] have been developed to deal with different types of cataracts: the trench technique for soft to moderately hard nuclei and the crater technique for moderately hard to very hard and even dense, brunescent nuclei.

Divide and Conquer

Following CCC, hydrodissection is used to facilitate divide and conquer nucleofractis phacoemulsification. Both phacoemulsification techniques incorporate four basic steps: (1) deep sculpting until a fracture is possible, (2) nucleofractis of the nuclear rim and posterior plate of the nucleus, (3) fracturing again and breaking away a wedge-shaped section of nuclear material for emulsification, and (4) rotation or repositioning of the nucleus for further fracturing and emulsification.

CRATER DIVIDE AND CONQUER

The deep sculpting of the nucleus was part of my first divide and conquer technique back in 1985. At that time, I sculpted out to the nuclear rim and removed as much of the right side of the lens as I could safely sculpt. I continued to stabilize the left side of the lens with the spatula and then, rather than just sculpting it, I broke away sections with radial fractures and emulsified them.

As I applied this technique to very hard lenses, I began using the fracturing technique for brunescent lenses after deep central sculpting. This technique became the *crater divide and conquer* (CDC) technique because of the large crater sculpted, leaving a dense peripheral rim to fracture into multiple sections (Figure 15-5). This required considerable patience as the nucleus was shaved progressively deeper. I also found that I could fracture the entire rim into sections and then bring these sections into the center in a manner similar to the way that sections were broken away in the earlier technique. A trench, trough, or groove is not used in these cases in which a dense, brunescent lens is present because it does not weaken the entire lens nucleus enough to easily fracture, and the resulting segments are too large to manage safely.

Before hydrodissection was introduced, the nucleus was mechanically broken away from the cortex by rocking clockwise and counterclockwise using two instruments, until the lens could be rotated within the cortical shell. As mentioned previously, complete hydrodissection is now routinely used because nuclear shifting or rotation is required for the nucleofractis technique. Hydrodissection has made this easier and safer by reducing stress on the zonular ligaments during rotation.

Some experience is required to enable the surgeon to judge how deeply the central coring may safely proceed without rupturing the posterior capsule. A safety mechanism built into the CDC technique is the maintenance of a peripheral nuclear

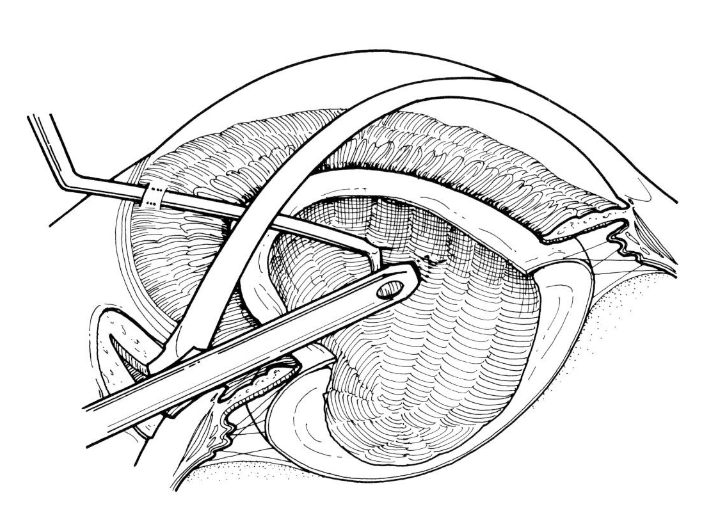

FIGURE 15-6 Cross-sectional view of sculpted crater.

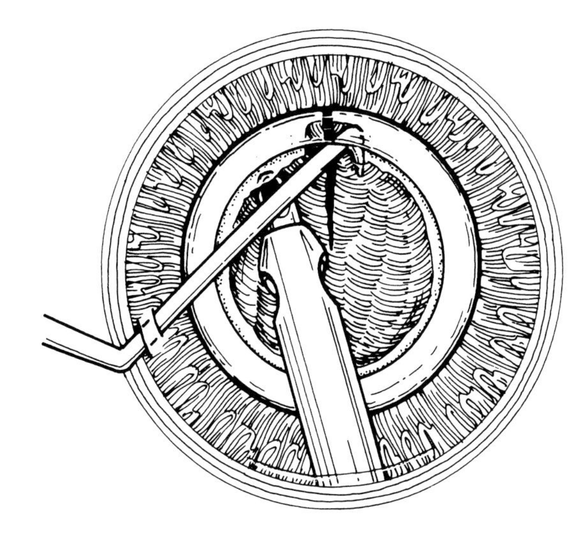

FIGURE 15-7 Using the cyclodialysis spatula and the phaco tip, the resultant peripheral nuclear rim is fractured.

rim after creation of the crater, which maintains distension of the capsular bag, keeping the posterior capsule deep and stretched during sculpting and nucleofractis. Once central coring is complete (Figure 15-6), the nuclear rim is fractured using the bimanual method, whereby the spatula and phaco tip create a counterpressure (Figure 15-7). The lens is rotated, and a second crack is made, isolating a pie-shaped section (Figure 15-8). The nuclear rim is then rotated clockwise for right-handed surgeons, facilitating systematic piece-by-piece nucleofractis. The harder the nuclear rim, the smaller the wedge-shaped sections should be to allow manageability of the individual pieces and to reduce the possibility of tearing the posterior capsule.

When using CDC and especially in very dense and brunescent cataracts, rather than immediately emulsifying each wedge-shaped section, the nuclear sections are generally left in place for capsular bag distension (Figure 15-9). Once the fracturing is complete, each pie-shaped wedge of the nuclear rim is brought to the center of the capsule, where phacoemulsification is safely accomplished (Figure 15-10). High flow, high vacuum, and low ultrasound power using a 15- or 30-degree tip keeps these segments fastened to the tip, reducing the chance of the segments tumbling into the chamber. The spatula is used to control what is coming to the tip and remains under the last segments being

TECHNICAL TIPS

The phaco tip itself may be more efficient for cutting through tissue in dense nuclei than the resistance of the phaco sleeve allows. That is why in very dense, brunescent lenses, deep burrowing is facilitated by retracting the sleeve to expose more of the tip. The extra amount exposed is conditional on the size of the pupil to minimize the potential for touching the edge of the iris with the metal part of the tip in small pupils. Usually, however, increasing the amount of tip exposed from the standard distance of 1.5 mm to 2 mm is advantageous in the denser lenses.

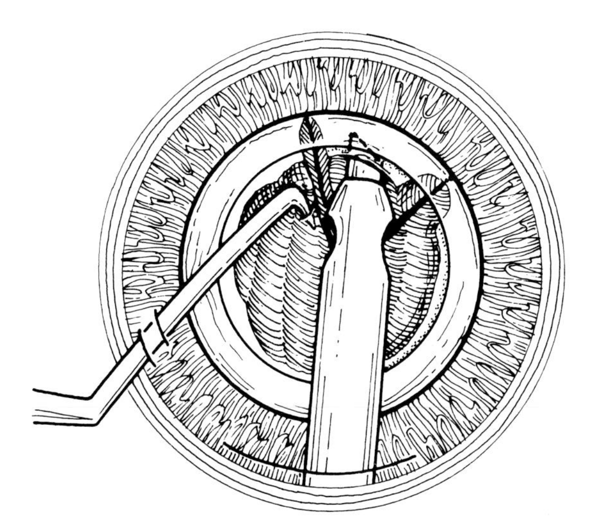

FIGURE 15-8 Nucleus is rotated, and a second fracture is made. The section is left in place, ensuring stabilization of the nucleus and capsule.

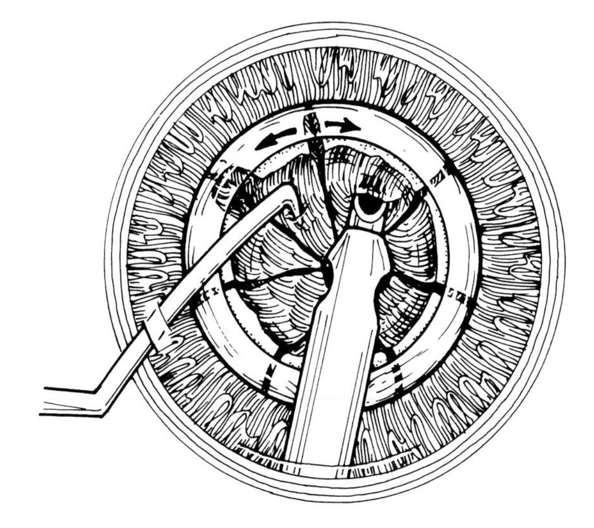

FIGURE 15-9 Remaining "donut" of nucleus is systematically fractured using the bimanual technique.

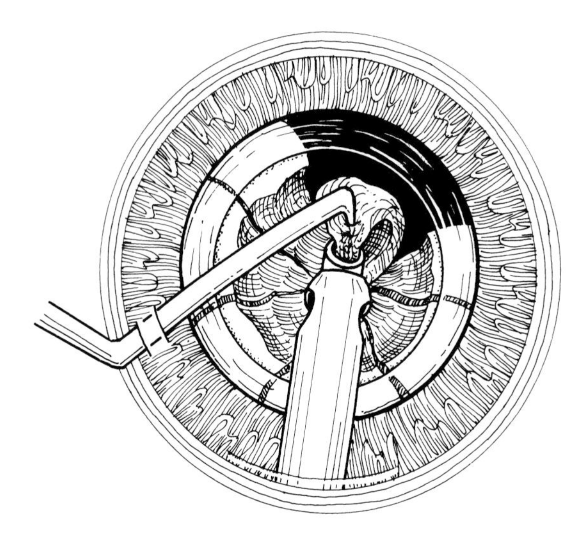

FIGURE 15-10 Individual sections are brought into the center for emulsification.

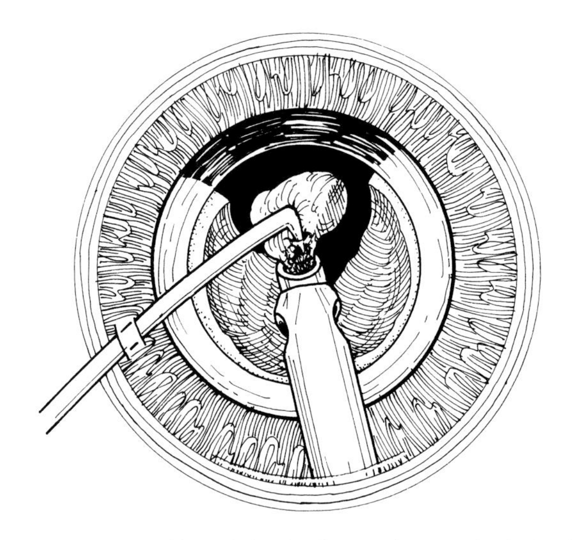

FIGURE 15-11 Alternatively, the first section may be isolated and emulsified to allow space for subsequent fracturing.

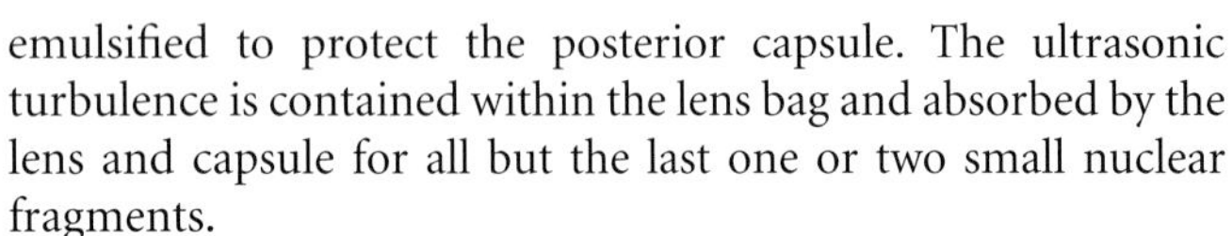

emulsified to protect the posterior capsule. The ultrasonic turbulence is contained within the lens bag and absorbed by the lens and capsule for all but the last one or two small nuclear fragments.

As an alternative during CDC, the first sector may be removed before performing additional nuclear fracturing to allow additional space for tissue separation (Figure 15-11). This technique is best performed in firm but easily fractured lenses such as in mature, white cataracts. Each section may be emulsified as it is broken away (Figure 15-12). This is analogous to the choice one has when serving pieces of birthday cake. One can either cut the entire cake into pieces before serving any piece or cut one only, serve it, and then cut the next piece and so forth.

TRENCH DIVIDE AND CONQUER

Realizing the efficiency of the fracturing maneuvers during CDC, I stopped sculpting the right side of soft lenses after making the central trench and instead made a central fracture. Then not only was the left side divided by fracturing but also the right side. I called these variations the *trench divide and conquer* (TDC) technique. For the purposes of these descriptions, a superior orientation of the incision with a subincisional area in the 12 o'clock position is assumed.

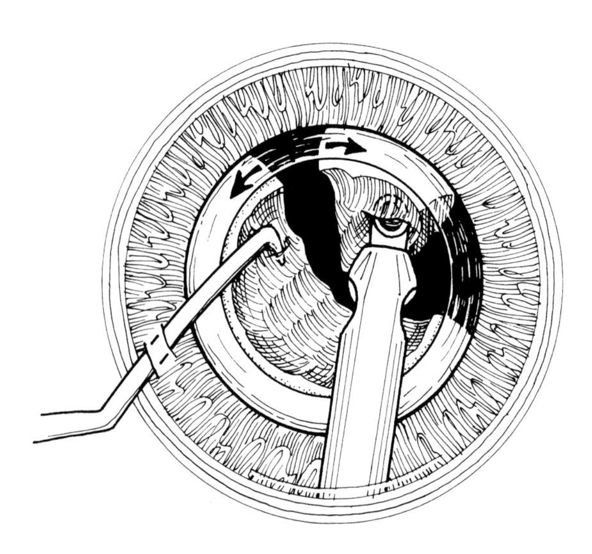

FIGURE 15-12 Remaining nuclear rim is individually fractured and emulsified.

TRENCH DIVIDE AND CONQUER WITH "DOWN SLOPE" SCULPTING

I appreciated a slight variation from the traditional sculpting method I had been employing with the nucleofractis techniques. By nudging the lens inferiorly with the second instrument, the upper central part of the nucleus can be sculpted very deeply, to the point of sculpting directly parallel and close to the posterior capsule. This allows the tip to remove more of the upper part of the nucleus during sculpting and to reach the posterior pole of the lens very early for effective fracturing. With the lens nucleus nudged toward the 6 o'clock position, the surgeon can sculpt very deeply down the slope of the posterior curvature of the upper part of the capsule. I have thus termed this method *TDC with "down slope" sculpting.*[104,105]

I first began using this nudging maneuver in small pupil cases out of necessity because of the limitations of the size of the pupil and capsule opening. I then began extending its applicability to almost all cases. This approach has greatly enhanced the speed and efficiency of the nucleofractis techniques and has increased the safety because the sculpting is parallel rather than somewhat perpendicular to the posterior capsule, as occurs when traditionally sculpting the inferior part of the lens.

Using a 30- or 45-degree tip, the TDC technique begins with a shallow trench or trough sculpted slightly to the right of the center of the lens surface (Figures 15-13 and 15-14). The lens is stabilized with the spatula or chopper through the paracentesis. Then, nudging the loosened lens nucleus inferiorly with the second instrument, down slope sculpting is accomplished, sculpting very deeply to the posterior pole of the lens (Figure 15-15). Hydrodissection is essential to achieve down slope sculpting because then the nucleus is not attached to the peripheral

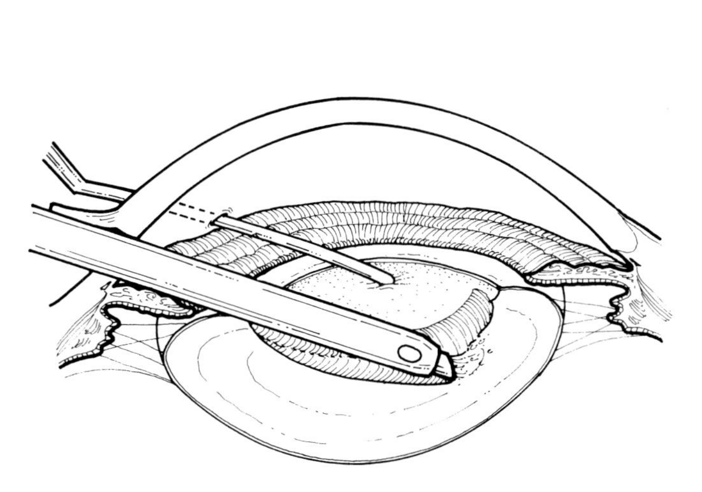

FIGURE 15-13 Cross-sectional view of initial sculpting of a trench or trough.

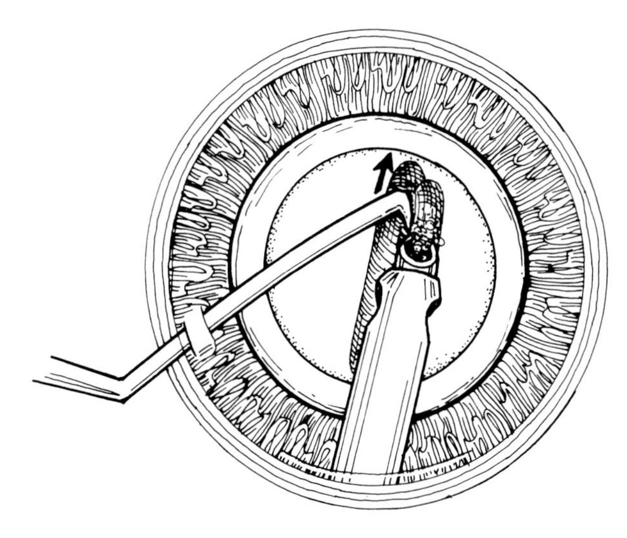

FIGURE 15-14 After nudging the lens inferiorly with the second instrument, the down slope technique starts with a trench or trough sculpted to just past the center of the lens surface.

cortex and capsule, and the nucleus can easily be displaced in the capsular bag.

Placing the instrument tips deep in the center of the lens, fracturing is accomplished by pushing toward the right with the phaco tip as the cyclodialysis spatula or chopper is pushed to the left (Figure 15-16). This accomplished in foot position 2 (irrigation/aspiration only and no ultrasound power). The lens usually splits from the center to the superior and inferior rim of the nucleus if the instruments are held deep in the center. If the split does not readily extend to the equator inferiorly or superiorly, moving the instruments away from the center can produce the mechanical advantage necessary to extend the fracture through the nuclear rim.

After this first crack has been obtained, the depth of the sculpted groove in the lens can be determined, and thus the surgeon can gauge how much deeper sculpting should be continued to facilitate further fracturing. In all but brunescent nuclei, usually three to five sculpting passes allow one to get deep enough into the lens to start fracturing.

Either before the first fracture or immediately afterward, the down slope technique may be used to sculpt the majority of the upper part of the lens. Keeping the probe deep in the tissue and close to the posterior cortex, the surgeon burrows deeply into the left hemisection and creates a second crack that intersects with the first, isolating a pie-shaped section of nucleus. In soft nuclei, this is usually performed about 60 degrees from the first fracture, but in hard nuclei, the crack is shortened to about 30 degrees away (Figures 15-17 and 15-18).

The isolated pie-shaped section can be either emulsified or left in place as the next crack is made in a similar fashion. The remaining right section of nucleus is maneuvered with the second instrument and brought to the midpupillary zone (Figure 15-19). A final split is made after impaling the tip with a short burst of ultrasound, pushing with the phaco tip toward

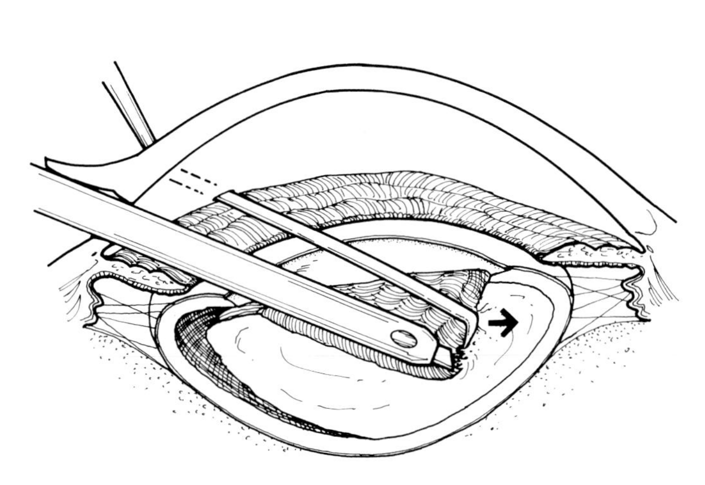

FIGURE 15-15 Cross-sectional view of nudging maneuver and down slope sculpting.

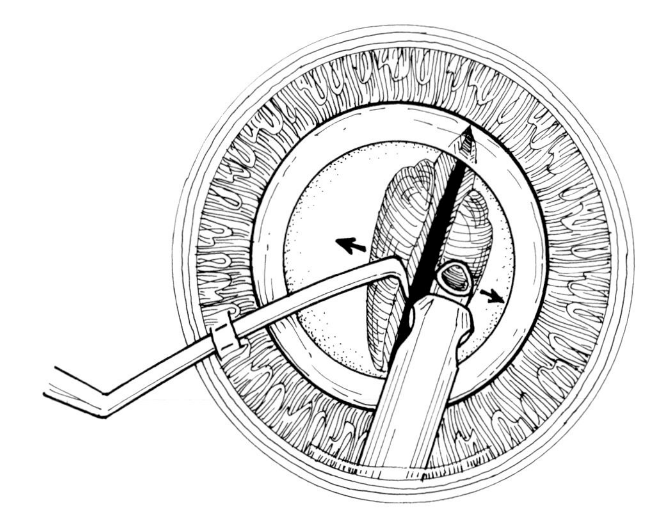

FIGURE 15-16 With the instrument tips deep in the center of the lens, a fracture can be obtained easily and early.

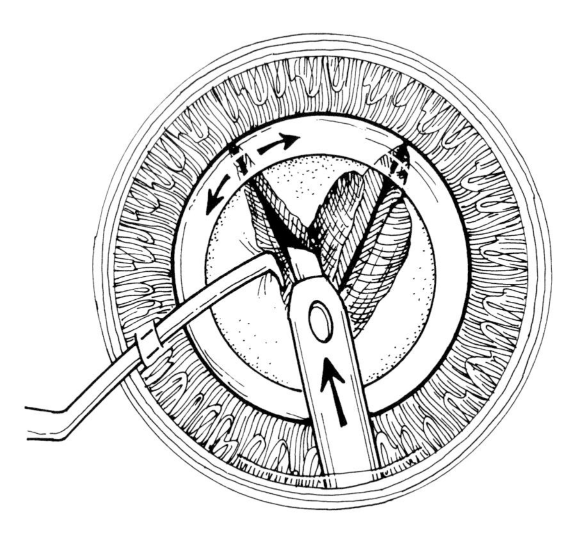

FIGURE 15-17 Using the bimanual technique again, a second crack is made and either emulsified or left in place for further fracturing.

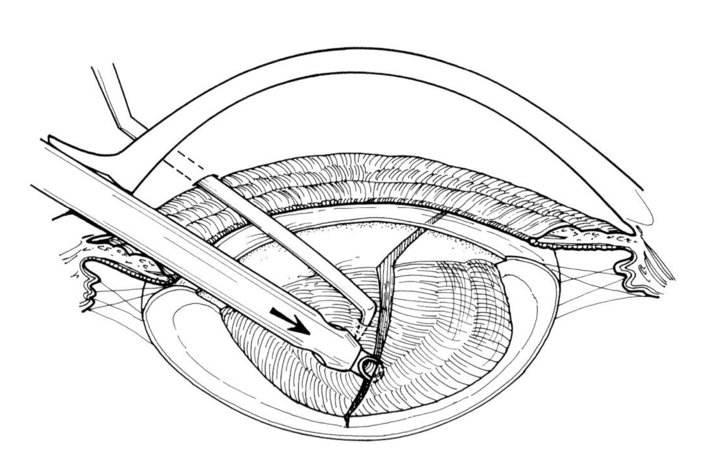

FIGURE 15-18 Cross-sectional view of second fracture.

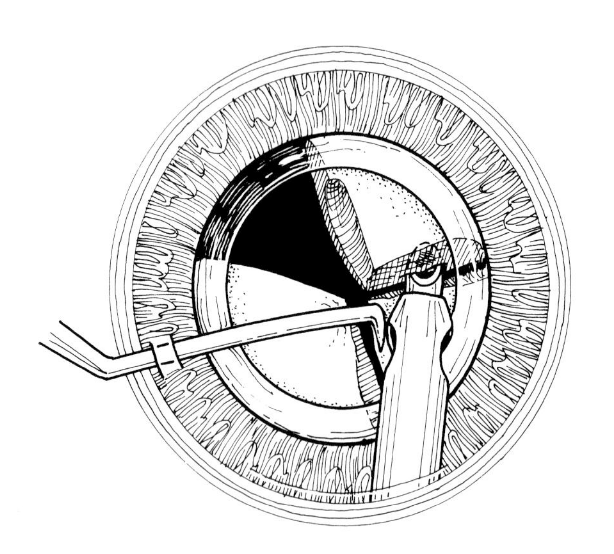

FIGURE 15-19 Right section is maneuvered into midpupillary zone for further nucleofractis.

the 6 o'clock position while stabilizing the upper portion. The piece can then be fractured into halves or thirds and emulsified as they are fractured. Alternatively, the right hemisection may be rotated to the left side and fractured in a way similar to the first hemisection (Figure 15-20).

The down slope method can also be used to remove a large portion of the upper part of the lens, creating a horizontal anterior-to-posterior wall in the nucleus. The phaco tip is used to stabilize the upper portion, while the second instrument pushes inferiorly against this wall, creating a horizontal fracture (Figure 15-21). The inferior hemisection is then divided into three or more sections by burrowing into the right side and breaking away a section for emulsification while stabilizing the left piece with the spatula. The thin upper hemisection is then brought to the center and divided similarly (Figure 15-22).

With traditional sculpting techniques, the deepest part of the sculpting inevitably ends up inferior to the center of the lens. If the surgeon rotates the lens 90 degrees after sculpting

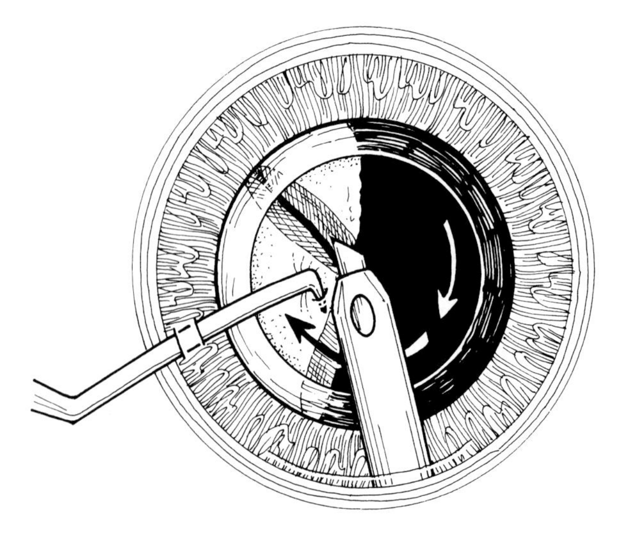

FIGURE 15-20 Alternatively, this section can be rotated to the left side and fractured.

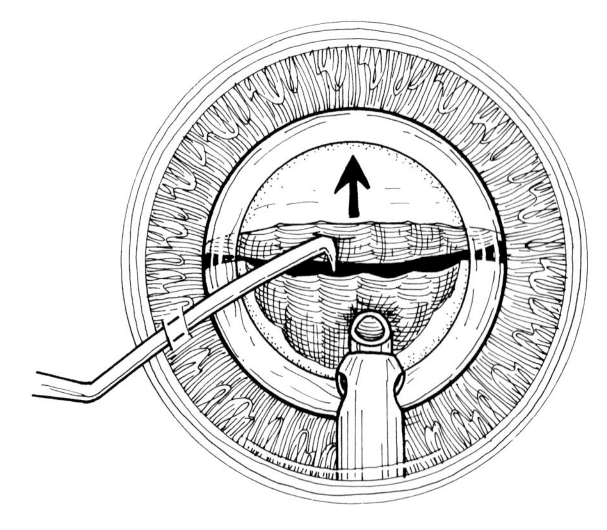

FIGURE 15-21 Using down slope sculpting and nucleofractis, a horizontal split can be created

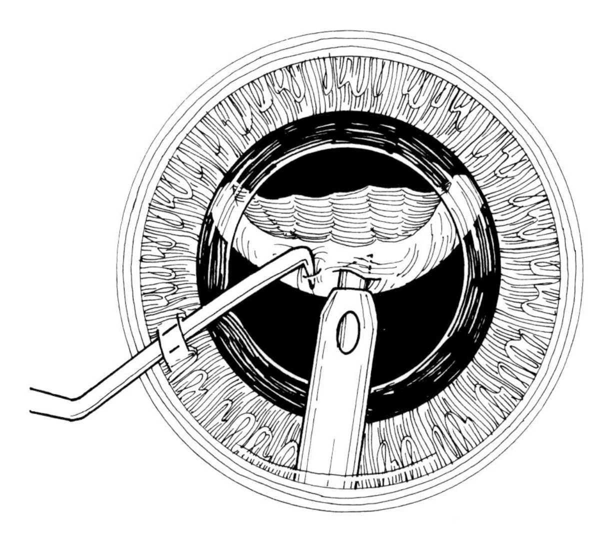

FIGURE 15-22 Inferior hemisection brought to center for division and emulsification.

each quadrant, then the nuclear material deep in the center or posterior pole of the nucleus may still impede complete fracturing to the center, and the sections will tend to hang together in the middle of the lens (Figure 15-23). However, with down slope sculpting, complete and efficient fracturing and subsequent emulsification can be accomplished by sculpting deeply and fracturing through the entire posterior plate of the nucleus. Rather than using grooves to start the fractures, the surgeon simply needs to get the instruments deep into the center of the lens to fracture through the naturally occurring radial fault lines of the lens. Formerly, phacoemulsification of brunescent nuclei was accomplished by sculpting the nuclear rim to create notches that facilitate manipulation of the nucleus with a spatula. Currently, brunescent and softer cataracts are removed without pre-grooving the nucleus through the down slope sculpting technique. Therefore, the principle advantage of the down slope sculpting technique is that pre-grooving the nucleus for subsequent fracturing is completely unnecessary and sculpting may be accomplished successfully without a chopper.

Down slope sculpting in the upper pole of the lens to just past the center reduces the chance of posterior capsule rupture with the phaco port. If the lens is nudged inferiorly by the second instrument and deep sculpting is done from just inside the CCC to the center of the lens, then the tip travel will be parallel to the concave slope of the posterior aspect of the nucleus and the posterior capsule. Although the surgeon cannot visualize the tip when going "down slope," the depth of the sculpting is determined by visualizing the depth of the groove and translucency of the remaining tissue.

With traditional techniques, if the nucleus is broken through unexpectedly when sculpting a deep, long trench toward 6 o'clock, the tip is more perpendicular to the inferior portion of the posterior capsule because of its concavity and is directly perpendicular to the equatorial capsule (Figure 15-24). With down slope sculpting, considerable nuclear material remains ahead of the tip at the end of each sculpting pass. Therefore breaking through is unlikely with this "cushion" present. The risk of engaging the capsule is thus minimized.

TECHNICAL TIPS

Occasionally, even without hydrodelineation, the nucleus spontaneously separates from the epinucleus during fracturing. Purposeful hydrodelineation ensures this separation and facilitates nucleofractis. Soft epinucleus can be removed as a bowl with low flow and low vacuum. Firm epinucleus usually fractures with the nucleus if hydrodelineation is not performed, but if separated, it may remain as sheets of rather firm material that must be teased to the center for emulsification. For this reason, I prefer not to attempt hydrodelineation in cases with very hard epinuclei. With complete hydrodissection, the typical soft epinucleus can be easily removed but must be approached gently with the phaco tip. Low settings of flow, vacuum, and ultrasound are safer and more effective. Any remaining sections of epinucleus in the subincisional zone can be dislodged with the help of the second instrument and maneuvered to the phaco port. Sliding the spatula under the anterior capsule and then pressing posteriorly into the material is more effective than engaging it directly in the equator of the epinucleus.

The position and number of cracks and the size of the resulting sections depend on the density of the lens, the manner in which it splits, and preference of the surgeon. As with CDC, the harder the lens, the smaller the pieces should be for greatest safety and manageability. In a moderate lens, two or three cracks usually are sufficient, and the surgeon can use the second instrument to control the larger sections. Probably the greatest challenge of the technique is gaining the confidence to sculpt very deep. By gaining confidence with the instruments in both hands, most surgeons should be able to be more assertive while sculpting.

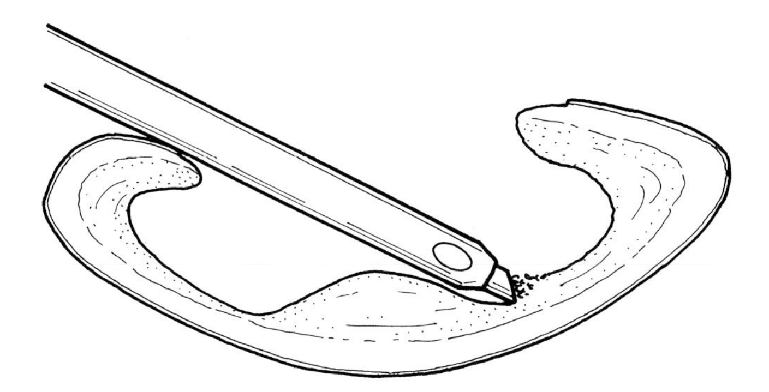

FIGURE 15-23 With traditional sculpting techniques, excessive central nuclear material may impede fracturing.

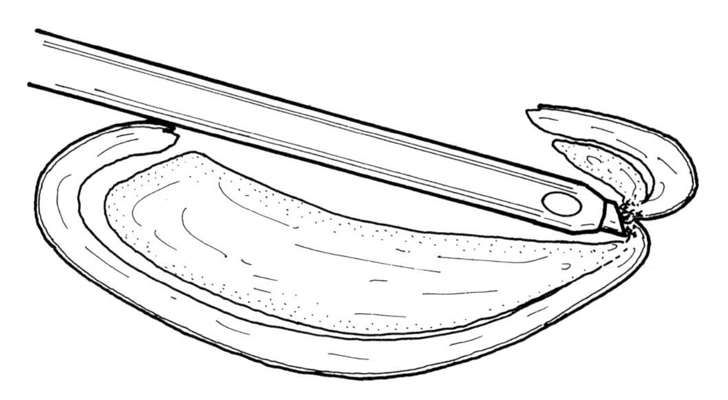

FIGURE 15-24 In addition, traditional shallow sculpting can create potential for direct contact with the posterior capsule.

The surgeon must be cautious when the CCC is small to avoid tearing the edge of the anterior capsule superiorly with the tip or the sleeve of the phaco instrument. In my experience, this is most likely to occur in cases with poor visualization, such as when hypermature, white cataracts are present. Ordinarily, the risk is low because one is not sculpting much past the center when first beginning the trench.

Care must also be exercised in displacing the nucleus within the capsular bag so that the whole bag is not displaced and the upper zonular ligaments are not unduly stretched and broken. Also, when tipping the handle of the phaco handpiece up to sculpt down toward the posterior pole, the surgeon must not push the tip posteriorly faster than the tip is chiseling its way through the lens material. The zonular ligaments may also be torn in such a manner. These risks are greatest in lenses with hard epinucleus and where the zonula are already weakened.

Limiting sculpting to the superior part of the nucleus adds safety because of the reduced risk of contacting the posterior capsule, and it adds efficiency because of the rapidity with which the posterior pole of the nucleus is reached with the phaco tip. With instruments this deep in the nucleus, the fracturing can be effectively initiated and safely completed.

Special Situations

Modifications to these general techniques may be necessary when a surgeon is confronted with any of a number of special, challenging situations. In *soft lenses,* Sinskey's technique of phacoemulsification[106] should be applied using basic sculpting without fracturing and without lifting the nucleus out of the bag. It is important to achieve hydrodissection in these lenses, but it may be difficult to achieve without prolapsing the nucleus out of the capsule. Therefore hydrodissection should be attempted with caution, and perhaps even only partial hydrodissection should be the goal. Hydrodissecting a small amount in a number of quadrants or using the technique of hydrofree dissection[104,107,108] may be applicable here. In addition, hydrodelineation can facilitate removing these softer lenses by achieving separation between nucleus and epinucleus. The epinucleus is often large and thick but also very soft. It folds and flips more readily if the central nucleus has been completely removed first.

In cases in which a history of *trauma exists,* a fibrotic anterior capsule may be present, or zonules may be missing in one quadrant or more, and the lens may be partially subluxated. In addition, an old perforating or penetrating capsule injury may be present and the capsule resealed. It is important to look for iridodonesis to confirm whether the zonules are weak, anticipating that intracapsular surgery may be required. If zonules are absent or very weak in one quadrant or hemisection, they may be strong in the other sections and allow standard techniques. It is important to recognize that traumatic cataracts may develop very quickly, necessitating surgery within days or weeks of the injury. If the zonules are weakened but no capsule puncture has occurred, complete hydrodissection and hydrodelineation are essential. If the capsule has been injured or damaged during pars plana vitrectomy, hydrodissection should not be attempted. Tedious, delicate sculpting, as described by Fine[109-111] and Koch,[112-114] should be used.

Phacoemulsification and Reverse Pupillary Block

On entering the anterior chamber with the phaco tip, particularly with high infusion sleeves and high bottles, reverse pupillary block or iris concavity may occur, resulting in patient discomfort especially in eyes under topical anesthesia. Although more common in the highly myopic or pediatric eye, iris concavity may occur without notice. Reverse pupillary block is the stretching or extension of the iris posteriorly, causing iris concavity and contact with the anterior lens capsule. This block can be immediately released by lifting the iris off from the top of the capsule with a spatula or any second instrument.

To prevent reverse pupillary block and avoid discomfort, it is preferable to have an instrument between the iris and capsule as the irrigation is turned on. This will allow fluid to circulate in behind the iris, thus preventing pupillary block. Another technique to help prevent reverse pupillary block is to turn the irrigation on with short staccato-like taps onto the foot switch. If reverse pupillary block should occur, with this technique one may interrupt the development of iris concavity before excessive deepening of the anterior chamber and minimize discomfort to the patient.

With *highly myopic cases,* the principal concern is the potential for lack of vitreous support. The lens iris diaphragm may be quite unstable and may fluctuate widely during on-and-off irrigation and even when shifting between foot positions 1 and 2. Machines with an adjustable flow rate are more advantageous in these cases and should be used to ensure more stable hydrodynamics.

Cases with a *shallow chamber* can be challenging, even with the use of viscoelastics, because it is difficult to achieve an average chamber depth in some of these cases with high hyperopia; very old, thick cataracts; and perhaps loose zonules as well. The most important consideration under these circumstances is to use a tunnel incision with a corneal entry, performed more anterior in location than usual. This helps to prevent iris prolapse through the wound during phacoemulsification. Even during the capsulotomy, the viscoelastic can potentially extrude from the eye, although the use of dispersive or noncohesive low-molecular-weight hyaluronate viscoelastic may minimize this problem. Maintaining the chamber for caspulorhexis is important because iris prolapse at this stage can lead to iris trauma when inserting the phaco probe. Iris trauma may occur just from the friction of the phaco sleeve passing over the iris.

TECHNICAL TIPS

A lower bottle position is advocated to allow the lens iris diaphragm not to be pushed far posteriorly as soon as irrigation is started. If the anterior chamber depth does fluctuate widely, the pupil is usually more dilated when the lens iris diaphragm is posterior and tends to be more constricted when the lens iris diaphragm is in a normal or anterior position (chamber collapse). Repeated episodes of chamber collapse can lead to a constricted pupil. In addition, a deep chamber should be avoided so that the phaco tip does not have to tip so far posteriorly. Simply stated, keeping the bottle low keeps the chamber at a normal depth and more stable.

TECHNICAL TIPS

It is also important to ensure proper wound size in these cases. Avoiding too large an incision is critical. Unless using a standard keratome, erring on the conservative side is recommended. In addition, the bottle may need to be raised for extra pressure to deepen the anterior chamber during phacoemulsification. As soon as possible, the phaco tip should be used to develop a trench rather than shaving more of the superficial anterior surface where turbulence can reach the cornea. By achieving depth into the lens early, the turbulence is dissipated.

Loose zonules can typically be detected on the first puncture of the capsule for capsulorhexis. The integrity of the zonules can be tested with the instrument being used to puncture the capsule: bent needle, cystotome, or forceps. If the lens is quite mobile and the zonules are very loose, an intracapsular tension ring may need to be used. To manage cases with lost or weak zonules in cataract surgery and to lower the incidence of postoperative capsular contraction, it is essential to maintain the circular contour of the capsular bag both intraoperatively and postoperatively. IOLs with loop shapes that conformed to that of the capsular bag or loopless IOLs that would exactly fit the capsular bag were initially used to achieve this goal. However, the large size of these IOLs required larger incisions, resulting in longer healing times and increased likelihood of significant postoperative astigmatism.

Clinically the capsular tension ring has been used in the management of patients with moderate loss of zonular support in cataract surgery. However, for cases with a significant loss of zonular support (more than a quadrant) the capsular tension ring and remaining zonules may be unable to provide enough support to stabilize the capsular bag. For these cases Cionni modified the conventional capsular tension ring by adding a polymethylmethacrylate (PMMA) hook on the loop. At the free end of the hook is an eyelet for manipulation and suture placement. When the ring is implanted in the capsular bag, a suture can be secured to this eyelet to allow scleral fixation without violating the integrity of the capsular bag. Clinical outcomes have shown that this ring provides excellent support and centration of the capsular bag and IOL both intraoperatively and postoperatively. Capsule tension rings are discussed extensively in Chapter 27.

Another set of conditions, such as coloboma, complete aniridia, or eye trauma that may result in loss of iris tissue or sphincter function, may be managed with an aniridia ring that creates an artificial iris diaphragm. Several types are commercially available. Iris repair and artificial iris segments are discussed in Chapter 29.

Capsular tension rings are indicated during any cataract surgery in which the stability of the capsular bag is compromised. An unstable capsular bag can result from previous trauma, pseudoexfoliation syndrome, floppy capsule syndrome, or various developmental or congenital syndromes. Instability of the capsular bag increases the risk of complications during or after cataract extraction and IOL implantation as discussed earlier. Capsular tension rings can significantly reduce this risk.

In many situations, inadequate capsular support is apparent before surgery. Placement of a capsular tension ring in these situations should be planned before surgery. There is debate as to weather to place a capsular tension ring in all eyes with pseudoexfoliation syndrome. Although this is not presently recommended in all cases, its use should be planned in all cases. In other situations, the need for a capsular tension ring may not be apparent until after the crystalline lens has been removed. For example, in the case of floppy capsule syndrome, the capsular bag is slowly stretched by a large crystalline lens. It is not until the lens is removed and the bag is released from this stretch that the floppy nature is apparent. In these cases a capsular tension ring may be placed at this time to prevent postoperative folds or wrinkles in the posterior capsule, which may transect in the visual axis. In other cases, there is no preoperative history or slit lamp biomicroscopic findings to suggest inadequate capsular support. In these cases, the attention to detail during surgery is paramount. If the surgeon performs a round CCC and then removes the crystalline lens and implants an IOL, the CCC should still be round if the capsular support is adequate. If the CCC becomes oval, it indicates inadequate capsular support in the meridian in which there is no IOL haptic support. In this situation a capsular tension ring may be placed, and the surgeon will note that the CCC is round once again. This should reduce the risk of late capsular bag subluxation. Late capsular bag subluxation may also be prevented by using capsular tension rings in cases of suspiciously unstable capsular bags after IOL implantation, especially in pseudoexfoliation syndrome.

In cases of zonular dehiscence involving one quadrant (i.e., less than 90 degrees), a capsular tension ring or a capsular edge ring is indicated. If two or less quadrants are involved (i.e., 90 to 180 degrees), a single-hook Cionni ring is indicated. A double-hook Cionni ring is indicated if the zonular dehiscence is greater than 180 degrees.

Capsular tension rings stabilize the capsular bag by exerting outward force on the bag; therefore the bag must be able to withstand this force for the tension ring to be safe and effective. A capsular tension ring cannot be placed into an eye that does not have a good quality CCC. If the CCC is torn, very eccentric, or very large, a tension ring may extend the tear and dislocate from its position within the bag.

If the posterior capsule is torn before inserting a tension ring, the ring can only be inserted if the surgeon is able to convert the torn posterior capsule into a posterior CCC. If this is accomplished, then a ring may be inserted safely. If the posterior capsule is torn after a ring has already been placed, it is not always necessary to remove the ring. All efforts should be made to convert the tear into a posterior CCC, but if this cannot be accomplished and the ring cannot be easily removed (i.e., via a safety suture), the ring may be left in place. However, there may be a higher likelihood of extension of the posterior capsule tear with resultant posterior dislocation of the ring and the IOL.

The lens nucleus and epinucleus act as an endoskeleton to the capsular bag. For this reason, if there is any suspicion of zonular dialysis, or if the bag starts collapsing during surgery, a capsular tension ring should be inserted into the bag before or during phacoemulsification to act as an alternate endoskeleton

TECHNICAL TIPS

When performing capsulorhexis, the lens can be inadvertently nudged to one side by the instrument. Centration of the CCC can be deceiving, but releasing the instrument from the anterior capsule as one is tearing it allows the lens to assume its natural position. Reinspecting is crucial to ascertain where the edge of the tear is progressing. The same recommendation applies in pediatric cases, in which very elastic zonules and a somewhat elastic capsule typically are present. During phacoemulsification, the two-handed technique is crucial for stabilizing the nucleus in cases with loose zonules.

to the bag before removing its own natural endoskeleton. In cases of severe zonular dehiscence and capsular dialysis, and when vitreous has prolapsed around the dehisced area, requiring anterior vitrectomy, the vitrectomy should be postponed until the ring is in place. The ring will exert an outward pressure on the capsular bag, thus preventing further vitreous from prolapsing anteriorly from around the edges of the dehisced capsular bag during the vitrectomy, which would cause further collapse of the capsular bag and further tearing of its zonular attachments, leading to a vicious cycle of vitreous prolapse and zonular dehiscence.

A *subluxated lens* is usually diagnosed before surgery by observation of iridodonesis, displaced Y sutures, and chamber angle abnormalities. As mentioned previously, however, preexisting zonular damage may first be detected during attempts to puncture the anterior capsule. Assuming the instrument is sharp, failure to puncture—with noticeable wrinkling of the capsule and movement of the lens—should suggest a loosened zonula.

Cataract surgery in patients with *pseudoexfoliation syndrome* carries a significantly higher risk of intraoperative postoperative complications.[115] Zonular dialysis, capsular rupture, vitreous loss, and late IOL dislocation have been reported to occur more frequently in the presence of pseudoexfoliation.[116-118] Also, fragile lens zonules, abnormal ciliary body interface, and poor papillary dilation have been implicated as a basis for more frequent complications.[119,120]

TECHNICAL TIPS

Hydrodissection is helpful to atraumatically loosen the nucleus but must be limited to avoid overhydrating the vitreous and expanding its volume. Low flow and vacuum reduce fluctuations in chamber depth and minimize lens movements that might further damage zonules.

Pharmacologic agents should be used to maintain maximal pupil dilation throughout the surgery. All contact with the iris must be strictly avoided during phacoemulsification to prevent additional constriction of the pupil. The bimanual in situ nucleofractis techniques with minimal zonular stress are ideally suited for safe phacoemulsification in cases with pseudoexfoliation, and their safety has been confirmed in a multicenter study.[121]

Variations

Since divide and conquer's inception, a number of popular variations have emerged. Shepherd[122,123] was one of the early advocates of fracturing and soon developed his in situ fracture technique, which also relies heavily on nuclear rotation. Using either a 30- or 45-degree tip, a groove two tip widths wide is sculpted from the 12 to 6 o'clock positions (Figure 15-25). The nucleus is then rotated by placing the phaco tip in the proximal and the spatula in the distal end of the groove and turning clockwise (Figure 15-26). Shepherd believes that this is most easily accomplished if no fracture has taken place. A second groove is carved, cross-hatched across the first, and carried slightly deeper (Figure 15-27). The phaco tip is pushed against

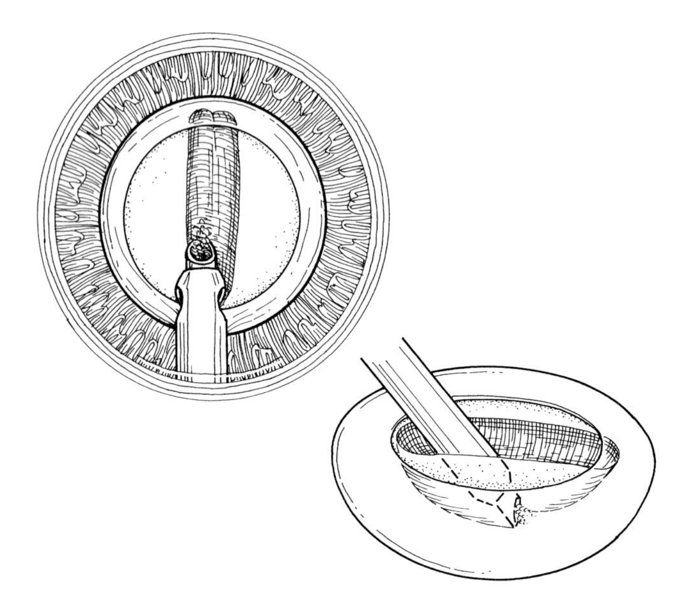

FIGURE 15-25 Shepherd's technique begins with a groove sculpted from 12 to 6 o'clock.

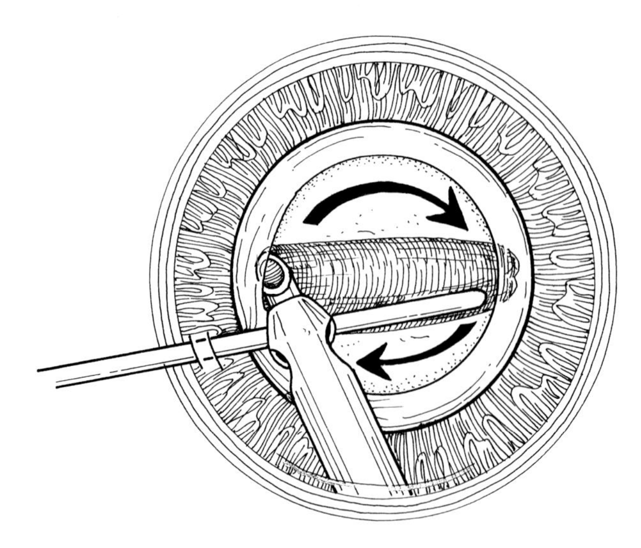

FIGURE 15-26 Clockwise pressure is exerted by both instruments to rotate the groove 90 degrees.

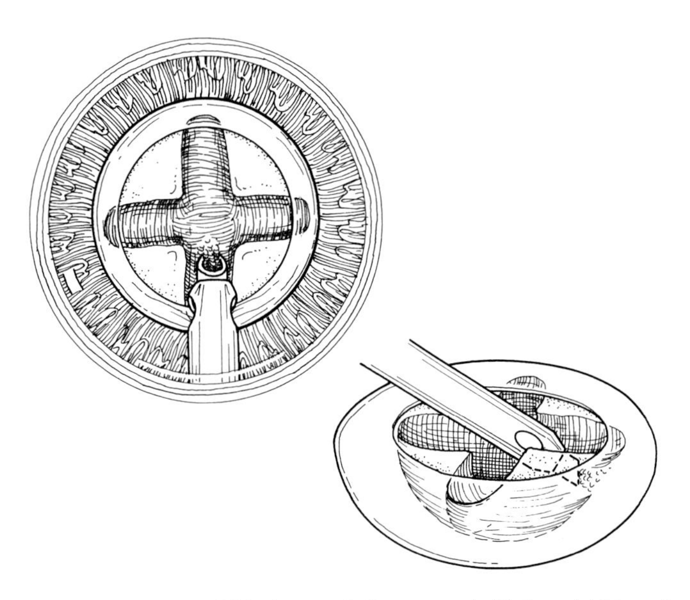

FIGURE 15-27 Original groove is then crossed with the establishment of a second groove.

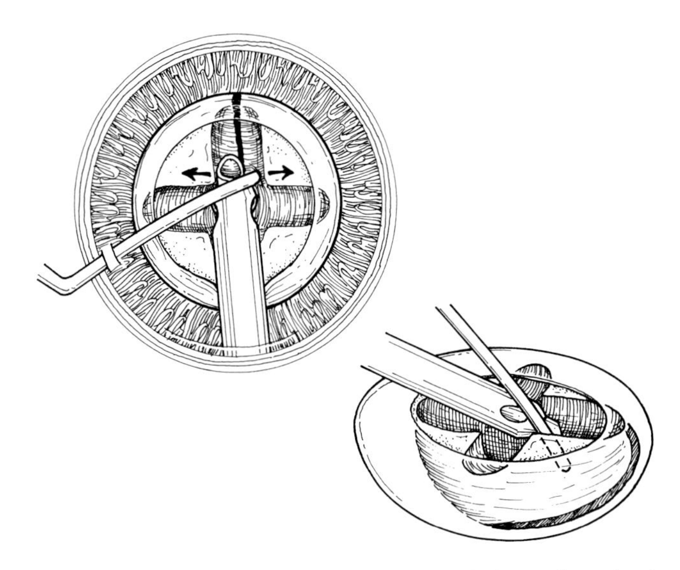

FIGURE 15-28 Spatula and phaco tip are pushed apart, fracturing the nucleus.

the left wall of the distal groove, the spatula is placed cross-action against the right wall, and the nuclear rim is gently separated (Figure 15-28). The nucleus is then rotated on quarter turn, and the fracturing procedure is repeated until all four grooves are broken (Figure 15-29). Shepherd uses a "tumble" rather than "follow" method for removing the segments. To initiate tumbling, a spatula is used to push down on the apex of an inferior fragment until the fragment flips over, and the piece is rotated centrally with the apex trailing (Figures 15-30 and 15-31). This quadrant can then be emulsified (Figure 15-32). Each quadrant is similarly manipulated into the central area and removed (Figure 15-33). Davison[124-127] has also developed a similar technique, in which the nuclear segments are managed using increased vacuum level settings.

One criticism of Shepherd's technique is that the tumbling maneuver may cause the central portion of the nuclear segments to point down toward the posterior capsule and possibly cause a tear.[128] In my opinion, this risk may be exaggerated. The base soon leaves the capsule and is displaced anteriorly, reducing pressure on the posterior capsule by the tip. Some surgeons have advocated engaging the apex and lifting it up to facilitate removal. A more practical and efficient method to avoid this situation would be to create more and smaller pieces that turn sideways on removal. Even if the segment starts to tumble, the top can be shaved off in one or two passes to reduce the thicker, equatorial portion of the lens. If the sculpting has been sufficiently wide and deep centrally, these apexes are thin, soft, and nonthreatening because one has reached the epinucleus during sculpting.

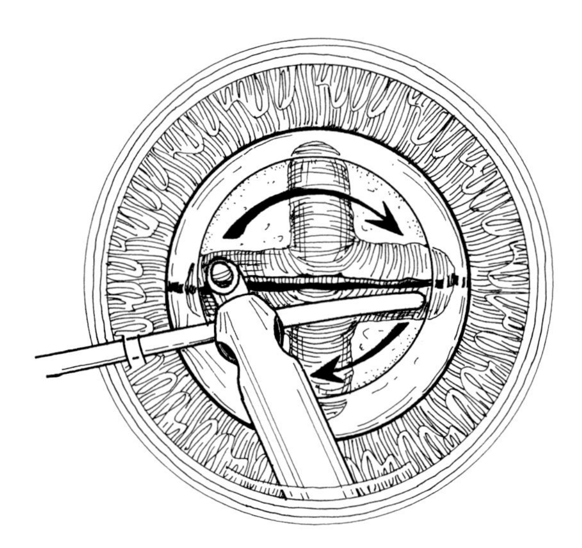

FIGURE 15-29 Following nuclear rotation, another groove is cracked, resulting in four quadrants of nucleus.

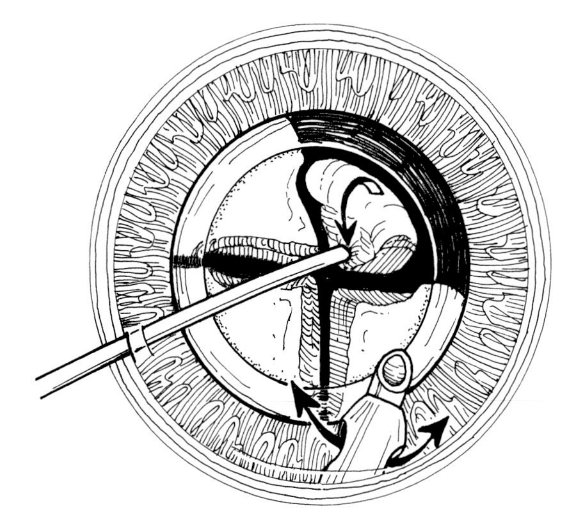

FIGURE 15-30 Spatula is used to depress the apex of a wedge and to tumble it into an upside-down position.

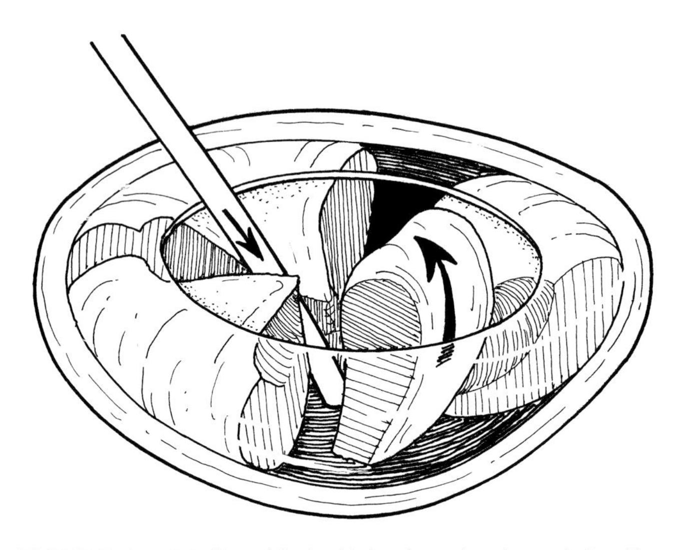

FIGURE 15-31 Base of the tumbled wedge ends up in a central position.

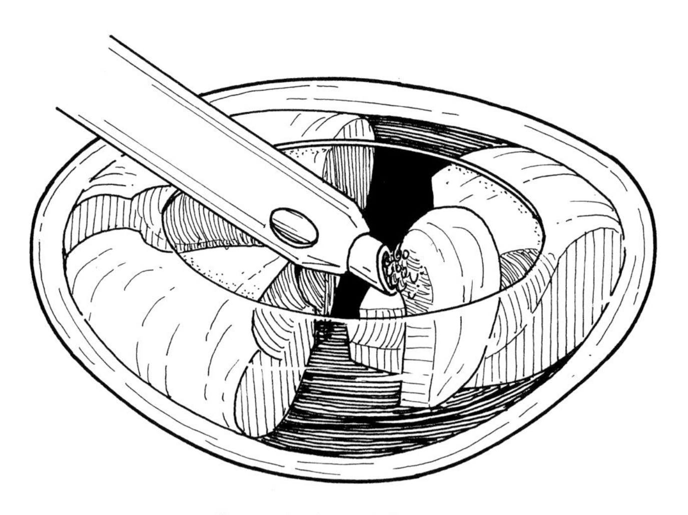

FIGURE 15-32 First wedge is emulsified.

To enhance the safety and control of quadrant management, Fine[109-111] attempted to create a central nuclear component and an outer epinuclear component and to perform phacoemulsification using the two zones. This became his "chip and flip" technique. Following hydrodelineation to create the zones, the chip and flip technique is initiated by performing central sculpting using a 30-degree tip (Figure 15-34). A Bechert nucleus rotator or cyclodialysis spatula is introduced, and the nucleus is pushed toward 12 o'clock (Figure 15-35). The rim of the inner nuclear bowl is removed at 5 to 6 o'clock, and the nucleus is rotated clockwise to sequentially facilitate each hour of rim being removed from the 5 to 6 o'clock region (Figure 15-36). Once the rim of the inner nuclear bowl is removed, the second handpiece is brought into the cleavage plane between the inner nuclear chip and the outer nuclear bowl and swept under the chip, elevating it into the center of the bag (Figure 15-37). Using the second handpiece to control the nuclear chip, the chip can then be quickly and safely removed (Figure 15-38).

In the late 1980s and early 1990s, Fine[97,109-111] described two endolenticular phacoemulsification techniques: the chip and flip and the chop and flip. The techniques used the pulse mode to remove nuclear material, which decreased chattering and increased holding power of the nuclear material. Many modulations in the delivery of power are now available. With these modulations, significantly less total ultrasound is delivered into the eye. The Alcon 20,000 Legacy has a bimodal option that allows the surgeon to use linear aspiration flow rate or vacuum in foot position 2. Fine[129,130] takes maximum advantage of the new technologies available with this system as described in his choo-choo chop and flip phacoemulsification technique. This uses the burst mode and bevel down technique with high vacuum and ultrasound power settings for enhanced efficiency.

The soft outer nuclear bowl, which has cushioned all previous phacoemulsification, is now displaced from the capsular fornix at 5 to 6 o'clock (Figure 15-39). The nuclear bowl is mobilized by pulling the rim at 5 to 6 o'clock toward 12 o'clock and

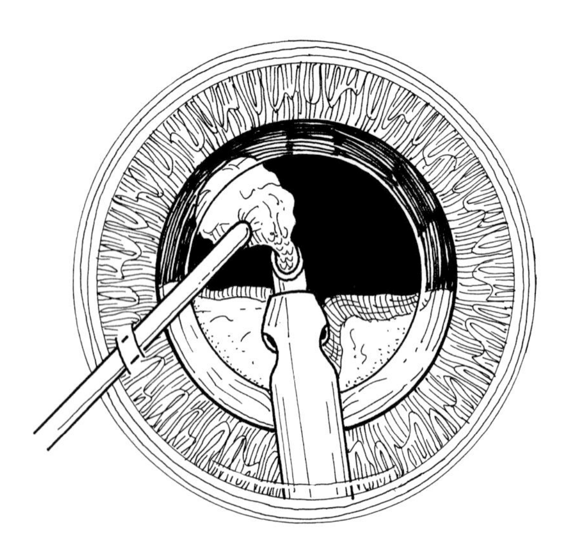

FIGURE 15-33 Remaining wedges are then similarly maneuvered within the bag and emulsified.

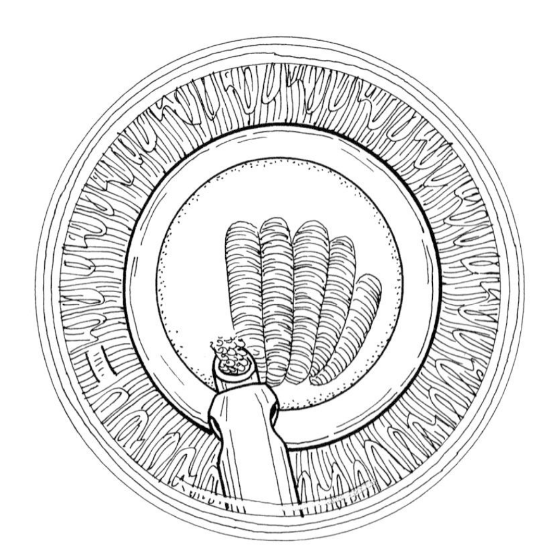

FIGURE 15-34 Fine's "chip and flip" technique begins with central sculpting of the nucleus.

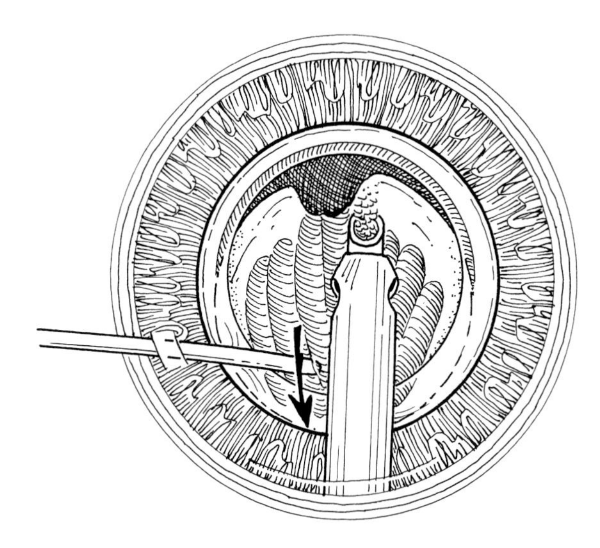

FIGURE 15-35 At the 5 to 6 o'clock position, the inner nuclear rim is removed.

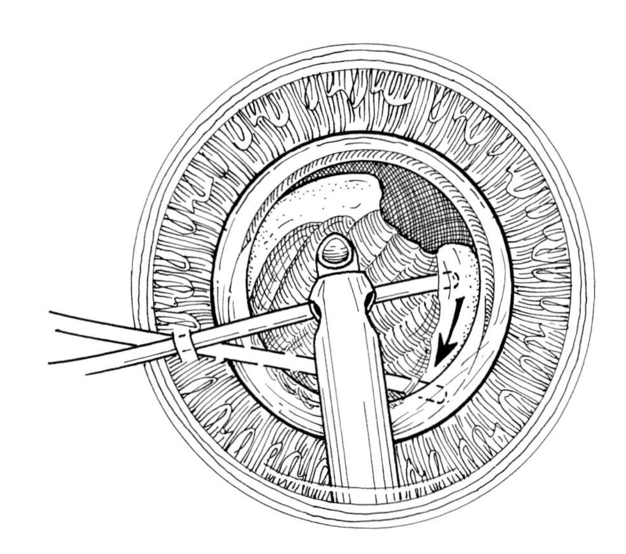

FIGURE 15-36 Second instrument is used below the phaco probe to rotate the nucleus and further facilitate removal in this region.

pushing with the second handpiece in the bottom of the nuclear bowl toward 5 to 6 o'clock to tumble or flip the soft outer nuclear bowl (Figure 15-40). By flipping the bowl away from the capsule, it can be removed safely, either with aspiration or with low-powered emulsification without jeopardizing the capsule (Figure 15-41).

A number of similar techniques for soft to moderate lenses have been published in the literature.[129,131-134] By necessity, these techniques are limited to lenses whose consistency is sufficiently soft to permit the creation of a cleavage plane within the nucleus by hydrodelineation.

Dillman and Maloney recognized the benefits of cracking and recently teamed with Fine to develop the "crack and flip" technique,[97] which is essentially a hybrid of Shepherd's in situ fracture, Fine's chip and flip, and Maloney and Dillman's fractional 2:4 phacoemulsification techniques.[135-137] With crack and flip, the sculpting starts centrally, and the first groove is made toward 6 o'clock (Figure 15-42). The sculpting takes place entirely within the central compact mass, and every effort is made to avoid actually reaching the golden hydrodelineation ring during sculpting. As one groove is completed, the nucleus is rotated clockwise 90 degrees, and the next groove is started (Figure 15-43).

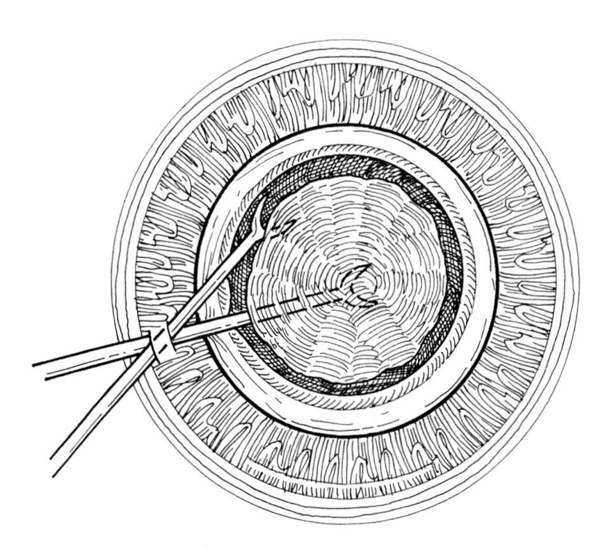

FIGURE 15-37 Bechert rotator is used to sweep under the nuclear chip and elevate it into the center of the bag.

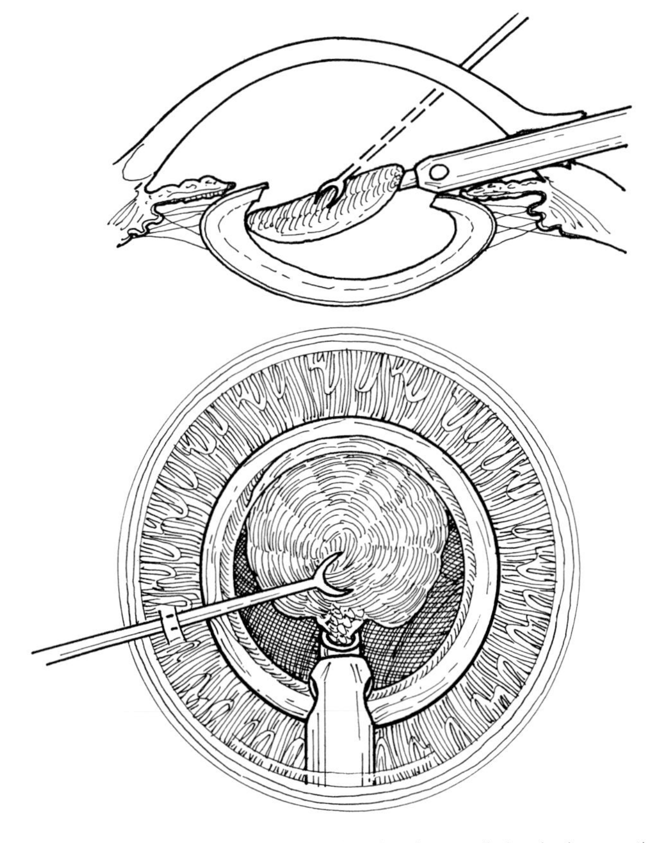

FIGURE 15-38 Remaining central nucleus is controlled and subsequently emulsified using a two-handed technique.

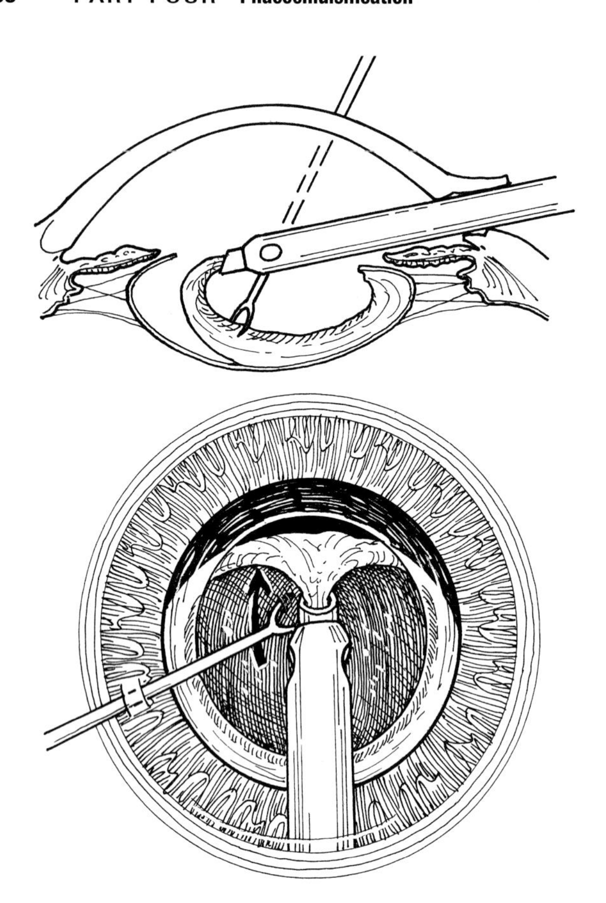

FIGURE 15-39 In the 5 to 6 o'clock position, the phaco tip engages the rim with aspiration only as the second instrument pushes the bottom of the bowl.

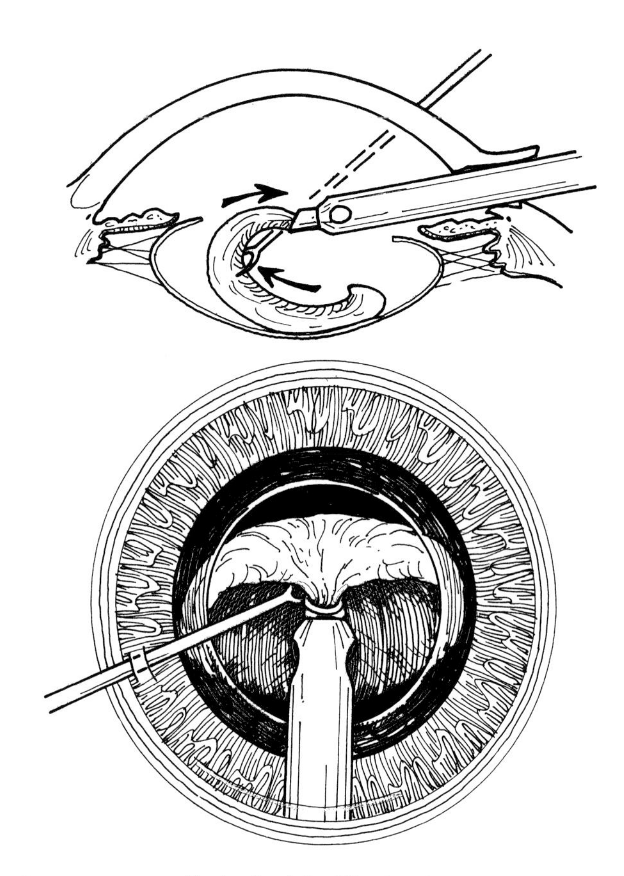

FIGURE 15-40 Nuclear bowl should begin to flip away from the posterior capsule.

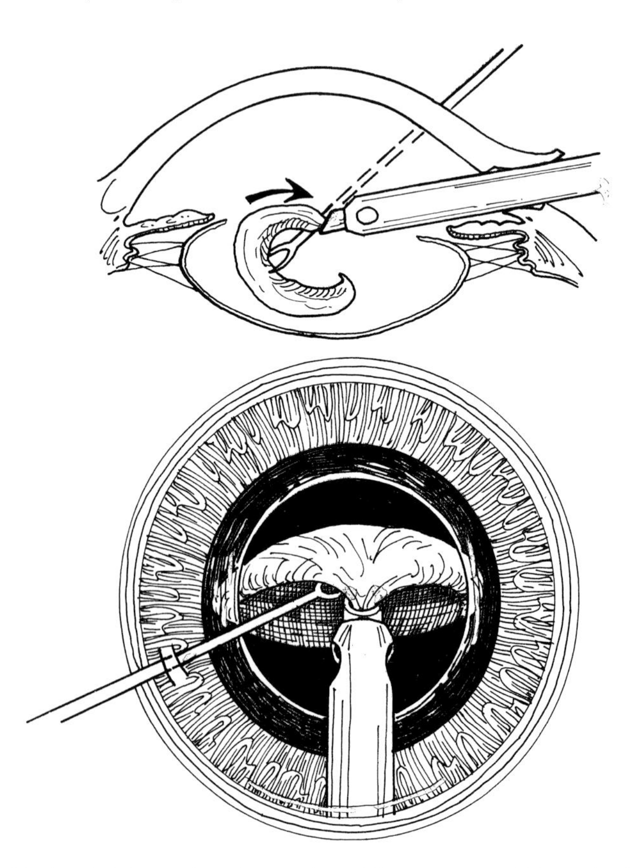

FIGURE 15-41 Bowl is worked out of the capsule and folded on itself.

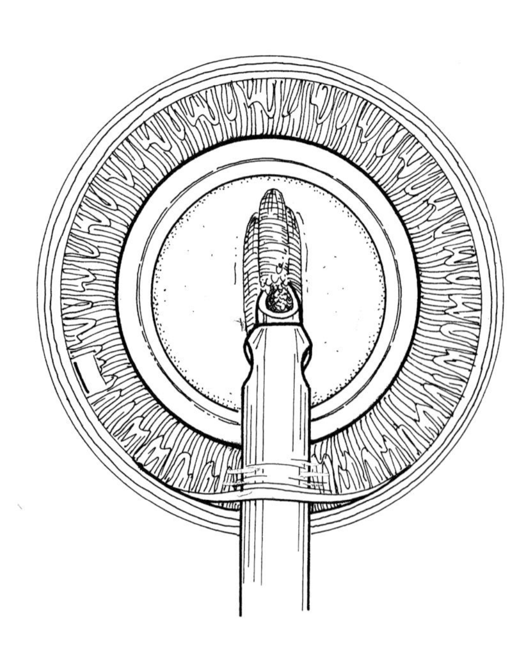

FIGURE 15-42 "Crack and flip" technique begins with a central groove toward 6 o'clock.

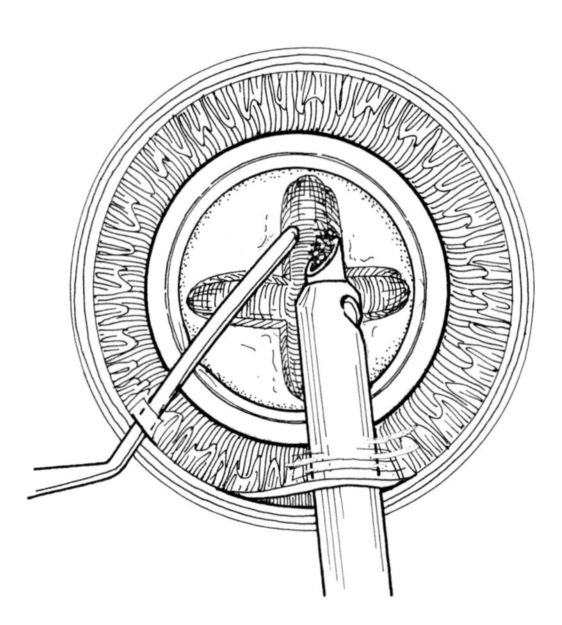

FIGURE 15-43 Nucleus is rotated 90 degrees, and a similar groove is created.

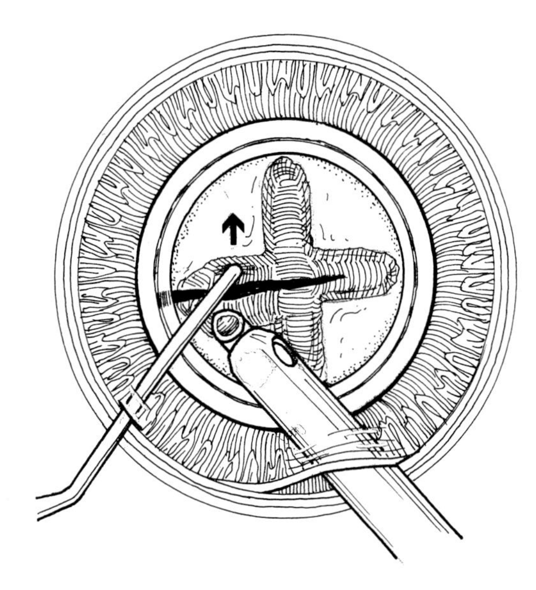

FIGURE 15-44 Following the formation of four grooves, the nucleus is split into quadrants.

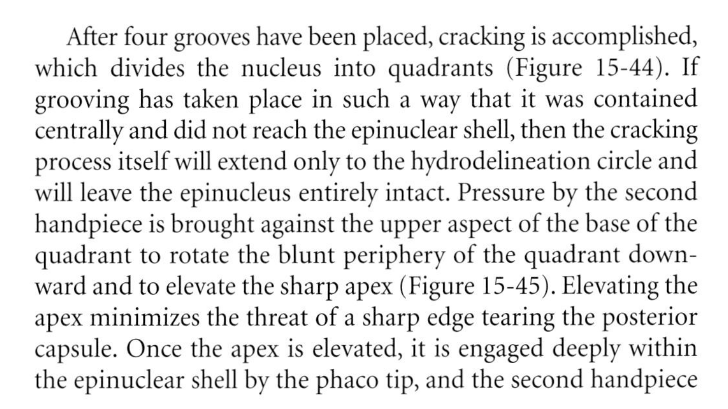

After four grooves have been placed, cracking is accomplished, which divides the nucleus into quadrants (Figure 15-44). If grooving has taken place in such a way that it was contained centrally and did not reach the epinuclear shell, then the cracking process itself will extend only to the hydrodelineation circle and will leave the epinucleus entirely intact. Pressure by the second handpiece is brought against the upper aspect of the base of the quadrant to rotate the blunt periphery of the quadrant downward and to elevate the sharp apex (Figure 15-45). Elevating the apex minimizes the threat of a sharp edge tearing the posterior capsule. Once the apex is elevated, it is engaged deeply within the epinuclear shell by the phaco tip, and the second handpiece is brought under the quadrant to support it until occlusion occurs (Figure 15-46). As occlusion occurs, the quadrant is brought toward the middle of the epinuclear shell, and the second handpiece can be used to either hold the quadrant down, to mash it toward the phaco tip, or to crack it into eighths. Once the quadrant is emulsified by the phaco tip, the second handpiece holds the remaining fragments deep within the epinucleus until they are sequentially removed by the phaco tip from within the epinuclear shell.

The remaining quadrants are rotated to bring another quadrant to the distal position for removal in the same manner. Each quadrant is sequentially removed in this way, working in

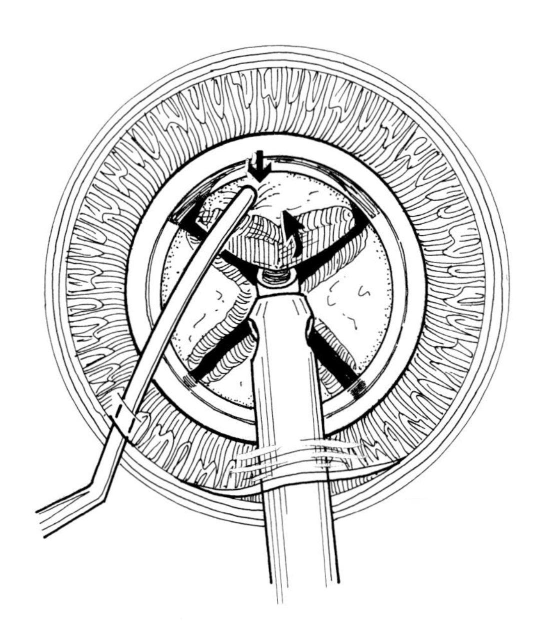

FIGURE 15-45 Second instrument is used to rotate the blunt periphery downward and to lift the sharp apex safely upward.

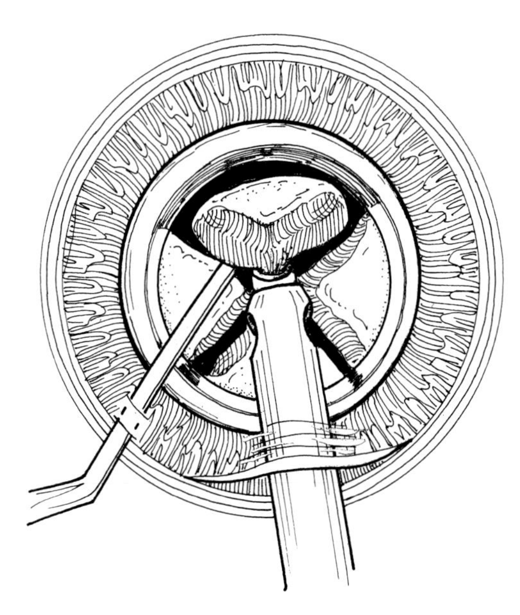

FIGURE 15-46 Once elevated, the apex is engaged and occluded using the second instrument as a maintenance tool.

the central portion of the epinucleus. Every attempt is made to keep a quadrant or any of its fragments from coming up into the anterior chamber. After removal of the quadrants, an empty but intact epinuclear shell remains.

Clearly, two schools of thought have emerged regarding hydrodelineation. Some surgeons believe that hydrodelineation detracts from the effectiveness and efficiency of the operation and prefer not to perform it. Others, including Dillman, Maloney, and Fine, use hydrodelineation to maintain the peripheral protective cushion of the outer nucleus. For my own technique, I do perform hydrodelineation on a frequent basis; however, under certain circumstances, as with a very dense lens, I prefer the option of fracturing right out to the periphery.

"Phaco chop" is an important variation in the method for nuclear disassembly. Originally described by Dr. Kunihiro Nagahara in 1993, phaco chop uses a chopping instrument to split the nucleus along natural cleavage planes. The details of this technique are described in Chapter 16.

The goal of the *endocapsular* phacoemulsification surgeon is to maximize the amount of anterior capsule in place during phacoemulsification. The anterior capsule is seen to serve as a physical barrier to protect the corneal endothelium during phacoemulsification and to limit the turbulence within the confines of the capsular bag. A number of endocapsular phacoemulsification techniques have been proposed in the literature but have not been integrated into current practice.[138-148]

Both Solomon[149-150] and Michelson[151] described what Michelson has termed a *minicapsulorhexis.* The minicapsulorhexis is small enough to maximize this barrier effect of the anterior capsule while being adequately large to allow lateral excursion of the phaco tip without creating undue stress on the margins of the capsulotomy (Figures 15-47 and 15-48). The technique facilitates near total compartmentalization of the emulsification process within the lens capsule, thereby providing significant protection to the iris and corneal endothelium. The minicap is typically 0.5 by 4 mm in size, made near the superior iris border. Reported advantages of this location include an enhanced barrier effect for the anterior chamber and better access to the 12 o'clock position. When emulsifying below the anterior capsule, visibility becomes extremely important, and the space-maintaining properties of viscoelastic materials should be used to their fullest potential.

Before commencing sculpting, working space may be created with several short bursts of low-power linear phacoemulsification under the leading edge of the anterior capsule. Solomon[149] recommends passing the handpiece through the anterior chamber in a "bevel down" position to prevent stripping Descemet's membrane and then rotating the tip to the "bevel up" position. The initial sculpting maneuver should be limited to half the nucleus, leaving the epinuclear rim intact. The depth of the sculpting should proceed to include at least two thirds to three fourths of the central nuclear thickness (Figure 15-49). The dislocation and rotation maneuver are accomplished by first impaling the phaco tip into the base of the superior ledge of the unsculpted rim of the nucleus. Gentle force is applied with the phaco tip to rotate the nucleus 90 degrees. The unsculpted nucleus is now inferiorly located (Figure 15-50). This remaining central material is thus sculpted, completing the nuclear bowl. The epinuclear rim may be emulsified under low phacoemulsification power (Figure 15-51). The residual nuclear plate is emulsified after it has been dislocated off the posterior capsule and floated anteriorly toward the iris plane (Figures 15-52 to 15-54).

Using this technique, Michelson claimed to observe no endothelial cell loss in between 40% and 65% of his cases and minimal cell loss (4% or less) in the remaining cases. Similar low cell loss levels have been reported by a number of surgeons using an endocapsular phacoemulsification method.[98,139,152,153]

Nishi[154,155] has also reported good results using a buttonhole capsulotomy opening, wherein a 3.5- to 4-mm horizontal capsulotomy is made in the superior portion of the capsule (Figure 15-55). The ends of the capsulotomy are then rounded

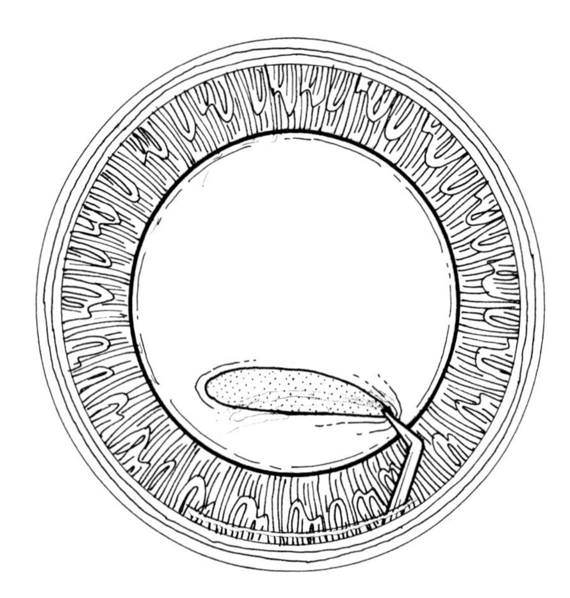

FIGURE 15-47 "Minicapsulorhexis" of endocapsular phacoemulsification is initiated with a puncture near the superior iris border in a well-dilated pupil.

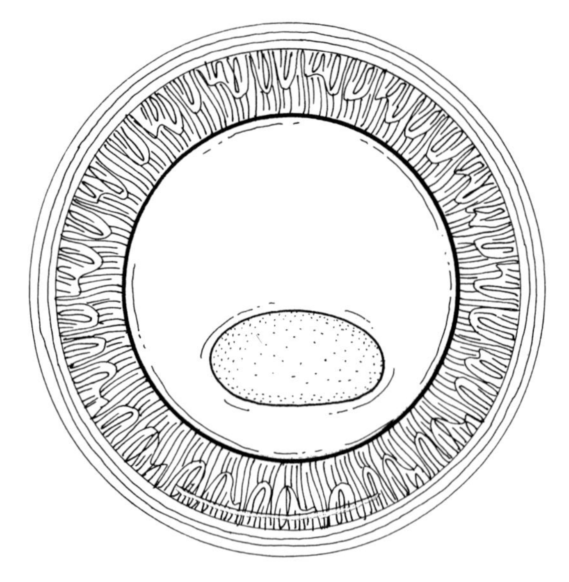

FIGURE 15-48 "Minicap" should be large enough to accommodate the phaco tip and sleeve while allowing easy access to the nucleus.

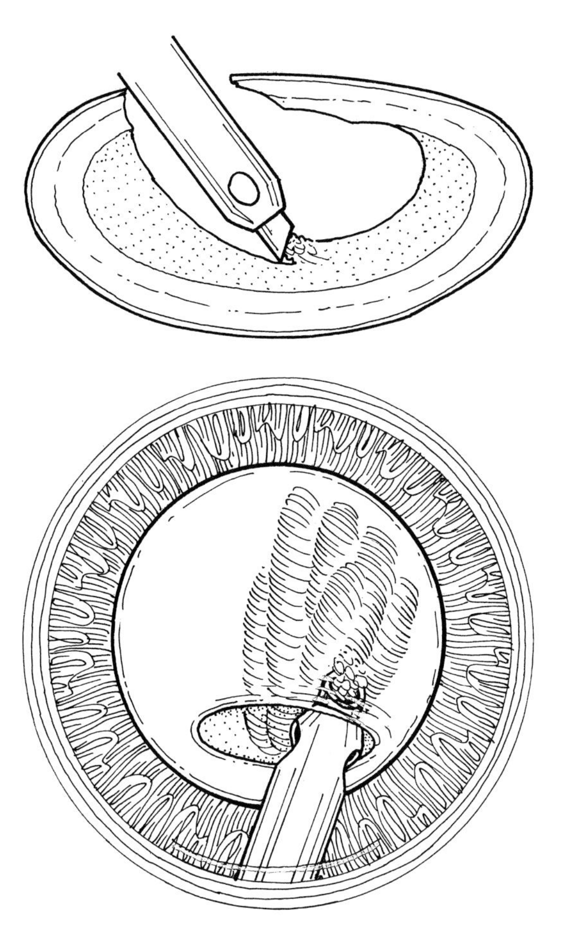

FIGURE 15-49 Initial sculpting includes at least two thirds to three fourths of the central nuclear thickness in depth. The epinuclear rim is left intact.

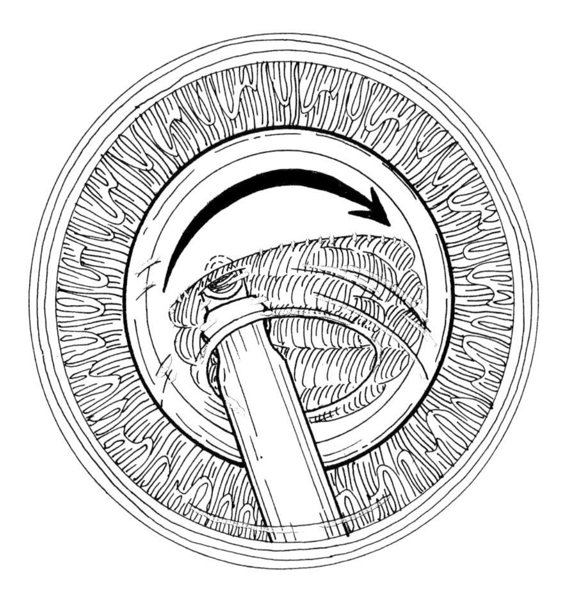

FIGURE 15-50 Phaco tip is used to rotate the nucleus 90 degrees, rendering the unsculpted portion in the easily accessible inferior position.

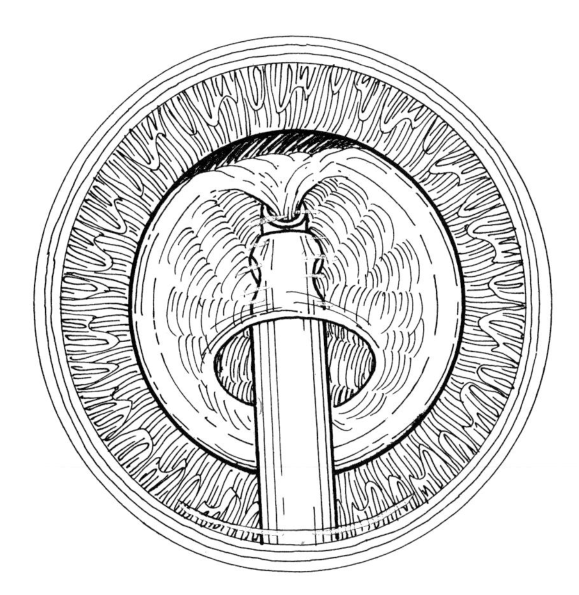

FIGURE 15-51 Following removal of the nuclear bowl, the epinuclear rim can be emulsified under low power.

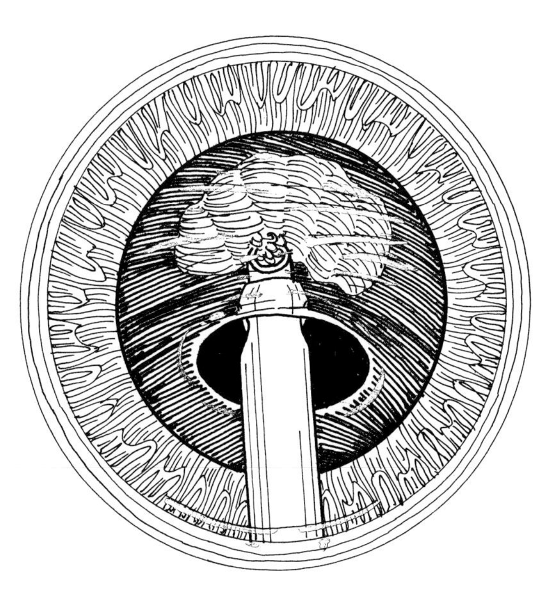

FIGURE 15-52 Residual nuclear plate is then dislocated off the posterior capsule, floated anteriorly toward the iris plane, and emulsified.

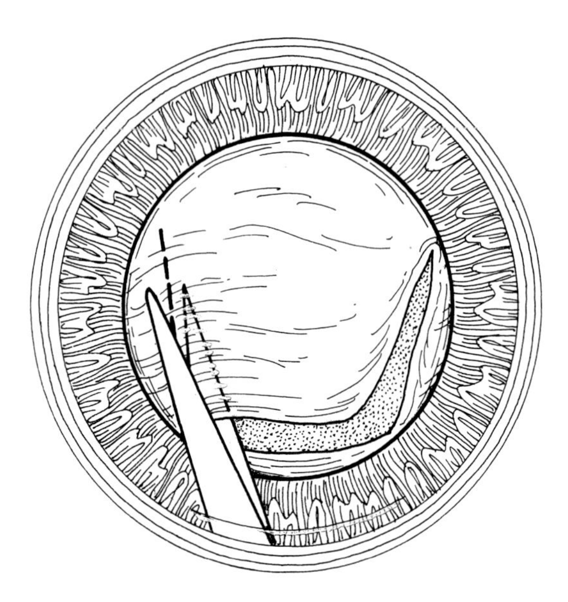

FIGURE 15-53 Following emulsification and before IOL implantation, capsule scissors are used to initiate a second-stage capsulorhexis.

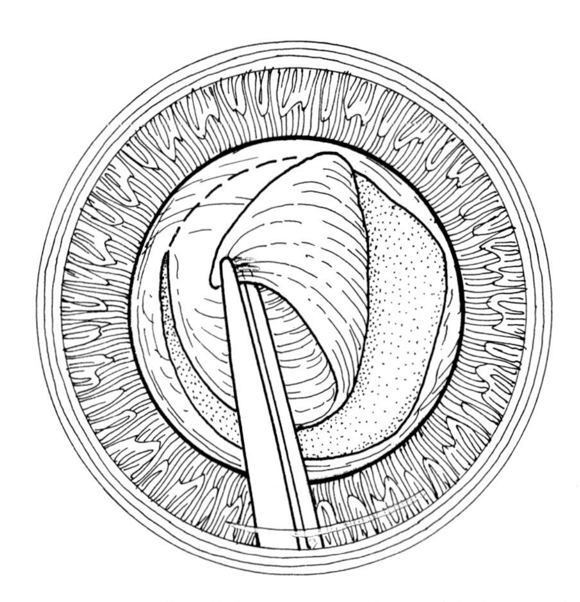

FIGURE 15-54 Capsule forceps are used to complete the second-stage capsulorhexis.

off, using forceps or a microcapsulopunch (Figure 15-56). Nishi reported that the buttonhole configuration reduces stress concentrations so that the capsulotomy does not easily tear.

Having a superiorly placed minicapsulotomy mandates a one-handed technique because the capsulotomy is not sufficiently large to introduce a second instrument. However, two-port endocapsular phacoemulsification has been proposed by Pop.[156] Under viscoelastic, a very small capsulorhexis for entrance of a spatula is created at the 2 o'clock position; a second capsulorhexis, about 3 mm in diameter, is made at about 11 o'clock for the phaco tip (Figure 15-57). The side port is created only after the initial capsulorhexis is performed to allow the incision line to be on the same plane as the port. The surgeon can then proceed with a bimanual phacoemulsification technique in up to 3+ density nuclei or more. Following phacoemulsification, the bridge between the two CCCs is incised (Figure 15-58). The IOL is implanted, a very small snip is made in the margin of the 3-mm CCC, and one large the original two is made (Figures 15-59 and 15-60). Pop reports that the procedure does not take much time and provides excellent protection to the corneal endothelium and anterior chamber. However, he concedes that the technique is not for beginners and requires excellent visualization.

In addition to the corneal protection afforded by the endocapsular phacoemulsification, many advocates of the technique report less stress on the zonules and assurance of a maintained

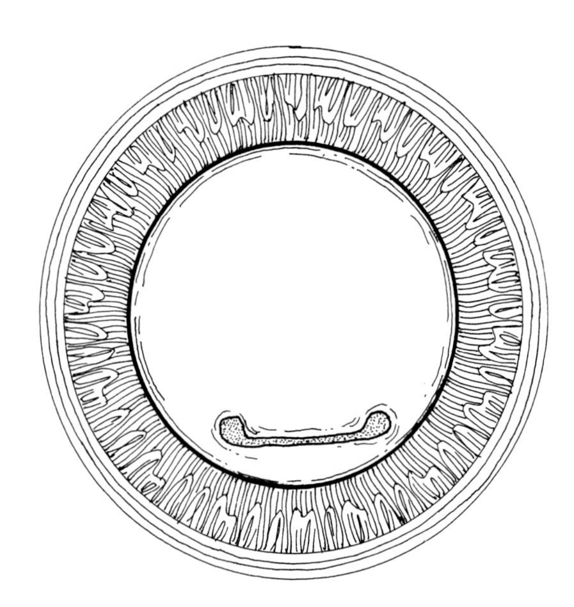

FIGURE 15-55 Nishi's buttonhole anterior capsulotomy for endocapsular phacoemulsification.

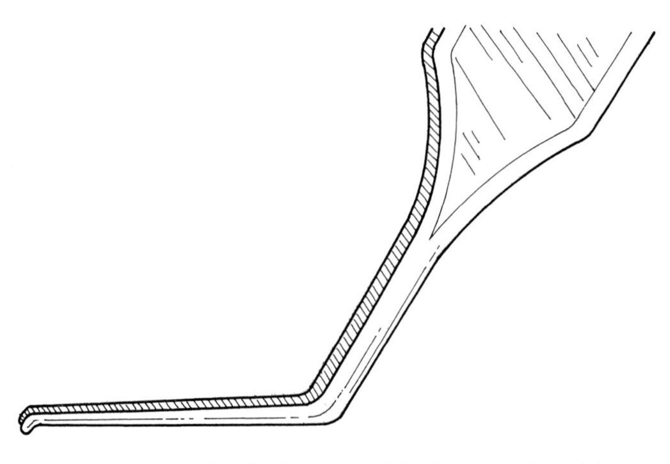

FIGURE 15-56 Angulated 60-degree Nishi-Utrata capsulorhexis forceps.

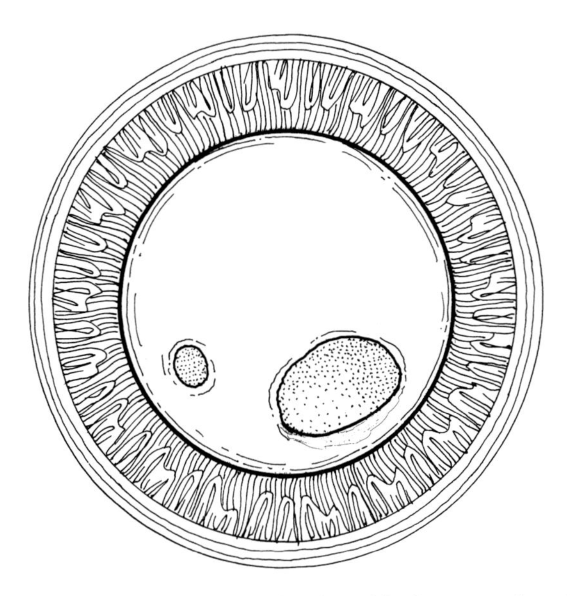

FIGURE 15-57 Respective locations of Pop's two capsule ports.

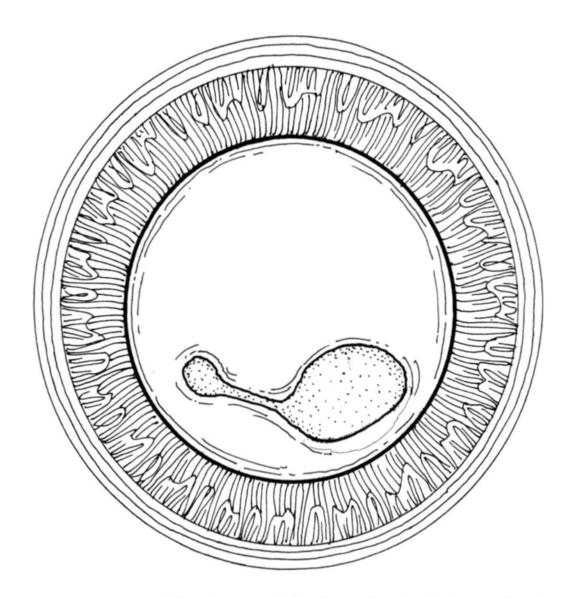

FIGURE 15-58 Following emulsification, a bridge between the two ports is created.

anterior capsule for IOL placement in the sulcus in the presence of a torn posterior capsule.[157,158] Furthermore, during anterior vitrectomy after a posterior capsule tear when prolonged infusion may occur, the anterior capsule provides a protective barrier against endothelial damage.

Certainly, the endocapsular technique provides less opportunity for fragments to come up against the corneal endothelium, but one must balance this against the increased potential for posterior capsule tears. A posterior capsule tear occurring during emulsification is more frequently associated with loss of nuclear material into the vitreous when a large part of anterior capsule is present. Anterior capsule tears may occur during manipulation of the instruments within the small CCC. Should the zonules be stretched or separated during emulsification, the zonular dehiscence may be worsened during the subsequent two-staged capsulotomy, resulting in a disinserted capsular bag.[102,104,159,160] The range of movement of the emulsification tip may be diminished or hindered by the limited nature of anterior capsule opening. This can challenge the surgeon's dexterity and create the possibility of extending an anterior capsular tear around the equator to the posterior capsule. Endolenticular phacoemulsification, with adequate experience, is a safe procedure and minimizes endothelial cell loss. In addition, any concerns regarding cell loss, for example, in patients with low endothelial cell counts preoperatively, can be alleviated to a great degree by using a more adhesive or viscous viscoelastic.

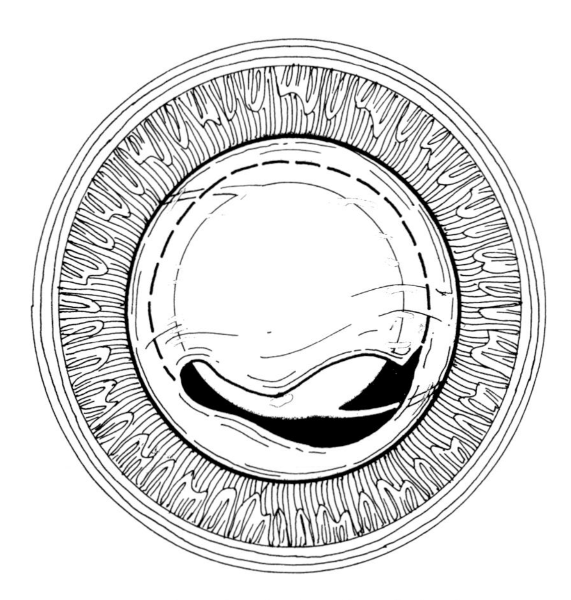

FIGURE 15-59 Following implantation of the lens, a complete capsulorhexis is performed.

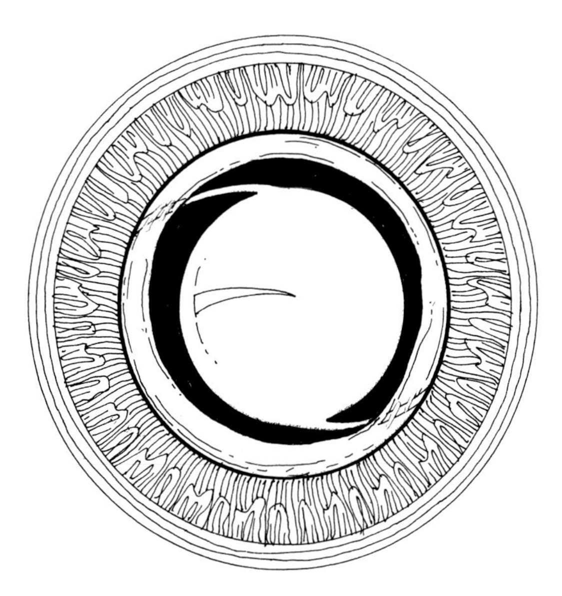

FIGURE 15-60 Appearance after completion of the capsulorhexis.

Endocapsular phacoemulsification is a technique that may provide the surgeon with an entry point into the future of ophthalmology and cataract surgery, given the research now taking place in the fields of injectable IOLs and endocapsular balloons, and in many other developing technologies.[141,142,146,161-163]

One-Handed Versus Two-Handed Phacoemulsification

Many surgeons have reported good results using a one-handed technique to perform central sculpting and removal of the nuclear rim and nuclear plate.[106,164-168] Pacifico[169] has developed a one-handed variation of my divide and conquer technique. Instead of bimanual cracking, the lens sections are cut, rotated, cut, and removed in sequence. The normal anatomic structures of the eye are used in a sense to act as a second instrument. Alternatively, sculpting can be performed with a one-handed technique, a viscoelastic can be injected, and a cracking device can be inserted and used for nucleofractis. Then emulsification is completed with the tip alone.

Typically, one-handed phacoemulsification is accomplished by sculpting a bowl and removing the bulk of the nuclear top, center, and rim (Figure 15-61). Pointing the phaco tip toward 9 o'clock and pushing counterclockwise toward 6 o'clock dislocates the nucleus to allow the equator to be aspirated into the tip (Figure 15-62). Pointing the tip toward 3 o'clock and pushing clockwise sometimes works better than using the 9 o'clock maneuver. The softer the nucleus, the harder this rotation maneuver is to accomplish; however, softer nuclei are easier to aspirate into the tip. For a hard nucleus, low power occludes the tip and emulsifies the nucleus more effectively than if power is simply increased. Once the tip is occluded, moving the tip toward 12 o'clock allows the nucleus to follow (Figure 15-63). The remaining posterior nuclear plate is sufficiently small to be freely attracted to the phaco tip for safe central emulsification in a circumferential manner in the posterior chamber (Figure 15-64). Again here, deep central sculpting to debulk the nucleus determines the ease with which the resultant nuclear plate can be removed.

One-handed techniques can be quite stressful to the lens capsule and zonules when the phaco handpiece is used as both manipulator and emulsifier. Movements against the lens capsule may be much more pronounced with one-handed techniques. In my experience, these techniques are not as efficient or safe as the bimanual methods. Nonetheless, for surgeons who feel more confident with a one-handed technique, these techniques are reasonably safe and can provide excellent results.

Machine Parameters

One commonly overlooked step in the mastery of phacoemulsification is a clear understanding of the equipment. A number of articles have been published that provide an elementary understanding of the basic dynamics of phacoemulsification energy and fluidics within the eye.[170-178] A familiarity with these principles should allow surgeons to better manage the mechanical energy and heat present.[179]

When the ultrasound tip impacts the nucleus, it mechanically slices, cuts, and emulsifies it. In addition, a physical effect known as cavitation occurs. With cavitation, a physical process creates microbubbles that implode as the sound waves expand and compress.[180] During the compression, a positive pressure is exerted on the liquid, which pushes the molecules together; during the expansion cycle, negative pressure pulls them apart. If the reaction is sufficiently intense, a cavity is formed, thus dissolving the nucleus in front of the phaco needle.

Variable surgeon control of phacoemulsification power or stroke has provided a great advantage to the cataract surgeon. Increasing the phacoemulsification power or stroke means that the to-and-fro thrust distance of each cycle of the phaco tip is

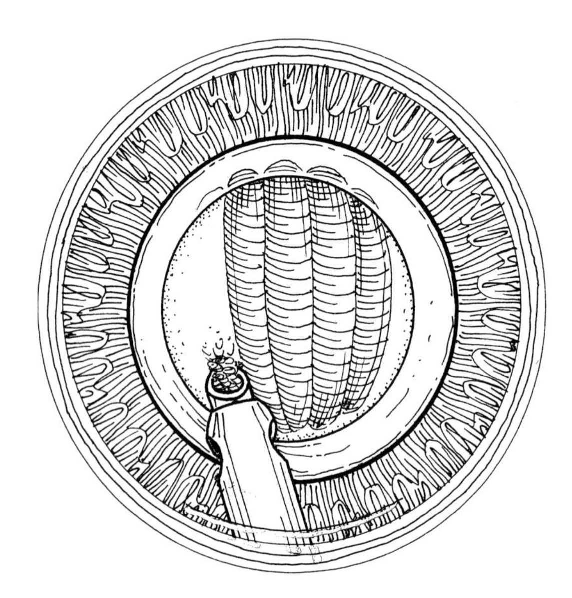

FIGURE 15-61 One-handed phacoemulsification. Very deep sculpting through the nucleus and into the soft transitional material.

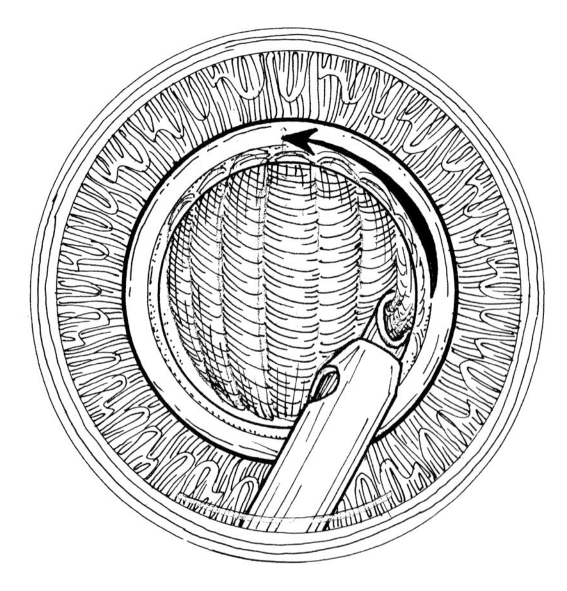

FIGURE 15-62 After maximum sculpting has been accomplished, the tip engages the nucleus at 9 o'clock and rotates that point to the 6 o'clock position.

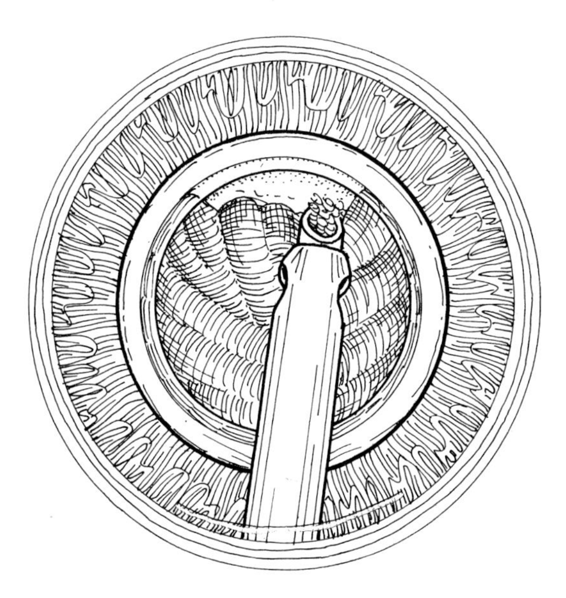

FIGURE 15-63 After a number of similar rotations, the entire nucleus has been sculpted in the 6 o'clock position.

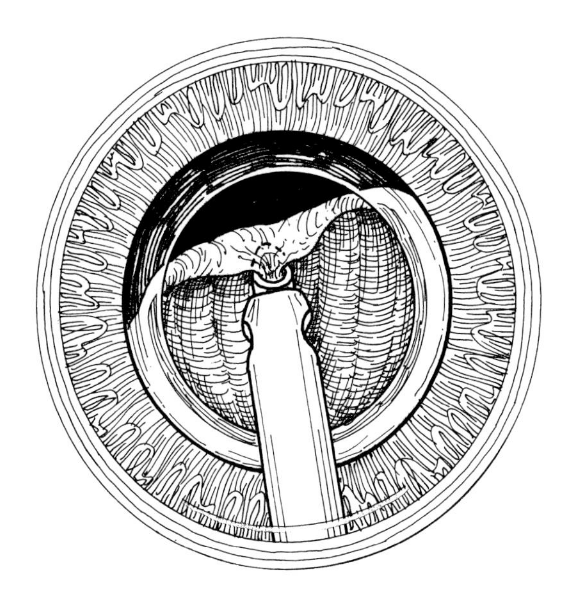

FIGURE 15-64 Phaco tip is used to engage and split the thin nuclear rim away from the capsule.

increased, whereas decreased phacoemulsification power or stroke results in a decrease in the distance that the phaco tip moves. Average phacoemulsification power is calculated by dividing cumulative delivered energy by total ultrasound time and multiplying it by 100.

Typically, four phaco cutting tip angles are available: 15, 30, 45, and 60 degrees.[181] The key to selecting a good tip angle is achieving a balance between occludability and burrowing effect, both of which are influenced by the lens type. With a standard lens that fractures quite easily and allows nuclear fragments to be emulsified as they are fractured, the 45-degree tip is probably more efficient. These sharper, more acutely angled tips are more useful in mobilizing the nucleus, cut more effectively at the same power level, and are much easier to observe when sculpting very deep in the nucleus. After cracking is complete, however, the emphasis changes to use more aspiration and less cutting. It can be difficult to completely occlude the broad 45-degree tip because of the larger elliptical area. To counter this, some surgeons change to a 30-degree tip, which more easily occludes and therefore builds vacuum on a peristaltic pump. In a dense, brunescent lens where a more delicate touch can be required to retrieve firmer epinuclear material out of the equatorial area, a smaller angle such as the 15- or 30-degree tip may be more advantageous. It is clear that one particular tip angle is not best for every surgeon on every case.

Many specialized tips have been designed. The minicobra tip is reported to allow the surgeon to emulsify cataracts with less ultrasound energy than conventional tips and can be inserted through a 2.5-mm incision.[182] Smaller port sizes are available as well, and this wider range certainly provides benefits to the surgeon.[183]

Soft nuclei can be better served by a smaller port, which assists with the sculpting portion. However, the smaller ports do not work as efficiently in very hard nuclei. Currently I use the modified 30-degree Kelman tip, which has a bend close to its distal end (Figure 15-65), which creates shear stresses on the lower edge and performs like a serrated knife. With this hook end, gripping and pulling are easily accomplished for fracturing purposes. This fingerlike effect additionally allows turning of the tip to work on either the left or right side of a central trench. In addition, the tip permits very effective and efficient down slope sculpting in the superior portion of the lens, allowing prompt access to the posterior pole for fracturing.

The cataract surgeon should choose the equipment that best responds to his or her needs and technique. For instance, two ways to move nuclear quadrants into the center of the lens exist. The first is to go to the periphery with the phaco tip, impale the nuclear quadrant, and physically tow it into the center. This technique is safest when used with low settings and a peristaltic pump. If the nucleus is not staying on the tip, a faster aspiration flow rate and higher vacuum are necessary to achieve more grabbing and holding power. Alternatively, Venturi or diaphragm pumps can increase the pulling power by increasing immediate vacuum levels and therefore the strength of fluid flow toward the phaco tip. An analogy has been made to a mountain stream. If the stream flows at a leisurely pace, it is unable to carry with it anything but the smallest pieces. However, if the stream is moving rapidly, the increased flow can carry larger objects.

For the past several years, I have used phaco machines with a peristaltic pump system that allows aspiration flow rates to be preset, that is, the rate in milliliters per minute at which the ultrasound needle aspirates fluid and lens material. The faster the flow, the more rapid the vacuum buildup is once the tip is occluded. I prefer this ability to adjust the rise time of vacuum

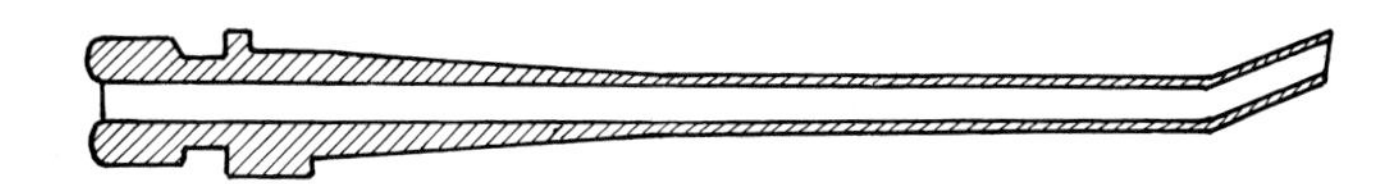

FIGURE 15-65 Cross-sectional schematic of the modified Kelman phaco tip.

buildup, as this dictates the safety margin or how fast materials come to the port. This can be invaluable in challenging cases such as those involving small pupils or in the presence of a loose capsule. The establishment of a different aspiration flow rate in foot positions 2 and 3 allows me to engage material with a safer vacuum level at foot position 2 and then change to position 3 for emulsification. This change of position can be monitored by the audio feedback that results from altering pump speeds.

In early 1993 I acquired an updated peristaltic pump unit that has improved efficiency of the system to be comparable with a Venturi/diaphragm pump while preserving the safety of the peristaltic pump system. This is a result of a number of upgrades, including the addition of more rollers in the pump and the incorporation of more direct channels rather than tubing to reduce compliance. A listing of my memory settings for the Legacy 20,000 is found in Table 15-1. Memory 1 is used for safety in cases with soft lenses, small pupils, or loose zonules. Memory 3 is used for maximum efficiency when fracturing is complete and segments are being emulsified in a deep chamber.

Several good articles are available in the literature surveying the available machines, and a number of ophthalmic newspapers usually run an annual feature highlighting the latest innovations in the phacoemulsification machine marketplace.[184-191] Because most units have their own unique advantages and disadvantages, manufacturers have been attempting to marry the best features of each system. By testing each type of pumps, the surgeon can determine which one best suits his or her technique and needs. It may be that in the future the surgeon will be able to switch between peristaltic and Venturi systems within the same unit. With this in mind, the consumer should consider the manufacturer's policy on future upgrades before purchase.

The Learning Curve

A small minority of cataract surgeons remain who do not perform phacoemulsification on a regular basis. Some experienced extracapsular cataract surgeons may delay converting to the phacoemulsification technique because of a perceived formidable "learning curve."[192,193] However, both prospective and retrospective studies of surgeons converting from extracapsular cataract extraction (ECCE) to phacoemulsification have demonstrated excellent results with no significant increase in the complication rate.[194,195] Pederson,[196] in a study of his first 125 unselected cases of phacoemulsification, found no significant increase in complication rates and attained a visual acuity of 20/40 or better in 98.4% of the patients.

Ophthalmology training programs are now routinely teaching phacoemulsification to residents under immediate supervision with excellent results. A number of papers have established that residents can learn to perform phacoemulsification safely with acceptable results when appropriately trained and supervised, and a good method for this type of teaching has been suggested by many authors.[197-201] A number of surgical training systems have been developed to assist with the learning process.[202,203] The particular technique being taught may be an important factor to consider as well. In two concurrent studies teaching phacoemulsification to residents, Allinson, Metrikin, and Fante[204] initially reported a 14.7% vitreous loss compared with previous studies that cited a 2.4% to 9% loss using ECCE.[205-207] In the follow-up study, in which a nuclear fracturing technique was taught, the complication rate dropped to 1.6%.[208]

In my opinion, phacoemulsification to this point has not been performed 95% or more of the time by 100% of the surgeons because of the risks related to capsule tears. If the

TABLE 15-1
Howard V. Gimbel's Personal Settings for Alcon Series 20,000 Legacy

	Phaco Memory Settings				BiModal Memory Settings			
Function	**Memory 1**	**Memory 2**	**Memory 3**	**Memory 4**	**Memory 1**	**Memory 2**	**Memory 3**	**Memory 4**
Power (%)	60	50	60	50	60	6	60	50
Aspiration (ml/min)								
FP 2	15	Up to 32	20	20	Up to 29	Up to 30	Up to 29	Up to 29
FP 3	15	35	20	20	30	34	30	30
Vacuum (mm Hg)	100	100	100	100	300	320	400	400
IV pole (cm)	55	55	95	100	100	100	100	100
I/A maximum-vacuum (mm Hg)	500+	500+	500+	500+	500+	500+	500+	500+
Aspiration rate (ml/min)	30	60	60	30	30	30	30	30
IV pole (cm)	80	80	80	55	100	65	65	45
I/A minimum-vacuum (mm Hg)	38	38	38	38	38	38	38	38
Aspiration rate (ml/min)	7	7	7	7	7	7	7	7
IV pole (cm)	65	65	65	45	45	45	45	45
I/A capsule/vacuum (mm Hg)	5	5	5	5	5	5	5	5
Aspiration rate (ml/min)	5	5	5	5	5	5	5	5
IV pole (cm)	42	42	42	45	45	42	42	45

FP, Foot position; *I/A*, irrigation/aspiration; *IV*, intravenous.

nucleus is pushed down at 6 o'clock, a tear can extend around to the posterior capsule and open it right up. This can also happen if sculpting is attempted too close to the equator at 6 o'clock. My suggestion is for those in transition or learning phacoemulsification in residency to start with a CCC and, if necessary, to make a relaxing incision for extracapsular conversion. Even if a tipping technique is going to be employed, the inferior capsule rim should be a continuous tear. In addition, it is important to remember that too small a CCC can make phacoemulsification quite difficult. Hence, attaining the properly sized and accomplished CCC is critical in learning phacoemulsification.

A familiarity with instrumentation can be achieved by initially practicing sculpting only and then converting to an extracapsular technique. Learning to work at higher magnification should also be a priority, as the increased stereopsis will assist in judging the depth of sculpting. It has helped me to have an assistant centering the microscope, allowing more attention to be paid to the microscope focus and zoom.

Although experience is the greatest teacher, continuing education through videotapes, journal articles, meetings, and textbooks such as this one can significantly contribute to this ongoing learning process. With thorough planning and attention to detail, proper patient selection, and adequate instruction, it is certainly possible to master phacoemulsification without compromising patients' welfare.

Physical and Mental Preparedness

Both the experienced and nonexperienced among us can form habits that will maximize our surgical abilities before we ever enter the operating room. The physical preparedness of the surgeon is comparable to that of the athlete. The literature on the benefits of a healthy personal lifestyle is voluminous, so this section is intended only as a brief overview.

In the area of nutrition, a number of studies indicate that eating too much food or high-fat foods can produce sluggish thinking.[209] The practice of eating balanced meals and having regular eating habits is seen as important to keep the level of glucose at a consistent, optimal level for critical thinking. Proper hydration is a must for peak performance. Pitts, at the Harvard University School of Health has established that an athlete's stamina is directly proportional to his or her level of hydration.[210] Aside from the general health benefits, temperance or abstinence from stimulants or depressants is extremely important. It has been demonstrated that nicotine interferes with muscle coordination and control, at least partly because of its ability to upset the acetylcholine balance in the nerve junctions. It has also been reported that caffeine causes a worsening of fine motor coordination because of increases in hand and arm tremors.[211] When I took my first course with Kelman, he advised us that if we wanted to do this surgery with an instrument vibrating at 40,000 cycles per second, we should not drink coffee and should not have alcohol for 24 to 48 hours beforehand. This advice confirmed my convictions on that subject.

Horne[212] has suggested that the loss of a night's sleep undermines creative thinking and the ability to deal with unfamiliar situations. We can all appreciate that a stable personal and professional life allows one optimal concentration, happiness, and positive outlook. The importance of regular exercise is attested to by the research of Rauhala[213] and colleagues in Finland. A lack of exercise allows some persistence of muscle activity at rest. The authors have established that regular exercise helps a person to relax muscles more completely, which seemingly would result in a steadier hand and, indeed, a steadier body. A study by Nieman[214] has established that exercise increases the size of mitochondria up to 40% and the number up to 120%, which gives one the capacity to produce much more energy. In addition, Neiman[215] reports that decreased anxiety and improved short-term cognition, as well as decreased depression and even an elevation of mood, are benefits of exercise. A final benefit that people often mention as a result of regular exercise is an increased feeling of self-confidence.

A healthy professional environment is also beneficial. By ensuring that one has proper equipment, systems, and staff with a cooperative "team" spirit, maximum attention can be allotted to surgery itself.

Conclusions

Avoiding "Formula" Phacoemulsification

In closing, the field of cataract surgery, like many others, is participating in an ongoing technological revolution. Keeping abreast of the rapid advances in our field is a challenge in and of itself. With every new technique, instrument, or application of technology, we are forced to modify our approach and adjust to changes in our routine. Perhaps more than ever before, we must develop problem-solving skills, as opposed to memorizing an established body of knowledge.

This chapter provides a summary of what has been accomplished in the past 30 years, a look at where we are today, and, perhaps, a preview of where we may be heading in the future. Certainly, each case should be approached with a strategy in mind, but an ability to adjust, interpret, modify, and improvise should be close at hand. It is my sincere hope that this text has assisted in stimulating this type of thinking and in nurturing these abilities.

REFERENCES

1. Heslin KB, Guerriero PN: Clinical retrospective study comparing planned extracapsular cataract extraction and phacoemulsification with and without lens implantation, *Ann Ophthalmol* 16:956-962, 1984.
2. Watson A, Sunderraj P: Comparison of small incision phacoemulsification with standard extracapsular cataract surgery: post-operative astigmatism and visual recovery, *Eye* 6:626-629, 1992.
3. Kraff MC, Sanders DR: Planned extracapsular extraction versus phacoemulsification with IOL implantation: a comparison of concurrent series, *J Am Intraocul Implant Soc* 8:38-41, 1982.
4. Neumann AC, McCarty GR, Sanders DR et al: Small incisions to control astigmatism during cataract surgery, *J Cataract Refract Surg* 15:78-84, 1989.
5. Polack FM, Sugar A: The phacoemulsification procedure II: corneal endothelial changes, *Invest Ophthalmol* 15:458-469, 1976.
6. Arentsen JJ, Rodriques MM, Laibson PR: Corneal opacification occurring after phacoemulsification and phacofragmentation, *Am J Ophthalmol* 83:794-804, 1977.
7. Binder PS, Sternberg H, Wickham MG et al: Corneal endothelial damage associated with phacoemulsification, *Am J Ophthalmol* 82:48-54, 1976.
8. Polack FM, Sugar A: The phacoemulsification procedure III: corneal complications, *Invest Ophthalmol* 16:39-46, 1977.

9. Sugar J, Mitchelson J, Kraff M: The effect of corneal endothelial cell density, *Arch Ophthalmol* 96:446-448, 1978.
10. Waltman SR, Cozean CH: The effect of phacoemulsification on the corneal endothelium, *Ophthalmic Surg* 10:31-33, 1979.
11. Abbott RL, Forster RK: Clinical specular microscopy and intraocular surgery, *Arch Ophthalmol* 97:1476-1479, 1979.
12. Yang HK, Kline OR Jr: Specular microscopy with intraocular implantations, *J Am Intraocul Implant Soc* 7:31-35, 1981.
13. Irvin AR, Kratz RP, O'Donnell JJ: Endothelial damage with phacoemulsification and intraocular lens implantation, *Arch Ophthalmol* 96:1023-1026, 1978.
14. Kraff MC, Sanders DR, Lieberman HL: Specular microscopy in cataract and intraocular lens patients, *Arch Ophthalmol* 98:1782-1784, 1980.
15. Colvard DM, Kratz RP, Mazzoco TR et al: Endothelial cell loss following phacoemulsification in the pupillary plane, *J Am Intraocul Implant Soc* 7:334-336, 1981.
16. Graether JM, Harris GW, Davison JA et al: A comparison of the effects of phacoemulsification and nucleus expression on endothelial cell density, *J Am Intraocul Implant Soc* 9:420-423, 1983.
17. Gwin RM, Warrant JK, Samuelson DA et al: Effects of phacoemulsification and extracapsular lens removal on corneal thickness and endothelial cell density in the dog, *Invest Ophthalmol Vis Sci* 24:227-236, 1983.
18. Davison JA: Endothelial cell loss during the transition from nucleus expression to posterior chamber: iris plane phacoemulsification, *J Am Intraocul Implant Soc* 10:10-13, 1984.
19. Hoffer KJ: Effects of extracapsular implant techniques on endothelial density, *Arch Ophthalmol* 100:791-792, 1982.
20. Holmberg AS, Philipson BT: Sodium hyaluronate in cataract surgery II: report on the use of Healon in extracapsular cataract surgery using phacoemulsification, *Ophthalmology* 91:53-57, 1984.
21. Bourne WM, Liesegang TJ, Waller RR et al: The effect of phacoemulsification on corneal endothelial cell density, *Am J Ophthalmol* 98:759-762, 1984.
22. Bleckman H, Vogt R: Experimental endothelial lesions by means of an ultrasound phacoemulsifier, *Graefes Arch Clin Exp Ophthalmol* 224:457-462, 1986.
23. Glasser DB, Katz HR, Boyd JE: Protective effects of viscous solutions in phacoemulsification and traumatic lens implantation, *Arch Ophthalmol* 107:1047-1051, 1989.
24. Craig MT, Olson RJ, Mamalis N et al: Air bubble endothelial damage during phacoemulsification in human eye bank eyes: the protective effects of Healon and Viscoat, *J Cataract Refract Surg* 16:597-601, 1990.
25. Glasser DB, Osborn DC, Nordeen JF et al: Endothelial protection and viscoelastic retention during phacoemulsification and intraocular lens implantation, *Arch Ophthalmol* 109:1438-1440, 1991.
26. Lane SS, Naylor DW, Kullerstarnd LJ et al: Prospective comparison of the effects of Occucoat, Viscoat, and Healon on intraocular pressure and endothelial cell loss, *J Cataract Refract Surg* 17:21-26, 1991.
27. Sheets JH: A step beyond ECCE, *CLAO J* 13:67-70, 1987.
28. Leaming DV: Practice styles and preferences of ASCRS members: 1992 survey, *J Cataract Refract Surg* 19:600-606, 1993.
29. Hattenhauer JM: To "phaco" or not? *Arch Ophthalmol* 109:315, 1991 (letter).
30. Prince RB, Tax RL, Miller DH: Conversion to small-incision phacoemulsification: experience with the first 50 eyes, *J Cataract Refract Surg* 19:246-250, 1993.
31. Landers JAG: Phacoemulsification in cataract surgery, *Med J Aust* 153:742, 1990 (letter).
32. Hodgkins PR, Luff AJ, Morrell AJ et al: Current practice of cataract extraction and anaesthesia, *Br J Ophthalmol* 76:323-326, 1992.
33. Miyajima H: Phacoemulsification surges forward in Japan, *Ocular Surg News* 10:38-39, 1992.
34. Oshika T, Amano S, Araie M et al: Current trends in cataract and refractive surgery in Japan: 1998 survey, *Jpn J Ophthalmol* 44:268-276, 2000.
35. Dada VK, Sindhu N: Management of cataract: a revolutionary change that occurred during last two decades, *J Indian Med Assoc* 97:313-317, 1999 (review).
36. Lee SY, Tan D: Changing trends in cataract surgery in Singapore, *Singapore Med J* 40:256-259, 1999.
37. Weiser M: Et voila! Phaco in France on the rise, *Ocular Surg News* 10:54, 1992.
38. Krootila K: Practice styles and preferences of Finish cataract surgeons: 1998 survey, *Acta Ophthalmol Scand* 77:544-547, 1999.
39. Masek P: Cataract surgery in the Czech Republic 1988-1997, *Cesk Slov Oftalmol* 55:117-122, 1999.
40. Ehrich C, Pham DT, Haberle H et al: Cataract surgery of the Berlin Virchow clinic: overview of the last 16 years, *Ophthalmologe* 95:427-431, 1998.
41. Gimbel HV, Neuhann T: Development, advantages and methods of the continuous circular capsulorhexis technique, *J Cataract Refract Surg* 16:31-37, 1990.
42. Neuhann T: Theorie und operationstechnik der kapsulorhexis, *Klin Monatsbl Augenheilkd* 190:542-545, 1987.
43. Gimbel HV, Neuhann T: Continuous curvilinear capsulorrhexis, *J Cataract Refract Surg* 17:110, 1991 (letter).
44. Apple DJ et al: Posterior chamber intraocular lens implantation in a series of 75 autopsy eyes. Parts I-III, *J Cataract Refract Surg* 12:358-371, 1986.
45. Kelman CD: Phacoemulsification and aspiration—a new technique of cataract removal: a preliminary report, *Am J Ophthalmol* 1967;64:23-35, 1967.
46. Kelman CD: Phacoemulsification and aspiration: a progress report, *Am J Ophthalmol* 67:464, 1969.
47. Kelman CD: Cataract emulsification and aspiration, *Trans Ophthalmol Soc UK* 90:13, 1970.
48. Kelman CD: Personal interview on phacoemulsification, *Highlights Ophthalmol* 13:40-61, 1970-1971.
49. Kelman CD: Summary of personal experience, *Trans Am Acad Ophthalmol Otolaryngol* 78:35-38, 1974.
50. Kelman CD: *Phacoemulsification and aspiration: the Kelman technique of cataract removal*, Birmingham, 1975, Aesculapius Publishing Co.
51. Kelman CD: Phacoemulsification and aspiration: a report of 500 consecutive cases, *Am J Ophthalmol* 75:764-768, 1973.
52. Kelman CD: Phacoemulsification and aspiration of senile cataracts: a comparative study with intracapsular extraction, *Can J Ophthalmol* 8:24, 1973.
53. Shock JP: Phacofragmentation and irrigation of cataracts: a preliminary report, *Am J Ophthalmol* 74:187, 1972.
54. Paton D: Phacoemulsification: trials and tribulations, *Invest Ophthalmol* 12:318, 1973.
55. Hiles DA, Hurite FG: Results of the first year's experience with phacoemulsification, *Am J Ophthalmol* 75:473-477, 1973.
56. Hurite FG, Kennerdel JS: Experiences with phacoemulsification, *Trans Pa Acad Ophthalmol Otolaryngol* 26:126-130, 1973.
57. Kratz RP: Difficulties, complications, and management. Symposium on phacoemulsification, *Trans Am Acad Ophthalmol Otolaryngol* 78:18, 1974.
58. Shock JP: Alternative techniques: phacofragmentation, phacocryolysis and irrigation of cataracts, *Trans Am Acad Ophthalmol Otolaryngol* 78:22, 1974.
59. Troutman RC: Preliminary report of the committee on phacoemulsification, *Trans Am Acad Ophthalmol Otolaryngol* 75:41-42, 1974.
60. Hurite FG: The contraindications to phacoemulsification and summary of personal experience, *Trans Am Acad Ophthalmol Otolaryngol* 78:14-17, 1974.
61. Emery JM, Paton D: Phacoemulsification: a survey of 2875 cases, *Trans Am Acad Ophthalmol Otolaryngol* 78:OP31-34, 1974.
62. Cleasaby GW, Fung WE, Wesbster RG: The lens fragmentation and aspiration procedure (phacoemulsification), *Am J Ophthalmol* 77:384-387, 1974.
63. Cleasby GW: The advantages and disadvantages of Kelman phacoemulsification (KPE), *Ophthalmology* 81:1973-1974, 1974.
64. Benolken RM, Emergy JM, Landis DJ: Temperature profiles in the anterior chamber during phacoemulsification, *Invest Ophthalmol* 13:71-74, 1974.
65. Dayton GO, Hulquist CR: Complications of phacoemulsification, *Can J Ophthalmol* 10:61-68, 1975.
66. Troutman RC, Clahane AC, Emery JM et al: Cataract survey of the cataract-phacoemulsification committee, *Trans Am Acad Ophthalmol Otolaryngol* 79:178-185, 1975.
67. Kline OR: Phacoemulsification visual results and complications: report of 800 cases, *Ophthalmic Surg* 8:94-97, 1976.
68. Fung WE: Phacoemulsification, *Ophthalmology* 85:46-51, 1978.
69. Emery JM: Phacoemulsification: cataract surgery of the future, *Int Ophthalmol Clin* 18:155-170, 1978.
70. Emery JM, Wilhelmus KA, Rosenburg S: Complications of phacoemulsification, *Ophthalmology* 85:141-150, 1978.
71. Kratz RP: Intracapsular versus extracapsular cataract extraction for intra ocular lens implantation, *Int Ophthalmol Clin* 19:179-194, 1979.
72. Ewing C: Phacoemulsification, *Can J Ophthalmol* 14:1-2, 1979.
73. Kraff MC, Sanders DR, Lieberman HL: Total cataract extraction through a 3 mm incision: a report of 650 cases, *Ophthalmic Surg* 10:46-54, 1979.
74. Emery JM, Little JH: *Phacoemulsification and aspiration of cataracts: surgical techniques, complications, and results,* St Louis, 1979, Mosby.
75. Knolle GE, Justice J, Spears WD: Discussion of presentation by Dr. Gilbert W. Cleasby, *Ophthalmology* 86:1975-1979.

76. Sinskey RM, Cain W: The posterior capsule and phacoemulsification, *J Am Intraocul Implant Soc* 4:206-207, 1978.
77. Little JH: *Outline of phacoemulsification for the ophthalmic surgeon,* ed 2, Oklahoma City, 1975, Samco Color Press.
78. Kratz RP: Teaching phacoemulsification in California and 200 cases of phacoemulsification. In Emery JM, Paton D, editors: *Current concepts in cataract surgery: selected proceedings of the Fourth Biennial Cataract Surgical Congress,* St Louis, 1976, Mosby, pp 196-200.
79. Kratz RP, Colvard DM: Kelman phacoemulsification in the posterior chamber, *Ophthalmology* 86:1983-1984, 1979.
80. Kratz RP, Mazzocco TR, Davidson B et al: The Shearing intraocular lens: a report of 1,000 cases, *J Am Intraocul Implant Soc* 7:55-57, 1981.
81. Maloney WF, Grindle L: *Textbook of phacoemulsification,* Fallbrook, Calif, 1990, Lasenda Publishers.
82. Gimbel HV: *Divide and conquer.* Presented at the European Intraocular Implantlens Council meeting, 1987 (video).
83. Gimbel HV: Divide and conquer nucleofractis phacoemulsification: development and variations, *J Cataract Refract Surg* 17:281-291, 1991.
84. Worgul BV: Lens. In Duane TD, Jaeger EA, editors: *Biomedical foundations of ophthalmology,* Philadelphia, 1983, Harper and Row.
85. Marshall J, Beaconsfield M, Rothery S: The anatomy and development of the human lens and zonules, *Trans Ophthalmol Soc UK* 102:423-440, 1982.
86. Drews RC: The lens capsule: a lens implant surgeon's understanding. The Mary Louise Prentice Lecture, *Trans Ophthalmol Soc UK* 105:265-272, 1986.
87. Worst J: A morphological description of human cataractous lenses by SEM, *Doc Ophthalmol* 67:197-207, 1987.
88. Worst J: Some aspects of cataract morphology: a SEM study, *Doc Ophthalmol* 70:155-163, 1988.
89. Duke-Elder S: Anatomy of the visual system. In *System of ophthalmology,* vol II, St Louis, 1961, Mosby, pp 320-323
90. Bron A, Smith G, Smith R et al: Changes in light scatter and width measurements from the human lens cortex with age, *Eye* 6:55-59, 1992.
91. Drews RC: YAG laser demonstration of the anatomy of the lens nucleus, *Ophthalmic Surg* 23:811-824, 1992.
92. Drews RC: Phacoemulsification without ultrasound, *Eur J Implant Refract Surg* 5:80-81, 1993.
93. Pisacano AM, Levy JH, Anello RD: New spatula to facilitate bimanual phacoemulsification, *J Cataract Refract Surg* 16:259-261, 1990.
94. Levy JH, Pisacano AM, Anello RD: A new endocapsular nucleus controller to facilitate nuclear splitting during bimanual endocapsular phacoemulsification, *Eur J Implant Refract Surg* 4:121-122, 1992.
95. Brauweiler P: Bimanual irrigation/aspiration, *J Cataract Refract Surg* 22:1013-1016, 1996.
96. Seibel BS: *Phacodynamics: mastering the tools and techniques of phacoemulsification,* Thorofare, NJ, 1993, Slack.
97. Fine IH, Maloney WF, Dillman DM: Crack and flip phacoemulsification technique, *J Cataract Refract Surg* 19:797-802, 1993.
98. Patel J, Apple D: Protective effect of the anterior lens capsule during extracapsular cataract extraction, *Ophthalmology* 96:598-602, 1989.
99. Krag S, Thim K, Corydon L: The stretching capacity of capsulorhexis: an experimental study on animal cadaver eyes, *Eur J Implant Refract Surg* 2:43-45, 1990.
100. Thim K, Krag S, Corydon L: Stretching capacity of capsulorhexis and nucleus delivery, *J Cataract Refract Surg* 17:31, 1991.
101. Ohrloff C, Oldendorp J, Puck A: Minimal endothelial cell loss following phacoemulsification and posterior chamber lens implantation, *Klin Monatsble Augentreilkd* 186:302-306, 1985.
102. Gimbel HV: Continuous curvilinear capsulorhexis and nucleus fracturing: evolution, technique and complications, *Ophthalmol Clin North Am* 4:235-249, 1991.
103. Gimbel HV: Trough and crater divide and conquer nucleofractis techniques, *Eur J Implant Refract Surg* 3:123-126, 1991.
104. Gimbel HV: Evolving techniques of cataract surgery: continuous curvilinear capsulorhexis, down-slope sculpting and nucleofractis, *Semin Ophthalmol* 7:193-207, 1992.
105. Gimbel HV: Down-slope sculpting, *J Cataract Refract Surg* 18:614-618, 1992.
106. Sinskey RM, Patel JV: *Manual of cataract surgery,* New York, 1987, Churchill Livingstone.
107. Gimbel HV: *Hydro-free dissection.* Presented at the ASCRS film festival, San Diego, 1992 (video).
108. Gimbel HV: Hydro dissection/hydrodelineation, *Int Ophthalmol Clin* 34:73-90, 1994.
109. Fine IH: The chip and flip phacoemulsification technique, *J Cataract Refract Surg* 17:366-371, 1991.
110. Fine IH: Two-handed phacoemulsification through a small circular capsulorhexis. In Koch P, Davison J, editors: *Phacoemulsification techniques,* Thorofare, NJ, 1991, Slack, Inc, pp 191-205.
111. Fine IH: The chip and flip phacoemulsification technique. In Yalon M, editor: *Techniques of phacoemulsification surgery and IOL implantation,* Thorofare, NJ, 1992, Slack, Inc, pp 3-23.
112. Koch PS: *Converting to phacoemulsification: a manual for the surgeon in transition,* Thorofare, NJ, 1988, Slack, Inc.
113. Koch PS: Spring surgery. In Koch P, Davison J, editors: *Phacoemulsification techniques,* Thorofare, NJ, 1991, Slack, Inc, pp 207-238.
114. Koch PS: A strategic approach to phacoemulsification based on nuclear density, *Semin Ophthalmol* 7:234-244, 1992.
115. Raitta C, Setala K: Intraocular lens implantation in exfoliation syndrome and capsular glaucoma, *Acta Ophthalmol (Copenh)* 64:130-133, 1986.
116. Guzek JP, Holm M, Cameron JA et al: Risk factors for intraoperative complications in 1000 extracapsular cataract cases, *Ophthalmology* 97:461-466, 1987.
117. Skuta G, Parrish RK, Hodapp E et al: Zonular dialysis during extracapsular cataract extraction in pseudoexfoliation syndrome, *Arch Ophthalmol* 105:532-534, 1987.
118. Dark A: Cataract extraction complicated by capsular glaucoma, *Br J Ophthalmol* 63:465-468, 1979.
119. Ghosh M, Speakman J: The ciliary body in senile exfoliation of the lens, *Can J Ophthalmol* 8:394-403, 1973.
120. Tarkkanen AHA: Exfoliation syndrome, *Trans Ophthalmol Soc UK* 105:233-236, 1986.
121. Osher RH, Cionni RJ, Gimbel HV et al: Cataract surgery in patients with pseudoexfoliation syndrome, *Eur J Implant Refract Surg* 5:46-50, 1993.
122. Shepherd JR: In situ fracture, *J Cataract Refract Surg* 16:436-440, 1990.
123. Shepherd JR: Shepherd phaco fracture. In Devine TM, Banko W, editors: *Phacoemulsification surgery,* 1991, Pergamon Press Canada Ltd, pp 67-72.
124. Davison JA: Minimal lift: multiple rotation technique for capsular bag phacoemulsification and intraocular lens fixation, *J Cataract Refract Surg* 14:25-34, 1988.
125. Davison JA: No-lift capsular bag phacoemulsification and dialing technique for no-hole intraocular lens optics, *J Cataract Refract Surg* 14:346-349, 1988 (letter).
126. Davison JA: Bimodal capsular bag phacoemulsification: a serial cutting and suction ultrasonic nuclear dissection technique, *J Cataract Refract Surg* 15:272-282, 1989.
127. Davison JA: Hybrid nuclear dissection technique for capsular bag phacoemulsification, *J Cataract Refract Surg* 16:441-450, 1990.
128. Johnson SH: Split and lift: nuclear quadrant management for phacoemulsification, *J Cataract Refract Surg* 19:420-424, 1993.
129. Fine IH, Packer M, Hoffman RS: Use of power modulations in phacoemulsification: choo-choo chop and flip phacoemulsification, *J Cataract Refract Surg* 27:188-197, 2001.
130. Fine IH: The choo-choo chop and flip phacoemulsification technique, *Operative Tech Cataract Refract Surg* 1:61-65, 1998.
131. Faust KJ: Hydrodissection of soft nuclei, *J Am Intraocul Implant Soc* 10: 75-77, 1984.
132. Krasnov MM, Makarov IA, Said Naim Iussef: Densitometric analysis of crystalline lens nucleus in the choice of strategy of surgical treatment of cataracts, *Vestn Oftalmol* 116:6-8, 2000.
133. Walkow T, Anders N, Klebe S: Endothelial cell loss after phacoemulsification: relation to preoperative and intraoperative parameters, *J Cataract Refract Surg* 26:727-732, 2000.
134. Corydon L, Krag S, Thim K: One-handed phacoemulsification with low settings, *J Cataract refract Surg* 23:1143-1148, 1997.
135. Maloney WF: Tutorial in phacoemulsification, *Eur J Implant Refract Surg* 2:125-133, 1990.
136. Maloney WF, Dillman D: Fractional 2:4 phaco. In Koch P, Davison J, editors: *Phacoemulsification techniques,* Thorofare, NJ, 1991, Slack, Inc, pp 241-255.
137. Maloney WF Dillman D: A comprehensive approach to phacoemulsification from beginning to advanced techniques, *Ophthalmol Clin North Am* 4:221-234, 1991.
138. Sakka Y: Phacoemulsification without anterior capsulectomy, *Folia Ophthalmol Jpn* 33:233-235, 1982.
139. Hara T, Hara T: Subcapsular phacoemulsification and aspiration, *J Am Intraocul Implant Soc* 10:333-337, 1984.
140. Gindi JJ, Wan WL, Schanzlin DJ: Endocapsular cataract surgery. I. Surgical technique, *Cataract* 2:6-10, 1985.
141. Hara T, Hara T: Recent advance in intracapsular phacoemulsification and complete in-the-bag intraocular lens implantation, *J Am Intraocul Implant Soc* 11:488-490, 1985.

142. Parel JM, Gelender H, Trafers WF et al: Phacoersatz: cataract surgery designed to preserve accommodation, *Graefes Arch Clin Exp Ophthalmol* 224:165-173, 1986.
143. Hara T, Hara T: Fate of the capsular bag in endocapsular phacoemulsification and complete in-the-bag intraocular lens fixation, *J Cataract Refract Surg* 12:408-412, 1986.
144. Hara T, Hara T: Clinical results of endocapsular phacoemulsification and complete in-the bag intraocular lens fixation, *J Cataract Refract Surg* 13:279-286, 1987.
145. Hara T, Hara T: Endocapsular phacoemulsification and aspiration (ECPEA): recent surgical technique and clinical results, *Ophthalmic Surg* 20:469-475, 1987.
146. Haeflinger E, Parel JM, Fantes F et al: Accommodation of an endocapsular silicone lens (phaco-ersatz) in the nonhuman primate, *Ophthalmology* 94:471-477, 1987.
147. Hara T, Hara T: Roundel phacoemulsification technique for in-the-bag intraocular lens fixation, *J Cataract Refract Surg* 13:441-446, 1987.
148. Hara T, Azuma N, Chiba K et al: Anterior capsular opacification after endocapsular cataract surgery, *Ophthalmic Surg* 23:94-98, 1992.
149. Solomon LD: Endocapsular phacoemulsification. In Solomon LD, editor: *Practical phacoemulsification: proceedings of the second annual workshop* [supplement to *Ophthalmic Practice*], pp 10-13, 1990.
150. Solomon LD: Endocapsular (intercapsular) phacoemulsification. In Solomon LD, editor: *Practical phacoemulsification: proceedings of the third annual workshop* [supplement to *Ophthalmic Practice*], pp 29-39, 1990.
151. Michelson MA: Endocapsular phacoemulsification with mini-capsulorhexis. In Koch P, Davison J, editors: *Phacoemulsification techniques,* Thorofare, NJ, 1991, Slack, Inc, pp 275-309.
152. Wan WL, Gindi JJ, Schanzlin DJ: Endocapsular cataract surgery. II. Effects on the corneal endothelium, *Cataract* 2:11-14, 1985.
153. Solomon KD, Gwin TD, O'Morchoe DJC et al: Protective effect of the anterior lens capsule during extracapsular cataract extraction. Part I: Experimental animal study, *Ophthalmology* 96:591-597, 1989.
154. Nishi O, Nishi K. Endocapsular phacoemulsification following buttonhole anterior capsulotomy: a preliminary report, *J Cataract Refract Surg* 16: 575-762, 1990.
155. Nishi O. Endo-intercapsular cataract surgery following buttonhole anterior capsulotomy. In Yalon M, editor: *Techniques of phacoemulsification and surgery and IOL implantation,* Thorofare, NJ, 1992, Slack, Inc, pp 249-266.
156. Pop M: Two-port endocap phaco: safe and quick, *Ocular Surg News* 9:1, 40, 1991.
157. Stark WJ, Streeten B: The anterior capsulotomy of extracapsular cataract extraction, *Ophthalmic Surg* 15:911-917, 1984.
158. Apple DJ, Kincaid MC, Mamalis N et al: *Intraocular lenses: evolution, designs, complications and pathology,* Baltimore, Williams & Wilkins, 1989, pp 141-143.
159. Gimbel HV: Two-stage capsulorhexis for endocapsular phacoemulsification, *J Cataract Refract Surg* 16:246-249, 1990.
160. Gimbel HV: Continuous circular, two-stage and posterior continuous circular capsulorhexis: description and analysis, *Ophthalmic Practice* 8:81-85, 1990.
161. Nishi O: Refilling the lens of the rabbit eye after intracapsular cataract surgery using an endocapsular balloon and an anterior capsule suturing technique, *J Cataract Refract Surg* 15:450-454, 1989.
162. Nishi O, Hara T, Hara T et al: Further development of experimental techniques for refilling the lens of animal eyes with a balloon, *J Cataract Refract Surg* 15:584-588, 1989.
163. Teichmann KD: Endocapsular closed chamber technique for disc lens implantation, *J Cataract Refract Surg* 16:253-256, 1989.
164. Arnold PN: One-handed method of posterior chamber phacoemulsification, *J Cataract Refract Surg* 16:646-648, 1990.
165. Fishkind WJ: In situ phacoemulsification. In Koch P, Davison J, editors: *Phacoemulsification techniques,* Thorofare, NJ, 1991, Slack, Inc, pp 143-152.
166. Arnold PN: Nuclear flip technique in small pupil phacoemulsification, *J Cataract Refract Surg* 17:225-227, 1991.
167. Kershner RM: Sutureless one-handed intercapsular phacoemulsification: the keyhole technique, *J Cataract Refract Surg* 17:719-725, 1991.
168. Klemen UM: V-style phacoemulsification, *J Cataract Refract Surg* 19: 548-550, 1993.
169. Pacifico RL: Divide and conquer phacoemulsification: one-handed variant, *J Cataract Refract Surg* 18:513-517, 1992.
170. Krey HF: Ultrasonic turbulences at the phacoemulsification tip, *J Cataract Refract Surg* 15:343-344, 1989.
171. Scleral and corneal burns during phacoemulsification with viscoelastic materials, *Health Devices* 17:377-379, 1988.
172. Shimmura S, Tsubota K, Oguchi Y et al: Oxiradical-dependent photoemission induced by phacoemulsification probe. *Invest Ophthalmol Vis Sci* 33:2904-2907, 1992.
173. Davis PL: Phaco transducers: basic principles and corneal thermal injury, *Eur J Implant Refract Surg* 5:109-112, 1993.
174. Wilbrandt HR, Wilbrandt TH: Evaluation of intraocular pressure fluctuations with differing phacoemulsification approaches, *J Cataract Refract Surg* 19:223-231, 1993.
175. Zetterstrom C, Laurell CG: Comparison of endothelial cell loss and phacoemulsification energy during endocapsular phacoemulsification surgery, *J Cataract Refract Surg* 21:55-58, 1995.
176. Hayashi K, Nakao F, Hayashi F: Corneal endothelial cell loss following phacoemulsification using the small-port phaco, *Ophthalmic Surg* 25: 510-513, 1994.
177. Pacifico RL: Ultrasonic energy in phacoemulsification: mechanical cutting and cavitation, *J Cataract Refract Surg* 20:338-341, 1994.
178. Probst LE, Nichols BD: Corneal endothelial and intraocular pressure changes after phacoemulsification with Amvisc Plus and Viscoat, *J Cataract Refract Surg* 19:725-730, 1993.
179. Strobel J, Jacobi KW: Phaco-emulsification and planned ECCE: intraoperative differences in intraocular heating, *Eur J Implant Refract Surg* 3:135-138, 1991.
180. Hunkeler JD: Peristaltic-based pump maximizes control, *Ocular Surg News* 11:22, 23, 1993.
181. Weiss IS: Aspiration pressure of phacoemulsification tips, *J Cataract refract Surg* 12:173, 1986.
182. Singer JA: Funnel shaped tip controls ultrasound energy during phaco, *Ocular Surg News* 10:48, 1992.
183. Zelman J: Small-port phacoemulsification. In Solomon LD, editor: *Practical phacoemulsification: proceedings of the third annual workshop* [supplement to *Ophthalmic Practice*], pp 40-42, 1991.
184. Heslin KB: Phacoemulsification with the Heslin/Mackool ocusystem: results of a retrospective study, *J Am Intraocul Implant Soc* 9:445-449, 1983.
185. Heslin KB, Guerriero PN: Phacoemulsification with the Heslin/Mackool ocusystem: a follow-up report, *Ann Ophthalmol* 17:601-603, 1985.
186. Neumann AC, Molyet E, Teal C et al: Phacoemulsification devices: a consumer's update, *J Cataract Refract Surg* 13:669-677, 1978.
187. Neumann AC, Molyet E, Teal C et al: Phacoemulsification devices: a consumer's report, *J Cataract Refract Surg* 13:70-75, 1987.
188. Davison JA: Personal correction of a phacoemulsification machine problem, *J Cataract Refract Surg* 14:456-458, 1988 (letter).
189. Eggleston RJ: One consumer's experience with a phacoemulsification device, *J Cataract Refract Surg* 14:232-233, 1988.
190. Phacoemulsification systems, *Health Devices* 18:377-404, 1989.
191. Ohneck JA: Comparative efficiency of current phacoemulsification units, *Ophthalmic Practice* 8:73-75, 1990.
192. Olson RJ: Is the phacoemulsification learning curve too steep? *Arch Ophthalmol* 109:1510, 1991 (letter).
193. Cotlier E: Phacoemulsification by residents, *Ophthalmology* 99:1481, 1992 (letter).
194. Hagan JC: A prospective study of the transition to phacoemulsification and small incision cataract surgery, *Mo Med* 89:663-667, 1992.
195. Prince RB, Tax RL, Miller DH: Conversion to small-incision phacoemulsification: experience with the first 50 eyes, *J Cataract Refract Surg* 19:246-250, 1993.
196. Pedersen O: Phacoemulsification and intraocular lens implantation in patients with cataract, *Acta Ophthalmol* 68:59-64, 1990.
197. Cotlier E, Rose M: Cataract extraction by the intracapsular methods and by phacoemulsification: the results of surgeons in training, *Trans Am Acad Ophthalmol Otolaryngol* 81:163-182, 1976.
198. Csordas JE: The surgeon's transition to phacoemulsification. In Solomon LD, editor: *Practical phacoemulsification: proceedings of the second annual workshop* [supplement to *Ophthalmic Practice*], pp 5-9, 1990.
199. Cruz OA, Wallace GW, Gay CA et al: Visual results and complications of phacoemulsification with intraocular lens implantation performed by ophthalmology residents, *Ophthalmology* 99:448-452, 1992.
200. Kreisler KR, Mortenson SW, Mamalis N: Endothelial cell loss following "modern" phacoemulsification by a senior resident, *Ophthalmic Surg* 23:158-160, 1992.
201. Goetz JS: Teaching phacoemulsification to residents, *Ophthalmic Practice* 10:219-222, 1992.
202. Maloney WF, Hall D, Parkinson DB: Synthetic cataract teaching system for phacoemulsification, *J Cataract Refract Surg* 14:218-221, 1988.
203. Zirm ME, Rosen ES: The high communication wetlab: a unique innovation in teaching ophthalmic surgery, *Eur J Implant Refract Surg* 4:145-148, 1992.

204. Allinson RW, Metrikin DC, Fante RG: Incidence of vitreous loss among third-year residents performing phacoemulsification, *Ophthalmology* 99:726-730, 1992.
205. Browning DJ, Cobo LM: Early experience in extracapsular cataract surgery by residents, *Ophthalmology* 92:1647-1653, 1985.
206. Pearson PA, Owen DG, Van Meter WS et al: Vitreous loss rates in extracapsular surgery by residents, *Ophthalmology* 96:1225-1227, 1989.
207. Sappenfield DL, Driebe WT Jr: Resident extracapsular surgery: results and a comparison of automated and manual technique, *Ophthalmic Surg* 20:619-624, 1989.
208. Allinson RW, Palmer ML, Fante R et al: Vitreous loss during phacoemulsification by residents, *Ophthalmology* 100:1181, 1993 (letter).
209. Spring B: Effects of food and nutrients on the behavior of normal individuals. In Wurtman RJ, Wurtman JJ, editors: *Nutrition and the brain,* New York, 1986, Raven Press, pp 1-41.
210. Pitts GL, Johnson RE, Consolzio FC: Work in the heat as affected by intake of water, salt and glucose, *Am J Physiol* 142:253-259, 1944.
211. Craig WJ: *Nutrition for the nineties,* Eau Claire, Wis, 1992, Golden Harvest Books, p 283.
212. Horne JA: Human sleep, sleep loss and behavior implications for the prenatal cortex and psychiatric disorders, *Br J Psychiatry* 162:413-419, 1993.
213. Rauhala E: Relaxation training combined with increased physical activity lowers the psychophysiological activation in community-home boys, *Int J Psychophysiol* 10:63-68, 1990.
214. Neiman DC: *Fitness and sports medicine,* Palo Alto, 1990, Bull Publishing Co, p 167.
215. Neiman DC: *Fitness and sports medicine,* Palo Alto, 1990, Bull Publishing Co, pp 389-392.

Phaco Chop*

16

Roger F. Steinert, MD

Over the past two decades, phacoemulsification has evolved from a simple "one-handed" technique to a number of variations, most of which involve use of instruments in both hands.

In 1993, Kunihiro Nagahara introduced the concept of a new technique for nuclear disassembly during phacoemulsification. His insight was that natural cleavage planes existed in the nucleus that had not been used previously (Figure 16-1, *A*). By impaling the nucleus with the phacoemulsification tip and thereby stabilizing it, the second "chopping" instrument could be pulled from the equatorial side of the outer nucleus toward the center. The nucleus was split readily by the chopping instrument, taking advantage of these natural cleavage planes. Nagahara made an analogy to the technique of chopping or, more accurately, splitting a log of wood with a wedge, taking advantage of the wood's grain, or cleavage planes (Figure 16-1, *B*).

Evolution of Phaco Chop

Stop and Chop

Several surgeons were stimulated by Nagahara's method and evolved techniques in an effort to improve the reliability and repeatability of phaco chop. Paul Koch found that the initial chop, intended to bisect the nucleus, was the most difficult. He reverted to creating an initial deep trough with the phaco tip and then cracking the trough with lateral pressure from the phaco tip and a second instrument, identical to the beginning of the quadrant cracking technique. At this point, however, Koch *stopped* the quadrant cracking approach and then began *chopping* the remaining pieces of nucleus; he labeled this technique as "stop and chop."[1] This technique (Figure 16-2) remains popular with many surgeons, and it is an important transition for almost anyone learning phaco chop because it eliminates the most difficult chopping step: the initial chop.

Chop and Debulk

To maximize the safety of the corneal endothelium and continue to perform phacoemulsification in the posterior chamber and iris plane, the surgeon should create some central space in order to use the chopping technique to disassemble the nucleus posterior to the iris. Similar to a multipiece jigsaw puzzle, taking pieces apart becomes easier once the initial piece is removed. In addition, the majority of ultrasound power is used to phacoemulsify the central hard nucleus, not the periphery. Steinert[2] described a technique that began identically to Nagahara's with an initial phaco chop to bisect the nucleus. Although perhaps more difficult to master, this initial chop is a more efficient maneuver than creating the trough and splitting it, as in the stop and chop technique. After the initial chop, however, the central hard nucleus is emulsified along the fault line of the initial crack before proceeding to chopping further pieces of nuclei. In softer nuclei, very little central material is removed at this step. In harder, larger nuclei, more central nucleus can be removed at this step; in very advanced cataracts, the center is bowled out to the midperiphery before beginning to chop further (Figure 16-3).

Circumferential Sequential Disassembly

Both Koch and Steinert found that the chop technique was better applied as a progressive chopping of small wedges in a circumferential direction, rather than chopping four full quadrants as originally described by Nagahara. The reason for this is that the progressive circumferential chopping of small wedges results in only one small piece at any given time. Because of the bulk, the large nuclear pieces remain stable within the posterior capsular sac. Therefore control of the phacoemulsification process is enhanced.

Howard Gimbel[3] earlier described several techniques of nuclear fracture whose principles have been incorporated in phaco chop as it has evolved. Gimbel pointed out the importance of debulking the central nucleus, forming a narrow trough for softer nuclei and a larger crater for hard nuclei. In addition, he demonstrated the ability to break off pieces of the peripheral nucleus with lateral separation movements after engaging them with the phacoemulsification tip, proceeding in a circumferential direction. Gimbel called this technique "nucleofractis." In essence, a phaco chop is the nucleofractis technique, greatly facilitated by the second "chopping" instrument instead of relying on forceful lateral movements of the phacoemulsification tip.

*Reprinted and modified from Spaeth GL, editor: *Ophthalmic surgery: principles and practice,* Philadelphia, 2003, WB Saunders.

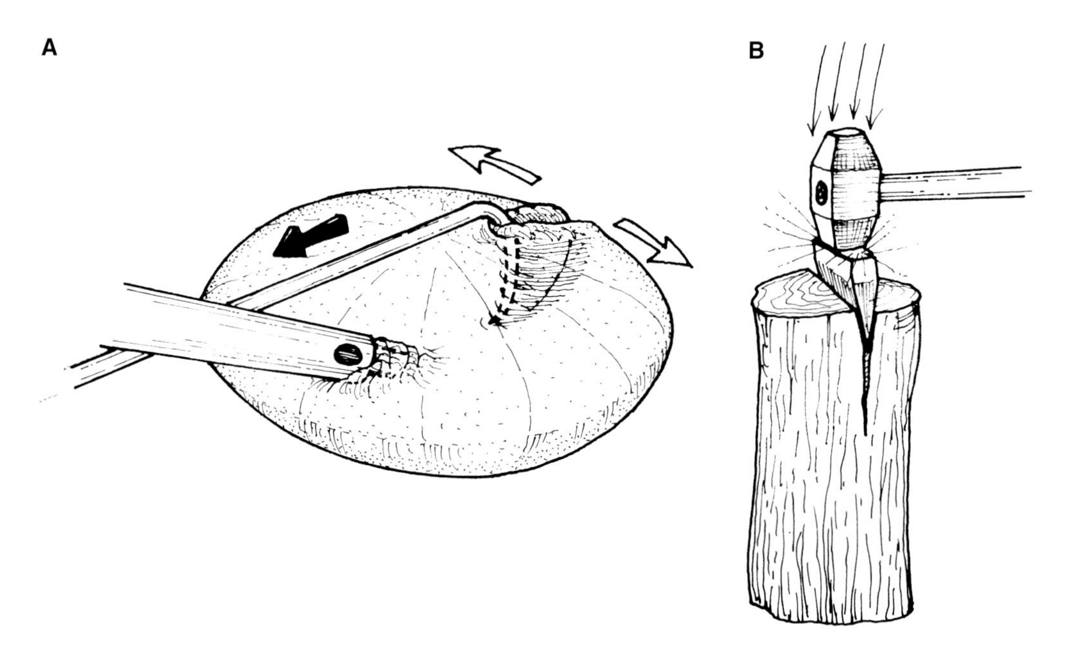

FIGURE 16-1 **A,** Nagahara's insight was to split the nucleus along its natural cleavage planes. **B,** The principle of chopping is the same as using a wedge to split a log along its natural planes.

High-Vacuum Phaco Chop

In addition to incorporating central debulking and using progressive circumferential chopping steps, Steinert recognized that using high vacuum during chopping further improves nuclear control and reduces the total ultrasound energy required. High vacuum allows the surgeon to grasp and hold the nuclear wedges and draw them toward the central zone of safety before completing the emulsification. Moreover, the manual energy input from the phaco chop, combined with the energy input from the high vacuum, reduces the total amount of ultrasonic energy required. Overall, the technique appears to be safer and more controlled. Because of its efficiency, the nuclear disassembly step of phacoemulsification cataract surgery is generally substantially faster than alternative techniques such as quadrant cracking.[4-6]

Phaco Quick Chop ("Vertical Phaco Chop")

Vladimir Pfeifer of Slovenia is generally credited for originating the fundamental concept of creating vertical forces that also fragment the nucleus. This technique has been developed and taught by David Dillman and Louis Nichamin as "phaco quick chop." Nagahara's fundamental concept is to stabilize the nucleus with the phaco tip and then pull the chopping

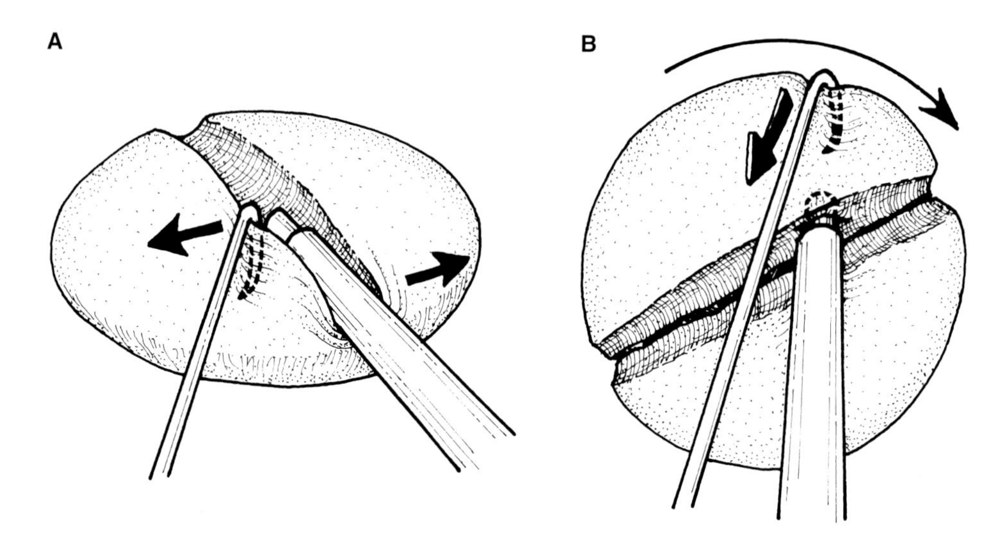

FIGURE 16-2 **A,** Paul Koch's "stop and chop" technique begins with a groove and cracking of the nucleus into two halves, identical to the start of "divide and conquer" nuclear fracture. **B,** Nucleus is rotated one to two clock hours, and the surgeon *stops* the "divide and conquer" technique and begins to "chop."

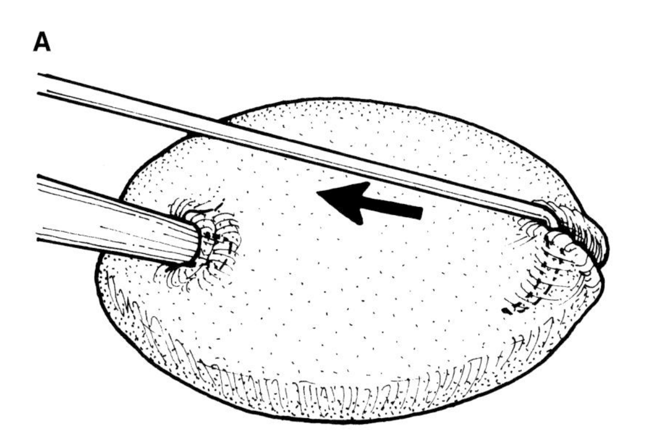

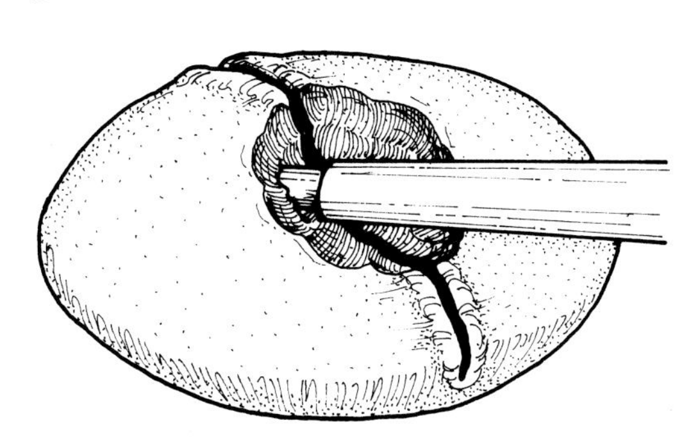

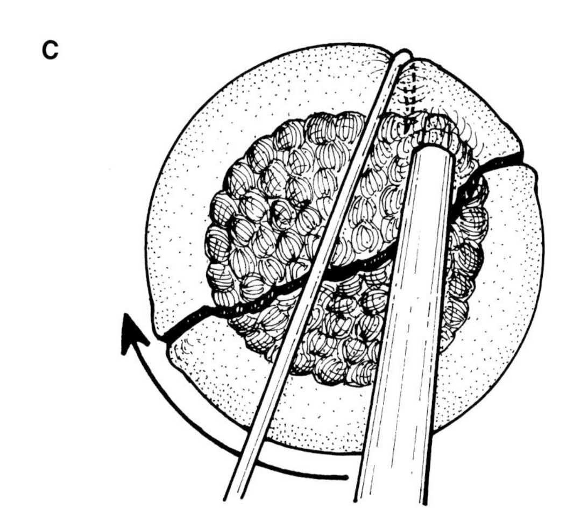

FIGURE 16-3 **A,** Full phaco chop approach uses the chopper to split the nucleus into two halves. **B,** Space is created, and the hardest central portion of the nucleus is removed, leaving enough peripheral nucleus to gain purchase by the phaco tip with a small amount of ultrasound and high vacuum. **C,** Nucleus is rotated clockwise (for a right-handed surgeon; a left-handed surgeon rotates counterclockwise and performs mirror-image maneuvers), and pie-shaped wedges are split off and removed with short bursts of ultrasound.

instrument in the *horizontal* plane from the equator toward the center. *Vertical* chop differs by embedding the phaco tip deeply into the nucleus and then impaling a sharp-tipped chopping instrument into the anterior nucleus in front and adjacent to the phaco tip. The chopper pushes downward sharply while the phaco tip lifts upward (Figure 16-4, *A*). Each instrument moves about one half of the total amount of vertical separation needed to generate a fissure. As soon as the vertical (anteroposterior) split begins to develop, the two instruments also spread horizontally slightly to complete the cleavage of the two sections (Figure 16-4, *B*). Vertical chop is then continued to break off smaller section of nucleus for emulsification, progressing circumferentially as in the technique described earlier (Figure 16-4, *C* and *D*).

The principal advantage of vertical chopping is the elimination of the need to pass the chopper under the anterior capsule out to the equator of the nucleus. Because neither the anterior capsule edge nor the equator can always be seen, some surgeons dislike the necessity to rely on tactile feedback and judgment of distances under the iris. On the other hand, vertical chopping works best in moderate-density nuclei. It often fails in softer nuclei, where the phaco tip and chopper pull through the nucleus, or in hard nuclei, where so much force is required that, when cleavage does occur, the abrupt movement threatens the integrity of the posterior capsule and/or zonules.

The "complete" phaco surgeon should be comfortable with both horizontal and vertical chopping maneuvers, as each has its place.

Detailed Technique of Phaco Chop

The basic concept of horizontal phaco chop, as it is usually practiced, is illustrated in Figure 16-5. The nucleus is stabilized with the phacoemulsification tip, which is impaled with moderate vacuum (typically 50 to 80 mm Hg) and low ultrasonic power, in a position near the center but decentered about 1 mm toward the incision. The irrigation sleeve should be retracted more than is customary for divide and conquer nuclear fracture, in order to permit the phaco tip to advance to the depth of midnucleus (1.5 to 2 mm). While impaling the nucleus, the phaco handpiece is markedly tipped in the vertical direction, as if aiming for the optic disc. The chopping instrument is passed through a paracentesis that is about one and a half clock hours away from the incision. The chopper can assist the proper location of the impaling of the phaco tip by pressing lightly on the nuclear surface and shifting the nucleus gently (about 1 mm) away from the incision.

The chopper is advanced under the anterior capsule until it can pass around the equator of the nucleus at the nucleus-epinucleus border, about 180 degrees opposite the paracentesis. If the nuclear equatorial border can be visualized as either a "golden ring" (smaller nucleus) or a dark ring (larger nucleus) as a result of effective hydrodelineation, the chopper can be placed into this ring under direct visualization (see Figure 16-5, *A* and *B*). If the nucleus is very large or the pupil does not adequately dilate, the surgeon will nevertheless be able to *feel* the abrupt change as the chopper tip passes from the hard

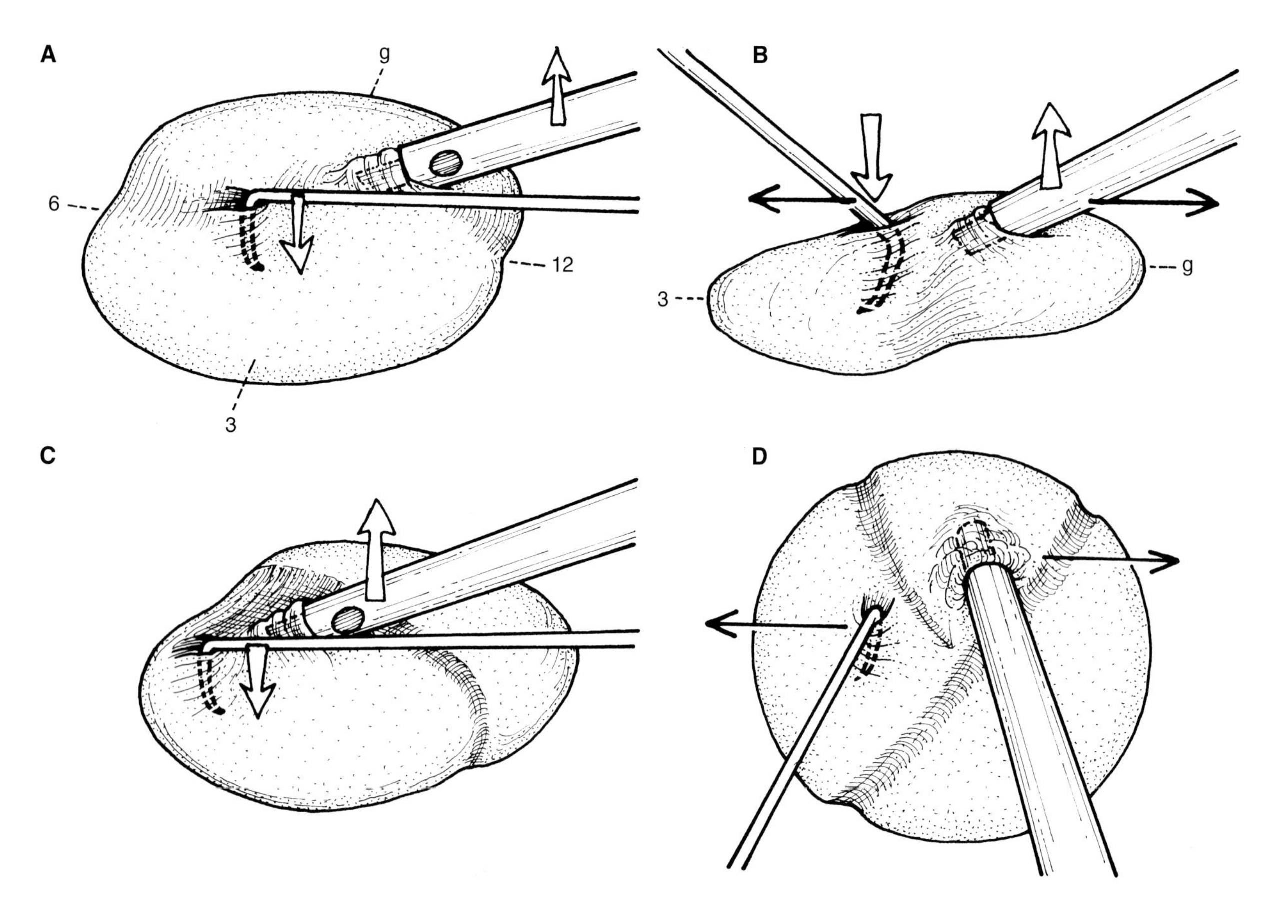

FIGURE 16-4 **A,** In vertical phaco chop ("phaco quick chop"), the deeply buried phaco tip is lifted up while a sharp-tipped chopper presses downward. **B,** Once the endonucleus starts to split, the instruments are separated slightly laterally as well to enhance full cleavage of the two sections of nucleus. **C** and **D,** Nucleus is rotated, and the vertical chop maneuver is repeated to create smaller nuclear fragments that can be removed with ultrasound and aspiration. (**C,** Side view; **D,** surgeon's view.)

nucleus to the relatively soft epinucleus. The chopping instrument will shift posteriorly by at least 1 mm when this border is encountered (see Figure 16-5, *C*).

The chopping instrument is then drawn across the center of the nucleus, moving from opposite the paracentesis in the direction toward the paracentesis (see Figure 16-5, *D*). Once the center of the nucleus is approached or fully transected, the nucleus fractures readily. To successfully split the nucleus, the chopper tip should be at least at half depth in the nucleus anteroposteriorly, as well as chopping across half of the nucleus radially. The impaled phaco tip will also have weakened the central nucleus and contributes to a successful chopping hemisection of the nucleus. This basic chop maneuver works well in nuclei ranging from low to high density.

The next step is to debulk the center of the nucleus. If the lens has mild to moderate density, the debulking is restricted to a zone no larger than a conventional trough. In that manner, the peripheral nuclear pieces retain enough integrity for the circumferential peripheral chopping maneuvers. On the other hand, if the lens is firmer, a crater or bowl is phacoemulsified to further debulk the center (see Figure 16-5, *E*). In all cases, it is important to leave sufficient firm peripheral nuclear material to allow the nucleus to be safely engaged and held by the phaco tip during the progressive circumferential chopping.

Circumferential peripheral nuclear chopping then proceeds. For a right-handed surgeon, the heminucleus being chopped should be located to the surgeon's left, and the nucleus rotated in a clockwise direction. The phacoemulsification tip engages the leading edge of the heminucleus, and then the chopper transects the peripheral wedge, leaving the wedge engaged in the phacoemulsification tip (see Figure 16-5, *F*). For a left-handed surgeon, the maneuvers are performed in a mirror-image fashion, with the direction of the nuclear rotation counterclockwise.

The size of the pie-shaped wedges of nucleus to be chopped depends on the density of the nucleus. The harder the nucleus, the smaller the fragment should be. The pie-shaped pieces can be created in virtually any size. For 2+ nuclear density, only three wedges should be created in each heminucleus; for a very dense 4+ nucleus, six to eight wedges should be created. If a piece is chopped and appears to be too large, it can be chopped once again. The goal is to create "bite-sized" pieces that are appropriate for the phacoemulsification tip.

Chopping Instruments

A large number of chopping instruments have been developed. Although this can perplex a novice, the variety of chopping

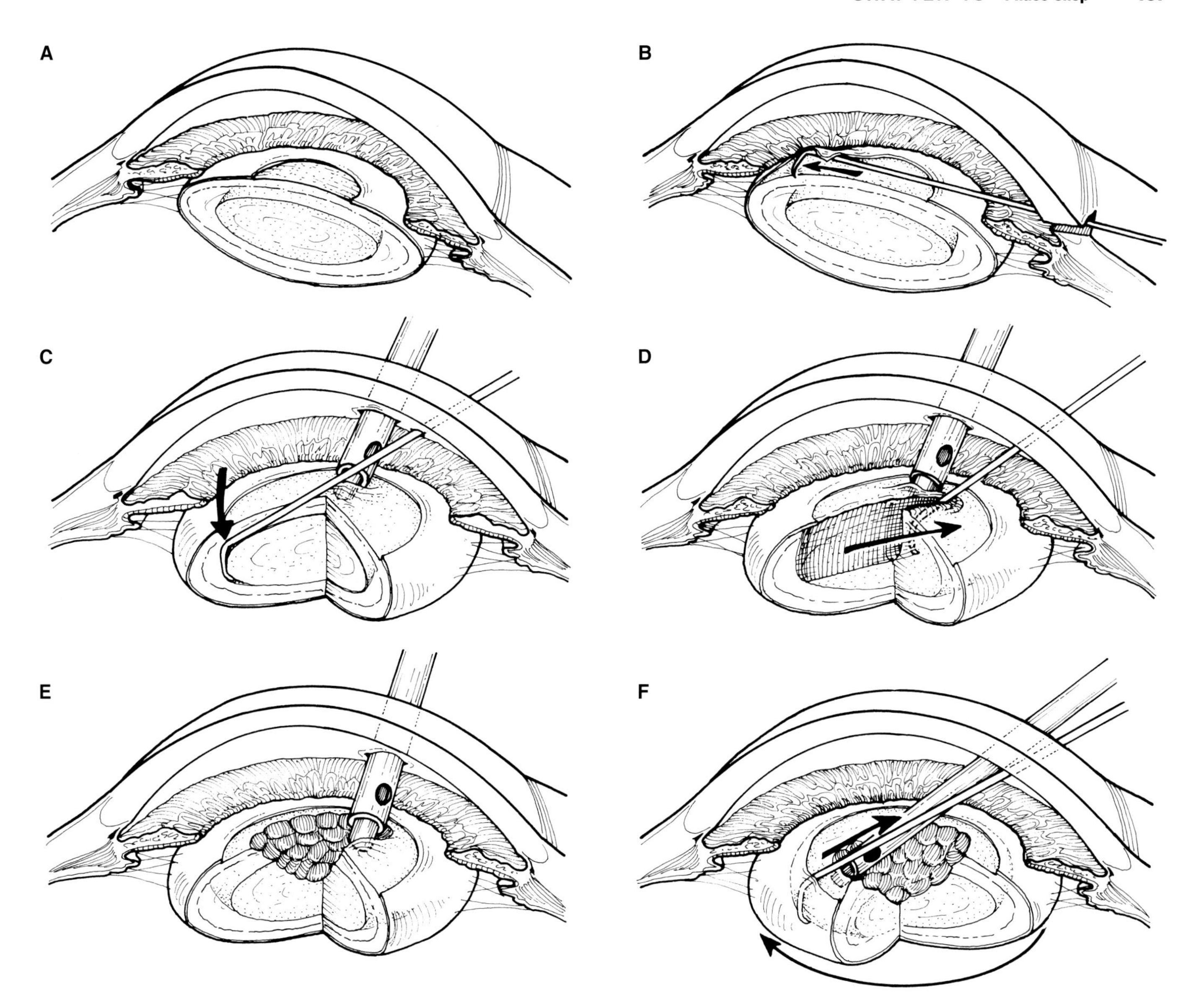

FIGURE 16-5 **A,** With a widely dilated pupil and small to moderate sized endonucleus, hydrodelineation will create a separation of the endonucleus from the epinucleus, seen as a golden ring or a black ring, depending on the illumination and red reflex. **B,** The surgeon directs the chopper under the anterior capsule and down into the ring. **C,** If the pupillary dilation is smaller than the size of the endonucleus, the surgeon must advance the tip of the chopper without being able to see the equator. The surgeon, with experience, will have a good sense of how much the chopper must be advanced to reach the zone of the ring and will be able to feel when the chopper tip reaches this point and is able to drop. **D,** The phaco tip impales the nucleus and is advanced to the depth of the midnucleus. The chopper pulls toward the phaco tip, splitting the nucleus in half. **E,** The central, hardest portion of the nucleus is removed. The harder the nucleus, the larger the area sculpted. Enough nuclear material must remain that the phaco tip can engage and become occluded on the periphery, while the chopper breaks off pie-shaped wedges for removal **(F).**

instruments gives the surgeon many options with which to solve technical problems. Once the surgeon becomes proficient with a specific design, however, there is little value in further change.

Original chopping instruments were fashioned out of Sinskey hooks, with the tip rebent to a length of approximately 1.5 mm. This type of instrument is generally inadvisable, however. The very-fine-gauge wire of a Sinskey hook can cut through a nucleus, but the absence of any bulk in the wire prevents the full realization of the potential of phaco chop. Recall that Nagahara's fundamental principle was that the chopping instrument should act like a wedge. Most models of chopping instruments have a thicker gauge than the Sinskey hook, often with sharp internal cutting surfaces, thus obtaining the desired wedge-splitting effect.

Sharp cutting surfaces in chopping instruments may be on only one surface, generally directed along the shaft of the chopper, or two or three surfaces may be sharpened, allowing more successful "lateral chopping" maneuvers. The shaft may also be angled for right- or left-hand approaches.

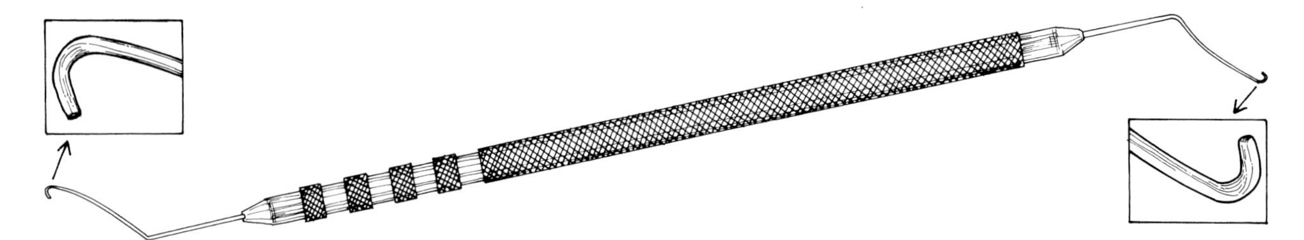

FIGURE 16-6 Steinert double-ended claw chopper. One end is 1.5 mm in length, for chopping most nuclei; the other end is 1.75 mm length, for chopping large, hard nuclei. (Courtesy Rhein Medical.)

Steinert designed a curved chopping instrument (Figure 16-6; Rhein Medical, Tampa, Fla.) to incorporate all of these principles and also to facilitate keeping the chopper engaged in the center of the nucleus. The curved distal element acts in the same manner as a cat's claw or a farmer's hoe. The chopper naturally engages the curved equator of the nucleus, which can be felt by the surgeon. The claw configuration then keeps the chopper engaged deeply into the nucleus, avoiding the tendency for straight choppers to rise up and out of the nucleus as they pass toward the center.

The Phacoemulsification Needle

For many years, phacoemulsification instrument manufacturers progressively increased the angle of the phacoemulsification tip to gain increased "cutting power." The phaco chop technique has reversed that trend, however. The greater the angle of the phacoemulsification tip, the larger the cross-sectional area of the phaco tip port. With a greater tip angle, more of the tip must be buried into the nuclear fragment to obtain occlusion, which is necessary for stabilizing the nucleus before the initial phaco chop and for engaging and controlling the peripheral circumferential wedges. In fact, Nagahara worked with one company to return to a true zero-degree phacoemulsification tip. The zero-degree tip greatly facilitates obtaining occlusion of the circumferential nuclear fragments and aiding their manipulation.

Why does this not reduce ultrasound power unacceptably? Phacoemulsification handpieces have greatly increased in power over recent years. More importantly, however, better understanding of ultrasonics had led to manipulations in the configuration of the phacoemulsification tip to improve the efficiency of ultrasonification of the nucleus through the creation of cavitation. For example, Nagahara's zero-degree tip (available from Allergan, Inc., Irvine, Calif.) has an internal bevel that vastly improves ultrasound power through internal cavitation, as well as reducing the cross-sectional area of the phacoemulsification needle tip.

Transition to Phaco Chop

The surgeon should first become proficient in anterior capsulorhexis, hydrodissection, and hydrodelineation. The nucleus must be freely mobile to allow easy rotation once chopping begins. An intact and well-defined circular-tear anterior capsulotomy provides a clear landmark for the surgeon, as well as the capsular strength for extra manipulation.[7] Hydrodelineation frees the nucleus from the epinucleus, which is necessary for chopped fragments to be removed, as well as disclosing the location of the nuclear equator.

The surgeon wishing to learn phaco chop should begin by chopping the second half of the nucleus in a case where the first half of the nucleus is removed with a conventional divide and conquer quadrant technique (Figure 16-7, *A*). The second half of the nucleus is usually quite mobile at that point, and the basic technique and tactile feel of phaco chop can be appreciated within several cases by chopping the second half of the heminucleus (Figure 16-7, *B*).

Once the surgeon feels comfortable with chopping the second heminucleus, the next step is to perform the stop and chop technique for both halves of the heminucleus, while still retaining the initial trough and split hemisection of traditional divide and conquer (see Figure 16-2).

The last step in the progress to full phaco chop is to bisect the nucleus with the phaco chopper (see Figures 16-3, *A*, and 16-5, *D*). Although some surgeons have found this to be the most challenging step in the technique, it also is the most rewarding. Full phaco chop markedly improves the efficiency of the disassembly of the nucleus, particularly because of the elimination of the multiple steps of rotation and trough creation in the standard quadrant cracking techniques.

Challenges in Phaco Chop

Small Pupils

A novice will be insecure about the inability to visualize the periphery during chopping maneuvers. Small pupil cases should only be undertaken with phaco chop after the surgeon has gained reasonable comfort in more straightforward cases with large pupils and moderate-density nuclei. However, once this basic skill is achieved, chopping is preferred over the quadrant cracking or divide and conquer technique because chopping does not require peripheral passes with the ultrasound tip, and it is not dependent on a good red reflex.[8-10]

The 4+ Nucleus

Chopping a 4+ hard nucleus can be particularly difficult, both because a hard nucleus is also a thick nucleus and because of the physical properties of a hard brunescent nucleus.[10] Nevertheless, chopping offers distinct advantages in phacoemulsification

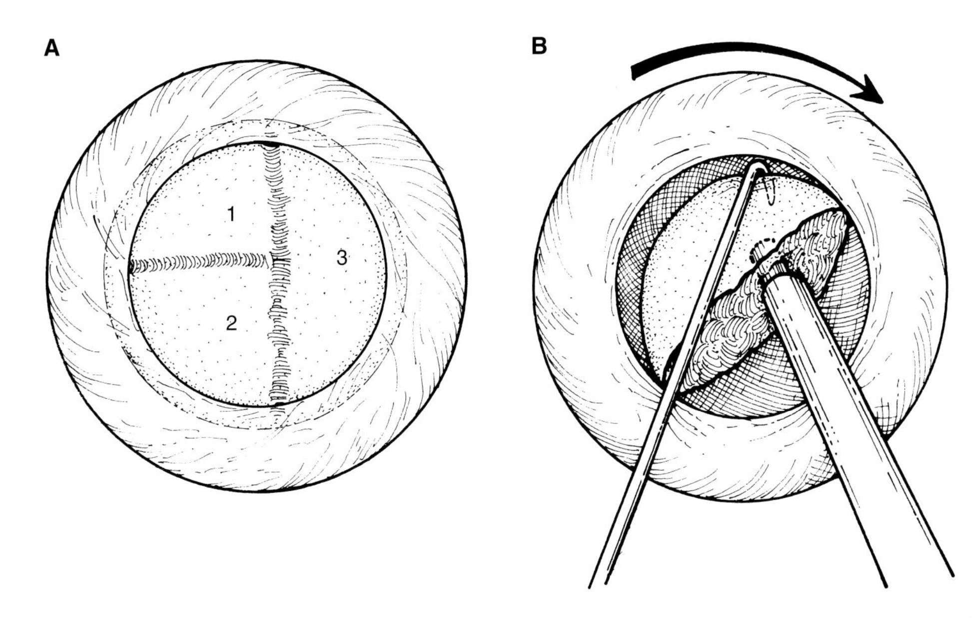

FIGURE 16-7 A, To begin learning phaco chop, the first half of the nucleus (pieces 1 and 2) is removed using standard divide and conquer technique; the second heminucleus (piece 3) remains undivided. **B,** The second half of the nucleus can now be chopped with good direct visualization.

of very advanced cataracts.[11] Because the nucleus is thick, a standard 1.5-mm-long phaco chopper will not have adequate length to pass through the center of a nucleus (Figure 16-8, *A*). As a result, a superficial vertical split will occur, but the deeper layer of the nucleus will tend to split in a more lateral fashion, creating a posterior plate (Figure 16-8, *B*). If this occurs, the surgeon must identify which half of the heminucleus is above the plate and which half is attached to the plate. The half of the nucleus that is above the plate should be removed first, which allows the larger fragment to be mobilized and chopped. Several chopping instruments are now available with longer tips, in the order of 1.75 to 2 mm, which greatly facilitates successful chopping of these thicker nuclei. These choppers, although longer, are still well short of endangering the posterior capsule, considering that a brunescent nucleus is at least 3.5 mm thick (Figure 16-8, *C*).

A very hard brunescent nucleus also tends to have a posterior "leathery" quality. Chopped fragments have posterior bridging strands that keep nuclear fragments attached to each other. These posterior strands represent posterior epinucleus that has partially hardened, with strong adhesion to the posterior nucleus and with a tough, strandlike quality. When these strands occur, they are seen against the red reflex as they bridge between two chopped nuclear fragments (see Figure 16-8, *D*). The surgeon can rotate the phaco chopper 90 degrees in his or her fingers, then carefully pass the chopper posterior to the nuclear fragment and transect the bridging fibers (see Figure 16-8, *E*). This maneuver has led to variations of phaco chop generally known as "posterior cracking."

Zonular Abnormalities

Once experience is gained with phaco chop, it is the preferred technique in the presence of weak or missing zonules. This situation occurs most commonly in pseudoexfoliation syndrome or after trauma.[12-15] Because horizontal chopping creates opposing forces between the two instruments, it minimizes forces on the zonules.[16]

Complications of Phaco Chop

Multiple Incomplete Chops

A surgeon inexperienced at phaco chop often tends to "scratch" the nucleus without accomplishing front-to-back cleavage. This usually occurs for two reasons. The first is not passing the chopper far enough into the periphery in order to allow the chopper to "hook" and engage the equator. The surgeon can test whether the chopper is around the equator by gently pulling on the chopper and verifying that the nucleus moves with it. The second common problem is allowing the chopper to ride up and out of the nucleus. The claw-shaped chopper was designed by Steinert to resist this tendency. For all chopper styles, the surgeon must learn to maintain appropriate posterior pressure on the chopping instrument.

When fragmented and incomplete chops do occur, the most important step is for the surgeon to remain patient. He or she should continue rotating and attempt to chop a new area, concentrating on proper technique. In addition, the chopper can act as a "finger" to hook around the equator of a fragment and help bring it toward the phaco tip in the central zone. This maneuver is particularly helpful when the vacuum is inadequate or complete occlusion cannot be achieved, and the nuclear fragment keeps "falling back," away from the phaco tip.

Posterior Capsule Rupture

The most feared complication for novice surgeons with phaco chop is rupture of the posterior capsule with the chopper. In fact, this is rare and should not occur at all with adherence to

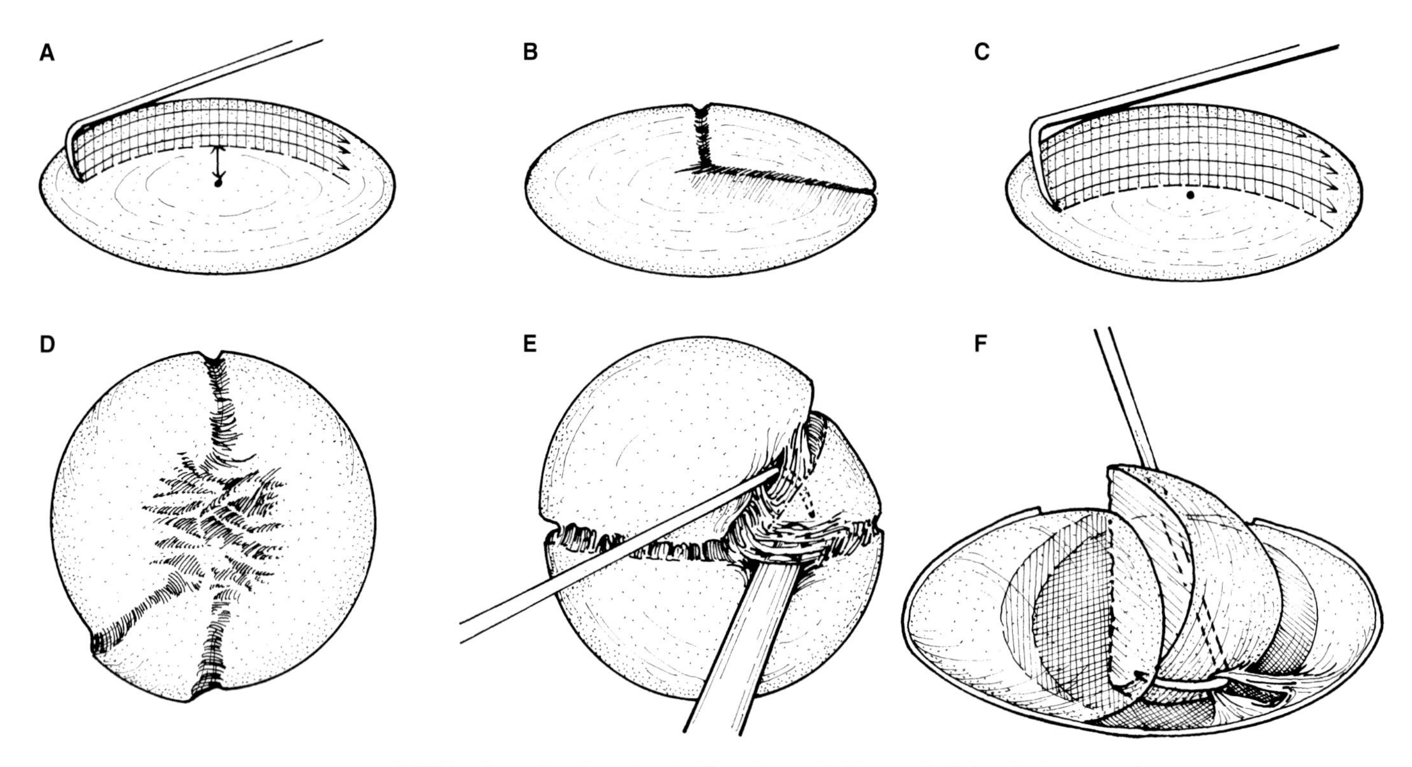

FIGURE 16-8 **A,** Thick, advanced nuclear cataract will not chop well with a standard chopping instrument because the length of the tip is inadequate to split the center of the nucleus. **B,** If the thick nucleus splits at all, a short-tip chopper will tend to split the upper portion of the nucleus, but the fracture line will lateralize, leaving a posterior nuclear plate attached to one portion of the two pieces of nucleus. **C,** A longer length chopper will have a better likelihood of cleanly splitting the nucleus. The extra length of the chopper tip is far from the posterior capsule. **D,** In advanced nuclear sclerosis, "leathery" posterior nuclear strands will bridge across a chopped wedge and interfere with its removal, particularly at the posterior apex. **E,** Chopper can be rotated 90 degrees, parallel to the posterior capsule, and used to snap across these strands and free the nuclear wedge.

the principles of phaco chop. The phaco chop instrument is typically only 1.5 mm long and, even with phaco chop instruments that have been elongated for dealing with a 4+ nucleus, the length never exceeds 2 mm (see Figure 16-8, *A* and *C*). The conventional lens is thicker than this in the periphery and increases to between 3 and 4 mm centrally (and sometimes even thicker). As a result, the phaco chopping instrument is well away from the posterior capsule. Many of the phaco chopping instruments have a blunted tip, which is also less likely to engage the posterior capsule.

Anterior Capsule/Zonular Rupture

A more common complication is misjudging the location of the anterior capsule, such that the phaco chopper is anterior to the peripheral anterior capsule rather than within the capsular bag (Figure 16-9, *A*). This mistake can be avoided by placing the phaco chopping instrument against the nucleus centrally, within the capsulorhexis, and keeping a small amount of posterior pressure against the nucleus as the chopper is passed peripherally. In a very hard nucleus with almost no anterior cortex, little space is present between the anterior capsule and the nucleus. In this case, the surgeon should rotate the phaco chopping instrument 90 degrees within the surgeon's fingers so that it can slip under the anterior capsule in a "flat" position (Figure 16-9, *B*). As the chopper passes out to the edge of the endonucleus, it is rotated back 90 degrees to the vertical chopping position (Figure 16-9, *C*).

Conclusion

With careful attention to detail in following the progressive learning technique suggested earlier, any two-handed phacoemulsification surgeon should be able to master the maneuvers of phaco chop. Phaco chop is faster, and, as a result, ultrasound time is reduced, with a reduction in corneal endothelial damage and the potential for rupture of the posterior capsule.

Moreover, because phaco chop is a technique that involves stabilizing the nucleus with a phaco instrument centrally and then applying centripetal forces with the phaco chopper against the ultrasound tip, there is much less zonular stress than in standard cracking techniques. After phaco chop is mastered, it becomes a central element in the phacoemulsification surgeon's technique.

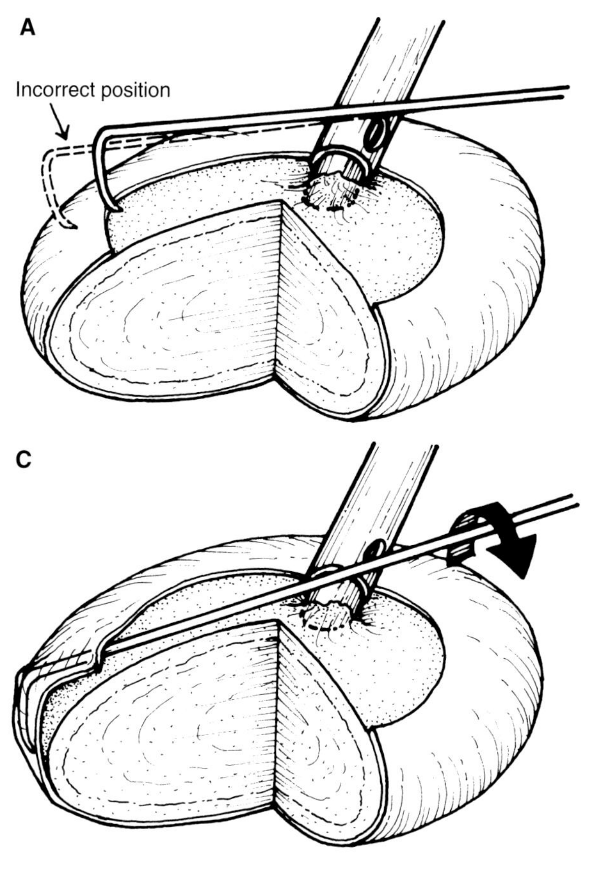

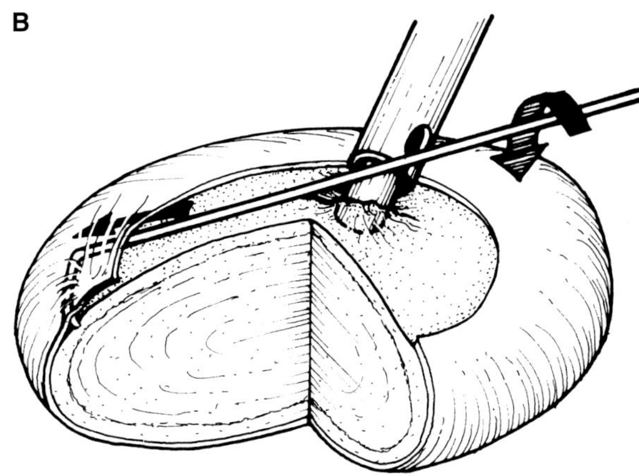

FIGURE 16-9 A, The surgeon must be careful to avoid passing the chopper over the anterior capsule instead of under it. This error is more likely in a large, dense cataract where little anterior cortex remains to separate the anterior capsule from the anterior nucleus. **B,** By rotating the chopper 90 degrees, in a horizontal position parallel to the iris plane, the tip can pass easily between the anterior capsule and the nucleus. **C,** As the chopper tip is advanced out to the level of the equator of the nucleus, the tip is then rotated back 90 degrees, from horizontal back to vertical, where it will pass around the nuclear equator and be positioned for chopping.

REFERENCES

1. Koch PS, Katzen LE: Stop and chop phacoemulsification, *J Cataract Refract Surg* 20:566-570, 1994.
2. Steinert RF: "Phaco chop." In Steinert et al, editors: *Cataract surgery: technique, complications, and management*, Philadelphia, 1995, WB Saunders.
3. Gimbel HV: Divide and conquer nucleofractis phacoemulsification: development and variations, *J Cataract Refract Surg* 17:281-291, 1991.
4. Pirazzoli G, D'Eliseo D, Ziosi M et al: Effects of phacoemulsification time on the corneal endothelium using phacofracture and phaco chop techniques, *J Cataract Refract Surg* 22:967-969, 1996.
5. DeBry P, Olson RJ, Crandall AS: Comparison of energy required for phacochop and divide and conquer phacoemulsification, *J Cataract Refract Surg* 24:689-692, 1998.
6. Ram J, Wesendahl TA, Auffarth GU et al: Evaluation of in situ fracture versus phaco chop techniques, *J Cataract Refract Surg* 24:1464-1468, 1998.
7. Gimbel HV, Neuhann T: Development, advantages, and methods of the continuous circular capsulotomy technique, *J Cataract Refract Surg* 16:31-37, 1990.
8. Lumme P, Laatikainen LT: Risk factors for intraoperative and early postoperative complications in extracapsular surgery, *Eur J Ophthalmol* 4:151-158, 1994.
9. Joseph J, Wang HS: Phacoemulsification with poorly dilated pupils, *J Cataract Refract Surg* 19:551-556, 1993.
10. Hayashi K, NakaoF, Hayashi F: Corneal endothelial cell loss after phacoemulsification using nuclear cracking procedures, *J Cataract Refract Surg* 20:44-47, 1994.
11. Vasavada A, Singh R: Step-by-step chop in situ and separation of very dense cataracts, *J Cataract Refract Surg* 24:156-159, 1998.
12. Lunne P, Laatikainen L: Exfoliation syndrome and cataract extraction, *Am J Ophthalmol* 116:51-55, 1993.
13. Osher RH, Cionni RJ, Gimbel HV et al: Cataract surgery in patients with pseudoexfoliation syndrome, *Eur J Implant Refract Surg* 5:45-50, 1993.
14. Fine IH, Hoffman RS: Phacoemulsification in the presence of pseudoexfoliation: challenges and options, *J Cataract Refract Surg* 23:160-165, 1997.
15. Moreno J, Duch S, Lajara J: Pseudoexfoliation syndrome: clinical factors related to capsular rupture in cataract surgery, *Acta Ophthalmol* 71:181-184, 1993.
16. Masket S, editor: Consultation section. *J Cataract Refract Surg* 24:1289-1298, 1998.

Technique of Tilt and Tumble Phacoemulsification

17

Elizabeth A. Davis, MD
Richard L. Lindstrom, MD

The technique of tilt and tumble was developed by Dr. Richard Lindstrom. Lindstrom was introduced to phacoemulsification in 1977 during a fellowship with William S. Harris, MD, in Dallas, Texas. At that time, phacoemulsification techniques were generally divided into anterior chamber phacoemulsification, as championed by Charles Kelman, MD; iris plane phacoemulsification, as championed by Richard Kratz, MD; and posterior chamber phacoemulsification, as championed by John Sheets, MD, and Robert Sinskey, MD. Under the tutelage of Dr. Harris, Lindstrom had the opportunity to try all of these techniques, and over time selected the iris plane phacoemulsification technique of Richard Kratz, MD, as his procedure of choice. What follows is Lindstrom's description of the evolution of the tilt and tumble procedure.

In this era before capsulorhexis and hydrodissection, a relatively large can-opener anterior capsulectomy was performed just inside the zonules. Following this, a portion of the central core nucleus was emulsified, leaving an inferior shelf of tissue. Then using a bimanual technique, the superior pole of the nucleus was tilted above the capsule and engaged by a beveled phacoemulsification tip. The nucleus was supported in the iris plane with a nucleus rotator and emulsified.

Occasionally the nucleus was subluxated into the anterior chamber, particularly when there was concern about a capsular tear. In addition, in some instances, posterior chamber phacoemulsification was the preferred technique, particularly in very soft nuclei in younger patients.

As the technique of continuous-tear anterior capsulectomy (capsulorhexis) was developed, it was incorporated into the procedure. Initially, a relatively small-diameter capsulorhexis in the range of 4 to 5 mm was constructed, especially when using 5.5-mm round optic polymethylmethacrylate intraocular lenses. This small continuous-tear anterior capsulectomy made it impossible to subluxate the nucleus safely into the iris plane or anterior chamber, and thus it was necessary to employ posterior chamber, endocapsular phacoemulsification techniques. With most nuclei a nuclear cracking technique was used, whereby the core nucleus was emulsified and the peripheral bowl of retained nuclear material and nuclear plate was infractured in a so-called one-handed technique. This technique was useful for soft nuclei in younger patients.

Soon thereafter, hydrodissection and hydrodelineation became a standard part of the technique to loosen the nucleus and allow it to be rotated easier. With a small continuous-tear anterior capsulectomy, the nucleus always remained localized in the posterior chamber. Although the endocapsular cracking techniques have many positive features, they were more difficult to teach and had a longer learning curve. Also, procedure times were somewhat longer than they had been with the iris plane technique. In addition, a mild increase in the capsular tear rate from approximately 1% to 1.8% was found. On the positive side, visual recovery was very rapid, especially when foldable intraocular lenses were used, and most patients had a clear cornea on the first postoperative day. In time the capsular tear rate was reduced to 1.3%, but the procedure required 10 to 15 minutes to complete. In addition, in some instances when the capsulorhexis was somewhat smaller, in the 4-mm range, particularly in patients with loose zonules (such as those with pseudoexfoliation), other undesirable side effects were possible, such as the capsular contraction syndrome.

Several Japanese investigators at the time suggested that retained subcapsular epithelium might play a role in postoperative inflammation and capsular opacity. Thus the procedure was modified to incorporate larger-diameter continuous-tear anterior capsulectomies. With a continuous-tear anterior capsulectomy of 5 to 6 mm, the nucleus would often inadvertently subluxate partially or totally anterior to the capsular rim. In such cases the nucleus could simply be pushed back into the capsular bag and the procedure completed using a nuclear fracture technique. It soon became obvious that the capability to subluxate the nucleus into the anterior chamber was advantageous, particularly in high-risk cases. With a large anterior segment, as in a myopic patient, a healthy cornea, and a relatively soft nucleus, the nucleus could be subluxated to a position anterior to the capsular bag, and then a deep anterior chamber phacoemulsification was performed while supporting the nucleus with a nucleus rotator. The larger anterior capsulectomy allowed an easier phacoemulsification, and no adverse effect was apparent in regard to intraocular lens centration. Fundus visibility was good, and the occasional case of capsular contraction syndrome disappeared. Capsular opacity rates appeared low, and a small randomized study suggested that they were somewhat lower than with the smaller anterior capsulectomy used in the past. The impact of capsulorhexis size on capsular opacity rate and postoperative inflammation remains controversial, with studies supporting both sides of the equation.

The next influence came from David Brown, MD, and William Maloney, MD, who have championed the concept of supracapsular phacoemulsification in which the nucleus is hydrodissected and tumbled before phacoemulsification. Although the technique was very efficient, it was not always easy to tumble the nucleus safely in all eyes. Also, more postoperative corneal edema occurred in these eyes compared with those treated with an endocapsular approach. However, use of this technique spurred the discovery that, rather than completing the tumbling of the entire nucleus, the nucleus could simply be supported in the plane of the iris and anterior capsular leaflet. Half of it could then be emulsified. With a much smaller nuclear remnant, the remaining half could be tumbled upside down and emulsified as in the classical supracapsular approach. The surgical technique was fast, simple, and safe. The following day the corneas of these patients were similarly clear compared with those treated with an endocapsular nuclear fracture approach. The author chose to call the technique "tilt and tumble" and refined it so that it could be taught effectively to residents, fellows, and other ophthalmologists with confidence. In the following paragraphs, this technique is described and illustrated in enough detail to allow an ophthalmologist to evaluate it for his or her own patients.

Indications

The indications for the tilt and tumble phacoemulsification technique are quite broad. It can be used with either a large or small pupil. Some surgeons favor it in small pupil settings where the nucleus can be tilted up such that the equator is resting in the center of a small pupil and then carefully emulsified away. It does require a larger continuous-tear anterior capsulectomy of at least 5 mm. If a small anterior capsulectomy is achieved, the hydrodissection step in which the nucleus is tilted can be dangerous, and the posterior capsule could be ruptured during the hydrodissection step. If a small anterior capsulectomy is created inadvertently, it is probably safest to convert to an endocapsular phacoemulsification technique or enlarge the capsulorhexis. If it is not possible to tilt the nucleus with either hydrodissection or manual technique, the surgeon should convert to an endocapsular approach. Occasionally the entire nucleus will subluxate into the anterior chamber. In this setting, if the cornea is healthy, the anterior chamber is roomy, and the nucleus is soft, then the phacoemulsification can be completed in the anterior chamber, supporting the nucleus away from the corneal endothelium. The nucleus can also be pushed back inferiorly over the capsular bag to allow the iris plane, tilt and tumble technique to be completed.

In patients with severely compromised endothelium, such as Fuchs' dystrophy or previous keratoplasty patients with a low endothelial cell count, endocapsular phacoemulsification is preferred to reduce endothelial trauma. In a normal eye, corneal clarity on the first postoperative day is excellent. Nevertheless, the tilting and tumbling maneuvers do increase the chance of endothelial cell contact of lens material, versus an endocapsular phacoemulsification. Therefore the endocapsular technique should be used in eyes with borderline corneas. This is a very good transition technique for teaching residents, fellows, and surgeons who are learning to phacoemulsification because it is easy to convert to a planned extracapsular cataract extraction with the nucleus partially subluxated above the anterior capsular flap at the iris plane.

Preoperative Preparation

The patient enters the anesthesia induction or preoperative area, and tetracaine drops are placed in both eyes. The placement of these drops increases the patient's comfort during the placement of the multiple dilating and preoperative medications, decreases blepharospasm, and also increases the corneal penetration of the drops to follow.

The eye is dilated with 2.5% neosynephrine and 1% cyclopentolate every 5 minutes for three doses. In addition, preoperative topical antibiotic and antiinflammatory drops are administered at the same time as dilation. We favor the combination of a preoperative topical antibiotic, topical steroid, and topical nonsteroidal agent. The rationale for this is to preload the eye with antibiotic and nonsteroidal drugs before surgery. The pharmacology of these drugs and the pathophysiology of postoperative infection and inflammation support this approach. An eye that is preloaded with antiinflammatories before the surgical insult is likely to demonstrate a much reduced postoperative inflammatory response. Topical steroids and nonsteroidal agents have been confirmed to be synergistic in the reduction of postoperative inflammation. In addition, the use of perioperative antibiotics appears to be supported by the literature as helpful in reducing the small chance of postoperative endophthalmitis. Because the patient will be sent home with the same drops used preoperatively, there is no additional cost.

The usual anesthesia is topical tetracaine reinforced with intraoperative intracameral 1% nonpreserved (methylparaben-free) Xylocaine. For patients with blepharospasm a "miniblock" O'Brien facial nerve anesthesia, using 2% Xylocaine with 150 units of hyaluronidase per 5 ml of Xylocaine, can be helpful in reducing squeezing. This block lasts 30 to 45 minutes and makes surgery easier for the patient and the surgeon. Patients are sedated before the block to eliminate any memory of discomfort. One way to determine when this facial nerve block might be useful is to ask the technicians to make a note in the chart when they have difficulty performing applanation pressures or an A-scan because of blepharospasm. In these patients a mini–facial nerve block can be helpful.

In younger anxious patients and in those with difficulty cooperating, a peribulbar block is performed. This decision is basically based on clinical impression. Naturally, general anesthesia is used for uncooperative patients and children. Although this is controversial, in some patients for whom general anesthesia is chosen and a significant bilateral cataract is present, Dr. Lindstrom will perform consecutive bilateral surgery, completely reprepping and starting with fresh instruments for the second eye. Again, this is a clinical decision weighing the risk-to-benefit ratio of operating on both eyes on the same day versus the risk of two general anesthetics.

In summary, in the induction area the patient's eye is dilated maximally and preloaded with antibiotic, steroid, and nonsteroidal antiinflammatory drops. Appropriate anesthesia is obtained. Ocular pressure can be used at the surgeon's discretion and may be performed even when using topical anesthesia. The patient is visited by the anesthetist, as well as the circulating nurse and the surgeon. Any questions are answered. The patient is then brought into the surgical suite.

On entering the surgical suite the patient table is centered on preplaced marks so that the bed is appropriately placed for microscope, surgeon, scrub nurse, and anesthetist access. We favor a wrist rest, and the patient's head is adjusted such that a ruler placed on the forehead and cheek will be parallel to the floor. The patient's head is stabilized with tape to the headboard to reduce unexpected movements, particularly if the patient falls asleep during the procedure and suddenly awakens. A second drop of tetracaine is placed in each eye. If the tetracaine is placed in each eye, blepharospasm is reduced. A periocular preparation with 5% povidone-iodine solution is completed. The ocular surface and fornices are prepped with povidone-iodine.

An aperture drape is helpful for topical anesthesia to increase comfort. When the drape is tucked under the lids, this often irritates the patient's eye and also reduces the malleability of the lids, decreasing exposure. Because it is important to isolate the meibomian glands and lashes, a reversible, solid blade speculum (Lindstrom-Chu speculum, Rhein Medical) may be used. With temporal and nasal approaches to the eye, the solid blades of the speculum are not in the way. In cases for which a superior approach is planned, a Tegaderm drape is used, tucking it under the lids. In these cases, a Kratz-Barraquer wire is useful because it enhances access to the globe. Nevertheless, we have been using a superior approach incision less often.

Balanced salt solution (BSS) is used in all cases. For the short duration of a phacoemulsification case, BSS Plus does not provide any clinically meaningful benefit. For assistance in dilation and perhaps hemostasis, 0.5 ml of the intracardiac nonpreserved (sodium bisulfate–free) epinephrine is placed in the bottle. Also, 1 ml (1000 units) of heparin sulfate is added to reduce the possibility of postoperative fibrin. This is also a good antiinflammatory and coating agent. At this dose there is no risk of enhancing bleeding or reducing hemostasis.

A final drop of tetracaine is placed in the operative eye, or the surface is irrigated with the nonpreserved Xylocaine. We do not like to use more than three drops of tetracaine or other topical anesthetic because excess softening of the epithelium can occur, resulting in punctate epithelial keratitis, corneal erosion, and delayed postoperative rehabilitation.

Operative Procedure

The patient is asked to look down. The globe is supported with a dry Merocel sponge, and a counterpuncture is performed superiorly at the 12 o'clock position with a Diamond stab knife (Osher/Storz). The incision is about 1 mm in length (Figure 17-1). Approximately 0.25 ml of 1% nonpreserved methylparaben-free Xylocaine is injected into the eye (Figure 17-2). Patients are advised that they will feel a "tingling" or "burning" for a second and then "the eye will go numb." This provides reassurance to patients that they will now have a totally anesthetized eye and should not anticipate any discomfort. They are told that they

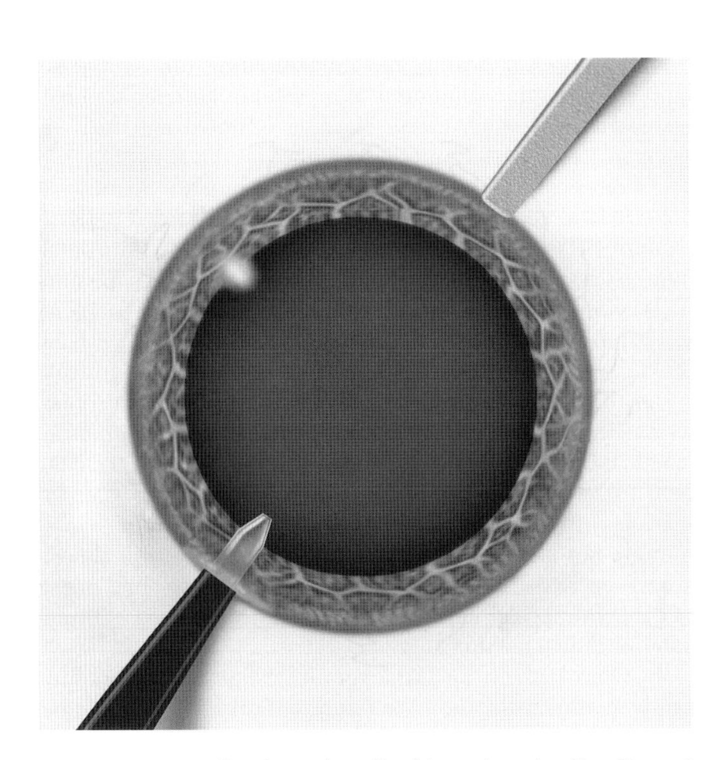

FIGURE 17-1 Counterpuncture site of 1 mm is made with a Diamond stab knife.

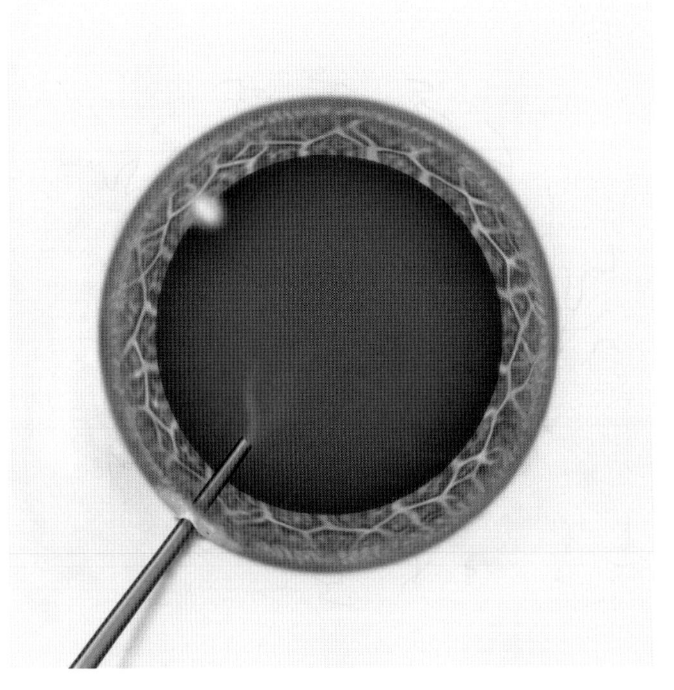

FIGURE 17-2 Preservative-free Xylocaine is injected intracamerally.

will feel some touch and fluid on the eye and will not feel anything sharp, and, if they do, supplemental anesthesia can be provided. This injection also firms up the eye for the clear corneal incision. We do not find it necessary to inject viscoelastic before constructing the corneal wound.

A temporal or nasal anterior limbal or posterior clear corneal incision is performed. Dr. Lindstrom performs a modified Langerman incision. A groove is made 400 to 500 μm deep into the perilimbal capillary plexus just anterior to the insertion of the conjunctiva. Care is taken not to incise the conjunctiva because this can result in ballooning during phacoemulsification and irrigation and aspiration. Some surgeons define this as a posterior clear corneal incision and others, as an anterior limbal incision. The anatomic landmark is the perilimbal capillary plexus and the insertion of the conjunctiva. When the groove is made, a small amount of capillary bleeding will occur. Because the incision is into a vascular area, long-term wound healing is expected to be stronger than it is with a true clear corneal incision. True clear corneal incisions, such as performed in radial keratotomy, clearly do not have the wound-healing capabilities that a limbal incision demonstrates when functioning blood vessels are present.

The anterior chamber is then entered parallel to the iris at a depth of approximately 300 μm or above the deepest portion of the groove. This creates a hinge-type or Langerman-type of incision (Figure 17-3). The preferred width of the incision is 1.75 to 2 mm, and Dr. Lindstrom has designed a keratome with Storz with two small black lines, which can serve as a guide to the surgeon in creating an appropriate width incision.

In right eyes the incision is temporal, and in left eyes, nasal. This allows the surgeon to sit in the same position for right and left eyes. The nasal cornea is thicker, has a higher endothelial cell count, and allows very good access for phacoemulsification. The nasal limbus is approximately 0.3 mm closer to the center of the cornea than the temporal limbus, and this can, in some cases where there is excess edema, reduce first-day postoperative vision more than one might anticipate with a temporal incision. In some patients, pooling can occur. For this reason, an aspirating speculum is useful. Tipping the head slightly to the left side is also helpful. Nonetheless, in left eyes a nasal, clear corneal approach is an excellent option, particularly for surgeons who find the left temporal position uncomfortable.

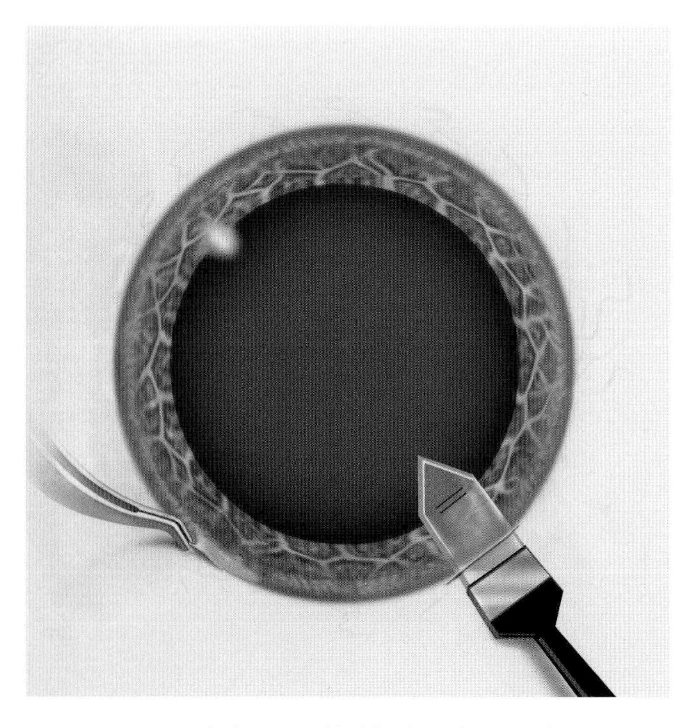

FIGURE 17-3 A clear corneal incision is made temporally in right eyes and nasally in left eyes.

The groove may be constructed by simply taking the keratome, tipping it up, and using the tip of the keratome. Some surgeons choose a guarded knife to create a consistently deep incision. An astigmatic keratotomy blade can be useful in this regard. This blade can also be helpful when patients have high astigmatism and an intraoperative astigmatic keratotomy is thought to be appropriate.

In some patients a corneal scleral incision may be safest, for example, in those who have had a previous radial keratotomy or demonstrate findings of peripheral corneal ulcerative keratitis; in some patients with very low endothelial cell counts; and in any case involving significant peripheral pathologic findings or thinning. The anterior limbal or posterior corneal incision described earlier can be made temporally, nasally, in the oblique meridian, or even superiorly without induction of significant corneal edema or endothelial cell loss.

With a corneal scleral incision, a small conjunctival flap is raised with a Westcott scissors. Before this step, anesthesia can be provided by holding a Merocel sponge soaked in tetracaine or nonpreserved Xylocaine in the area of the limbus where the conjunctival flap will be raised for 30 to 60 seconds. Mild cautery can be applied, or a Merocel sponge soaked in thrombin 1/1000 in BSS can be applied to effect hemostasis. If there is minimal capillary oozing, the mild bleeding can simply be ignored. Thrombin solution is also useful in anterior segment reconstructions when excess bleeding is noted and may be safely injected into the anterior chamber if diluted in BSS.

All clear corneal incisions larger than 4 mm are closed with a horizontal mattress, X, or single radial suture. The least amount of astigmatism will be induced with the horizontal mattress suture. A corneal scleral incision greater than 5.5 mm is also closed with one horizontal mattress suture. The incision, if 3 mm in length, tends to cause an induction of 0.25 ± 0.25 diopters of astigmatism. If it is placed on the steeper meridian, it can therefore be expected to reduce the astigmatism somewhere between 0 and 0.50 diopter. If the incision is 4 mm in length, there usually is a reduction in astigmatism of 0.50 ± 0.50 or 0 to 1.00 diopter if the incision is placed on the steeper meridian. In routine cataract surgery, incisions larger than 4 mm are not used. An incision in the 3-mm range will almost always be self-sealing. With modern injector systems, most foldable intraocular lenses can be implanted through a 3-mm anterior limbal incision.

In select patients an intraoperative astigmatic keratotomy can be performed at the 7- to 8-mm optical zone. This can be done at the beginning of the operation. The patient's astigmatism axis is marked carefully using an intraoperative surgical keratometer, which allows one to delineate the steeper and flatter meridian and not be concerned about globe rotation. One 2-mm incision at a 7- to 8-mm optical zone will correct 1 diopter of astigmatism, and two 2-mm incisions will correct 2 diopters of astigmatism in a patient who is of the age when cataracts develop. One 3-mm incision will correct 2 diopters, and two 3-mm incisions, 4 diopters. One can combine a 3 mm and 2 mm, correcting 3 diopters. Larger amounts of astigmatism can also be corrected using the Arc-T nomogram. Depending on the age of the patient, up to 8 diopters of astigmatism can be corrected with two 90-degree arcs. Many surgeons have moved to a more peripheral, corneal limbal arcuate incision, but Dr. Lindstrom favors the 7- to 8-mm optical zone because of his years of experience with this approach. Certainly a variation in response is seen, but there have not been any significant induced complications with this approach. The outcome goal is 1 diopter or less of astigmatism in the preoperative axis. It is preferable to undercorrect rather than overcorrect. The key in astigmatism surgery is "axis, axis, axis." If one is not careful in preoperative planning and the incisions are placed more than 15 degrees off axis, one is better avoiding this approach.

The anterior chamber is constituted with a viscoelastic. Our studies have not found any significant difference between one viscoelastic and another in regard to postoperative endothelial cell counts. Ocucoat has proved to be an excellent viscoelastic, which can also be used to coat the epithelial surface during surgery. This eliminates the need for continuous irrigation with BSS. It gives a very clear view and is also economically a good choice in most settings. Amvisc Plus also works well and 0.8 ml of it can be obtained at a fair price.

Next a relatively large-diameter continuous-tear anterior capsulectomy is fashioned (Figures 17-4 and 17-5). This can be made with a cystotome or forceps. The optimal size is 5 to 6 mm in diameter and inside the insertion of the zonules (usually at 7 mm). Larger is better than smaller because there is less subcapsular epithelium and thus lower risk of capsular opacification. In addition, a larger capsulorhexis makes for an easier cataract operation. With this technique there has not been any change in the incidence of intraocular lens decentration. With some intraocular lenses the capsule will seal down to the posterior capsule around the loops rather than being symmetrically placed over the anterior surface of the intraocular lens. These eyes do extremely well, and this might be preferable to having the capsule anterior to the optic. This is also a controversial position.

Hydrodissection is then performed using a Pearce hydrodissection cannula on a 3-cc syringe filled with BSS. Slow continuous hydrodissection is performed, gently lifting the anterior capsular rim until a fluid wave is seen. At this point, irrigation is continued until the nucleus tilts on one side, up and out of the capsular bag (Figure 17-6). If the capsule is retracted at approximately the 7:30 position with the hydrodissection cannula, usually the nucleus will tilt superiorly. If it tilts in another position, it is simply rotated until it is facing the incision (Figure 17-7).

Once the nucleus it tilted, some additional viscoelastic can be injected under the nucleus, pushing the iris and capsule back. Also, additional viscoelastic can be placed over the nuclear edge to protect the endothelium. The nucleus is emulsified outside-in while supporting the nucleus in the iris plane with a second instrument, such as a Rhein Medical or Storz-Lindstrom Star or Lindstrom Trident nucleus rotator (Figure 17-8). Once half the nucleus is removed, the remaining half is tumbled upside down and attacked from the opposite pole (Figure 17-9). Again it is supported in the iris plane until the emulsification is

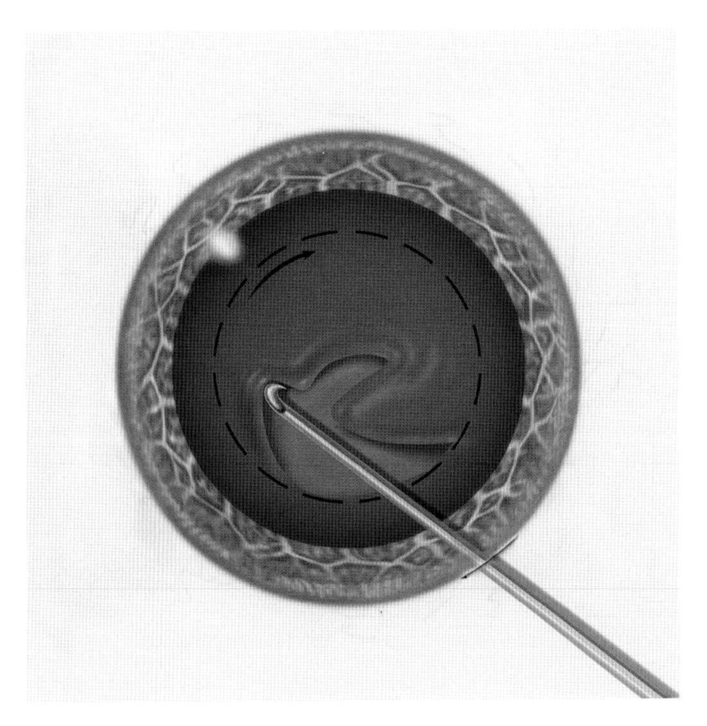

FIGURE 17-4 Continuous curvilinear capsulotomy is made with a cystotome.

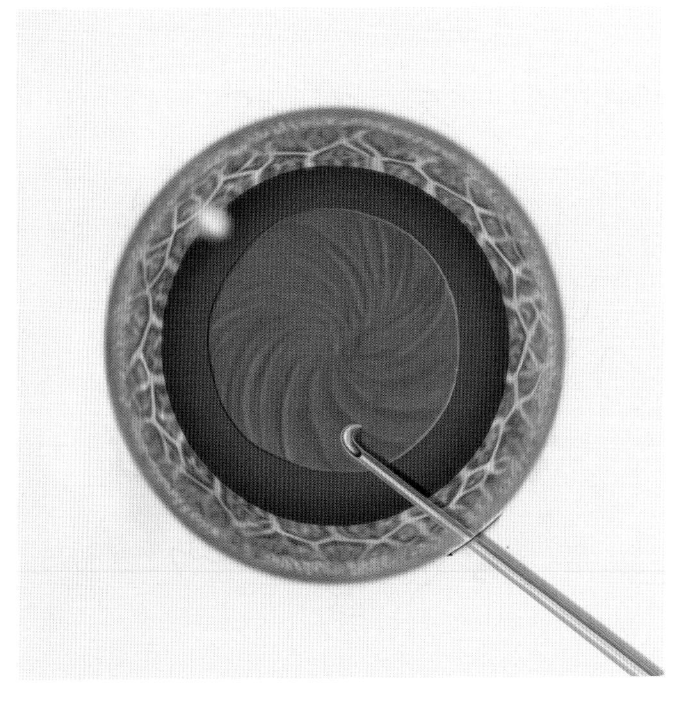

FIGURE 17-5 Capsulotomy is optimally 5 to 6 mm in diameter.

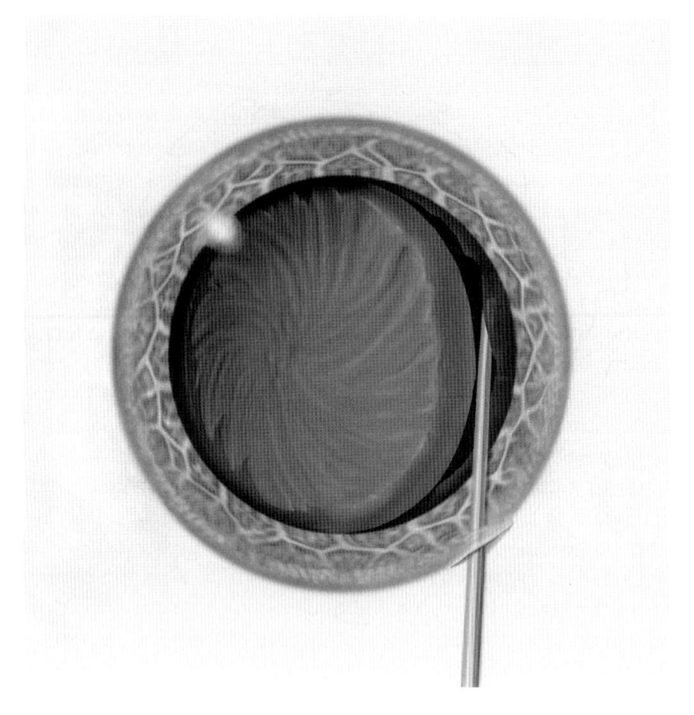

FIGURE 17-6 Continuous slow hydrodissection leads to tilting of the nucleus out of the bag.

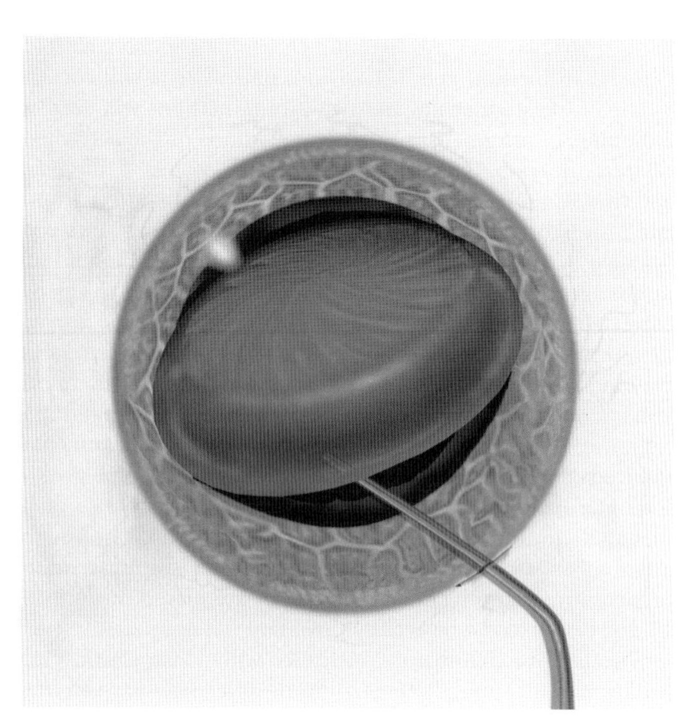

FIGURE 17-7 Nucleus is rotated to face the incision.

completed (Figure 17-10). Alternatively the nucleus can be rotated and emulsified from the outside edge in, in a carousel or cartwheel type of technique. Finally, in some cases, the nucleus can be continuously emulsified in the iris plane if there is good "followability" until the entire nucleus is gone.

This a very fast and safe technique, and as mentioned before, it is a modification of the iris plane technique taught by Richard Kratz, MD, in the late 1970s and 1980s. Surgery times now range between 5 and 10 minutes with this approach rather than 10 to 15 minutes for endocapsular phacoemulsification. In addition,

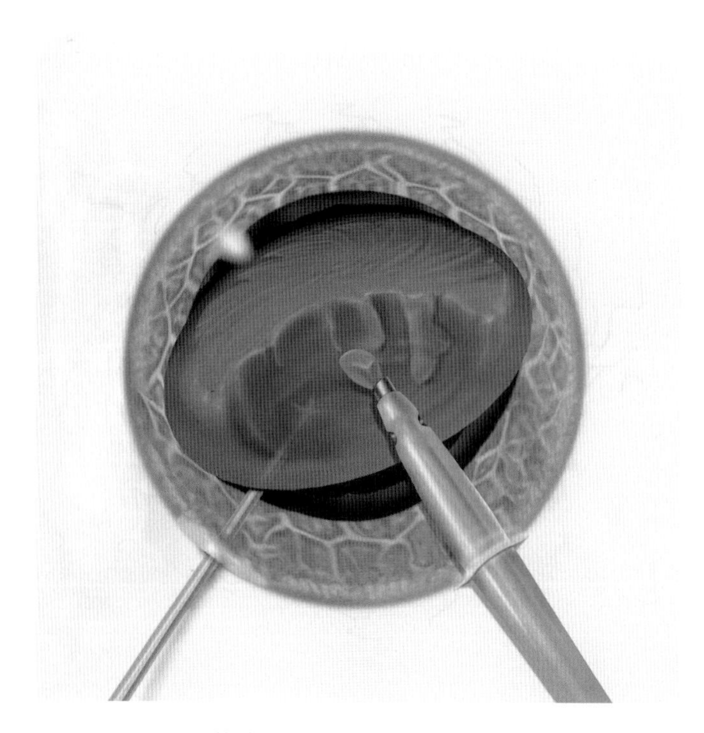

FIGURE 17-8 Nucleus is supported during phacoemulsification with a second instrument.

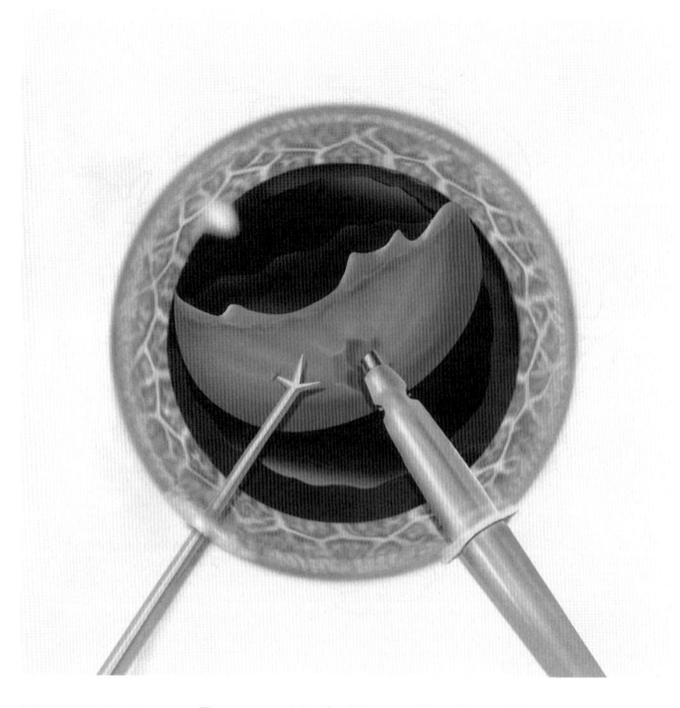

FIGURE 17-9 The second half of the nucleus is tumbled upside down.

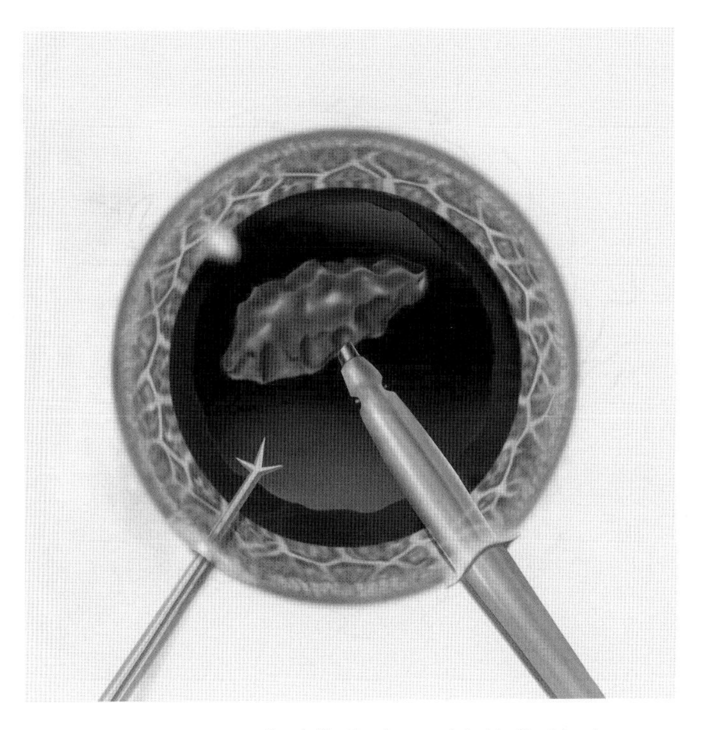

FIGURE 17-10 Emulsification is completed in the iris plane.

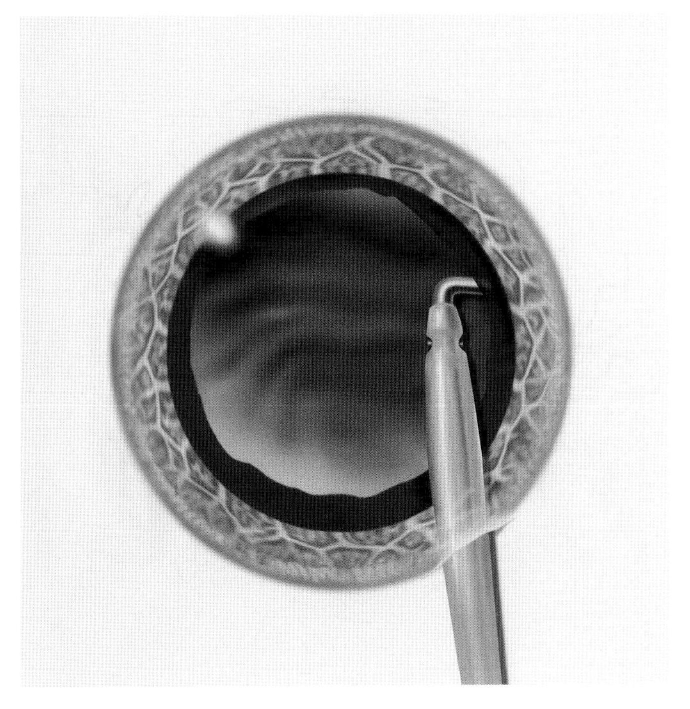

FIGURE 17-11 Subincisional cortex is removed with a right-angled tip.

our capsular tear rate is now less than 1%. Therefore we find this technique to be easier, faster, and safer. In this technique the phacoemulsification tip is closer to the iris margin and also somewhat closer to the corneal endothelium; however, the margin of error is significantly greater in regard to the posterior capsule. Care must be taken to position the nucleus away from the corneal endothelium and away from the iris margin when using this approach.

If the nucleus does not tilt with simple hydrodissection, it can be tilted with viscoelastic or a second instrument such as a nuclear rotator, Graether collar button, or hydrodissection cannula.

When using this approach of phacoemulsification with the Storz Premier instrument, we use a vacuum of 60 mm Hg and an anterior chamber maintainer pressure of 60 mm Hg. We favor the Storz MicroFlow Plus needle with a 30-degree bevel.

When using a peristaltic machine, a slightly higher vacuum in the range of 80 to 100 mm of Hg is used. It is best to maintain a relatively high bottle with some overflow of fluid. Again a 30-degree bevel needle is appropriate for this approach. When using tilt and tumble, very high vacuum settings are not necessary and may be inappropriate. The reason is that the iris margin is in the vicinity of the phacoemulsification tip, and it is possible to core through the nucleus and aspirate the iris margin if very high vacuums are used.

The dual-function Bausch & Lomb Millennium is also excellent for all cataract techniques, including tilt and tumble. The vacuum is set with a range of 60 to 100 mm Hg and the ultrasound power from 10% to 50% with the Storz Millennium. The foot pedal is arranged so that the surgeon has control over ultrasound on the vertical or pitch motion of the foot pedal; then on the yaw or right motion of the foot pedal, the surgeon will have vacuum control. This allows efficient emulsification, and the Millennium is currently our preferred machine. The MicroFlow Plus needle with a 30-degree angle tip works well with the Millennium.

Following completion of nuclear removal, the cortex is removed with the irrigation-aspiration handpiece. A 0.3-mm tip and the universal handpiece with interchangeable tips are preferred. A curvilinear tip is used for most cortex removal. Subincisional cortex can be aspirated with a Lindstrom right-angle sand-blasted tip currently manufactured by Rhein and Storz (Figure 17-11). If there is significant debris or plaque on the posterior capsule, some polishing and vacuum cleaning can be attempted but not so aggressively as to risk capsular tears. Many times an unexpected small burr or sharp defect on the irrigation-aspiration tip results in a capsular tear after a case that was otherwise well done.

The anterior chamber is reconstituted with viscoelastic, and the intraocular lens is inserted using an injector system (Figures 17-12 and 17-13). We prefer the three-piece silicone lenses, which are injectable through a 3-mm incision. In select cases an acrylic implant is chosen, such as in patients with diabetic retinopathy.

Excess viscoelastic is removed with irrigation and aspiration. Pushing back on the intraocular lens and slowly turning the irrigation and aspiration to the right and left two or three times allow a fairly complete removal of viscoelastic under the intraocular lens.

We favor injection of a miotic and tend to prefer carbachol over Miochol at this time because it is more effective in reducing postoperative intraocular tension spikes and has a longer duration of action. It is best to dilute the carbachol 5 to 1 or an excessively small pupil may be obtained, which results

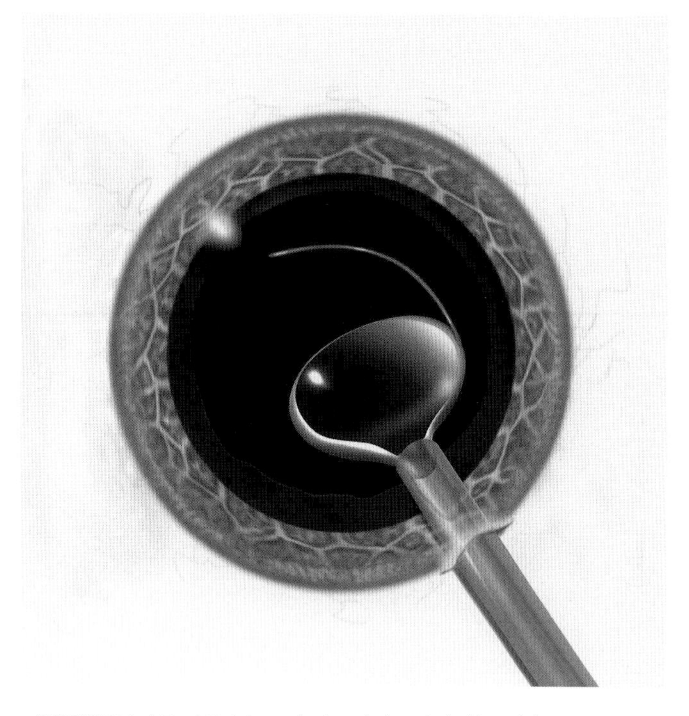

FIGURE 17-12 Intraocular lens is inserted with an injector system.

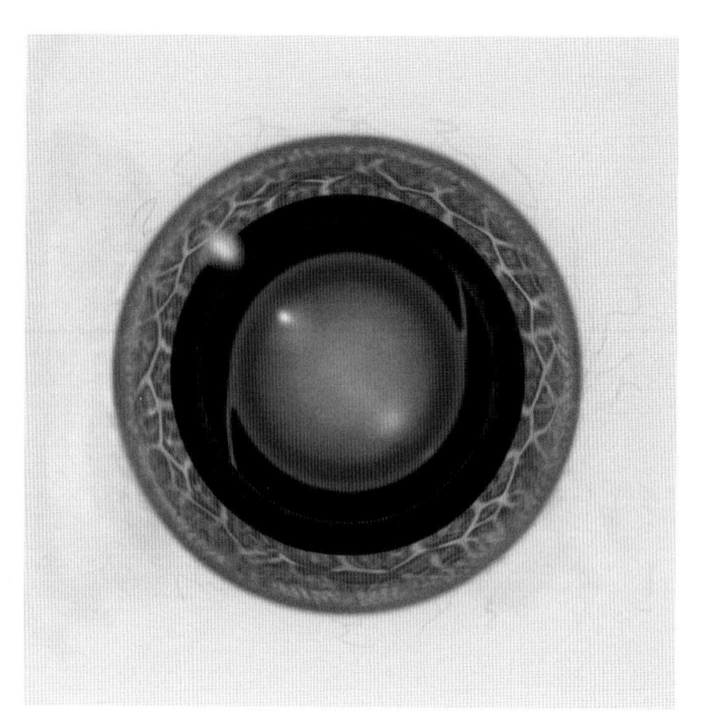

FIGURE 17-13 Lens is centered in the capsular bag.

in dark vision for the patient at night for 1 to 2 days. The anterior chamber is then refilled through the counterpuncture, and the incision is inspected. If the chamber remains well constituted and there is no spontaneous leak from the incision, wound hydration is not necessary. If there is some shallowing in the anterior chamber and a spontaneous leak, wound hydration is performed by injecting BSS peripherally into the incision and hydrating it to push the edges together. We suspect that within a few minutes these clear corneal or posterior limbal incisions seal, much as a LASIK flap will stick down, through the negative swelling pressure of the cornea and capillary action. It is important to leave the eye slightly firm at 20 mm Hg or so to reduce the side effects of hypotony and also help the internal valve incision appropriately seal.

At completion of the procedure, another drop of antibiotic, steroid and nonsteroidal agent, is placed on the eye. In addition, one drop of an antihypertensive such as levobunolol (Betagan) or brimonidine (Alphagan) is applied to reduce postoperative intraocular tension spikes.

Postoperative Care

No patch is routinely used for the topical and intracameral approach. If a miniblock of the lids has been performed, it will wear off in 30 to 45 minutes, and usually lid function is adequate for a normal blink at the completion of the procedure. Patients are advised that they will have some erythropsia, meaning that they will see a pink afterimage for the rest of the day, but usually this resolves by the next morning. They are also told that their vision may be a little dark at night from the miotic and not to be concerned if they wake up at night and their vision seems dimmer.

The patient is seen on the first postoperative day and at approximately 2 to 3 weeks after the operation. At this time a refraction, slit lamp, and funduscopic examination is performed. If no inflammation is present, patients are seen again in 1 year. If at 3 weeks inflammation still persists, additional postoperative antiinflammatory medications are recommended, and the patient is asked to return again at 2 to 3 months after the operation.

Topical antibiotic, steroid, and nonsteroidal agents are used twice a day, usually requiring a 5-ml bottle and 3 to 4 weeks of therapy. Occasionally a second bottle of steroid and nonsteroidal drops is necessary if flare and cell persist at the 3-week examination. There are minimal restrictions, including a request to avoid swimming and avoid very heavy lifting for 2 weeks. Many patients are given half-glasses the first postoperative day, allowing functional vision at distance and near. The ideal postoperative refractive spherical equivalent for a monofocal lens is –0.62 diopters with less than 0.50 diopters of astigmatism in the same axis as existed preoperatively. Most patients can see 20/30+ and J3+ with this type of correction. Monovision can be used in the appropriate settings. Good results can also be obtained with the Allergan ARRAY multifocal intraocular lens. In this setting we target plano to –0.25 diopter with minimal astigmatism.

The second eye is done at 1 month or greater postoperatively except in rare situations. Any neodymium:yttrium-aluminum-garnet (Nd:YAG) lasers are deferred for 90 days to allow the blood-aqueous barrier to become intact and capsular fixation to be firm.

Conclusion

In summary, the key points of tilt and tumble phacoemulsification are listed in Table 17-1. We hope other surgeons will find this approach to cataract surgery useful. These techniques must be personalized, and every surgeon will find that slight variations in technique are required to achieve optimum results for their own individual patients in their own individual environment. Continuous efforts at incremental improvement result in meaningful advances in our ability to help the cataract patient obtain rapid, safe, visual recovery following surgery.

TABLE 17-1

Key Points in the Technique of Tilt and Tumble Phacoemulsification

1. The procedure may be performed with a clear cornea, topical anesthetic approach.
2. A medium to large capsulorrhexis is necessary.
3. Gentle continuous hydrodissection will prolapse the nucleus out of the bag.
4. The nucleus is phacoemulsified in the iris plane while being supported from beneath with a second instrument.
5. Phacoemulsification is performed away from the capsule, significantly decreasing the risk of capsular rupture.

Pars Plana Lensectomy for Primary Extraction and Retained Lens Fragments

18

Michael G. Morley, MD
Gregory M. Sulkowski

The two most common indications for pars plana lensectomy are (1) a significantly subluxated crystalline lens and (2) retained nuclear fragments in the vitreous after incomplete cataract extraction.

Management of the Subluxated Crystalline Lens

Trauma is the most common cause of a subluxated crystalline lens. A subluxated lens (Figure 18-1) may also occur in isolation or as part of a systemic condition such as Marfan's syndrome, homocystinuria, and the Weill-Marchesani syndrome. Less commonly, a subluxated lens may be associated with uveitis, pseudoexfoliation, aniridia, Rieger's syndrome, megalocornea, syphilis, Ehlers-Danlos syndrome, inherited retinal disorders, and, finally, idiopathic causes.[1-3] The detection of lens subluxation involves careful examination in both dilated and undilated states. In the undilated state, iridodonesis and phacodonesis may be more apparent than in the dilated state because of ciliary body and iris retraction during cycloplegia. In the dilated state, displacement of the lens from the visual axis confirms the diagnosis of a subluxated crystalline lens. If surgery is planned, *examination in the prone position* is essential to determine the extent of zonular damage. Gravity may pull the lens more posteriorly into the vitreous cavity. A lens that may initially appear approachable from the anterior segment may sink deeply into the vitreous in the prone position and be best handled from the pars plana approach.

Following the detection of a subluxated lens, a search must be made to determine the underlying cause of the subluxation. Uncovering the cause of the subluxation is not a matter of academic interest alone. Patients with Marfan's syndrome require perioperative cardiovascular evaluations and antibiotics for prophylaxis against endocarditis. Patients with homocystinuria are prone to life-threatening thrombotic events, especially with general anesthesia, and require anticoagulation to reduce morbidity and mortality. Although trauma is the most common cause, a history of past trauma may be incidental, and other causes should be considered. The patient's history and family history may provide clues. Specific questions regarding any history of trauma, seizures, or systemic disease should be asked. The direction and laterality of the dislocation may also provide diagnostic clues (up-and-out lens dislocation in Marfan's syndrome, down-and-in lens subluxation in homocystinuria). Musculoskeletal evaluation and aortic and cardiac echocardiograms may be performed to rule out Marfan's syndrome. A sodium nitroprusside test of the urine will rule out homocystinuria. An FTA-ABS test may be obtained to rule out syphilis (Table 18-1).

Treatment Options

Treatment of a substantially subluxated clear crystalline lens generally involves one of four strategies (Table 18-2). The first treatment option involves correcting the optical defects associated with the subluxation. A subluxated lens may cause a myopic shift as a result of the increased radius of the lens from loss of zonular traction. Also, astigmatism and prism effect may contribute to visual disturbance. Careful refraction through either the phakic or aphakic portion of the pupil is the first and simplest treatment method.[4] Partially occluding contact lenses have also been developed, which can be used to occlude either the phakic or aphakic portion of the lens to minimize diplopia.

The second treatment modality uses a medical approach of either mydriasis or miosis.[4] Mydriatics are used to enlarge the aphakic portion of the pupil to allow the aforementioned optical corrections. However, the dilator muscle may be absent or weakened in some patients with syndromes associated with subluxated lenses, and this method is not always fruitful.[5] Miosis may sometimes be used to minimize diplopia and reduce the pupillary aperture to confine the visual axis to a purely phakic or aphakic portion.

The third category of treatment involves the use of laser. The argon or neodymium: yttrium-aluminum-garnet (Nd:YAG) lasers may be used to create an optical iridotomy or iridoplasty that enlarges the aphakic portion of the pupillary aperture.[6] Alternatively, Nd:YAG laser zonulysis has been described as a technique to further displace a partially subluxed lens with the goal being to enlarge the aphakic portion of the pupillary opening.[7,8] The Nd:YAG laser zonulysis may result in 1- to 3-mm movement of the crystalline lens out of the visual axis. Formed vitreous may prevent shifting of the lens despite laser zonulysis. The lens movement may not be apparent for a week or more after laser treatment. The data describing results following

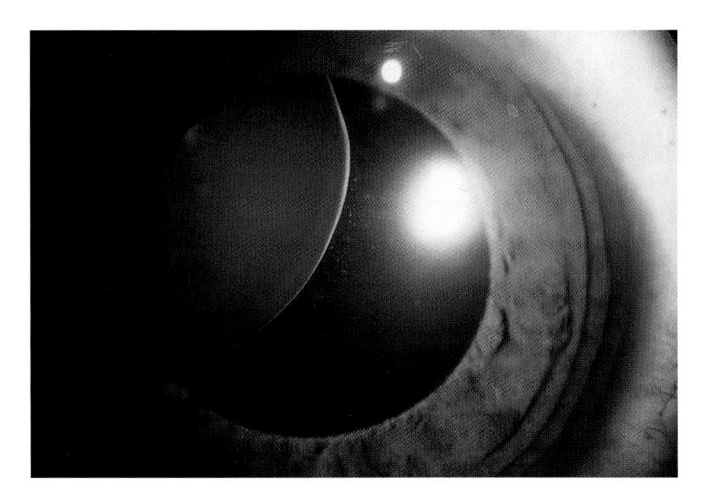

FIGURE 18-1 Clinical photograph of subluxed crystalline lens.

Nd:YAG laser zonulysis is sparse and with limited follow-up.[7,8] Only seven patients (10 eyes) have been reported. Laser iridoplasty and iridotomy also have very limited data and follow-up reporting.

Surgical removal of the subluxated lens is the fourth treatment modality available. Surgery is recommended when dislocation causes unacceptable symptoms not amenable to optical, medical, or laser therapy.

TABLE 18-1

Systemic Conditions Commonly Associated with Subluxed Crystalline Lenses

MARFAN'S SYNDROME

- Up-and-out lens dislocation
- Tall stature
- Arachnodactyly
- Aortic aneurysm and cardiomyopathy
- Retinal detachment
- Autosomal dominant inheritance

HOMOCYSTINURIA

- Down-and-in lens subluxation
- Marfanoid habitus
- Mental retardation
- Thrombosis
- Retinal detachment
- Autosomal recessive inheritance

WEILL-MARCHESANI SYNDROME

- Microspherophakia
- Short fingers and stature
- Myopia
- Seizures
- Autosomal recessive inheritance

Phacoemulsification of a Subluxated Lens from the Anterior Segment

A minimally subluxated cataract (i.e., less than one quadrant of zonular disruption or less than 1- to 2-mm displacement) can be successfully removed with phacoemulsification with delicate technique, and an intraocular lens (IOL) can be placed.[9,10] This decision depends on the surgeon's experience in dealing with phacoemulsification in the presence of subluxation and the amount of subluxation. A relatively large capsulorhexis should be made so that the nucleus can be tilted anteriorly if necessary. Hydrodissection and reduced vacuum and irrigation levels can help reduce zonular stress. Iris retractors may be used to fix the anterior capsulorhexis relative to the sclera, which stabilizes the capsular bag.[11] Alternatively, a capsular tension ring may help stabilize the capsule during phacoemulsification of a lens with zonular dehiscence or dialysis.[12,13] The phacoemulsification may be performed either "in the bag" or "out of the bag" depending on the surgeon's preference. Prolapsing the nucleus in the anterior chamber with gentle hydrodissection will allow phacoemulsification in the iris plane or deep anterior chamber while the corneal endothelium is protected by abundant viscoelastic solution. A 7-mm IOL optic should be used to minimize symptoms if any decentration occurs. The IOL can be placed in the bag or in the sulcus, and rotation should be avoided. Some surgeons advocate placing the haptics in the sulcus where there is zonular support and inserting the optic through the capsulorhexis (like a button through a button hole). In some cases, an anterior chamber (AC) IOL or scleral-sutured posterior chamber (PC) IOL will be needed. A vitrectomy should be performed if the vitreous presents to the anterior chamber.

TABLE 18-2

Four Treatment Options for Subluxed Clear Crystalline Lens

1. Correction of optical defects
   - Aphakic spectacles; correction of myopic shift, astigmatism, or prism caused by lens subluxation
   - Occluding contact lens
2. Medical intervention
   - Mydriatics
   - Miotics
3. Laser therapy
   - Argon or Nd:YAG optical iridotomy
   - Nd:YAG zonulolysis
4. Surgical removal of subluxed lens
   - Anterior approach phacoemulsification
   - Pars plana lensectomy

Nd:YAG, Neodymium:yttrium-aluminum-garnet.

Pars Plana Lensectomy for Subluxated Lens

A pars plana approach should be considered if there is enough zonular disruption or subluxation to make an anterior approach unsafe.

The pars plana approach involves a standard three-port vitrectomy with an infusion port in the inferotemporal quadrant and two superior sclerotomies to allow for the illumination source and either a vitreous cutter or a pars plana phacoemulsification

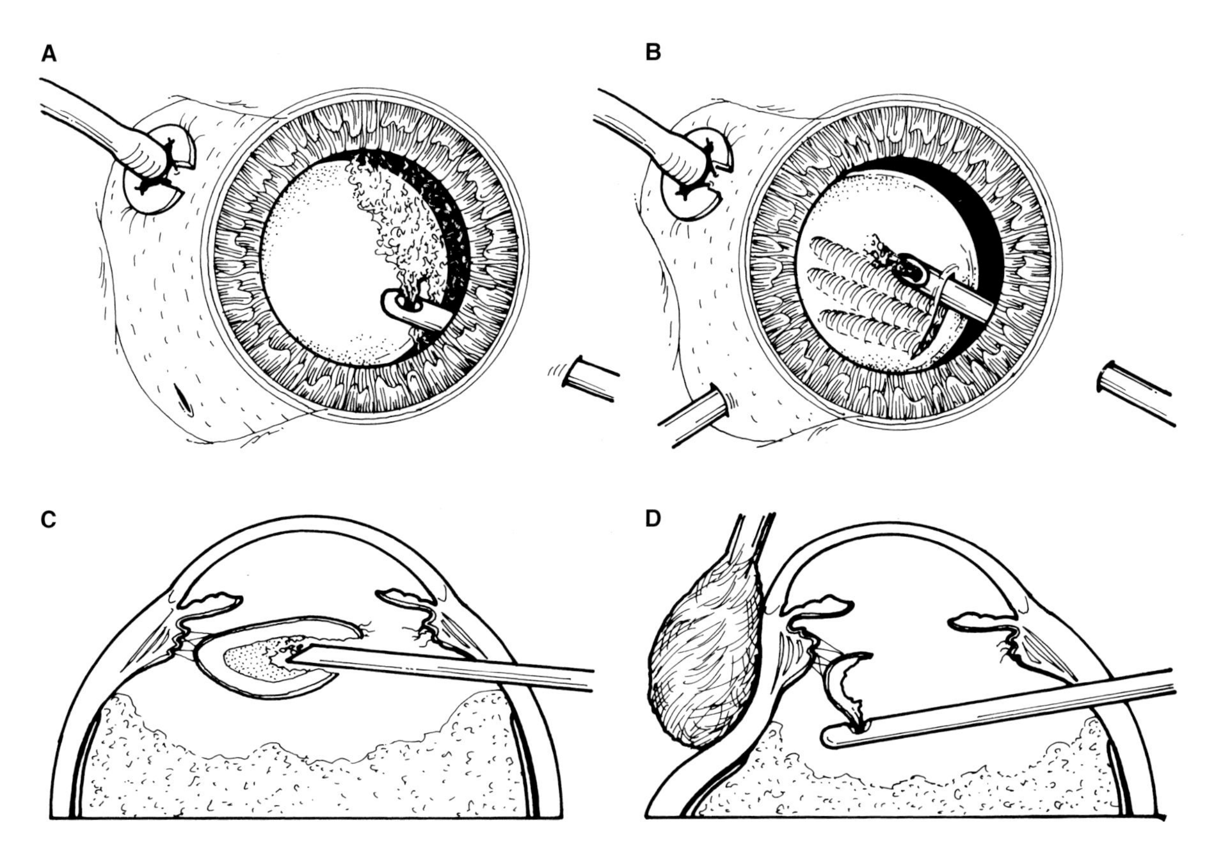

FIGURE 18-2 Drawing of pars plana lensectomy. **A,** Pars plana vitrectomy to remove loose vitreous humor in the anterior chamber. **B,** Ultrasonic fragmentation of the lens nucleus as viewed from the operating microscope. **C,** Cross-sectional diagram of pars plana phacoemulsification of the nucleus. **D,** Scleral depression used to bring peripheral capsular and cortical remnants into view.

tip (Figure 18-2). Depending on the density of the nucleus, the lens may be phacoemulsified or aspirated with the vitreous cutter. The limbal approach involves an anterior chamber infusion cannula and a second limbal incision to allow for a suction cutter (Figure 18-3). The disadvantage of the limb approach is that if any fragments should fall posteriorly, they are not retrievable without converting to a standard pars plana approach. Vitreous to the wound is more likely to occur with the limbal approach as well. With either approach, an IOL may be placed, that is, an AC IOL, a sulcus-fixed PC IOL, or a capsular fixated PC IOL depending on the circumstances and capsular support.

Associated Considerations

Patients with Marfan's syndrome and homocystinuria are predisposed to the development of retinal detachments.[1] The retina must be carefully examined preoperatively, and any retinal breaks must be treated before surgical removal of the subluxed lens. Following surgery, the retina must be reexamined and any breaks treated with cryopexy or laser photocoagulation.

Many patients with subluxated lenses are children.[14] The pars plana does not attain its full adult size until the age of 7. Thus surgical intervention must keep pediatric ocular anatomy in mind. A subluxated lens in a young patient may be associated with amblyopia. Patching for amblyopia should be initiated when necessary.

Glaucoma may also be seen in association with subluxed crystalline lenses, and careful measurement of the intraocular pressure and observation of the optic nerve are necessary. Pupillary block may occur with lens subluxation. This is treated with a peripheral iridotomy as in aphakic pupillary block glaucoma.

Results

The early studies reporting the surgical results following intracapsular cataract extraction and other methods showed a high rate of postoperative complications, including a retinal detachment rate of 20%.[15] In the past decade, techniques have improved, so surgical removal of a subluxated lens is a reasonable option[16-19] (Table 18-3).

Vitrectomy for Dislocated Nuclear Fragments Following Cataract Surgery

The second major indication for the anterior segment surgeon to consider a pars plana lensectomy is retained nuclear fragments following cataract surgery (Figure 18-4). Dislocation of nuclear fragments during the phacoemulsification is an uncommon but potentially serious complication.[20]

Retained nuclear fragments in the vitreous cavity almost invariably incite an inflammatory response, which can result in

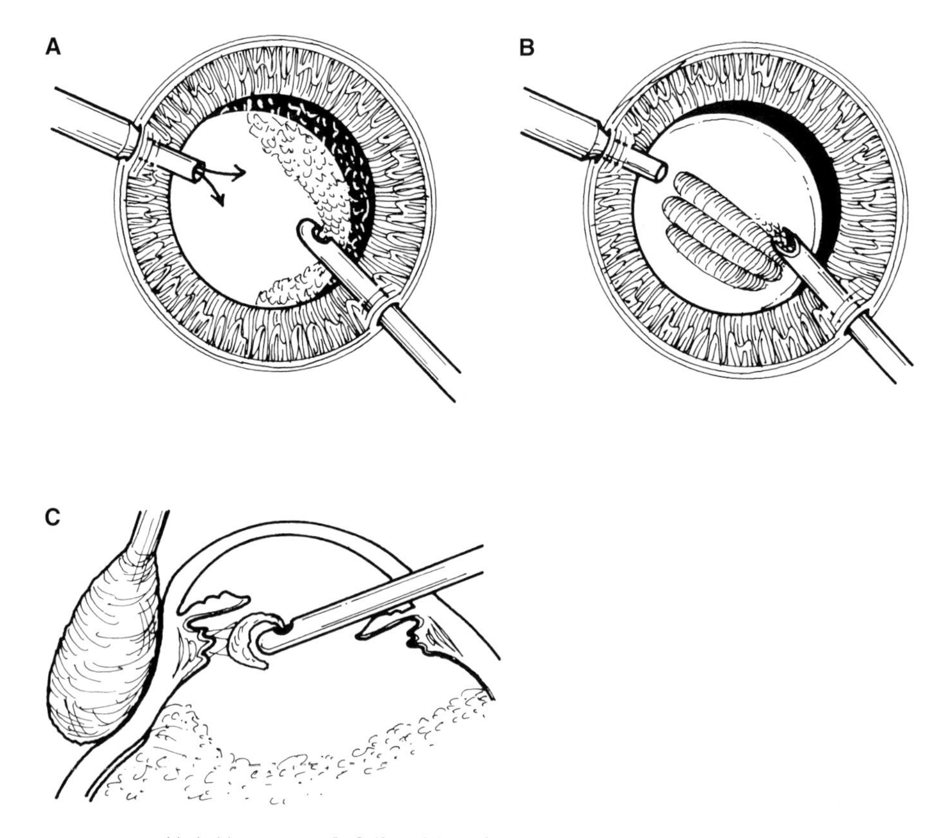

FIGURE 18-3 Limbal lensectomy. **A,** Self-retaining infusion line is placed through the peripheral limbus, and the vitreous cutter is used to remove loose vitreous humor in the anterior chamber. **B,** Phacoemulsification is performed. For soft lenses, a vitreous cutter can be used. **C,** Scleral depression is used to bring peripheral capsular and cortical remnants to the vitreous cutter.

cystoid macular edema, uveitis, corneal decompensation, glaucoma, and retinal detachment. Left untreated, blindness often results.[21] However, recent advances in vitreoretinal surgical techniques and instrumentation make a good visual outcome possible following this complication.[22-27]

All cataract surgeons will eventually encounter a ruptured capsule and vitreous admixed with cataract fragments. Lens fragments may dislocate at almost any point during the cataract procedure, including viscoelastic insertion, capsulorhexis, hydrodissection, and phacoemulsification. Wisely managing this complication will maximize the opportunity for a good visual outcome (Table 18-4).

Small amounts of cortical material in the vitreous cavity will resorb with time and can be safely observed. Large amounts of

TABLE 18-3

Subluxed Lenses

1. Examine dilated, undilated, and prone.
2. Consider systemic workup to rule out Marfan's syndrome and homocystinuria. Trauma may be a "red herring."
3. Use optical and pharmacologic methods first, if appropriate.
4. If less than one quadrant of zonular dehiscence, can use phacoemulsification or extracapsular cataract extraction, depending on the surgeon's comfort. If more than one quadrant, usually use a pars plana approach.
5. Place an AC or PC IOL, depending on capsular support.
6. Use pars plana approach for more significantly subluxed lenses.
7. Subluxed lenses are associated with conditions that have a high incidence of retinal detachment, so check retina before and after surgery.
8. Because patients with subluxed lenses are often children, keep anatomy and amblyopia in mind.

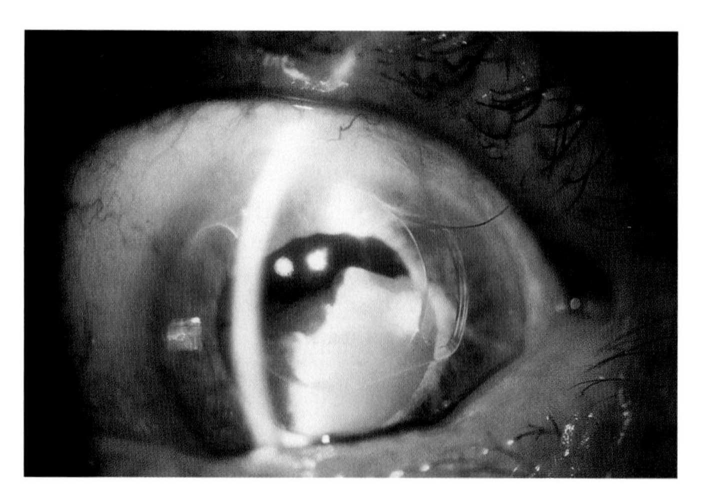

FIGURE 18-4 Slit lamp photograph of dislocated nuclear fragment resting behind an anterior chamber intraocular lens.

TABLE 18-4

What To Do When a Nucleus Is Lost

1. First, do no harm! Avoid aggressive pursuit of dislocated nuclear fragments.
2. If posterior dislocation of nuclear material occurs:
   a. Clean anterior segment of cortex and vitreous.
   b. Place an IOL.
   c. Close wound securely.
3. Use an AC IOL, capsule-fixated PC IOL, sulcus-fixed PC IOL, or transscleral sutured PC IOL.
4. Make a prompt referral to a vitreoretinal surgeon. Do not procrastinate if significant lens fragments remain in the eye.

AC, Anterior chamber; *IOL,* intraocular lens; *PC,* posterior chamber.

TABLE 18-5

Mistakes to Avoid with Dislocated Cataract Fragments

1. Do not go fishing for retained fragments intraoperatively.
2. Do not wait too long for cataract fragments to resorb when inflammation and increased IOP are present. Make a timely referral if indicated, especially if increased IOP and inflammation are present.

IOP, Intraocular pressure.

cortex can incite a prolonged inflammatory response, which can have adverse sequelae such as cystoid macular edema, and are often best removed with vitrectomy. Nuclear fragments, however, will not resorb but will incite a severe and prolonged inflammatory response. In general, nuclear fragments must be removed. Failure to remove nuclear fragments results in a very poor visual outcome.[21]

Intraoperative Management of Dislocation of Nuclear Fragments

The disturbing sight of cataract fragments floating in the vitreous cavity may induce a surgeon to perform extraordinary maneuvers to retrieve the fragments at the potential expense of creating vitreoretinal complications (Table 18-5). Aggressive use of the lens loop, phaco probe, or cryoprobe or vigorous irrigation of the vitreous cavity should be avoided.[27]

The patients with the worst visual outcomes are those with retinal detachments.[28] Aggressive pursuit of the dislocated nucleus can result in retinal tears, giant retinal tears, and retinal detachments.[29] These patients have a dramatically poorer visual outcome.[30]

Cortical remnants in the anterior vitreous can be removed with the vitreous cutter by the anterior segment surgeon. However, nuclear fragments in the vitreous cannot be phacoemulsified because of vitreous occlusion of the suction port, and neither can the hard nuclear fragment be aspirated adequately to be cut with a mechanical vitrector. If the nuclear fragment is in the anterior chamber, microinstruments or viscoelastic substance may be used to deliver the fragments. A nuclear fragment that remains in the anterior chamber postoperatively will cause uveitis and corneal edema and must be removed surgically.[31]

If the nucleus has sunk posteriorly, the goal should be to clear the anterior chamber of the vitreous and cortex, place an IOL, if possible, and close the eye. The nucleus should not be pursued posteriorly with a limbal approach because of potential vitreoretinal complications. A pars plana extraction of the fragments is a safer and more effective technique for removing the fragments, and the outcomes are generally good.

The type of IOL placed will depend on the remaining capsular support. If sufficient residual capsular support and good zonular integrity are present, a PC IOL should be inserted either in the bag or in the sulcus. Alternatively, if capsular support is not sufficient, a sulcus-sutured PC IOL or an AC IOL may be used. After the vitreous to the wound has been cleared and the lens has been placed, the cataract wound should be closed in routine fashion. A good visual outcome is likely if a dislocated nucleus is managed properly.

The timing of the vitreoretinal intervention has been debated in the literature.[25,26] Some investigators have noted that early intervention is helpful as evidenced by a lower incidence of postoperative glaucoma and a better visual outcome. Others advocate medical management of inflammation and intraocular pressure before surgical intervention. Most studies do not find a significant difference between early (<1 week) and late (>1 week) vitrectomy. Urgent, but not emergent, referral is probably indicated in cases with dislocated nuclear fragments. Vitreoretinal referral is best made within several days following cataract surgery. It is not necessary that the retained nuclear fragments be removed on the same day as cataract surgery.

More than one third of patients with retained lens fragments have an intraocular pressure greater than 30 mm Hg. Vitrectomy is curative for most of those patients, but a small number will require ongoing medical therapy for glaucoma.[32]

Techniques for Removing Intravitreal Lens Fragments

A standard three-port vitrectomy is carried out to remove all the vitreous within the vitreous cavity (Figure 18-5). Any vitreous strands to the nuclear fragments should be cut so that manipulations will not result in vitreoretinal traction and the fragments are freely mobile (Figure 18-6, *A* and *B*). Following a complete vitrectomy, the mobile lens fragments are aspirated and withdrawn away from the retinal surface into the middle of the vitreous cavity (see Figure 18-6, *C*). In the safety of the midvitreous cavity, they are phacoemulsified. Low-power, high-suction rates and support from the light pipe can help reduce the nuclear fragments from being propelled away from the phacoemulsification into the retina (see Figure 18-6, *D*). The retina should be examined with the indirect ophthalmoscope and scleral depression to be sure that all fragments have been removed (see Figure 18-6, *E*). Small fragments may occasionally become stuck far anteriorly in the vitreous base only to be found postoperatively.

Some vitreoretinal surgeons use perfluorocarbon liquids to float the nuclear fragments up from the retinal surface.[33] This has the theoretical benefit of minimizing retinal trauma from the nuclear fragments propelled by the phacoemulsifier.

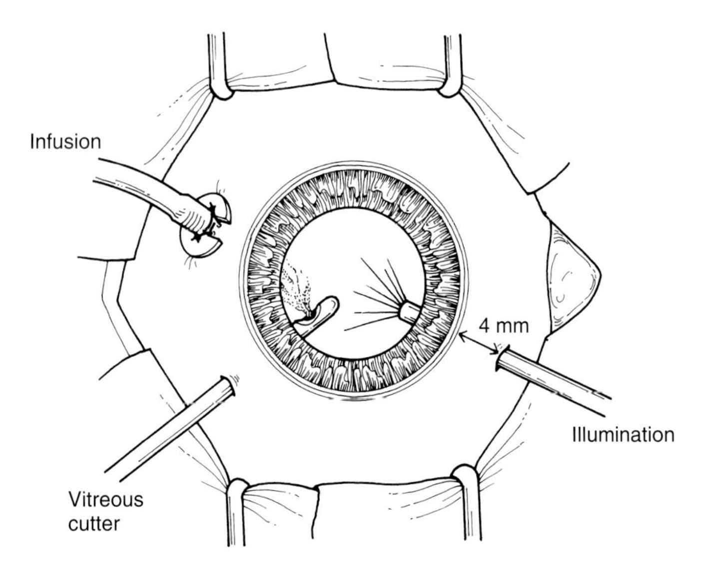

FIGURE 18-5 Standard three-port vitrectomy with an infusion cannula in the inferotemporal quadrant 4 mm from the limbus. Two additional sclerotomies are made in the superotemporal and superonasal quadrants for the vitreous cutter and the endoillumination probe.

Results

Approximately half to two thirds of patients undergoing vitrectomy-lensectomy for dislocated nuclear fragments will have a final visual acuity of 20/40 or better. Poorer outcomes are associated with retinal detachment, corneal decompensation, chronic inflammation, cystoid macular edema, and glaucoma.[22-27,30] Patients who receive an IOL tend to do slightly better than those left aphakic, and those with a PC IOL tend to do best of all. In the past, some vitreoretinal surgeons desired an aphakic eye to deliver nuclear fragments into the anterior chamber and through the limbal wound, but this is no longer necessary in most cases. Advances in pars plana phacoemulsification techniques now permit most surgeons to primarily place an IOL even when subsequent pars plana nuclear removal is anticipated.

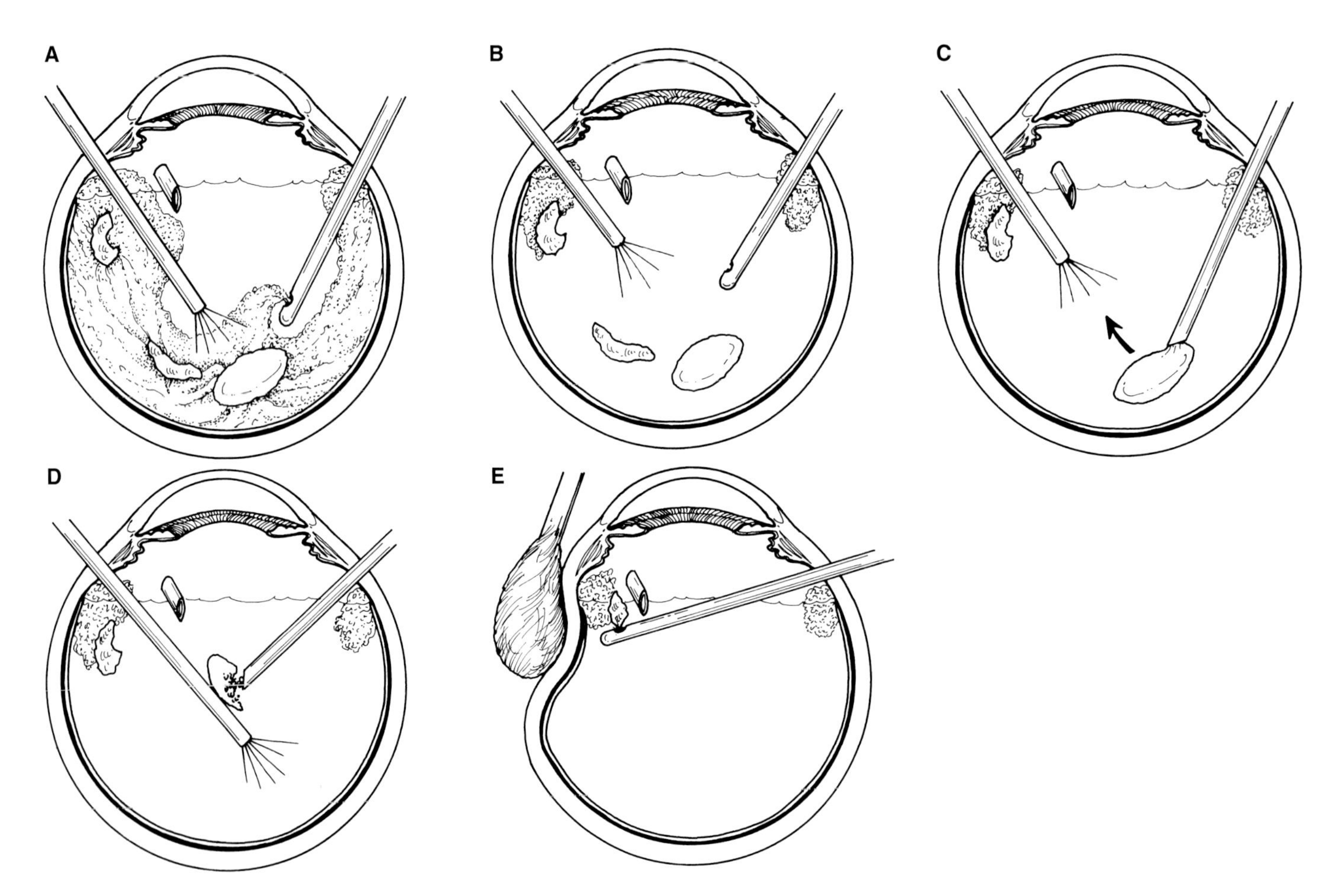

FIGURE 18-6 A, Vitreous cutter used to perform a thorough vitrectomy and to relieve any vitreous attachments to the nuclear fragments. **B,** Nuclear fragments should be completely mobile and free of vitreous attachments. **C,** Nuclear fragment is aspirated with the ultrasonic tip and moved into the midvitreous cavity. **D,** High suction, low power, and the light pipe are used to minimize propulsion of the nucleus away from the phacoemulsifier. The nucleus is emulsified in the vitreous cavity. **E,** Scleral depression is used to remove any cortical fragments trapped in the vitreous base.

REFERENCES

1. Nelson LB, Maumenee IH: Ectopia lentis, *Surv Ophthalmol* 27:143-160, 1982.
2. Bartholomeu RS: Lens displacement associated with pseudocapsular exfoliation, *Br J Ophthalmol* 54:744, 1970.
3. Jofe M: Detection of lens subluxation in pseudoexfoliation, *Arch Ophthalmol* 106:1032, 1988.
4. Nelson LB, Szmyd SM: Aphakic correction in ectopia lentis, *Ann Ophthalmol* 17:445-447, 1985.
5. Goldberg MF: Clinical manifestations of ectopia lentis et pupillae in 16 patients, *Ophthalmology* 95:1080, 1988.
6. Straatsma BR, Allen RA, Pettit TH et al: Subluxation of the lens treated with iris photocoagulation, *Am J Ophthalmol* 61:1312-1324, 1966.
7. Tchah H, Larson RS, Nichols BD et al: Neodymium:YAG laser zonulysis for treatment of lens subluxation, *Ophthalmology* 96:230-234, 1989.
8. Rosen PH, Dart JK, Turner GS: Neodymium:YAG laser zonulotomy, *Arch Ophthalmol* 105:892-894, 1987.
9. Bleckmann H, Hanuschik W, Vogt R: Implantation of posterior chamber lenses in eyes with phakodonesis and lens subluxation, *J Cataract Refract Surg* 15:485-489, 1990.
10. Cross HE, Jensen AD: Ocular manifestations in the Marfan syndrome and homocystinuria, *Am J Ophthalmol* 75:405-420, 1973.
11. Merriam JC, Zheng L: Iris hooks for phacoemulsification of the subluxated lens, *J Cataract Refract Surg* 23:1295-97, 1997.
12. Gimbel HV, Sun R, Heston JP: Management of zonular dialysis in phacoemulsification and IOL implantation using the capsular tension ring, *Ophthalmic Surg Lasers* 28:273-281, 1997.
13. Cionni RJ, Osher RH: Endocapsular ring approach to the subluxated cataractous lens, *J Cataract Refract Surg* 21:245-249, 1999.
14. Reese PD, Weingeist TA: Pars plana management of ectopia lentis in children, *Arch Ophthalmol* 105:1202-1204, 1987.
15. Jarrett WH: Dislocation of the lens: a study of the 166 hospitalized cases, *Arch Ophthalmol* 78:289, 1967.
16. Hakin KN, Jacobs M, Rosen P et al: Management of the subluxated crystalline lens, *Ophthalmology* 99:542-545, 1992.
17. Girard LJ, Canizales R, Esnaola N et al: Subluxated (ectopic) lenses in adults, *Ophthalmology* 97:462-465, 1990.
18. Peyman GA, Richard M, Goldberg MF: Management of the subluxated and dislocated lenses with the vitrophage, *Br J Ophthalmol* 63:771, 1979.
19. Omulecki W, Nawrocki J, Palenga-Pydyn D et al: Pars plana vitrectomy, lensectomy, or extraction in transscleral intraocular lens fixation for management of dislocated lenses in a family with Marfan's syndrome, *Ophthalmic Surg Lasers* 29:375-379, 1998.
20. Michels RJ, Shacklet RDE: Vitrectomy techniques for removal of retained lens material, *Arch Ophthalmol* 95:1767, 1977.
21. Blodi BA, Flynn HW, Blodi CF et al: Retained nuclei after cataract surgery, *Ophthalmology* 99:41-44, 1992.
22. Gilliland GD, Hutton WL, Fuller DG: Retained intravitreal lens fragments after cataract surgery, *Ophthalmology* 99:1263-1269, 1992.
23. Lambrou FH Jr, Stewart MW: Management of dislocated lens fragments during phacoemulsification, *Ophthalmology* 99:1260, 1992.
24. Watts P, Hunter J, Bunce CJ: Vitrectomy and lensectomy in the management of posterior dislocation of lens fragments, *J Cataract Refract Surg* 26:832-837, 2000.
25. Margherio R, Margherio A, Pendergast SP et al: Vitrectomy for retained lens fragments after phacoemulsification, *Ophthalmology* 104:1426-1432, 1997.
26. Kim JC, Flynn JW Jr, Smiddy WE et al: Retained lens fragments after phacoemulsification, *Ophthalmology* 101:1827-1832, 1994.
27. Fastenberg D, Schwartz PL, Shakin JL et al: Management of dislocated nuclear fragments after phacoemulsification, *Am J Ophthalmol* 112:535, 1991.
28. Smiddy WE, Flynn HW Jr, Kim JE: Retinal detachment in patients with retained lens fragments or dislocated PC IOLs, *Ophthmic Surg Lasers* 27:856-861, 1996.
29. Aaberg JM Jr, Rubsanen PE, Flynn HW Jr et al: Giant retinal tear as a complication of attempted removal of intravitreal lens fragments during cataract surgery, *Am J Ophthalmol* 174:222-226, 1997.
30. Borne MJ, Tasman W, Regillo C et al: Outcomes of vitrectomy for retained lens fragments, *Ophthalmology* 103:971-976. 1996.
31. Bohegian GM, Wexler SA: Complications of retained nuclear fragments in anterior chamber after phacoemulsification with posterior chamber lens implant, *Am J Ophthalmol* 123:546-547, 1997.
32. Vilar NF, Flynn HW Jr, Smiddy WE et al: Removal of retained lens fragments after phacoemulsification reverses secondary glaucoma and restores visual acuity, *Ophthalmology* 104:787-791, 1997.
33. Liu KR, Peyman GA, Chen MS et al: Use of high-density vitreous substitutes in the removal of posteriorly dislocated lenses or intraocular lenses, *Ophthalmic Surg* 22:503-507, 1991.

Phacoemulsification in the Presence of a Small Pupil

19

I. Howard Fine, MD
Mark Packer, MD
Richard S. Hoffman, MD

The pupil that dilates poorly or is fibrosed or hyalinized is frequently associated with complications during cataract surgery and is, on occasion, the determining factor in the decision not to proceed with phacoemulsification.

With newer endolenticular techniques, especially with nucleofractis procedures and chop techniques,[1-4] pupils do not have to be as large as previously required. This is because much of the procedure takes place in the endolenticular space, within the center of the capsulorhexis, rather than at the equator of the lens as in anterior chamber phacoemulsification[5] and nuclear tilt pupillary plane phacoemulsification techniques.[6] However, there still are numerous instances in which the pupil is inadequate to allow the surgeon to proceed, and some form of manipulation or surgery is required.

Techniques That Depend on Manipulation of the Pupil

The surgeon may tailor the initial pharmacologic intervention for pupillary mydriasis in cataract surgery to achieve greater dilation. The use of phenylephrine 10% and cyclopentolate 2% will sometimes produce more effective mydriasis than lower concentrations of these or other agents, especially when administered in multiple doses over 1 hour. The use of preoperative nonsteroidal antiinflammatory agents, such as flurbiprofen sodium (Ocufen) 0.03% or suprofen (Profenal) 1% mitigates any intraoperative pupillary constriction. In addition, preservative-free epinephrine 1:10,000 may increase the diameter of the pupil when injected into the anterior chamber at the start of surgery.

A viscoelastic device, particularly a high-molecular-weight product, can increase mydriasis by applying direct mechanical pressure on the pupillary margin during instillation. In particular, we have found Healon 5 (Pharmacia) to produce stable mydriasis during phacoemulsification. When poor mydriasis is caused by the presence of posterior synechiae and there is adequate zonular support, the surgeon may introduce the viscoelastic cannula between the anterior capsule and the pupillary margin and then inject viscoelastic to disrupt the iridocapsular adhesions. The cannula is angled in a tangential fashion to create a wave of viscoelastic, which will dissect the synechiae. Multiple injection sites may be used to fully free the pupil. Following dissection of the synechiae, additional dispersive viscoelastic may be injected in the center of the pupil to achieve even greater dilation of the pupillary margin.

Often the pupil can be manipulated with the phacoemulsification handpiece. The surgeon can retract the proximal portion of the pupil through the incision with the sleeve on the phacoemulsification handpiece and effectively enlarge its size (Figure 19-1). This technique requires a great deal of skill and may result in thermal injury with chafing of the pupil and focal depigmentation of the iris. Additional advantage can be obtained by using the second handpiece in such a way as to stretch the pupil in advance of the phacoemulsification tip, once again enlarging the pupil for adequate visualization of structures just under the margin of the pupil (Figure 19-2).

In other circumstances, a portion of the lens may be manipulated through the pupil to maintain the pupil in a semidilated state. The protruding portion of the nucleus can then be consumed by the phacoemulsification handpiece before repositioning the nucleus within the pupil (Figure 19-3). The surgeon may accomplish mechanical stretching of the pupil with a variety of instruments. Frye[7] has taught a technique that he attributes to Keener of Indianapolis, Ind. Two hooks are used to engage the pupillary margin at opposite points, and steady, gentle pressure is applied across the full extent of the anterior chamber to produce a pupillary diameter of 5 to 6 mm. A second stretch placed orthogonal to the first increases the diameter further. Viscoelastic protects the anterior lens capsule during this maneuver.

Alternatively, the Beehler pupil dilator (Moria No. 19009) is uniformly applicable in the presence of small pupils. Inserted through a 2.5-mm single-plane clear corneal incision, it usually stretches the pupil to 6 to 7 mm while creating tiny microsphincterotomies circumferentially around the pupil (Figure 19-4). The pupil can then be mechanically reduced at the end of the procedure with a Lester hook supplemented with an intraocular miotic agent. Pupils enlarged in this manner maintain a good cosmetic appearance and an ability to react to light but may require a miotic agent for some time after cataract surgery to prevent the formation of iridocapsular synechiae.

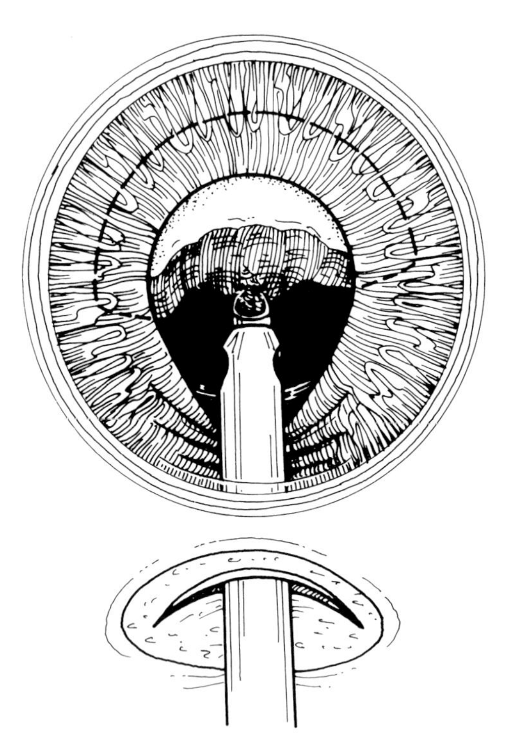

FIGURE 19-1 Retraction of the proximal pupil with the silicone sleeve of the phaco handpiece.

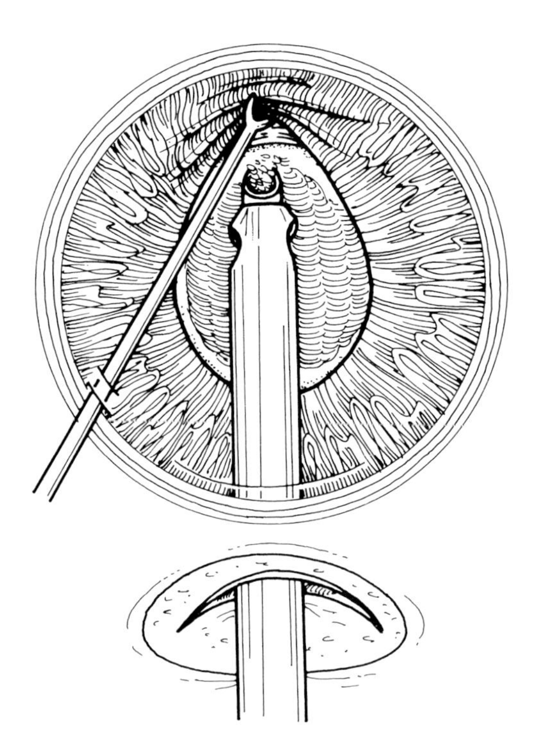

FIGURE 19-2 Stretching the distal pupil with an instrument through the side-port incision.

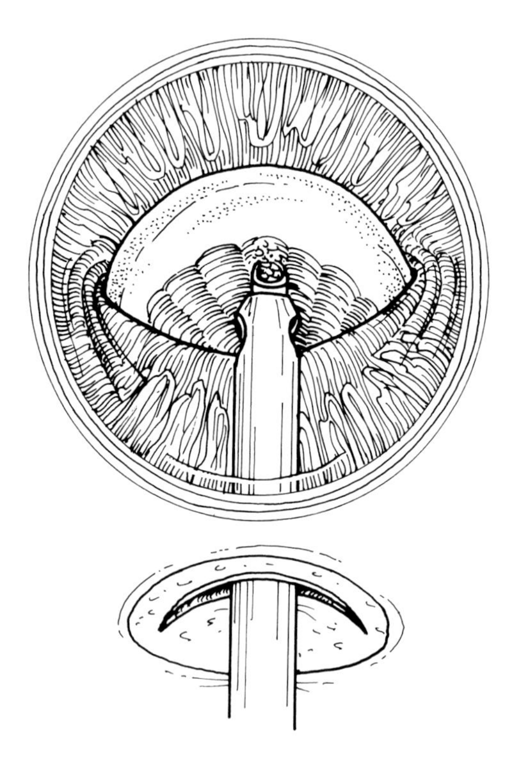

FIGURE 19-3 Expanding the pupil with nuclear material.

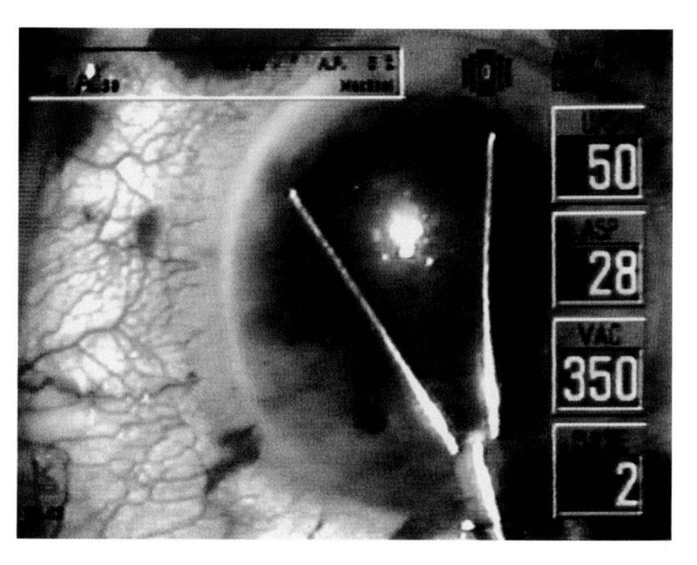

FIGURE 19-4 The Beehler pupil dilator effectively stretches the pupil to a diameter of 6 to 7 mm by creating tiny microsphincterotomies.

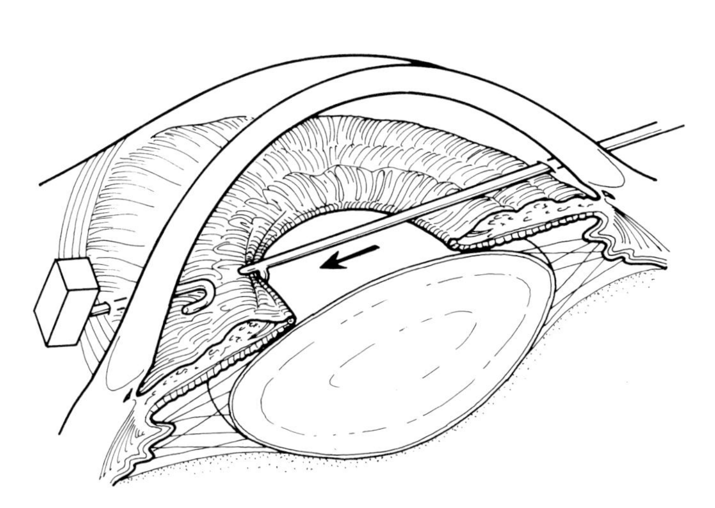

FIGURE 19-5 Stretching the pupil with an iris repositor in the process of engaging the pupil by the iris hook.

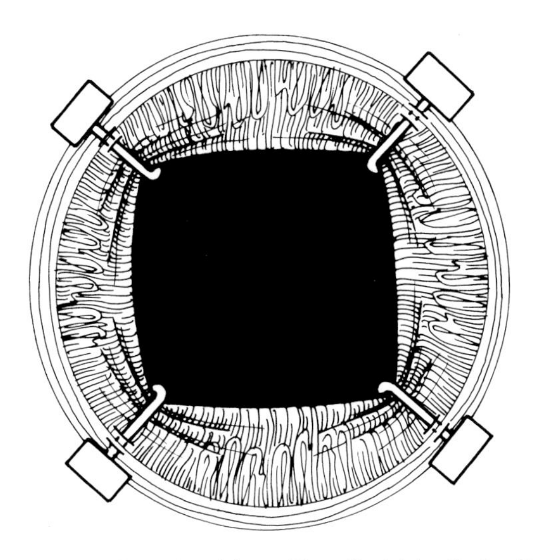

FIGURE 19-6 Retraction of the pupil by self-retaining titanium iris hooks.

Recently we have seen a renewed interest in the use of iris hooks as described by McReynolds.[8] Mackool[9] has designed self-retaining titanium hooks that can be placed through paracenteses so that the pupil can be positioned and held in a widely dilated state in a triangular or square shape to adequately perform phacoemulsification regardless of the initial size of the pupil (Figures 19-5 and 19-6). Although this procedure is somewhat time consuming and results in considerable fluid loss from the eye because of leakage through the paracenteses during phacoemulsification, it is an effective method of pupillary dilation and visualization of the structures for phacoemulsification. De Juan designed disposable nylon hooks with an adjustable silicone retaining sleeve that can be used through smaller paracenteses (Figures 19-7 and 19-8). Although more costly per case, they may offer some additional advantages as reported by Nichamin,[10] particularly facilitation of removal of the hooks through the paracentesis incisions.

Pupil ring expanders represent another option in the surgical armamentarium for small pupil cases. The Hydroview Iris Protector Ring (Grieshaber) forms a compressed oval in its dehydrated state (Figure 19-9). It can then be placed in the anterior chamber through a 3-mm incision and inserted into the small pupil. This hydrogel device expands with hydration (Figure 19-10) and captures the pupillary margin by means of flanges (Figure 19-11). The ring can be manipulated to expand the pupil as it hydrates. The device then remains in place for the entire surgical procedure, including implantation of the intraocular lens (Figure 19-12), and can then be removed through the same small incision (Figure 19-13). The Morcher pupil dilator Type 5S is a solid polymethylmethacrylate ring that is placed at the pupillary margin and expands the pupil through 300 degrees of even tension, thus reducing the likelihood of iris sphincter tears and postoperative pupillary deformity. The ring may be introduced into the anterior

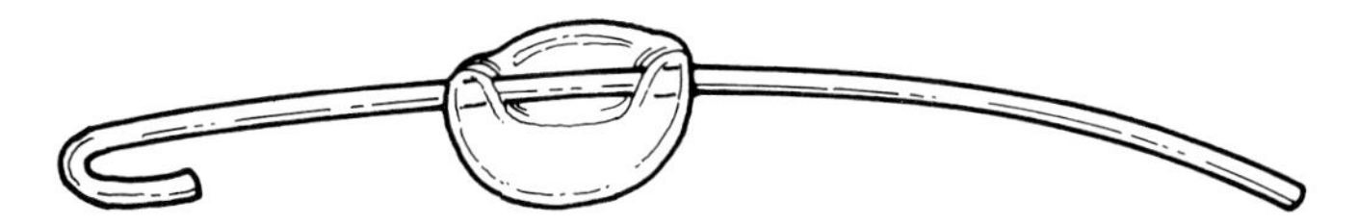

FIGURE 19-7 Disposable nylon hook with adjustable silicone retaining sleeve.

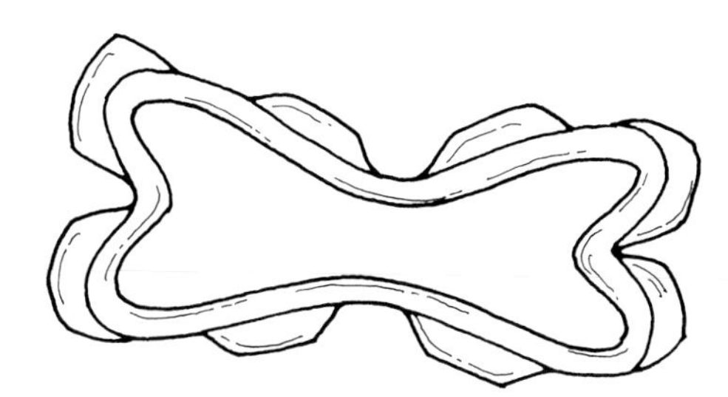

FIGURE 19-9 Dehydrated iris protector ring.

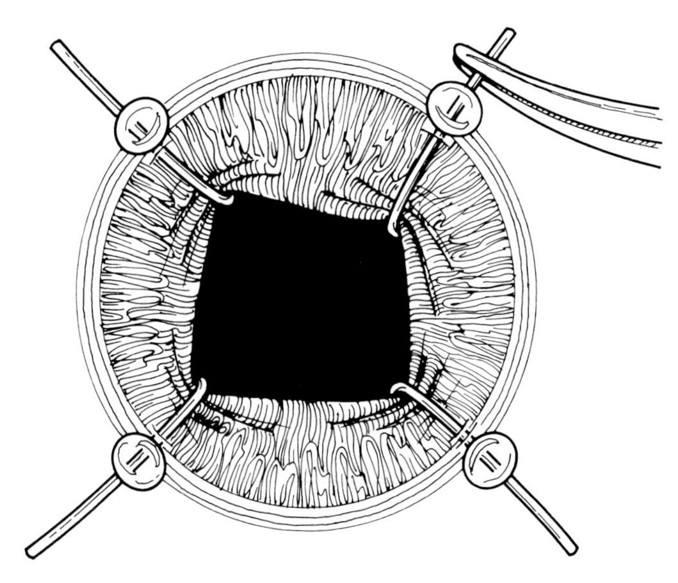

FIGURE 19-8 Tightening the sleeve on the retractor to adjust pupillary aperture.

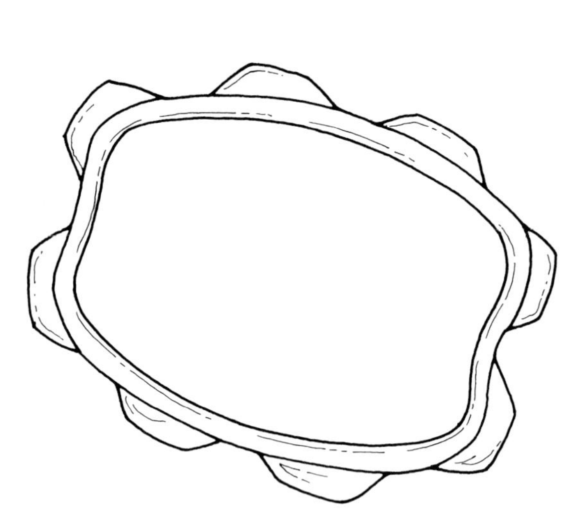

FIGURE 19-10 Iris protector ring expanding as it hydrates.

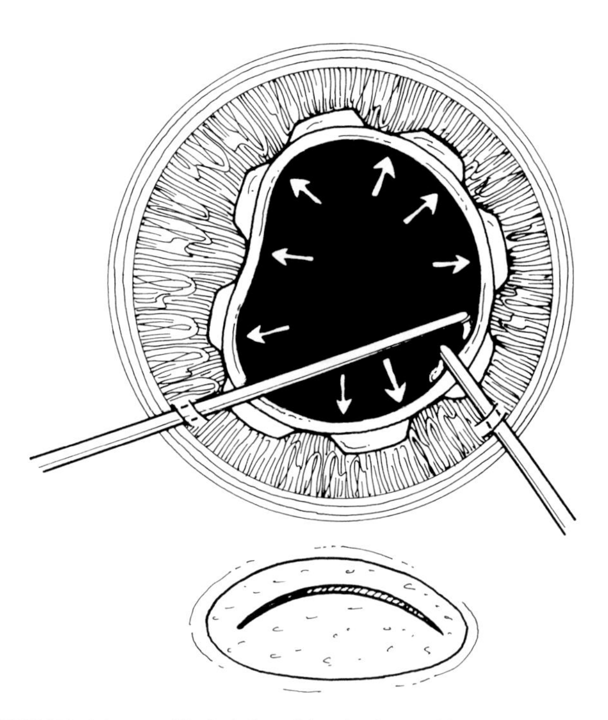

FIGURE 19-11 Manipulation of the ring into position and dilation of the pupil as the ring expands.

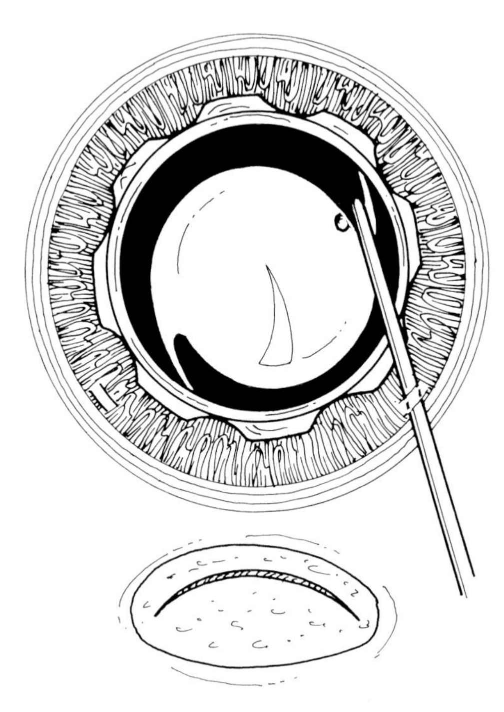

FIGURE 19-12 Implantation of intraocular lens through iris protector ring.

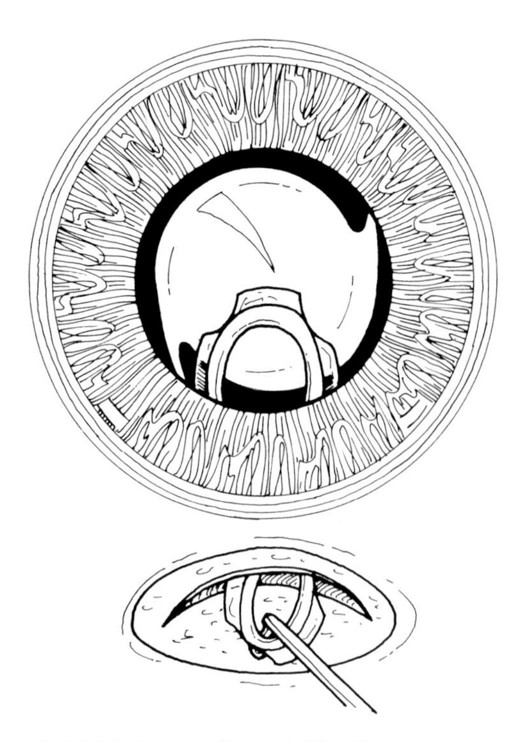

FIGURE 19-13 Removal of the iris protector ring.

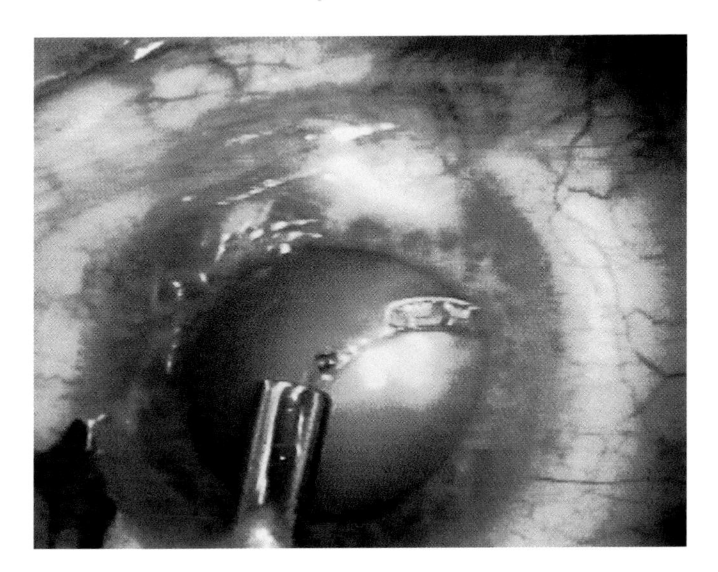

FIGURE 19-14 The Morcher pupil dilator may be injected via a device available from Geuder, as seen in this case of floppy iris.

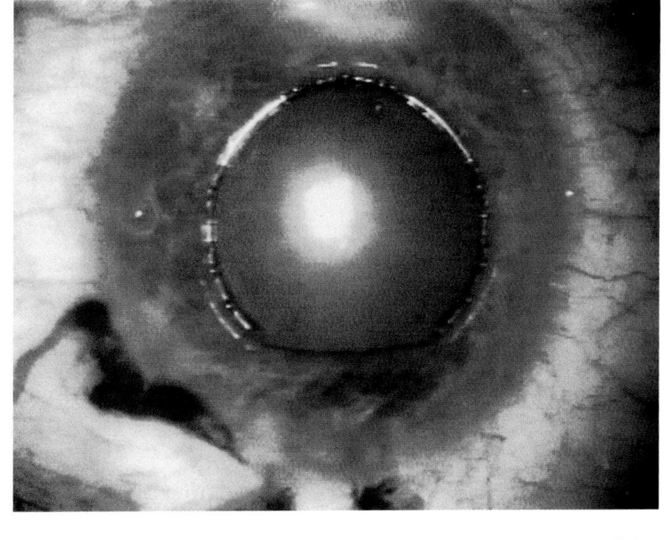

FIGURE 19-15 The Morcher pupil dilator in place, permitting capsulorhexis and completion of the surgery.

chamber with forceps and then placed within the pupillary margin with a small hook. The central segment of the ring is manipulated into position first in apposition to the distal pupillary margin, and the ends of the ring are placed with the aid of eyelets on the ring. Following implantation of the intraocular lens the ring is removed by first freeing the ends from their point of apposition with the pupil by means of the small hook, again placed in each eyelet. The ring may then be withdrawn from the anterior chamber with forceps. An injection device is also available for the ring from Geuder (Figures 19-14 and 19-15).

The Perfect Pupil (Becton-Dickinson) represents a new and effective option for both maintaining mydriasis and protecting the pupillary margin during surgery. This polyurethane device features a 7.0-mm internal diameter and an available injection device.

Iris Surgery

A variety of techniques using iris surgery enable enlargement of the pupil. A proximal sphincterotomy can be performed by grasping the superior sphincter and pulling it out of the incision. A small segment of the sphincter can be excised, after which the iris is repositioned (Figure 19-16).[11] Although this procedure results in a permanently enlarged pupil that may be

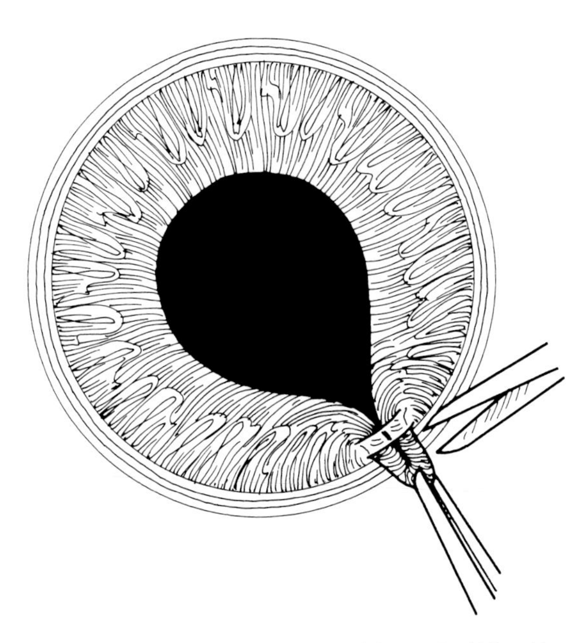

FIGURE 19-16 Excising a portion of the proximal iris sphincter.

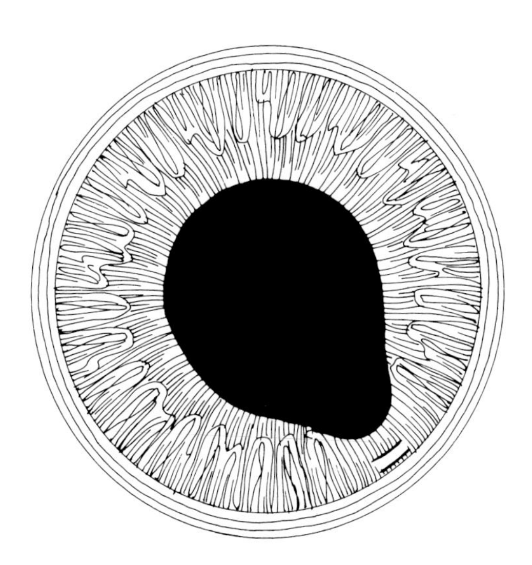

FIGURE 19-17 Enlargement of the pupil following partial sphincterectomy.

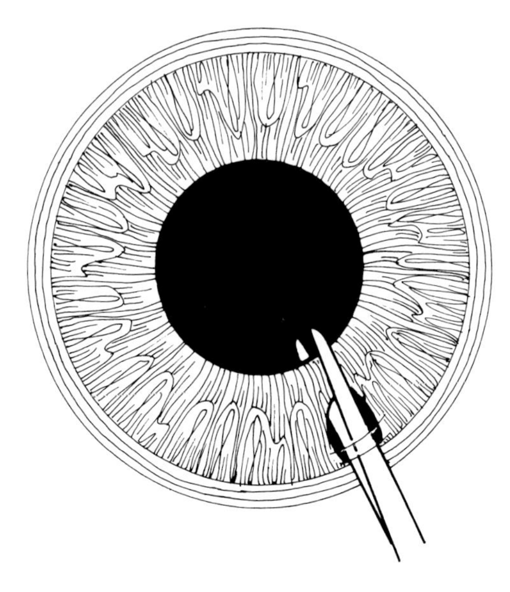

FIGURE 19-18 Midiris iridectomy.

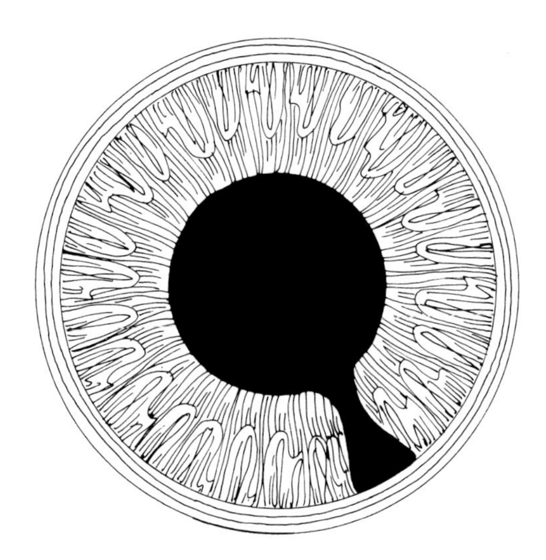

FIGURE 19-19 Appearance of sector iridotomy following sphincterotomy through midiris iridotomy.

somewhat oval (Figure 19-17), it often achieves adequate dilation for completion of the surgery. This has been found especially useful in glaucoma patients undergoing cataract surgery and may be combined with a small inferior sphincterotomy.

Performing a superior sector iridectomy is often used for pupillary enlargement. However, this technique subjects the patient to glare and other undesirable retinal images postoperatively because of the permanently enlarged pupil and the potential for edge effects from lenses and haptics uncovered by the prominently enlarged pupils.

A modification of the superior sector iridectomy, which tends to give adequate dilation for surgery and yet is less of a problem postoperatively, is the superior midiris iridectomy followed by sphincterotomy. This allows the pillars of the iris to come together more closely following completion of the surgery than does a sector iridectomy (Figures 19-18 and 19-19).

Many surgeons use a suture to close the sphincterotomy at the completion of surgery, hoping to avoid potential sources of glare and trying to achieve a more cosmetically acceptable appearance postoperatively. These sutures may be preplaced

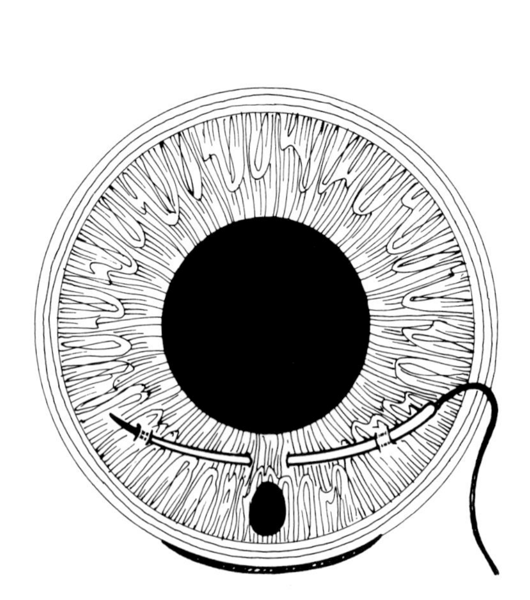

FIGURE 19-20 Needle is passed through clear cornea through each of the iris pillars and back out through cornea on the other side.

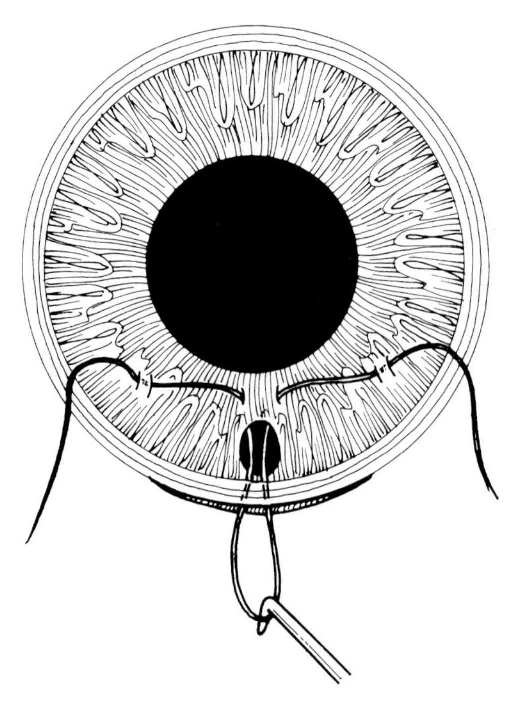

FIGURE 19-21 Central loop pulled through the peripheral iridotomy out of the incision before sphincterotomy.

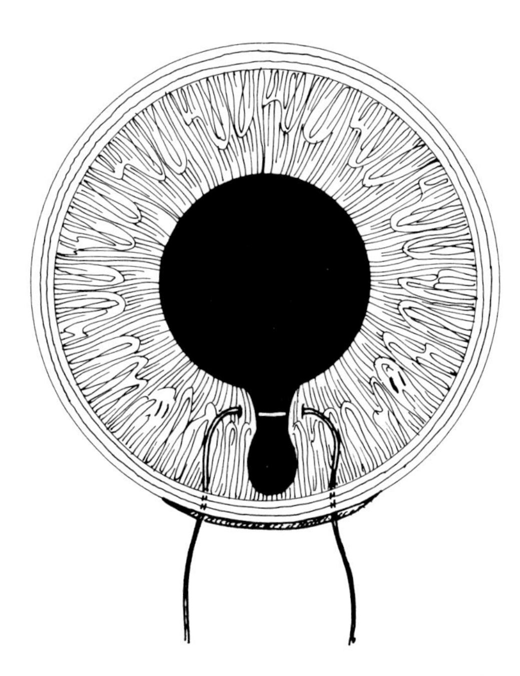

FIGURE 19-22 Suture is cut from the needle, and both ends are brought out of the incision for tying after lens implantation.

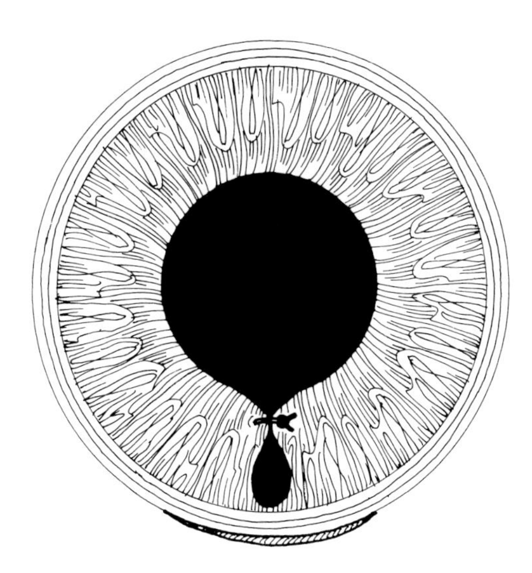

FIGURE 19-23 Appearance of the iris following tying of the suture to close the sphincterotomy.

through the clear cornea. The posterior loop is drawn out of the peripheral iridectomy with a hook before sphincterotomy (Figures 19-20 through 19-23). Alternatively, the suture may be placed through clear cornea at the end of the surgical procedure. The ends are drawn out of the cataract incision and tied in the same way as originally described by Worst and reported by Drews.[12]

Masket[13] has described a technique for using a preplaced suture in the inferior or distal portion of the iris (Figure 19-24), drawing a loop of the central segment of the suture out of the incision (Figure 19-25) and then performing a sphincterotomy inferiorly or distally (Figure 19-26). After implantation of the intraocular lens, the ends of the suture are drawn out of an inferior or distal limbal self-sealing paracentesis and tied (Figure 19-27). This can dramatically increase exposure to the area in which most of the phacoemulsification takes place. Exposure is increased specifically at the distal portion of the capsulorhexis and the capsular bag just under the distal capsular flap (Figure 19-28). This suture can restore an acceptable cosmetic appearance to the pupil postoperatively and remove

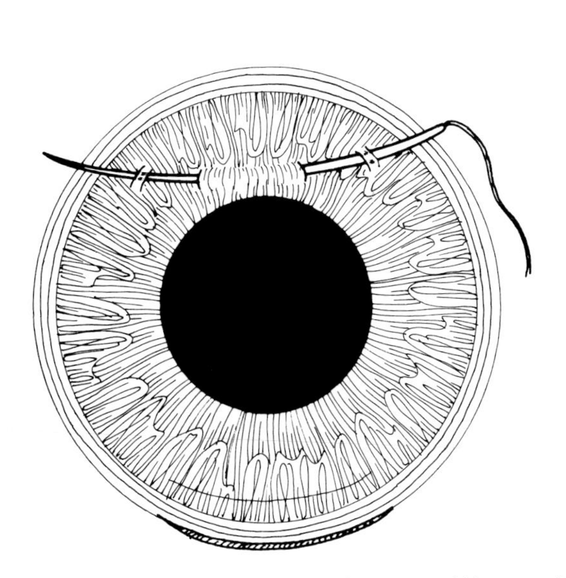

FIGURE 19-24 Preplacement through clear cornea of iris suture distally.

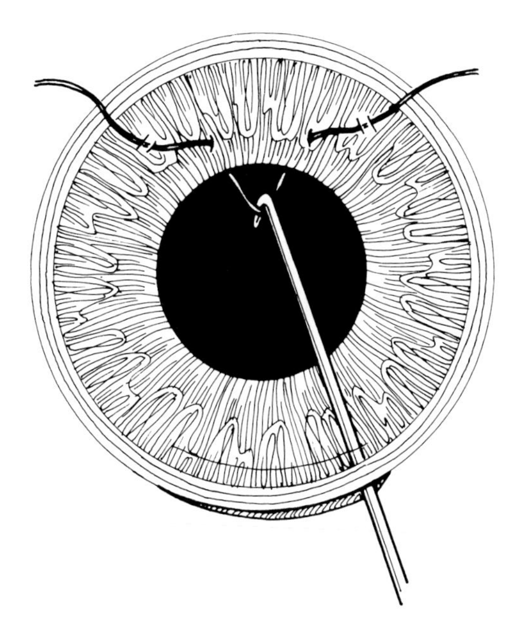

FIGURE 19-25 Retrieval of central loop of suture from under the iris and through the incision.

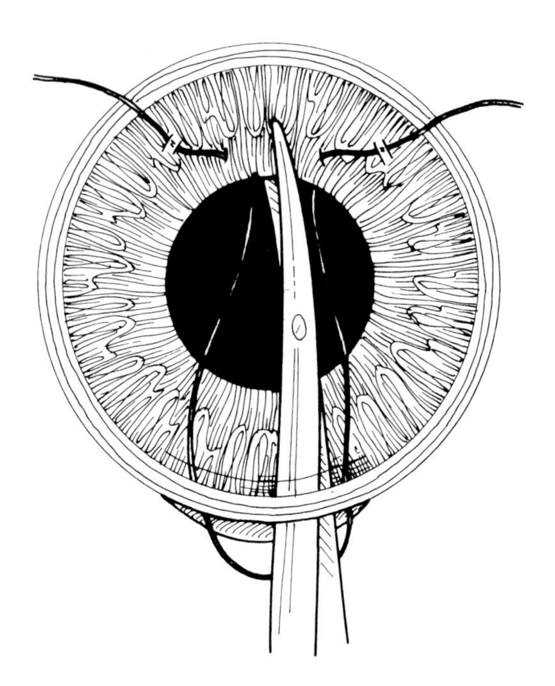

FIGURE 19-26 Inferior sphincterotomy.

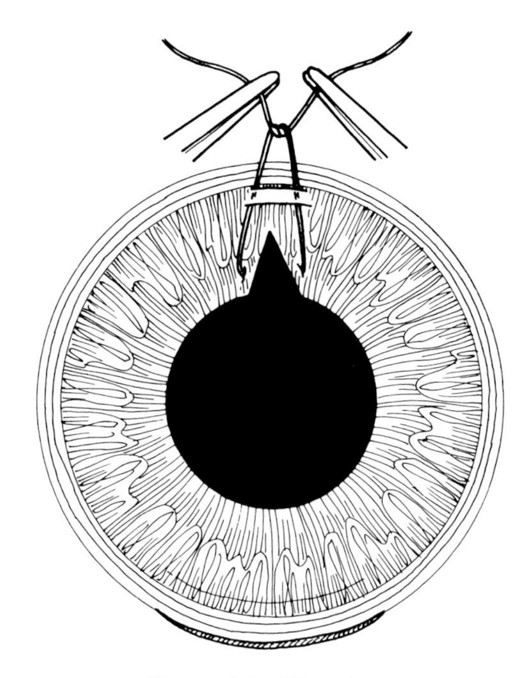

FIGURE 19-27 Closure of distal iris sphincter after lens implantation.

the potential for unwanted glare (Figure 19-29). An additional iris surgical procedure for pupillary enlargement is the pupilloplasty technique of Fine.[14] After lysing synechiae, partial-thickness sphincterotomies are made using Rappazzo scissors (Storz Instruments, E-1961-A) through the paracentesis or through the cataract incision (Figures 19-30 and 19-31). The sphincterotomies cut full thickness through approximately half the width of the musculus sphincter pupillae (Figure 19-32) at each of eight sites (Figure 19-33). Following sphincterotomies, each of the sites is stretched to the root of the iris. We believe that this results in fracturing of the hyalinized fibrotic portions of the pupil but only stretching of the residual circular muscle in the pupil that was not transected. This technique usually achieves 6- to 7-mm pupil diameters, regardless of the initial size of the pupil (Figure 19-34). At the completion of the phacoemulsification and implantation procedure, a Lester-type hook is used to mechanically return the pupil to as small a configuration as possible (Figures 19-35 and 19-36). The patient uses miotic drops and ointments postoperatively to keep the pupil small and to avoid synechiae from the sphincterotomy sites to the anterior edge of the capsulorhexis. This technique tends to achieve an excellent cosmetic appearance postoperatively

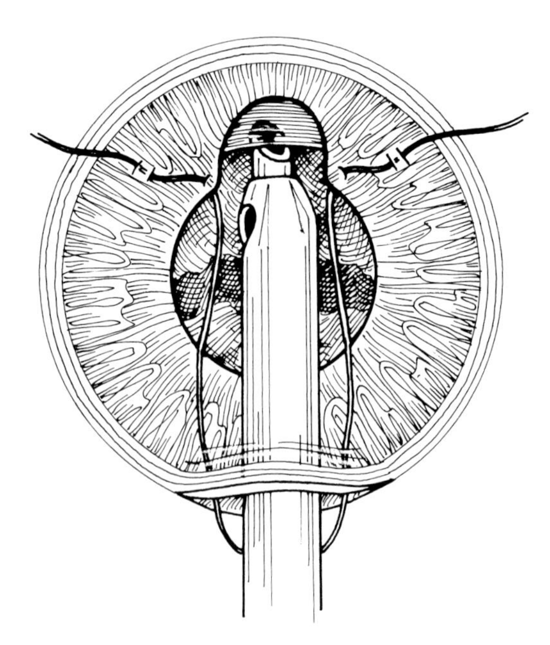

FIGURE 19-28 Maximum exposure under the distal capsulorhexis.

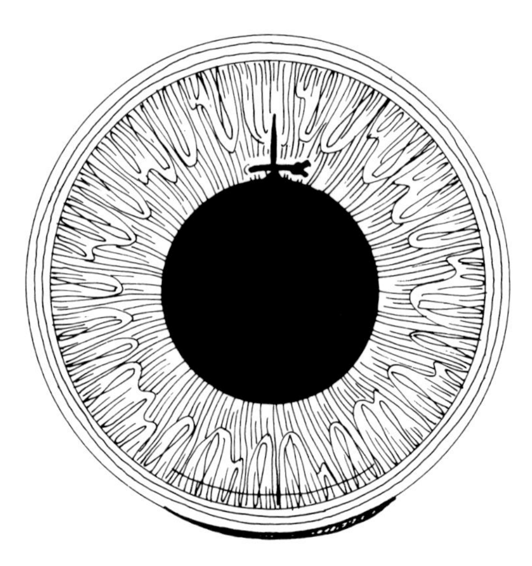

FIGURE 19-29 Undilated view of the patient postoperatively.

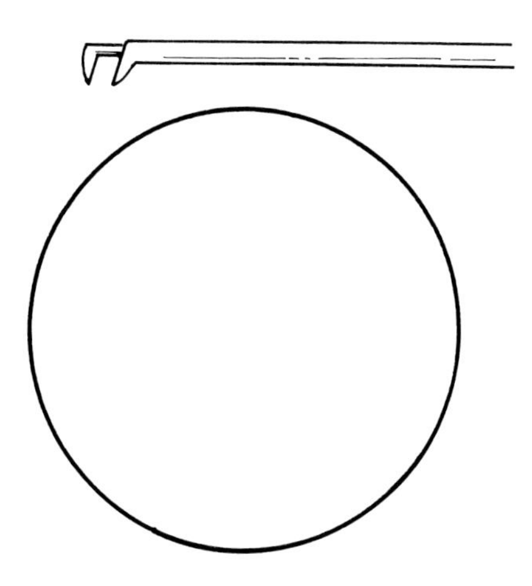

FIGURE 19-30 Rappazzo scissors relative to size of a U.S. Government dime.

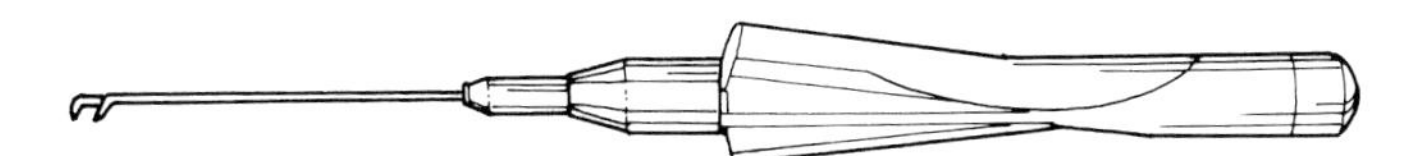

FIGURE 19-31 Rappazzo scissors showing squeeze-action handles that cause opposing blades to shear.

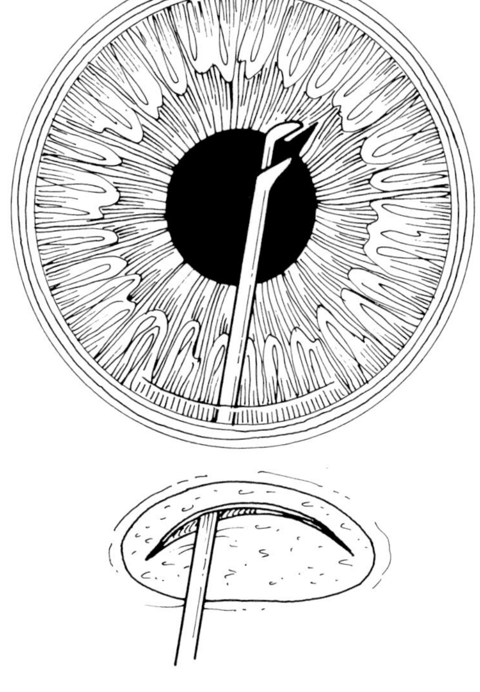

FIGURE 19-32 Half-width sphincterotomy.

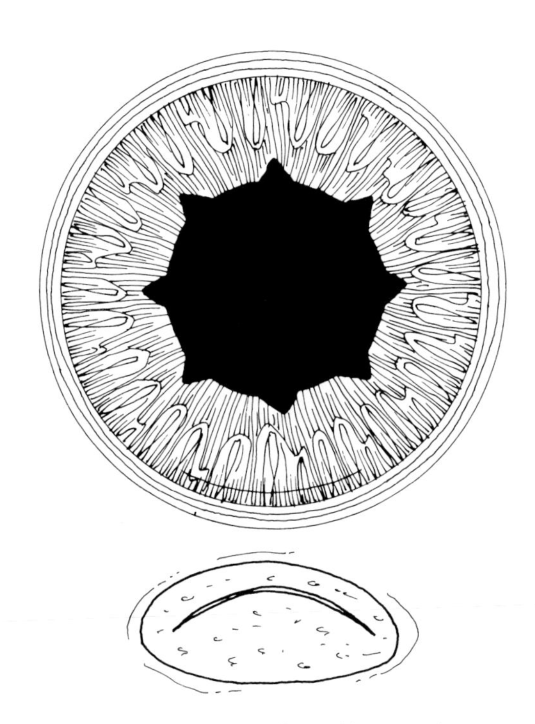

FIGURE 19-33 Eight sphincterotomies.

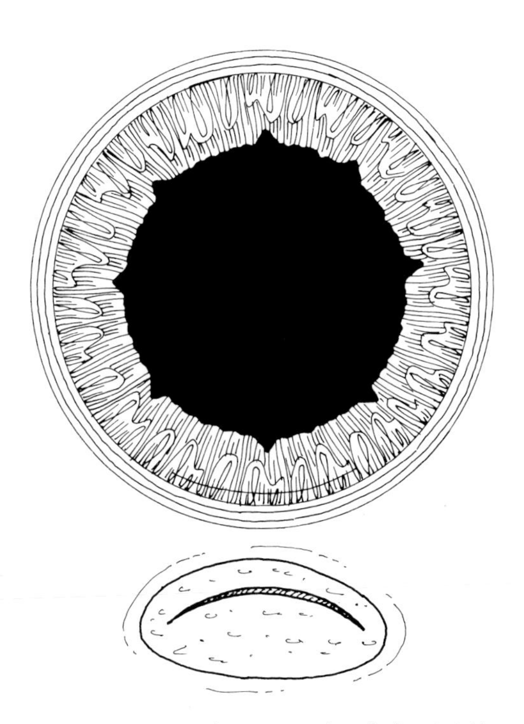

FIGURE 19-34 Appearance of pupil after stretching.

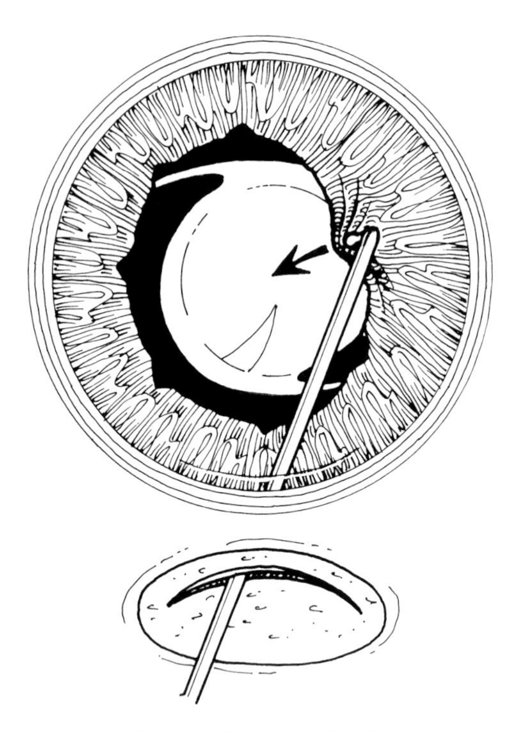

FIGURE 19-35 Mechanical reduction of pupil size using Lester hook.

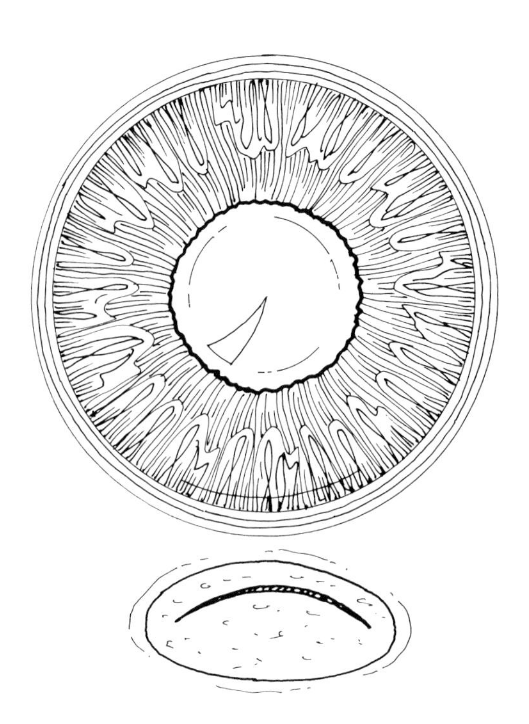

FIGURE 19-36 Appearance of pupil immediately postoperatively.

(Figures 19-37 and 19-38) and also allows more normal and physiologic behavior of the pupil.

Osher[15] has described pupillary membrane dissection as a technique to allow dilation of the pupil to an adequate diameter. This procedure involves meticulous dissection with a bent needle or microforceps to free and remove a fibrotic pupillary membrane (Figures 19-39 and 19-40). This technique is time consuming and may produce some bleeding, but it has proved a valuable aid in the management of some cases of small pupil.

In conclusion, phacoemulsification in the presence of a small pupil continues to pose a challenge to the surgeon. However, the diverse techniques for management of these pupils present us with options for reducing complications in these cases to the standard low complication rate.

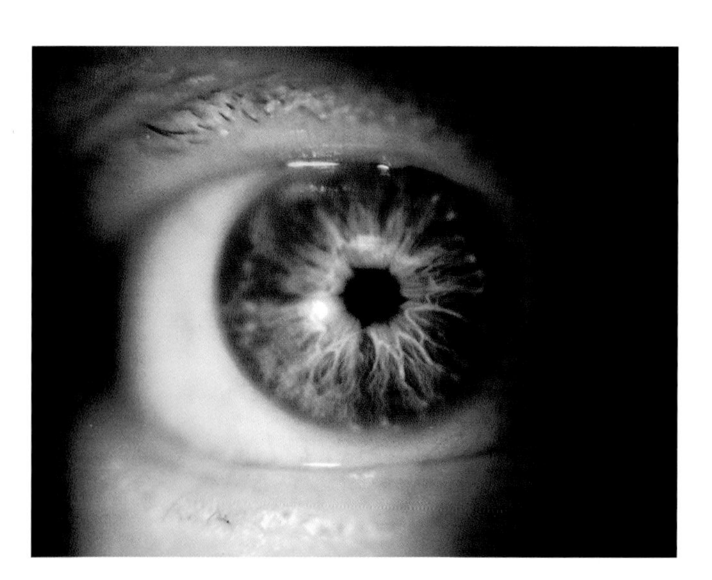

FIGURE 19-37 Late postoperative appearance of sphincterotomized and stretched light brown pupil.

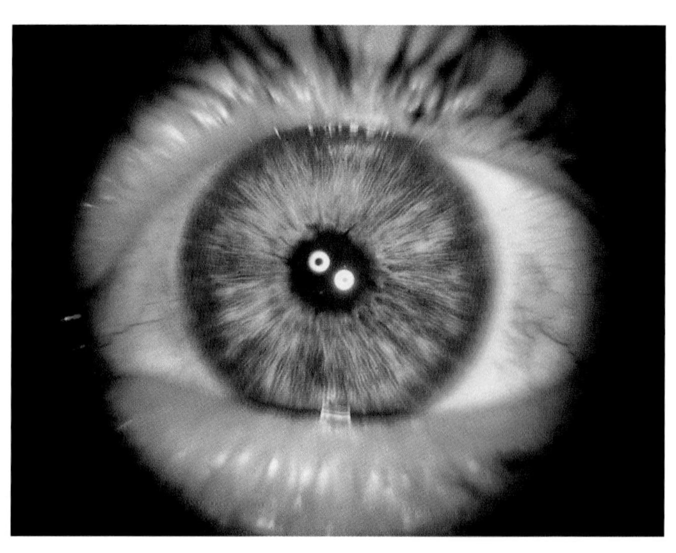

FIGURE 19-38 Late postoperative appearance of sphincterotomized and stretched blue pupil.

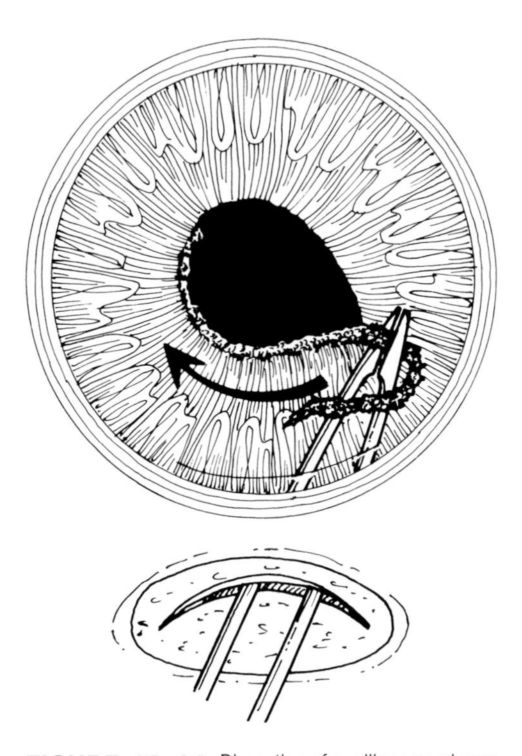

FIGURE 19-39 Dissection of pupillary membrane.

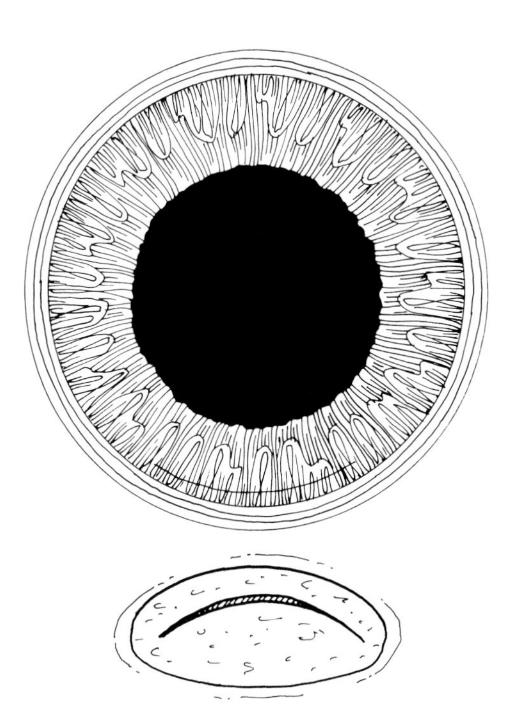

FIGURE 19-40 Dilation of pupil after dissection and peeling of pupillary membrane.

REFERENCES

1. Gimbel HV: Divide and conquer nucleofractis phacoemulsification: development and variations, *J Cataract Refract Surg* 17:281-291, 1991.
2. Shepherd JF: In situ fracture, *J Cataract Refract Surg* 16:436-440, 1990.
3. Fine IH, Maloney WF, Dillman DM: Crack and flip phacoemulsification technique, *J Cataract Refract Surg* 19:797-802, 1993.
4. Fine IH: The choo-choo chop and flip phacoemulsification technique, *Operative Techniques Cataract Refract Surg* 1:61-65, 1998.
5. Kelman CD: Phacoemulsification in the anterior chamber, *Ophthalmology* 86:1980-1982, 1979.
6. Kratz RP, Colvard DM: Kelman phacoemulsification in the posterior chamber, *Ophthalmology* 86:1983-1984, 1979.
7. Frye LL: Pupil stretch maneuver. Course No. 454 (Modern Phaco/ECCE Implant Surgery: XII, Wed, Nov 11, 1992). Dallas, Tex, American Academy of Ophthalmology.
8. McReynolds WU: Pupil dilator for phacoemulsification. In Emery JM, Paton D, editors: *Current concepts in cataract surgery: selected proceedings of the First Biennial Cataract Surgery Congress,* St Louis, 1976, Mosby.
9. Mackool RJ: Small pupil enlargement during cataract extraction: a new method, *J Cataract Refract Surg* 18:523-526, 1992.
10. Nichamin LD: Enlarging the pupil for cataract extractions using flexible nylon iris retractors, *J Cataract Refract Surg* 19:795-796, 1993.
11. Fishkind WA, Koch PS: Managing the small pupil. In Koch PS, Davison JA, editors: *Textbook of advanced phacoemulsification techniques,* Thorofare, NJ, 1991, Slack, Inc, pp 79-90.
12. Drews RC: Straight needle technique. In Emery JM, Jacobson AC, editors: *Current concepts in cataract surgery: selected proceedings of the Eighth Biennial Cataract Surgical Congress.* Norwalk, Conn, 1984, Appleton-Century-Crofts.
13. Masket S: Preplaced inferior iris suture method for small pupil phacoemulsification, *J Cataract Refract Surg* 18:518-522, 1992.
14. Fine IH: Pupilloplasty for small pupil phacoemulsification, *J Cataract Refract Surg* 20:192-196, 1994.
15. Osher RH: Pupillary membranectomy, *Audiovisual J Cataract implant Surg* 7(3), 1991.

Combined Cataract Implant and Filtering Surgery

20

John S. Cohen, MD
Anup K. Khatana, MD
Robert H. Osher, MD

History

The indications for combined surgery have evolved full circle during the past several decades. In the 1970s and early 1980s, cataract surgery alone was thought to have a beneficial effect on long-term glaucoma control.[1-3] Although the precise mechanism for this is not known, large incisions and large sutures often resulted in unintentional filtering blebs in some eyes and probable subclinical filtration in others, which had beneficial effects on intraocular pressure (IOP) in glaucoma eyes. Combined surgery at that time was technically more complex than present techniques and was associated with greater risks and limited success. To avoid the increased risks of this more complex surgery, patients often underwent staged surgery with performance of one procedure and then the other, resulting in a longer total period of rehabilitation.

In the 1980s, with newer techniques of extracapsular surgery and safer intraocular lenses (IOLs), cataract surgery was performed earlier with improved visual results. In the late 1980s and 1990s, more secure closure of surgical incisions and concern about the risks of postoperative IOP elevations prompted greater interest in combined cataract and glaucoma surgery.[4-8] Enthusiasm, however, was dampened with clinicians' belief that the more extensive combined procedure resulted in less filtration than trabeculectomy surgery when performed alone. With the ability to increase filtration after combined surgery by modifying wound healing with antimetabolite therapy, the indications became more liberal. Expectations increased that short- and long-term IOP control would be improved, many patients would be able to discontinue glaucoma medications altogether, and both cataract and glaucoma would be effectively managed with one surgical procedure. Several studies showed the benefits of this approach with minimal complications.[9-11] In time, however, it became evident that antimetabolite use was associated with a small but troubling incidence of complications such as leaking blebs, hypotony, "blebitis," and endophthalmitis, which represented a significant contrast to the infrequent incidence of complications of cataract surgery alone. In addition, with the development of small-incision surgery, clear corneal incisions, foldable IOLs placed in the capsular bag, improvements in techniques of anesthesia, and virtually same-day rehabilitation, cataract surgery alone became much more desirable if it could be performed without risk of glaucoma damage from perioperative IOP elevation.

With the realization that IOP elevations were uncommon (although still possible) following the present atraumatic technique of phacoemulsification and IOL implantation, cataract surgery alone is becoming the procedure of choice in many patients with diagnoses of ocular hypertension, glaucoma suspects, and patients with early to moderate glaucoma. Combined surgery may rarely be considered in eyes with ocular hypertension and in eyes of glaucoma suspects when IOP is significantly elevated despite the use of multiple medications. (This may also be a situation in which combined surgery with nonpenetrating trabeculectomy can be considered. See Nonpenetrating Trabeculectomy and Combined Surgery later in text.) Combined surgery is advisable when glaucoma is uncontrolled with maximum medical therapy, glaucoma control requires two or more medications (or fewer if unused medications are contraindicated), and damage is advanced with visual field loss threatening or involving fixation even if IOP is controlled.

Surgical Options in Patients with Cataract and Glaucoma

Before any surgical procedure is performed, advantages and disadvantages must be considered, taking into account severity of disease, condition of the fellow eye, availability and affordability of medications, compliance with medication schedules, and so on. As with most surgical procedures, the precise indications for combined surgery vary among surgeons depending on the level of comfort, experience, and skill. The surgeon and patient must balance the benefits and risks of performing combined cataract and glaucoma surgery with those of performing either procedure alone.

Cataract Surgery Alone (Phacoemulsification)

Cataract surgery alone can be performed efficiently with rapid if not immediate visual recovery in most cases. Postoperative elevation of IOP is a risk in all eyes. Its occurrence must be considered when choosing a surgical procedure in eyes with ocular hypertension, pigment dispersion syndrome, pseudo-exfoliation, primary open-angle glaucoma, postoperative pressure spike in the fellow eye, and a family history of glaucoma. One study measured IOP after phacoemulsification performed with clear corneal and sclerocorneal incisions in eyes without glaucoma. Peak elevations were higher for sclerocorneal than clear corneal incisions, measuring 43 and 37 mm Hg 6 hours postoperatively for each group, respectively, and 30 mm Hg for both groups 24 hours postoperatively. At 15 months, peak IOP measured 19 mmHg in both groups. Eyes with glaucoma would be expected to have a greater risk of IOP elevation.[6,12-14]

Although no formal surveys have polled surgeons regarding approaches to coexisting cataract and glaucoma, as a general rule of thumb, cataract surgery alone will be considered if the glaucoma is adequately controlled with two or fewer medications (with no contraindications or allergy to the remaining available medications) and visual field loss does not involve fixation (Table 20-1). The surgeon must anticipate the possibility of an acute and/or chronic postoperative elevation of IOP that could require an increase in medical therapy. Perioperative beta-blocker and carbonic anhydrase inhibitor therapy should be considered to reduce this risk. Postoperative IOP elevation may be more likely in the presence of coexisting uveitis, when iris manipulation or posterior synechialysis is required, if peripheral anterior synechiae are present, when cortex or viscoelastic are incompletely removed, and so on. In addition, there may be a relative contraindication to the use of prostaglandin analogues and miotics postoperatively because of the potential increased risk of inflammation and cystoid macular edema. If visual field loss involves or threatens fixation, delay in lowering a postoperative IOP spike could result in progression of glaucoma damage with increased visual disability. These risks warrant consideration of combined surgery. We favor a conservative approach and, when in doubt, consider combined surgery.

Cataract surgery employing techniques other than small-incision clear corneal phacoemulsification (such as extracapsular cataract extraction, which usually requires a larger incision and may be associated with more extensive inflammation) may have a greater risk of postoperative IOP elevation and glaucoma damage.

TABLE 20-1
Indications for Cataract Surgery

PHACOEMULSIFICATION

Indications

Presence of a cataract that impairs visual function or prevents adequate view of the optic nerve, with:

- IOP controlled with fewer than two medications
- Ability to use remaining available medications
- Mild to moderate visual field loss that does not involve fixation

TRABECULECTOMY

Indications

Cataract does not decrease visual function or impair view of optic nerve, and progression that would require surgery is not anticipated (surgeon's judgment), with:

- Uncontrolled IOP with maximum tolerated medical therapy
- Extreme IOP elevation (e.g., with corneal edema, even if cataract is present) unless glaucoma is lens induced

COMBINED SURGERY

Indications

Cataract decreases visual function or prevents view of optic nerve or is likely to do so if trabeculectomy alone were performed (surgeon's judgment), and

- Uncontrolled IOP with two or more medications
- Uncontrolled IOP with less than two medications with others ineffective or contraindicated
- Unable to use medications because of cost, compliance, physical limitations, and so on
- Pupil stretch or extensive posterior synechialysis required (with resulting debris potentially blocking trabecular outflow and increasing IOP postoperatively)
- Extensive peripheral anterior synechia (increasing potential for postoperative IOP elevation)
- Visual field loss is moderate to advanced or involves fixation

IOP, Intraocular pressure.

Trabeculectomy Surgery

Trabeculectomy surgery alone may be considered when the IOP is uncontrolled despite maximum medical therapy and the cataract does not decrease visual function. Even with uneventful trabeculectomy surgery, however, a cataract can progress. If cataract surgery is necessary in the near future, even a clear corneal approach may result in scarring of the filtering bleb with elevation of IOP, requiring additional medical therapy or glaucoma surgery.[15,16] The surgeon's judgment must be used in determining the best procedure for these patients (see Table 20-1).

In cases of marked IOP elevation (e.g., with corneal edema, neovascular glaucoma, traumatic glaucoma) with coexisting cataract, trabeculectomy with mitomycin C (MMC) or tube implant surgery may be the safest and best choice, deferring consideration of the cataract to a future, more controlled time. Alternatively, if lens-induced glaucoma is suspected, combined surgery may be the best approach.

Combined Cataract and Trabeculectomy Surgery

Combined surgery attempts to manage both cataract and glaucoma with one surgical procedure. The choice of this procedure should be determined on an individual basis for each patient (see Table 20-1). Although combined surgery has been considered controversial in the past, it is now accepted as an indicated procedure in selected eyes with coexisting cataract and glaucoma. (For this discussion, *combined surgery* is defined as phacoemulsification with posterior chamber IOL implantation and trabeculectomy or possibly nonpenetrating trabeculectomy.)[7]

Glaucomatous eyes have compromised trabecular meshwork and reduced aqueous outflow. There is a greater risk of postoperative IOP elevation that may further increase when posterior synechialysis or pupil manipulation is required. Although visual recovery after combined surgery may be delayed compared with cataract surgery alone, it is more rapid than when the glaucoma and cataract are managed separately in a two-stage approach. Combined surgery decreases the incidence and facilitates the management of postoperative IOP elevations versus cataract surgery alone.[17] However, early postoperative elevations of IOP have been reported even when combined surgery is performed.[8,18] Use of releasable sutures with combined surgery permits secure wound closure, minimizing risk of a flat or shallow anterior chamber, and permits suture removal to increase aqueous flow and lower IOP postoperatively when the eye is stable.[9] (Laser suture lysis can be used in place of releasable sutures.)[19]

Although most filtering blebs function successfully, those that fail are likely to do so within 6 months, with the remaining failing years later.[20] Although the use of antimetabolites decreases the incidence of bleb failure, it is important to preserve conjunctiva for possible future filtering surgery. Conjunctival dissection in combined surgery should be restricted to a single superior quadrant (the superotemporal quadrant provides the greatest exposure), leaving the remaining superior quadrant for future glaucoma surgery if needed.

Combined surgery with MMC has been reported to reduce IOP from 13.4% to 34% with 1.2 to 1.4 fewer glaucoma medications. These results were statistically better than both combined surgery with 5-fluorouracil (5-FU) and with no antimetabolite use, which were the same.[9,11] Lack of efficacy of MMC in an additional study may have been due to surgical technique or the risk factors in the patient population studied.[21]

Combined phacoemulsification, IOL implantation, and trabeculectomy surgery with MMC is most applicable in eyes that have uncontrolled glaucoma with maximum medical therapy and a cataract that impairs vision. Eyes requiring more than two glaucoma medications, eyes controlled on fewer than two medications with others contraindicated or ineffective, and eyes with visual field damage that is advanced or involves fixation are also good candidates for combined surgery with MMC to minimize the possibility of potentially damaging postoperative IOP elevation. Combined surgery will permit better management of postoperative IOP elevation and provide a high probability of improved short-term and long-term IOP control with fewer medications. In these eyes, it is safer to perform one combined procedure than two separate procedures. Although trabeculectomy with MMC performed alone has the potential for greater reduction of IOP and glaucoma medications than combined surgery with MMC, the success of combined surgery with MMC more than justifies its use in appropriate patients. In addition, the techniques presently employed in combined surgery do not increase risk more than performing the procedures separately and may even reduce the risk with only one trip to the operating room.

If the glaucoma is controlled with fewer than two medications, with the ability to add others, and visual field loss is mild in an eye with a visually disabling cataract, combined surgery with MMC may not be required. Phacoemulsification with IOL alone may be performed to avoid some of the potential complications of combined surgery, such as bleb dysesthesia, bleb infection, and endophthalmitis. Although unlikely, significant IOP elevation can occur. One study showed that 1 of 17 eyes with stable open-angle glaucoma requiring one or two medications for control had an IOP elevation to 30 mmHg 1 day following clear corneal phacoemulsification surgery.[22] If postoperative elevation of IOP does occur, significant glaucoma progression is unlikely.

Eyes with a functioning filtering bleb and controlled IOP also require special decision making when planning cataract removal. Present techniques of clear corneal phacoemulsification have a decreased risk of early postoperative elevations of IOP. In 69 eyes undergoing small-incision clear corneal phacoemulsification with a functioning filtering bleb, two eyes required subsequent additional glaucoma surgery. Sixteen eyes required more glaucoma medications postoperatively than preoperatively. If preoperative IOP was less than 15 mm Hg, the chance of needing more medications was 27.6%, and if greater than 15 mm Hg, the chance of needing more was 41.7%. Thus the surgeon must be aware that, even in this situation, dangerous elevations of IOP could occur with cataract surgery alone and that there is a risk that increased glaucoma therapy will be required.[15,16] If a previously filtered eye contains a questionably functioning filtering bleb with a significant cataract and IOP is uncontrolled or controlled with multiple medications in the presence of advanced glaucoma damage, combined surgery should be performed. Internal or external revision of the existing trabeculectomy combined with phacoemulsification could also be considered.

Antimetabolites

Daily postoperative subconjunctival 5-FU injections enhanced filtration success when trabeculectomy was performed alone.[23-25] Although in an early report, 5-FU mildly improved filtration success in combined surgery, other studies found no benefit.[26-29]

Chen's pioneering work with MMC,[30] a stronger antimetabolite than 5-FU that could be applied topically at the time of filtering surgery, offered the potential of improved filtration success with combined surgery. The initial report of combined surgery with MMC showed improved IOP control with fewer glaucoma medications at 1-year follow-up. Subsequent investigations have supported these results.[9,30-32]

Although MMC improves the success of filtration in combined surgery, it also may increase the risk of complications such as hypotony maculopathy, bleb leaks, bleb infection, and endophthalmitis. As a result, the concentration of MMC and duration of application have decreased since its initial use. Although MMC appears to have a fairly flat dose-response curve, reduced exposure seems to decrease the incidence of complications.[26,27,33,34]

Many variables are associated with MMC use. Surgeons using similar concentrations and exposure times of MMC may get different results, and surgeons using different concentrations and exposure times may get similar results. The choice of sponge material may be one of these variables. Different cellulose spears, instrument wipes, and corneal caps may each absorb different amounts of MMC and, when placed in contact with tissue, result in different antimetabolite effect. Surgeons may choose materials that will not tear or fragment during application, cut variable-sized pieces of the material to be placed in contact with the tissue, place pressure on the material containing MMC through the overlying conjunctiva to squeeze MMC into the tissues, or use a cellulose spear to absorb any MMC containing liquid that seeps out from beneath the conjunctival flap and threatens to contact the edges of the conjunctival incision. In addition, many surgeons wipe the subconjunctival space lateral and posterior (the space posterior to the conjunctival incision in limbus-based flaps) to the bleb area for about 20 to 30 seconds with the hope that a more diffuse, lower-profile filtering bleb will form, which may be less likely to become localized and cystic with less potential to develop a late leak through a thinned wall.

Each surgeon should develop his or her own technique, starting with conservative MMC exposure times to minimize the risk of complications. The surgeon should consider the risk/benefit ratio of MMC use and err on the side of less rather than more antimetabolite exposure to avoid complications, realizing that additional glaucoma surgery could be required. When the surgeon is comfortable with the technique and the results, the exposure times can be modified and individualized depending on the severity of glaucoma, risk factors for failure, ability to perform additional glaucoma surgery in the future, and so on (See Application of Mitomycin later in text for specific parameters of one technique of MMC use.)

Application of Mitomycin Before or After Entering the Anterior Chamber

When MMC was first used in combined surgery, many surgeons applied the antifibrotic agent near the end of the procedure, after watertight closure of the scleral flap. The area was irrigated with balanced salt solution (BSS), and the conjunctiva was closed. No clinically evident adverse effects were noted. Concern subsequently developed over the possibility of toxicity to corneal endothelial cells and the ciliary body epithelium. Experiments in rabbits showed that MMC penetrated the sclera and resulted in detectible aqueous levels. A reversible decrease in aqueous production followed application of MMC to the scleral surface in monkey eyes. However, the dose of MMC used in these studies was larger than that used clinically in humans.[35-38]

MMC can be applied before entering the anterior chamber or after removing the cataract and securely closing the wound to prevent MMC entry into the eye. Cohen[26] provided evidence that topical application of MMC at the end of the procedure after secure closure of the scleral incision does not cause loss of corneal endothelial cells. This method permits the surgeon to abort the use of MMC if a defect occurred in the conjunctiva or in the scleral wound that would contraindicate its use and therefore might be safer for the surgeon who is less experienced with combined surgery. When the surgeon is comfortable with the surgical technique, if desired, MMC can be applied before entering the anterior chamber. (See Applications of Mitomycin.)

Subconjunctival or Sub-Tenon's Injection of Antimetabolite Postoperatively

Based on the work by Gressel, Parrish, and Folberg,[23] which initially showed that daily postoperative subconjunctival injections of 5-FU improve success of trabeculectomy surgery, many surgeons will augment intraoperative antimetabolite therapy with postoperative 5-FU if bleb failure is threatened (increased bleb vascularization, decreased filtration, etc.).

Results Following Combined Surgery

Several prospective and retrospective studies, using varying techniques of MMC application in varying concentrations, found significantly lower IOP with fewer glaucoma medications. Mean IOP decreased 5 mm Hg in the MMC group versus 3 mm Hg in the placebo group. The mean number of medications required for IOP control decreased 0.5 to 2.7 in the MMC groups versus 0.7 to 0.9 in the placebo groups. Fifty percent to 100% of eyes in the MMC groups versus 10% to 67% in the placebo groups were controlled without medications.[9-11,39]

Complications Following Combined Surgery

Complications and their frequency were listed in several prospective and retrospective studies and included vitreous loss (2% to 7%), wound leak (1% to 30%), iris incarceration in sclerostomy (2%), shallow anterior chamber (7% to 14%), serous choroidal detachment (14% to 27%), hypotony (6% to 18%), and fibrin formation in the anterior chamber (7% to 19%). With improved surgical techniques and modified methods and durations of MMC application, complications have been significantly reduced.

(The management of complications is discussed under Postoperative Management and Complications.)

Combined Surgery Method

Preoperative Preparations

MEDICATIONS

Topical corticosteroid eyedrops are used every 2 hours starting the day before surgery. Topical antibiotic eyedrops are used every 2 hours starting the evening before surgery. A combination antibiotic-steroid ointment is applied to the eyelashes at bedtime the evening before surgery. A nonsteroidal antiinflammatory eyedrop is applied twice the morning of surgery. Cyclopentolate 1%, phenylephrine 2.5%, and homatropine 2% eyedrops are applied every 5 to 10 minutes for four applications before surgery. One drop of betaxolol (Betoptic) is applied ½ hour before surgery. One drop of 5% povidone-iodine (Betadine) solution is administered immediately before the facial prep.[40]

Topical antiglaucoma therapy has been shown to have an adverse effect on the conjunctival cellular profile and on filtering surgery success. This is why corticosteroid eyedrops are started preoperatively.[41] Consideration should be given to discontinuing IOP-lowering agents that compromise the blood aqueous barrier and increase the risk of iritis (such as miotics and prostaglandin analogues) several days to a week before surgery. (This should not be done if other glaucoma medications cannot be substituted to blunt possible IOP elevation in eyes with advanced glaucoma.)

ANESTHESIA

Although topical anesthesia is used by many surgeons for combined surgery, we usually use either a short- or long-acting retrobulbar block. The short-acting block is performed with 3 to 4 ml of 2% lidocaine (Xylocaine) with 150 units of hyaluronidase without a postoperative eye patch. The long-acting retrobulbar block is performed with 3 to 4 ml of 4% lidocaine (Xylocaine) and 0.75% bupivacaine (Marcaine) in a 1:2 mixture, with 150 units of hyaluronidase combined with a Van Lint block using the same anesthetic mixture and requiring a patch postoperatively. Preoperative discussion with the patient of anesthetic options may be helpful.

The long-acting block is especially helpful in more difficult cases when pupil stretch or posterior synechialysis are required and phacoemulsification and cortex removal will be done through a small pupil and capsulorhexis.

Operative Technique

CONJUNCTIVAL FLAP

We prefer a limbus-based conjunctival flap. Although a limbus-based flap requires more manipulation and is technically more cumbersome than a fornix-based flap, it provides greater certainty of watertight closure and avoidance of postoperative incision leak. In contrast, the fornix-based flap provides easier and better surgical exposure but has a greater risk of postoperative wound leak. Although there is evidence that limbus- and fornix-based flaps result in the same long-term IOP results, we believe that an incision leak in a fornix-based flap is counterproductive to bleb formation.[18,42] When antimetabolites are used with the surgery, leaks may heal more slowly and be more difficult to repair with a fornix-based flap.[9,23] However, we will usually perform a fornix-based flap if significant subconjunctival scar tissue exists from previous surgery.

Limbus-based conjunctival flap. Dissection is performed in the superotemporal quadrant to minimize the anatomic restrictions from the brow and the superior orbital rim. The initial incision should be made 8 to 9 mm posterior to the limbus and penetrate conjunctiva and Tenon's capsule to expose sclera, using sharp scissors and toothed forceps. Blunt scissors and nontoothed forceps (e.g., Pearce forceps, instrument #2-136, Duckworth & Kent, St. Louis, Mo.) extend the incision parallel to the limbus and laterally in both directions to permit adequate exposure. The incision width usually approximates 12 mm (Figure 20-1). The incision should remain about 8 to 9 mm from the limbus along the entire length to minimize the limitation of filtration from the incision scar and to avoid the thinner and more delicate conjunctiva that is sometimes present closer to the limbus. Tenon's tissue is bluntly pushed anteriorly with a dry cellulose sponge or curved edge of a blade to expose the limbus. (Sometimes the insertion of Tenon's tissue must be cut to provide adequate exposure. If at all possible, Tenon's capsule insertion should be left intact to provide extra integrity to the bleb.) Blunt dissection is also performed beneath the edge of the conjunctival incision posteriorly with scissors.

Fornix-based conjunctival flap. In the superotemporal quadrant, a toothed forceps and sharp scissors are used to create a limbal conjunctival incision several millimeters wide. A nontoothed forceps and blunt scissors extend the incision laterally in both directions and then bluntly dissect posteriorly to provide adequate exposure for the scleral incision and a potential space for filtration (Figure 20-2).

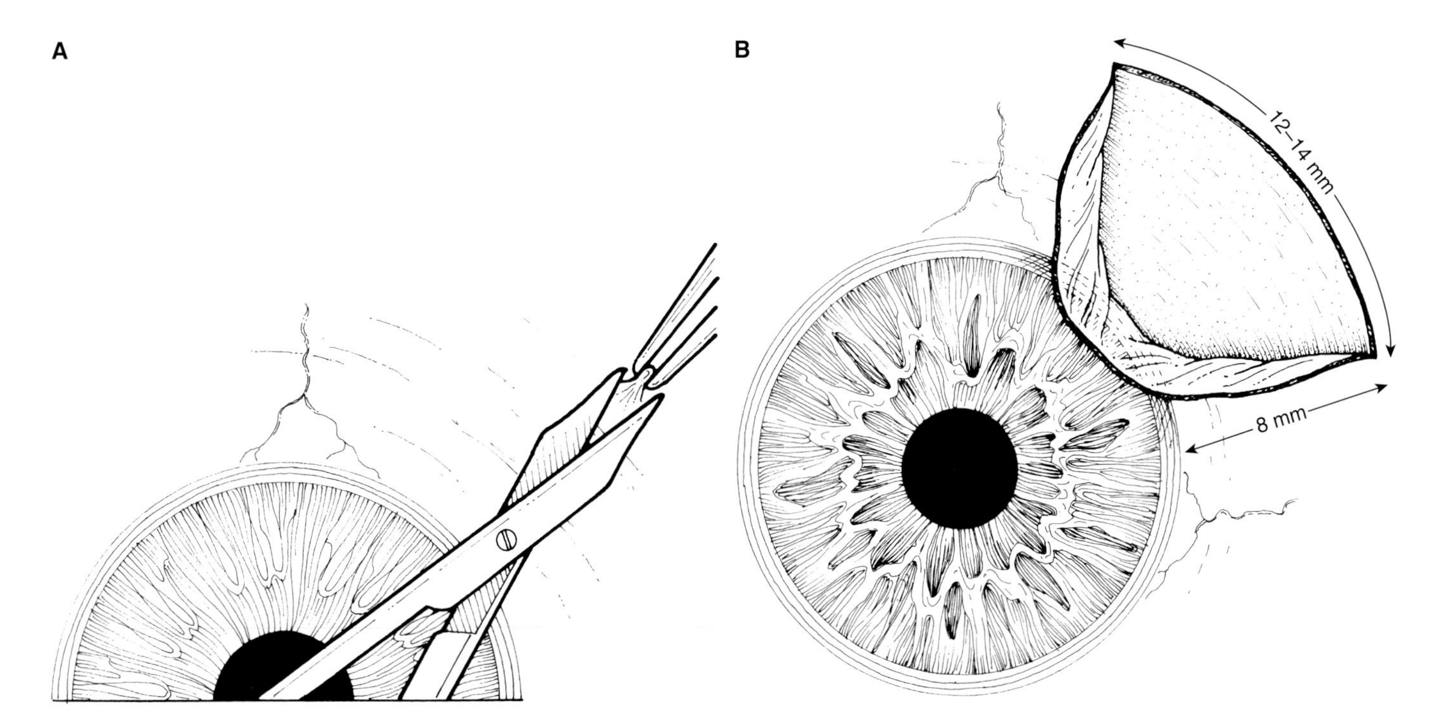

FIGURE 20-1 **A,** Initial incision for limbus-based conjunctival flap is made with sharp scissors and toothed forceps, 8 to 9 mm posterior to the limbus, exposing sclera. **B,** Limbus-based flap should be about 12 mm wide to provide adequate exposure.

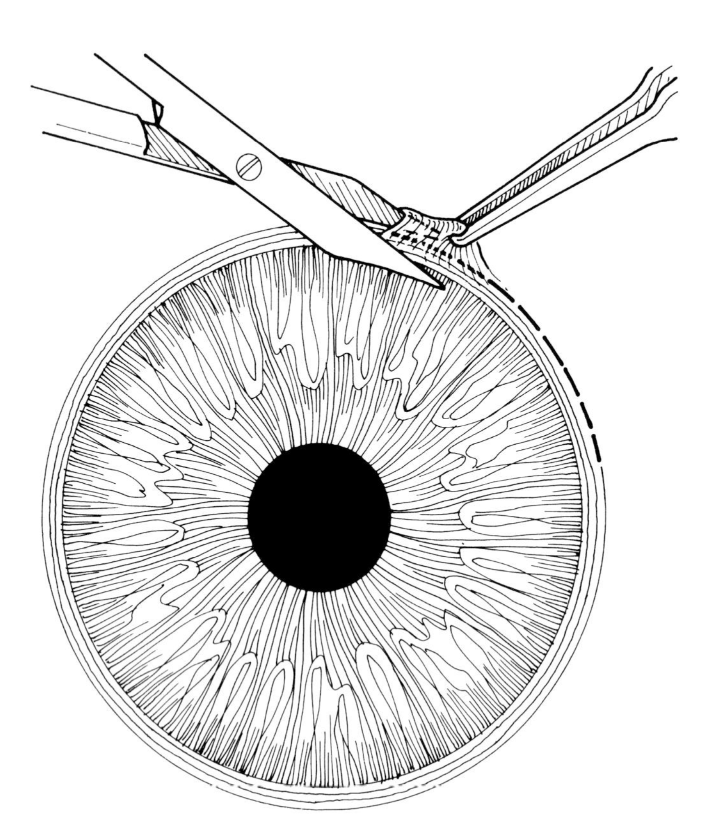

FIGURE 20-2 Limbal conjunctival incision is made to create a fornix-based conjunctival flap.

SCLERAL INCISION AND PARACENTESIS

A three-stage tunnel incision is made with the initial vertical incision approximately 2 mm posterior to the limbus. The first-stage vertical incision is performed at about one-half scleral depth and the necessary width for insertion of the desired IOL (we use a 0.37-mm preset diamond blade) (Figure 20-3, *A*). The second stage of the incision is made horizontally, parallel to Descemet's membrane (we use a crescent steel blade), and extends approximately 1 to 2 mm anterior to the limbus. MMC is now used. (See Application of Mitomycin later in text.) A keratome blade (appropriate for the size of the phacoemulsification tip) makes the vertical third stage of the incision and enters the anterior chamber (see Figure 20-3, *B*). A narrow, sharp-pointed blade is then used to make a small peripheral paracentesis opening in the cornea, at a position about 3 clock hours to the left of the scleral incision (right-handed surgeon) for insertion of a manipulating instrument. A viscoelastic agent is then injected to fill and maintain the anterior chamber.

APPLICATION OF MITOMYCIN

Two small pieces of a cellulose spear (we use i-Spear ophthalmic sponge, Alcon, Fort Worth, Tex.), each the approximate size of the scleral flap, are soaked in MMC (0.4 mg/ml). These two pieces are then placed on the scleral surface, overlying and extending beyond the scleral tunnel on both sides (Figure 20-4, *A*). This will spread the MMC effect beyond the area overlying the scleral tunnel and hopefully extend the area of filtration laterally in both directions. The conjunctiva is brought down over the

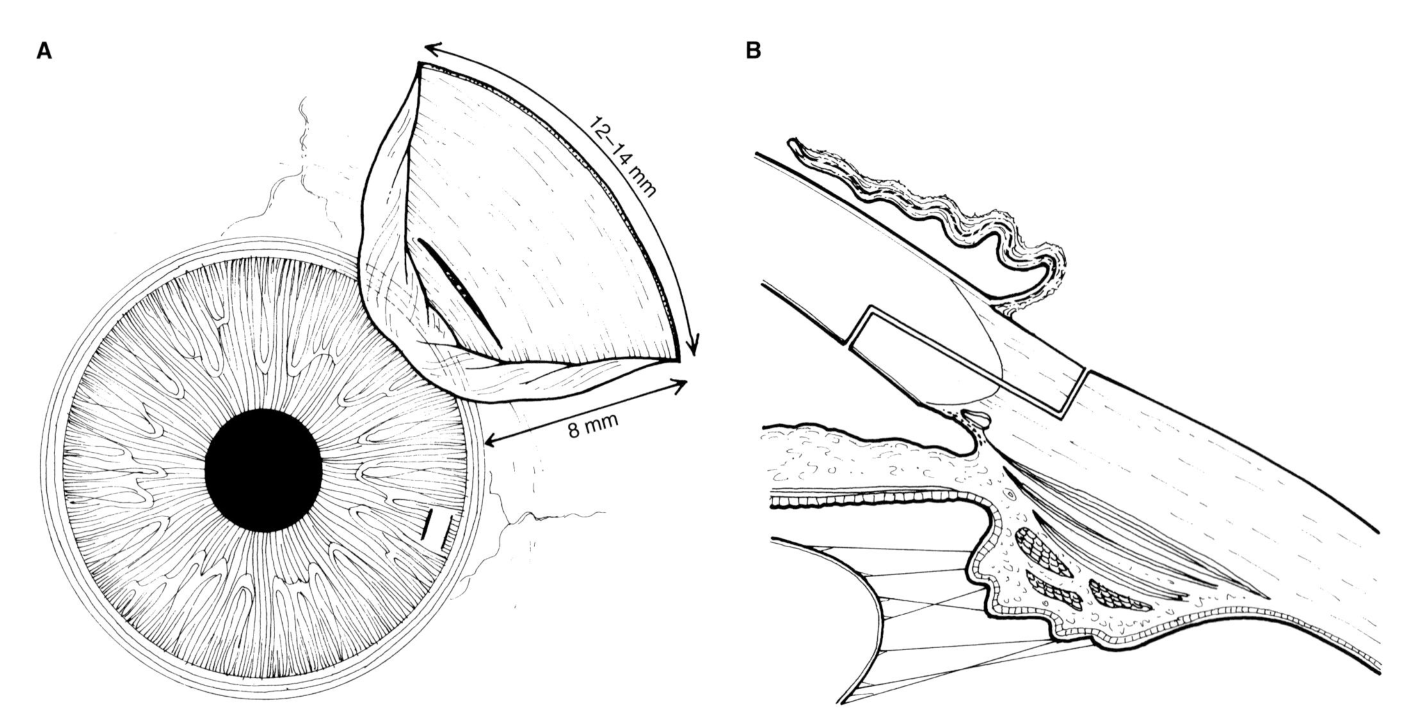

FIGURE 20-3 **A,** First-stage vertical incision is performed at about one-half scleral depth and the necessary width for insertion of the desired intraocular lens. **B,** Three-stage scleral incision is made into the anterior chamber.

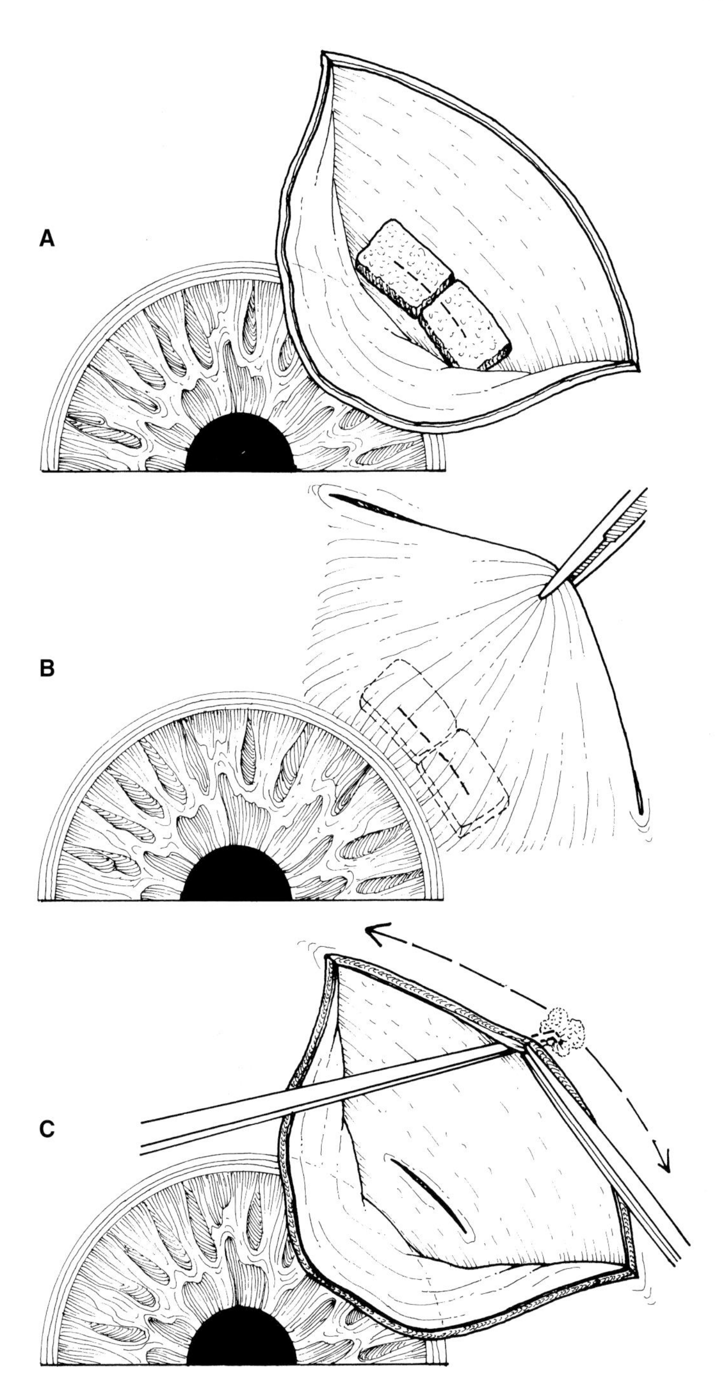

FIGURE 20-4 A, Two pieces of cellulose sponge are placed on the scleral surface, overlying and extending beyond the scleral tunnel on both sides. **B,** Conjunctiva is brought down over the sponges. **C,** An intact piece of cellulose sponge, about 2 × 3 mm in size, is securely grasped by toothed forceps and wiped beneath the previously dissected posterior subconjunctival space.

sponges (see Figure 20-4, *B*). The edges of the conjunctival incision should not touch the sponges or any liquid containing MMC. A cellulose sponge should be used to absorb any excess liquid that flows out from under the conjunctival flap. After 1 minute of tissue exposure, one of the sponges is removed, and the remaining sponge is positioned centrally on the scleral flap. After an additional minute, the second sponge is removed, and the conjunctival and corneal surfaces, the tissues beneath the edges of the conjunctiva laterally, and the scleral tunnel are irrigated with 15 ml of BSS. An intact piece of cellulose sponge, about 2 × 3 mm in size, is securely grasped by toothed forceps and wiped beneath the previously dissected posterior subconjunctival space (limbus-based flap) for 15 to 30 seconds (see Figure 20-4, *C*). This area is also irrigated with 15 ml of BSS. (When a fornix-based flap is used, a similar maneuver can be performed deeper than the area previously exposed.)

A total of 2 minutes of MMC exposure time beneath the limbus-based conjunctival flap is used for most eyes. The duration of exposure may be decreased by $\frac{1}{2}$ to 1 minute if the need for IOP reduction is less because of less severe glaucoma, a reduced tendency for healing related to older age, systemic use of corticosteroids or other immunocompromising drugs, and so on. The duration may be increased by $\frac{1}{2}$ to 1 minute if there are risk factors for failure such as previous surgery, African-American race, or history of uveitis. Evidence has shown that the dose-response curve of MMC is fairly flat but that longer exposure times may have an increased incidence of complications.[33]

MANAGEMENT OF THE SMALL PUPIL AND POSTERIOR SYNECHIA

Long-term use of glaucoma (especially miotic) eyedrops may limit the effectiveness of pupillary dilation in preparation for phacoemulsification. If the patient is using miotic eyedrops and the IOP and stage of glaucoma permit, discontinuation of the miotics and, if possible, substitution of other glaucoma drops may enhance the mydriasis. The minimum acceptable and comfortable pupil size may vary depending on the specific type and severity of the cataract. A "soft" cataract may not require surgical enlargement of the pupil even if dilation is poor. A brunescent cataract, however, may require surgical enlargement of the pupil even if it dilates moderately. Although manipulation of the pupil may result in decreased sphincter function, patients rarely complain of any problems and are far better off avoiding more serious events such as a capsule defect or vitreous loss. Each surgeon must determine what pupil size is adequate.

The dilated preoperative examination helps predict whether pupil manipulation will be necessary. Stripping a pupillary membrane or lysis of posterior synechia may significantly enhance pupil size. "Viscodilation" with a cohesive viscoelastic may be all that is required to enlarge the pupil to a comfortable size for capsulorhexis. If further enlargement is required, we have found pupil stretch to be successful virtually 100% of the time. Although iris hooks, pupil ring expanders, and minisphincterotomies will enhance pupil size, they are rarely required because of the success of pupil stretch, improved techniques of phacoemulsification, and newer viscoelastics. (See Chapter 19, Phacoemulsification in the Presence of a Small Pupil.)

If pupil enlargement is required, we employ a bimanual stretch maneuver. Two instruments designed for iris manipulation are used (Osher Y-hook, E0577, Storz, Claremont, Calif.; Kuglen Iris Hook and IOL Manipulator, 6-400 and 6-402, Duckworth & Kent, St. Louis, Mo.). One instrument is placed in the anterior chamber through the paracentesis opening while the other enters through the phacoemulsification incision, and the pupil is stretched by simultaneously pushing and pulling the pupillary edge of the iris in opposite directions in the same meridian (6 clock hours apart) (Figure 20-5, *A*).[43-45] For additional enlargement, a second stretch maneuver can be performed in a meridian about 90 degrees from the first (see Figure 20-5, *B*), or the two stretch instruments can be placed less than 6 clock hours apart before stretching. A slow and gradual stretch will minimize the risk of an atonic pupil. Self-limited bleeding may occur from the tears in the pupillary margin of the iris. Elevation of the IOP by filling the anterior chamber with BSS or viscoelastic can help tamponade the bleeding.

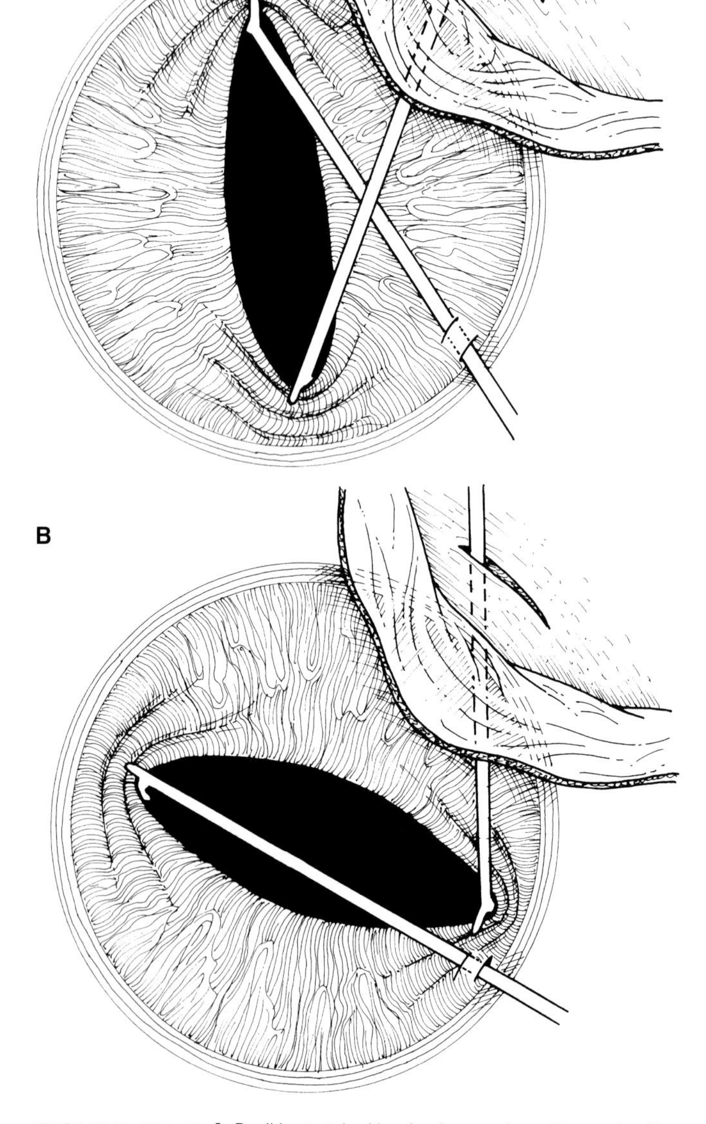

FIGURE 20-5 **A,** Pupil is stretched by simultaneously pushing and pulling the pupillary edge of the iris in opposite directions in the same meridian (six clock hours apart). **B,** Additional enlargement can be achieved by performing a second stretch maneuver 90 degrees away from the first.

In the rare cases when bimanual stretch inadequately dilates the pupil, multiple small sphincterotomies performed with fine intraocular scissors or iris retraction hooks can be helpful.

CAPSULORHEXIS

Continuous circular capsulorhexis is performed using a 22-gauge needle with a right-angle bend made about 1 mm from the tip. An alternate method using capsule forceps is preferred by many surgeons. The size of the capsulorhexis is often limited by suboptimal pupillary dilation and may require enlargement later in the procedure when the chamber has been deepened by a viscoelastic agent. (See earlier section, Management of the Small Pupil and Posterior Synechia.) Too small a capsulorhexis may compromise phacoemulsification and cortical aspiration, increase the risk of a radial extension of the capsulorhexis, and result in intraoperative and postoperative complications. (Also see Chapter 13, Capsulorrhexis.)

HYDRODISSECTION, HYDRODELINEATION, AND VISCODISSECTION

The nuclear and cortical lens layers are hydrodissected from the lens capsule by gently injecting BSS just beneath the edge of the capsulorhexis with a blunt 27-gauge cannula, using moderate infusion pressure. The pupil is observed for passage of a fluid wave across the red reflex. When dense cataracts preclude observation of the fluid wave, slight anterior movement of the nucleus confirms hydrodissection. Injection of fluid into the cataractous lens can achieve hydrodelineation by separating the nuclear, epinuclear, and cortical layers. (A 27-gauge J-shaped cannula can direct the hydrodissection to the cortex beneath the scleral incision and achieve better mobilization of the more difficult-to-remove cortex in this area.) Successful hydrodissection is crucial in poorly dilated pupils. It is helpful to test for adequate hydrodissection by rotating the nucleus (with viscoelastic in the anterior chamber) using one or two manipulating instruments. The injection of a viscoelastic may also be used to dissect cortex or nucleus away from the lens capsule when normal irrigation-aspiration techniques may be dangerous (e.g., with a small pupil or capsulorhexis, capsule defect). (Also see Chapter 14, Hydrodissection and Hydrodelineation.)

PHACOEMULSIFICATION AND CORTICAL ASPIRATION

Phacoemulsification is performed using the preferred technique of the surgeon. We usually create a central groove greater than two thirds of the depth of the lens and use a second instrument to help crack the nucleus into two halves. Each half is then rotated and chopped into smaller pieces, which permit easier and safer phacoemulsification in the posterior chamber.

Aspiration of the cortex is performed in the usual manner. This can be more challenging in the presence of a small pupil and capsulorhexis. An iris manipulating hook should be used to push the iris peripherally and expose the peripheral capsular bag, when it is inadequately seen, to ensure removal of hidden cortex. Use of a separate aspiration cannula (Surgical Design Corporation, Long Island City, NY; Oasis Medical Inc., Glendora, Calif.) that is small enough to be passed through the paracentesis opening can be extremely helpful in removing cortex from the capsular bag opposite the paracentesis and beneath the area of the scleral incision (Figure 20-6, *A*). A J-shaped cannula on a

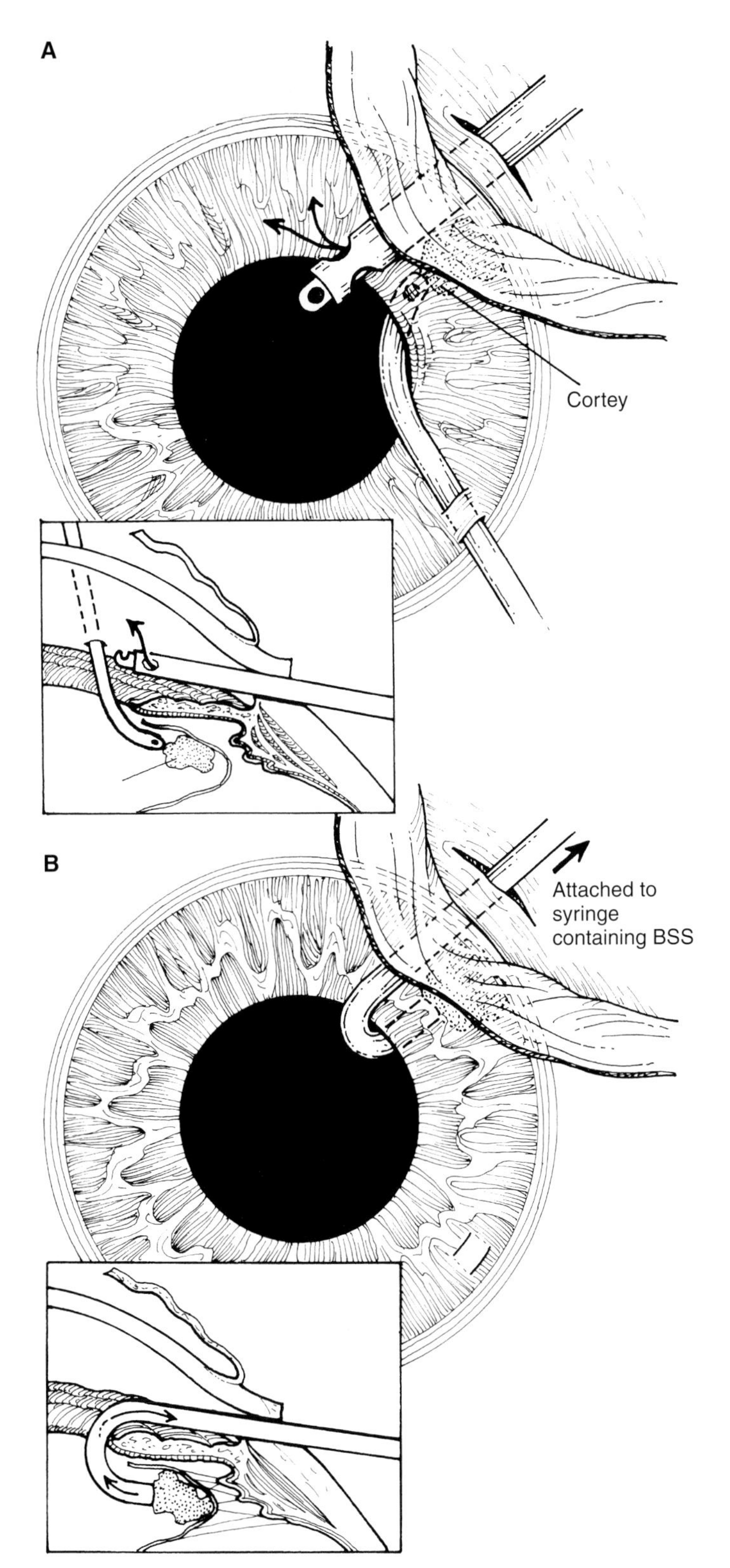

FIGURE 20-6 A, Separate aspiration canula, small enough to be passed through the paracentesis opening, can be extremely helpful in removing cortex from beneath the area of the scleral incision. **B,** J-shaped cannula on a syringe containing BSS can also be used to remove the subincisional cortex after inflating the capsular bag with viscoelastic.

syringe containing BSS can also be used to remove the subincisional cortex after having inflated the bag and anterior chamber with viscoelastic (see Figure 20-6, *B*). (Also see Chapter 15, Principles of Nuclear Phacoemulsification, and Chapter 16, Phaco Chop.)

INTRAOCULAR LENS IMPLANTATION

The tunnel incision is enlarged to the required size for IOL implantation. Use of IOL injectors may require little or no enlargement, depending on the specific IOL and injector used. (Also see Part VI, Intraocular Lenses.)

TRABECULECTOMY OR SCLERECTOMY

The left side of the scleral tunnel is cut anteriorly to permit elevation of the corner and exposure of the tunnel floor (Figure 20-7, *A*). A nontoothed forceps is used to elevate the roof of the scleral tunnel to perform the trabeculectomy or sclerectomy.

A sharp blade is used to make an incision in the scleral floor of the tunnel, parallel to the limbus, about 0.5 to 1 mm anterior to the posterior edge of the tunnel (see Figure 20-7, *B*). A Kelly punch (instrument #E-2798, Storz, Claremont, Calif.) is used to create a 1 × 2 mm opening into the anterior chamber on the left side of the tunnel (Figures 20-7, *C*, and 20-8, *A*). Trabecular meshwork or peripheral cornea anterior to the trabeculum is removed. (Alternatively, the punch can be passed into the phacoemulsification incision and punch posteriorly; see Figure 20-8, *B*.) If preferred, a freehand dissection is performed by making the same incision in the tunnel floor. Radial incisions are made anteriorly with a fine scissors (e.g., Vannas, instrument #E3389, Storz, Claremont, Calif.) on both sides of this incision. While the deep scleral tissue is grasped with toothed forceps, the scissors are used to cut the anterior edge, excising the tissue and creating a 1- × 2-mm filtration opening (Figure 20-9). An assistant can elevate the roof of the tunnel with nontoothed forceps or a cellulose sponge, or the surgeon can use the edge of the Vannas scissors to elevate the scleral flap during this dissection.

It is important to avoid extending the sclerectomy to the posterior edge of the tunnel floor to prevent simulation of a "full-thickness filtering procedure" with free access of aqueous flow through the incision to the scleral surface. Leaving a portion (0.5 to 1 mm) of the scleral floor intact forces the aqueous humor to percolate from the trabeculectomy or sclerectomy opening, across a short portion of the scleral floor, and through the incision to the scleral surface, resulting in slight resistance to flow. If the trabeculectomy or sclerectomy opening is inadvertently created over the ciliary body and uvea, the dissection should be extended anteriorly over the iris. If required, a fine needle tip cautery can be used at low power to control bleeding.

PERIPHERAL IRIDECTOMY

Although some surgeons have suggested that an iridectomy is not necessary, it is safest to perform one. Without an iridectomy, a shallow anterior chamber or application of digital pressure could result in occlusion of the trabeculectomy or sclerectomy opening.

The iridectomy is performed by grasping the peripheral iris through the trabeculectomy or sclerectomy opening with a fine-toothed forceps. The peripheral iris is elevated with a slight

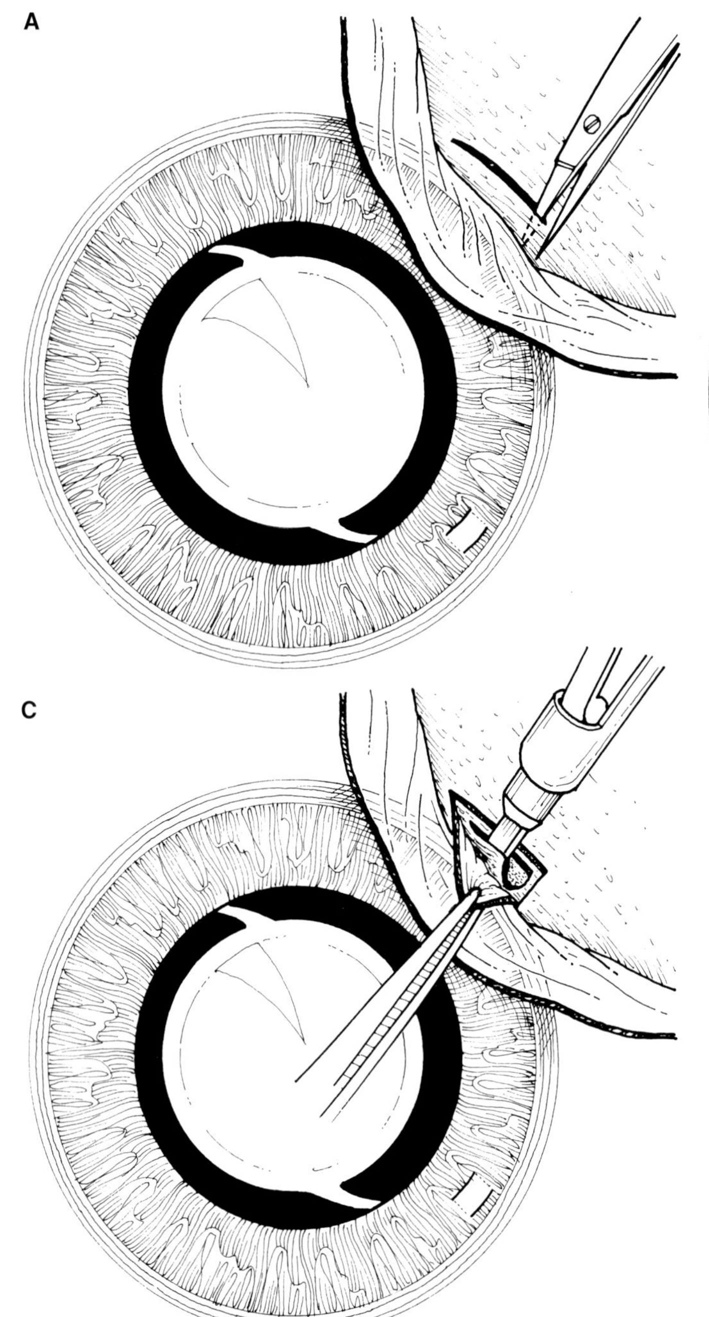

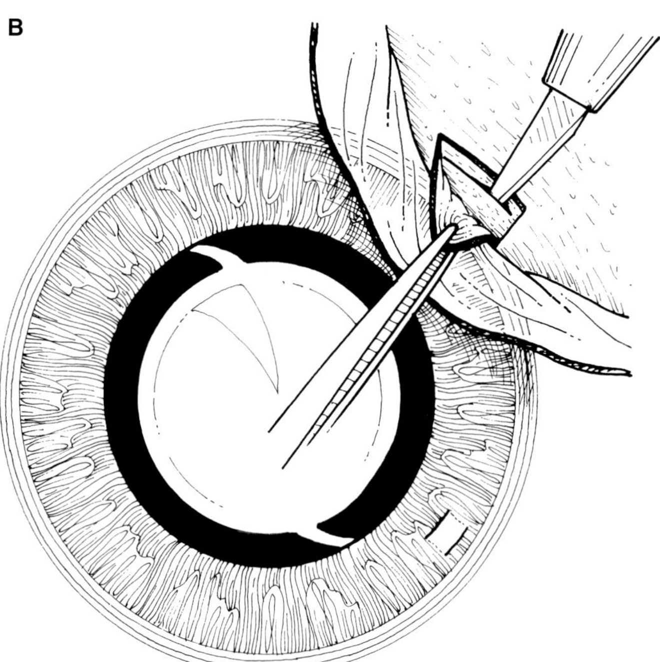

FIGURE 20-7 **A,** Left side of the scleral tunnel is cut anteriorly to permit elevation of the corner and exposure of the tunnel floor. **B,** Sharp blade is used to make an incision in the scleral floor of the tunnel, parallel to the limbus, about 0.5 to 1 mm anterior to the posterior edge of the tunnel. **C,** Kelly punch is used to create a sclerectomy on the left side of the tunnel.

side-to-side pulling motion, and Vannas scissors create the iridectomy opening (Figure 20-10, *A*). The size of the iridectomy should approximate the size of the trabeculectomy or sclerectomy opening. Prolapsed iris tissue should be irrigated or gently massaged into the anterior chamber by bluntly rubbing centrally on the corneal surface over the iridectomy. Aqueous humor will pass through the sclerectomy opening and the scleral incision into the subconjunctival space (Figure 20-10, *B*). A fine needle tip cautery can be used at low power to control bleeding from the iridectomy edge.

SCLERAL FLAP CLOSURE WITH RELEASABLE SUTURES

The scleral flap is closed with releasable sutures. These will secure the wound and provide nearly watertight closure, preventing early postoperative hypotony, flat anterior chamber, and associated complications. Three releasable sutures are usually used, placing one at the corner and two along the scleral incision. When the anterior chamber has stabilized and bleb healing has produced some resistance to aqueous flow, the sutures can be released to increase aqueous flow and help reach the target IOP.

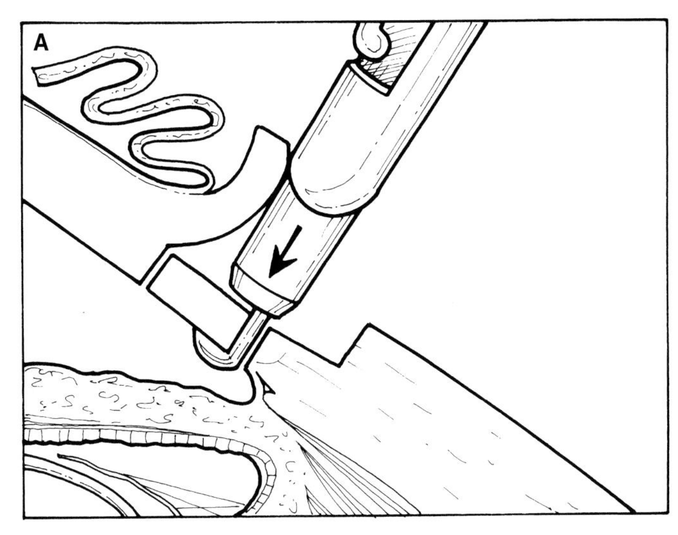

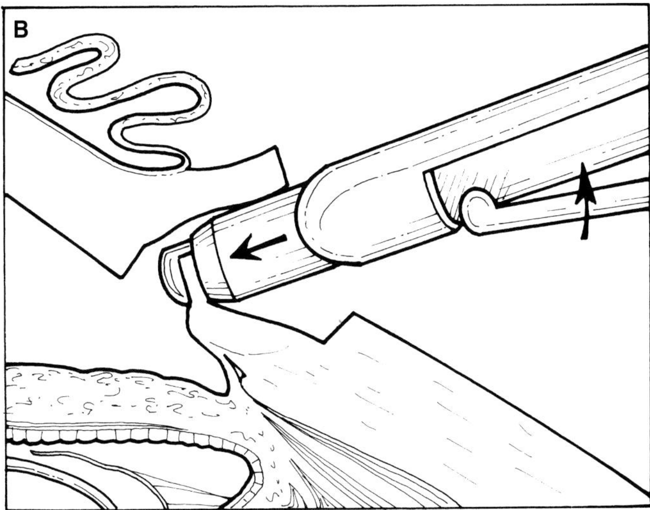

FIGURE 20-8 A, Kelly punch creates a sclerectomy (side view of Figure 20-7, *C*). **B,** Alternatively, the punch can be passed into the phacoemulsification incision and punch posteriorly.

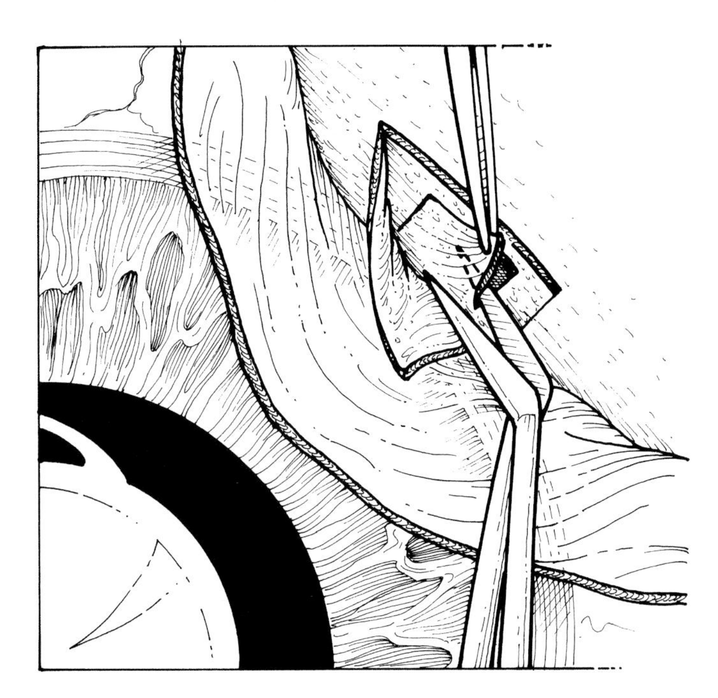

FIGURE 20-9 Sclerectomy can be created freehand with scissors and forceps.

The releasable sutures are placed in three steps. Using a narrow cutting needle on a 9-0 nylon suture (#7760, Ethicon, Sommerville, NJ) the first bite is placed through partial-thickness cornea, about 2 mm central and parallel to the limbus (Figure 20-11, *A* and *B*). The second bite is placed radial to the limbus (approximately 90 degrees to the first bite), passing through partial-thickness cornea beneath the conjunctival insertion at the limbus and exiting on the scleral side of the limbus (see Figure 20-11, *C* and *D*). (In the early postoperative period, epithelial cells grow over the suture lying on the corneal surface between the first and second bites.) The third bite is placed across the scleral flap incision (see Figure 20-11, *E* and *F*). Before tying the releasable sutures, the viscoelastic is aspirated from behind and in front of the IOL. After placing the first suture, the second and third sutures are also placed (see Figure 20-11, *G*).

The releasable sutures are tied by grasping the suture exiting the sclera from the third bite and passing three throws around a tying forceps (see Figure 20-11, *H*). The tying forceps then is used to grasp the suture on the scleral flap surface between the second bite and the third bite (across the scleral incision) (see Figure 20-11, *I*), and the three throws are brought down over the grasped suture, creating a loop knot that secures the scleral incision (see Figure 20-11, *J*). The suture is trimmed long enough so that it lies flat on the scleral surface (see Figure 20-11, *K*). The suture lying on the corneal surface is trimmed where it entered the cornea for the first bite (see Figure 20-11, *L*). Forceps are used to pull gently on the suture, and scissors are used to push gently on the cornea so that when the suture is cut at the corneal surface, it retracts into the corneal tissue.

After placement of the releasable sutures, acetylcholine (Miochol-E) is injected through the paracentesis tract to deepen the anterior chamber and to constrict the pupil. Slight pressure is placed on the posterior edge of the scleral incision to ensure that it does not leak. An elevated IOP on the first post-operative day is preferable to hypotony. It is easier to manage the former. (Management of IOP and release of sutures are discussed later in this chapter.)[46-48]

The technique of laser suture lysis and three other releasable suture techniques have been described by Hoskins and Migliazzo,[49] Savage et al.,[50] McAllister and Wilson,[51] Shin,[52] and Johnstone[53] and can be researched if desired.

CONJUNCTIVAL FLAP CLOSURE

The limbus-based conjunctival flap is closed with a 9-0 or 10-0 absorbable suture on a taper (noncutting) needle. Using a running suture technique, the deeper Tenon's layer is closed with locking stitches, and the superficial conjunctival layer is closed with a nonlocking stitch. Widely spaced stitches are used in the deeper Tenon's layer, and stitches 0.5 to 1 mm from the

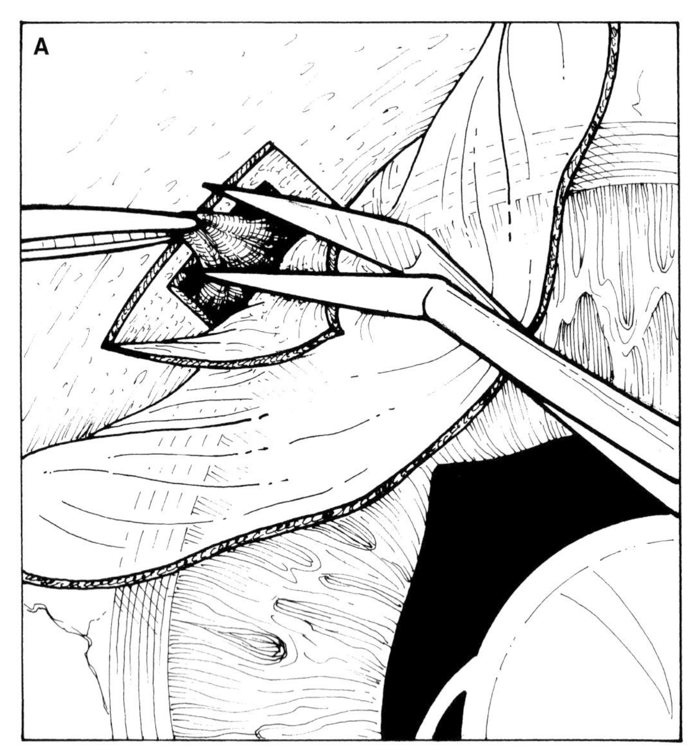

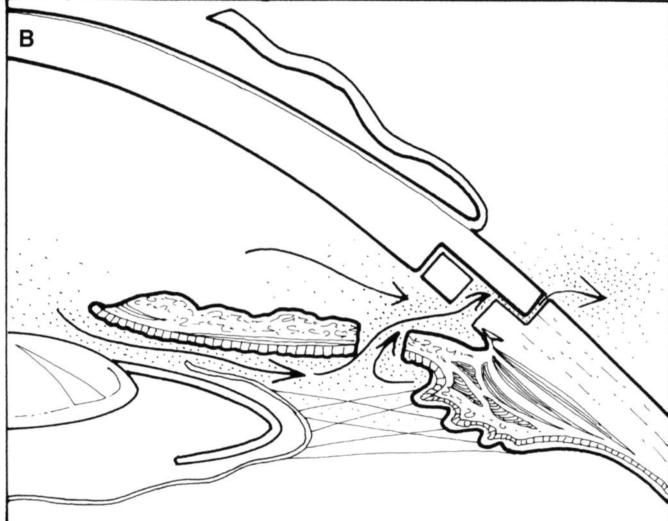

FIGURE 20-10 A, Peripheral iris is elevated with a slight side-to-side pulling motion, and Vannas scissors are used to create the iridectomy opening. **B,** Aqueous passes through the sclerectomy opening and the scleral incision into the subconjunctival space.

incision edge and separated by 1 to 2 mm are used in the conjunctival layer (Figure 20-12, *A*).

A fornix based conjunctival flap is closed with 9-0 Vicryl (Ethicon V439, Sommerville, NJ) by securing one side of the conjunctival flap to the peripheral cornea with a mattress suture. The other side of the conjunctival flap incision is then pulled, stretching the conjunctival edge against the peripheral cornea, and another mattress suture is placed. The limbal edge of conjunctiva is inspected, and additional mattress sutures are placed as necessary for secure closure. The surgeon must be sure that the exposed "elbow" of the releasable suture, between the first and second bites (the place where the suture is grasped when removed postoperatively), is not covered by the conjunctival flap. A running (noncutting needle on 9-0 or 10-0 absorbable) suture closes the conjunctiva laterally (see Figure 20-12, *B*). It is helpful to start this closure with a bite of episclera at the limbus. An overlapping running suture, using 9-0 nylon (Ethicon 2890) can also be used to close the conjunctiva at the limbus (see Figure 20-12, *C*).

An alternative closure of a fornix-based conjunctival flap has been reported by Wise,[54] using a 9-0 nylon suture on a vascular needle (Ethicon 2890, Ethicon, Inc., Somerville, NJ).

PHACOEMULSIFICATION AND TRABECULECTOMY AT SEPARATE SITES

Combined surgery with separate-site temporal clear corneal phacoemulsification and superonasal trabeculectomy has been advocated by some surgeons. This approach requires the surgeon to change positions and move the microscope when switching from one surgical site to the other. The benefit of this technique is uncertain. Although one study suggested slight benefit in IOP control, another study did not confirm this finding.[55,56] We only use this approach when superotemporal scarring requires superonasal filtration or when the presence of extremely thin conjunctiva increases the risk of a defect from the added manipulation.

Intraoperative Medications

At the completion of the procedure, aqueous betamethasone (Celestone) is injected subconjunctivally. (At the time of writing of this chapter, betamethasone is unavailable. Many surgeons are substituting triamcinolone acetonide [Kenalog] to achieve the antiinflammatory effect.) An antibiotic preparation may also be injected subconjunctivally at the surgeon's discretion. In addition, one drop of 5% povidone-iodine solution (Betadine) is placed in the fornix at the conclusion of the procedure. If the anesthetic block requires postoperative patching, antibiotic-steroid ointment is also applied.

Postoperative Management

FREQUENCY OF EXAMINATIONS

The early postoperative period is critical to the success of combined surgery. This is when elevated IOP is most likely to occur and when it can most effectively be managed. Examinations

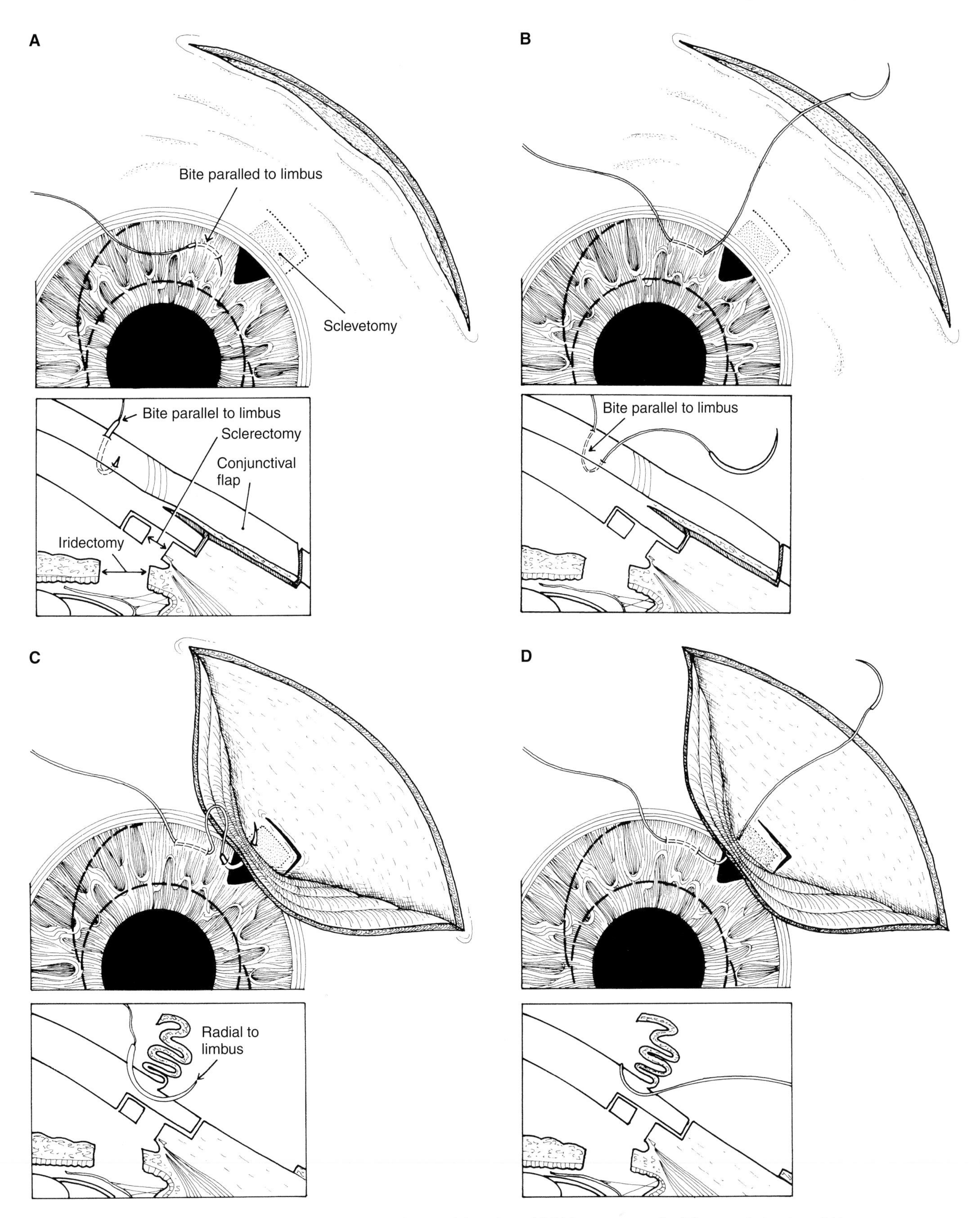

FIGURE 20-11 **A** and **B,** First bite is passed through partial-thickness cornea, about 2 mm central and parallel to the limbus. **C** and **D,** Second bite is placed radial to the limbus (approximately 90 degrees to the first bite), passing through partial-thickness cornea beneath the conjunctival insertion at the limbus and exiting on the scleral side of the limbus.

(Continued)

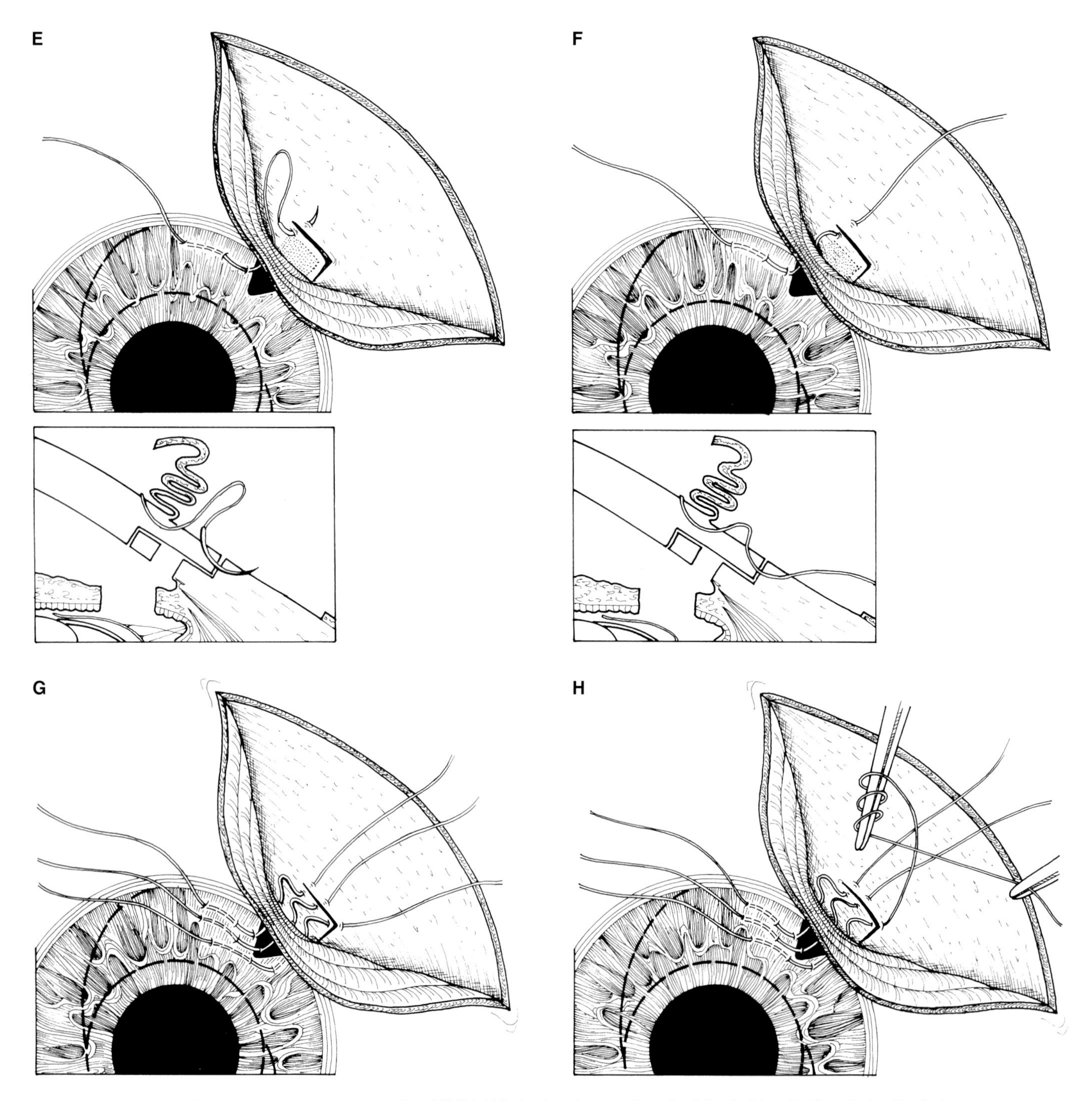

FIGURE 20-11, cont'd **E** and **F,** Third bite is placed across the scleral flap incision. **G,** After placing the first suture, the second and third sutures are also placed. **H,** Releasable sutures are tied by grasping the suture exiting the sclera from the third bite and passing three throws around a tying forceps.

(Continued)

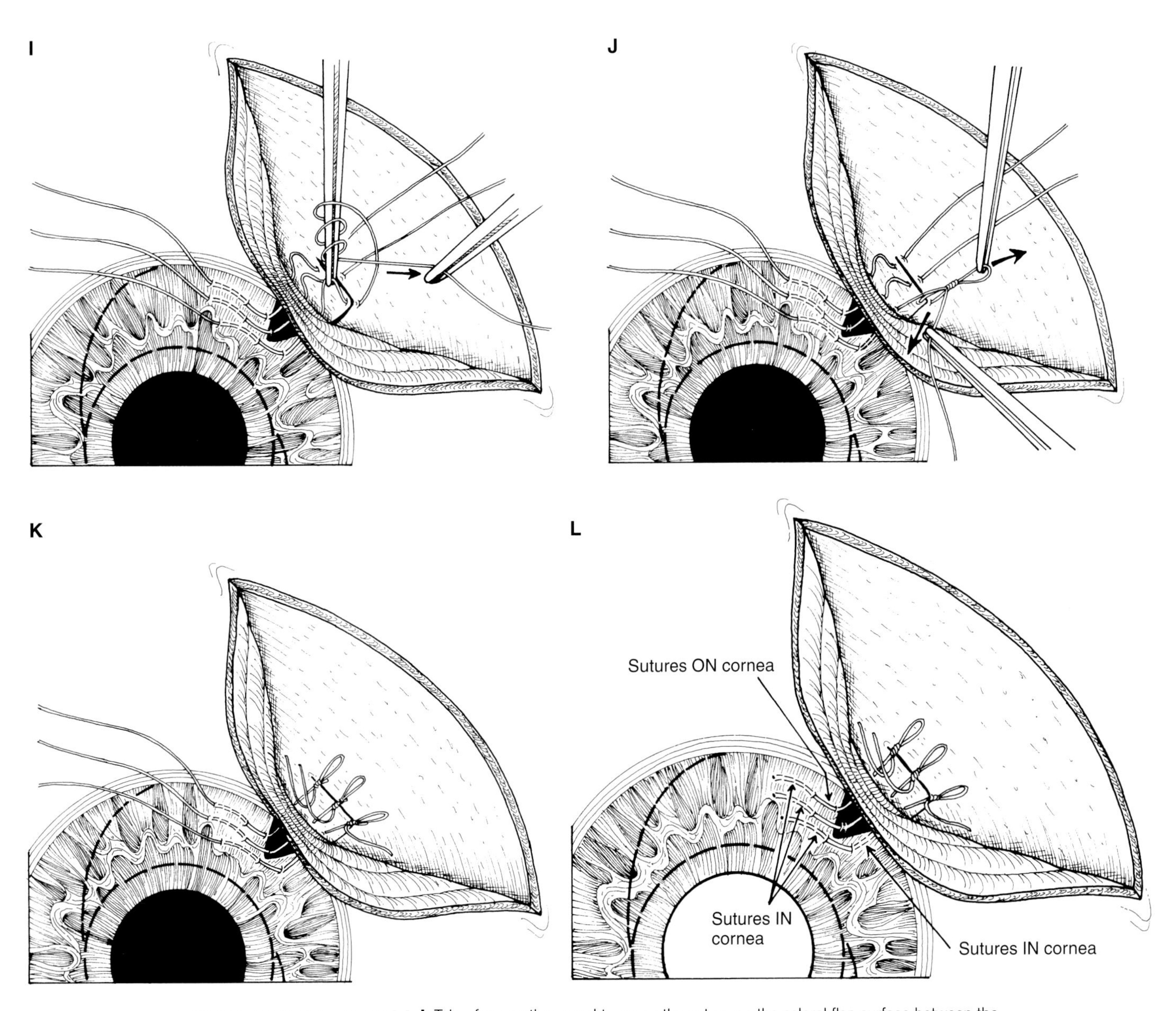

FIGURE 20-11, cont'd I, Tying forceps then used to grasp the suture on the scleral flap surface between the second bite and the third bite. **J,** Three throws are brought down over the grasped suture, creating a loop knot that secures the scleral incision. **K,** Suture is trimmed long enough so that it lies flat on the scleral surface. **L,** Suture lying on corneal surface is trimmed where it entered the cornea for the first bite.

should be performed 1 day after surgery and at least weekly during the first postoperative month.

POSTOPERATIVE MEDICATIONS

Topical (maximum strength) corticosteroid eyedrops are used every 2 hours during the first week following surgery and are then gradually tapered and discontinued at the end of the third postoperative month. Topical antibiotic eyedrops (we use a quinolone eyedrop) are used four times a day during the first 7 to 10 days and then discontinued. If releasable suture removal is anticipated, the antibiotic drops are continued. Topical non-steroidal antiinflammatory eyedrops are used three times a day for about 3 weeks.

Postoperative subconjunctival injections of 5-FU may be administered for augmentation of intraoperative antifibrosis effect.

Postoperative Management and Complications

Postoperative Elevated IOP

DETERMINING THE CAUSE OF ELEVATED IOP

Elevation of IOP often occurs in the early postoperative period. It is important to proceed through a stepwise logical evaluation of potential causes along the path of aqueous filtration from the anterior chamber to the subconjunctival space. Careful

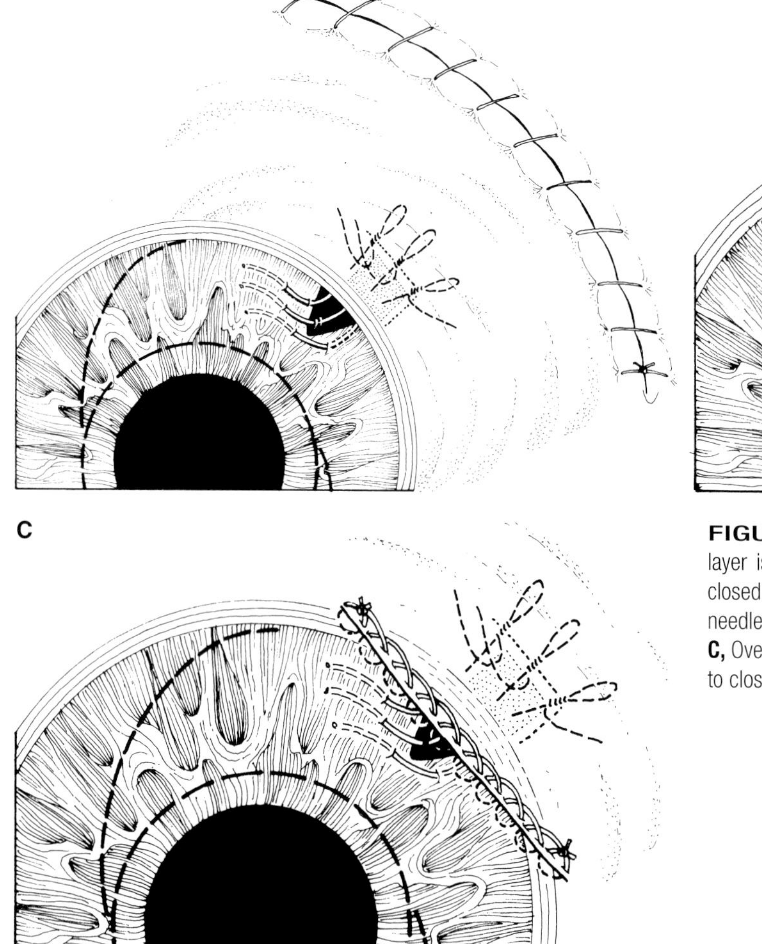

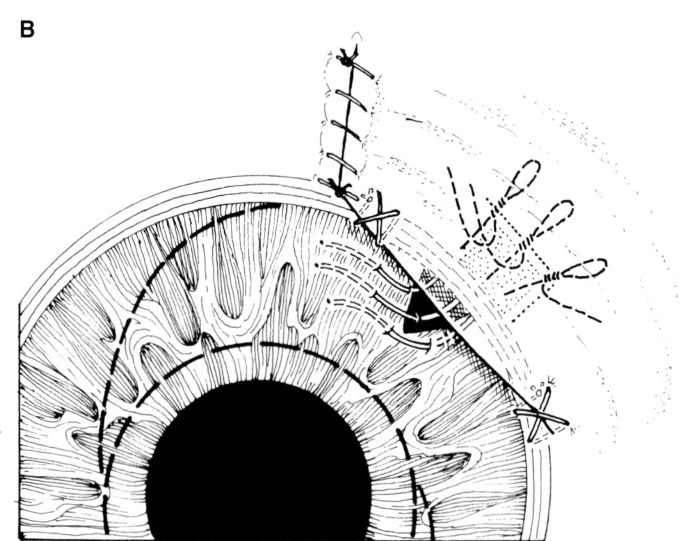

FIGURE 20-12 **A,** Using a running suture technique, the deeper Tenon's layer is closed with locking stitches, and the superficial conjunctival layer is closed with a nonlocking stitch. **B,** Mattress and a lateral running (noncutting needle on 9-0 or 10-0 absorbable) suture closes the conjunctiva laterally. **C,** Overlapping running suture, using 9-0 nylon (Ethicon 2890) can also be used to close the conjunctiva at the limbus.

examination of the anterior chamber may reveal the presence of noncirculating cells, indicating retained viscoelastic material that interferes with flow at the trabeculectomy or sclerectomy opening. Gonioscopy will rule out obstruction of the trabeculectomy or sclerectomy opening by vitreous, iris, fibrin, or a blood clot or incompletely removed Descemet's membrane, sclera, or cornea. Examination of the filtering bleb may reveal a shallow or flat bleb from tight wound closure and inadequate filtration, an encysted filtering bleb, a subconjunctival hemorrhage, or blood clot blocking filtration through the scleral incision. Hemorrhage in the filtering bleb may occur intraoperatively from bleeding associated with tissue dissection; from anesthetic, antibiotic, or steroid injection; or postoperatively from suture release or laser lysis.

Late postoperative elevation of IOP is almost always due to episcleral scarring in the filtering bleb. This may occur gradually over time or may be precipitated by episodes of inflammation from uveitis, subsequent eye surgery, and so on.

TREATMENT OF EARLY POSTOPERATIVE ELEVATION OF IOP

Blockage of internal filtration opening. If the internal sclerectomy is blocked by a blood clot or fibrin, injection of tissue plasminogen activator into the anterior chamber may correct the obstruction.[57] If iris, vitreous, Descemet's membrane, or lens capsule is preventing aqueous outflow, Nd:YAG or argon laser treatment may open the obstruction, but surgical intervention and wound revision will probably be required.

Tight wound closure and technique of removal of releasable sutures. If the elevated IOP is due to inadequate filtration from tight scleral flap closure, removing releasable sutures can loosen the scleral flap and increase filtration. (Similar principles also apply to laser lysis of conventional sutures.) The surgeon, however, must use a reasoned and rational approach (Table 20-2). If the sutures are released before adequate healing has occurred, hypotony and overfiltration can result. If suture release is delayed too long and too much healing has occurred, increased filtration and lowered IOP will not be achieved. Virtually all combined procedures are now performed with adjunctive antimetabolite therapy. In most patients, this will slow wound healing and delay suture release compared with when antimetabolite therapy is not used.

The vascularity of the filtering bleb serves as a helpful indication of the extent of underlying wound healing. Highly vascularized filtering blebs indicate a high probability of more rapid healing and should prompt consideration of earlier suture removal. Avascular or relatively avascular filtering blebs suggest

TABLE 20-2
Removal of Releasable Sutures*

- A. Surgery performed with antimetabolites
  - 1. Elevated IOP first postoperative week
    - a. Try to avoid suture removal because of risk of:
      - Hypotony and flat anterior chamber
      - Wound leak (and potential bleb failure) in fornix-based conjunctival flap
    - b. Lower IOP by
      - IOP-lowering medications (beta-blocker or CAI preferred to avoid hyperemia)
      - Mild digital or instrument pressure on edge of incision in limbus-based conjunctival flap
      - Decompression through paracentesis
      - Recheck IOP after 20 minutes
  - 2. Elevated IOP after first postoperative week
    - a. Trial of digital or instrument pressure
      - Recheck IOP after 20 minutes
    - b. Remove one releasable suture if needed
      - If no IOP decrease, augment with instrument or digital pressure
      - Remove only one suture on any day (usually)
      - Depending on IOP, recheck in 1 day
  - 3. Effect of bleb appearance on decision to remove suture
    - a. Can remove suture earlier if bleb is vascular
    - b. Delay removal if bleb is avascular
    - c. If bleb is avascular with low IOP
      - Permit healing (2 or 3 months)
      - Consider tapering steroids more rapidly
      - Then trim suture at the corneal surface
- B. Surgery performed without antimetabolites
  - 1. Healing is more rapid
  - 2. Effort is made to avoid removal during first week
  - 3. Removal after second week usually has minimal or no effect

*These principles also apply to laser suture lysis.
IOP, Intraocular pressure.

slower healing and should prompt consideration of delayed suture removal. (It is advisable to discuss with the patient the pros and cons of suture removal or laser suture lysis so that they are aware of the possible complications.)

During the first postoperative week, every effort should be made to avoid suture removal because of the increased risk of overfiltration, hypotony, chamber flattening, and associated complications. An IOP in the 20s for a short period will usually not cause progression of glaucoma damage. If a limbus-based conjunctival flap was used, digital, cotton swab, or instrument pressure can be applied while observing the bleb for enlargement.[53,58] If a fornix-based conjunctival flap was used, digital pressure or instrument pressure could cause a bleb leak and should be avoided during this period. Topical and, if needed, oral therapy (including acetazolamide and hyperosmotic) can be administered, and, if necessary, paracentesis can be performed at the slit lamp examination (preceded by a drop of topical anesthetic, topical antibiotic, and 5% povidone-iodine solution [Betadine]). IOP should be monitored for 30 to 60 minutes and then rechecked the following day to ensure stability.

During the second postoperative week, healing has progressed and removal of releasable sutures is safer. It is preferable to first apply gentle and then stronger digital pressure to stimulate filtration. Sometimes this maneuver will dislodge a fibrin clot or disrupt initial wound healing and result in lasting IOP control. IOP should be rechecked in 20 to 30 minutes to determine if the effect is lasting. If the IOP has returned to an undesirable level, and depending on the stage of glaucoma damage and the risk factors for failure (previous surgery, race, type of glaucoma, etc.), suture release can be performed. The surgeon should realize that complications of suture release can still occur.

During the third postoperative week, suture removal is usually safe, unless the filtering bleb is thin and contains few or no vessels. If suture removal is performed, the principles of adjunctive digital pressure, reevaluation of IOP in 30 minutes, and avoidance of multiple suture removal in one day should be followed.

Although increasing filtration by removal of sutures becomes less likely beyond the third postoperative week, the use of antimetabolites may result in a filtering bleb that will permit IOP reduction from suture removal months postoperatively.

The technique of suture release involves elevation of the upper eyelid (an assistant is helpful but not required) and use of a fine forceps to grasp the suture where it changes direction between the first (intracorneal) and the second (sublimbal) bites of the releasable suture. If necessary, the superficial layers of the corneal epithelium (which have grown over this portion of suture that was on the epithelial surface at the time of surgery) are penetrated to grasp the suture. The intracorneal segment of suture is teased out of the tissue and then pulled to release the loop knot and remove the suture (Figure 20-13, *A* and *B*). The bleb is observed for enlargement during suture removal, and the IOP is measured. If the IOP is unchanged, gentle digital pressure can be applied to initiate or promote filtration. If IOP decreased, it is checked again in about 20 minutes to determine if the effect is lasting. Follow-up can be planned for the next day or in 1 week, depending on the surgeon's preference. As a general rule, only one suture should be released on any day, and the sutures are removed from left to right, with the corner suture removed last.

If the surgeon decides that suture removal will not be necessary, the sutures can remain (the 9-0 nylon will dissolve over the next 2 to 3 years) or can be trimmed by teasing the intracorneal portion (the first of the three bites) out of the tissue, pulling it slightly with forceps while depressing the cornea with scissors so that the cut end will retract into the tissue (see Figure 20-13, *C*).

Laser suture lysis. Argon laser suture lysis can be very useful in the postoperative management of trabeculectomy surgery. The timing of suture lysis is similar to the removal of releasable sutures. If available, the Hoskins or the Ritch lens (Ocular Instruments, Bellevue, Wash.) can compress the overlying conjunctiva (and its blood vessels) and aid in visualization of the scleral flap sutures. If these lenses are not available, the corner of a four-mirror Posner goniolens (Ocular Instruments,

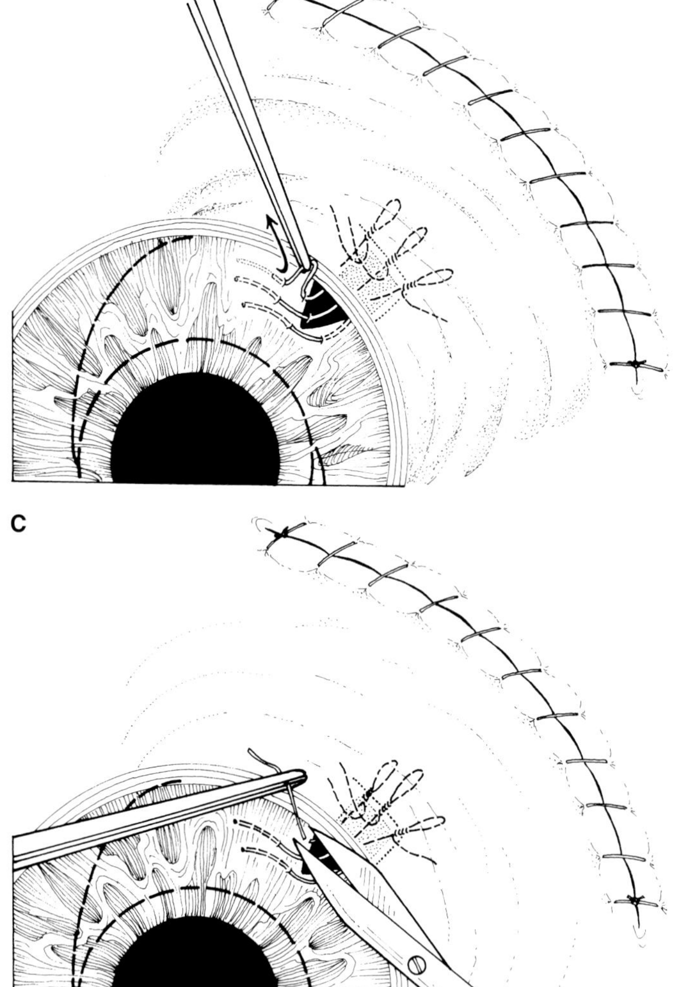

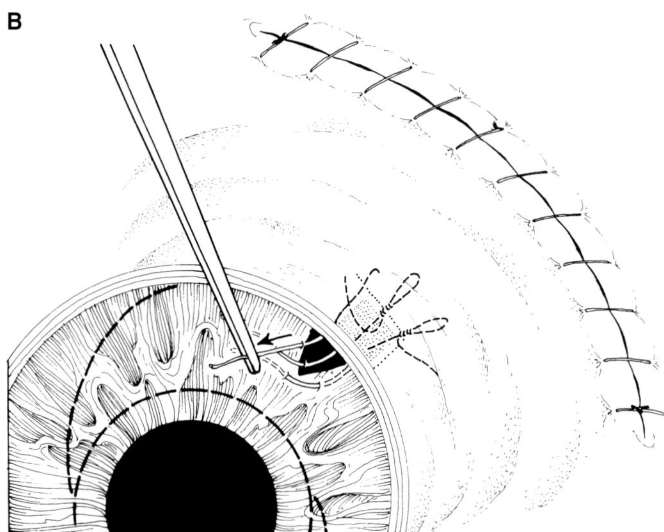

FIGURE 20-13 A, Intracorneal segment of suture is teased out of the tissue. **B,** Suture is pulled to release the loop knot and remove the suture. **C,** If suture removal is not needed, the sutures can be trimmed by teasing the intracorneal portion out of the tissue, pulling slightly with forceps and depressing the cornea with scissors so that the cut end will retract into the tissue.

Bellevue, Wash.) can serve the same purpose. If visualization is difficult because of thick or boggy overlying tissue or engorged blood vessels, topical phenylephrine may be helpful.

In eyes with residual subconjunctival blood overlying the scleral flap sutures, use of the argon or blue-green wavelength risks absorption of the laser energy by the blood and the overlying conjunctiva and could result in a conjunctival defect that may not heal. Laser lysis with a krypton or red wavelength laser permits selective treatment of the suture and minimizes risk to the conjunctiva.

TABLE 20-3

Laser Suture Lysis Settings

Spot size: 50 μm
Burn duration: 70 to 100 ms
Power: 300 to 350 mW

Laser suture lysis settings are 50-mm spot size, 70- to 100-ms burn duration, and 300 to 350 mW of power (Table 20-3). Ideally, one should attempt to cut the suture at one end to allow the short end to retract into the sclera and the long end to lay flat to avoid perforation of the conjunctiva. If necessary, the other end can also be cut to ensure that the long episcleral piece of suture lays flat.

MANAGEMENT OF SUBCONJUNCTIVAL HEMORRHAGE

Subconjunctival hemorrhage in the filtering bleb may increase the risk of bleb failure. More aggressive use of topical corticosteroid eyedrops is usually adequate to preserve the filtering bleb. Earlier suture release, subconjunctival injection of corticosteroids adjacent to the filtering bleb, and subconjunctival 5-FU injections may be considered.

ENCYSTED FILTERING BLEB

An encysted filtering bleb is characterized by localized filtration that is demarcated by a thickened bleb wall. It is usually evident within the first postoperative month and may develop as early as several weeks following surgery. Conservative management with addition of IOP-lowering agents is usually successful in controlling IOP. Needling the filtering bleb at the slit lamp examination (preceded by topical anesthetic, broad-spectrum topical antibiotic, and 5% povidone-iodine solution [Betadine]) or in the operating room may restore diffuse filtration and lower IOP. The conjunctiva is slightly elevated by a subconjunctival injection of sterile BSS or anesthetic such as 1% lidocaine (Xylocaine) with epinephrine for vasoconstriction, administered about 1 cm from the bleb. A cotton-tipped applicator is used to push the BSS toward the bleb. A needle knife is passed into the subconjunctival space through the same entry point used for the BSS injection. The knife is passed beneath the elevated conjunctiva to the bleb where the wall is punctured and cut. If the nature of the bleb permits, the knife can also be passed across the bleb to cut the opposite wall. This procedure can be augmented with daily subconjunctival injections of 5-FU to prevent healing. Hypotony can result from this procedure.

TREATMENT OF LATE POSTOPERATIVE IOP ELEVATION

Scarring of the filtering bleb, the most common cause of late IOP elevation, may be managed by needling the bleb and scleral flap. This technique is best performed when the scleral flap edges can be seen through the conjunctiva by slit lamp examination. (IOP reduction may first be attempted by addition of eyedrops to avoid the risks of subconjunctival hemorrhage and hypotony.) Although some surgeons prefer to perform this at the slit lamp examination, where the scleral flap can be transilluminated, others may prefer the operating room.

Late scleral flap needling (and injection of antimetabolite). The eye is prepared by several applications of a topical anesthetic eyedrop and a drop of 5% povidone-iodine solution (Betadine). A subconjunctival injection of BSS separates scar tissue and creates a plane for safer passage of the needle. The needle or needle knife is passed into the subconjunctival space 1 cm from the bleb and is passed beneath the conjunctiva to the scarred filtering bleb or the scleral flap incision. A back-and-forth motion is used to disrupt the scar tissue, elevate the scleral flap, and, if necessary, penetrate the sclerostomy. Restoration of aqueous flow is indicated by elevation of the filtering bleb. After removal of the needle, the entry point is observed for aqueous leakage. If necessary, careful light cautery can be applied to shrink the conjunctiva surrounding the leak to achieve closure. Suture closure is rarely necessary.

Antimetabolite can be injected before needling. A mixture of bupivacaine 0.75% with epinephrine (Marcaine) or lidocaine 1% with epinephrine (Xylocaine), and MMC 0.4 mg/ml is prepared for injection by aspirating 0.01 ml of the MMC into a 30-gauge needle on a 1-ml syringe, followed by 0.02 ml of bupivacaine (or lidocaine). This small volume only partially fills the hub of the needle. The needle is inserted into the subconjunctival space 1 cm from the bleb, and the mixture is injected near the site of revision, elevating the tissue. A sterile cotton swab is used to spread the mixture in the subconjunctival space. After 15 or 20 minutes, a second needle (or "Stiletto" knife, Becton-Dickinson), passed through the same entry point as the first, is used to revise the bleb, scleral flap, and, if necessary, the sclerostomy.[59]

A similar technique has been reported, employing a needle revision of the filtering bleb with postoperative injections of 5-FU.[60]

OTHER CAUSES OF IOP ELEVATION

Rare causes of postoperative elevation of IOP may include aqueous misdirection (malignant glaucoma, ciliary block glaucoma), suprachoroidal hemorrhage, choroidal effusion, and so on. Management of these entities is complex. Publications and texts should be consulted to develop appropriate strategies of treatment.

Postoperative Hypotony—Mechanisms. Hypotony may result from excessive outflow or inadequate production of aqueous. In the early postoperative period, excessive outflow from a wound leak or bleb leak is more common than overfiltration with a large bleb, aqueous flow through a cyclodialysis cleft or aqueous underproduction from iridocyclitis, choroidal detachment, or rarely from a previous cyclodestructive procedure. (Hyposecretion of aqueous from iridocyclitis may be clinically diagnosed by noting stagnant or slowly moving cells in the anterior chamber after residual viscoelastic has been ruled out.)

An aqueous leak can usually be identified by applying fluorescein solution and patiently observing the bleb surface under blue light for an interruption in the fluorescein pattern. Painting the area of interest with a fluorescein strip will sometimes detect aqueous leaks that may be difficult to identify with liquid fluorescein. Sometimes hypotonous eyes will not demonstrate a leak without application of gentle digital pressure to the globe.

Overfiltration with leak. A bleb leak should prompt consideration of the potential management options. Bleb leaks are of great concern because of the increased risk of bleb failure (especially if they occur in the early postoperative course) and future bleb infection and endophthalmitis. If there is no evidence of blepharitis or other factors that might predispose to endophthalmitis, there has been no previous occurrence of blebitis, and the IOP is relatively high (in the teens), the leak may be observed after educating the patient about signs and symptoms of infection and instructions to contact the doctor immediately if they occur. The patient may be given a prescription for a broad-spectrum antibiotic to use until the doctor can be seen.

Conservative attempts to close bleb leaks have limited success. (Leaks at the site of the incision in a fornix-based flap will usually close spontaneously.) Some techniques, however, are worth consideration. A large bandage contact lens may tamponade the leak and permit healing. Application of tissue glue and use of a large bandage contact lens to prevent discomfort can be helpful with a small, slow leak.[61,62] Compression sutures are sometimes successful in localizing a conjunctival defect and closing the aqueous leak.[63] Late leaks, which are usually associated with devitalized conjunctival tissue, most often require extensive bleb revision with creation of a new bleb surface.

Overfiltration without leak: Extensive bleb. Overfiltration may occur in the first few days following surgery as a result of inadequate scleral flap closure. (Most surgeons will ensure tight scleral flap closure, realizing that postoperative elevations of IOP can be treated with medications, paracentesis, or suture release rather than risk hypotony, which is more difficult to manage.) If overfiltration results in complications, such as choroidal detachment, shallow or flat anterior chamber, or hypotony maculopathy, management should include decreasing frequency of topical corticosteroids, restoration of the anterior chamber by pressure patch (with "torpedo" on the eyelid in the area of the filtering bleb) or injection of viscoelastic, resuturing of the scleral flap, and so on.[64] The method and nature of management should be determined by the associated risks and the potential benefits of the treatment.

If hypotony is present beyond the normal period of resolution, and if reversible causes such as choroidal detachment and more permanent causes such as cyclodialysis cleft have been excluded, several management possibilities may be considered. Injection of autologous blood into the bleb, application of trichloroacetic acid, and treatment with cryotherapy have been effective in decreasing filtration.[65] Placement of a barrier suture across the filtering bleb can also limit the area of filtration and decrease bleb size.[63] Rarely, return to the operating room to place additional scleral flap sutures may be required.

In the absence of a bleb leak, hypotony may be observed without definitive treatment, as long as there are no complications. Many eyes will tolerate an IOP below 6 mm Hg indefinitely. Others may develop a choroidal detachment with an IOP as high as 10 to 12 mm Hg.

Overfiltration without leak: Cyclodialysis cleft. Management of a cyclodialysis cleft may initially be attempted by use of topical cycloplegic eyedrops but may require laser treatment, cryotherapy, or transscleral suturing.[66,67]

Decreased ciliary body production of aqueous. This can be one of the most challenging problems associated with hypotony. Aggressive antiinflammatory therapy may be helpful. Reopening the conjunctival flap and resuturing the scleral flap to reduce or stop filtration may be necessary.

Large uncomfortable bleb. Uncommonly, even though filtration provides excellent IOP control, the bleb size will cause discomfort or interfere with tear lubrication and result in dellen formation or punctate corneal staining. This can be one of the most frustrating challenges for both the patient and the physician. Topical lubricants (drops during the day and ointment at bedtime) and topical nonsteroidal antiinflammatory eyedrops may be helpful. Specialized techniques of laser treatment, use of trichloroacetic acid, and surface cryotherapy may improve comfort with some risk of creating a bleb leak. Compression sutures have also been helpful. If all else has failed, bleb revision surgery can be considered with the risk that filtration will be compromised.[20,68-70]

Blebitis and endophthalmitis. Significant risk factors for blebitis and endophthalmitis include the presence of a thin-walled bleb, an avascular bleb, and a bleb leak. Patients should be alerted to the signs and symptoms of bleb infection, which are redness, discharge, pain, photophobia, and reduced vision, and advised to contact their ophthalmologist immediately if they occur. If infection is limited to the bleb, a culture of the lids, conjunctiva, and bleb may be helpful in determining the etiologic agent. Intensive topical broad-spectrum antibiotic therapy may be curative. Evidence of more severe infection with hypopyon or vitreous involvement warrants more aggressive therapy that may include vitreous tap or vitrectomy and intraocular injection of antibiotics.[70]

Nonpenetrating Trabeculectomy and Combined Surgery

Although nonpenetrating trabeculectomy has been advocated and abandoned in the past, modifications have resulted in a resurgence of this technique in the form of viscocanalostomy and deep sclerectomy with and without scleral implant. Most observers have described less IOP reduction but fewer complications with nonpenetrating surgery.[71] The long-term prospects for these new techniques are uncertain, but many surgeons are enthusiastic about their potential.

Nonpenetrating trabeculectomy in combination with phacoemulsification may offer the possibility of improved long-term IOP control with decreased complications. The consensus among glaucoma specialists remains that the final level of IOP achieved with nonpenetrating trabeculectomy is higher than that seen with conventional trabeculectomy. Penetrating trabeculectomy therefore provides a better chance of lowering IOP and stabilizing glaucoma. However, such conclusions may be premature, pending the results of additional prospective, randomized, masked studies with long-term follow-up.[72,73]

INDICATIONS AND CONTRAINDICATIONS OF NONPENETRATING TRABECULECTOMY

At this time, nonpenetrating trabeculectomy may be indicated for patients with early primary open-angle glaucoma (with definite glaucomatous cupping and little or no visual field damage) who have uncontrolled IOP or require multiple medications for IOP control. These patients have a high probability of maintaining vision even if the IOP is not lowered to the most desirable levels. At this time, patients who are at increased risk of glaucoma damage have the best chance for preservation of vision with combined surgery using a penetrating trabeculectomy with antimetabolite therapy.

A potential but significant contraindication to nonpenetrating trabeculectomy is the presence of a narrow angle. Because a peripheral iridectomy is not performed with nonpenetrating surgery, a narrow angle increases the risk that the iris will obstruct the site of filtration or prolapse into an inadvertent or unrecognized microperforation of the juxtacanalicular trabecular meshwork or Descemet's membrane. When performed in combination with phacoemulsification, this is not likely to be a risk except in eyes with short axial lengths and small anterior segments (e.g., nanophthalmos).

MECHANISM OF FUNCTION OF NONPENETRATING TRABECULECTOMY

The mechanism of IOP lowering with nonpenetrating trabeculectomy surgery has not been conclusively determined. Viscoelastic dilation of Schlemm's canal with resulting enhanced filtration of aqueous into the outflow channels has been proposed by some authors. Alternative possibilities may be egress of aqueous through exposed Descemet's membrane or inadvertent microdefects in the inner wall of Schlemm's canal and the juxtacanalicular trabecular meshwork. Removal of the deep scleral flap in both the deep sclerectomy and viscocanalostomy procedures is believed by some surgeons to create a deep reservoir for the accumulation of aqueous. Many reports have identified shallow filtering blebs in these patients, suggesting that aqueous accumulates in the subconjunctival space similar to but perhaps not as much as in conventional penetrating trabeculectomy surgery.[74]

TECHNIQUE OF NONPENETRATING TRABECULECTOMY COMBINED WITH PHACOEMULSIFICATION

Nonpenetrating trabeculectomy can be performed at the same site as the phacoemulsification in the superior temporal quadrant or at separate sites with the nonpenetrating trabeculectomy in the superior nasal quadrant and the phacoemulsification through clear cornea temporally. Performing the two procedures at separate sites ensures that any bleb formation is resulting from the nonpenetrating trabeculectomy and not from the phacoemulsification wound. Many surgeons perform this procedure at one site.[75]

Both limbus- and fornix-based conjunctival flaps can be used. Some surgeons prefer to use a fornix-based conjunctival flap for greater exposure and because the decreased aqueous flow is less likely to result in a leak at the limbal conjunctival closure. If inadvertent perforation and entry into the anterior chamber occur and the procedure is converted to a penetrating trabeculectomy, the risk of a leak at the limbus will be greater.

The scleral flap is created one-third to one-half scleral thickness and dissected anteriorly to the limbus (Figure 20-14, *A*). A deep scleral flap is then dissected about two thirds of the distance to the limbus, leaving a very thin layer of sclera on the choroid (see Figure 20-14, *B*). Phacoemulsification and IOL placement are performed through a temporal clear corneal incision (see Figure 20-14, *C*). Viscoelastic is left in the eye. The deep scleral flap is now completed (see Figure 20-14, *D*). It is dissected anteriorly, unroofing Schlemm's canal and exposing Descemet's membrane anterior to Schwalbe's line. Viscoelastic is removed from the capsular bag and the anterior chamber. The deep scleral flap is excised. The surgeon should see aqueous percolation through the juxtacanalicular trabecular meshwork and Descemet's membrane. When the distal tip of a cellulose sponge touches these tissues, it should expand as it absorbs aqueous humor that is filtering through (see Figure 20-14, *E*). If aqueous percolation through the deep trabecular layers and Descemet's membrane is not adequate, fine-toothed forceps, capsule forceps, or the edge of a sharp blade can be used to debride the surface of the tissue to enhance flow. If a collagen implant is used, it is sutured to the scleral floor, and the outer scleral flap is sutured over it. If viscocanalostomy is preferred, Healon is injected into the cut ends of Schlemm's canal with a special cannula, after which the scleral flap is sutured closed. Some surgeons will use neither a collagen implant nor injection of viscoelastic. Others will use antimetabolite therapy but with no consensus about the best method. Some will apply the antimetabolite after dissecting the superficial scleral flap but before dissecting the deep scleral flap, and others will apply the antimetabolite after excising the deep scleral flap and suturing closed the superficial scleral flap.

We presently prefer a limbus-based conjunctival flap. MMC is administered, as described in Application of Mitomycin, after dissecting the superficial scleral flap and before dissecting the deep scleral flap. A shorter exposure time (usually 1 to 1½ minutes) is employed because we presently perform this procedure when less IOP reduction is required and lower risk of complications is desired.

Conjunctival closure and administration of postoperative corticosteroids and antibiotics are performed as previously described for combined surgery with a penetrating trabeculectomy.

Nonpenetrating trabeculectomy (with or without phacoemulsification) represents a new technique that must be learned by the surgeon.[76] If the anterior chamber is inadvertently entered while attempting a nonpenetrating trabeculectomy, the surgeon should be prepared to convert to a conventional trabeculectomy procedure to avoid risk of iris incarceration postoperatively.

Intraoperative complications specific to the nonpenetrating trabeculectomy procedure have included inadvertent perforation of the anterior chamber (33%) and exposure of the choroid while dissecting the deep scleral flap anteriorly.[76]

Postoperative complications are similar in nature to trabeculectomy surgery but are generally less common.[74-78] If filtration through the intact inner trabecular meshwork and Descemet's membrane is inadequate, Nd:YAG goniopuncture has been used to increase aqueous flow and lower IOP.[79]

Conclusion

Combined phacoemulsification and trabeculectomy is an excellent surgical technique for management of coexisting glaucoma and cataract. The patient can benefit from decreased disability and morbidity by having one rather than two procedures performed. However, the surgeon must understand the appropriate indications and the special techniques required for intraoperative and postoperative care of these patients. This approach represents an exciting challenge for the surgeon with great potential for preserving visual function, increasing visual acuity, and improving quality of life.

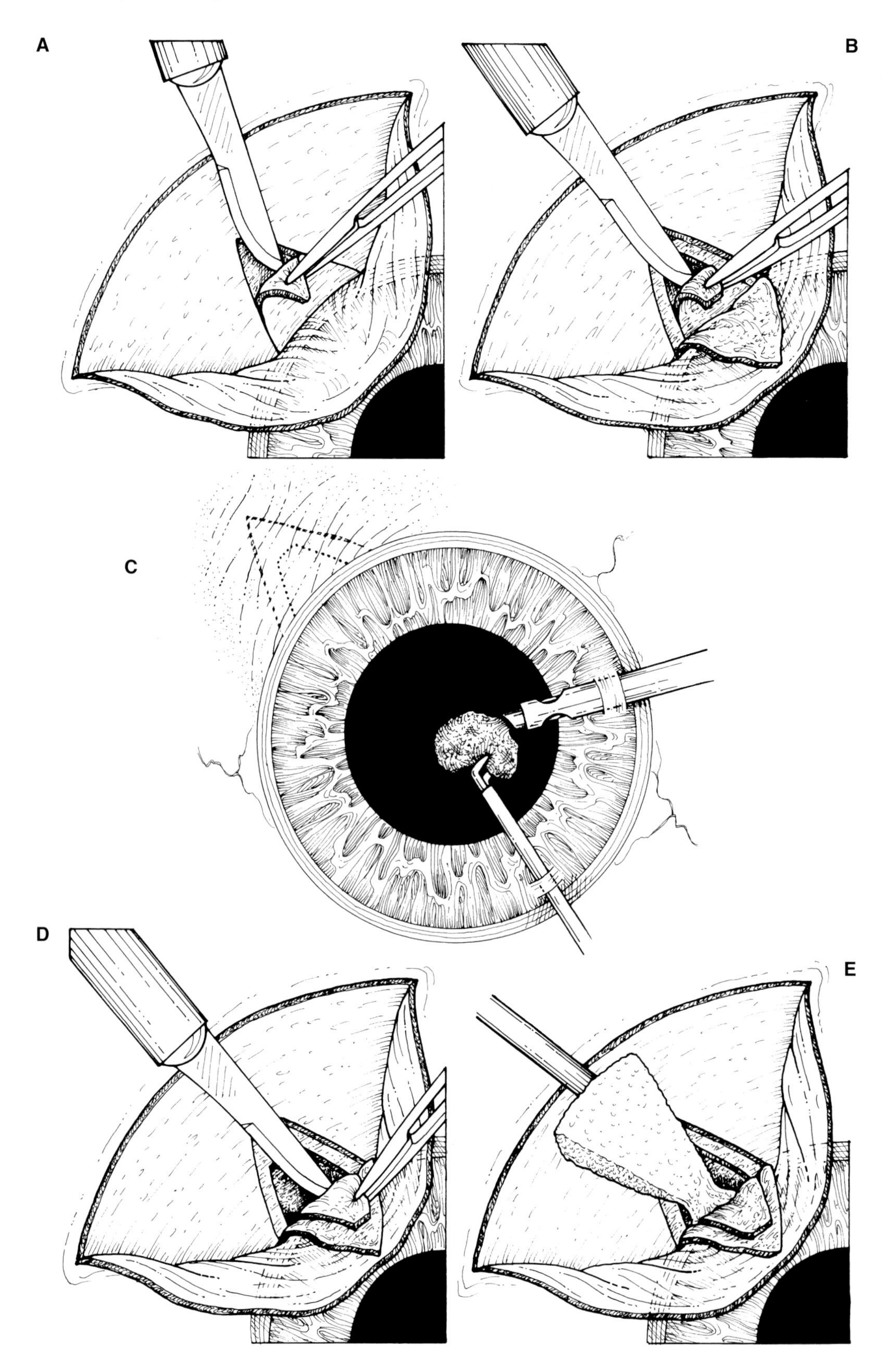

FIGURE 20-14 **A,** Scleral flap is created one-third to one-half scleral thickness and dissected anteriorly to the limbus. **B,** Deep scleral flap is then dissected about two thirds of the distance to the limbus, leaving a very thin layer of sclera on the choroid. **C,** Phacoemulsification and IOL placement are performed through a temporal clear corneal incision. **D,** Deep scleral flap is completed. **E,** Deep scleral flap is excised. Aqueous percolation should be seen through the juxtacanalicular trabecular meshwork and Descemet's membrane. When the distal tip of a cellulose sponge touches these tissues, it should expand as it absorbs aqueous.

REFERENCES

1. Spaeth GL, Sivalingam E: The partial-punch: a new combined cataract glaucoma operation, *Ophthalmic Surg* l7:53, 1976.
2. Levene R: Triple procedure of extracapsular cataract surgery, posterior chamber lens implantation, and glaucoma filter, *J Cataract Refract Surg* 12:385, 1986.
3. Shields MB: Combined cataract extraction and guarded sclerectomy: reevaluation in the extracapsular era, *Ophthalmology* 93:366, 1986.
4. Shields M: Combined cataract extraction and glaucoma surgery, *Ophthalmology* 89:231, 1982.
5. Savage JA, Thomas JV, Belcher CDIII et al: Extracapsular cataract extraction and posterior chamber intraocular lens implantation in glaucomatous eyes, *Ophthalmology* 92:1506, 1985.
6. Vu MT, Shields MB: The early postoperative pressure course in glaucoma patients following cataract surgery, *Ophthalmic Surg* 19:467, 1988.
7. McCartney DL, Memmen JE, Stark WJ et al: The efficacy and safety of combined trabeculectomy, cataract extraction, and intraocular lens implantation, *Ophthalmology* 95:754, 1988.
8. Krupin T, Feitl ME, Bishop KI: Postoperative intraocular pressure rise in open-angle glaucoma patients after cataract or combined cataract-filtration surgery, *Ophthalmology* 96:579, 1989.
9. Cohen JS, Greff LJ, Novack G et al: A placebo-controlled double-masked evaluation of mitomycin-C in combined glaucoma and cataract procedures, *Ophthalmology* 103:1934, 1996.
10. Carlson DW, Alward WLM, Barad JP et al: A randomized study of mitomycin augmentation in combined phacoemulsification and trabeculectomy, *Ophthalmology* 104:719, 1997.
11. Budenz DL, Pyfer M, Singh K et al: Comparison of phacotrabeculectomy with 5-fluorouracil, mitomycin-C, and without antifibrotic agents, *Ophthalmic Surg Lasers* 30:367, 1999.
12. Savage JA, Thomas JV, Belcher CD et al: Extracapsular cataract extraction and posterior chamber intraocular lens implantation in glaucomatous eyes, *Ophthalmology* 92:1506, 1985.
13. McGuigan LJB, Gottsch J, Stark WJ et al: Extracapsular cataract extraction and posterior chamber lens implantation in eyes with preexisting glaucoma, *Arch Ophthalmol* 104:1301, 1986.
14. Schwenn O, Burkhard Dick H, Krummenauer et al: Intraocular pressure after small incision surgery: temporal sclerocorneal versus clear corneal incision, *J Cataract Refract Surg* 27:421, 2001.
15. Crichton ACS, Kirker AW: Intraocular pressure and medication control after clear corneal phacoemulsification and AcrySof posterior chamber intraocular lens implantation in patients with filtering blebs, *J Glaucoma* 10:38, 2001.
16. Seah SKL, Jap A, Prata JA Jr, et al: Cataract surgery after trabeculectomy, *Ophthalmic Surg Lasers* 27:587, 1996.
17. Murchison JF, Shields MB: An evaluation of three surgical approaches for coexisting cataract and glaucoma, *Ophthalmic Surg* 20:383, 1989.
18. Simmons ST, Litoff D, Nichols DA et al: Extracapsular cataract extraction and posterior chamber intraocular lens implantation combined with trabeculectomy in patients with glaucoma, *Am J Ophthalmol* 104:465, 1987.
19. Hoskins HD Jr, Migliazzo C: Management of failing filtering blebs with the argon laser, *Ophthalmic Surg* 15:731, 1984.
20. Cohen JS, Shaffer RN, Hetherington J Jr et al: Revision of filtration surgery, *Arch Ophthalmol* 95:1612, 1977.
21. Shin DH, Hughes BA, Song MS et al: Primary glaucoma triple procedure with or without adjunctive mitomycin, *Ophthalmology* 103:1925, 1996.
22. Shingleton BJ, Wadhwani RA, O'Donoghue MW et al: Evaluation of intraocular pressure in the immediate period after phacoemulsification, *J Cataract Refract Surg* 27:524, 2001.
23. Gressel MG, Parrish RK II, Folberg R: 5-Fluorouracil and glaucoma filtering surgery. I. An animal model, *Ophthalmology* 91:378-383, 1984.
24. Heuer DK, Parrish RK II, Gressel MG et al: 5-Fluorouracil and glaucoma filtering surgery. II. A pilot study, *Ophthalmology* 91:384-393, 1984.
25. Heuer DK, Parrish RK II, Gressel MG et al: 5-Fluorouracil and glaucoma filtering surgery. III. Intermediate follow-up of a pilot study, *Ophthalmology* 93:1537-1546, 1986.
26. Cohen JS: Combined cataract implant and filtering surgery with 5-fluorouracil, *Ophthalmic Surg* 21:181-186, 1990.
27. Budenz DL, Pyfer M, Singh K et al: Comparison of phacotrabeculectomy with 5-fluorouracil, mitomycin-C, and without antifibrotic agents, *Ophthalmic Surg Lasers* 30:367, 1999.
28. Hennis HL, Stewart WC: The use of 5-fluorouracil in patients following combined trabeculectomy and cataract extraction, *Ophthalmic Surg* 22:451, 1991.
29. Wong PC, Ruderman JM, Krupin T: 5-Fluorouracil after primary combined filtration surgery, *Am J Ophthalmol* 117:149, 1994.
30. Chen C-W: Enhanced intraocular pressure controlling effectiveness of trabeculectomy by local application of mitomycin-C, *Trans Asia-Pacific Acad Ophthalmol* 9:172, 1983.
31. Palmer SS: Mitomycin as adjunct chemotherapy with trabeculectomy, *Ophthalmology* 98:317, 1991.
32. Carlson DW, Alward WLM, Barad JP et al: A randomized study of mitomycin augmentation in combined phacoemulsification and trabeculectomy, *Ophthalmology* 104:719, 1997.
33. Cohen JS, Novack GD, Zhang LL: The role of mitomycin treatment duration and previous intraocular surgery on the success of trabeculectomy surgery, *J Glaucoma* 6:3, 1997.
34. Greenfield DS, Suner IJ, Miller MP et al: Endophthalmitis after filtering surgery with mitomycin, *Arch Ophthalmol* 114:943, 1996.
35. Nuyts RM, Pels E, Greve EL: The effects of 5-fluorouracil and mitomycin C on the corneal endothelium, *Curr Eye Res* 11:565, 1992.
36. Sarraf D, Eezzuduemhoi RD, Cheng Q et al: Aqueous and vitreous concentration of mitomycin C by topical administration after glaucoma filtration surgery in rabbits, *Ophthalmology* 100:1574, 1993.
37. Heaps RS, Nordlund JR, Gonzalez-Fernandez F et al: Ultrastructural changes in rabbit ciliary body after extraocular mitomycin C, *Invest Ophthalmol Vis Sci* 39:1971, 1998.
38. Kee C, Pelzeki C, Kaufman PL: Mitomycin C suppresses aqueous humor flow in cynomolgus monkeys, *Arch Ophthalmol* 113:239, 1995.
39. Lederer CM Jr: Combined Cataract extraction with intraocular lens implantation and mitomycin augmented trabeculectomy, *Ophthalmology* 103:1025, 1996.
40. Apt L, Isenberg SJ, Yoshimori R et al: The effect of povidone-iodine solution applied at the conclusion of ophthalmic surgery, *Am J Ophthalmol* 119:701, 1995.
41. Broadway DC, Chang LP: Trabeculectomy, risk factors for failure and the preoperative state of the conjunctiva, *J Glaucoma* 10:237, 2001.
42. Tezel G, Kolker AE, Kass MA et al: Comparative results of combined procedures for glaucoma and cataract. II. Limbus-based versus fornix-based conjunctival flaps, *Ophthalmic Surg Lasers* 28:551, 1997.
43. Frye LL: Pupil stretch maneuver, course #454 (Modern phacoemulsification/ECCE implantation surgery: XII, Nov 11, 1992), Dallas, Tex, AAO.
44. Miller KV, Keener GT Jr: Stretch pupilloplasty for small pupil phacoemulsification, *Am J Ophthalmol* 117:107, 1994.
45. Osher RH, editor: *Video journal of cataract and refractive surgery*, vol 11, no 1, Cincinnati, Ohio, 1995, Cincinnati Eye Institute.
46. Cohen JS, Osher RH: Releasable scleral flap sutures. In Krupin T, Wax MB, editor: *Ophthalmology Clinics of North America, new techniques in glaucoma surgery*, Philadelphia, 1988, WB Saunders, 1:187.
47. Kunesh MT, Cohen JS, Kunesh JC et al: Releasable suture for trabeculectomy, *Glaucoma* 15:185, 1993.
48. Kolker AE, Kass MA, Rait JL: Trabeculectomy with releasable sutures, *Arch Ophthalmol* 112:62, 1994.
49. Hoskins HD, Migliazzo C: Management of failing filtering blebs with the argon laser, *Ophthalmic Surg* 15:731, 1984.
50. Savage JA, Condon GP, Lytle RA et al: Laser suture lysis after trabeculectomy, *Ophthalmology* 95:1631, 1988.
51. McAllister JA, Wilson RP: *Glaucoma*, Boston, 1986, Butterworths, p 243.
52. Shin DH, Removable-suture closure of the lamellar scleral flap in trabeculectomy, *Ann Ophthalmol* 19:51, 1987.
53. Johnstone MS, Wellington DP, Ziel CJ: A releasable scleral flap suture for guarded filtration surgery, *Arch Ophthalmol* 111:398, 1993.
54. Wise JB: Mitomycin-compatible suture technique for fornix-based conjunctival flaps in glaucoma filtration surgery, *Arch Ophthalmol* 111:992, 1993.
55. Wyse T, Meyer M, Ruderman JM et al: Combined trabeculectomy and phacoemulsification: a one-site vs a two-site approach, *Am J Ophthalmol* 125:334, 1998.
56. Sayyad FE, Helal M, El-Maghraby A et al: One-site versus two-site phacotrabeculectomy: a randomized study, *J Cataract Refract Surg* 25:77, 1999.
57. Lundy DC, Sidoti P, Winarko T et al: Intracameral tissue plasminogen activator after glaucoma surgery, *Ophthalmology* 103:274, 1996.
58. Traverso CE, Greenidge KC, Spaeth GL et al: Focal pressure: a new method to encourage filtration after trabeculectomy, *Ophthalmic Surg* 15:62, 1984.
59. Mardelli PG, Lederer CM, Murray PL et al: Slit-lamp needle revision of failed filtering blebs using mitomycin-C, *Ophthalmology* 11:1946, 1996.
60. Ewing RH, Stamper RL: Needle revision with and without 5-fluorouracil for the treatment of failed filtering blebs, *Am J Ophthalmol* 110:254, 1990.

61. Awan KJ, Spaeth PG: Use of Isobutyl-2-cyanoacrylate tissue adhesive in the repair of conjunctival fistula in filtering procedures for glaucoma, *Ann Ophthalmol* 6:851, 1974.
62. Weber PA, Baker ND: The use of cyanoacrylate adhesive with a collagen shield in leaking filtering blebs, *Ophthalmic Surg* 20:284, 1989.
63. Furgason TG, Perkins TW: A "clothesline" suture technique for the repair of a conjunctival tear during trabeculectomy, *Ophthalmic Surg Lasers* 28:772-773, 1997.
64. Osher RH, Cionni RJ, Cohen JS: Reforming the flat anterior chamber with Healon, *J Cataract Refract Surg* 22:411, 1996.
65. Wise J: Treatment of chronic postfiltration hypotony by intrableb injection of autologous blood, *Arch Ophthalmol* 111:827, 1993.
66. Stamper RL, Lieberman MF, Drake MV: Aqueous humor outflow. In *Becker-Shaffer's diagnosis and therapy of the glaucomas*, ed 7, St Louis, 1999, Mosby, p 52.
67. Stamper RL, Lieberman MF, Drake MV: Complications and failure of Filtering Surgery. In *Becker-Shaffer's diagnosis and therapy of the glaucomas*, ed 7, St Louis, 1999, Mosby, p 632.
68. Budenz DL, Chen PP, Yaffa KW: Conjunctival advancement for late-onset filtering bleb leaks, *Arch Ophthalmol* 117:1014, 1999.
69. Wadhwani RA, Bellows AR, Hutchinson BT: Surgical repair of leaking filtering blebs, *Ophthalmology* 107:1681, 2000.
70. Catoira Y, WuDunn D, Cantor LB: Revision of dysfunctional filtering blebs by conjunctival advancement with bleb preservation, *Am J Ophthalmol* 130:574, 2000.
71. Gianoli F, Schnyder CC, Bovey E et al: Combined surgery for cataract and glaucoma: phacoemulsification and deep sclerectomy compared with phacoemulsification and trabeculectomy, *J Cataract Refract Surg* 25:340, 1999.
72. Zimmerman TJ, Kooner KS, Ford VJ et al: Trabeculectomy vs. nonpenetrating trabeculectomy: a retrospective study of two procedures in phakic patients with glaucoma, *Ophthalmic Surg* 15:734-739, 1984.
73. Ophthalmic Technology Assessment Committee Glaucoma Panel, Netland P (primary author), Nonpenetrating glaucoma surgery, *Ophthalmology* 108:416, 2001.
74. Johnson DH, Johnson M: How does nonpenetrating glaucoma surgery work? Aqueous outflow resistance and glaucoma surgery, *J Glaucoma* 10:55, 2001.
75. Gimbel HV, Penno EEA, Ferensowicz M: Combined cataract surgery, intraocular lens implantation, and viscocanalostomy, *J Cataract Refract Surg* 25:1370, 1999.
76. Carassa RG, Bettin P, Fiori M et al: Viscocanalostomy: a pilot study, *Eur J Ophthalmol* 8:57, 1998.
77. Mermoud A, Schnyder C, Sickenberg M et al: Comparison of deep sclerectomy with collagen implant and trabeculectomy in open-angle glaucoma, *J Cataract Refract Surg* 25:323, 1999.
78. Stegmann R, Pienaar A, Miller D: Viscocanalostomy for open angle glaucoma in black African patients, *J Cataract Refract Surg* 25:316, 1999.
79. Mermoud A, Karlen ME, Schnyder CC et al: Nd:YAG goniopuncture after deep sclerectomy with collagen implant, *Ophthalmic Surg Lasers* 30:120, 1999.

Combined Cataract Extraction and Corneal Transplantation

21

Roger F. Steinert, MD

Successful combined cataract extraction and corneal transplantation requires appropriate preoperative assessment of suitable candidates[1-7] and attention to several specific surgical details of the combined procedure. This chapter reviews these particular issues. Mastery of corneal transplantation techniques, cataract surgery, and intraocular lens (IOL) implantation is assumed. This chapter emphasizes only those areas in which these techniques interact during the combined procedure.

Decision Making

When a patient has a potentially optically significant corneal disorder simultaneous with a potentially optically significant cataract, the surgeon must assess the relative contribution of each.[8]

Assessment of the Cataract

In the presence of an abnormal cornea, visualization of the cataract is impaired. Moderate corneal, epithelial, and stromal edema can be transiently cleared for diagnostic purposes with the application of several drops of 10% glycerin. This must be preceded with topical anesthetic drops to minimize patient discomfort. Some of the usual landmarks used to assess the optical significance of the cataract are reduced or eliminated. For example, the ability to see fundus details with a direct ophthalmoscope or the appearance of the media on red reflex does not distinguish between the contributions from the cornea and those from the lens. The status of the lens in the fellow eye is a useful clue if it can be visualized and if the patient has not had an ocular condition that might be expected to lead to unilateral cataract acceleration, such as inflammation or trauma. Pupillary dilation is mandatory to maximally visualize the lens. The surgeon must guard against extraction of a minimally brunescent but optically clear lens. The prognosis for rapid recovery of excellent vision is often best in a phakic eye. Moreover, cataract extraction performed after healing of the penetrating keratoplasty allows the surgeon the opportunity to adjust the refractive status with more accurate IOL power determination.[4,5] Conversely, a moderate cataract often will accelerate after uncomplicated penetrating keratoplasty.[9,10] Both the patient and the surgeon are frustrated when visual recovery after penetrating keratoplasty is progressively impaired by cataract progression just as the corneal optics improve. No study has been able to adequately resolve the relative stress to the corneal endothelium by cataract extraction following penetrating keratoplasty compared with a simultaneous combined procedure.

Assessment of the Cornea

Corneal opacity itself can be assessed by the degree to which visualization of iris and crystalline lens detail is impaired. Surface irregularity is more deceptive. Slit lamp biomicroscopy often will not disclose optically significant surface distortions. Corneal topography evaluation with a Placido disc, photokeratoscope, or computer-assisted topographic analysis will disclose the presence of irregularities but not their relative contribution to the visual impairment. A diagnostic hard contact lens refraction is invaluable in identifying and quantifying the extent of surface irregularity and its relationship to the total visual impairment. A frequent clinical dilemma is the decision about combining cataract extraction with corneal transplantation in a patient with dense corneal guttae in the absence of clinically evident microcystic epithelial edema or stromal edema. Many patients who exhibit severe central guttate changes in the central cornea can nonetheless undergo successful cataract extraction without subsequent corneal decompensation. Although dense guttae can sometimes cause a mild visual impairment, it is generally best to attempt cataract surgery alone in the absence of signs or symptoms of physiologic corneal endothelial corneal decompensation. Recovery from cataract extraction alone is much more rapid, and the patient is spared the lifelong problems associated with a corneal homograft. The patient and surgeon must have a frank discussion about the markedly increased chance of corneal decompensation postoperatively from the underlying corneal dystrophy to prevent later misunderstanding.

Conversely, if endothelial decompensation is inevitable after atraumatic cataract extraction, proceeding immediately to a combined procedure is warranted. Assessment of the endothelial reserve in a patient with significant guttate change is an inexact science at best. In taking the patient's history, the surgeon must be particularly alert to symptoms of early morning blur. Edema after lid closure throughout the night is often the first sign of frank decompensation. Slit lamp biomicroscopic visualization of endothelial stria or microcystic edema is definite evidence of early decompensation. Subtle microcystic edema can be particularly difficult to visualize in the presence of dense central guttae. Application of fluorescein will help demonstrate early microcystic epithelial changes.

Two special tests can be employed. Specular microscopy is often used in these circumstances, but it can be misleading. First, corneal endothelial decompensation occurs over a wide range of endothelial cell densities because endothelial pump function depends not only on the number of cells but also on the number of pump sites per cell and the integrity of the cell membrane junctions, neither of which is assessed by specular microscopy. Second, in guttate dystrophy, interpretation of specular microscopy is impeded by masking of the endothelial cells that occurs because of the guttae. Corneal guttae appear dark on specular microscopy and prevent visualization of endothelium that may be covering the back of the excrescences of the Descemet's membrane. It has not been established whether endothelial cell density in the clearer corneal periphery can predict the status of the central endothelium.

The only readily available objective measure of physiologic endothelial pump function is pachymetry, either optical or ultrasonic. Normal corneas have a bell-shaped distribution of thickness and occasionally exceed 600 μm in thickness. As a general rule, pachymetry readings less than 600 μm indicate an adequately functioning endothelium for most patients, although a *disparity* between the same areas of the patient's two corneas exceeding 20 μm would raise suspicion of early edema in the thicker cornea. Pachymetry readings exceeding 650 μm strongly suggest the onset of physiologic endothelial decompensation, making combined penetrating keratoplasty and cataract extraction advisable even in the absence of frank corneal edema. Table 21-1 outlines the diagnostic steps in evaluating corneal endothelial function.

TABLE 21-1

Evaluation of Corneal Endothelial Function

MORPHOLOGIC EVALUATION
Specular microscopy
Confocal microscopy (research)
PHYSIOLOGIC FUNCTION
Corneal thickness
Ultrasonic pachymetry
Light pachymetry
Evaluation of the diurnal curve (research) or recovery after patching (research)
Fluorophotometry
HISTORY
Morning blur
Glare complaints
Symptoms of variable contrast sensitivity impairment

Special Techniques for Combined Penetrating Keratoplasty and Cataract Extraction

Preoperative Preparation

Obtaining a soft eye is critical to the success of an "open-sky" procedure. In addition to the administration of the usual dilating and antibiotic regimen employed for cataract surgery, softening of the globe and orbit begins with application of gentle pressure over the closed eyelids after administration of the peribulbar or retrobulbar block. An instrument such as the Honan balloon at 30 mm Hg should be applied for at least 20 minutes before beginning the procedure. Intravenous mannitol is administered over 1 to 2 minutes at the time of preparing and draping the patient. The dose should be adjusted according to the patient's body weight and medical status, taking particular care to avoid the patient with potential congestive heart failure. A typical dose for most adults is 50 ml of 25% mannitol. When administered at this time interval, the maximal hyperosmotic effect will occur at the time of opening the eye, in about 10 to 15 minutes. If the mannitol is administered earlier, the maximal pressure-lowering effect is sometimes lost.

Technique for Cataract Removal

Some surgeons employ a phacoemulsification technique through a scleral tunnel limbal wound before the transplantation.[11] This has the advantage of the control inherent in a closed-chamber technique. It does require a separate wound and incurs the cost of the phacoemulsification tubing and tip. In many cases warranting a combined procedure, the corneal pathologic condition will impair the clear visualization necessary for phacoemulsification. In particular, visualization of the posterior capsule can be difficult.

Because open-sky extracapsular cataract extraction can be used routinely in conjunction with penetrating keratoplasty, it does carry the risk of an open-sky procedure without protection against an expulsive suprachoroidal hemorrhage. Management of this potential complication is discussed later in the section on complications. An open-sky extracapsular extraction begins with the anterior capsulotomy. Manual retraction of the iris with an iris hook is often necessary because of an associated pathologic condition preventing wide dilation. A can-opener capsulotomy is usually satisfactory, as is a scissors capsulotomy. However, continuous curvilinear capsulorhexis is ideal in terms of retaining a defined anterior capsular edge, facilitating cortical aspiration, and reliably implanting the IOL within the capsular bag. Obtaining an adequately sized anterior capsulotomy is critical to delivering the entire nucleus. In general, a diameter of 7 mm or larger is needed. Control of a capsulorhexis tear at this diameter can be difficult. Because of the open-sky wound, some degree of positive pressure is inevitable. The posterior pressure on the nucleus tends to cause the capsulorhexis to extend toward the equator. In addition to the critical decompression of the eye preoperatively (described earlier), positive pressure can be counteracted by using a spatula in the nondominant hand to apply posterior pressure on the center of the nucleus while the capsulorhexis is being performed (Figure 21-1). If the tear

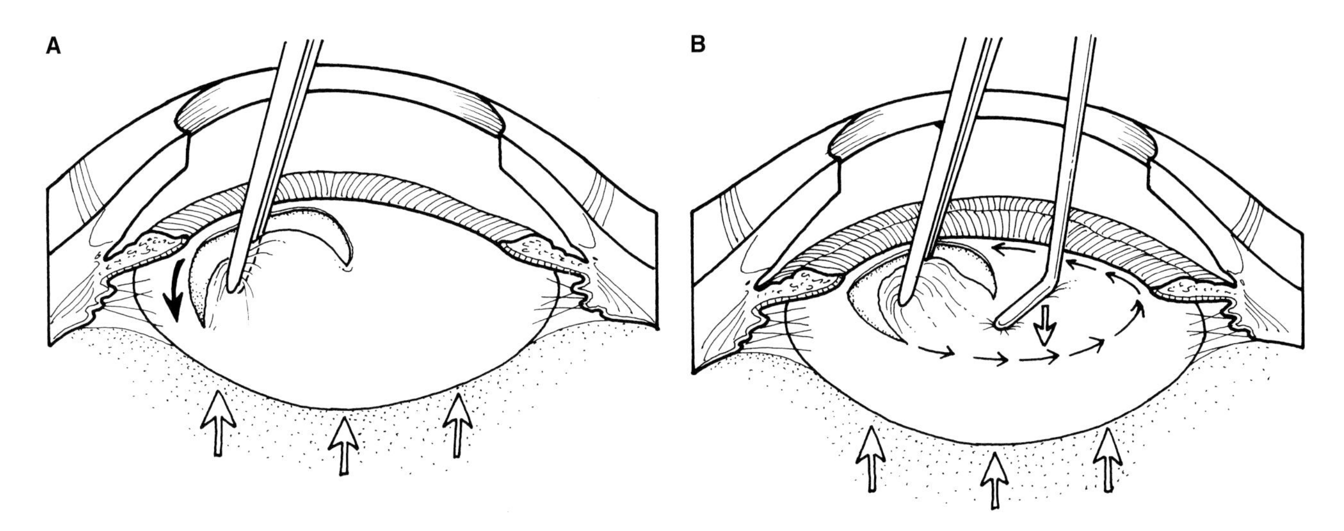

FIGURE 21-1 A, In the setting of penetrating keratoplasty, vitreous pressure is particularly likely to cause a circular tear capsulotomy to extend toward the equator and potentially around to the posterior capsule. **B,** In addition to preoperative maneuvers to soften the globe and to dehydrate the vitreous fluid, positive pressure intraoperatively can be counteracted by applying downward pressure on the nucleus itself while completing the circular tear anterior capsulotomy.

begins to extend beyond 8 mm and cannot be recovered, it is best to discontinue the tearing maneuver and convert to a scissors capsulotomy to prevent further extension of the tear out to the equator and beyond.

The nucleus can be removed through several maneuvers. If the anterior capsular tear is continuous, hydrodissection can be safely employed. Hydrodissection is helpful in loosening the nucleus. If a fluid stream is directed under the anterior capsule, cortical cleaving hydrodissection may occur, greatly facilitating the later cortical cleanup (see Chapter 14). In the absence of hydrodissection, the nucleus can usually be loosened readily by rocking it with an impaled sharp instrument such as a 23-gauge hypodermic needle or the end of a fine dialysis spatula (Figure 21-2). When one edge of the nuclear equator can be visualized, a microsurgical loop is passed under the nucleus, and the nucleus is delivered though the center of the anterior

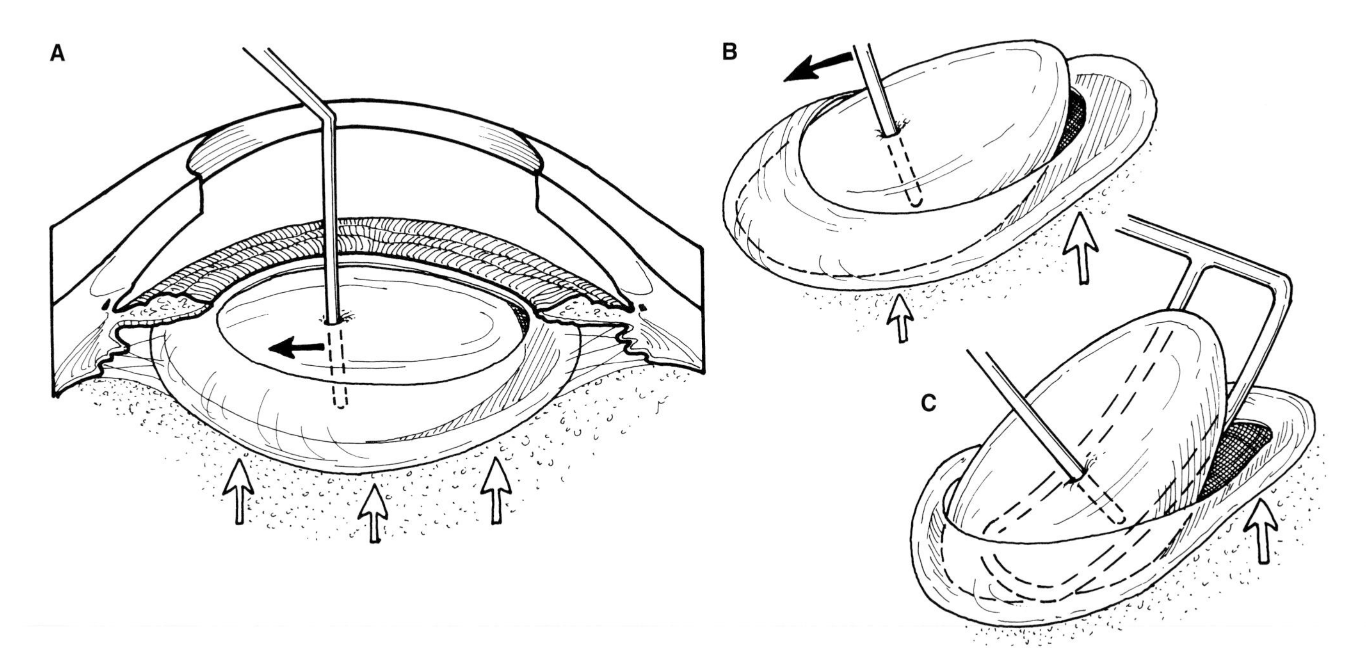

FIGURE 21-2 A, First step in delivering the nucleus is to rock the nucleus with an instrument such as a cyclodialysis spatula until one pole of the equator presents. Positive vitreous pressure usually facilitates this step; if the eye is particularly soft, gentle pressure on the sclera to create positive vitreous pressure can be helpful. **B,** Nucleus is tilted once the equatorial pole becomes exposed. **C,** Microsurgical lens loop can then be safely passed behind the nucleus and the nucleus delivered in its entirety.

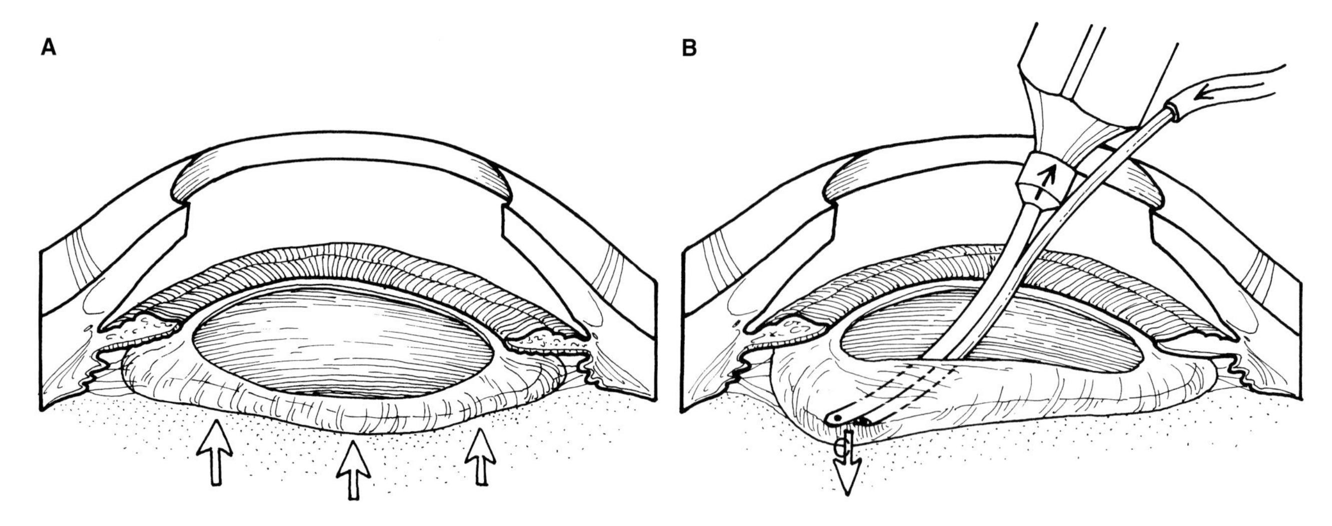

FIGURE 21-3 **A,** After nucleus delivery, the vitreous pressure flattens the capsular bag with apposition of the anterior and posterior capsules. **B,** Cortical cleanup can be performed with a variety of instruments. One device that is particularly well suited to the open-sky situation is the relatively flat and thin "reverse Simcoe" irrigation-aspiration needle. The tip can be gently slid between the anterior and posterior capsules, and then slight downward pressure separates the anterior and posterior capsules, allowing the equatorial cortex to be engaged and stripped safely.

capsulotomy. If the nucleus tends to fall back, *very gentle* placement of a small volume of viscoelastic agent behind the lens nucleus can lift it forward. Care must be taken not to create pressure posteriorly that would extend a capsular tear. Another alternative for delivering the lens nucleus is to place a cryoprobe on the central nucleus after removing as much loose anterior cortex as possible. If good adhesion is obtained, the nucleus is delivered in a "lollipop" maneuver.

Residual epinucleus and cortex are then aspirated. A conventional automated irrigation-aspiration unit can be used. In the open-sky situation, however, aspiration of air with resultant variation in pump function is inevitable. The large volumes of infusion fluid typical of automated units can be problematic in an open-sky setting. Furthermore, avoidance of aspiration of anterior capsular flaps and tearing of zonules can be difficult, particularly when there is any posterior pressure.

For these reasons, it is helpful to become comfortable with a manual irrigation-aspiration system such as the Simcoe or McIntyre systems. The so-called reverse Simcoe unit combines the advantages of each concept. An aspirating 3-ml syringe is attached to the unit directly. Because the irrigation-aspiration tip is flat and gently curved, it is particularly well suited to aspirating cortex in the presence of positive pressure with apposition of the anterior and posterior capsules (Figure 21-3).

Great care must be taken to avoid aspiration of the anterior capsule and tearing of zonules in the open-sky situation. All cortex must be cleaned to minimize postoperative inflammation that will be injurious to corneal transplantation.

After full removal of cortex, and polishing of the posterior capsule if needed, a posterior chamber IOL is placed. When placement within the capsular bag is ensured in an intact capsulorhexis, my personal preference is a one-piece all-polymethylmethacrylate posterior chamber IOL with a haptic diameter of 12 mm. When sulcus fixation is possible or probable, a 13- to 14-mm haptic diameter is preferred to better ensure stability in the sulcus. A patient with a normal pupil can accept a 6 mm-diameter optic; if there is any pupillary abnormality, a 6.5- or 7-mm diameter optic without any positioning holes is used.

The selection of an IOL power is problematic.[4,5,12,13] Axial length can be measured preoperatively, but penetrating keratoplasty will affect the keratometric contribution to the total optics. Some surgeons employ the patient's preoperative keratometry values to calculate IOL power. My personal preference is to use my "typical" value for corneal curvature after keratoplasty, which averages 45 diopters for all patients. Each surgeon must determine his or her postoperative "personalized" keratometric value after corneal grafting. If a consistent surgical technique is employed, a keratoplasty surgeon will usually obtain repeatable results. Only occasionally will the postoperative power be sufficiently inaccurate that the anisometropia becomes symptomatic.

Complications

Positive Pressure and Vitreous Loss

Positive pressure in the form of a bulging posterior capsule, but with maintenance of a normal red reflex, can be due to a variety of causes. The most common cause is transmitted lid and drape pressure through the lid speculum. To maximize the ability to resist such pressure on the open globe, a Schott or Smirmaul lid speculum provides excellent exposure while controlling pressure transmission to the eye. Wire lid specula are the most likely to transmit pressure to the globe. Whatever lid speculum is used in the presence of positive pressure, the surgeon must immediately check the lid speculum. Countersupport is provided if lifting or repositioning a lid speculum relieves the positive pressure.

If the positive pressure is extreme and threatens rupture of the posterior capsule or zonules, or both, the surgeon can attempt vitreous aspiration. With the open eye, however, a simple needle stab through the pars plana will generate even more positive pressure and ensure vitreous loss. Only an extremely delicate cutdown through the sclera with a sharp knife, such as a diamond knife, can minimize this risk. In many cases, the rapid progression of the positive pressure will not give the surgeon adequate time for this type of dissection.

The surgeon must always be alert for evidence of suprachoroidal hemorrhage or effusion. This much more threatening complication is discussed further on. Without signs of this additional complication, vitreous loss must be definitively addressed with vitrectomy. Automated mechanical vitrectomy with a guillotine-type cutter is preferred to minimize traction on the vitreous base. If a mechanical vitrectomy is not possible, an open-sky vitrectomy with cellulose sponge and scissors can be performed, taking care to minimize vitreous traction. At the completion of the vitrectomy, the anterior chamber must be carefully inspected, including wiping the pupillary aperture and iris face with a cellulose sponge, to ensure removal of all vitreous. Residual vitreous in the anterior chamber will tend to become incarcerated in the keratoplasty wound, distorting the pupil, at a minimum, and often leading to further complications, such as cystoid macular edema.

Suprachoroidal Hemorrhage and Effusion

With the corneal button removed, the eye is vulnerable to devastating suprachoroidal effusion and hemorrhage. The surgeon must always be alert to this possible complication and be prepared to deal with it immediately. Signs of suprachoroidal hemorrhage and effusion in an open-sky setting include positive pressure on an intact posterior capsule, rupture of the posterior capsule and zonules with vitreous loss, alteration in the red reflex, or a combination of these factors. If the patient is aphakic before the placement of the IOL, the retina may be directly visualized in detail through the operating microscope. An advancing smooth "roll" of elevated retina or normal color may represent effusion; if the advancing elevation is dark, suprachoroidal hemorrhage is likely. A slow hemorrhage will likely lead to expulsion of intraocular contents if immediate action is not taken.

As soon as the suprachoroidal mass is recognized, the surgeon should immediately place a gloved index finger over the corneal opening. It is an excellent idea to have a clear lens available to maintain the globe when a suprachoroidal event is recognized. One such lens is the Cobo temporary keratoprosthesis, available from Ocular Instruments (Figure 21-4). This tapered lens can fit a wide range of trephine openings. This will stabilize the globe while the surgeon proceeds to a cutdown into the suprachoroidal space to remove the pressure.

One of the causes of suprachoroidal hemorrhage during penetrating keratoplasty is a lightly anesthetized patient under general anesthesia straining against the endotracheal tube. Because penetrating keratoplasty is relatively painless, little general anesthesia is needed, and many anesthesiologists progressively reduce the amount of general anesthetic during the procedure to avoid hypotension. To avoid this complication, the anesthesiologist should be specifically instructed by the surgeon to use a paralytic agent.

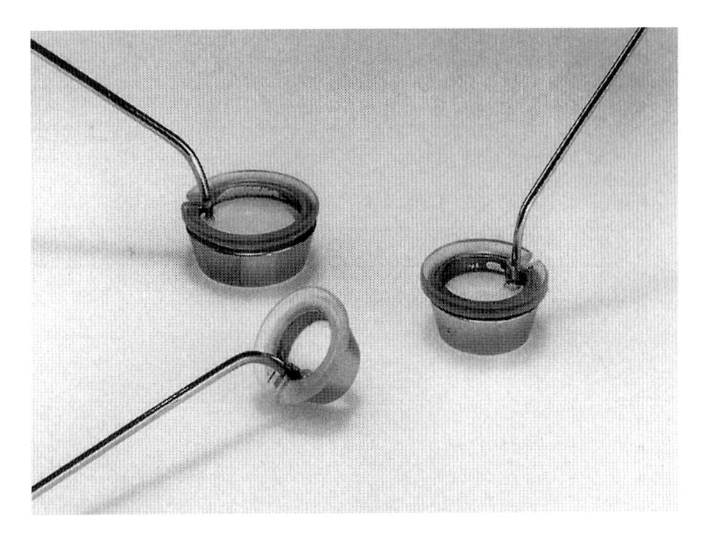

FIGURE 21-4 Cobo temporary keratoprosthesis (Ocular Instruments, Inc.) is highly valuable in controlling suprachoroidal effusion or hemorrhage in the vulnerable open-sky setting. (Courtesy Ocular Instruments, Inc., Bellevue, Wash.)

Intraocular Lens Implantation After Vitreous Loss

If vitreous loss has occurred, and the ability of the residual posterior capsule to support a posterior chamber IOL is in doubt, the surgeon faces three choices for IOL implantation: an anterior chamber IOL, an iris-sutured posterior chamber IOL, or a scleral suture-fixed posterior chamber IOL.

The literature does not show a clear-cut difference in outcomes among these three alternatives. If a posterior chamber IOL is desired, dissection of scleral flaps for scleral fixation is extremely difficult once the corneal button is absent. The surgeon can iris-fixate a posterior chamber IOL with midperipheral sutures or, with a technique first described by Lane, use a scleral cutting technique that does not require dissecting scleral flaps. The latter can be performed using a posterior chamber IOL with a suturing hole in the haptic. A loop of permanent suture such as 10-0 or 9-0 polypropylene is passed through the positioning hole, and then each arm of the double-arm suture is passed through the sclera approximately 1 mm apart through the ciliary sulcus region. The suture is tied and cut. The knot is then rotated beneath the sclera. Conjunctiva is closed over the smooth loop of polypropylene. The smooth loop of external suture material will not erode through the conjunctiva. This technique is illustrated for a closed-chamber procedure in Figure 37-1.

REFERENCES

1. Lindstrom RL, Harris WS, Doughman DJ: Combined penetrating keratoplasty, extracapsular cataract extraction, and posterior chamber intraocular lens implantation, *J Am Intraocul Implant Soc* 7:130-132, 1981.
2. Hunkeler JD, Hyde LL: The triple procedure: combined penetrating keratoplasty, extracapsular cataract extraction, and posterior chamber intraocular lens implantation: an expanded experience, *J Am Intraocul Implant Soc* 9:20-24, 1983.

3. Kramer SG: Penetrating keratoplasty combined with extracapsular cataract extraction, *Am J Ophthalmol* 100:129-133, 1985.
4. Binder PS: The triple procedure: refractive results. 1985 Update, *Ophthalmology* 93:1482-1488, 1986.
5. Crawford GJ, Stulting RD, Waring GO et al: The triple procedure: analysis of outcome, refraction, and intraocular lens calculation, Ophthalmology 93: 817-824, 1986.
6. Busin M, Arffa RC, McDonald MB et al: Combined penetrating keratoplasty, extracapsular cataract extraction, and posterior chamber intraocular lens implantation, *Ophthalmic Surg* 18:272-275, 1987.
7. Meyer RF, Musch DC: Assessment of success and complications of triple procedure surgery, *Am J Ophthalmol* 104:233-240, 1987.
8. Fine M: Therapeutic keratoplasty and Fuchs' dystrophy, *Am J Ophthalmol* 57:371-378, 1964.
9. Payant JA, Gordon LW, VanderZwaag R et al: Cataract formation following corneal transplantation in eyes with Fuchs' endothelial dystrophy, *Cornea* 9:286-289, 1990.
10. Martin TP, Reed JW, Legault C et al: Cataract formation and cataract extraction and penetrating keratoplasty, *Ophthalmology* 101:113-119, 1984.
11. Malbran ES, Malbran E, Buonsanti J et al: Closed-system phacoemulsification and posterior chamber implant combined with penetrating keratoplasty, *Ophthalmic Surg* 24:403-406, 1993.
12. Binder PS: Intraocular lens implantation after penetrating keratoplasty, *Refractive Corneal Surg* 5:224-230, 1989.
13. Flowers CW, McLeod SD, McDonnell PJ et al: Evaluation of intraocular lens power calculation formulas in the triple procedure, *J Cataract Refract Surg* 22:116-122, 1996.

Control of Astigmatism in the Cataract Patient

22

Richard L. Lindstrom, MD
Douglas D. Koch, MD
Robert H. Osher, MD
Li Wang, MD, PhD

For over a century, it has been recognized that cataract incisions influence astigmatism.[1-3] Only in the past 15 years, however, have cataract surgeons mounted serious investigations aimed at measuring and minimizing astigmatism induced by cataract surgery. These efforts have paralleled but, until recently, have lagged behind the success of intraocular lenses (IOLs) in correcting the spherical refractive error precipitated by removal of the crystalline lens.

The term *refractive cataract surgery* has entered general ophthalmic usage. The term implies a coordinated and encompassing attention to both spherical and astigmatic components of refraction. The current goal of refractive cataract surgery may or may not be emmetropia; for some patients, the postsurgical target may be slight residual astigmatism, which contributes to depth of field. The critical difference between modern refractive cataract surgery and cataract surgery of a decade ago is the very existence of a target. Today's refractive cataract surgeon determines the starting point (the preexisting astigmatic condition of the patient), knows the astigmatic effects of various approaches, and selects a surgical plan that optimizes the refractive outcome for the individual patient. It is a degree of precision that was previously unattainable, requiring a depth of surgical planning that was previously unnecessary.

In addition to the cataract incision, whose size, location, and configuration help determine the astigmatic effects of surgery, the cataract surgeon now has two additional options in his or her armamentarium for correcting astigmatism: (1) corneal relaxing incisions (CRIs) and (2) toric IOLs. CRIs can be characterized as those made in the corneal midperiphery (e.g., 6- to 8-mm zone), so-called astigmatic keratotomy (AK), and those made peripherally, so-called peripheral or limbal corneal relaxing incisions (PCRIs). CRIs, particularly AK, were first studied purely for their corneal refractive effects.[2,4,5] In terms of both its nomenclature and the actual clinical practices that it incorporates, *refractive cataract surgery* therefore represents a true marriage of refractive and cataract surgical specialties.

This chapter describes the astigmatic effects of various cataract incisions, the techniques of PCRIs, two different approaches to AK, and toric IOLs. The reader will find no hard-and-fast rules herein. Depending on the cataract extraction technique employed, the degree and meridian of preexisting astigmatism, and a host of other variables, the same patient might find effective treatment in a variety of ways. We hope to convey a sense of the general principles involved and to sketch out treatment approaches to the range of astigmatic errors that most cataract surgeons commonly encounter.

Patient Selection and Evaluation

People with over 0.5 to 0.75 diopters (D) of astigmatism usually require some kind of optical correction. Astigmatic errors of 1 to 2 D may reduce uncorrected visual acuity to the 20/30 or 20/50 level, whereas an astigmatic error of 2 to 3 D may correspond to visual acuity between 20/70 and 20/100.[6]

Up to 95% of eyes have some degree of naturally occurring astigmatic error. The incidence of clinically significant astigmatism reported in the literature varies between 7.5% and 75%.[6] From 3% to 15% of eyes may have astigmatic refractive errors greater than 2 D.[7] The incidence of postcataract surgery astigmatism greater than 2 D may be as high as 25% to 30%.[8,9]

In a patient with little or no preexisting astigmatism, cataract surgery should be designed to be as astigmatically neutral as possible. For patients with significant degrees of preexisting astigmatism, two types of approaches can be employed as a function of the type of cataract incision. The surgeon can (1) operate on the steep corneal meridian and select the type of cataract incision that will produce the desired amount of against-the-wound flattening or (2) make a small incision at a favored location (e.g., clear corneal temporal incision), factor in the small amount of astigmatic change induced by this decision, and supplement it with either CRIs or implantation of a toric IOL. Obviously, CRIs can also be used postoperatively to further modify the result.

Careful patient selection is crucial in avoiding postoperative surprises and unhappy patients. As a rule of thumb, some form of astigmatic surgery should be considered in patients in whom a standard cataract operation will result in 1 D or more of postoperative astigmatism and whose fellow eye (1) has 1.5 D or less of astigmatism, (2) has astigmatism at a different meridian than that of the operative eye, or (3) has a similar amount and meridian of astigmatism and is itself an imminent surgical candidate.[10]

The rationale, surgical methods, and risks are discussed with the patient preoperatively. As noted previously, the target may be a slight undercorrection of the preexisting astigmatism because some patients are bothered by the shift in astigmatic meridian brought about by an overcorrection, and a small amount of residual astigmatism can provide pseudophakic patients with reasonably good uncorrected near and distance vision.

The sections that follow address the cataract incision, CRIs (PCRIs and AK), and toric IOLs separately and in greater detail. However, cataract incision manipulation and these other approaches are dual partners in the treatment of a wide range of astigmatism in people with varied personalities and lifestyle requirements.

Alignment

Accurate astigmatic surgery is highly sensitive to precise meridional alignment. Vector analysis demonstrates that a misalignment of only 15 degrees results in a 50% reduction in the astigmatic correction. A 30-degree misalignment results in no change, but there is a large shift in the astigmatic axis. Misalignment errors in excess of 30 degrees actually result in a net increase in the magnitude of the astigmatism.[11]

Various approaches can be taken to minimize alignment errors. Whenever possible, we make small drawings of the patient's eyes when they are seen in the office preoperatively. The patient's head is carefully positioned to ensure that it is vertically oriented in the slit lamp. We then look for prominent conjunctival, corneal, or iris features that are likely to be visible when the patient is dilated as seen in the operating room (Figure 22-1). It is particularly helpful to indicate landmarks that provide a clear indication of the 90- and 180-degree meridians because these can be easily identified relative to the position of the vertical or horizontal slit lamp beam.

An alternative approach is to mark the eye before entering the operating room. Topical anesthetic drops are administered, and the patient is asked to sit upright on the surgical stretcher. A marking pen is used to indicate either the 6:00 and 12:00 o'clock or 3:00 and 9:00 o'clock positions.

A third option is to mark the eyes as the patient is lying on the operating room table. For the majority of patients, this approach works extremely well. However, a small percentage of eyes rotate as the patient moves from an upright to a supine position. Swami et al.[12] demonstrated that 8% of eyes (20/240) had a deviation of greater than 10 degrees.

A fourth option is to perform intraoperative keratoscopy to identify the major meridian and quantitate the amount, which should be consistent with the preoperative keratometry measurements and corneal topography. This can be achieved with a device like the Hyde-Osher ruler manufactured by Ocular Instruments, which is accurate for identifying 1.5 D or more.

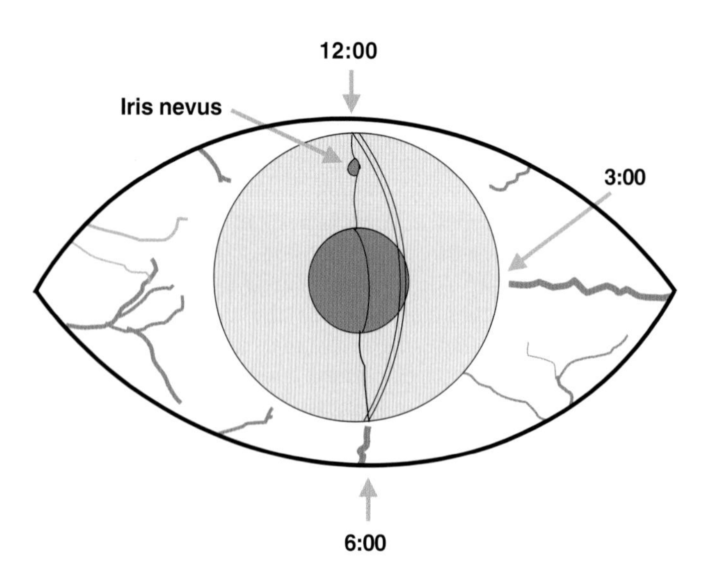

FIGURE 22-1 Identifying the steep meridian: find on the cornea, iris, or conjunctiva one or more landmarks that are likely to be visible in surgery.

The Cataract Incision

An incision of the cornea or sclera creates tissue gape. This gape causes corneal flattening along the meridian of the incision and steepening in the meridian 90 degrees away (Figure 22-2), with the magnitude of this determined by several factors (see following two paragraphs). To compensate, wounds can be closed with

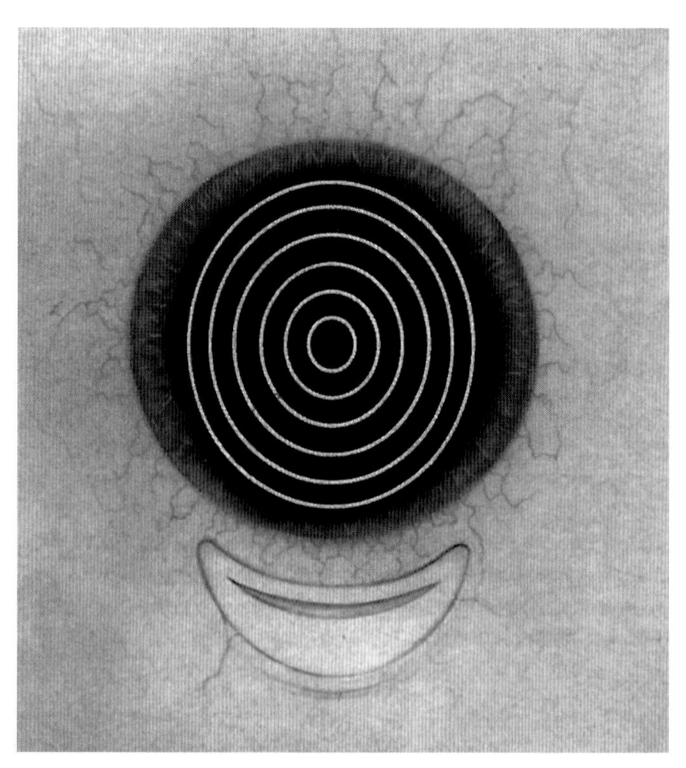

FIGURE 22-2 Following a limbal incision, tissue gape produces flattening along the meridian of the incision and steepening 90 degrees away. (From Koch DD, Lindstrom RL: Controlling astigmatism in cataract surgery, *Semin Ophthalmol* 7:224-233, 1992.)

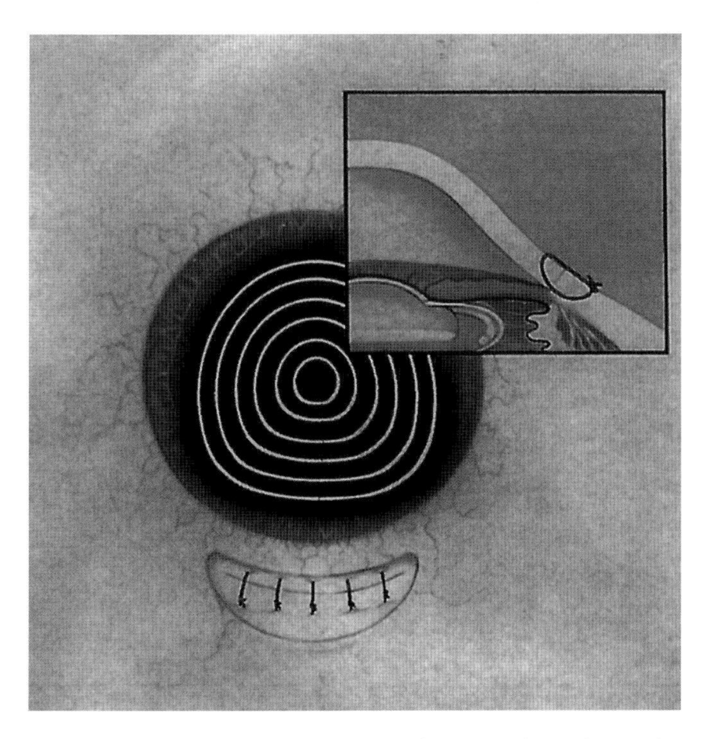

FIGURE 22-3 Sutures create peripheral flattening and central steepening along the meridian of the incision and steepening 90 degrees away. (From Koch DD, Lindstrom RL: Controlling astigmatism in cataract surgery, *Semin Ophthalmol* 7:224-233, 1992.)

sutures. Sutures produce local tissue compression, resulting in peripheral flattening and central steepening along the meridian of the incision and flattening 90 degrees away (Figure 22-3).

The suture-induced net steepening persists for several months postoperatively. Over several years, however, progressive flattening occurs. The net result is an against-the-wound astigmatism.

Factors that affect the astigmatic change produced by a cataract incision include its length, meridional location, radial location (e.g., corneal, limbal, or scleral), construction, and wound damage, such as thermal injury. With larger incisions, intrinsic patient factors can be important, as variations in wound healing can lead to markedly different astigmatic effects. Sutures have a temporary affect but rarely produce changes that persist beyond 2 years, with the possible exception being those instances in which tissue is actually damaged or displaced by the sutures and heals in this new configuration.

Using scleral flap recessions of varying widths in eyebank eyes, Samuelson, Koch, and Kuglen[13] have shown the direct relationship that exists between incision length and against-the-wound corneal flattening (Table 22-1). Notably, clinically significant flattening (0.5 D or more) occurred only in incisions longer than 3 mm.

Suture Versus Sutureless

Properly constructed scleral incisions up to 7 mm wide can be self-sealing in the absence of sutures. The key to watertightness is the anterior entry into the anterior chamber, which creates a valve effect as intraocular pressure compresses the mouth of the incision closed. However, we suspect that sutured scleral incisions heal more rapidly and perhaps more completely than unsutured incisions. It is therefore possible that sutureless incisions are more prone to late wound sliding.

For corneal incisions, the majority can be left sutureless. We recommend suturing these incisions if they are greater than 4 mm in length or if the incision is not watertight at the conclusion of surgery.

TABLE 22-1

Induced Corneal Flattening Along Meridian of Incision (Scleral Pocket Incision) in Eyebank Eyes

Incision Length (mm)	Mean Flattening (Standard Deviation, D)
2.0	0.07 (0.10)
2.5	0.10 (0.17)
3.0	0.24 (0.17)
3.5	0.47 (0.35)
4.0	0.74 (0.45)
4.5	1.00 (0.46)
5.0	1.07 (0.41)
5.5	1.40 (0.56)

From Samuelson SW, Koch DD, Kuglen CC: Determination of maximal incision length for true small-incision surgery, *Ophthalmic Surg* 22:204-207, 1991.

Incision Location

As a general rule, for any given incision size and construction, the further the incision is from the center of the cornea, the less the surgically induced astigmatism. For small incisions, most surgeons have adopted the clear or near-clear corneal approach. Fortunately, these incisions are typically sufficiently small that they induce little astigmatism despite their anterior location. For incisions longer than 4 mm, the limbal and, particularly, scleral incisions offer greater astigmatic stability. Conversely, if against-the-wound drift is desired, these larger incisions can be placed more anteriorly to attempt to achieve the desired astigmatic change.

Incision Size

PLANNED EXTRACAPSULAR INCISIONS

Curved scleral incisions concentric with the limbus and closed with interrupted 10-0 nylon or polyester sutures are recommended for planned extracapsular surgery.[10] Interrupted sutures are probably more prone to inducing excessive early steepness on the meridian of the incision, compared with continuous sutures. However, for these large incisions, interrupted sutures have two advantages: (1) they reduce the risk of excessive flattening along the meridian of the incision, and (2) they offer the opportunity to cut single sutures, which gives greater latitude in modifying astigmatism postoperatively. These incisions can typically drift 1 to 3 D in the first few years after surgery, and against-the-wound flattening of up to 5 D can rarely occur.

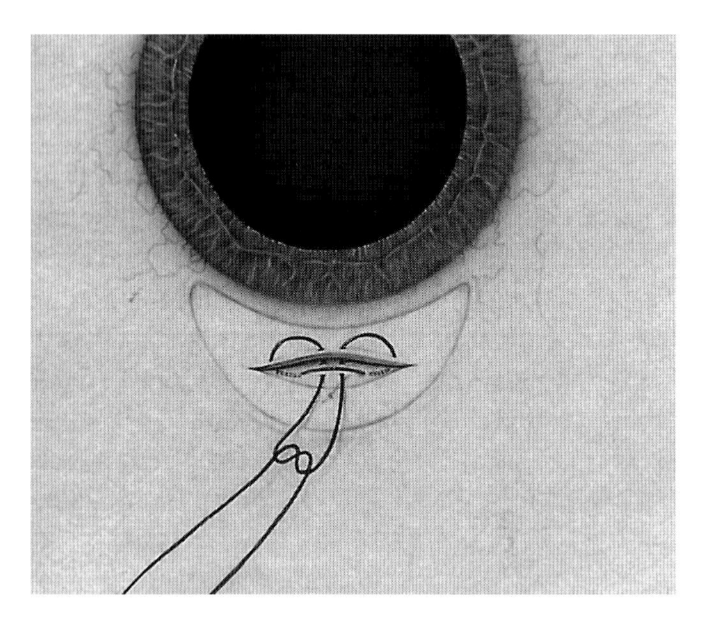

FIGURE 22-4 The Masket continuous horizontal suture closure consists of a posterior radial bite, two right-to-left bites concentric with the limbus, and an anterior-posterior radial bite. (From Koch DD, Lindstrom RL: Controlling astigmatism in cataract surgery, *Semin Ophthalmol* 7:224-233, 1992.)

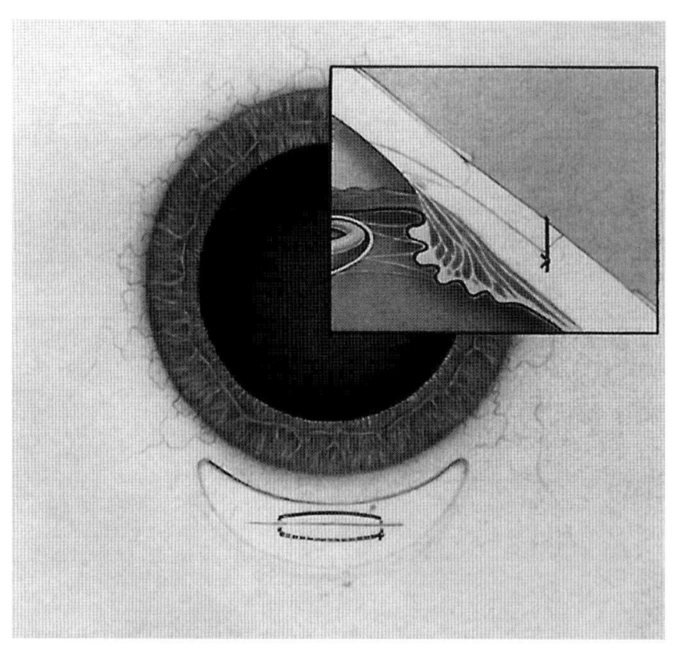

FIGURE 22-5 Technique for single vertical mattress suture. (From Koch DD, Lindstrom RL: Controlling astigmatism in cataract surgery, *Semin Ophthalmol* 7:224-233, 1992.)

ENLARGED PHACOEMULSIFICATION INCISIONS

Incisions 6.5 to 7.5 mm wide are used for implantation of 6- to 7-mm polymethylmethacrylate (PMMA) optic lenses after phacoemulsification. The incisions may be curved, as with the extracapsular incision, or straight. An incision of this size can be expected to drift 1 to 2 D against the wound. If properly constructed, these incisions can be left unsutured, or they are closed with running shoelace suture, interrupted sutures, or a continuous horizontal suture. The advantage of a continuous horizontal suture is that it can be tightened sufficiently to provide watertight closure and perhaps to minimize late wound sliding without inducing excessive astigmatism. Long-term follow-up is needed to assess the stability of incisions closed in this manner.

The horizontal-suture closure described by Masket is especially clever. Suture of 9-0 or 10-0 nylon is used; 9-0 may be preferred for its extra strength. A unique feature of the Masket suture is its small radial component; however, its main advantage may be in the ease of insertion and tightening. The first bite is passed backhanded, posteriorly to anteriorly, in the bed of the incision (Figure 22-4). After two right-to-left passes, the final bite is again radial, front-handed this time, through the anterior lip of the incision and the bed of the flap. The suture is tied with a 3-1-1 knot.

Appropriately constructed scleral incisions 5 mm and smaller can be left unsutured, or they can be closed with interrupted or a single horizontal (vertical mattress) suture (originally described by John Shepherd, *Video Journal of Cataract and Refractive Surgery,* volume V, issue 3) (Figure 22-5). Osher modified the continuous horizontal suture by posteriorly offsetting the bite through the bed to achieve two radial components. In placing the suture, the needle enters the right lateral extent of the groove at its base. The suture bite begins at the junction of the groove and the forward dissection; the bite is angled 45 degrees posteriorly, thereby passing through a greater amount of sclera. The needle is passed along the base of the groove, entering and exiting about 0.5 mm from the edge of the groove. The total length of the bite is thus about 3 mm. The needle is then passed up through the undersurface of the overlying flap, across to the original right side of the incision, and down through the flap, where the suture ends can be tied and are covered by the overlying flap. Incisions of this type can be expected to drift 0.5 to 1 D against the wound.

"SMALL-INCISION" CATARACT SURGERY

Incisions of 4 mm or less are used for insertion of foldable small-incision lenses after phacoemulsification. These incisions were originally made in the sclera or limbus, but clear or near-clear corneal incisions are now the most popular choice.

We have reviewed the ophthalmic literature regarding the astigmatic change induced by small scleral limbal and corneal incisions, and the summaries of these results are shown in Tables 22-2 and 22-3.[14-27] Interestingly, the results from these clinical studies mirror the results that were found in the cadaver eye study previously performed by Samuelson and Koch.

TABLE 22-2
Surgically Induced Astigmatism by Scleral Tunnel Incisions

Incision Length (mm)	Surgically induced astigmatism (D)
3.0-3.5	0.20-0.40
4.0	0.42-0.72
5.0-5.5	0.35-0.89

TABLE 22-3
Surgically Induced Astigmatism by Clear Corneal Incisions

Incision Length (mm)	Surgically induced astigmatism (D)
3.0-3.5	0.20-0.68
4.0	0.36-0.56
5.0-5.5	0.46-1.24

If we define true "small-incision" surgery on an astigmatic basis such that less than 0.5 D is induced, then this definition would pertain to scleral incisions measuring 4 mm and corneal incisions measuring 3 to 3.5 mm.

Incision Configuration and Manipulation

The configuration of the incision may also influence wound stability and eventual against-the-wound drift. A straight or frown-shaped incision appears to induce less against-the-wound astigmatic change than the traditional curved incision parallel to the limbus (Figure 22-6).

Preexisting astigmatism can be reduced through the use of scleral flap recession on the steep corneal meridian. The approach has the advantages of (1) requiring only one incision (AK may be obviated), thereby minimizing wound-healing variables, and (2) avoiding the potential complications of corneal incisions, such as irregular astigmatism and glare.

To perform the technique, a trapezoidal scleral flap is made, centered meticulously on the steep meridian (Figure 22-7). The curvilinear base of the flap is located 2 mm behind the limbus, and the lateral walls of the flap are cut to within 0.5 mm of the cornea. The width of the flap at the limbus should slightly exceed the anticipated size of the incision into the anterior chamber (e.g., for a 6-mm incision, the flap measures 7 mm at the limbus and 8 mm posteriorly). The flap should be approximately two-thirds depth. As with standard incisions, the flap is dissected into clear cornea to enhance watertightness.

The flap is recessed and secured with a running 9-0 nylon suture anchored at each end and tied centrally. The suture pattern shown in Figure 22-7 forms a barrier that prevents posterior migration of the flap and ensures its stable fixation in the recessed position.[28]

With this technique, up to 4 to 5 D of astigmatism can be corrected. Each 0.25 mm of recession produces about 1 D of astigmatic correction; the maximum recession is about 1 mm. The goal is to slightly overcorrect at surgery, as measured by qualitative or quantitative intraoperative keratometry. In the presence of significant undercorrection, the suture can be removed and the flap advanced an additional amount.

Corneal Relaxing Incisions

The combination of CRI with cataract surgery (Figure 22-8) is fundamental to the current definition of *refractive cataract surgery*. A number of surgeons in the early 1980s, among them Fenzl, Lindstrom, Martin, Neumann, Nordan, Tate, Terry, and Thornton, began investigating surgical techniques to correct naturally occurring astigmatism. In 1983, Osher began a study that addressed the correction of preexisting astigmatism by

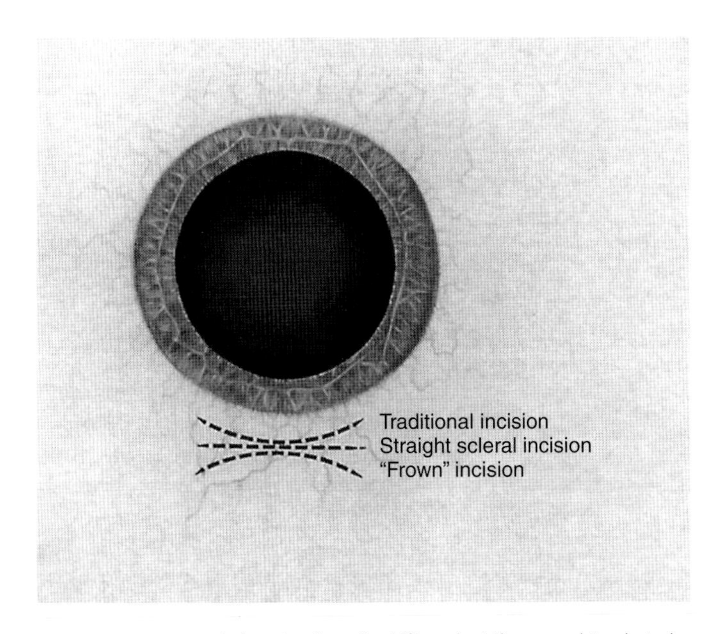

FIGURE 22-6 Induced astigmatic drift against the wound tends to be greatest with traditional curved incisions and least with frown-shaped incision configurations. (From Koch DD, Lindstrom RL: Controlling astigmatism in cataract surgery, *Semin Ophthalmol* 7:224-233, 1992.)

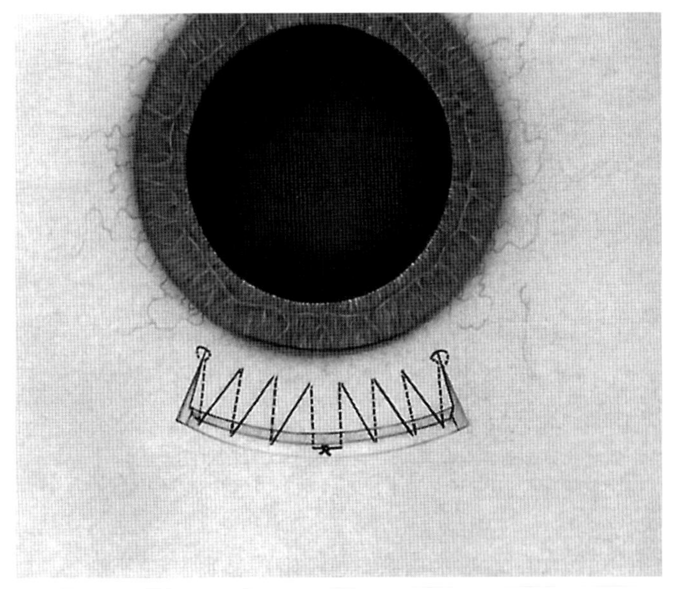

FIGURE 22-7 Configuration of the trapezoidal scleral flap and running suture closure for scleral flap recession. Note that the anterior edges of the flap are slightly lateral to the intended incision into the anterior chamber. Each suture bite exits in the bed of the flap to create a barrier that prevents posterior migration of the flap. (From Koch DD, Lindstrom RL: Controlling astigmatism in cataract surgery, *Semin Ophthalmol* 7:224-233, 1992.)

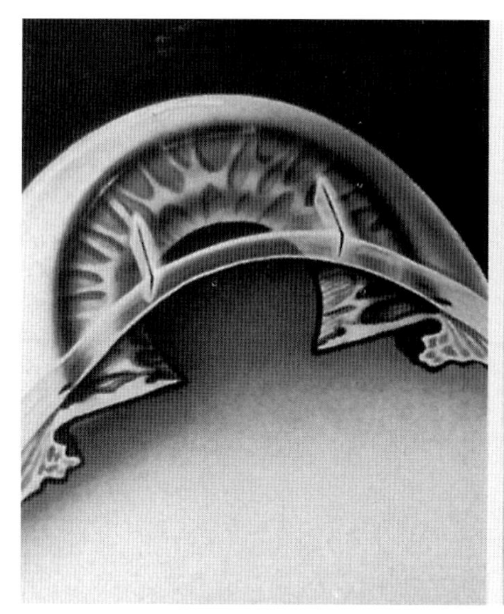

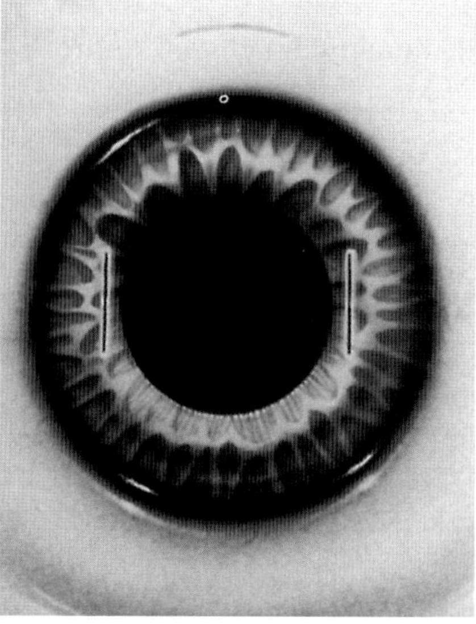

FIGURE 22-8 Transverse astigmatic keratotomy combined with cataract surgery. (From Osher RH: Transverse astigmatic keratotomy combined with cataract surgery, *Ophthalmol Clin North Am* 5:717-725, 1992.)

combining transverse relaxing incisions with cataract surgery. He presented preliminary results at general meetings from 1984 to 1990.[29]

Osher's original technique consisted of placing a single straight CRI in the periphery perpendicular to the steep meridian at the end of surgery and then adding a second parallel incision on a 7- to 10.5-mm-diameter optical zone. Maloney (Refractive cataract replacement: a comprehensive approach to maximize refractive benefits of cataract extraction, Annual Meeting of the American Society of Cataract and Refractive Surgery, Los Angeles, 1986) described a more aggressive approach in which he placed two pairs of transverse incisions before phacoemulsification. Other surgeons attempted to quantify the effect of adding transverse corneal incisions to cataract surgery by varying incision length,[30] number of incisions,[31] optical zone size,[32] or incision depth.[33] Merlin[34] introduced arcuate incisions, and Thornton[35] and Lindstrom[36] became leading advocates while refining diamond blade technology.

Lindstrom[36] found that the *coupling ratio,* the amount of flattening in the incised meridian divided by the amount of steepening in the opposite meridian, was approximately 1:1 when a straight 3-mm keratotomy or a 45- to 90-degree arcuate keratotomy was used at 5- to 7-mm-diameter optical zones. The maximal effect of either straight or arcuate incisions occurred when incisions were placed around a 5- to 7-mm-diameter optical zone. Although most of the effect was achieved with the first pair of incisions, a 20% to 30% additional effect could be attained with a second pair of incisions. The effect could not be increased by placing more than four relaxing incisions in the cornea.

Thornton[35] described what he believed was the geometric advantage of arcuate incisions, the use of which seems to be growing in popularity. He stated that true 1:1 coupling can occur only when the corneal circumference is unchanged, which is achieved only with short, concentric arcuate incisions. A straight transverse incision increases the overall corneal circumference, creating a flatter cornea and necessitating a compensatory addition of power to the IOL. Furthermore, a shorter arcuate incision achieves the same result as a longer straight incision.

Peripheral or Limbal Corneal Relaxing Incisions

Hollis and Gills first investigated the use of limbal relaxing incisions centered along the steep corneal meridian to correct preexisting astigmatism during cataract surgery. As the single or paired relaxing incisions are placed just inside the limbal vessels, they are actually more appropriately called "peripheral corneal relaxing incisions" (PCRIs). Because they are placed at the peripheral cornea, a potential advantage of the incisions over AK is the minimal risk of inducing irregular astigmatism.

The criterion for PCRIs in conjunction with a temporal clear corneal incision is preexisting with-the-rule keratometric astigmatism of ≥0.75 D or preexisting against-the-rule keratometric astigmatism of ≥1.25 D. This criterion was derived from a study of the astigmatic effect of a standard 3.2- to 3.5-mm temporal clear-corneal incision, which produces approximately 0.3 D of with-the-rule change. The length and number of PCRIs are determined according to a nomogram based on age and preoperative corneal astigmatism (Table 22-4). This nomogram is designed for use in combination with 3.2- to 3.5-mm temporal clear-corneal incision with PCRIs made near the end of the cataract surgery, and it is conservative in order to minimize the risk of overcorrections. PCRIs typically cause a mild hyperopic shift of approximately 0.2 D, and this should be taken into account when selecting IOL power.

The location of the steep meridian is carefully determined as noted earlier in this chapter. Intraoperatively, the intended incision site is marked using one of many commercially available markers or even standard surgical calipers. The incision is made just inside the limbal vessels with a guarded diamond

TABLE 22-4

Nomogram for Peripheral Corneal Relaxing Incisions to Correct Keratometric Astigmatism During Cataract Surgery (Temporal 3.2- to 3.5-mm Clear Corneal Incision)

Preoperative Astigmatism (D)	Age (year)	Number	Length
WITH-THE-RULE			
0.75-1.00	<65	2 (or 1 × 60°)	45°
	≥65	1	45°
1.01-1.50	<65	2	60°
	≥65	2 (or 1 × 60°)	45°
>1.50	<65	2	80°
	≥65	2	60°
AGAINST-THE-RULE			
1.00-1.25*	—	1	35°
1.26-2.00	—	1	45°
≥2.00	—	2	45°

From Wang L, Misra M, Koch DD: Peripheral corneal relaxing incisions combined with cataract surgery, *J Cataract Refract Surg* (in press).
*Especially if cataract incision is not directly centered on steep meridian.

knife set at a depth of 600 μm (Figure 22-9). In eyes receiving paired incisions along the horizontal meridian (i.e., in eyes with preexisting against-the-wound astigmatism), the groove of the temporal clear corneal incision is enlarged at the end of surgery to serve as the second peripheral relaxing incision, or the temporal peripheral relaxing incision can be made first by grooving at 600-μm depth to planned length and then entering the anterior chamber at the 50% to 75% depth of this incision. A PCRI at the cataract incision site can slightly destabilize the wound, so it is important to ensure that the incision is water-tight at the conclusion of surgery.

Early studies with a small number of cases showed that the PCRIs were an effective method to reduce preexisting astigmatism during cataract surgery.[37,38] Recently, Wang, Misra, and Koch[39] reported the results in a large series of patients (93 eyes) who underwent combined clear corneal phacoemulsification and PCRIs. PCRIs significantly decreased preexisting astigmatism, and the percentages of the eyes with keratometric astigmatism of ≤1 D increased from 6% preoperatively to 51% at 4 months postoperatively. Overcorrections of 1 D or more occurred in two eyes of two patients; both were over 80 years old. One of the two eyes had a corneal diameter of 10.5 mm, which might contribute to the overcorrection because of both the shorter distance between the PCRI and the center of the cornea and the longer arc length relative to the corneal circumference. For this reason, we recommend measuring PCRI length by degrees instead of millimeters. There were no ocular perforations in our series, suggesting a good safety profile for using a guarded diamond knife set at a depth of 600 μm when PCRIs are performed at the conclusion of cataract surgery.

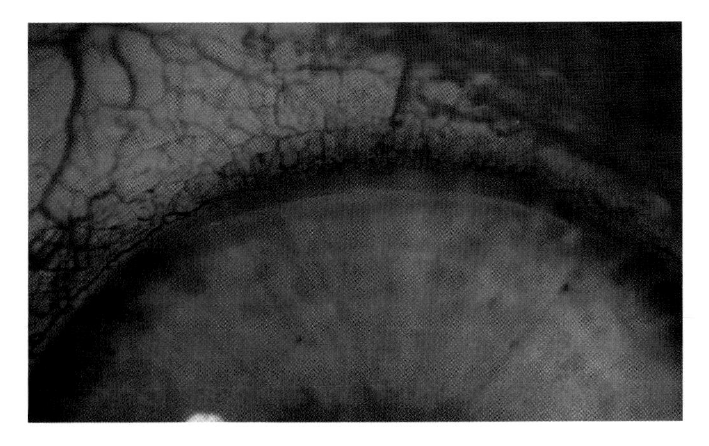

FIGURE 22-9 A view of a superior PCRI centered along 90-degree meridian on an eye 1 day after surgery.

We place PCRIs at the conclusion of the surgery because we had good success with this approach in our early cases and developed our first nomogram based on the results with these eyes. An advantage of performing the incisions at the conclusion of surgery is that these incisions can be omitted if there is some need to enlarge or change the site of the cataract incision. An obvious disadvantage is that there might be greater variability in corneal thickness and intraocular pressure at the conclusion of surgery, which could affect the depth of the incisions. We presume that incisions placed early in the surgery might have a greater effect and might also pose a greater risk of corneal perforation, particularly in older eyes with thinner corneas in the region of the limbus.

Astigmatic Keratotomy

Lindstrom and Koch's Technique

Manifest refraction, keratometry, and computerized video-keratography are performed preoperatively. For cataract patients, the surgical plan is formulated based on the intended incision and the preexisting corneal astigmatism.

The standard nomograms shown in Tables 22-5 and 22-6 are used. The technique employs either a straight or arcuate keratotomy at the 6- and/or 7-mm zones. The nomogram, if adopted by others, must be adjusted to each surgeon's particular technique.

AK is performed at the end of the cataract procedure with the eye inflated. A smaller (5 mm or less) self-sealing incision is preferred when AK is combined with cataract surgery. When planning the AK, the surgeon must factor in the expected against-the-wound drift of the particular incision used.

Equipment includes an operating microscope, a Sinskey hook, 0.12 Colibri corneal fixation forceps, and various zone and incision markers. The Lindstrom arcuate marker (Katena Products, Denville, NJ) is preferred for arcuate incisions. Round 3-, 5-, and 7-mm radial keratotomy optical zone markers and 8-, 12-, and 16-cut radial keratotomy incision markers can be used to localize the incision location and length. A skin-marking pencil or stencil ink pad is used to clarify the marks. An ultrasonic pachymeter is used to measure corneal thickness intraoperatively. A surgical keratometer is useful but not essential for intraoperative monitoring.

TABLE 22-5
Arcuate Keratotomy 6-mm Optical Zone Nomogram*

	Surgical Option												
Age (year)	**1 × 30°**	**2 × 30° or 1 × 45°**	**1 × 60°**	**2 × 45° or 1 × 90°**	**2 × 60°**	**2 × 90°**	**Age (year)**	**1 × 30°**	**2 × 30° or 1 × 45°**	**1 × 60°**	**2 × 45° or 1 × 90°**	**2 × 60°**	**2 × 90°**
20	0.60	1.20	1.80	2.40	3.60	4.80	50	1.05	2.10	3.15	4.20	6.30	8.40
21	0.62	1.23	1.85	2.46	3.69	4.92	51	1.07	2.13	3.20	4.26	6.39	8.52
22	0.63	1.26	1.89	2.52	3.78	5.04	52	1.08	2.16	3.24	4.32	6.48	8.64
23	0.65	1.29	1.94	2.58	3.87	5.16	53	1.10	2.19	3.29	4.38	6.57	8.76
24	0.66	1.32	1.98	2.64	3.96	5.28	54	1.11	2.22	3.33	4.44	6.66	8.88
25	0.68	1.35	2.03	2.70	4.05	5.40	55	1.13	2.25	3.38	4.50	6.75	9.00
26	0.69	1.38	2.07	2.76	4.14	5.52	56	1.14	2.28	3.42	4.56	6.84	9.12
27	0.71	1.41	2.12	2.82	4.23	5.64	57	1.16	2.31	3.47	4.62	6.93	9.24
28	0.72	1.44	2.16	2.88	4.32	5.76	58	1.17	2.34	3.51	4.68	7.02	9.36
29	0.74	1.47	2.21	2.94	4.41	5.88	59	1.19	2.37	3.56	4.74	7.11	9.48
30	0.75	1.50	2.25	3.00	4.50	6.00	60	1.20	2.40	3.60	4.80	7.20	9.60
31	0.77	1.53	2.30	3.06	4.59	6.12	61	1.22	2.43	3.65	4.86	7.29	9.72
32	0.78	1.56	2.34	3.12	4.68	6.24	62	1.23	2.46	3.69	4.92	7.38	9.84
33	0.80	1.59	2.39	3.18	4.77	6.36	63	1.25	2.49	3.74	4.98	7.47	9.96
34	0.81	1.62	2.43	3.24	4.86	6.48	64	1.26	2.52	3.78	5.04	7.56	10.08
35	0.83	1.65	2.48	3.30	4.95	6.60	65	1.28	2.55	3.83	5.10	7.65	10.20
36	0.84	1.68	2.52	3.36	5.04	6.72	66	1.29	2.58	3.87	5.16	7.74	10.32
37	0.86	1.71	2.57	3.42	5.13	6.84	67	1.31	2.61	3.92	5.22	7.83	10.44
38	0.87	1.74	2.61	3.48	5.22	6.96	68	1.32	2.64	3.96	5.28	7.92	10.56
39	0.89	1.77	2.66	3.54	5.31	7.08	69	1.34	2.67	4.01	5.34	8.01	10.68
40	0.90	1.80	2.70	3.60	5.40	7.20	70	1.35	2.70	4.05	5.40	8.10	10.80
41	0.92	1.83	2.75	3.66	5.49	7.32	71	1.37	2.73	4.10	5.46	8.19	10.92
42	0.93	1.86	2.79	3.72	5.58	7.44	72	1.38	2.76	4.14	5.52	8.28	11.04
43	0.95	1.89	2.84	3.78	5.67	7.56	73	1.40	2.79	4.19	5.58	8.37	11.16
44	0.96	1.92	2.88	3.84	5.76	7.68	74	1.41	2.82	4.23	5.64	8.46	11.28
45	0.98	1.95	2.93	3.90	5.85	7.80	75	1.43	2.85	4.28	5.70	8.55	11.40
46	0.99	1.98	2.97	3.96	5.94	7.92							
47	1.01	2.01	3.02	4.02	6.03	8.04							
48	1.02	2.04	3.06	4.08	6.12	8.16							
49	1.04	2.07	3.11	4.14	6.21	8.28							

*Find patient age, then move right to find result closest to refractive cylinder without going over.
From Richard L. Lindstrom, MD, Phillips Eye Institute, Minneapolis, Minn, and Chiron IntraOptics, Irvine, Calif.

A vertical-blade (push) diamond micrometer knife allows the surgeon good visibility while pushing through the length of the keratotomy. The knife is calibrated with the Mastel Retiscope (Mastel, Rapid City, SD) or a similar device. Extreme care should be taken in knife selection, calibration, and maintenance to ensure reproducible cuts. Balanced salt solution and an irrigation cannula are used to keep the cornea moist and to irrigate incisions.

Topical anesthesia is particularly helpful in these patients, as it permits them to fixate the filament of the surgical microscope. This permits centration, as demonstrated in Figure 22-10. For cataract patients who have been anesthetized with peribulbar or retrobulbar injection, the surgeon can accurately estimate the center of the pupil with the patient's eye adjusted to be perpendicular to the microscope. As with the method shown in Figure 22-10, the pupillary center is marked with a Sinskey hook or similar device.

The keratotomy optical zone is marked with a 7-mm marker (Figure 22-11). The steep meridian is marked with a skin-marking pen using intraoperative keratometry or preoperative landmarks and an axis marker (Figure 22-12). To mark the length of a 3-mm transverse keratotomy, a 3-mm circular zone

TABLE 22-6
Arcuate Keratotomy Nomogram for Males with 7-mm Optical Zone*

	Surgical Option						
Age (year)	1 × 45°	2 × 30°	1 × 60°	1 × 90°	2 × 45°	2 × 60°	2 × 90°
20	0.32	1.62	0.92	2.02	2.22	2.72	3.82
21	0.36	1.66	0.96	2.06	2.26	2.76	3.86
22	0.39	1.69	0.99	2.09	2.29	2.79	3.89
23	0.40	1.73	1.03	2.13	2.33	2.83	3.93
24	0.46	1.76	1.06	2.16	2.36	2.86	3.96
25	0.50	1.80	1.10	2.20	2.40	2.90	4.00
26	0.54	1.84	1.14	2.24	2.44	2.94	4.04
27	0.57	1.87	1.17	2.27	2.47	2.97	4.07
28	0.61	1.91	1.21	2.31	2.51	3.01	4.11
29	0.64	1.94	1.24	2.34	2.54	3.04	4.14
30	0.68	1.98	1.28	2.38	2.58	3.08	4.18
31	0.72	2.02	1.32	2.42	2.62	3.12	4.22
32	0.75	2.05	1.35	2.45	2.65	3.15	4.25
33	0.79	2.09	1.39	2.49	2.69	3.19	4.29
34	0.82	2.12	1.42	2.52	2.72	3.22	4.32
35	0.86	2.16	1.46	2.56	2.76	3.26	4.36
36	0.90	2.20	1.50	2.60	2.80	3.30	4.40
37	0.93	2.23	1.53	2.63	2.83	3.33	4.43
38	0.97	2.27	1.57	2.67	2.87	3.37	4.47
39	1.00	2.30	1.60	2.70	2.90	3.40	4.50
40	1.04	2.34	1.64	2.74	2.94	3.44	4.54
41	1.08	2.38	1.68	2.78	2.98	3.48	4.58
42	1.11	2.41	1.71	2.81	3.01	3.51	4.61
43	1.15	2.45	1.75	2.85	3.05	3.55	4.65
44	1.18	2.48	1.78	2.88	3.08	3.58	4.68
45	1.22	2.52	1.82	2.92	3.12	3.62	4.72
46	1.26	2.56	1.86	2.96	3.16	3.66	4.76
47	1.29	2.59	1.89	2.99	3.19	3.69	4.79
48	1.33	2.63	1.93	3.03	3.23	3.73	4.83
49	1.36	2.66	1.96	3.06	3.26	3.76	4.86
50	1.40	2.70	2.00	3.10	3.30	3.80	4.90
51	1.44	2.74	2.04	3.14	3.34	3.84	4.94
52	1.47	2.77	2.07	3.17	3.37	3.87	4.97
53	1.51	2.81	2.11	3.21	3.41	3.91	5.01
54	1.54	2.84	2.14	3.24	3.44	3.94	5.04
55	1.58	2.88	2.18	3.28	3.48	3.98	5.08
56	1.62	2.92	2.22	3.32	3.52	4.02	5.12
57	1.65	2.95	2.25	3.35	3.55	4.05	5.15
58	1.69	2.99	2.29	3.39	3.59	4.09	5.19
59	1.72	3.02	2.32	3.42	3.62	4.12	5.22
60	1.76	3.06	2.36	3.46	3.66	4.16	5.26
61	1.80	3.10	2.40	3.50	3.70	4.20	5.30
62	1.83	3.13	2.43	3.53	3.73	4.23	5.33
63	1.87	3.17	2.47	3.57	3.77	4.27	5.37
64	1.90	3.20	2.50	3.60	3.80	4.30	5.40
65	1.94	3.24	2.54	3.64	3.84	4.34	5.44
66	1.98	3.28	2.58	3.68	3.88	4.38	5.48
67	2.01	3.31	2.61	3.71	3.91	4.41	5.51
68	2.05	3.35	2.65	3.75	3.95	4.45	5.55
69	2.08	3.38	2.68	3.78	3.98	4.48	5.58
70	2.12	3.42	2.72	3.82	4.02	4.52	5.62
71	2.16	3.46	2.76	3.86	4.06	4.56	5.66
72	2.19	3.49	2.79	3.89	4.09	4.59	5.69
73	2.23	3.53	2.83	3.93	4.13	4.63	5.73
74	2.26	3.56	2.86	3.96	4.16	4.66	5.76
75	2.30	3.60	2.90	4.00	4.20	4.70	5.80

*Subtract 0.37 from each predicted value for females.

marker is placed over the 7-mm zone mark (and also over the 5-mm zone mark if four cuts are planned) in the steep meridian (Figure 22-13). If arcuate keratotomy is preferred, the Lindstrom arcuate marker guides the performance of 45-, 60-, and 90-degree arcuate cuts (Figures 22-14 and 22-15). The use of a 16-, 12-, or 8-ray RK marker, respectively, can provide similar guidance (Figure 22-16). Arcuate incisions of more than 90 degrees are not recommended.

Intraoperative pachymetry is used at the appropriate optical zone in the steep meridian on one (for a single incision) or both sides of the cornea (Figure 22-17). The blade depth of the calibrated diamond knife is set at 100% of the thinnest paracentral pachymetry. If pachymetry is not available, setting the knife at 0.6 mm for a 7-mm optical zone incision appears to be safe and effective.

With the corneal fixation forceps held in the nondominant hand and used to grasp tissue at the limbus, the knife in the dominant hand is set into the cornea, pausing for 1 second. The knife is then guided slowly through the incision (Figure 22-18).

The completed incision is irrigated with balanced salt solution (Figure 22-19), and several drops of gentamicin or tobramycin are placed on the eye. Patching or cycloplegia is not routinely

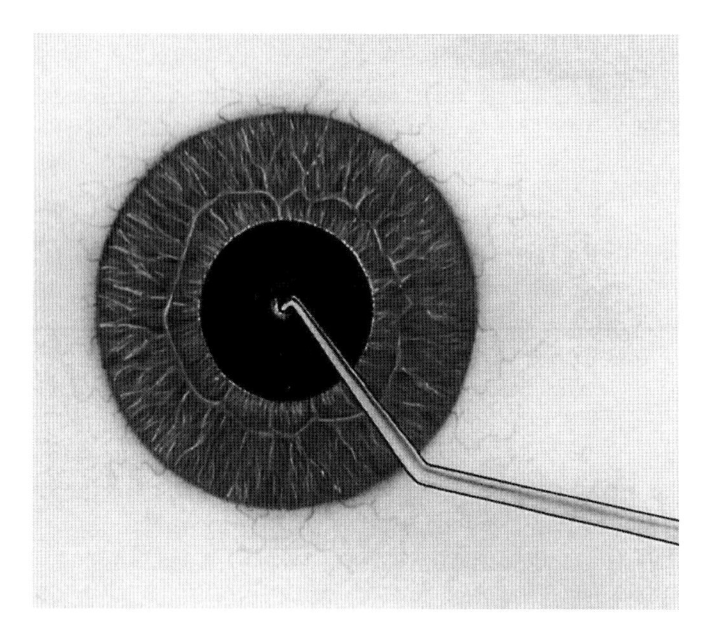

FIGURE 22-10 The center of the optical zone is determined by asking the patient to fixate on the microscope light, on a mark placed directly between the two oculars, or on the Mastel Aximeter (Mastel, Rapid City, SD). While the patient is properly fixating, the center of the entrance pupil is marked with a Sinskey hook. (From Koch DD, Lindstrom RL: Controlling astigmatism in cataract surgery, *Semin Ophthalmol* 7:224-233, 1992.)

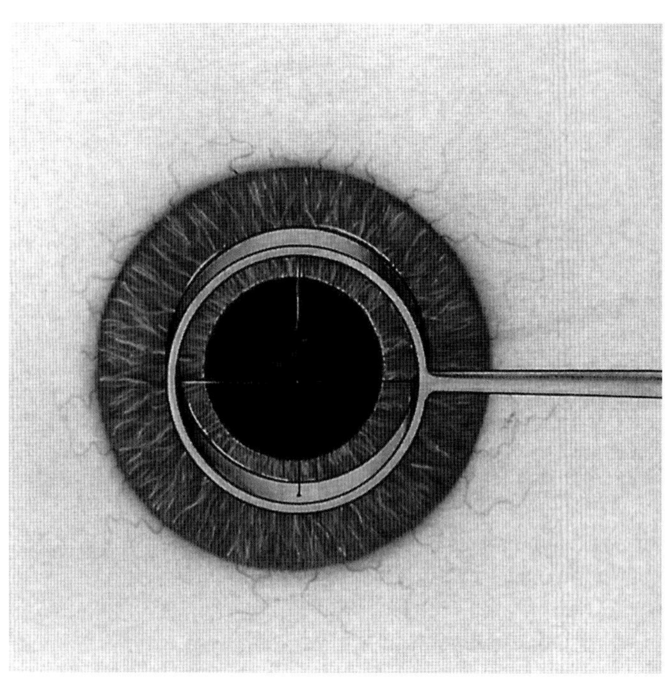

FIGURE 22-11 Marking the optical zone with a 7-mm zone marker. (From Koch DD, Lindstrom RL: Controlling astigmatism in cataract surgery, *Semin Ophthalmol* 7:224-233, 1992.)

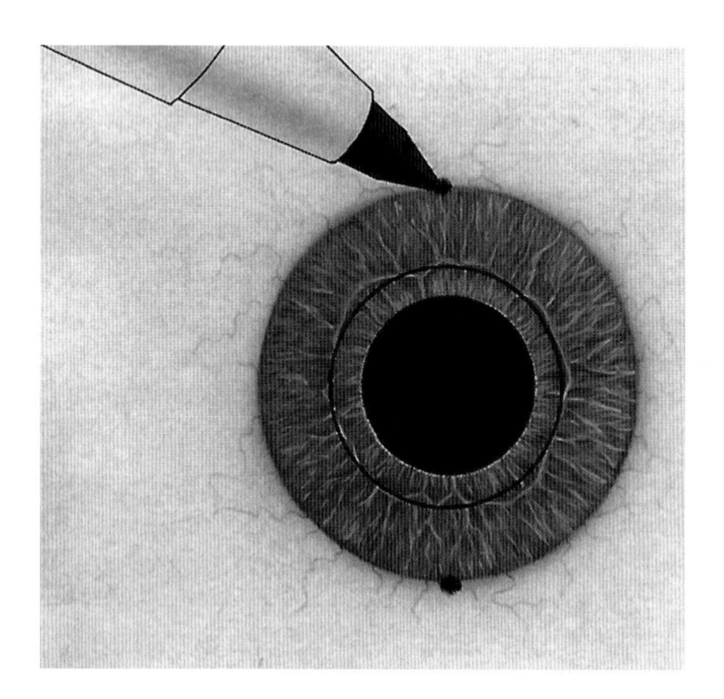

FIGURE 22-12 Marking the steep meridian. (From Koch DD, Lindstrom RL: Controlling astigmatism in cataract surgery, *Semin Ophthalmol* 7:224-233, 1992.)

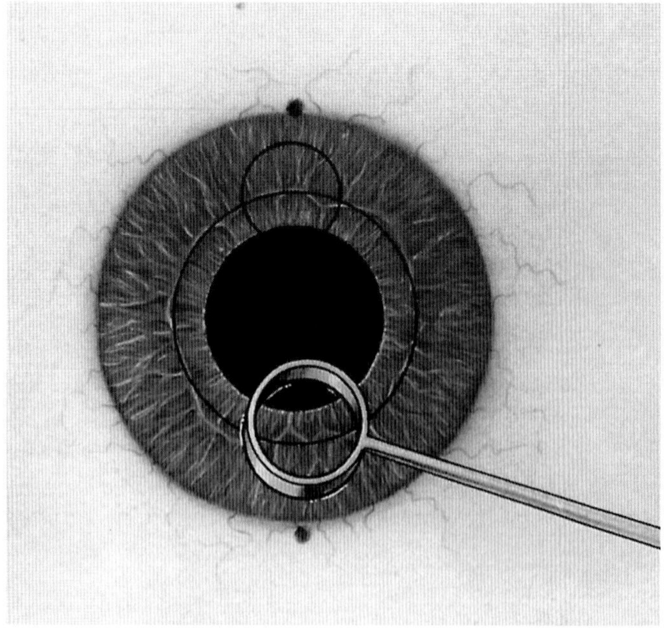

FIGURE 22-13 Use of a 3-mm zone marker to delineate the incision length. (From Koch DD, Lindstrom RL: Controlling astigmatism in cataract surgery, *Semin Ophthalmol* 7:224-233, 1992.)

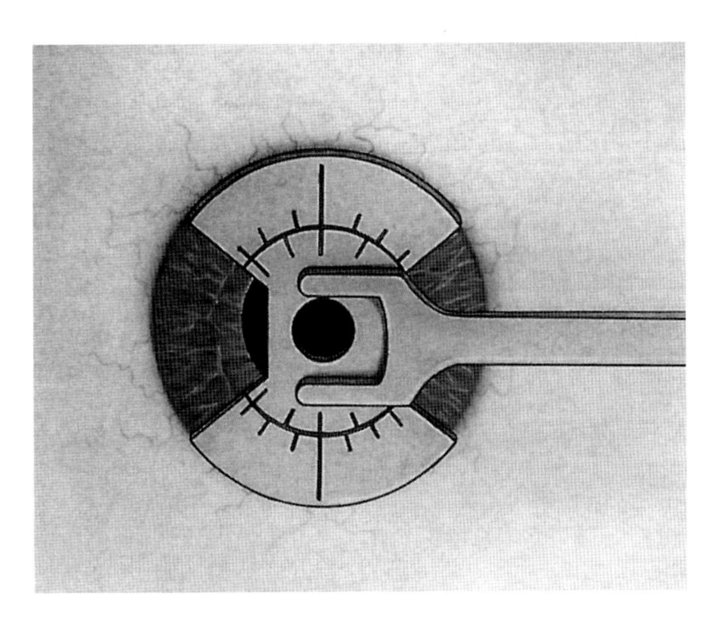

FIGURE 22-14 The Lindstrom arcuate marker (Katena Products) is placed on the cornea aligned with the steep meridian. (From Koch DD, Lindstrom RL: Controlling astigmatism in cataract surgery, *Semin Ophthalmol* 7:224-233, 1992.)

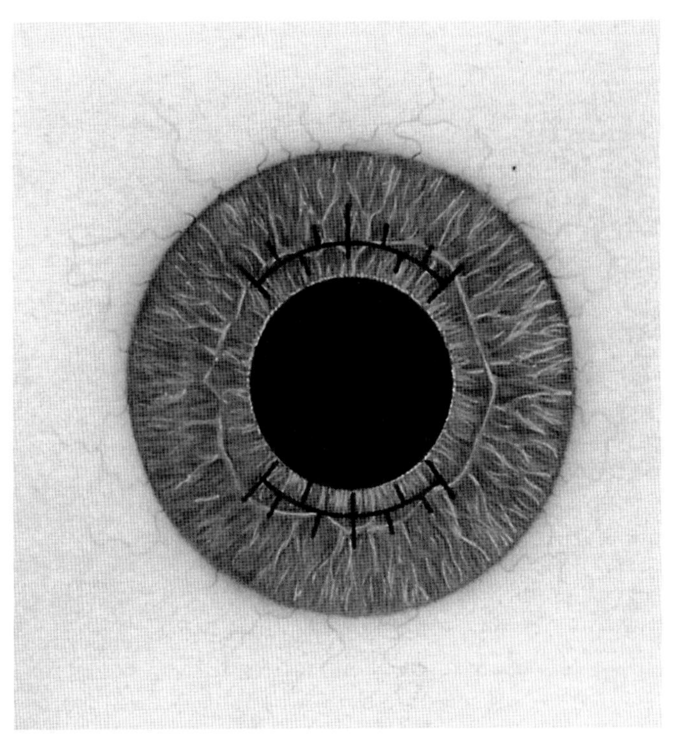

FIGURE 22-15 Cornea marked before astigmatic keratotomy. Perpendicular lines mark 45, 60, and 90 degrees for arcuate cuts. (From Koch DD, Lindstrom RL: Controlling astigmatism in cataract surgery, *Semin Ophthalmol* 7:224-233, 1992.)

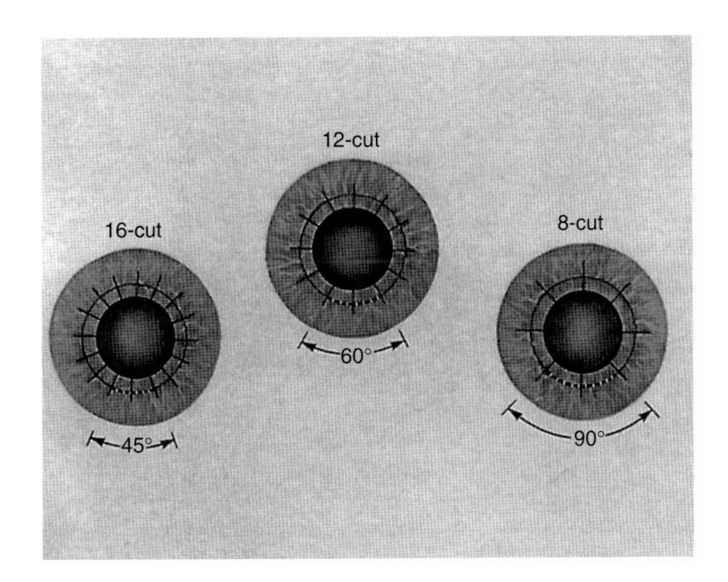

FIGURE 22-16 *Left,* 16-ray RK marker is useful to delineate 45-degree arcuate keratotomy. *Center,* 12-ray RK marker is useful to delineate 60-degree arcuate keratotomy. *Right,* 8-ray RK marker is useful to delineate 90-degree arcuate keratotomy. (From Koch DD, Lindstrom RL: Controlling astigmatism in cataract surgery, *Semin Ophthalmol* 7:224-233, 1992.)

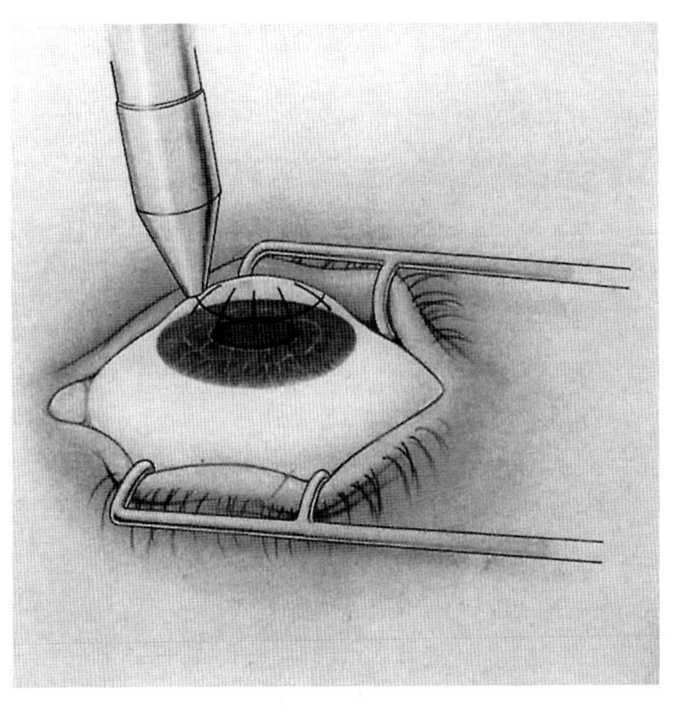

FIGURE 22-17 Corneal pachymetry is measured directly over the incision site; the blade is set at 90% to 100% of the thinnest pachymetry reading. (From Koch DD, Lindstrom RL: Controlling astigmatism in cataract surgery, *Semin Ophthalmol* 7:224-233, 1992.)

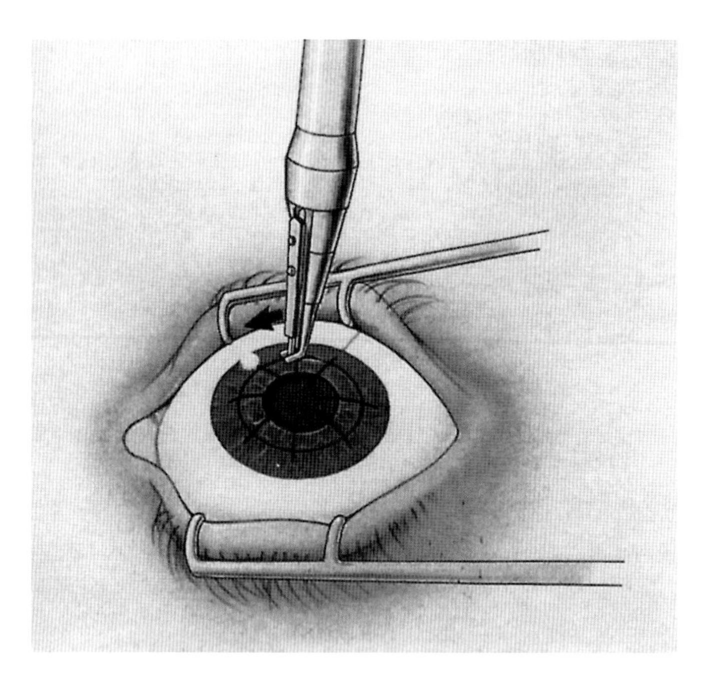

FIGURE 22-18 Marking the incision. (From Koch DD, Lindstrom RL: Controlling astigmatism in cataract surgery, *Semin Ophthalmol* 7:224-233, 1992.)

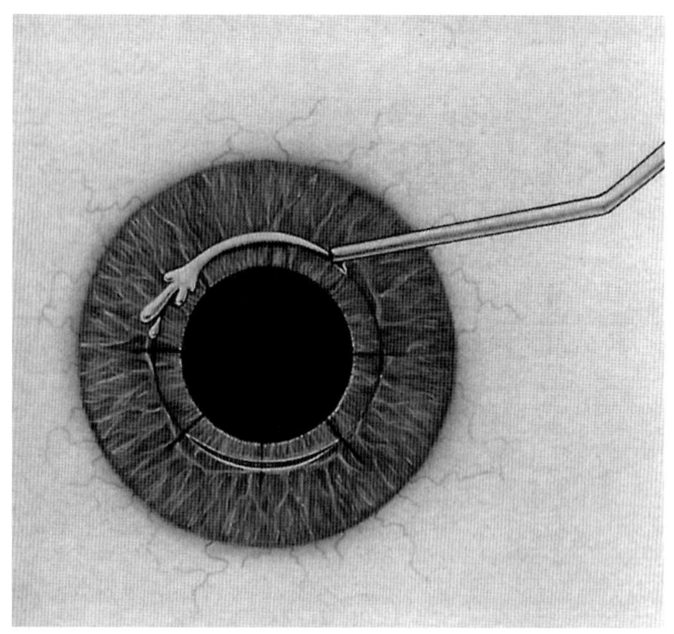

FIGURE 22-19 Irrigation with balanced salt solution. (From Koch DD, Lindstrom RL: Controlling astigmatism in cataract surgery, *Semin Ophthalmol* 7:224-233, 1992.)

used. If a significant perforation occurs, subconjunctival antibiotic, topical cycloplegia, and a pressure patch are used; obviously, if chamber depth cannot be maintained, then the incision with the perforation is sutured. Perforations are extremely rare with the technique described.

Osher's Technique

Since beginning astigmatic keratometry combined with cataract surgery for the reduction of preexisting astigmatism in 1983, Osher's technique has gone through several revisions. The initial examination had always included careful keratometry, and each new generation of corneal topography has been added. The amount of phakic or pseudophakic astigmatism in the fellow eye must be considered in determining candidacy. Patients with significant anterior membrane dystrophy or severe Fuchs' endothelial dystrophy are excluded. An explanation of the surgical plan to reduce the astigmatism is given, and the patient is informed that this procedure is elective and inexact and may result in more ocular irritation than normal for several days following surgery (although this is usually not the case). Permission to perform the astigmatic keratometry is part of the routine informed consent form for cataract surgery.

Following the initial evaluation, an operative plan is formulated. The optical zone is selected, primarily based on the Osher nomogram (Table 22-7) while keeping the length, depth, and shape of the incisions constant.[40] Principles gained through experience, such as the greater response in eyes having against-the-rule cylinder, a large corneal diameter, increasing patient age, and the perceived effect of intraocular pressure, are taken into consideration. The nomogram will need to be adjusted according to each surgeon's particular technique. Because AK does not change *average* preoperative keratometric power, no change is needed in IOL power. After arriving at the optimal approach for the patient, a drawing is made on the chart, which is hung from the microscope next to the topography for easy reference. The drawing shows the size of the optical zone and the location of the incisions to ensure proper orientation.

In the early years of performing this procedure, the major meridians of the eye were marked in the holding room before surgery with a drop of topical anesthetic and a cautery while the eye was in the primary position of gaze for distance fixation. This method has been replaced by quantitative intraoperative keratoscopy. A Hyde-Osher ruler made by Ocular Instruments has a series of spherical and astigmatic circles cut out of a metallic bar. This is held between the eye and the microscope and easily identifies the steep meridian of curvature, which is marked at the limbus with two spots 180 degrees from each other using the coaptation cautery. With the eye coaxial with the microscope, the amount of cylinder is quantitated by

TABLE 22-7

Osher Nomogram for 3-mm T-cuts

Cylinder (D)	Optical Zone (mm)
1.5	8.5
2.0	8.0
2.5	7.0-7.5
3.0	6.0-6.5
3.5	2 pair: 6.0 and 8.5

From Osher RH: Transverse astigmatic keratotomy combined with cataract surgery, *Ophthalmol Clin North Am* 5:717-725, 1992.

neutralizing the progressive astigmatic openings in the bar until a circular reflex is observed. The measurements of the axis and amount of cylinder are usually consistent with the preoperative data. If the axis is off by several degrees, the intraoperative observations are favored. If a disparity greater than 10 or 15 degrees exists, AK is not performed—a decision that is rarely necessary.

Although initially blade depth was determined by intraoperative pachymetry, for many years Osher has simply set the blade at 690 μm for an optical zone of 6 mm or greater. Formerly, AK was performed at the conclusion of the procedure to maximize visualization during the cataract surgery, but currently the incisions are made at the beginning of the procedure. The advantages include a firmer globe with a better epithelium, yielding more accurate intraoperative keratoscopy and incision depth. In addition, the healthier epithelium results in many fewer corneal abrasions, so the eye does not require patching.

The incision length is 3 mm. The globe is stabilized with a multiple dull-toothed forceps held in the fellow hand. Increasing experience has resulted in consistent incision depth between 80% and 95%, which is important in achieving effective results. A second pair of incisions is reserved for cylinder greater than 3.5 D. After the incisions are made, a 30-gauge cannula is used to confirm that the depth is adequate; it is then used to gently irrigate a stream of balanced salt solution into the incision to remove any trapped air bubbles or cellular debris. Complications include corneal abrasion in about 5% and microperforation in less than 1%. If a superficial abrasion occurs, a double pressure patch is applied at the conclusion of the procedure.

Astigmatic keratometry is performed in approximately those 20% of patients with preexisting cylinder of 1.5 D or greater. In a study of this conservative approach to AK using the same nomogram in which only the optical zone was varied, all eyes except one with amblyopia enjoyed a best-corrected visual acuity comparable to that of a controlled population not receiving AK.[29] However, the uncorrected vision was outstanding with acuity of 20/40 or better achieved in 76%. Certainly only a fraction of these patients would have achieved this visual result had their cylinder not been reduced by AK. Comparison of preoperative and postoperative keratometry measurement showed that the IOL selected would have been unchanged in 87% of eyes. Although 13% showed a power change between 0.5 and 1 D, it was reassuring to find that the surgical change in the cornea influenced the IOL power less than 1 D in all cases.

Toric Intraocular Lens

The toric IOL was devised by Shimizu, Misawa, and Suzuki[41] and has been used clinically since 1992. The first toric IOL introduced was a nonfoldable three-piece posterior chamber lens; foldable toric single-piece IOLs are available currently. Advantages of astigmatism correction with toric IOLs over CRIs are reversibility and excellent optical quality with no induction of irregular astigmatism.

STAAR toric IOL models (STAAR Surgical Company, Monrovia, Calif.) have a toric anterior surface, spherical posterior surface, two positioning marks along the long axis on the anterior surface, and two 1.15-mm fenestrations at the opposite ends (Figure 22-20). The lens is available with cylindrical adds of 2 D and 3.5 D, which theoretically correct 1.4 D and 2.3 D of astigmatism at the corneal plane, respectively. Thus patients with 1.5 to 3.5 D of regular preexisting astigmatism are candidates for this lens implantation.

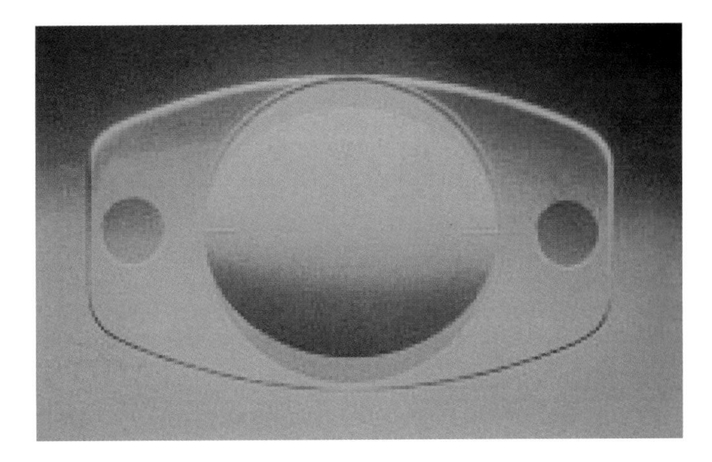

FIGURE 22-20 STAAR toric IOL.

The surgical technique of toric IOL implantation involves careful preoperative marking of the correct meridian for IOL alignment and intraoperative rotation of the toric IOL to orient the IOL axis markings along the steep corneal meridian.

Postoperative rotation of the toric IOL is a significant problem. Leyland et al.[42] reported that 18% (4 of 22) IOLs rotated more than 30 degrees. Sun et al.[43] reported that 18% rotated between 20 and 40 degrees, and 7% rotated more than 40 degrees. In the study by Till et al.,[44] 6% of IOLs rotated more than 31 degrees. This presumably results in a greater than 10% incidence of surgical reintervention to reposition the implants. Modifications in toric IOL designs are needed to address this problem. An additional drawback in the use of toric IOLs is that the only cylindrical adds currently available are 2 D and 3.5 D.

New toric IOL designs are under clinical investigation, including a one-piece acrylic model (Alcon Surgical, Inc.) that may have excellent rotational stability, thereby reducing the incidence of IOL rotation postoperatively. A new concept from Calhoun Vision is a silicone IOL that can be laser irradiated postoperatively to modify both the spherical and astigmatic outcome. A lens of this type could potentially offer exquisite refractive accuracy.

Conclusions

Refractive cataract surgery requires meticulous planning and surgical technique to optimize the spherical and astigmatic refractive outcomes. Patient expectations are increasing; for many, excellent uncorrected visual acuity is a primary goal of surgery.[45] The development of multifocal and accommodating IOLs heightens the clinical mandate for precision in reaching targeted refractive goals. The practitioner who has mastered the current tools and philosophies in dealing with astigmatism in cataract surgery may be in the best position to incorporate new technologies as they emerge.

Although no single best approach to astigmatism correction in cataract surgery has yet been established, it is likely that evolving toric and adjustable IOL designs will ultimately provide the most consistent refractive results and superior optics. However, by incorporating the general principles outlined in this chapter, surgeons will be able to transition into the new subspecialty of refractive cataract surgery and greatly enhance their surgical outcomes using current technology. By paying meticulous attention to results, each surgeon will inevitably create his or her own nomograms, tailored not only to the technical aspects of a preferred surgical approach but also to the visual demands of the individual patient.

REFERENCES

1. Schiotz HA: Ein Fall von hochgradigem hornhautastigmatismus nach starrextraction. Besserung auf operativem wege, *Arch Augenheilkunde* 15:178-181, 1885.
2. Faber E: Operative behandelingf van astigmatisme, *Ned Tijdschr Geneeskd* 2:495-496, 1895.
3. Lans LJ: Experimentelle untersuchugen uber entstehung von astigmatismus durch nich-perforirende corneawunden, *Albrect Con Graef's Arch Ophthalmol* 45:117-152, 1898.
4. Bates WH: A suggestion of an operation to correct astigmatism, *Arch Ophthalmol* 23:9-13, 1894.
5. Frranks JB, Binder PS: Keratotomy procedures for the correction of astigmatism, *J Refract Surg* 1:11-17, 1985.
6. Duke-Elder SS, Abrams D: Ophthalmic optics and refraction. In *System of ophthalmology,* vol 5, St Louis, 1970, Mosby, pp 274-295.
7. Buzard K, Shearing S, Relyea R: Incidence of astigmatism in a cataract practice, *J Refract Surg* 4:173, 1988.
8. Axt JC: Longitudinal study of postoperative astigmatism, *J Cataract Refract Surg* 13:381-388, 1987.
9. Jampel HD, Thompson JR, Baker CC et al: A computerized analysis of astigmatism after cataract surgery, *Ophthalmic Surg* 17:786-790, 1986.
10. Koch DD, Lindstrom RL: Controlling astigmatism in cataract surgery, *Semin Ophthalmol* 7:224-233, 1992.
11. Stevens JD: Astigmatic excimer laser treatment: theoretical effects of axis misalignment, *Eur J Implant Ref Surg* 6:310-318, 1994.
12. Swami AU, Steinert RF, Osborne WE et al: Rotational malposition during laser in situ keratomileusis, *Am J Ophthalmol* 133:561-562, 2002.
13. Samuelson SW, Koch DD, Kuglen CC: Determination of maximal incision length for true small-incision surgery, *Ophthalmic Surg* 22:204-207, 1991.
14. Pfleger T, Scholz U, Skorpik C: Postoperative astigmatism after no-stitch, small incision cataract surgery with 3.5 mm and 4.5 mm incisions, *J Cataract Refract Surg* 20:400-505, 1994.
15. Lyhne N, Corydon L: Two year follow-up of astigmatism after phacoemulsification with adjusted and unadjusted sutured versus sutureless 5.2 mm superior scleral incisions, *J Cataract Refract Surg* 24:1647-1651, 1998.
16. Huang FC, Tseng SH: Comparison of surgically induced astigmatism after sutureless temporal clear corneal and scleral frown incisions, *J Cataract Refract Surg* 24:477-481, 1998.
17. Dam-Johansen M, Olsen T: Induced astigmatism after 4 and 6 mm scleral tunnel incision: a randomized study, *Acta Ophthalmol Scand* 75:669-674, 1997.
18. Mendivil A: Frequency of induced astigmatism following phacoemulsification with suturing versus without suturing, *Ophthalmic Surg Lasers* 28:377-381, 1997.
19. Olsen T, Dam-Johansen M, Bek T et al: Corneal versus scleral tunnel incision in cataract surgery: a randomized study, *J Cataract Refract Surg* 23:337-341, 1997.
20. Haubrich T, Knorz MC, Seiberth V et al: Vector analysis of surgically-induced astigmatism in cataract operation with 4 tunnel incision techniques, *Ophthalmologe* 93:12-16, 1996.
21. Gross RH, Miller KM: Corneal astigmatism after phacoemulsification and lens implantation through unsutured scleral and corneal tunnel incisions, *Am J Ophthalmol* 121:57-64, 1996.
22. Beltrame G, Salvetat ML, Chizzolini M et al: Corneal topographic changes induced by different oblique cataract incisions, *J Cataract Refract Surg* 27:720-727, 2001.
23. Lyhne N, Krogsager J, Corydon L et al: One year follow-up of astigmatism after 4.0 mm temporal clear corneal and superior scleral incisions, *J Cataract Refract Surg* 26:83-87, 2000.
24. Pfleger T, Skorpik C, Menapace R et al: Long-term course of induced astigmatism after clear corneal incision cataract surgery, *J Cataract Refract Surg* 22:72-77, 1996.
25. Kohnen T, Dick B, Jacobi KW: Comparison of the induced astigmatism after temporal clear corneal tunnel incisions of different sizes, *J Cataract Refract Surg* 21:417-424, 1995.
26. Nielsen PJ. Prospective evaluation of surgically induced astigmatism and astigmatic keratotomy effects of various self-sealing small incisions, *J Cataract Refract Surg* 21:43-48, 1995.
27. Vass C, Menapace R, Rainer G, Findl O et al: Comparative study of corneal topographic changes after 3.0 mm beveled and hinged clear corneal incisions, *J Cataract Refract Surg* 24:1498-1504, 1998.
28. Koch DD, Del Pero RA, Wong TC et al: Scleral flap surgery for modification of corneal astigmatism, *Am J Ophthalmol* 104:259-264, 1987.
29. Osher RH: Paired transverse relaxing keratotomy: a combined technique for reducing astigmatism, *J Cataract Refract Surg* 15:32-37, 1989.
30. Shepherd JR: Induced astigmatism in small incision surgery, *J Cataract Refract Surg* 15:85-88, 1989.
31. Davison JA: Transverse astigmatic keratotomy combined with phacoemulsification and intraocular lens implantation, *J Cataract Refract Surg* 15:38-44, 1989.
32. Hall GW, Campion M, Sorenson CM et al: Reduction of corneal astigmatism at cataract surgery, *J Cataract Refract Surg* 17:407-414, 1991.
33. Gills, JP: Relaxing incisions reduce postop astigmatism, *Ophthalmology Times* November 15, 1991, p 11.
34. Merlin U: Corneal keratotomy procedure for congenital astigmatism, *J Refract Surg* 3:92-97, 1987.
35. Thornton SP: Theory behind corneal relaxing incision/Thornton nomogram. In Gills JP, Martin RG, Sanders DR, editors: *Sutureless cataract surgery,* Thorofare, NJ, 1992, Slack, pp 123-144.
36. Lindstrom RL: The surgical correction of astigmatism: a clinician's perspective, *J Cataract Corneal Surg* 6:441-454, 1990.
37. Budak K, Friedman NJ, Koch DD: Limbal relaxing incisions with cataract surgery, *J Cataract Refractive Surg* 24:503-508, 1998.
38. Müller-Jensen K, Fischer P, Siepe U: Limbal relaxing incisions to correct astigmatism in clear corneal cataract surgery, *J Refract Surg* 15:586-589, 1999.
39. Wang L, Misra M, Koch DD: Peripheral corneal relaxing incisions combined with cataract surgery, *J Cataract Refractive Surg* (in press).
40. Osher RH: Transverse astigmatic keratotomy combined with cataract surgery. In Stamper R, editor: *Ophthalmology clinics of North America: contemporary refractive surgery,* Philadelphia, Pa, 1992, WB Saunders, 5:717-725.
41. Shimizu K, Misawa A, Suzuki Y: Toric intraocular lenses: correcting astigmatism while controlling axis shift, *J Cataract Refractive Surg* 20:523-526, 1994.
42. Leyland M, Zinicola E, Bloom P et al: Prospective evaluation of a plate haptic toric intraocular lens, *Eye* 15:202-205, 2001.
43. Sun XY, Vicary D, Montgomery P et al: Toric intraocular lenses for correcting astigmatism in 130 eyes, *Ophthalmology* 107:1776-1781, 2000.
44. Till JS, Yoder PR Jr, Wilcox TK et al: Toric intraocular lens implantation: 100 consecutive cases, *J Cataract Refract Surg* 28:295-301, 2002.
45. Osher, RH: Evolution of refractive cataract surgery. In Wallace RB, editor: *Refractive cataract surgery and multifocal IOLs,* Thorofare, NJ, 2001, Slack, Inc.

Cataract Surgery in Uveitis Patients

23

Michael B. Raizman, MD

Most of the medical literature on cataract extraction in patients with uveitis dates from the 1960s, 1970s, and 1980s.[1] Predictably, the tone of these articles is pessimistic and cautionary. Since the late 1980s, there has been a shift in belief and a new consensus has arisen, one that recognizes the utility and safety of cataract extraction and intraocular lens (IOL) implantation in the majority of patients with uveitis.[1-6] This change is largely a result of improvements in surgical techniques and, to some extent, a greater recognition of the need to aggressively control inflammation in the eyes of these patients before and after surgery.

Only a small portion of the cataract extractions performed in an average practice will be in eyes with uveitis. However, nearly every ophthalmologist faces such cases periodically. Cataracts may be induced by the inflammation or the corticosteroid therapy prescribed to control the inflammation. Of course, patients with uveitis may also experience age-related (not uveitis-related) cataracts that require removal. In certain conditions—especially intermediate uveitis (pars planitis), Fuchs' heterochromic iridocyclitis, and juvenile rheumatoid arthritis with uveitis—the majority of eyes will acquire cataract.[7-9] Cataract extraction in such situations can be challenging. The careful strategies outlined in this chapter will allow consistently successful management of cataracts in uveitis patients.

Patient Selection

Given the greater inherent risks of operating on an eye with uveitis, cataract surgery is generally deferred longer in these cases than in a case of uncomplicated cataract. In many cases, the posterior pole cannot be seen to assist in determining visual potential. Current techniques for assessing visual potential, such as a potential acuity meter, laser interferometry, or entoptic phenomena can be helpful but are limited.[10] Fluorescein angiography and ultrasonography can occasionally provide useful information. Before surgery, patients must realize that visual potential may be restricted by the preexisting complications of uveitis, such as cystoid macular edema (CME), epiretinal membranes, or glaucomatous optic neuropathy.

The cause of the inflammation should be ascertained whenever possible. This can help in determining a prognosis and whether to implant an IOL. In some conditions, clinical findings will permit a diagnosis (e.g., heterochromia in Fuchs' iridocyclitis or pars planitis "snowbanks" in intermediate uveitis). Other cases will require laboratory evaluations. Depending on the clinical setting, useful laboratory studies may include a complete blood count, a fluorescent treponemal antibody absorption test, a chest x-ray study, screening for angiotensin-converting enzyme and HLA-B27, and a urinalysis.

Cataract surgery may be performed successfully regardless of the cause of the uveitis. However, some conditions pose a relative contraindication to lens implantation.[1-4] In general, patients with juvenile rheumatoid arthritis, Vogt-Koyanagi-Harada or Harada syndrome, sympathetic ophthalmia, or recurrent granulomatous uveitis of any cause with extensive synechia formation are poor candidates for lens implantation (Figure 23-1).[11,12] Some controversy exists regarding the placement of an IOL in patients with juvenile rheumatoid arthritis, but the preponderance of the literature suggests that IOLs should be avoided in most of these eyes.[13-17] IOL implantation may also present a problem in patients with any form of uveitis that is difficult to control (Figure 23-2). Certain uveitis patients do especially well after cataract extraction with lens implantation. In particular, patients with Fuchs' heterochromic iridocyclitis almost always have a good outcome,[8,18] as do patients whose uveitis has been quiet for more than 1 year without the use of medication. In one study, after posterior chamber IOL implantation in eyes with uveitis, uveitis recurred in 41%, CME in 33%, and posterior synechiae in 8%.[19] In every case, good clinical judgment is needed to determine whether lens implantation is appropriate.

Some patients with uveitis and glaucoma may do well with combined cataract extraction, lens implantation, and filtering surgery. Glaucoma should be controlled as well as possible before surgery. The use of antimetabolites is common in eyes with uveitis and may reduce the chance of filter failure.[20] Some surgeons prefer to place a seton in eyes with uveitis and glaucoma.

Preoperative Management

One of the most important determinants of successful cataract extraction in a patient with uveitis is the ability to control the inflammation before surgery. Elimination of intraocular inflammation for at least 3 months (and preferably longer) before surgery is desirable. Elimination of flare may be impossible in

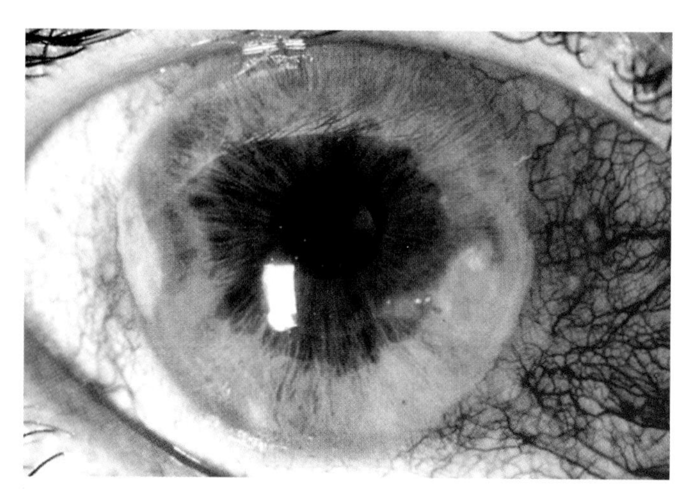

FIGURE 23-1 This cataract, in a patient with chronic iritis associated with juvenile rheumatoid arthritis, is probably best removed in combination with a vitrectomy. Eyes such as these usually do poorly with an IOL. Note the band keratopathy and posterior synechiae, characteristic ocular features of juvenile rheumatoid arthritis with uveitis.

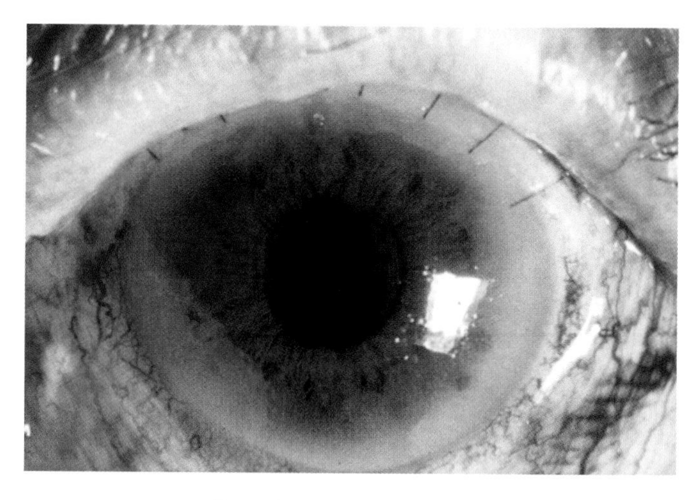

FIGURE 23-2 Excessive postoperative inflammation with fibrinous membranes across the intraocular lens are apt to occur when surgery is performed in an eye with chronic, uncontrolled inflammation, as in this case.

patients with long-standing inflammation, so the emphasis should be on the absence of cells in the anterior chamber and the absence of "active," mobile cells in the vitreous. The mainstay of preoperative antiinflammatory therapy is topical corticosteroids. Potent topical corticosteroids, such as prednisolone acetate or sodium 1% or dexamethasone 0.1%, should be used as often as needed for the months before surgery to reduce all inflammation. A typical patient might require one drop two to four times a day. For patients with severe uveitis that requires more intensive therapy, cataract surgery should be postponed.

In unusual situations, cataract surgery may be required despite active uveitis. Such cases arise, for example, when surgical intervention for vitreoretinal diseases cannot be accomplished without cataract removal. In these circumstances, intraorbital injections of corticosteroids or oral prednisone may be used. Rarely, other immunosuppressive agents such as cyclosporine, methotrexate, azathioprine, or cyclophosphamide are required to control inflammation. This therapy should be coordinated with a rheumatologist, hematologist, or other practitioner experienced in the use of these drugs.

It is helpful to treat all uveitis patients with oral prednisone for 3 to 7 days before surgery. A daily dose of 60 mg is reasonable for most individuals. The risks of this therapy must be discussed with the patient, although short-term use of prednisone is relatively safe. The use of oral nonsteroidal agents has been advocated in the preoperative period, but their efficacy has not been clearly demonstrated.

Cataract Extraction

Surgical Approach

Phacoemulsification is the preferred approach to the removal of most cataracts in eyes with uveitis. The small incision, reduction of iris trauma from prolapse into the wound, reduction of iris stretch with nucleus expression, and capsulorhexis all favor phacoemulsification. Studies confirm the reduction in inflammation with a smaller incision,[21-22] but the issue has not been well studied specifically in eyes with uveitis. Nevertheless, excellent results can be obtained with nucleus expression, and surgeons may use either approach.

There are advocates for removal of the cataract through a limbal approach and advocates of a pars plana approach. Pars plana vitrectomy and lensectomy are preferable when posterior segment disease must be addressed surgically and complete removal of the cataract and capsule is desired.[23-27] In such cases, lens implantation is not performed. The most common setting for this surgery is in a patient with juvenile rheumatoid arthritis.[28,29] These eyes often do poorly with IOLs. In addition, leaving the posterior capsule in place may provide a scaffold for cyclitic membrane formation. For these individuals, pars plana vitrectomy and lensectomy are preferred.

When vitreous debris is present along with the cataract, limiting vision, a reasonable approach is to perform cataract extraction via the limbus and vitrectomy through the pars plana, allowing the placement of an IOL in the capsular bag.[30] Vitrectomy may be performed at the same sitting or as a second surgical procedure. It is possible that removal of the vitreous may reduce subsequent inflammation in the posterior segment.[31] This is hard to confirm, and vitrectomy probably should not be performed unless the vitreous opacity limits vision.

In the special circumstance of lens-induced uveitis following trauma or resulting from a hypermature lens, extracapsular surgery by phacoemulsification or expression is safe and effective. IOLs are well tolerated in most of these eyes. Intracapsular extraction is not longer the treatment of choice.

Clear corneal incisions may produce less inflammation than scleral tunnel incisions,[32,33] but this advantage has not been well documented in eyes with uveitis.

Management of the Pupil

Poor dilation can be a problem in eyes with uveitis. The pupil may be held in place by synechiae to the lens at the pupil or

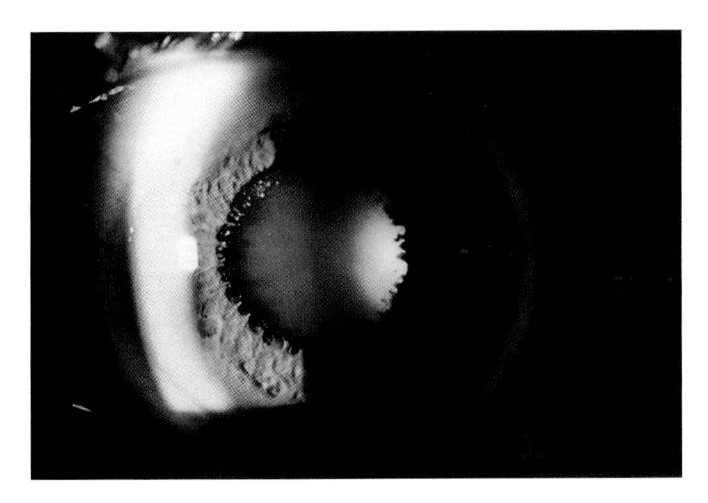

FIGURE 23-3 Posterior synechiae can usually be easily lysed with a spatula or hook, providing adequate visualization for capsulotomy and phacoemulsification.

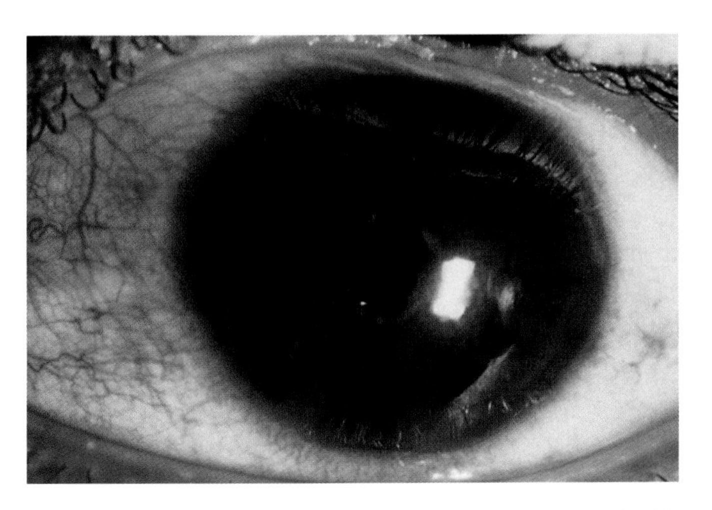

FIGURE 23-4 With some cases of chronic inflammation, as in this example of uveitis with Vogt-Koyanagi-Harada disease, a fibrous band forms at the pupil. This must be excised or transected to allow dilation of the pupil. Stretching maneuvers or the use of iris hooks do not succeed until the integrity of the fibrous ring is disrupted.

anywhere on the posterior surface of the iris (Figures 23-3 and 23-4). In addition, fibrous bands on the pupil and around the sphincter may prevent dilation. On occasion, fibrous bands at the pupil can be stripped off with a forceps or gently excised with scissors, allowing dilation. Any of the techniques mentioned in Chapter 19 can be used in these individuals. Whatever technique is used to enlarge the pupil, it is important to minimize trauma to the iris and to avoid cutting iris vessels if possible. Synechiae should be gently lysed with a spatula placed under the iris through the pupil. A collar button or similar hook can be used to push and pull the pupil to free synechiae. Stretching the pupil with two instruments placed 180 degrees apart at the pupil margin can help break circumferential fibrous bands. Injection of balanced salt solution containing epinephrine can help, as can placement of viscoelastic material in the anterior chamber and under the iris. At this point the pupil may be large enough to permit the capsule to be opened.

If the pupil is still too small, iris hooks may be inserted. They provide good visualization and are less likely to transect iris vessels than are multiple sphincterotomies or a radial iridotomy. Excessive stretch from the iris hooks can lead to postoperative inflammation and permanent distortion of the pupil. Just enough dilation for adequate exposure should be achieved.

Peripheral iridectomies are not needed in most patients with uveitis, although controversy about this exists. Creating a peripheral iridectomy increases inflammation but reduces the risk of postoperative iris bombé and angle-closure glaucoma. Most cases of iris bombé can be managed with yttrium-aluminum-garnet (YAG) laser iridectomy. Given the low rate of iris bombé after cataract surgery, even in patients with uveitis, routine iridectomies are probably not needed. Certainly, in cases of severe inflammation or narrow angles, performing an iridectomy is prudent.

Capsulorhexis and Cataract Extraction

A round capsulorhexis is preferred in patients with uveitis. Synechiae are less likely to form with a smooth capsulorhexis edge than with a ragged, torn capsular edge. In addition, a rhexis smaller than the optic diameter prevents adhesions from the iris to the posterior capsule, a problem with capsule tears that extend beyond the optic. With a rhexis of 4 to 5 mm, the pupil may be kept dilated after surgery, significantly reducing the formation of posterior synechiae. Another alternative is to create a 7-mm rhexis and avoid dilation after surgery.

Removal of the nucleus and cortex is the same as in an eye without uveitis. However, it is crucial to remove all cortical material to prevent postoperative phacogenic inflammation. The bag should be carefully inspected, with retraction of the iris to ensure complete cortical removal.

After placement of the posterior chamber IOL in the capsular bag, the pupil may be pharmacologically constricted or dilated, depending on size of the capsulorhexis and the degree of anticipated inflammation. Topical and subconjunctival corticosteroids administered at the conclusion of the case are helpful.

Intraocular Lens Implantation

There may be a theoretical advantage to lenses made wholly of polymethylmethacrylate (PMMA) over those with Prolene haptics. Prolene may induce complement activation and has been associated with a slightly higher rate of endophthalmitis, including anaerobic infections.[34-36] Prolene haptics are no longer present on most IOLs. Silicone lenses with silicone or PMMA haptics have been used in patients with uveitis. Acrylic lenses appear to be well tolerated, as well. Surface modification of lenses holds some promise for reduction of inflammation and synechiae. Several controlled studies support their effectiveness, though the clinical significance remains unclear.[37-41]

Every effort should be made to place the lens in the capsular bag. This eliminates contact of the lens with other ocular structures, especially the iris and ciliary body. Contact of the lens with these structures in an eye with preexisting uveitis can lead to uncontrollable inflammation, deposition of inflammatory debris on the implant, and, rarely, hyphema and glaucoma, even with posterior chamber placement.[42,43] Many patients do well despite placement of the lens in the ciliary sulcus, and at least one study suggests that there may be an advantage to sulcus placement.[44] Problems with anterior chamber lenses in eyes with uveitis occur frequently enough to contraindicate their use in such cases. If complications arise during surgery and it is not possible to place the implant in the capsular bag, it is probably best to leave the eye aphakic. In some cases of mild uveitis, including eyes that have been quiet without medication for more than a year, sulcus placement or suturing the lens to the sclera may be acceptable. This should be performed with caution, bearing in mind that it is possible to return at a later date for secondary lens placement in the same site if the patient does not tolerate aphakic spectacles or a contact lens.

Postoperative Management and Complications

Topical corticosteroids should be used as often as every hour if necessary to control inflammation after surgery. Prednisone should be tapered over 7 to 10 days after surgery. If hourly corticosteroid drops are inadequate to control inflammation, prednisone should be continued. Alternatively, intraorbital injections of 1 ml triamcinolone (Kenalog) 40 mg/ml may be performed weekly or as needed. Systemic immunosuppression besides prednisone is rarely necessary, but occasionally a patient who is intolerant of prednisone or who has uncontrollable pressure elevation from corticosteroids will benefit from agents such as methotrexate, azathioprine, cyclosporine, or cyclophosphamide.

Cycloplegia need not be routine but can be useful in eyes with fibrin in the anterior chamber and in any eye with even a hint of synechia formation.

Patients with uveitis are more likely to experience inflammatory glaucoma and iris bombé. It is best to avoid pilocarpine therapy in these eyes. YAG laser iridectomy is usually effective in eyes with iris bombé. Treatment first with argon laser to close vessels, followed by a large YAG laser iridectomy, is most likely to ensure patency. In some eyes, repeat closure of laser iridectomies will be best managed by surgical iridectomy.

Prophylactic therapy of CME is controversial. Many of these eyes have preexisting macular edema from long-standing uveitis. Some argue for the use of topical or oral nonsteroidal agents following cataract extraction in all patients with uveitis. When CME develops, standard therapy as outlined in Chapter 47 applies, but it is also essential to eliminate all intraocular inflammation.

Hypotony and cyclitic membrane formation after cataract extraction are quite unusual and usually require pars plana vitrectomy and membranectomy. Macular pucker and membranes can be treated surgically in selected cases. Pupillary membranes or membranes around the IOL that do not respond to corticosteroids and recur following YAG laser therapy necessitate removal of the IOL.

Iris capture of an IOL with excessive lens deposits and inflammation can be managed in some cases by repositioning the lens and eliminating iris contact. However, some cases require lens removal.[45] Other postoperative problems are discussed in Chapters 39 through 50 (in particular, see Chapter 50, Prolonged Intraocular Inflammation).

REFERENCES

1. Hooper PL, Rao NA, Smith RE: Cataract extraction in uveitis patients, *Surv Ophthalmol* 35:120-144, 1990.
2. Foster CS, Fong LP, Singh G: Cataract surgery and intraocular lens implantation in patients with uveitis, *Ophthalmology* 96:281-288, 1989.
3. Foster RE, Lowder CY, Meisler DM et al: Extracapsular cataract extraction and posterior chamber intraocular lens implantation in uveitis patients, *Ophthalmology* 99:1234-1241, 1992.
4. Chung YM, Yeh TS: Intraocular lens implantation following extracapsular cataract extraction in uveitis, *Ophthalmic Surg* 21:272-276, 1990.
5. Anderson W: IOLs in uveitis patients, *Ophthalmology* 101:625-626, 1994.
6. Alio JL, Chipont E: Surgery of cataract in patients with uveitis, *Dev Ophthalmol* 31:166-174, 1999.
7. Michelson JB, Friedlander MH, Nozik RA: Lens implant surgery in pars planitis, *Ophthalmology* 97:1023-1026, 1990.
8. Rutzen AR, Raizman MB: Fuchs' heterochromic iridocyclitis. In Albert DM, Jakobiec FA, editors: *Principles and practice of ophthalmology,* Philadelphia, 1994, WB Saunders, pp 503-516.
9. Wolf MD, Lichter PR, Ragsdale CG: Prognostic factors in the uveitis of juvenile rheumatoid arthritis, *Ophthalmology* 94:1242-1248, 1987.
10. Palestine AG, Alter GJ, Chan CC et al: Laser interferometry and visual prognosis in uveitis, *Ophthalmology* 92:1567-1569, 1985.
11. Akova YA, Foster CS: Cataract surgery in patients with sarcoidosis-associated uveitis, *Ophthalmology* 101:473-479, 1994.
12. Moorthy RS, Rajeev B, Smith RE et al: Incidence and management of cataracts in Vogt-Koyanagi-Harada syndrome, *Am J Ophthalmol* 118:197 204, 1994.
13. Harris DJ Jr: Causes of reduced visual acuity on long-term follow-up after cataract extraction in patients with uveitis and juvenile rheumatoid arthritis, *Am J Ophthalmol* 115:682-684, 1993.
14. Probst LE, Holland EJ: Intraocular lens implantation in patients with juvenile rheumatoid arthritis, *Am J Ophthalmol* 122:161-170, 1996.
15. Holland GN: Intraocular lens implantation in patients with juvenile rheumatoid arthritis-associated uveitis: an unresolved management issue, *Am J Ophthalmol* 122:255-257, 1996.
16. BenEzra D, Cohen E: Cataract surgery in children with chronic uveitis, *Ophthalmology* 107:1255-1260, 2000.
17. Lundvall A, Zetterstrom C: Cataract extraction and intraocular lens implantation in children with uveitis, *Br J Ophthalmol* 84:791-793, 2000.
18. Avramides S, Sakkias G, Traianidis P: Cataract surgery in Fuchs' heterochromic iridocyclitis, *Eur J Ophthalmol* 7:149-151, 1997.
19. Estafanous MF, Lowder CY, Meisler DM et al: Phacoemulsification cataract extraction and posterior chamber lens implantation in patients with uveitis, *Am J Ophthalmol* 131:620-625, 2001.
20. Patitsas CJ, Rockwood EJ, Meisler DM et al: Glaucoma filtering surgery with postoperative 5-fluoracil in patients with intraocular inflammatory disease, *Ophthalmology* 99:594-599, 1992.
21. Chee S-P, Ti S-E, Sivakuma M et al: Postoperative inflammation: extracapsular cataract extraction versus phacoemulsification, *J Cataract Refract Surg* 25:1280-1285, 1999.
22. Dowler JG, Hykin PG, Hamilton AM: Phacoemulsification versus extracapsular cataract extraction in patients with diabetes, *Ophthalmology* 107:457-462, 2000.
23. Diamond JG, Kaplan HJ: Lensectomy and vitrectomy for complicated cataract due to uveitis, *Arch Ophthalmol* 96:1798-1804, 1978.
24. Dangel ME, Stark WJ, Michels RG: Surgical management of cataract associated with uveitis, *Ophthalmic Surg* 14:145-149, 1983.
25. Nobe JR, Kokoris N, Diddle KR, et al: Lensectomy-vitrectomy in chronic uveitis. *Retina* 3:71-76, 1983.
26. Petrilli AM, Belfort R Jr, Abre MT et al: Ultrasonic fragmentation in of cataract in uveitis, *Retina* 6:61-65, 1986.
27. Girard LJ, Rodriguez J, Mailman ML et al: Cataract and uveitis management by pars plana lensectomy and vitrectomy by ultrasonic fragmentation, *Retina* 5:107-114, 1985.
28. Flynn HW Jr, Davis JL, Culbertson WW: Pars plana lensectomy and vitrectomy for complicated cataracts in juvenile rheumatoid arthritis, *Ophthalmology* 95:1114-1119, 1988.
29. Fox GM, Flynn HW Jr, Davis JL et al: Causes of reduced visual acuity on

long-term follow-up after cataract extraction in patients with uveitis, *Am J Ophthalmol* 114:708-714, 1992.

30. Foster RE, Lowder CY, Meisler DM et al: Combined extracapsular cataract extraction, posterior chamber intraocular lens implantation, and pars plana vitrectomy, *Ophthalmic Surg* 24:446-452, 1993.
31. Diamond JG, Kaplan HJ: Uveitis: Effect of vitrectomy combined with lensectomy, *Ophthalmology* 86:1320-1327, 1979.
32. Dick HB, Schwenn O, Krummenauer F et al: Inflammation after sclerocorneal versus clear corneal tunnel phacoemulsification, *Ophthalmology* 107:241-247, 2000.
33. Rauz S, Stavrou P, Murray PI: Evaluation of foldable intraocular lenses in patients with uveitis, *Ophthalmology* 107:909-919, 2000.
34. Tuberville AW, Galin MA, Perez HD et al: Complement activation by nylon- and polypropylene-looped prosthetic intraocular lenses, *Invest Ophthalmol Vis Sci* 22:727-733, 1982.
35. Mondino BJ, Nagata S, Glovsky MM: Activation of the alternative complement pathway by intraocular lenses, *Invest Ophthalmol Vis Sci* 26:905-908, 1985.
36. Menikoff JA, Speaker MG, Marmor M et al: A case-control study of risk factors for postoperative endophthalmitis, *Ophthalmology* 98:1761-1768, 1991.
37. Rose GE: Fibrinous uveitis and intraocular lens implantation: surface modification of polymethylmethacrylate during extracapsular cataract surgery, *Ophthalmology* 99:1242-1247, 1992.
38. Lin CL, Wang AG, Chou JC et al: Heparin-surface-modified intraocular lens implantation in patients with glaucoma, diabetes, or uveitis, *J Cataract Refract Surg* 20:550-553, 1994.
39. Lardenoye CW, van der LA, Berendschot TT et al: A retrospective analysis of heparin-surface-modified intraocular lenses versus regular polymethylmethacrylate intraocular lenses in patients with uveitis, *Doc Ophthalmol* 92:41-50, 1996.
40. Trocme SD, Li H: Effect of heparin-surface-modified intraocular lenses on postoperative inflammation after phacoemulsification: a randomized trial in a United States patient population: Heparin-Surface-Modified Lens Study Group, *Ophthalmology* 107:1031-1037, 2000.
41. Ravalico G, Baccara F, Lovisato A et al: Postoperative cellular reaction on various intraocular lens materials, *Ophthalmology* 104:1084-1091, 1997.
42. Van Liefferinge T, Van Oye R, Kestelyn P: Uveitis-glaucoma-hyphema syndrome: a late complication of posterior chamber lenses, *Bull Soc Belge Ophthalmol* 252:61-66, 1994.
43. Aonuma H, Matsushita H, Nakajima K et al: Uveitis-glaucoma-hyphema syndrome after posterior chamber intraocular lens implantation, *Jpn J Ophthalmol* 41:98-100, 1997.
44. Holland GN, Van Horn SD, Margolis TP: Cataract surgery with ciliary sulcus fixation of intraocular lenses in patients with uveitis, *Am J Ophthalmol* 128:21-30, 1999.
45. Foster RE, Stavrou P, Zafirakis P et al: Intraocular lens removal from patients with uveitis, *Am J Ophthalmol* 128:31-37, 1999.

Surgical Management of Pediatric Cataracts

24

Howard V. Gimbel, MD, MPH, FRCSC
Brian M. DeBroff, MD, FACS

Cataract extraction with lens implantation in children has undergone dramatic changes during the past 40 years, largely as a result of advances in technology and microsurgical techniques.[1-7] The management of cataracts in infants and very young children is, by far, more complex than the management of cataracts in adults. The timing of surgery, the surgical technique, the choice of the intraocular lens (IOL), and the management of amblyopia are of utmost importance for achieving good visual results in children.[3,8-11] Other challenges in the management of cataracts in infants and children include the difficulties in examining infants and young children, the risks of general anesthesia, poor preoperative pupillary dilation, and the management of postoperative inflammation and fibrin formation. Children are at higher risk for postoperative pupillary capture, posterior synechiae, IOL precipitates, fibroid uveitis, correctopia, pupillary block glaucoma, and peripheral iris erosion.[12] Because pediatric cataracts are relatively rare, many ophthalmologists lack surgical experience with this particular group of patients. The development of continuous curvilinear capsulorhexis (CCC)[13] and viscoelastic agents, advances in posterior chamber IOL designs, and the use of the neodymium:yttrium-aluminum-garnet (Nd:YAG) laser have brought the pediatric cataract surgical technique closer to the adult procedure.

There are many nuances of pediatric surgery—including preoperative evaluation, timing of surgery, operative technique, and postoperative management—which this chapter attempts to elucidate. The evolution of techniques in pediatric cataract surgery are emphasized, including the trend toward CCC, placement of posterior chamber lenses in the capsular bag, and methods to reduce the formation of secondary cataracts.

Preoperative Evaluation

A preoperative assessment is essential to adequately evaluate the size, density, location, and visual impact of the cataract; to evaluate for other ocular abnormalities; and to properly plan the surgical procedure. A history from the parents is often helpful in clarifying whether the cataract is congenital, developmental, or traumatic and to ascertain if there was any maternal drug use, infections, or exposure to ionizing radiation during pregnancy. Infants with bilateral congenital cataracts demonstrate decreased visual interest and may have delayed developmental milestones.[14] Past or present illness and a history of medication use may give a clue to the cause of the cataract. Past ocular history and a family history of ocular diseases may reveal other possible causes.

Complete examination of infants or young children may require sedation or even general anesthesia. Although there may be variations in the baseline ophthalmic assessment because of the age and compliance of the pediatric cataract surgery patient, a full anterior and posterior segment examination is essential in all patients preoperatively. An assessment of the best corrected visual function is performed by testing the patient's ability to fix and follow (in infants), progressing to picture cards, illiterate *E*'s, and Snellen letter charts in older children. Cycloplegic refraction by retinoscopy, autorefractor, or even trial lens is important to determine the best correction. Binocularity, fusion, and stereopsis preoperatively give the ophthalmologist an idea of how well the eyes function together. Strabismus evaluation should involve cover-uncover and alternative cover testing for both distance and close up. Any restrictions of extraocular movements should be noted. The presence of nystagmus is an ominous sign, indicating poor vision resulting from sensory deprivation.[15] Pupils should be evaluated for the presence of an afferent pupillary defect.

An anterior segment examination, preferably by slit lamp microscopy, may reveal potential challenges to surgery, including iris deformities, synechiae, zonulolysis, posterior lentiglobus, intumescent cataract, anterior or posterior capsule plaques, or evidence of past trauma. The extent and location of the cataract must be evaluated. Small anterior polar cataracts often do not require lens extraction, whereas nuclear and posterior opacities tend to be more visually significant.

When the clarity of the media permits, indirect ophthalmoscopy will reveal any posterior segment abnormalities or pathologic condition that may have an impact on postoperative vision. Axial length and corneal curvature are essential measurements for IOL power determination. To measure the axial length of an eye in a child as young as 2 years old, a handheld A-scan and keratometry should be performed without sedation so that the child can fixate on a target object. However, both A-scan and keratometry may be performed in the operating room under general anesthesia before cataract extraction or during an examination under anesthesia. In the event of a traumatic cataract in which the A-scan is unattainable, the patient's other eye may be used for proxy measurements on which to base IOL power calculations. Corneal diameter measurement helps rule out microcornea and microphthalmos. Measurement of intraocular pressure can be accomplished by Tonopen, Shiotz tonometry, or pneumotonometry under anesthesia in infants or by applanation tonometry in older children. If the cataract is very dense with no view of the fundus, a B-scan will help evaluate any posterior segment abnormalities. Also, electrophysiologic testing, including electroretinography and visual evoked potential, may be performed to assess the neurologic function of the retina and to detect stimulus deprivation and amblyopia.[16]

Consultation with a pediatrician is essential for infants with congenital cataracts. Some laboratory tests that may be considered include urine evaluation for reducing substances; toxoplasmosis, rubella, cytomegalovirus, and herpes simplex titer; serum screen for galactosemia, and a serum calcium screen to evaluate for hypoparathyroidism.[17] Also, it is important to observe for any systemic processes that may be coexistent, especially in children with bilateral cataracts. Genetic testing should be considered for infants with congenital cataracts.[18]

Timing of Surgery

The timing for surgical intervention in pediatric cataracts was profoundly influenced by the work of Hubel and Weisel and later by von Noorden,[9] who established that sensory deprivation in the first few months of life is the critical period for visual development and that sensory deprivation during this period results in both irreversible anatomic changes in the lateral geniculate bodies and decreased activity in the occipital cortex on visual stimulation.[18,19] Congenital monocular complete cataracts should be removed within the first few months of life and preferably in the first few days or weeks of life.[20-22] If surgery is performed within the first 4 months of life, deprivation amblyopia can still be reversed.[10,17,23] Bilateral complete congenital cataracts should be removed within the first few months of life, first in the eye with the more opaque lens opacity and approximately a week later in the other eye. In children who are of an age at which they are at risk for the development of amblyopia, a monocular cataract should be operated on when the best corrected visual acuity is 20/70 or worse.[24] Recommendation for surgery in children with bilateral cataracts is often made when the vision in the worse eye is 20/70 or poorer. In children older than 8 years, who are no longer at risk for amblyopia, cataract surgery is recommended when the child has difficulty functioning in school or in sports or has problems with normal daily activities. Although surgical removal is the definitive therapy for the majority of congenital cataracts when visual function is jeopardized, visual acuity in many children with small cataracts may be improved by first maintaining dilation of the pupil. When cycloplegia is used, however, photophobia is often aggravated, and reading glasses are often necessary.[15,25]

Review of Pediatric Surgical Techniques

The Early Years

Several different surgical techniques for the management of cataracts in pediatric patients have been advocated in the past, including discission or needling, linear extraction, or a combination of discission and displacement of lens fragments into the anterior chamber by irrigation without IOL implantation.[26-29] In the early 1960s the aspiration procedure as popularized by Scheie, Rubenstein, and Kent[30] with the widespread use of the operating microscope became the accepted technique for extracting cataracts in infants and children.[31] With the aspiration technique, the lens material was suctioned by a push-pull technique using a needle with a syringe attached. Using this method, surgical complications associated with earlier techniques were dramatically reduced. Significant intraoperative risks, however, such as anterior chamber collapse and vitreous loss remained prevalent.[30,31] The Scheie technique, which leaves the posterior capsule intact, led to an extremely high incidence of secondary membranes and the development of synechiae between the iris and the remaining capsular bag. A sector iridectomy was necessary to prevent iris bombé and secondary glaucoma.[26,30,32-35] Often, additional operations using general anesthesia were required. The delay in amblyopia therapy became significant and was undoubtedly part of the poor visual results seen in patients with unilateral bilateral congenital cataracts.

In the mid-1960s, the next development that changed pediatric cataract surgery was the introduction of a double-barreled cannula, one for aspiration and one for irrigation.[36] The irrigation-aspiration technique enabled the ophthalmologist to maintain anterior chamber depth during cataract aspiration while keeping the posterior capsule intact. Unfortunately, in many pediatric cases, the lens epithelium would still grow in from the periphery relentlessly and cover the posterior capsule surface, resulting in a translucent membrane.[32] The incidence of postoperative secondary membrane formation with aspiration techniques remained high,[32,37] necessitating a secondary surgical procedure weeks or months later to open the posterior lens capsule.[38]

The 1970s witnessed the introduction of phacoemulsification in pediatric cataract surgery.[39,40] Although many pediatric cataracts can be removed using the irrigation-aspiration handpiece alone or by using the phacoemulsification handpiece with no ultrasound power, in some cases short bursts of phacoemulsification may be required. Pediatric cataracts vary dramatically in type, ranging from the very soft to the very hard and calcified. Nuclei that are too hard to be simply aspirated can be fragmented using phacoemulsification. Thus phacoemulsification in pediatric surgery allows a wider application of the basic aspiration technique.[41,42] In addition, the closed phacoemulsification system incorporates the principles of controlled infusion to maintain intraocular pressure and variable and controlled suction or aspiration. Even with phacoemulsification and meticulous polishing of the anterior and posterior capsule, however, the incidence of posterior capsule opacification remained significantly high.[43-45]

Pharmacologic Method to Reduce the Incidence of Secondary Cataract Formation

Tissue plasminogen activator can be used to decrease fibrin formation following cataract surgery.[46,47] Experimentally, hirudin has been evaluated for preventing postoperative fibrin formation.[48] Heparin-surface–modified IOLs and even heparin infusion at a concentration of 5 IU/ml of fluid may help prevent a secondary membrane.[49,50] Other experimental methods to reduce secondary membrane formation include antimetabolites, including mitomycin and caffeine acid; phenyl ester; immunotoxins, including one in a phase III clinical trial; antigrowth factor agents; agents that inhibit binding of lens epithelial cells to the capsule; and even a gene therapy involving a replication-defective recombinant adenovirus. If toxicity issues can be overcome and these agents can be shown to affect lens epithelial cells (proliferation, migration, adhesion to the capsular bag, and fibrous metaplasia) without collateral damage to ocular tissues, this approach may represent the future in prevention of secondary membranes. Such agents may in the future be given by single injections, combined with viscoelastic, by sustained relapse, or via coating the IOL. The most promising are either gene therapy or specific monoclonal antibodies that selectively target lens epithelial cells.

New Techniques to Reduce the Incidence of Secondary Cataract Formation

One of the major concerns in pediatric IOL implantation surgery has been the high incidence of postoperative opacification of the posterior capsule and retropseudophakic membrane formation in children.[32,51,52] Residual lens capsule epithelial cells transform to fibroblasts and Elschnig pearls, which proliferate using the posterior capsule, anterior vitreous face, and anterior and posterior surfaces of the IOL as a scaffold.[53,54] Secondary membranes form, reocclude the visual axis, and can lead to irreversible deprivation amblyopia. In general, with decreasing age there is an increasing aggressiveness of secondary cataract formation.[55] Different techniques to avoid or reduce postoperative fibrosis or Elschnig pearl formation have been proposed, including primary posterior capsulotomy and anterior vitrectomy, pars plana posterior capsulotomy, and posterior continuous curvilinear capsulorhexis (PCCC) with posterior optic capture.[27-29,36,56-59]

With the development of automated vitrectomy instruments in the 1970s, cutting and aspirating capabilities added a new dimension to the treatment of pediatric cataracts.[60] By performing a posterior capsulotomy and anterior vitrectomy at the time of cataract extraction, a clear optical axis resulted, whereas the need for secondary surgical procedures was minimized. Controversy exists regarding the advisability of performing a primary posterior capsulotomy and anterior vitrectomy versus a posterior capsulotomy at a later date.[38,61]

The eye in children older than 5 years of age responds to surgery with less inflammation and posterior capsule opacification than does the infant's eye.[44] Also, with the development of modern microsurgical techniques and the availability of the Nd:YAG laser, routine primary posterior capsulotomy openings are unnecessary in this population. Leaving the posterior capsule intact for posterior chamber in-the-bag IOL implantation with the option of Nd:YAG posterior capsulotomy at a later date may be the best approach in older children and provides the best visual results with the least risk.[62] Secondary Nd:YAG capsulotomy has been demonstrated to be successful in children older than 6 years of age with posterior capsular opacity.[63,64]

For children younger than 5 or 6 years of age, less cooperative children, and infants, an Nd:YAG laser vertically mounted in the operating room can be used to perform posterior capsulotomies either at the time of surgery or weeks to months after the cataract procedure. Laser capsulotomy in the pediatric population, however, requires high energy, and some membranes are too dense to allow the creation of large enough openings. General anesthesia is required, and the recurrence of the membrane is possible because the anterior vitreous face remains as a scaffold for secondary membrane formation.

Studies have demonstrated an inevitable development of secondary cataracts in younger children unless the posterior capsule is opened generously and an anterior vitrectomy is performed at the time of cataract extraction and IOL implantation.[65-67] Many pediatric ophthalmologists currently perform a posterior capsulotomy and a shallow anterior vitrectomy routinely at the time of cataract extraction, before insertion of the IOL.[68,69] Special instruments have been developed to perform posterior capsulotomy underneath a posterior chamber IOL.[70] Higher viscous viscoelastics, including Healon 5, make this a safer and technically less difficult procedure. A recent modification involves removing the cataract through a scleral tunnel incision with implantation of a posterior chamber IOL and then, during the same procedure, performing a pars plana posterior capsulotomy and pars plana anterior vitrectomy.[55,71] In such a manner, proper positioning of the IOL is ensured before performing the capsulotomy, and it is possible to achieve large capsular openings.

One disadvantage of primary capsulotomy and anterior vitrectomy is dislocation of the IOLs, which has been demonstrated in 3% to 20% of cases.[55,72-74] In addition, there have been reports of cystoid macular edema following pediatric cataract extraction with anterior vitrectomy.[75] Subsequent studies, however, have found the risk of this complication to be quite minimal.* Anterior vitrectomy may also be associated with vitreous incarceration in the wound and vitreous adhesions that increase the risk of retinal detachment.[80] Finally, even after primary posterior capsulectomy with vitrectomy, many children's visual axes still become reoccluded by secondary membranes,[55,64,81] necessitating repeated capsulotomies and sometimes pars plana membranectomy.[44,82]

Other techniques have been proposed to prevent posterior capsular and vitreous face membrane formation while reducing the risk of dislocation of the IOL. One such technique involves placing the IOL anterior to the entire capsular bag. This creates

*References 12, 44, 45, 66, 67, 76-79.

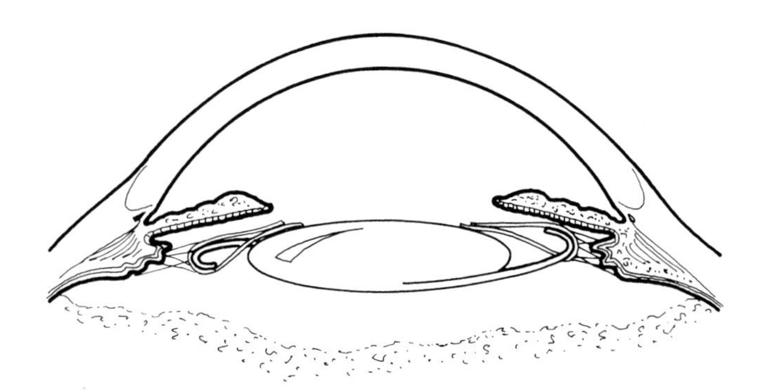

FIGURE 24-1 Posterior capsulorhexis with optic capture.

a tight adhesion between the anterior and posterior capsule and helps prevent lens epithelial cells from migrating, proliferating, and forming Elschnig pearls.[41-44] Another new technique described by Marie-José Tossignon[83] and performed in a limited number of cases with excellent results involves a newly designed IOL that fits within an anterior and posterior CCC and sandwiches the capsule leaflets in peripheral concavity of the IOL. To further reduce or eliminate opacification of the posterior capsule in pediatric cases while reducing the need for anterior vitrectomy, a technique of posterior capsulorhexis with optic capture has been shown to be beneficial.[56-59] This technique involves primary PCCC and placement of the optic of the IOL through the posterior capsulorhexis opening with resultant optic capture while the haptics remain in the bag.[40,42] This technique has been used in pediatric cases since April 1993 with promising results. The technique for performing posterior capsulorhexis with optic capture is described later under Current Surgical Techniques.

Primary PCCC with posterior capsule optic capture helps to maintain a clear visual axis, reducing the need for subsequent intervention because of the apposition of anterior and posterior capsule leaflets anterior to the IOL. These capsule leaflets are apposed 360 degrees except at the haptic-optic junctions. This seals the bag, causing release of Elschnig pearls to occur anterior to the IOL, where they will be removed by the aqueous humor (Figure 24-1). Any adhesion of protein on the anterior surface of the IOL may be cleared away with the Nd:YAG laser. The benefit of this technique is that it provides excellent IOL fixation and ensures centration of the IOL. The tight barrier that is created prevents vitreous from moving forward. The disadvantages are that the procedure is technically challenging, requires precise and controlled capsulotomies, and makes IOL exchange difficult.[84,85] Piggyback IOL placement, however, is possible. Koch and Kohnen[84] have described that performing this technique in conjunction with anterior vitrectomy is beneficial in preventing posterior capsule opacifications. Primary PCCC with posterior capsule optic capture represents a technique that serves to keep the optical axis clear while maintaining excellent support and centration of the implant. In our experience, using the Gimbel PCCC with optic capture technique, 19 consecutive pediatric eyes have shown no secondary opacification in the long term. The mean follow-up was 4 years (range, 1 year to 8.25 years). The mean age of the children at the time of surgery was 6 ± 3.8 (range, 2 to 12 years of age).

Pars Plana Versus Limbal Approach

In addition to successfully managing secondary membranes and vitreous loss, vitrectomy instruments have allowed surgeons to perform cataract procedures via a pars plana approach.[86-88] Both the limbal and pars plana approach have their advocates and opponents.[68,89-91] The main advantages of the pars plana approach are the reduced incidence of vitreous disturbance and retinal traction when performing an anterior vitrectomy,[92] the facilitation of reaching lenticular material in the periphery, and less damage to corneal endothelium and iris tissue.[90,93] The principal disadvantage of the pars plana approach is the loss of integrity of the capsular bag. Removal of the entire cataract by a pars plana approach takes away the majority of capsular bag support for IOL placement and virtually eliminates the possibility of in-the-bag IOL placement.[90,94] Implantation of a posterior chamber lens in the sulcus, although possible after pars plana lensectomy, is less advantageous.[95] An IOL placed in the sulcus has the disadvantage of contact with vascular tissue and the possibility of inducing a chronic inflammatory response. Thus the pars plana approach limits the safety of IOL placement and decreases the options for optical rehabilitation if contact lenses cannot be worn or if epikeratophakia fails. The pars plana approach also increases the risk for iatrogenic retinal dialysis or ciliary body detachment.[86]

The risk of retinal detachment, however, has persuaded many ophthalmologists to use the limbal approach.[96] Keech, Tongue, and Scott[96] reported one case of retinal detachment 6 years after translimbal lensectomy and anterior vitrectomy. Recent studies, however, have shown no statistically significant differences between the limbal and pars plana approach.[97] Increasing preference for the limbal surgical approach for pediatric cataract extraction also occurred with the introduction of higher viscosity viscoelastic agents, including Healon GV and Healon 5. These agents have facilitated the maintenance of the anterior chamber, the performance of anterior and posterior capsulotomies, the manipulation of instruments within the anterior chamber, and the placement of IOLs into the capsular bag, while protecting the corneal endothelium.[5] The limbal approach allows CCC, complete removal of the cataract, implantation of an IOL in the capsular bag, PCCC, optic capture, and anterior vitrectomy. As pediatric surgical techniques and intraocular implants have continued to be refined, more interest has shifted to posterior chamber IOLs placed through a limbal incision into the capsular bag as a means of aphakic correction in children of younger and younger ages.

Pediatric Intraocular Lens Implantation

Aphakic spectacles are severely debilitating visually, cosmetically, and psychologically. Epikeratophakia requires intensive postoperative management and may be associated with decreased lenticular clarity, irregular astigmatism, spherical error, and a prolonged period until visual rehabilitation is achieved.[94,98,99] Contact lenses are successful in a relatively small number of pediatric cases over a long period, are emotionally stressful both for the child and the family, and are economically beyond the reach of many patients, particularly those in developing countries.[68,100] Such difficulties with aphakic spectacles, epikeratophakia, and contact lenses, combined with more

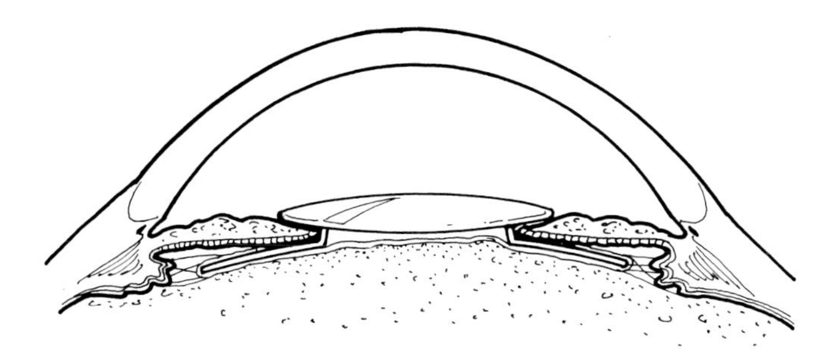

FIGURE 24-2 Capsule-fixated Binkhorst two-loop iridocapsular lens.

experience with IOLs, viscoelastics, improved IOL design, and improved surgical techniques, have increased the popularity of and diminished the controversy over IOL implantation. Pseudophakia offers the method of optical correction that requires the least compliance and induces minimal aniseikonia and astigmatism.[80]

IOL implants were first advocated by anterior segment surgeons as early as 1955.[1,101-104] Early IOL implantation in children involved anterior chamber and iris-supported lense.[103] The first published implantation of an IOL in a child was by Choyce[105] in 1955, using an anterior chamber lens. Anterior chamber lenses invariably stimulate an inflammatory response as a result of their contact with vascular tissues and are associated with long-term complications in adults.[2,62] Endothelial cell loss over many years is a concern, especially with children who tend to rub their eyes frequently. Trauma to an eye with an anterior chamber lens may lead to iris or ciliary body rupture. Binkhorst and Gobin[51] implanted an iridocapsular fixated IOL in 1959 (Figure 24-2). When fixed and stable in the capsule, the iridocapsular IOLs were very successful. Some, however, were associated with complications, including iris sphincter erosion, hyphema, anterior synechiae, iris bombé, iritis, and pupillary fibrotic membranes. Also, lens dislocation, pseudophakodonesis, and corneal endothelial trauma were possible when capsule fixation was not achieved.

These complications, which were secondary to inferior lens design and primitive microsurgical techniques, had at one point made IOL implantation in children a very controversial subject. Additional negative opinion toward implantation of IOLs in children resulted from the concern of the possible long-term risk of the eye reacting to polymethylmethacrylate. The observation times in most pediatric IOL series are short in relation to a child's life expectancy.[1,5,100,106-110] Also, many ophthalmologists were concerned that an intense inflammatory reaction might be incited by placement of implants in infants. Histopathologic studies, however, have subsequently revealed that the eyes of children could tolerate IOLs in a manner similar to that of adult eyes.[111] Work by Hiles[2,112] in the 1970s and 1980s helped demonstrate the safety and effectiveness of aphakic rehabilitation of children with IOLs, especially in cases of traumatic or unilateral infantile cataracts.

IOL implantation is now becoming the preferred method of pediatric aphakic rehabilitation, especially for children over 1 year of age.* With IOL implantation, there is almost immediate postoperative visual rehabilitation, which maximizes the treatment of amblyopia. In addition, the technique of CCC developed in the 1980s providing assurance of in-the-bag placement of the IOL, and the development of improved lens designs have helped avoid many complications associated with early lens implantation in children. Relative contraindications do exist for IOL implantation. They include glaucoma, persistent or recurrent uveitis, aniridia, severe microphthalmia, other ophthalmic defects that preclude useful vision, and cases of inadequate capsular support.[2] Recent studies have shown that good results can be achieved in microphthalmic eyes, and this problem is now becoming less of a concern.[119,120] Capsular tension rings with artificial irides may provide improved quality of vision in patients with aniridia.

Some ophthalmologists consider patient age of less than 1 year to be a relative contraindication for IOL implantation. The youngest age at which implants can be safely and effectively used has not yet been clearly established. Many ophthalmologists prefer aphakia for bilateral congenital cataracts with the plan of secondary implants within a couple of years. In children older than 2 years of age, lens implantation into the capsular bag may be routinely achieved in monocular or bilateral congenital, developmental, or traumatic cases using current surgical techniques, including CCC, and viscoelastic materials. Experts in the field of infantile cataract extraction recently have been implanting posterior chamber IOLs in infants as early as the first 2 months of life.[69,122] Proponents of IOL implantation for treatment of unilateral infantile aphakia claim that this is the best available method to reduce the incidence of irreversible amblyopia.[69,121,123] Recent studies have shown the effectiveness of bilateral implants in children over the age of 2,[123] and other studies have demonstrated excellent results in children between the ages of 4 to 6 months of age.[124] More recently, O'Keefe, Mulvihill, and Yeoh[125] found bilateral IOL implantation safe and produced good visual results in children of all ages, including infants. Peterseim and Wilson[126] have also published encouraging results. Because the infant eye has a rapidly changing refraction during the first year of life, controversy surrounds the proper power lens to choose for implants in infants.[121]

The development of the eye necessitates initial undercorrection to avoid permanent overcorrection. The growth of the anterior segment of the eye is generally completed at the end of the second year of life.[127] Therefore little adaptation of the size and power of the IOL is needed in the eyes of children older than 2 years. Hyperopic undercorrection is often desired in younger children, although anisometropia should be minimized to promote binocular function. The final hyperopia desired should be correlated to the child's age. Because the greatest change in axial length and keratometry readings occurs in the first 2 years of life, it is wiser to choose an IOL that will initially correct only 80% of the aphakia in infants. To minimize the need to exchange IOLs, it is preferable to undercorrect young children by 10% to 20%. In infants, greater degrees of initial hypermetropia are required because the greatest degree of eye growth occurs before 2 years of age. Over 6 diopters (D) of average myopic shift have been documented in pseudophakic infants over a minimum 2-year follow-up.[128] Aiming for emmetropia in infants would create a large myopic shift that can be amblyogenic itself and may require an IOL exchange.[129,130]

*References 2, 21, 44, 80, 82, 100, 102, 113-118.

An infant should receive 80% of the IOL power needed for emmetropia.[128] The initial hypermetropia can be corrected with spectacles or contact lenses and adjusted as the eye grows, to prevent amblyopia. Dr. M. Edward Wilson has developed a technique of piggyback IOL for infants with a planned removal of an IOL later in life after eye growth.[131] The permanent IOL is placed within the capsular bag, and the temporary IOL is placed within the ciliary sulcus. On average, a 26.5-diopter IOL is placed in the bag and an 11-D lens in the sulcus. Dr. Wilson believes that this approach may be most appropriate for families less likely to comply with scheduled follow-up visits or with wearing glasses full time. In children aged 2 to 5 years, a postoperative hyperopic spherical equivalent of +2.5 D is desired. Preschoolers are usually able to tolerate small amounts of residual hyperopia and astigmatism quite well without the need for spectacle correction. Higher residual refractive errors can be corrected with glasses, which are adjusted as necessary during childhood. Using this method, the patients are initially hyperopic. As the eye grows, emmetropia is approached, and by adolescence, moderate myopia is common. Eye growth with progressively decreasing hyperopia appears to run its normal course in the eye with an IOL, provided that the eye attains sufficient visual acuity.[127,132] In children who have already started school, the desired postoperative refraction should approach emmetropia. Bifocal lenses are often required for near vision.

Compared with all other currently available methods, postoperative amblyopic therapy is best maximized by the immediate visual rehabilitation afforded by IOL implantation.[44,45,63] Better visual outcomes in children with IOLs are probably related to the uninterrupted and permanent optical correction provided by the lens implant. Strict compliance with amblyopic treatment, however, is still necessary.[89] It is undeniable that in young children in need of amblyopic treatment, implantation of IOLs has far-reaching advantages, including immediate correction of the major portion of the refractive error. IOL implantation with patching of the nonoperated eye is most readily accepted by children and parents, and it maximizes postoperative visual acuity.[68]

Current Surgical Techniques

Surgical Technique for Cataracts in Infants

Two corneolimbal incisions are made at the 10 o'clock and 2 o'clock positions: one to allow the insertion of a chamber maintainer connected to an infusion of balanced salt solution (BSS) containing adrenaline, 1:500,000, and the other for an irrigation-aspiration cannula, a phacoemulsification probe, or an anterior vitrector, depending on the density of the nucleus. The chamber maintainer allows intraocular manipulations in a well-formed globe, thus minimizing iatrogenic trauma to the iris. A central circular anterior capsulotomy 4 to 6 mm in diameter is started with a cystotome with high-viscosity viscoelastic material (Figure 24-3). The lens material is aspirated, with care being taken to preserve the posterior capsule and an intact rim of anterior capsule (Figure 24-4).

Following the complete removal of lens material, an elective central posterior capsulotomy of not less than 4 mm in diameter is performed using the vitrectomy probe. A smaller posterior capsulotomy can close, especially in infants. Unlike that in an adult, a central posterior capsulotomy in a child will not ensure permanently clear visual axis unless a generous anterior vitrectomy is performed with a vitrectomy instrument (Figure 24-5). The aim is to remove at least the anterior one third of the vitreous gel, thus eliminating vitreous remnants near the posterior capsule, which can serve as a scaffold for lens fibers to grow on and occlude the posterior capsule opening. When implantation of an IOL is not intended (as in cases of bilateral congenital cataracts), the operation is completed at this stage by suturing the two limbal wounds with tight 10-0 nylon or Vicryl sutures. Aphakic correction can be achieved using contact lenses or glasses.

When IOL implantation is planned, as in unilateral congenital cataracts, uneven developmental cataracts, or traumatic cataracts, one-piece polymethylmethacrylate lenses or acrylic foldable lenses are recommended. In order to insert a posterior chamber IOL in the bag remnants, viscoelastic material is

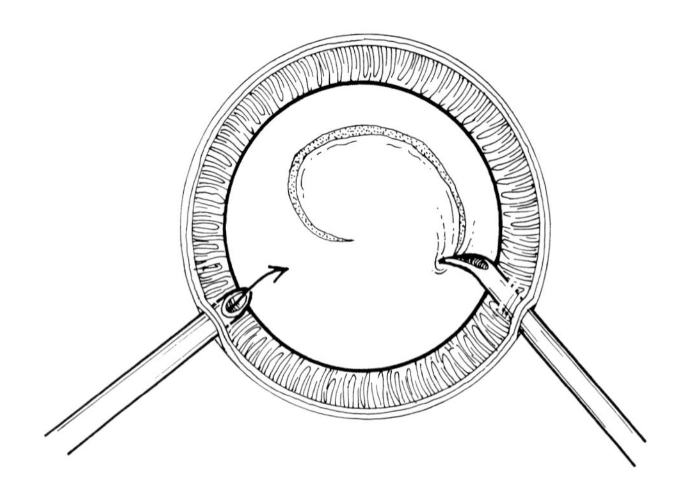

FIGURE 24-3 Continuous curvilinear capsulorhexis using a chamber maintainer and cystotome.

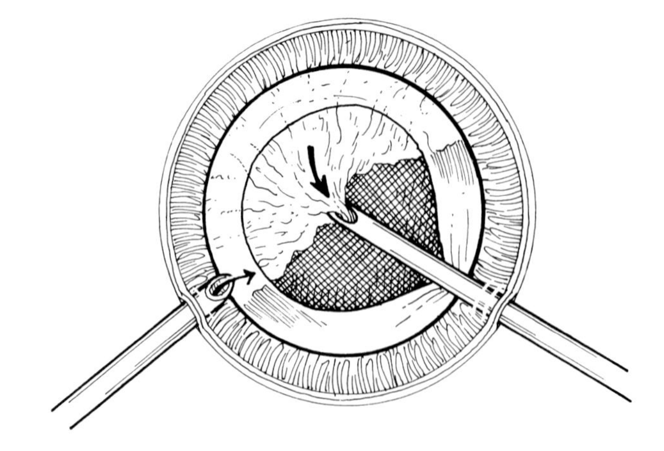

FIGURE 24-4 Lens material aspiration using a chamber maintainer and an Anis cannula with a 0.4-mm port.

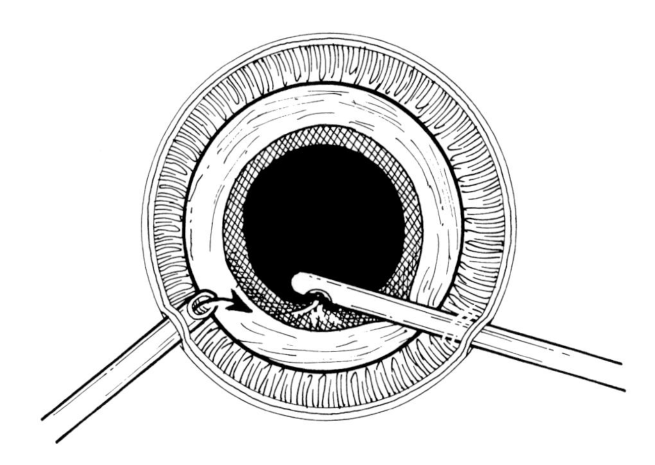

FIGURE 24-5 Elective posterior capsulotomy and anterior vitrectomy using a chamber maintainer and a guillotine-type vitrectomy probe.

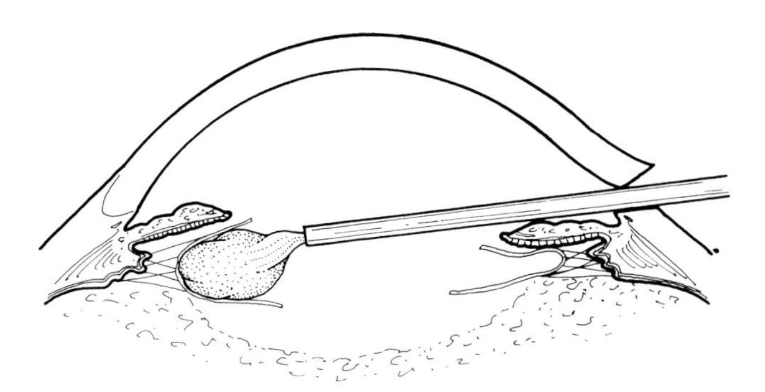

FIGURE 24-6 Viscoelastic is injected into the bag fornices (side view).

injected into the bag fornices (Figures 24-6 and 24-7). The corneolimbal wound is enlarged to allow insertion of the IOL. The limbal wounds are closed with tight interrupted sutures to prevent dehiscence of the wound, which is a common postoperative complication in children. The viscoelastic material in the anterior chamber is aspirated and replaced with BSS.

Surgical Technique for Cataracts in Children Older Than 2 Years of Age

The surgical preparation and technique for cataract extraction and posterior chamber IOL implantation in children older than 2 years is similar to standard adult procedures performed by one of the authors (HVG). Currently advocated is a limbal-based conjunctival flap, scleral tunnel incision, capsulorhexis under viscoelastic material, and irrigation-aspiration of the cataract material using the phacoemulsification handpiece or an irrigation-aspiration handpiece, or both. After an IOL is placed in the capsular bag, a posterior capsulorhexis and possibly an anterior vitrectomy (if vitreous herniates despite the viscoelastic material) are performed if the child is younger than 6 years of age. The posterior capsulotomy is performed using the technique of PCCC. Capture of the IOL optic through the circular opening in the posterior capsule without performing a vitrectomy may also be considered. A more detailed description of these techniques follows, with emphasis on particular differences from the standard adult procedure.

RECTUS SUTURE AND CONJUNCTIVAL INCISION

A lid speculum is placed over a sterile drape, and a superior rectus suture is secured. A limbal-based conjunctival flap is made, and cautery is used to control bleeding from episcleral vessels.

PARACENTESIS INCISION

A small, long-tunnel paracentesis incision is made temporally at the limbus through which a 0.5-mm cyclodialysis spatula and a 30-gauge cannula may be passed. Use of a second instrument may be helpful for breaking anterior synechiae and for assisting in the placement of an IOL. Because it is essential in children to remove all cortical material to reduce the incidence of postoperative inflammation and secondary cataract formation, the paracentesis can often aid in removal of cortical remnants at the 12 o'clock position. This is performed by using a bent 30-gauge cannula to strip cortex from the capsular bag (Figure 24-8).

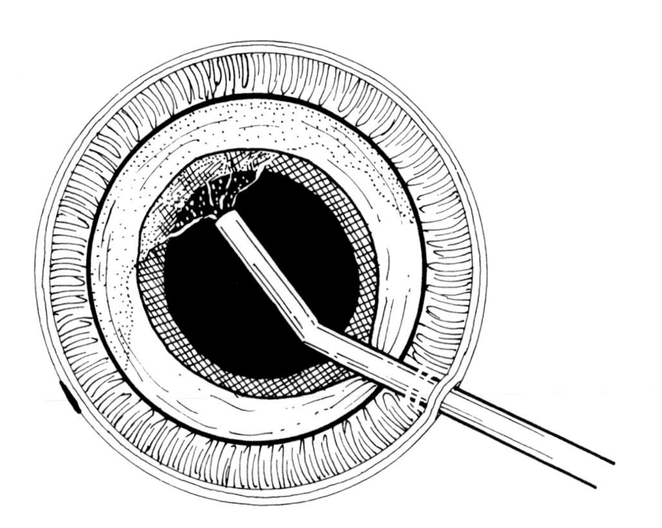

FIGURE 24-7 Viscoelastic is injected into the bag fornices.

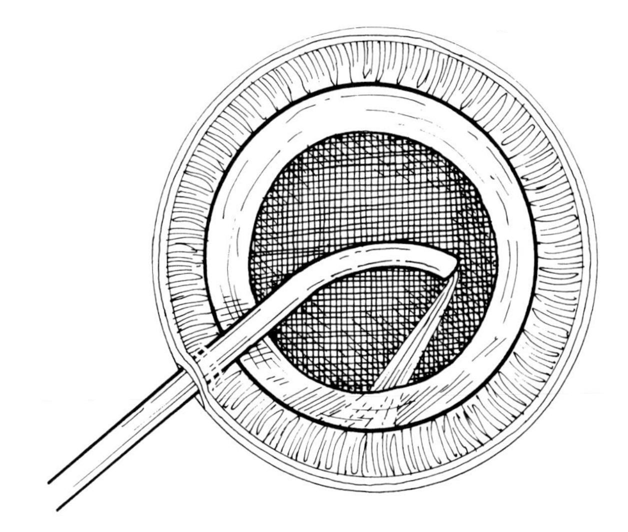

FIGURE 24-8 A 30-gauge cannula is passed through the paracentesis incision to strip adherent cortex at 12 o'clock location.

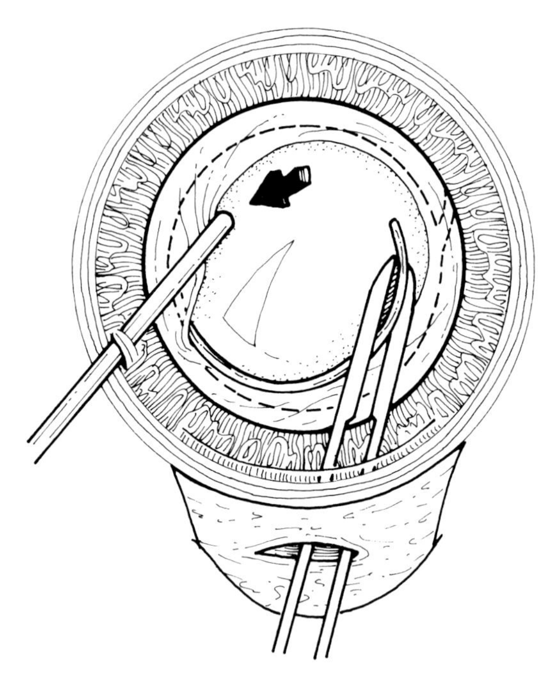

FIGURE 24-9 Use of second instrument through paracentesis incision to facilitate lens implantation.

Because there is a tendency in pediatric patients for the paracentesis to leak, some surgeons attempt to eliminate its use. Most pediatric lenses are soft and can be aspirated using a one-handed technique. Even if this technique is used, however, a paracentesis may still facilitate lens implantation (Figure 24-9) and removal of cortical debris. A paracentesis is also necessary to re-form the anterior chamber and test the seal of the main incision.

LIMBAL INCISION

The sclera in a young child is elastic, encouraging the use of the smallest possible incision, which also helps to prevent iris prolapse. A small scleral scratch incision is made approximately 2.5 mm from the limbus and is dissected as a 3.0-mm or 5.5- to 6.5-mm wide scleral tunnel, depending on the IOL selected, using a crescent blade (Figures 24-10 and 24-11). Viscoelastic material is placed in the anterior chamber to maintain anterior chamber depth.

CAPSULORHEXIS

Achieving an intact and identifiable continuous capsular rim with the CCC technique is an important step in pediatric implantation procedures because it facilitates lens extraction and ensures in-the-bag placement of the IOL. A high-viscosity viscoelastic, preferably Healon GV or Healon 5, is used to counteract the intralenticular forces that cause the CCC to tend to turn toward the equator. CCC may be achieved using a bent needle, cystotome, or forceps. A forceps is often necessary for control of the elastic capsule encountered in children. Because of the increased elasticity of the pediatric capsule,[133] any discontinuity that occurs in the rim during a capsulotomy can easily extend as a tear out to the equator. When this happens, the edges of the capsule may retract, making it extremely difficult to ascertain with confidence that the lens loops are positioned in the capsular bag. Also, anterior capsule tears that extend into the posterior capsule present the greatest intraoperative challenge for nucleus removal, and they compromise in-the-bag or even sulcus IOL placement.

When attempting CCC in a pediatric patient, the tip of an irrigating cystotome, bent needle, or capsulorhexis forceps is used to make a small central puncture (Figure 24-12). The elastic pediatric lens capsule requires a distinct pressure point to achieve a central puncture. Once the central puncture is made, the cystotome guides the tear radially out to the periphery at the 3 o'clock position (Figure 24-13). If the tear is not easily guided because of the elasticity of the capsule, forceps are used to grasp at the leading edge of the tear (Figure 24-14). To overcome the stretchability of the capsule, several repeated grasps at the leading edge of the tear are recommended for maximal control of the tear. With these small regrasping maneuvers at the leading edge of the tear, capsulorhexis is directed to achieve the desired diameter. Viscoelastic material is added as required. The capsulorhexis should be kept as small as possible because

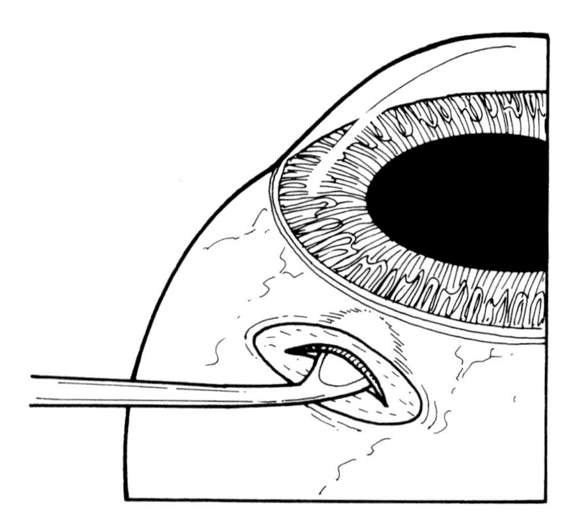

FIGURE 24-10 Scleral tunnel incision (technique).

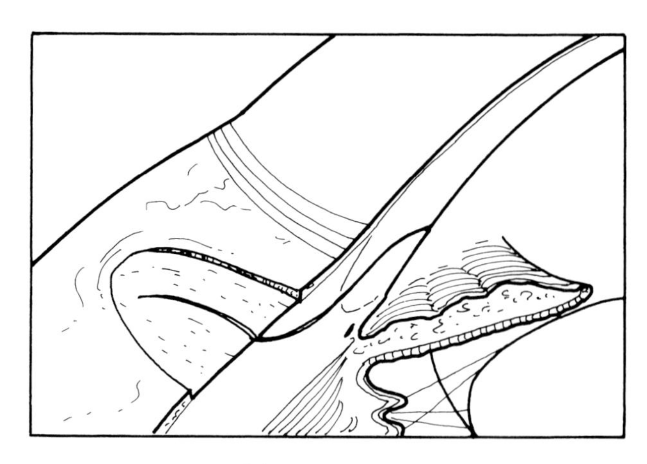

FIGURE 24-11 Scleral tunnel incision (cross-sectional view).

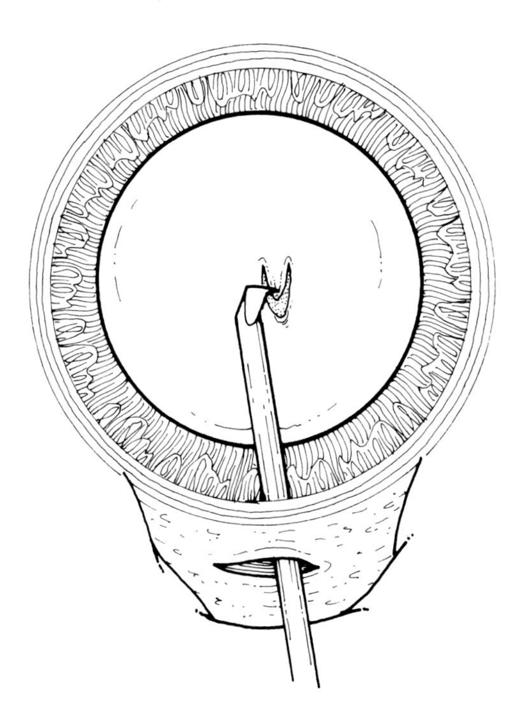

FIGURE 24-12 Cystotome makes a central puncture in anterior capsule.

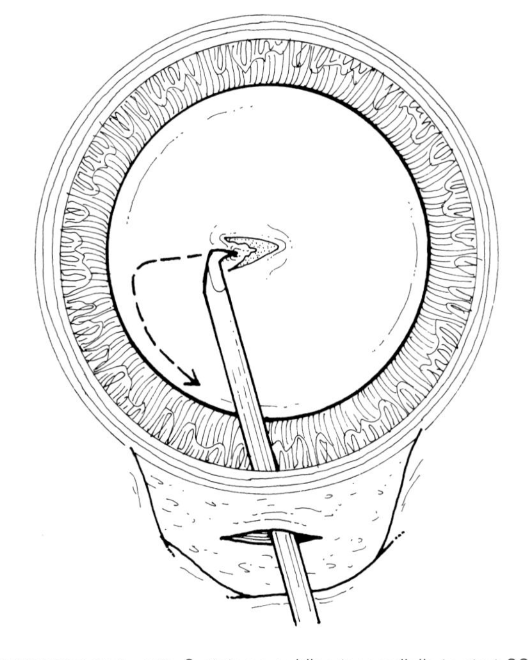

FIGURE 24-13 Cystotome guiding tear radially to start CCC.

the elasticity of the child's lens capsule can create a capsular opening that is larger than expected or desired. The pediatric capsule acts like a thin rubber sheet that retracts toward the periphery after anterior capsulotomy. This elasticity necessitates frequent regrasping of the leading edge of the capsular tear with careful observation and direction of vector forces to ensure that radial extensions are prevented. During capsulorhexis, the internal pressure or anterior chamber depth must be well maintained by injecting a viscous viscoelastic agent such as Healon GV or Healon 5.

If the cataract is intumescent, a sharp needle is used to make the central puncture in the capsule (Figure 24-15), and any liquid cortex is aspirated before capsulorhexis (Figure 24-16). If poor visualization prevents a CCC from being performed, a can-opener capsulotomy is best achieved using several small bites with a needle or a cystotome (Figure 24-17). Liquid lens

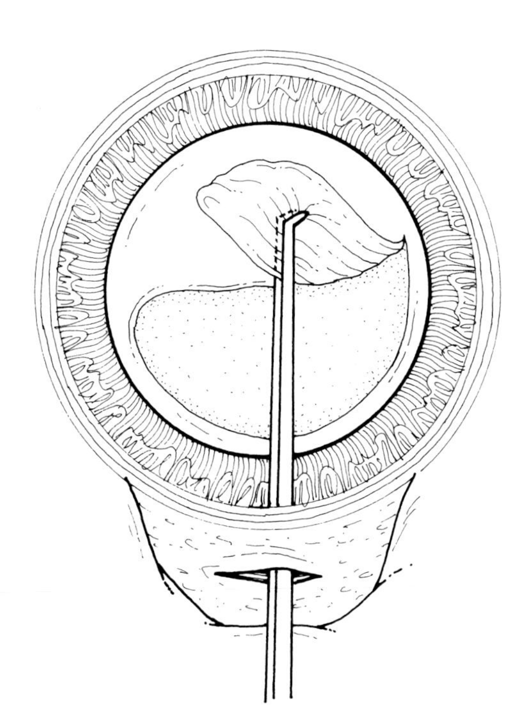

FIGURE 24-14 Capsulorhexis forceps is used for better control of progressing curvilinear tear.

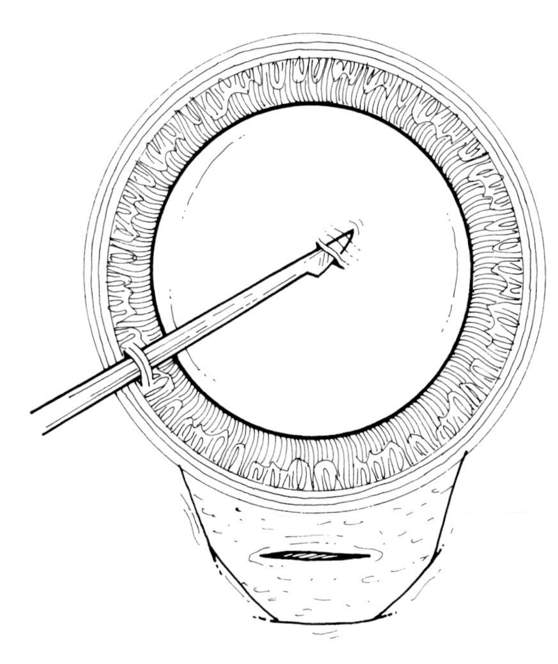

FIGURE 24-15 Sharp needle is used to make central puncture in anterior capsule of intumescent lens.

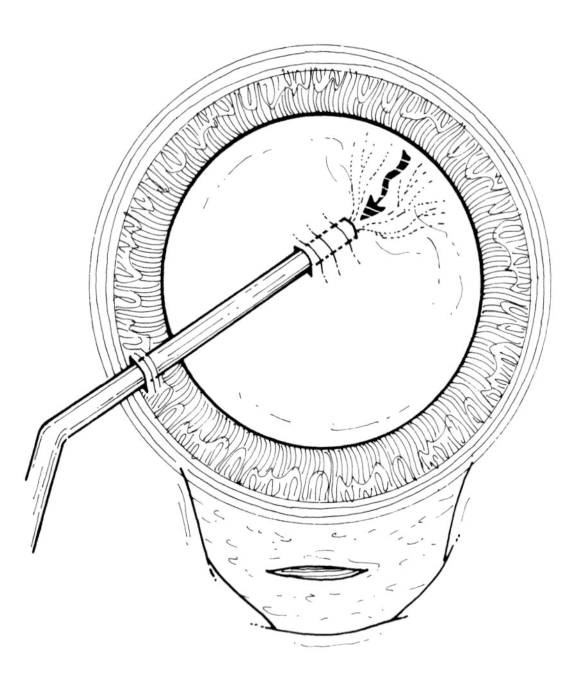

FIGURE 24-16 Liquid cortex is aspirated from capsular bag of intumescent lens.

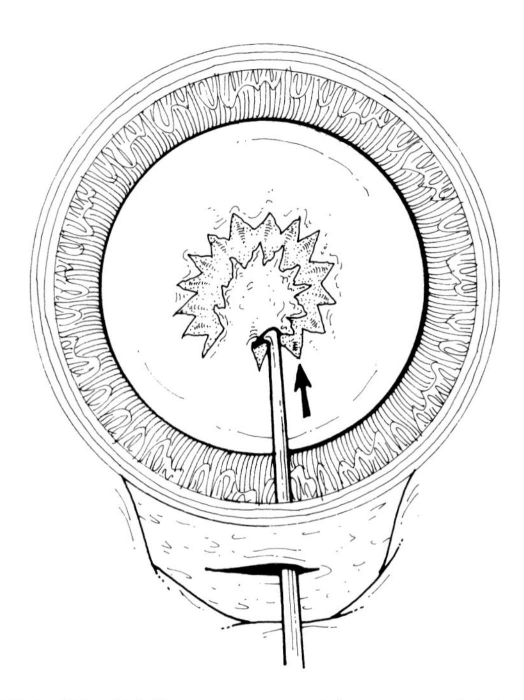

FIGURE 24-17 Can-opener capsulotomy necessitated by poor visualization in intumescent lens.

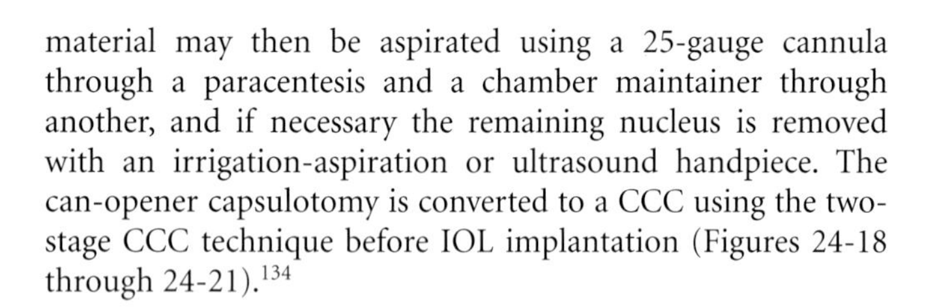

material may then be aspirated using a 25-gauge cannula through a paracentesis and a chamber maintainer through another, and if necessary the remaining nucleus is removed with an irrigation-aspiration or ultrasound handpiece. The can-opener capsulotomy is converted to a CCC using the two-stage CCC technique before IOL implantation (Figures 24-18 through 24-21).[134]

IRRIGATION-ASPIRATION AND ULTRASOUND

Aspiration of the lenticular material can often be performed in pediatric patients with the irrigation-aspiration handpiece alone through a limbal incision. Harder nuclei may require short bursts of ultrasound energy using the phacoemulsification handpiece. Most nuclei are too soft to be fractured, and the maneuver can be performed using the one-handed technique.

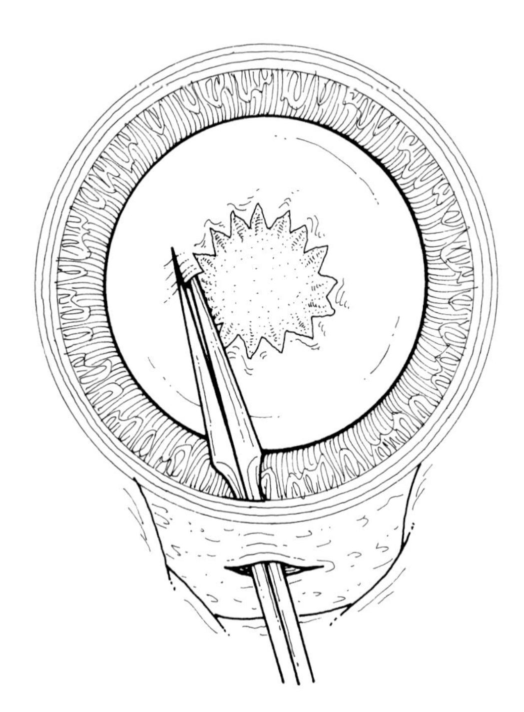

FIGURE 24-18 A scissor cut begins the two-stage CCC technique to convert can-opener capsulotomy to CCC.

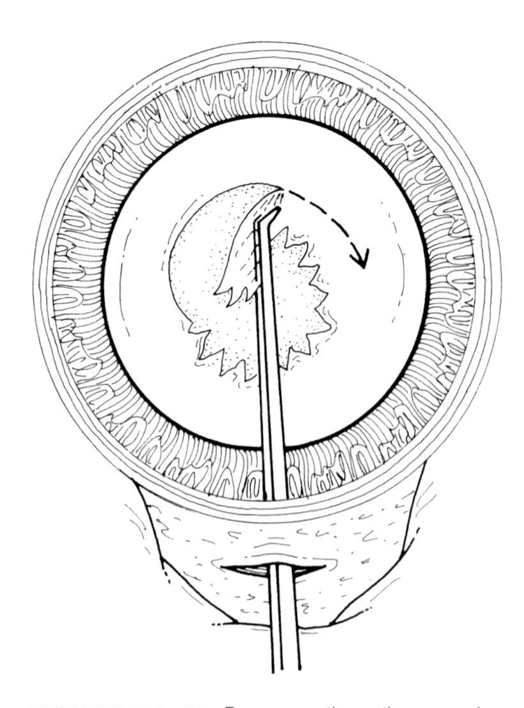

FIGURE 24-19 Forceps continues the conversion.

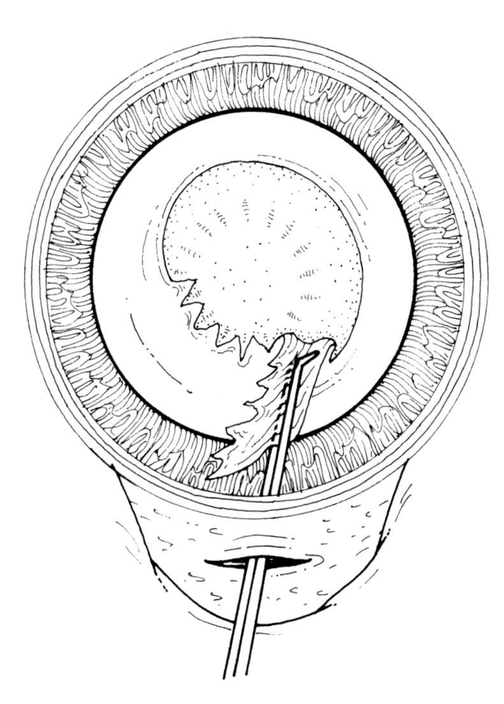

FIGURE 24-20 CCC progresses.

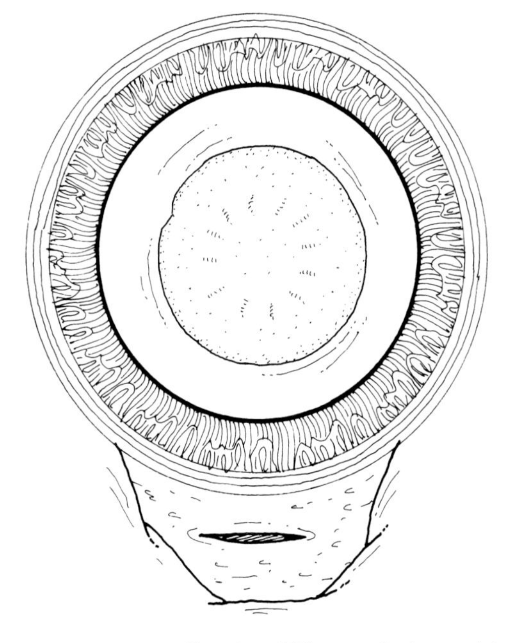

FIGURE 24-21 Two-stage CCC conversion is completed.

INTRAOCULAR LENS IMPLANTATION

Foldable acrylic is the preferred IOL for implantation. Often a 5.5- or 6-mm diameter IOL is implanted through an approximate 3.5-mm incision. Also, one-piece biconvex ultraviolet-blocking polymethylmethacrylate IOLs with an overall diameter between 10.5 and 12 mm and with an optic diameter between 5.5 and 6.5 may be used. Heparin-coated IOLs may be advantageous in decreasing the intense postoperative inflammatory response often seen in pediatric patients.

Recently, multifocal IOLs have been recommended for pediatric implants with potential benefits of compensation for presbyopia, functional vision over a broader range of distances, and greater spectacle independence.[135] Patient satisfaction was high, and visual function remained within acceptable levels in this study of 35 eyes of 26 pediatric patients aged 2 to 14 years of age. Posterior capsulotomy was performed in 68% of patients and was mostly accompanied by anterior vitrectomy and posterior optic capture.

Some concerns with the placement of multifocal IOLs in children include centration problems. IOL power calculations, the use of silicone IOLs, the amblyopiagenic effect of multiple overlapping images and decreased contrast, and the tolerability of glare.[136] Caution should be used when considering the insertion of multifocal IOLs in children outside of research protocols at the present time.

POSTERIOR CONTINUOUS CURVILINEAR CAPSULORHEXIS

A planned primary posterior capsule opening, created in an attempt either to prevent inevitable secondary cataract formation (in children younger than 6 years of age) or to remove a posterior plaque, should be achieved using the PCCC technique. PCCC can also be used as a method to prevent extension of a tear when a small linear or triangular posterior capsular rupture inadvertently occurs. Posterior capsulorhexis requires the use of viscoelastic agents and may be performed before or after posterior chamber IOL in-the-bag implantation.[137]

In creating a primary posterior capsule opening in pediatric eyes, PCCC is started by using a cystotome or bent needle to make a small central puncture in the posterior capsule (Figure 24-22). Healon GV or Healon 5 is injected through the opening. The circular tear is accomplished by using CCC principles and strategies. Additional viscoelastic material is placed through the

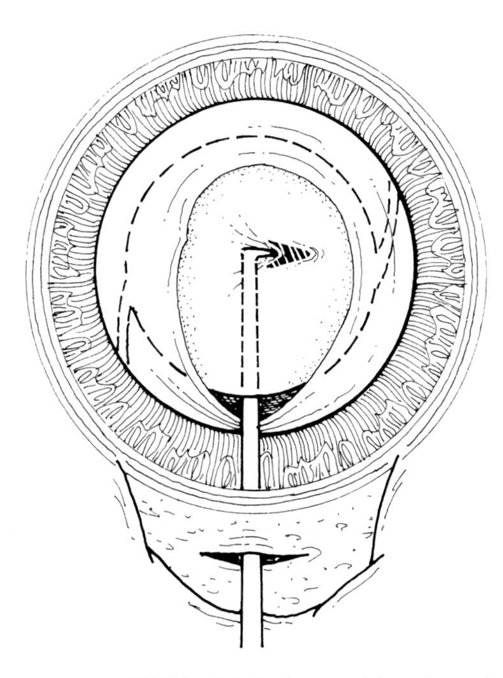

FIGURE 24-22 PCCC is started using a cystotome to create a central puncture of the posterior capsule posterior to the posterior chamber IOL.

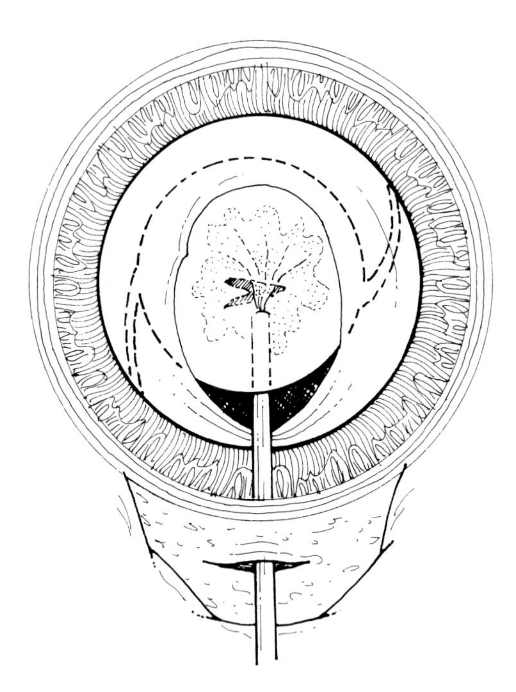

FIGURE 24-23 Viscoelastic is placed through the posterior capsule opening to push vitreous humor posteriorly

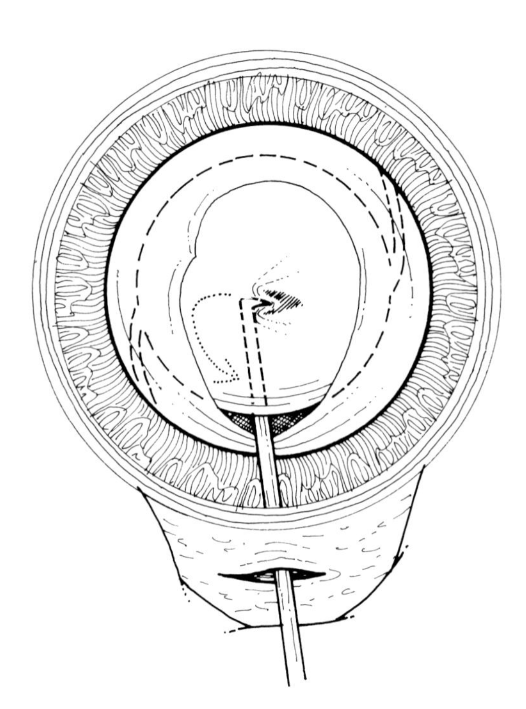

FIGURE 24-24 PCCC is extended toward 3 o'clock; this technique is similar to that used with CCC.

central puncture of the posterior capsule to push the vitreous face away (Figure 24-23). Care should be taken so that the viscoelastic agent does not push the flap posteriorly, thus making it difficult to grasp the posterior capsule tag. Also, if too much viscoelastic material is pushed through the opening, it may extend the tear in an unpredictable fashion. The tear is directed radially to the 3 o'clock position before being turned and continued counterclockwise for 360 degrees (Figure 24-24). Optional control of the progressing tear in the posterior capsule is achieved by using elongated Kelman-McPherson or pointed capsulorhexis forceps. The capsule flap is grasped near the point of tearing, and the tear is turned in the desired direction (Figure 24-25). The end result should be a well-centered PCCC concentric to and smaller than the CCC (Figure 24-26).

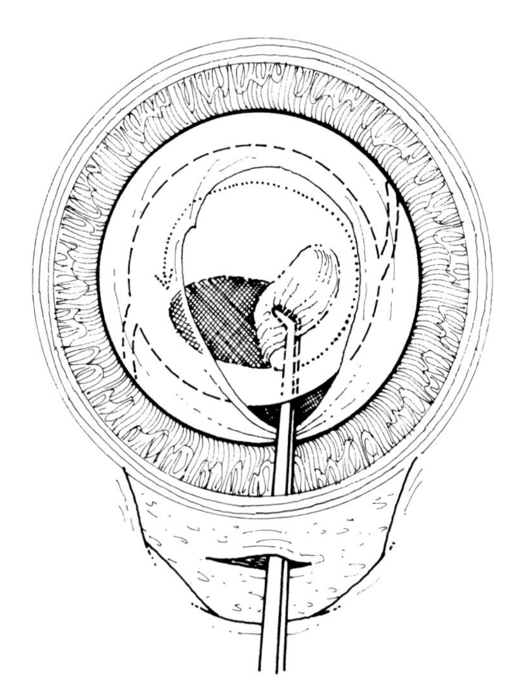

FIGURE 24-25 Capsule forceps are used for better control in directing and completing PCCC.

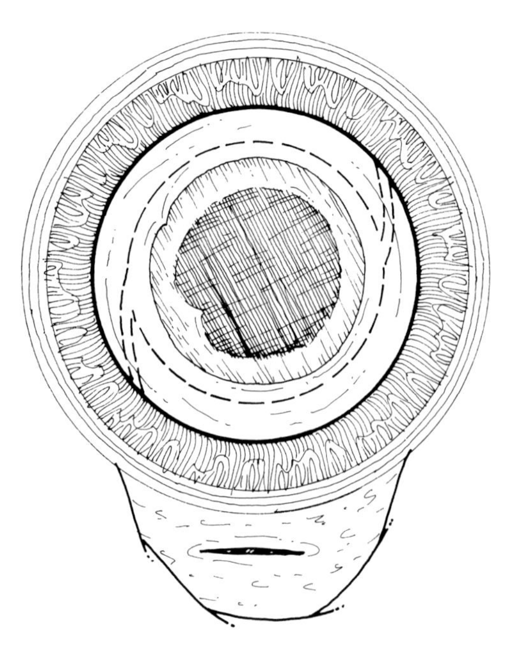

FIGURE 24-26 Well-centered PCCC, concentric and smaller than the CCC.

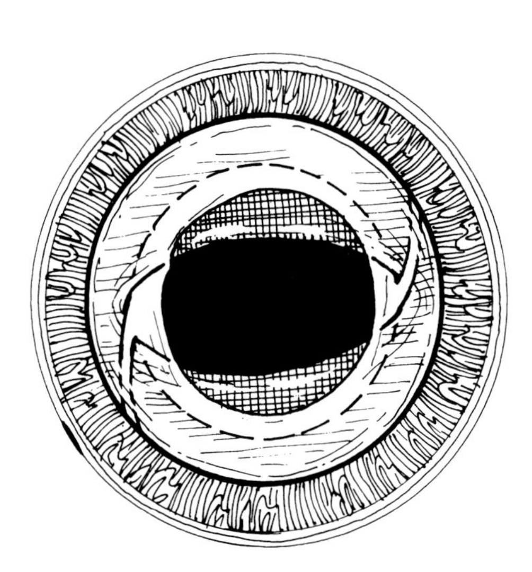

FIGURE 24-27 Posterior capsulorhexis with optic capture.

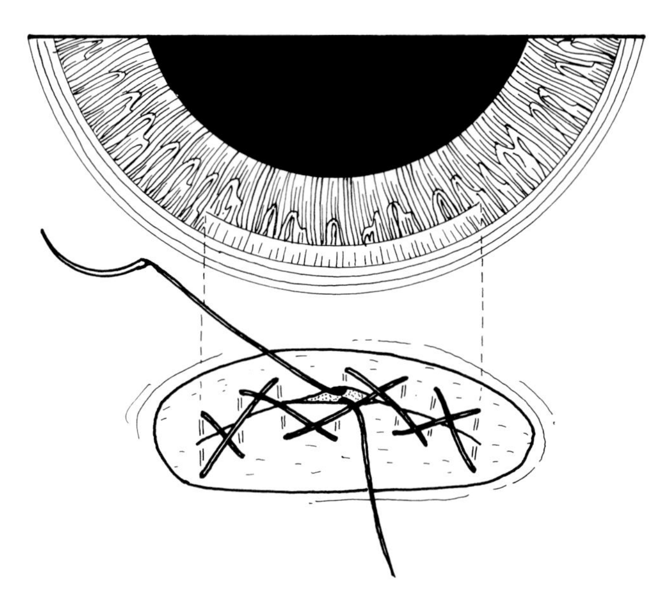

FIGURE 24-28 Shoelace suturing techniques.

POSTERIOR CAPSULE CAPTURE

Posterior capture of the IOL optic may be carried out after suturing of the scleral wound but before the viscoelastic material is removed. Under and through the viscoelastic, the IOL optic is slipped inferiorly and then superiorly through the PCCC by means of a spatula or cannula (Figure 24-27). Viscoelastic material behind the IOL is left in place, whereas that remaining in the anterior chamber is slowly and carefully removed. Simultaneous irrigation of BSS is performed while aspirating the viscoelastic material to maintain a deep chamber and prevent vitreous and the IOL from moving forward. An anterior vitrectomy may be necessary if vitreous herniates at the time of PCCC.

Posterior capsulorhexis with posterior capsular optic capture is a technically challenging procedure. The posterior capsule is thinner than the anterior capsule, adding to the difficulty of achieving a circular opening that is small and concentric to the pupil. In order to have a well-positioned posterior capsulorhexis captured optic, the PCCC must be well centered. The vaulting of the intraocular optic through the PCCC requires cautious manipulation as the posterior capsule is thin. The PCCC seems to have the same stretching capacity as the anterior CCC.[60,86] The disadvantage of this technique is that it requires skill to avoid peripheral tears in the posterior capsule, which could destroy the integrity of the capsular bag. In addition, the safety and long-term efficacy of the procedure have yet to be established.

CLOSURE

Scleral closure of a 5.5- to 6-mm incision for one-piece IOLs usually involves the continuous shoelace suturing technique or a combination of continuous and horizontal sutures using either absorbable or permanent sutures (Figure 24-28). Small incisions for foldable IOLs may still require a suture in very young eyes to obtain a watertight closure or to ensure that the wound does not reopen with blinking or eye rubbing. Currently, the most popular suture material for closing corneoscleral incisions in children is 10-0 nylon, followed by 7-0 polyglactin.[138] One or more interrupted 10-0 nylon sutures may be required to close the paracentesis site. Conjunctival incisions are closed with 9-0 or 10-0 Vicryl. No peripheral iridectomy is performed unless the IOL is placed in the sulcus. The chamber is redeepened after scleral closure, and the wound is checked for water tightness. The internal portion of the wound is also checked for gaping or fish-mouthing with a sterile Posner gonioscopy mirror (Figure 24-29). Full-thickness corneal sutures of 10-0 nylon are placed as necessary to close the internal wound (Figure 24-30). The viscoelastic material is replaced with BSS, and the conjunctiva is closed with an absorbable running suture knotted under the conjunctiva or with interrupted sutures. Conjunctival closure may include a running temporary absorbable or nonabsorbable suture, which is left untied.

Postoperative Treatment

Postoperatively, a child's eye tends to react with more inflammation than that of an adult.[2,68,139,140] The inflammatory response can usually be managed well with intensive topical steroid therapy and cycloplegic drops. After cataract surgery in

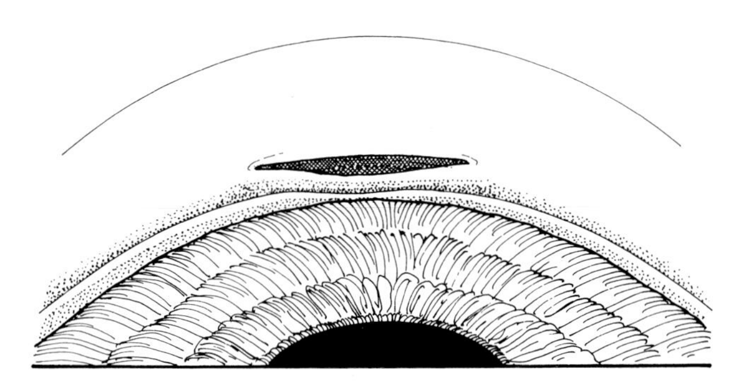

FIGURE 24-29 Internal would demonstrating fish-mouthing.

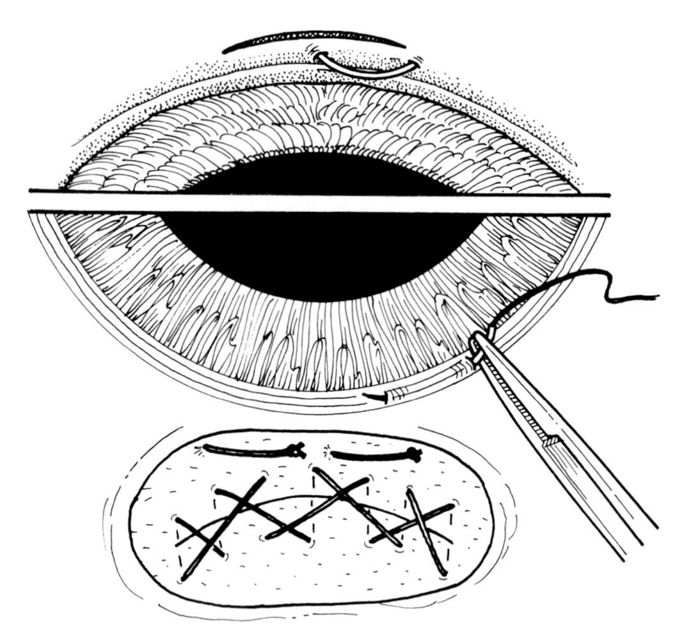

FIGURE 24-30 Suture technique for repair of fish-mouthing of internal wound.

infants, topical steroids and antibiotic drops should be administered four times a day. The pupils are dilated with atropine, which is gradually tapered off over the ensuing weeks. By 4 to 6 weeks postoperatively, the child is no longer receiving any eye medication. Suture removal is performed within 2 to 3 months postoperatively using general anesthesia. The refractive status can be evaluated at the same time. Amblyopia treatment starts within a week postoperatively when the media is clear. Close follow-up by a pediatric ophthalmologist is mandatory until the patient is 10 years of age.

Postoperative treatment in children older than 2 years of age should begin immediately at the end of surgery with the instillation of a combination ointment of antibiotic and corticosteroids. Atropine (1%) or homatropine (5%) is also instilled, and the eye is patched until the child fully recovers from the anesthesia. Cycloplegia is continued for up to 1 month after surgery to minimize fibrin deposition.[25] Also, corticosteroid drops are used postoperatively on a tapering schedule for up to 3 months.

In both infants and children, the peak inflammatory reaction does not appear until a day or two after surgery. The surgeon should not be deceived by a very quiet eye the first day after surgery but should remain vigilant in the management of postoperative inflammation in pediatric patients. Because the inflammatory response may be subtle, with few symptoms and only mild ciliary congestion, frequent postoperative visits are recommended.[62] Postoperative synechiae formation is also possible, even though the eye may appear to be quiet. The Nd:YAG laser may be used to break up fibrin strands and to disperse anterior and posterior keratoprecipitates on the IOL.

Despite recent advances in pediatric surgical techniques, inadequate preoperative evaluation and postoperative treatment of amblyopia may limit the ultimate visual success in pediatric cases, especially those involving monocular cataract.[140-143] Vigorous occlusion therapy is instituted as early as possible in all cases of unilateral cataract extraction in infancy. Alternate patching may be recommended in patients with bilateral correction.

Complications

Posterior Capsule Opacity

Posterior capsule opacification is one of the most serious complications because it can lead to irreversible deprivation amblyopia caused by the insidious formation of retropseudophakic membranes. The management and prevention of secondary cataracts, including the proposal of a new technique, were discussed in the section Review of Pediatric Surgical Techniques.

Endophthalmitis

Endophthalmitis is the most serious eye complication after surgery. The incidence has been reported to be 0.07%, which is similar to that reported in the adult population.[144] This complication is the strongest argument against synchronous bilateral surgery in children with bilateral cataracts.[145] Absolute sterility must be maintained and excellent wound closure achieved. Upper respiratory tract infection and nasolacrimal duct obstruction should be treated before cataract surgery.[145] Careful follow-up of the patient is necessary to observe for any signs of infection, especially in cases of cataracts induced by trauma. Because children and infants are often unable to appreciate or recognize the importance of sudden decreased vision, careful follow-up is essential.

Wound Leak

Children often rub their eyes and are involved in activities of physical contact that can lead to eye trauma. It is important to tightly suture the wound and have the child wear an eye shield until the wound is well healed.

Glaucoma

If excessive inflammation occurs, causing extensive peripheral anterior synechiae, or if pupillary block leads to iris bombé, an acute rise in intraocular pressure may occur. It is important to control postoperative inflammation as much as possible to prevent this sequela. Also, certain eye diseases are associated with both cataracts and glaucoma (e.g., Lowe syndrome and congenital rubella). Open-angle glaucoma develops in 3% to 41% of eyes after surgery for congenital or developmental cataracts. Placement of an IOL may lead to lower rates of postoperative glaucoma than that observed with aphakia.[146]

Strabismus

Strabismus is the most common complication following pediatric cataract extraction.[17] The interruption of fusion caused by the lens opacification and possible anisometropia and aniseikonia that follows aphakic correction leads to a 66% to 86% incidence of strabismus in children who are treated for cataracts.[147,148] Approximately one quarter of pediatric patients undergoing cataract surgery may require strabismus surgery.[17]

Amblyopia

Amblyopia is more often associated with monocular than bilateral cataracts. Occlusion therapy during the postoperative period is essential.

Nystagmus

The presence of nystagmus indicates poor vision resulting from sensory deprivation[13] and usually will be present if a congenital cataract is not removed by the fourth month of life. If nystagmus is present, the best visual acuity after cataract surgery will usually be less than 20/50.

Retinal Detachment

The incidence of retinal detachment after pediatric cataract surgery has been found to be between 1% and 1.5%.[96,149] With older techniques such as lens needling, the incidence was as high as 10%.[150] Although the pathogenesis of retinal detachment in pseudophakic patients is not fully understood, secondary changes of the vitreoretinal interface may be an important factor.[151,152] Retinal detachment may occur many years after surgery. The mean age in one series was 31.9 years.[153]

Challenges

Small Pupil

Even with mydriatics such as 1% cyclopentolate and 2.5% phenylephrine, the pupils of children, especially infants, may remain small. This is especially true with cataracts caused by rubella.[92] Difficulties in performing CCC may be encountered with small pupils. A smooth-edged capsular border can be made larger than the diameter of the small pupil by guiding the tear under the iris while observing the folded edge of the capsular flap. To improve visualization during this procedure, the surgeon may stretch the iris in the quadrant of the advancing tear by using the shaft of the cystotome or a bent needle or by using a second instrument such as a cyclodialysis spatula (Figure 24-31).[154] If emulsification of the cataract is necessary, it should be performed in the central part of the small pupil where visualization is adequate and where the risk of touching the iris or capsule with the tip of the instrument is minimized.

Maintaining the Intraocular Lens Centration

A precise CCC that preserves the architecture of the capsular bag is proving to be one of the most important advances in small-incision cataract and lens implantation surgery, including pediatric cases. The CCC technique increases the probability of safe and secure in-the-bag IOL placement because it maintains the relative integrity of the capsular bag. The visible, flexible rim of CCC always makes it possible to verify the placement of IOL haptics within the bag and therefore guarantees centration (Figure 24-32). Performing CCC in the pediatric population is more challenging than in adults because of the elastic nature of the child's capsule and zonules. Because of the zonules' elasticity, centration of the CCC may be deceiving. It may be necessary to release the forceps from the anterior capsule as the tear is progressing to allow the lens to assume its natural position. Reinspection is important to ascertain if the tear is progressing in a manner that will create a central capsulorhexis opening.

Late decentration of in-the-bag posterior chamber IOL implants is a potential problem with pediatric lens implants. Some contraction of the bag always occurs postoperatively,

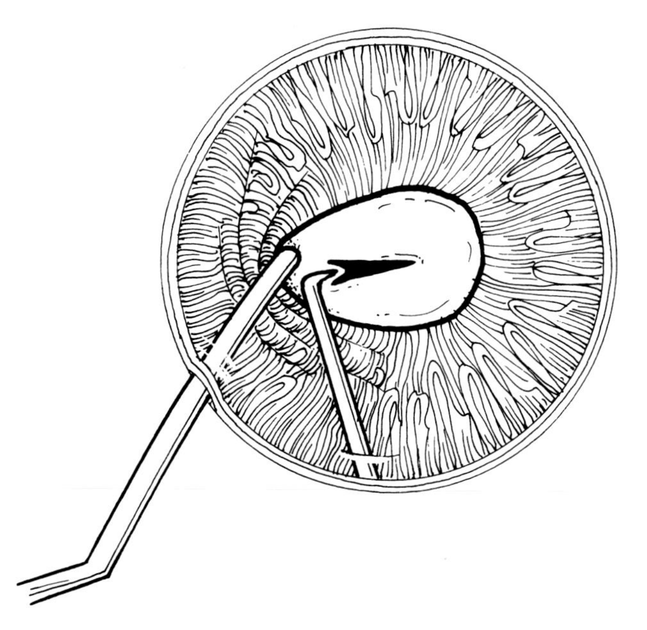

FIGURE 24-31 Improving visualization for CCC in a small pupil case by stretching the iris with a second instrument.

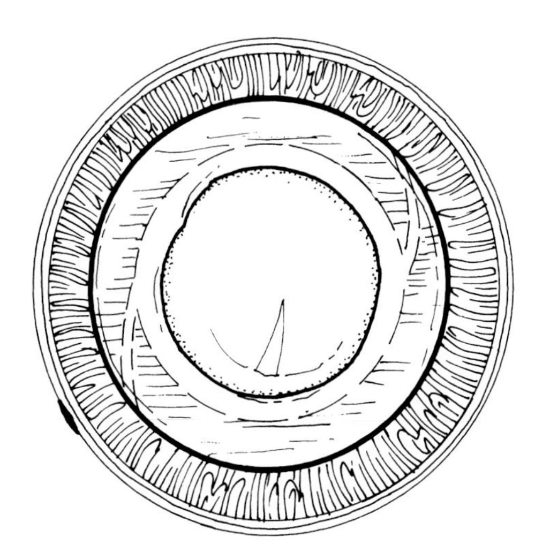

FIGURE 24-32 CCC ensures centration and verification of the IOL haptics in the bag.

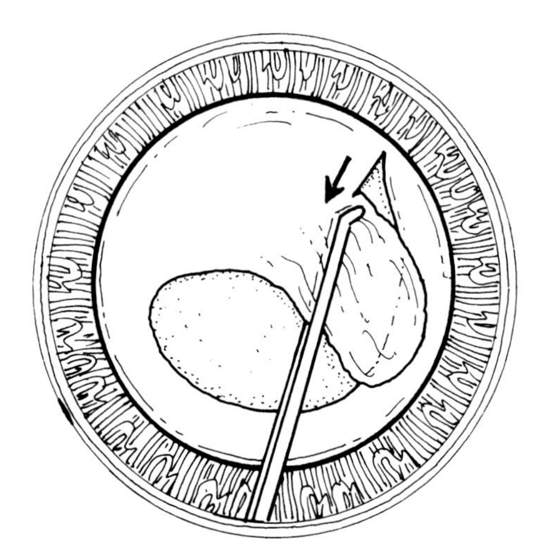

FIGURE 24-33 Turning back a radial extension of the CCC tear.

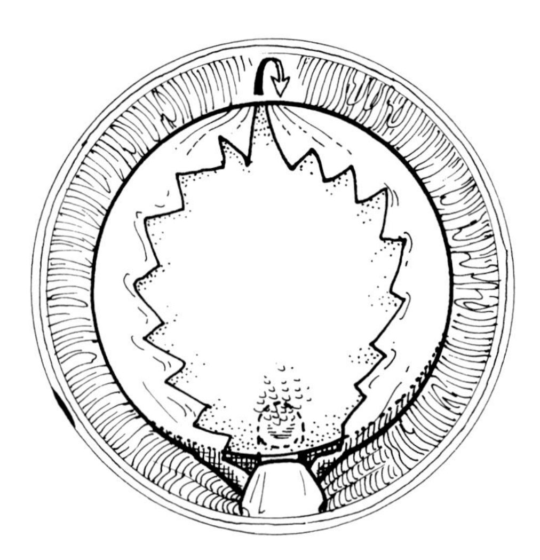

FIGURE 24-34 Pressure during phacoemulsification in the presence of an anterior capsular radial tear causing extension of the tear.

primarily along the torn edge of the anterior capsule because of fibrous metaplasia of lens epithelial cells and the subsequent contracture of the fibrous membrane attached to the capsule. Anterior capsulectomy techniques, such as the can-opener capsulotomy, the Christmas tree technique, the scissors technique, or any opening that has edge discontinuity, increase the chances of an asymmetric contracture of the rim. Uneven tension on the capsular bag and zonules results. Significant decentration is likely to occur if one loop is in the bag and the other is in the sulcus. With CCC, the contracture is symmetric if the capsular opening is circular, central, and smaller than the optic of the IOL.

If a short anterior capsule tear occurs in the pediatric anterior capsule CCC border without extension to the equator, it can be blunted or turned back toward the CCC by using forceps (Figure 24-33). The opening will be eccentric, but the smooth continuous rim prevents radial extensions of tears in elastic pediatric capsules. If a longer anterior capsule tear occurs, care must be taken during cataract removal to prevent excessive pressure that could extend the tear past the equator and into the posterior capsule (Figure 24-34). In such cases, the irrigation-aspiration or ultrasound should be carried out with the handpiece kept centrally over the capsulotomy, avoiding stress to the anterior capsule rim. The irrigation-aspiration should be slow with fewer movements for vacuuming of cortical material. Careful selection of IOL design is important in the presence of an anterior capsule tear; one-piece C-loop designs and IOLs no longer than 11 mm cause the least capsular stress.

When an anterior capsule tear occurs, viscoelastic agents may be useful to help avoid an extension around to the posterior capsule during IOL insertion. However, the viscoelastic agent should be injected carefully, adding a little above and then below the torn edge to sandwich it within the viscoelastic material. If the capsular bag is filled without significant viscoelastic material above the capsule, the pressure within the bag can extend the tear. The IOL haptics should be oriented perpendicular to the tear. In addition, the anterior capsule tear should be matched by creating a second anterior capsule tear 180 degrees away from the first. This precaution ensures symmetric tension on the anterior capsule rim as the capsule contracts postoperatively (Figure 24-35). Consistent in-the-bag IOL centration can be achieved by analyzing the configuration and location of anterior capsule defects.

Anterior Capsule Ring Contracture

Although there are multiple advantages of CCC, there is one potential complication peculiar to the technique. In adults with weakened zonules or after trauma in any age-group, significant contraction of the capsule may occur along the edge of the tear a few months postoperatively. Unlike the situation after irregularly torn capsulotomies, this contracture rarely leads to any significant degree of IOL decentration, as there is usually a symmetric contracture of the CCC. Anterior capsule ring contracture can be released using the Nd:YAG laser. Radial peripheral placement of Nd:YAG pulses in the contracted anterior capsule

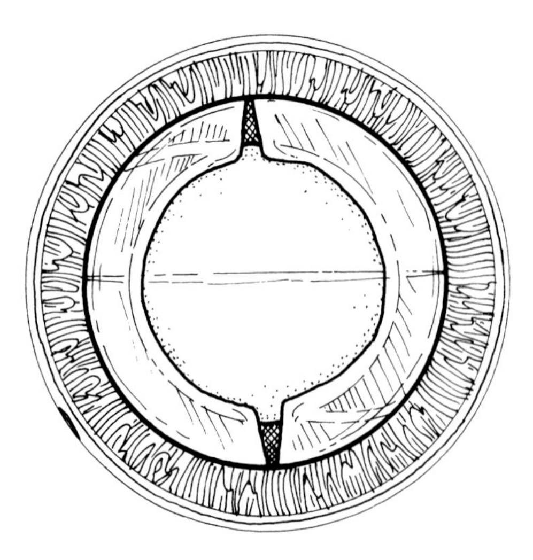

FIGURE 24-35 Anterior capsular tear matched with second anterior capsular tear 180 degrees away to ensure symmetric tension on the anterior capsular rim.

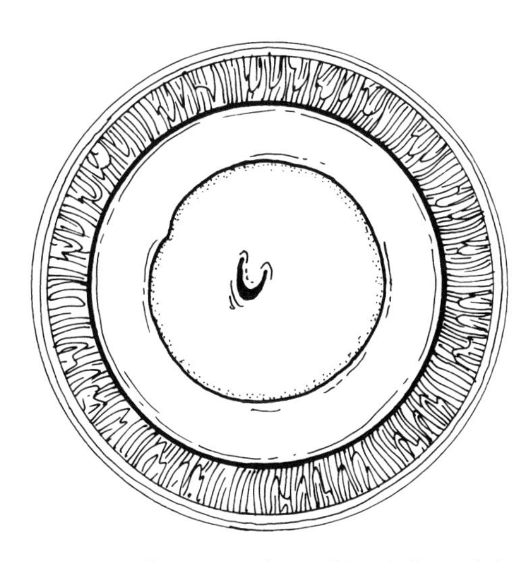

FIGURE 24-36 Appearance of a small tear in the posterior capsule.

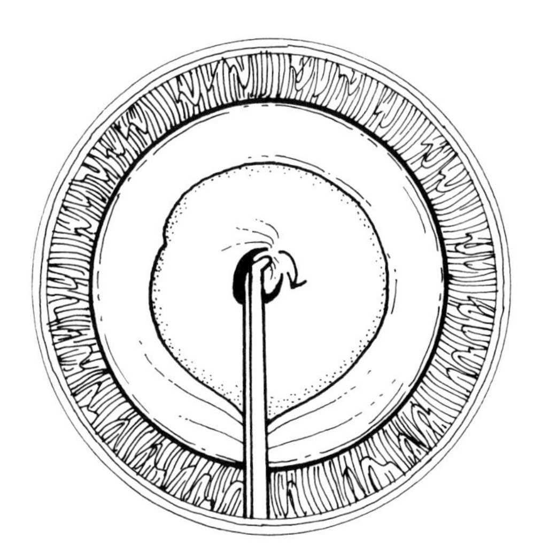

FIGURE 24-37 PCCC technique for blunting small tears in the posterior capsule is identical to anterior CCC.

releases the contracture of the capsule and prevents early or late decentration of the IOL. The Nd:YAG successfully releases this anterior capsule purse-string effect.[44]

Posterior Capsular Tears

PCCC may be employed in the making of a primary posterior capsulectomy as previously described. It may also be used when a small linear or triangular tear inadvertently occurs in the posterior capsule. Even though the posterior capsule is thinner than the anterior capsule, a smooth continuous circular capsulorhexis in the posterior capsule is resistant to radial tears and thus maintains capsular bag integrity.[155] Tears of the posterior capsule that have not extended as far as the capsular equator are candidates of PCCC. The rounding off of a posterior capsule tear or completing it full circle usually prevents extension of the tear, which can frequently occur during anterior vitrectomy or lens placement. Thus PCCC should be performed before anterior vitrectomy or lens insertion when a small posterior capsule tear has occurred. Also, if a stalk of a persistent hyaloid membrane is present, Vannas scissors can be used to sever it after completing PCCC.

The goal is to direct the advancing tear into a circle that encompasses the entire extent of the tear. Alternatively, one or both ends of a linear tear may be rounded and blunted by means of PCCC techniques. For maximal control when redirecting a tear of the posterior capsule, elongated Kelman-McPherson or Kraff-Utrata forceps are used to grasp the capsule flap near one point of the tear and to turn the tear in the desired direction (Figures 24-36 through 24-38). The PCCC is kept as small as possible to preserve maximal integrity of the posterior capsule.

Preexisting Posterior Capsule Defects (Posterior Lentiglobus)

Posterior lentiglobus tends to distort the preoperative retinoscopy reflex—a condition that makes optical correction of refractive errors difficult.[6,156-158] Early detection of these patients is recommended, and cataract extraction should be performed as soon as any decrease in visual acuity occurs that is unamenable to optical correction and amblyopia therapy.[78] Because the posterior capsule in these patients is thinned and weakened centrally, hydrodissection should never be performed, as this can create a posterior capsule rupture. "Hydro-free" fluidless dissection can be used to aid in dissection of the cortex from the capsule before aspiration or phacoemulsification of the lens (Figures 24-39 and 24-40).[159,160]

Preexistent defects or splits in the posterior capsule (as in posterior lentiglobus or perforating trauma) may also be managed by PCCC. Complete PCCC may not be possible, depending on the configuration and extent of the split of the lentiglobus. However, the technique can still be used to round off the points of the leading tears. If one is unable to blunt a slitlike tear, sometimes an IOL may be placed in the bag with its loops perpendicular to the tear. If the IOL is not stable and secure in the capsular bag with this method, it should be removed from the bag and placed in the sulcus. To ensure centration following this maneuver, the optic can then be pushed through the anterior CCC into the bag.[161]

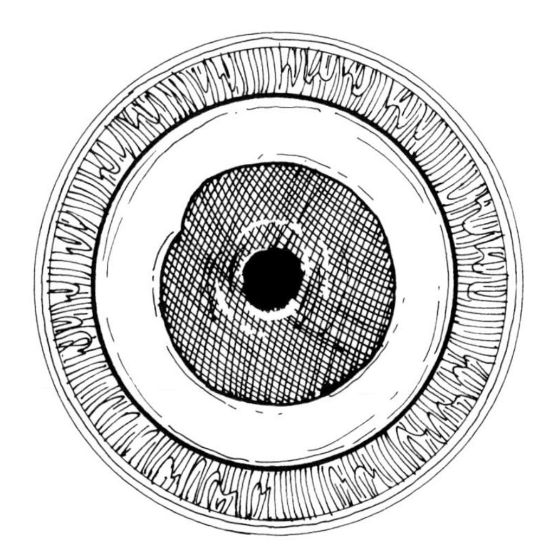

FIGURE 24-38 Posterior tear cannot enlarge after completion of PCCC.

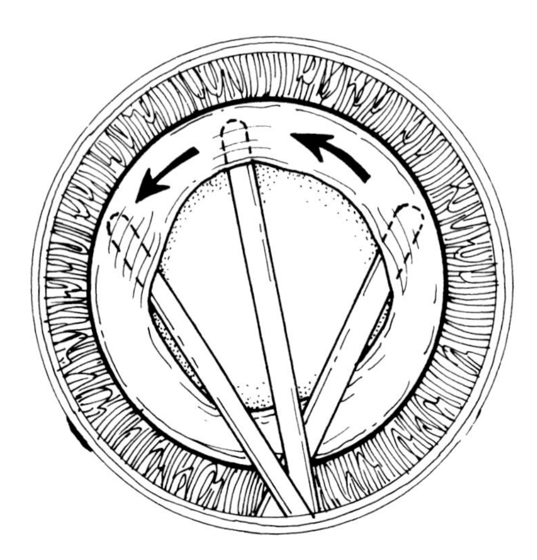

FIGURE 24-39 Hydro-free dissection: achieving dissection of the cortex from the capsule without injecting fluid inferiorly.

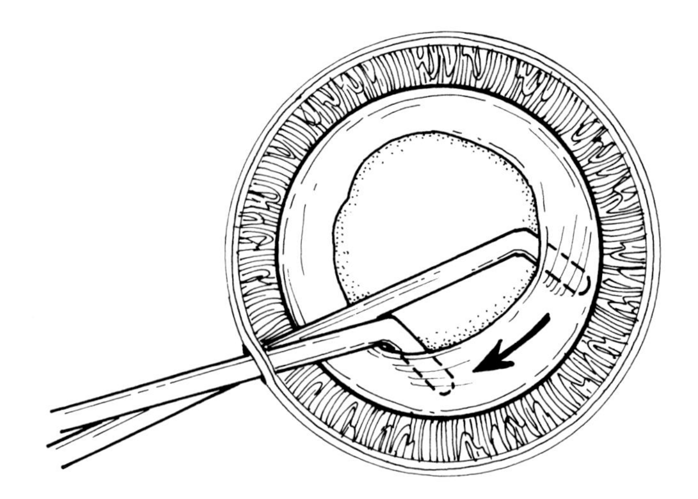

FIGURE 24-40 Hydro-free dissection superiorly through the paracentesis wound.

Posterior Capsule Plaques

PCCC can also be employed for the removal of thickened fibrotic posterior capsule plaques. In these cases, the PCCC is made as a controlled circle that encompasses the central opacity and results in a posterior capsule opening that resists extension to the equator. This capsular opening can be made after the IOL is implanted in the capsular bag. By nudging the IOL eccentrically and slipping a barbed needle on a syringe of viscoelastic material under the lens, PCCC is achieved. This technique was first used in 1987 for the removal of dense plaque from the posterior capsule of a 7-year-old boy who had acquired a cataract secondary to irradiation for rhabdomyosarcoma.[134]

Conclusions

Given the qualities characteristic of children's eyes, pediatric cataract surgery is technically challenging. Tissue elasticity, a propensity for postoperative inflammation, and a high rate of secondary cataract formation are matters of concern. The surgical techniques are more demanding, and there is less room for error. Also, diligent preoperative and postoperative management is essential for satisfactory visual results. The timing of surgery is often crucial to prevent deprivational amblyopia and to attempt the preservation or restoration of binocular vision. The surgeon must be cognizant of the many complications that may occur in pediatric cataract surgery and must be prepared to manage any that arise.

Longer-term follow-up of larger IOL series should continue to support the safety and efficacy of posterior chamber IOL implantation after cataract extraction in infants and children. With continued improvements in surgical and laser techniques, IOL designs, antiinflammatory agents, and amblyopia therapy, the refractive and visual outcomes in pediatric cataract surgery should continue to improve, whereas the need for secondary procedures should diminish.

REFERENCES

1. Maida JW, Sheets JH: Pseudophakia in children: a review of results of eighteen implant surgeons, *Ophthalmic Surg* 10:61-66, 1997.
2. Hiles DA: Intraocular lens implantation in children with monocular cataracts 1974-1983, *Ophthalmology* 91:1231-1237, 1984.
3. Juler F: Visual acuity after traumatic cataract in children, *Trans Ophthalmol Soc UK* 41:129, 1921.
4. McKinna AJ: Results of treatment of traumatic cataract in children, *Am J Ophthalmol* 52:43, 1961.
5. Menezo JL, Taboada JF, Ferrer E: Complications of intraocular lenses in children, *Trans Ophthalmol Soc UK* 104:546-552, 1985.
6. Crouch ER, Parks MM: Management of posterior lenticonus complicated by unilateral cataract, *Am J Ophthalmol* 85:503-508, 1978.
7. Nelson LB: Diagnosis and management of cataracts in infancy and childhood, *Ophthalmic Surg* 15:688-697, 1984.
8. Wiesel TVN, Hubel DH: Effects of visual deprivation on morphology and physiology of cells in the cat's lateral geniculate body, *J Neurophysiol* 26:978-993, 1963.
9. von Noorden GK: Experimental amblyopia in monkeys: further behavioral observations and clinical correlations, *Invest Ophthalmol Vis Sci* 12:721-726, 1973.
10. Vaegan Taylor D: Critical period for deprivation amblyopia in children, *Trans Ophthalmol Soc UK* 99:432-439, 1979.
11. Robb RM, Mayer DI, Moore BD: Results of early treatment of unilateral congenital cataracts, *J Pediatr Ophthalmol Strabismus* 24:178-181, 1987.
12. Sharma N, Pushker N, Dada T et al: Complications of pediatric cataract surgery and intraocular lens implantation, *J Cataract Refract Surg* 12:1585-1588, 1999.
13. Gimbel HV, Neuhann T: Development, advantages, and methods of the continuous circular capsulorhexis technique, *J Cataract Refract Surg* 16:31-37, 1990.
14. Parks MM: Visual results in aphakic children, *Am J Ophthalmol* 441-449, 1982.
15. Crawford JS, Morin JD: The lens. In Crawford JS, Morin JD, editors: *The eye in childhood,* New York, 1982, Grune & Stratton, pp 259-287.
16. Ohzeki T: The value of electro-physiological testing in assessment of visual function in children, *Eur J Implant Refract Surg* 2:249-252, 1990.
17. Del Monte MA: Diagnosis and management of congenital and developmental cataracts, *Ophthalmol Clin North Am* 3:205-219, 1990.
18. Awaya S: Stimulus vision deprivation amblyopia in humans. In Reinecke RD, editor: *Strabismus. Proceedings of the Third Meeting of the International Strabismological Association.* May 10-12, 1978, Kyoto, Japan. New York, 1978, Grune & Stratton, pp 31-44.
19. Beller R, Hoyt CS, Marg E et al: Good visual function after neonatal surgery for congenital monocular cataracts, *Am J Ophthalmol* 91:599-565, 1981.

20. Hoyt CS: Treatment of congenital cataracts. In Davidson SI, editor: *Recent advances in ophthalmology,* New York, 1987, Churchill Livingstone.
21. Gelbert SS, Hoyt CS, Jastrebski G et al: Long-term visual results in bilateral congenital cataracts, *Am J Ophthalmol* 93:615-621, 1982.
22. Stark WJ, Taylor HR, Michels RG et al: Management of congenital cataracts, *Ophthalmology* 86:1571-1578, 1979.
23. Taylor D: Choice of surgical technique in the management of congenital cataract, *Trans Ophthalmol Soc UK* 101:114-117, 1981.
24. Nelson LB, Ullman S: Congenital and developmental cataracts. In Tasman W, Jaeger EA, editors: *Duane's clinical ophthalmology,* vol 1, Philadelphia, 1992, JB Lippincott, pp 1-10.
25. Palmer EA: How safe are ocular drugs in pediatrics? *Ophthalmology* 93:1038-1040, 1986.
26. Moncreiff WF: Contributions to the surgery of congenital cataract. I. Modification of discission in the preschool age group, *Am J Ophthalmol* 29:1513-1522, 1946.
27. Chandler PA: Surgery of congenital cataracts, *Am J Ophthalmol* 65: 663-674, 1968.
28. Jones IS: The treatment of congenital cataracts by needling, *Am J Ophthalmol* 52:347-355, 1961.
29. Dordes FH: A linear extraction of congenital cataract surgery, *Am J Ophthalmol* 52:355-360, 1961.
30. Scheie HG, Rubenstein RA, Kent RB: Aspiration of congenital or soft cataracts: further experience, *Am J Ophthalmol* 63:3-8, 1967.
31. Scheie HG: Aspiration of congenital or soft cataracts: a new technique, *Am J Ophthalmol* 50:1048-1056, 1960.
32. Parks MM, Hiles DA: Management of infantile cataracts, *Am J Ophthalmol* 63:10-19, 1967.
33. Francois J: Late results of congenital cataract surgery, *Trans Am Acad Ophthalmol Otolaryngol* 86:1586-1598, 1979.
34. Francois J: Glaucoma and uveitis after congenital cataract surgery, *Ann Ophthalmol* 3:131-135, 1971.
35. Phelps CD, Arafat NJ: Open angle glaucoma following surgery for congenital cataracts, *Arch Ophthalmol* 95:1985-1987, 1977.
36. Ferguson AC: A modified instrument for aspiration and irrigation of congenital and soft cataract, *Am J Ophthalmol* 57:596-600, 1964.
37. Sheppard RW, Crawford JS: The treatment of congenital cataracts, *Surv Ophthalmol* 17:340-347, 1973.
38. Parks MM: Posterior lens capsulectomy during primary cataract surgery in children, *Ophthalmology* 90:344-345, 1983.
39. Hiles DA, Hurite FG: Results of the first year's experience with phacoemulsification, *Am J Ophthalmol* 75:473, 1973.
40. Hiles DA, Wallan PH: Phacoemulsification versus aspiration in infantile cataract surgery, *Ophthalmic Surg* 5:13-26, 1974.
41. Hiles DA, Carter DT, Chotnier D: Phacoemulsification of infantile cataracts, *Trans Pa Acad Ophthalmol Otolaryngol* 31:30-37, 1978.
42. Callahan MA: Technique of congenital cataract surgery with the Kelman cavitron phaco emulsifier, *Ophthalmology* 86:1994-1998, 1979.
43. Hiles DA: Phacoemulsification of infantile cataracts, *Int Ophthalmol Clin* 17:83-102, 1977.
44. Gimbel HV: Implantation in children, *J Pediatr Ophthalmol Strabismus* 30:69-79, 1993.
45. Sinskey RM, Stoppel JO, Amin P: Long-term results of intraocular lens implantation in pediatric patients, *J Cataract Refract Surg* 19:405-408, 1993.
46. Lesser GR, Osher RH, Whipple D et al: Treatment of anterior chamber from fibrin following cataract surgery with tissue plasminogen activator, *J Cataract Refract Surg* 19:301-305, 1993.
47. Klais CM, Hattenbach L, Steinkamp GWK et al: Intraocular recombinant tissue-plasminogen activator fibrinolysis of fibrin formation after cataract surgery in children, *J Cataract Refract Surg* 25:357-362, 1999.
48. Mittra RA, Dev S, Nasir MA et al: Recombinant hirudin prevents postoperative fibrin formation after experimental cataract surgery, *Ophthalmology* 104:558-561, 1997.
49. Johnson RN, Blankenship GA: A prospective, randomized clinical trial of heparin therapy for postoperative intraocular fibrin, *Ophthalmology* 95:312-317, 1988.
50. Basti S, Aasuri M, Reddy MK et al: Heparin-surface-modified intraocular lenses in pediatric cataract surgery: prospective randomized study, *J Cataract Refract Surg* 25:782-787, 1999.
51. Binkhorst CD, Gobin MH: Injuries to the eye with lens opacity in young children, *Ophthalmologica* 148:169-183, 1964.
52. Binkhorst CD: Iris-clip and irido-capsular lens implants (pseudophakoi): personal techniques of pseudophakia, *Br J Ophthalmol* 51:767-771, 1967.
53. Cobo LM, Ohsawa E, Chandler D et al: Pathogeneses of capsular opacification after extracapsular cataract extraction: an animal model, *Ophthalmology* 91:857, 1984.
54. Nishi O: Fibrinous membrane formation on the posterior chamber lens during the early post-operative period, *J Cataract Refract Surg* 14:73-77, 1988.
55. Buckley E, Kombers L, Seaber J et al: Management of posterior capsule during pediatric intraocular lens implantation, *Am J Ophthalmol* 115: 722-728, 1993.
56. Gimbel HV, DeBroff BM: Posterior capsulorhexis with optic capture: maintaining a clear visual axis after pediatric cataract surgery, *J Cataract Refract Surg* 20:658-664, 1994.
57. Gimbel HV: Posterior capsulorhexis with optic capture in pediatric cataract and intraocular lens surgery, *Ophthalmology* 103:1871-1875, 1996.
58. Gimbel HV: Posterior continuous curvilinear capsulorhexis and optic capture of the intraocular lens to prevent secondary opacification in pediatric cataract surgery, *J Cataract Refract Surg* 23:652-656, 1997.
59. Gimbel HV, DeBroff BM: Management of lens implant and posterior capsular with respect to prevention of secondary cataract, *Operative Techniques Cataract Refractive Surg* 1:185-190, 1998.
60. Machamer R, Parel J, Buettner H: A new concept for vitreous surgery: instrumentation, *Am J Ophthalmol* 73:1-7, 1972.
61. France TD: Management of the posterior capsule in congenital cataracts, *J Pediatr Ophthalmol Strabismus* 21:116-117, 1984.
62. Sinskey RM, Karel F, Dal Ri E: Management of cataracts in children, *J Cataract Refract Surg* 15:196-200, 1989.
63. Kora Y, Inatomi M, Yoshinao F et al: Long-term study of children with implanted intraocular lenses, *J Cataract Refract Surg* 18:485-488, 1992.
64. Hiles DA, Hered RW: Modern intraocular lens implants in children with new age limitations, *J Cataract Refract Surg* 13:493-497, 1987.
65. McDonnell PJ, Zarbin MA, Green WR: Posterior capsule opacification in pseudophakic eyes, *Ophthalmology* 90:1548-1553, 1983.
66. Hiles DA, Johnson DL: The role of the crystalline lens epithelium in postpseudophakos membrane formation, *J Am Intraocul Implant Soc* 6:141-147, 1980.
67. Morgan KS, Karcioglu ZA: Secondary cataracts in infants after lensectomies, *J Pediatr Ophthalmol Strabismus* 24:45-48, 1987.
68. Hemo Y, BenEzra D: Traumatic cataracts in young children: correction of aphakia by intraocular lens implantation, *Ophthalmic Paediatr Genet* 8:2032-207, 1987.
69. Dahan E, Salmenson BD: Pseudophakia in children: precautions, technique and feasibility, *J Cataract Refract Surg* 16:75-82, 1990.
70. Lischetti P: New technique for posterior capsulotomy, *Eur J Implant Refract Surg* 2:77-79, 1990.
71. Mackool R, Chhatiawala H: Pediatric cataract surgery and intraocular lens implantation: a new technique for preventing or excising postoperative secondary membranes, *J Cataract Refract Surg* 17:62-66, 1991.
72. Hiles DA, Watson BA: Complications of implant surgery in children, *J Am Intraocul Implant Soc* 5:24-32, 1979.
73. Burke JP, Willshaw HE, Young JDH: Intraocular lens implants for uniocular cataracts in childhood, *Br J Ophthalmol* 73:860-864, 1989.
74. Dutton JJ, Baker JD, Hiles DA et al: Visual rehabilitation of aphakic children, *Surv Ophthalmol* 34:365, 1990.
75. Hoyt CS, Nickel B: Aphakic cystoid macular edema: occurrence in infants and children after transpupillary lensectomy and anterior vitrectomy, *Arch Ophthalmol* 100:746-749, 1982.
76. Morgan KS, Franklin RM: Oral fluorescein angioscopy in aphakic children, *J Pediatr Ophthalmol Strabismus* 21:33-36, 1984.
77. Poer DV, Helveston EM, Ellis FD: Aphakic cystoid macular edema in children, *Arch Ophthalmol* 99:249-252, 1981.
78. Cheng KP, Hiles DA, Biglan AW et al: Management of posterior lenticonus, *J Pediatr Ophthalmol Strabismus* 28:143-149, 1991.
79. Rao SK, Ravishankar K, Sitalakshmi G et al: Cystoid macular edema after pediatric intraocular lens implantation: fluorescein angioscopy results and literature review, *J Cataract Refract Surg* 27:432-436, 2001.
80. Koenig SB, Ruttum MS, Lewandowsit MF et al: Pseudophakia for traumatic cataracts in children, *Ophthalmology* 100:1218-1224, 1993.
81. Wright KW, Christensen LE, Noguchi BA: Results of late surgery for presumed congenital cataracts, *Am J Ophthalmol* 114:409-415, 1992.
82. Gimbel HV, Ferensowicz M, Ranaan M et al: Implantation in children, *J Pediatr Ophthalmol Strabismus* 19:405-408, 1993.
83. Tossignon M: A new technique for the prevention of posterior capsule opacification. Canadian Ophthalmological Society (COS) Annual Meeting, Toronto, 2001.
84. Koch DD, Kohnen T: Retrospective comparison of techniques to prevent secondary cataract formation after posterior chamber intraocular lens

implantation in infants and children, *J Cataract Refract Surg* 23:657-663, 1997.
85. DeVaro JM, Buckley EG, Awner S et al: Secondary posterior chamber intraocular lens implantation in pediatric patients, *Am J Ophthalmol* 123:24-30, 1997.
86. Calhoun JH, Harley RD: The roto-extractor in pediatric ophthalmology, *Trans Am Ophthalmol Soc* 73:292-305, 1975.
87. Peyman GA, Raichand M, Goldberg MF: Surgery of congenital and juvenile cataracts: a pars plicata approach with the vitrophage, *Br J Ophthalmol* 62:780-783, 1978.
88. Calhoun JH: Cataracts. In Harley RD, editor: *Pediatric ophthalmology,* ed 2, Philadelphia, 1983, WB Saunders, p 558.
89. BenEzra D, Paez JH: Congenital cataract and intraocular lenses, *Am J Ophthalmol* 96:311-314, 1983.
90. BenEzra D: The surgical approaches to paediatric cataract, *Eur J Implant Refract Surg* 2:241-244, 1990.
91. BenEzra D, Rose L: Intraocular versus contact lenses for the correction of aphakia in unilateral congenital and developmental cataract, *Eur J Implant Refract Surg* 2:303-307, 1990.
92. Cheah WM: A review of the management of congenital cataract, *Asia-Pacific J Ophthalmol* 1:22-26, 1989.
93. Green BF, Morin JD, Grant HP: Pars plicata lensectomy/vitrectomy for developmental cataract extraction: surgical results, *J Pediatr Ophthalmol Strabismus* 27:229-232, 1990.
94. Morgan KS, McDonald MB, Hiles DA, et al: The nationwide study of epikeratophakia for aphakia in children, *Am J Ophthalmol* 103:366-374, 1987.
95. Tablante RT, Cruz EDG, Lapus JV, et al: A new technique of congenital cataract surgery with primary posterior chamber intraocular lens implantation, *J Cataract Refract Surg* 14:139-157, 1988.
96. Keech RV, Tongue AC, Scott WE: Complications after surgery for congenital and infantile cataracts, *Am J Ophthalmol* 108:136-141, 1989.
97. Ahmadieh H, Javadi MA, Ahmady M et al: Primary capsulectomy, anterior vitrectomy, lensectomy, and posterior chamber lens implantation in children: limbal versus pars plana, *J Cataract Refract Surg* 25:768-775, 1999.
98. Steinert RF, Grene RB: Postoperative management of epikeratoplasty, *J Cataract Refract Surg* 14:255-264, 1988.
99. Kelley CG, Keates RH, Lembach RG: Epikeratophakia for pediatric aphakia, *Arch Ophthalmol* 104:680-682, 1986.
100. Hiles DA: Indications, techniques and complications associated with IOL implantation in children. In Hiles DA, editor: *Intraocular lens implants in children,* New York, 1980, Grune & Stratton, p 189.
101. Binkhorst CD, Gobin MH: Treatment of congenital and juvenile cataract with intraocular lens implants (pseudophakos), *Br J Ophthalmol* 54: 759-765, 1970.
102. Binkhorst CD, Gobin MH: Congenital cataract and lens implantation, *Ophthalmologica* 164:392-397, 1972.
103. Hiles DA: The need for intraocular lens implantation in children, *Ophthalmic Surg* 8:162-169, 1977.
104. Binkhorst CD: The irido-capsular (two-loop) lens and the iris-clip (four-loop) lens in pseudophakia, *Trans Am Acad Ophthalmol Otolaryngol* 77:589-617, 1973.
105. Choyce DP: Correction of uni-ocular aphakia by means of anterior chamber acrylic implants, *Trans Ophthalmol Soc UK* 78:459-470, 1958.
106. Hiles DA: Intraocular lens implantations in children, *Ann Ophthalmol* 9:789-797, 1977.
107. Binkhorst CD, Greaves B, Kats A et al: Lens injury in children with irido-capsular supported intraocular lenses, *J Am Intraocul Implant Soc* 4:34, 1978.
108. Choyce DP: Anterior chamber lens implantation in children under eighteen years. In Hiles DA, editor: *Intraocular lens implants in children,* New York, 1980, Grune & Stratton, p 179.
109. Fyodorov SN: The results of intraocular lens correction of aphakia in children. In Hiles DA, editor: *Intraocular lens implants in children,* New York, 1980, Grune & Stratton, p 41.
110. Helveston EM, Saunders RA, Ellis FD: Unilateral cataracts in children, *Ophthalmic Surg* 11:102-108, 1980.
111. Reynolds JD, Hiles DA, Johnson BL et al: A histopathological study of bilateral aphakia with a unilateral intraocular lens in a child, *Am J Ophthalmol* 93:289-293, 1982.
112. Hiles DA: Visual acuities of monocular IOL and non-IOL aphakic children, *Ophthalmology* 87:1296-1300, 1980.
113. van Balen ATM: Binkhorst's method of implantation of pseudophakoi in unilateral traumatic cataract, *Ophthalmologica* 165:490-494, 1972.
114. Sinskey RM Patel J: Posterior chamber intraocular lens implants in children: report of a series, *J Am Intraocul Implant Soc* 9:157-160, 1983.
115. Fyodorov SN, Egorova EV, Zubareva LN: 1004 cases of traumatic cataract surgery with implantation of an intraocular lens, *J Am Intraocul Implant Soc* 7:147-153, 1981.
116. Sheets JH: *Indications for intraocular lens implantations in children,* New York, 1980, Grune & Stratton, pp 31-40.
117. Aron JJ, Aron-Rosa D: Intraocular lens implantation in unilateral congenital cataract: a preliminary report, *J Am Intraocul Implant Soc* 9:306-308, 1983.
118. Gupta AK, Grover AK, Gurha N: Traumatic cataract surgery with intraocular lens implantation in children, *J Pediatr Ophthalmol Strabismus* 29:73-78, 1992.
119. Dahan E: Lens implantation in microphthalmic eyes of infants, *Eur J Implant Refract Surg* 1:9-11, 1989.
120. Sinskey RM, Stoppel J: Intraocular lens implantation in microphthalmic patients, *J Cataract Refract Surg* 18:480-484, 1992.
121. Dahan E, Welsh NH, Salmenson BD: Posterior chamber implants in unilateral congenital and developmental cataracts, *Eur J Implant Refract Surg* 2:295-302, 1990.
122. Lambert SR, Lynn M, Drews-Botsch C et al: A comparison of grading visual acuity, strabismus, and reoperation outcomes among children with aphakia and pseudophakia after unilateral cataract surgery using the first six months of life, *J Pediatr Ophthalmol Strabismus* 5:70-75, 2001.
123. Gimbel HV, Basti S, Ferensowicz M et al: Results of bilateral cataract extraction with posterior chamber intraocular lens implantation in children, *Ophthalmology* 104:1737-1743, 1997.
124. Metge P, Cohen H, Chemila JF: Intercapsular implantation in children, *Eur J Implant Refract Surg* 2:319-328, 1990.
125. O'Keefe M, Mulvihill A, Yeoh PL: Visual outcome and complication of bilateral intraocular lens implantation in children, *J Cataract Refract Surg* 26:1758-1764, 2000.
126. Peterseim MW, Wilson ME: Bilateral intraocular lens implantation in the pediatric population, *Ophthalmology* 107:1261-1266, 2000.
127. van Balen AT, Koole FD: Lens implantation in children, *Ophthalmic Pediatr Genet* 9:121-125, 1988.
128. Dahan E, Drusedau MUH: Choice of lens and dioptric power in pediatric pseudophakia, *J Cataract Refract Surg* 23(suppl):S618-S623, 1997.
129. Koro Y, Shimisu K, Inatomi M et al: Eye growth after cataract extraction and intraocular lens implantation in children, *Ophthalmic Surg* 24:467-475, 1993.
130. Huber C: Increasing myopia in children with intraocular lenses (IOL): an experiment in form deprivation myopia? *Eur J Implant Refract Surg* 5:154-158, 1993.
131. Yashar AG: 'Polypseudophakia' may be an option in first year of life, *Ophthalmology Times,* Jan 15, 2001, p 44.
132. Rabin J, Van Sluyters RC, Malach R: Emmetropization: a vision dependent phenomenon, *Invest Ophthalmol Vis Sci* 20:561-564, 1981.
133. Andreo LK, Wilson E, Apple DJ: Elastic properties and scanning electron microscopic appearance at manual continuous curvilinear capsulorhexis and vitrectorhexis in an animal model of pediatric cataract, *J Cataract Refract Surg* 25:534-539, 1999.
134. Gimbel HV: Two-stage capsulorhexis for endocapsular phacoemulsification, *J Cataract Refract Surg* 16:246-249, 1990.
135. Jacobi PC, Dietlein TS, Konen W: Multifocal intraocular lens implantation in pediatric cataract surgery, *Ophthalmology* 108:1375-1380, 2001.
136. Hunter DG: Multifocal intraocular lenses in children, *Ophthalmology* 108:1373-1374, 2001 (guest editorial).
137. Gimbel HV: Posterior capsule tears using phacoemulsification: causes, prevention and management, *Eur J Implant Refract Surg* 2:63-69, 1990.
138. Lavrich JB, Goldberg DS, Nelson LB: Suture use in pediatric cataract surgery: a survey, *Ophthalmic Surg* 24:554-555, 1993.
139. Blumenthal M, Yalon M, Treister G: Intraocular lens implantation in traumatic cataract in children, *J Am Intraocul Implant Soc* 9:40-41, 1983.
140. Maltzman BA, Wagner RS, Caputo AR: Neodymium:YAG laser surgery: the treatment of pediatric cataract disease, *Ann Ophthalmol* 18:245-246, 1986.
141. Catalano RA, Simon JW, Jenkins PL et al: Preferential looking as a guide for amblyopia therapy in monocular infantile cataracts, *J Pediatr Ophthalmol Strabismus* 24:56-63, 1987.
142. Cheng KP, Hiles DA, Biglan AW et al: Visual results after early surgical treatment of unilateral cataracts, *Ophthalmology* 98:903-910, 1991.
143. Pratt-Johnson JA, Tillson G: Unilateral congenital cataracts: binocular status after treatment, *J Pediatr Ophthalmol Strabismus* 26:72-75, 1989.
144. Wheeler DT, Stager DR, Weakley DR: Endophthalmitis following pediatric intraocular surgery for congenital cataracts and congenital glaucoma, *J Pediatr Ophthalmol Strabismus* 29:139-141, 1992.

145. Lloyd IC, Goss-Sampson M, Jeffrey BG et al: Neonatal cataract: aetiology, pathogenesis, and management, *Eye* 6(pt 2):184-196, 1992.
146. Asrani S, Friedman S, Hasselblad V et al: Does primary intraocular lens implantation prevent "aphakic" glaucoma in children? *J Pediatr Ophthalmol Strabismus* 4:33-39, 2000.
147. France TD, Frank JW: The association of strabismus and aphakia in children, *J Pediatr Ophthalmol Strabismus* 21:223-226, 1984.
148. Lambert SR, Amaya L, Taylor D: Detection and treatment of infantile cataracts, *Int Ophthalmol Clin* 29:51-56, 1989.
149. Chrousos GA, Parks MM, O'Neill JF: Incidence of chronic glaucoma, retinal detachment and secondary membrane surgery in pediatric aphakic patients, *Ophthalmology* 91:1238-1241, 1984.
150. Shephard CD: Retinal detachment in aphakia, *Trans Ophthalmol Soc UK* 54:176, 1934.
151. Jagger JD, Cooling RJ, Fison LG et al: Management of retinal detachment following congenital cataract surgery, *Trans Ophthalmol Soc UK* 103: 103-107, 1983.
152. DeJuan E Jr: The treatment of pediatric retinal detachments, *Arch Ophthalmol* 111:599, 1993.
153. Toyofuku H, Hirose T, Schepens CL: Retinal detachment following congenital cataract surgery. I. Preoperative findings in 114 eyes, *Arch Ophthalmol* 98:669-675, 1980.
154. Gimbel HV: Nucleofractis phacoemulsification through a small pupil, *Can J Ophthalmol* 27:115-119, 1992.
155. Castaneda VE, Ulrich FC, Legler MD et al: Posterior continuous curvilinear capsulorrhexis, *Ophthalmology* 99:45-50, 1992.
156. Butler TH: Lenticonus posterior. *Arch Ophthalmol* 3:425-436, 1930.
157. Franceschetti A, Rickli H: Posterior (eccentric) lenticonus, *Arch Ophthalmol* 51:499-508, 1954.
158. March EJ: Slit-lamp study of posterior lenticonus, *Arch Ophthalmol* 56:128-136, 1927.
159. Gimbel HV: Hydro-free dissection. Video presentation at the 1992 ASCRS film festival in San Diego.
160. Gimbel HV: Evolving techniques of cataract surgery: continuous curvilinear capsulorhexis, down-slope sculpting and nucleofractis, *Semin Ophthalmol* 7:193-207, 1992.
161. Neuhann T, Neuhann TH: The rhexis-fixation lens (film), American Society of Cataract Refractive Surgery, Boston, 1991.

The Intumescent Cataract

25

Roger F. Steinert, MD

Surgical removal of an intumescent lens presents several special challenges to the surgeon. An intumescent lens is a lens that has begun to lose structural integrity; the protein is denatured to the point that the lens is becoming hydrating. The capsule is thinner and more fragile, the red reflex is absent, zonules may be weakened or absent, and the nucleus is often large and hard if the intumescence occurs in an age-related cataract.

Clinical Presentation

A crystalline lens in which the cortex has become extensively hydrated, with white opacification, is historically known as a *mature* cataract. A mature lens that is swollen to the point of obstructing aqueous flow through the pupil and/or physically crowding the anterior chamber and angle is causing *phacomorphic glaucoma*. If the nucleus has sunk off-center in the lens as a result of liquefaction of the cortex, it is known as *morgagnian*. If the process is so advanced that some hydrated and denatured protein has begun to slowly leave the capsular bag, resulting in wrinkles in the no longer distended bag, the cataract is called *hypermature*. If the capsule loses integrity so that macrophages are attracted to scavenge the lens protein that has been released out of the capsular bag, *phacolytic glaucoma* may result from obstruction of the trabecular outflow. Severe inflammation caused by the released lens protein is called *phacoanaphylaxis*.

Some cases of intumescent cataract are due to physical damage to the capsule. A frank traumatic break in the capsule will result in rapid hydration and opacification of the cortex. A small break, particularly a puncture, will occasionally seal itself and result in only a local opacity. Physical damage to the capsule usually occurs in the setting of a perforating or severe blunt trauma or from intraocular surgery, particularly pars plana vitrectomy. Zonules are often damaged in this same process.

In mature and hypermature cataracts, the anterior capsule may undergo degeneration, with deposition of calcium or development of focal dense plaques. Dense postinflammatory plaques are particularly common after blunt trauma that triggers an intumescent cataract (Figure 25-1). If present, these areas will interfere with a normal capsulorhexis tear. The surgeon will need to direct the tear around these abnormalities, if possible, or use another technique, such as a Gills-Vannas scissors, to cut across these densities.

As part of the preoperative evaluation of a patient with an intumescent cataract, the surgeon should ask about past ocular history that might alter the surgical approach, obtain past medical records if possible, perform further nonroutine preoperative testing, and discuss with the patient that the potential for surgical complications is increased and the prognosis for full recovery of vision is uncertain. In particular, the surgeon must try to answer the questions: "Why did the patient wait so long before presenting?" Is the eye densely amblyopic, or was useful vision lost years earlier to a process such as a retinal vascular occlusion or retinal detachment? Did the patient suffer traumatic maculopathy or optic neuropathy? In most cases of an intumescent lens, where the fundus cannot be seen, a B-scan ultrasound is indicated. Other helpful evaluations include testing for entoptic imagery, perception of colored lights, gross visual field examination with a point light source, and bright flash visual evoked response. Usually these tests do not provide a highly accurate prognosis of visual potential, but they may help determine the potential value of surgery in patients with questionable past histories.

Absence of the Red Reflex

The largest challenge in removal of the intumescent cataract is the absence of a red fundus reflex when the cataract is viewed through the operating microscope.[1] If the surgeon intends to perform phacoemulsification with placement of an intraocular lens (IOL) in the capsular bag, an intact capsulorhexis is critical in maintaining structural integrity.[2] If the surgeon's intention is to perform an extracapsular cataract extraction and express the nucleus, then a can-opener style of anterior capsulotomy may be acceptable. Even then, however, it is nearly impossible to avoid large capsule flaps and the potential for equatorial and posterior tears unless the anterior capsule can be visualized.

Surgeons have used several approaches to improve visualization of the anterior capsule in the absence of the red reflex, most notably employing oblique illumination from another instrument such as a fiberoptic light pipe.[3] In addition, when the anterior capsule is opened and white cortex clouds the surgeon's view, the surgeon should pause the capsulotomy and improve the view, either by adding more viscoelastic or using the irrigation-aspiration device to remove the obscuring cortex while taking care not to engage the capsule.

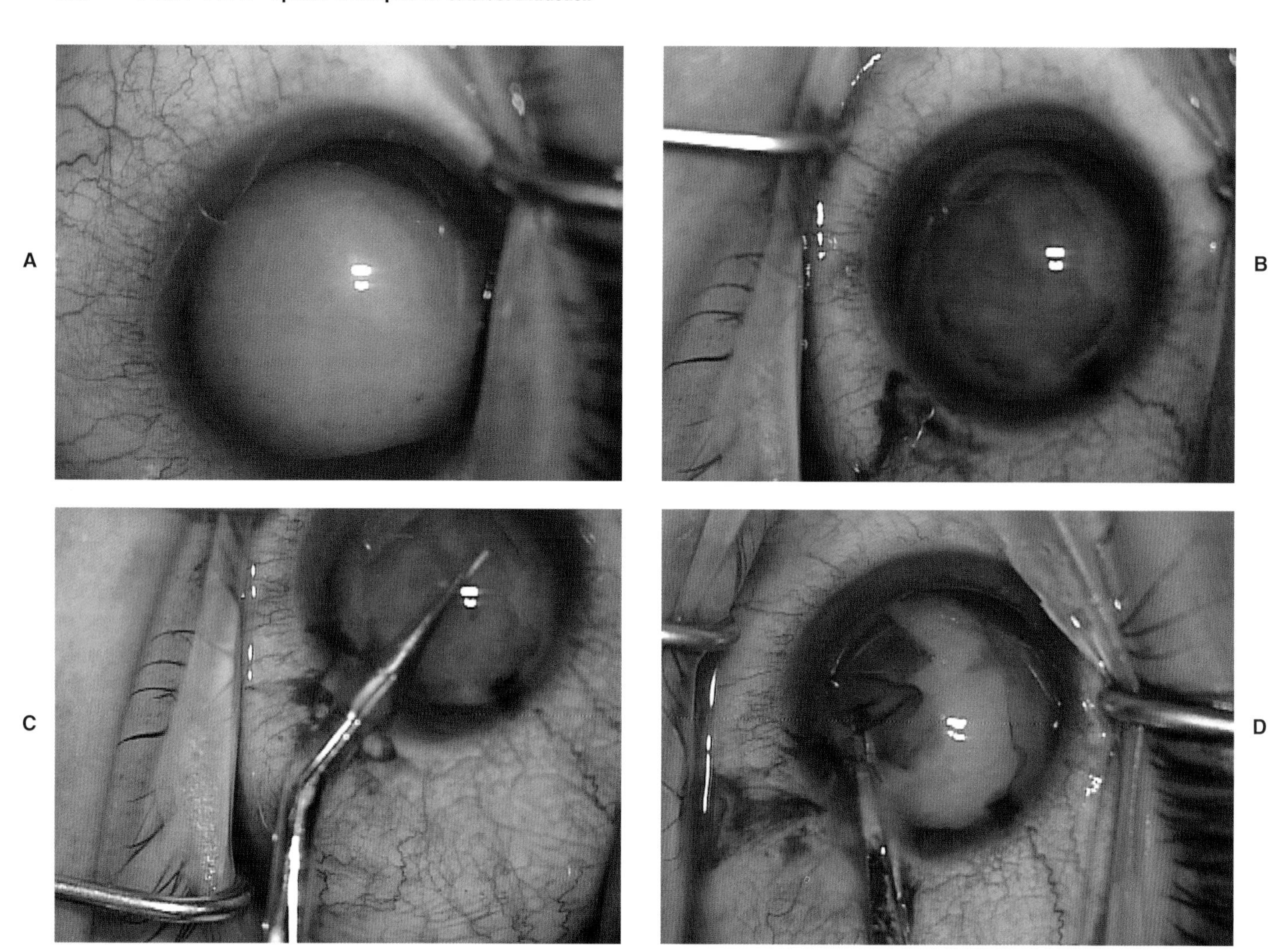

FIGURE 25-1 **A,** Intumescent traumatic cataract. Note the loss of zonules in the upper right. **B,** Trypan blue staining of the anterior capsule reveals a dense, darker staining plaque on the anterior capsule that will not tear with a conventional capsulorhexis technique. **C** and **D,** Gills-Vannas scissors must be used to cut through the anterior capsular plaque.

The most important advance in managing the anterior capsule in the absence of a red reflex is the use of an anterior capsule stain. Surgeons have attempted to stain the anterior capsule with a variety of substances. Fluorescein sodium 2% weakly stains the anterior capsule on the exterior surface and has slightly stronger uptake on the inner (epithelial) surface if it is injected after an initial opening into the capsular bag.[4] Cobalt blue illumination, not generally available on most operating microscopes, may be necessary to visualize the stain.[5] Some other commonly available stains, such as methylene blue and gentian violet, are toxic to the endothelium, at least in many common formulations.[6] The patient's own blood has been applied to the capsule as a method of staining as well.[7]

Two dyes are now available that have been proven safe and effective for staining the anterior capsule. Horiguchi et al.[8] elegantly demonstrated both the endothelial safety and also the effective technique for safely dissolving, diluting, and applying indocyanine green to the anterior capsule. Melles et al.[9] have developed a commercial preparation of trypan blue (VisionBlue, DORC, Zuidland, Holland) that is also safe and effective. In the original version of these techniques, the dye is applied under an air bubble that fills the anterior chamber, in order not to dilute the dye. The dye is applied as one or two microdrops wiped across the anterior capsule under the air bubble from a 27- or 30-gauge cannula. The air bubble itself, although preventing dye dilution by aqueous humor in the anterior chamber, prevents the dye from contacting the anterior capsule; therefore the cannula is used to wipe the dye under the air bubble and across the anterior capsule. The air bubble is then replaced with viscoelastic, and the capsulotomy is performed in the usual manner (Figure 25-2).

An alternative to the air bubble technique is the use of Healon 5 (Pharmacia). The surgeon must avoid injection of more than the minimum amount of dye necessary to stain the capsule. Otherwise, free dye in the anterior chamber surrounding the bolus of Healon 5 may obscure visualization of the

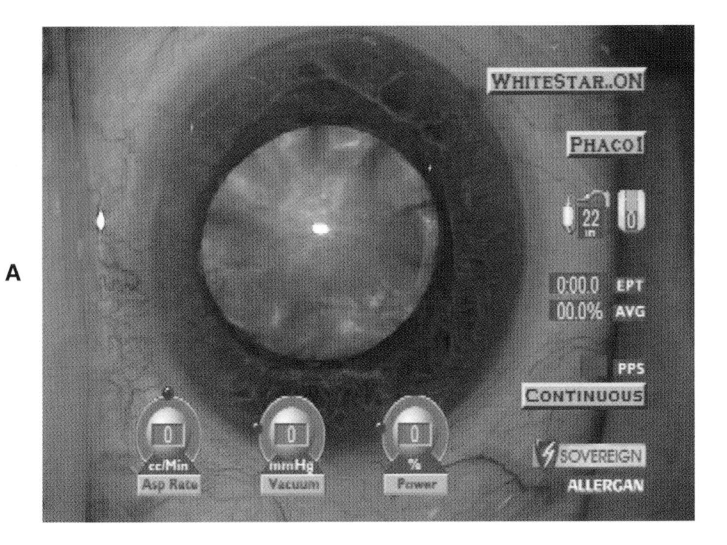

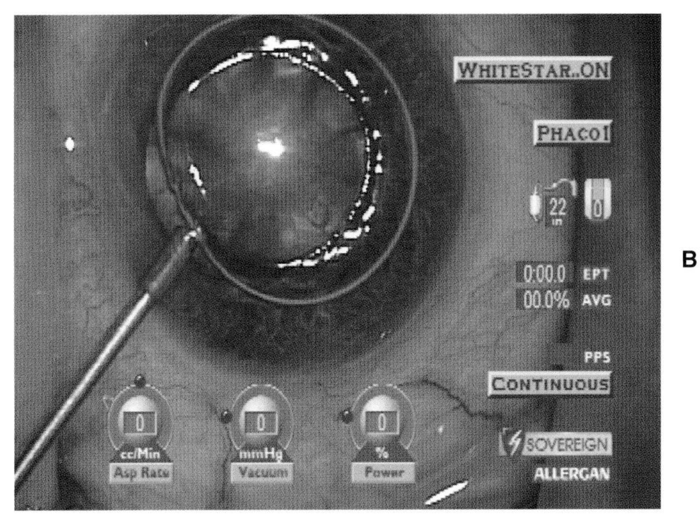

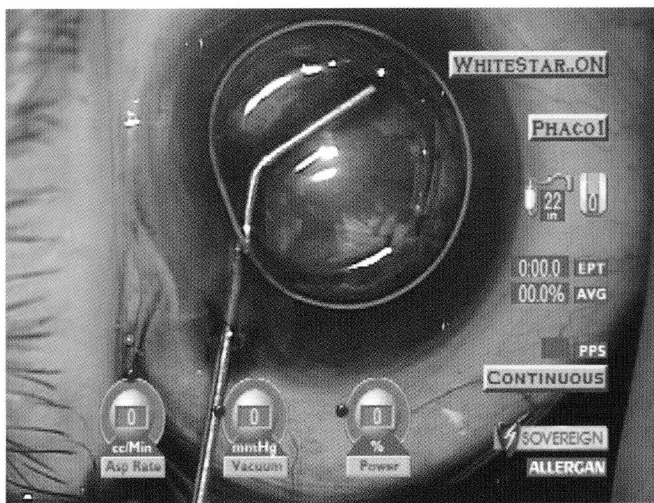

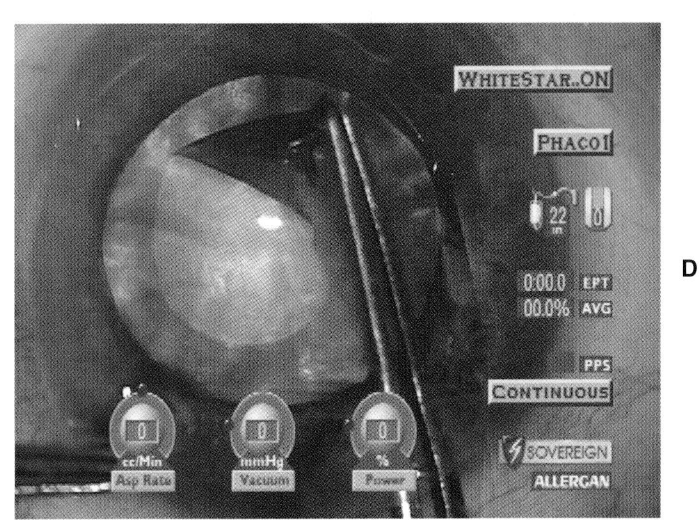

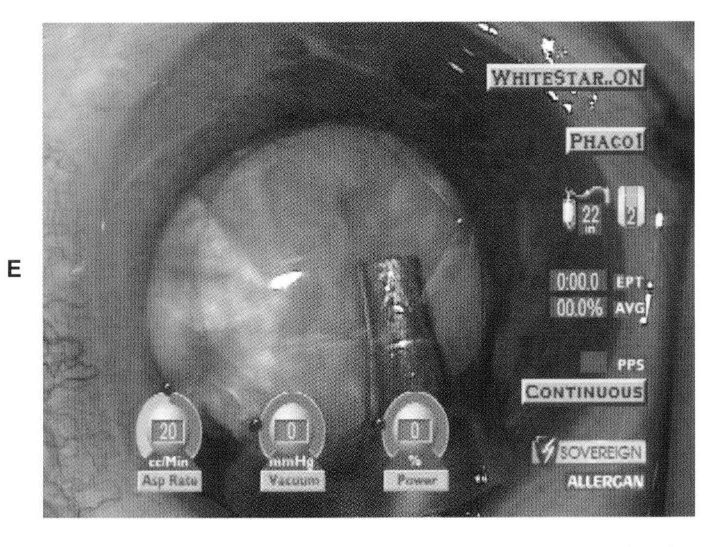

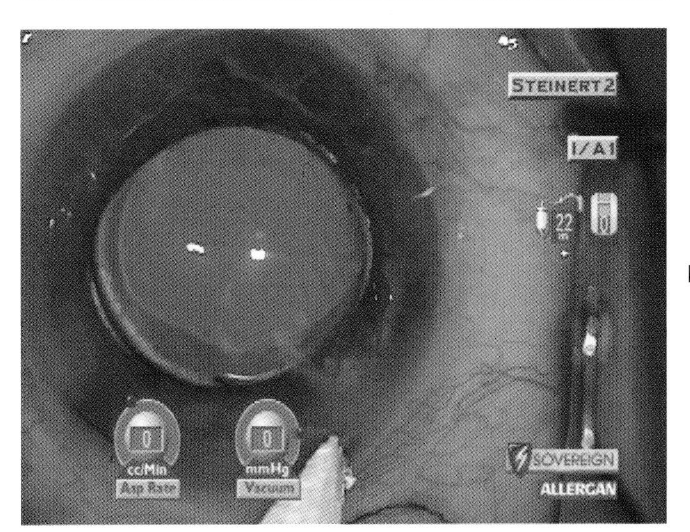

FIGURE 25-2 A, Intraoperative photographs of a mature white cataract with anterior capsule staining by trypan blue. **B,** Injection of air bubble through paracentesis. **C,** Trypan blue dye is applied under an air bubble filling the anterior chamber, using a blunt-tip cannula to inject and wipe the stain across the anterior capsule. **D,** Capsulorhexis proceeds normally, with clear visualization as a result of the staining. **E,** During phacoemulsification, the surgeon can visualize the stained anterior capsule edge, reducing the potential for inadvertent damage by the phaco tip. **F,** After IOL implantation, the stained anterior capsule can be seen overlying the IOL optic.

anterior capsule and require washout of the anterior chamber and reinstillation of viscoelastic to perform the capsulorhexis. However, in my experience, Healon 5 allows better contact of the dye with the anterior capsule compared with an air bubble (Figure 25-3). More intense anterior capsule staining results. In addition, there is no need to perform the steps of injecting air and later exchanging the air bubble for the viscoelastic agent to perform the anterior capsulotomy.

With either the air bubble or Healon 5 technique, the dye should be left in contact with the anterior capsule for at least 1 minute before performing the anterior capsulotomy to obtain adequately intense staining of the anterior capsule.

In addition to facilitating the capsulotomy, the dye-enhanced visualization of the capsule often proves helpful in avoiding operative trauma to the capsulorhexis edge by the phacoemulsification instruments (see Figure 25-2, *E* and *F*).

Thinning and Weakening of the Posterior Capsule

Many clinicians have the clinical impression that the posterior capsule presents increased challenges in the surgery of an intumescent lens. More prolonged phacoemulsification time and manipulation of a large and hard nucleus explain only part of the reason for increased frequency of posterior capsule complications.

The posterior capsule is often thinned and stretched by the expanded intumescent lens. As a result, the surgeon is faced with a posterior capsule that is not only weak but also flaccid, with wrinkles and a laxity that makes it prone to come up to the phaco tip and be ruptured. This problem is worsened by the absence of any epinucleus that protects the posterior capsule. A useful step is to inject a dispersive, noncohesive viscoelastic behind the nucleus one or more times during the phacoemulsification. This will provide an artificial epinucleus to keep the posterior capsule back from the operative plane and also stabilize the nucleus against tumbling.

Weak or Absent Zonules

Zonular weakness or frank absence of zonules sometimes presents a challenge during surgery of an intumescent cataract. Usually this occurs either because the patient is elderly, when zonules typically weaken as part of the aging process, or because the cataract has been induced by trauma.

As soon as clinically significant zonular weakness is suspected, placement of a Witschell capsular tension ring (Morcher GmbH) is advised. If the loss of zonules is severe, with major instability of the capsular bag, then the Cionni modification of the capsule tension ring allows the surgeon to directly add stabilization with an ab interno polypropylene transscleral suture (see Chapter 27).

If the capsular bag and/or sulcus is compromised to the point where the ability to support an IOL long term is uncertain, then a transscleral sutured posterior chamber IOL or an anterior chamber IOL should be implanted (see Chapter 37).

The Nucleus

In a relatively young patient with an intumescent lens, the hydration that opacifies the cortex will also lead to softening of the immature nucleus. The nucleus will then aspirate or require minimal ultrasound for removal. In elderly patients, however, the nucleus is often quite sclerotic and large. Because the cortex is already hydrated, hydrodissection and hydrodelineation are unnecessary. The removal of a large, hard nucleus is covered in Chapter 26 and is not discussed here. Caution must be taken in view of the weak posterior capsule and zonules.

A
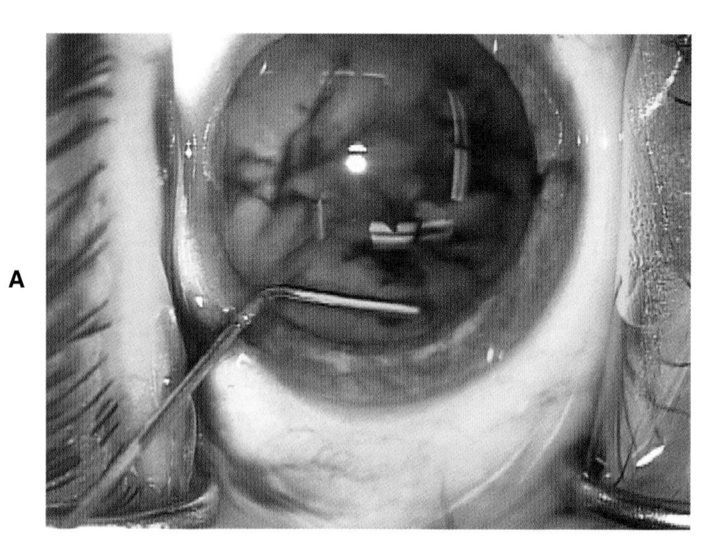

B
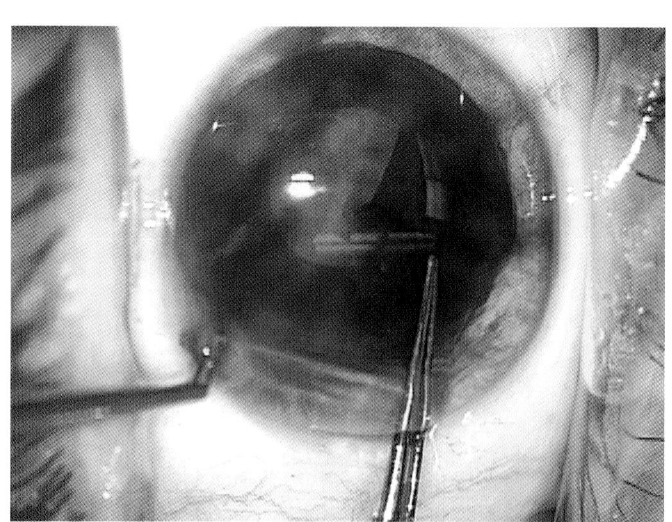

FIGURE 25-3 Application of trypan blue stain under a dome of Healon 5. **A,** Cannula is wiped across the anterior capsule while the stain is injected into the space created between the capsule and the Healon 5. **B,** If the dye does not mix with the solid mass of Healon 5 and the surgeon avoids injecting excess dye, visualization is adequate to proceed with the capsulorhexis without washing out the Healon 5 and replacing it.

In some advanced cases of intumescence, the nucleus itself will begin to hydrate slightly. These mildly hydrated nuclei typically have a characteristic golden haze rather than the dark brown, cola color of a dense and aged nucleus Although the nucleus will not soften to the point of being removable with aspiration alone, it will split more readily with chopping or cracking techniques and not be encumbered by a leathery posterior epinucleus, unlike a dark brown nucleus.

Conclusion

The intumescent cataract presents some special surgical challenges, most notably in visualizing the anterior capsule and protecting potentially weakened zonules and posterior capsule.

With the advent of staining of the anterior capsule to ensure visibility during surgery and with increasingly atraumatic phacoemulsification techniques, supplemented by use of viscoelastics, capsule tension rings, and transscleral sutures, the removal of an intumescent cataract is a surgical challenge that frequently has a successful outcome.

REFERENCES

1. Gimbel HV, Willerscheidt AB: What to do with a limited view: the intumescent cataract, *J Cataract Refract Surg* 19:657-661, 1993.
2. Gimbel HV, Neuhann T: Development, advantages, and methods of the continuous circular capsulorhexis technique, *J Cataract Refract Surg* 16: 31-37, 1990.
3. Mansour AM: Anterior capsulorhexis in hypermature cataracts, *J Cataract Refract Surg* 19:116-117, 1993 (letter).
4. Hoffer KJ, McFarland JE: Intracameral subcapsular fluorescein staining for improved visualization during capsulorhexis in mature cataracts, *J Cataract Refract Surg* 19:566, 1993 (letter).
5. Fritz WL: Fluorescein blue light-assisted capsulorhexis for mature or hypermature cataract, *J Cataract Refract Surg* 24:19-20, 1998.
6. Perez AR, Vainer AI: "Capsular Dyes" Video presentation at the Symposium on Cataract, IOL, and Refractive Surgery, April 1998, San Diego, Calif.
7. Cimetta DJ, Gatti M, Lobianco G: Haemocoloration of the anterior capsule in white cataract CCC, *Eur J Implant Refract Surg* 7:184-185, 1995.
8. Horiguchi M, Miyake K, Ohta I et al: Staining of the lens capsule for circular continuous capsulorhexis in eyes with white cataract, *Arch Ophthalmol* 116:535-537, 1998.
9. Melles GRJ, de Waard PWT, Pameyer JH et al: Trypan blue capsule staining to visualize the capsulorhexis in cataract surgery, *J Cataract Refract Surg* 25: 7-9, 1999.

Dense Brunescent Cataract

26

Roger F. Steinert, MD

A darkly brunescent nucleus, with the color of molasses or a cola soft drink, presents special surgical challenges. First the surgeon must select the basic surgical strategy. Depending on a surgeon's experience, the details of the patient's pathologic condition, and the treatment goals, the patient may be best served by phacoemulsification, by extracapsular cataract extraction, or by referral to a surgeon with experience and good results in phacoemulsification of dense nuclei.

Paradoxically, patients with particularly strong indications for small-incision phacoemulsification are often the patients who present with these advanced, technically challenging cataracts. A common clinical scenario is a patient with one functional eye who was told by an eye doctor decades earlier, "Don't let anyone touch your good eye." Today, such a patient is often better served by small-incision phacoemulsification surgery under topical anesthesia, retaining the use of the good eye. Other patients with a particular indication for small-incision cataract surgery include high myopes, at risk for scleral collapse or with liquefied vitreous inhibiting nuclear expression in extracapsular extraction, and high hyperopes who may have microphthalmos or nanophthalmos, with increased risk for positive pressure vitreous loss and/or choroidal effusion (see Chapter 31).

If phacoemulsification is thought to be the best alternative for the lens extraction, several special aspects of cataract surgery in this setting are important to maximize the probability of a successful outcome in the presence of a densely brunescent cataract.

Anterior Capsular Staining

Staining the anterior capsule is a critical step in performing successful phacoemulsification cataract surgery in situations in which the red reflex is insufficient to allow adequate visualization of the anterior capsule edge. In addition, a stained peripheral anterior capsule facilitates later phacoemulsification. The surgeon who can see the anterior capsule edge is less likely to nick it with the ultrasound tip or misplace a phaco chopping instrument on top of the anterior capsule.

The technique for anterior capsule staining is illustrated in detail in the chapter on the intumescent cataract (see Chapter 25).

Protecting the Endothelium and the Posterior Capsule

The protection of the corneal endothelium is especially important in phacoemulsification of dense nuclei, for which the surgery is prolonged, more manipulation is required, and more ultrasound power is employed. The corneal endothelium in such cases is often clinically "stressed" on the first postoperative day, with striae of Descemet's membrane and stromal edema.

In addition to meticulous surgical technique, protection of the endothelium is best achieved by a dispersive, retentive viscoadaptive device (see Chapter 5). Cohesive viscoadaptive devices, typically high-molecular-weight hyaluronic acid, often are flushed out of the anterior chamber within several seconds of initiating phacoemulsification. The dispersive agents (most commonly Viscoat [Alcon] and Vitrax [AMO]) are more likely to be retained as a protective layer against the endothelium.

Dispersive, retentive viscoadaptive agents can also be used to create an artificial epinucleus to protect the posterior capsule. A dense brunescent cataract usually has little to no epinucleus; the epinucleus has stiffened and become part of the nucleus. The posterior capsule therefore has no protective layer to guard against laceration from the sharp and bulky nuclear fragments. In addition, the posterior capsule is usually thinner and more vulnerable because the advanced cataract has stretched the capsule as the cataract expanded.

A helpful maneuver is to pause the phacoemulsification once enough nucleus has been removed to expose a small portion of the posterior capsule, heralded by the appearance of a "window" of bright red reflex. The viscoadaptive agent is injected between the posterior capsule and remaining nucleus. This creates an artificial epinucleus, physically separating the posterior capsule from the nucleus undergoing phacoemulsification. In addition, the viscoadaptive agent stabilizes the remaining nucleus, reducing tumbling of the nuclear fragments (Figure 26-1).

The "Leathery" Posterior Nucleus

A frequent surgical observation during phacoemulsification of a dense brunescent nucleus, whether by quadrant cracking or phaco chop technique, is that split fragments will nevertheless resist being drawn into the midanterior chamber for complete

A

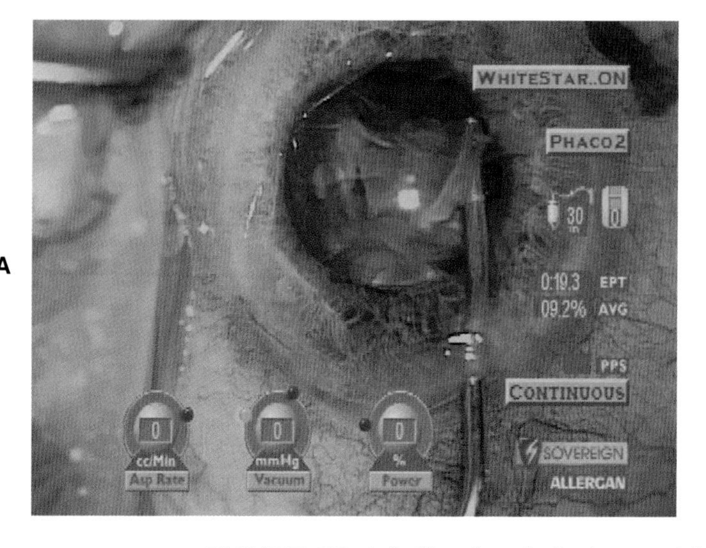

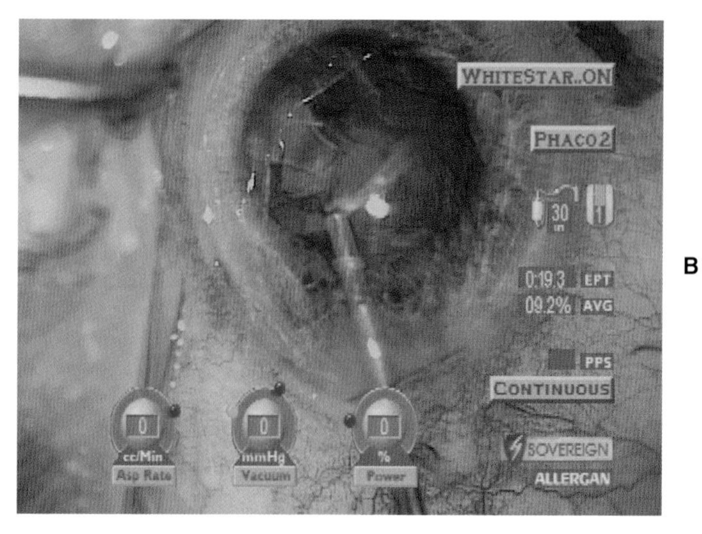

B

FIGURE 26-1 A, When the red reflex becomes visible, injection of a retentive viscoadaptive device behind the remaining nucleus will create an artificial epinucleus, protecting the posterior capsule and stabilizing the remaining nucleus. **B,** Later in the procedure, injection of further retentive viscoadaptive agent behind the nucleus helps preserve the protection of the posterior capsule.

destruction and aspiration by the ultrasound needle. The reason for this problem is that tough elastic strands, with a "leathery" quality and appearance, span across and connect the split nuclear fragments on their posterior surface.

These leathery strands emanate from the epinuclear layer, which, in advanced brunescence, is stiffening and becoming more tightly adherent to the nucleus.

These strands on the posterior surface will challenge the surgeon attempting to mobilize nuclear pieces in a controlled manner. The best technique to address these strands is to transect them with an instrument. The nuclear fragment is engaged and stabilized by the vacuum of the phaco tip. While the nuclear fragment is partially drawn anteriorly, but not to the point of breaking the vacuum hold, the second instrument is used to transect the strands. I prefer the phaco chopper as the second instrument. The handle is rotated so that the chopper is parallel to the posterior capsule, and the chopper is drawn across the strands. As long as the chopper is parallel to the posterior capsule and the surgeon maintains infusion of balanced salt solution (phaco foot position 1 or higher), the posterior capsule will not be endangered (Figure 26-2).

The surgeon must be patient in dealing with these many strands, but ultimately the nucleus can be successfully divided and emulsified.

A

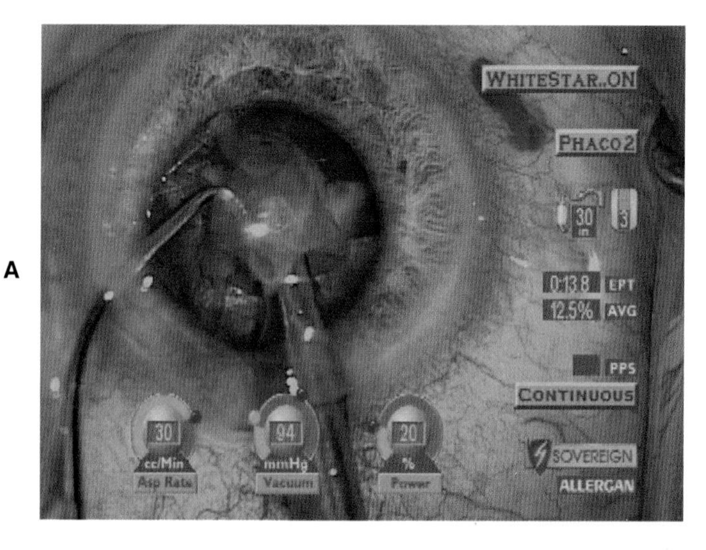

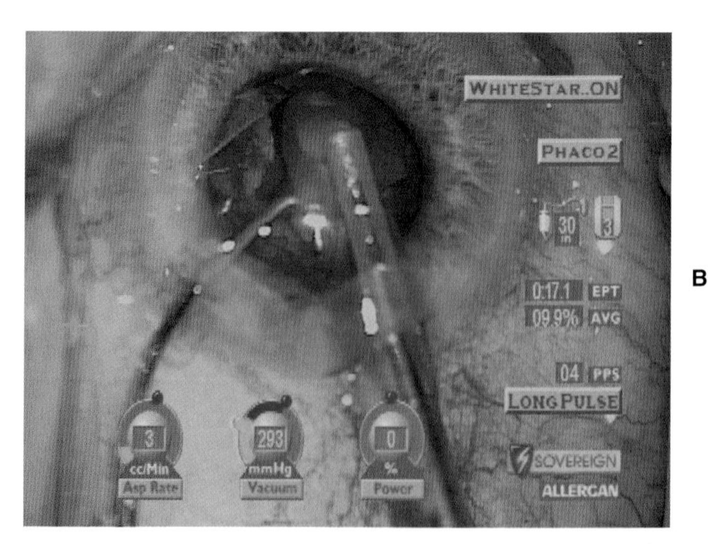

B

FIGURE 26-2 A, Chopping instrument can be oriented horizontally and used to cut across posterior leathery nuclear strands. **B,** Posterior strand cutting must continue across the apex of the nuclear wedge centrally.

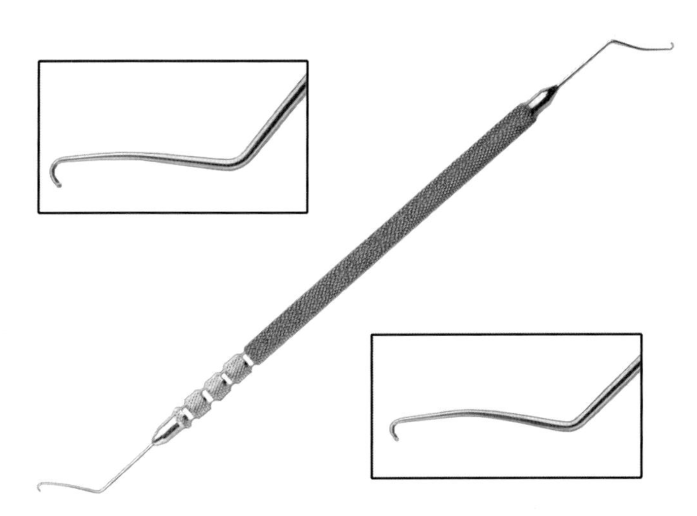

FIGURE 26-3 Chopping a dense, 4-plus nucleus is facilitated by a longer chopping tip, such as 1.75 mm *(top left),* compared with the more common 1.5-mm length chopping tip used for average-sized nuclei *(bottom right).* (Photo courtesy Rhein Medical, Tampa, Fla.)

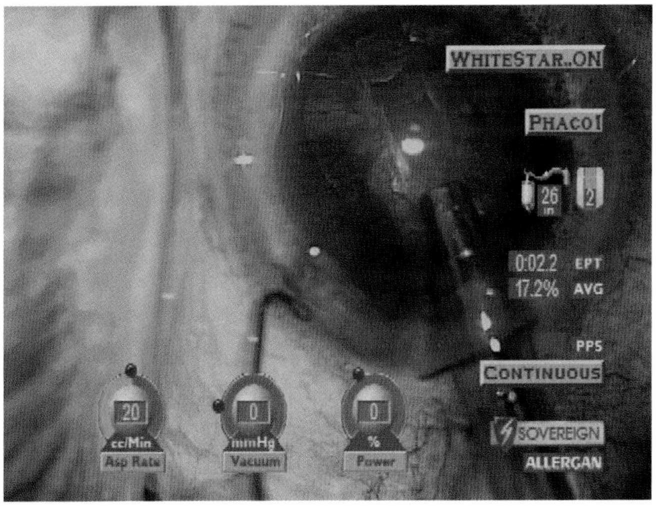

FIGURE 26-4 Creation of a groove in a dense nucleus facilitates chopping by thinning the nucleus and creating a weak zone, similar to the grooves that facilitate cracking a chocolate candy bar.

The surgeon must be patient in dealing with these many strands, but ultimately the nucleus can be successfully divided and emulsified.

Special Instruments

When confronted with a particularly challenging case, the surgeon generally should not attempt a new, unfamiliar technique. However, for surgeons who routinely employ phaco chop (see Chapter 16), a small adjustment can be helpful. Most phaco chopping instruments have a distal tip length of 1.25 to 1.5 mm. This is sufficient to reach the middle of an average nucleus. Having the tip of the chopper reach the middle of the nucleus is important in achieving a reliable chop.

Some choppers have a longer tip for use with dense nuclei. Elongating the tip to only 1.75 mm is sufficient to dramatically improve the reliability of successfully transecting a thicker, dense nucleus. Although such an instrument will look large inside the eye, the nuclear thickness that often approaches 4 mm or more means that the posterior capsule is not endangered (Figure 26-3). Alternatively, creation of a preparatory groove will reduce the nuclear thickness and create a weak zone more likely to crack (Figure 26-4).

Manufacturers are devoting increased attention to modulation of the delivery of ultrasound energy and control of fluidics (see Chapter 7). These advances enhance the surgeon's ability to deal with challenging dense nuclei, as well as more routine cataracts.

SUGGESTED READINGS

Mehta KR: Simplified and safe phacoemulsification of supra hard cataracts. In Agarwal A, Agarwal S, Sachdev MS et al., eds: *Phacoemulsification, laser cataract surgery, and foldable IOLs.* New Delhi, 1998, Jaypee, pp 210-211.

Vanathi M, Vajpayee RB, Tandon R et al: Crater-and-chop technique for phacoemulsification of hard cataracts, *J Cataract Refract Surg* 27:659-661, 2001.

Vasavada A, Singh R: Surgical techniques for difficult cataracts, *Curr Opin Ophthalmol* 10:46-52, 1999.

Surgical Management of the Congenitally Subluxed Crystalline Lens Using the Modified Capsular Tension Ring

27

Robert J. Cionni, MD

Subluxation of the crystalline lens may occur as an ocular manifestation of a hereditary disorder as in Marfan syndrome, homocystinuria, Weill-Marchesani syndrome, hyperlysinemia, or sulfite oxidase deficiency (Figure 27-1). Progressive subluxation of the crystalline lens commonly induces large refractive errors and anisometropia. In addition, movement of the dislocated lens can cause an intermittent phakic or aphakic visual axis, leading to marked visual disturbances. Such disturbances in a child undergoing visual development will often result in amblyopia. Therefore intervening quickly in young children with significant lenticular subluxation is important so that amblyopia can be prevented or amblyopia therapy can be started. However, many of these lenses may remain centered long enough to allow the child to develop and maintain normal vision well beyond the amblyogenic years. If so, the timing of intervention is less critical.

Historically, surgical removal of the congenitally subluxated lens has been undertaken with great caution because of numerous reports of complications and poor visual outcomes.[1-3] Until recently, the surgical management was limited to iridectomy, laser iridotomy, discission, or intracapsular extraction.[4] After intracapsular surgery, the patients were usually left aphakic, requiring aphakic spectacles or aphakic contact lenses. Alternatively, these eyes received epikeratophakia or, in older patients, an anterior chamber intraocular lens (AC IOL). These patients often ended up with graft rejection, retinal detachments, glaucoma, vitreous loss, and poor visual outcomes after surgery.

Many advances have been made in the ability to surgically manage these patients. With the introduction of small-incision cataract surgery and vitreous cutting devices, the success rate has dramatically increased. Pars plana vitrectomy and lensectomy, combined with aphakic contact lens wear or in the older patient an AC IOL, is a viable surgical option. The ability to suture a posterior chamber intraocular lens (PC IOL) into the ciliary sulcus provides yet another option. Some surgeons are favoring sutured PC IOLs even in children.[5] Even more recently, capsular tension rings (CTRs) have provided the opportunity to perform small-incision phacoemulsification and in-the-bag implantation of a PC IOL.[6]

Capsular Tension Rings

In 1993, Legler and Witschel[7] showed us that the CTR could provide both intraoperative and postoperative stabilization of the capsular bag and IOL in patients with zonular dialysis. Since its introduction, many surgeons have come to depend on the CTR for their patients with zonular compromise. These polymethylmethacrylate (PMMA) rings can be inserted into the capsular bag at any point after the capsulorhexis has been completed. The effect is a dramatic expansion and stabilization of the capsular bag.

Although the CTR has helped surgeons manage patients with a moderate loss of zonular support, eyes with profound zonular compromise or lens subluxation may still not obtain adequate stabilization or centration despite CTR placement. In addition, long-term stability of the bag and IOL is uncertain in eyes with progressive zonular loss, as in patients with Marfan syndrome. Several surgeons have devised techniques for suturing the CTR to the scleral wall for better support and centration. Osher[8] demonstrated the technique of suturing the CTR to the scleral wall by straddling the CTR with 10-0 Prolene suture, double-armed with CIF-4 needles. This technique may work well yet involves passing needles through the peripheral capsular bag, risking rupture of the bag because it is under stretch from the presence of the CTR. Pfeifer[9] preferred to fashion a small peripheral capsulorhexis through which a similar passage of suture could be made. Both techniques provide a solution to the bag that remains displaced after insertion of the CTR. However, both involve violating the integrity of the peripheral capsular bag and may risk rupture of the bag after placement of the CTR.

The modified CTR (MCTR), designed by Dr Robert Cionni, incorporates a unique fixation hook to provide scleral fixation without violating the integrity of the capsular bag[10] (Figure 27-2). The MCTR is manufactured by Morcher GmbH (Stuttgart, Germany). Like the original CTR, it consists of an open, flexible PMMA filament. However, the MCTR has a fixation hook that courses anteriorly and centrally in a second plane. The hook wraps around the capsulorhexis edge and rests on the residual anterior capsular rim. At the free end of the hook is an eyelet

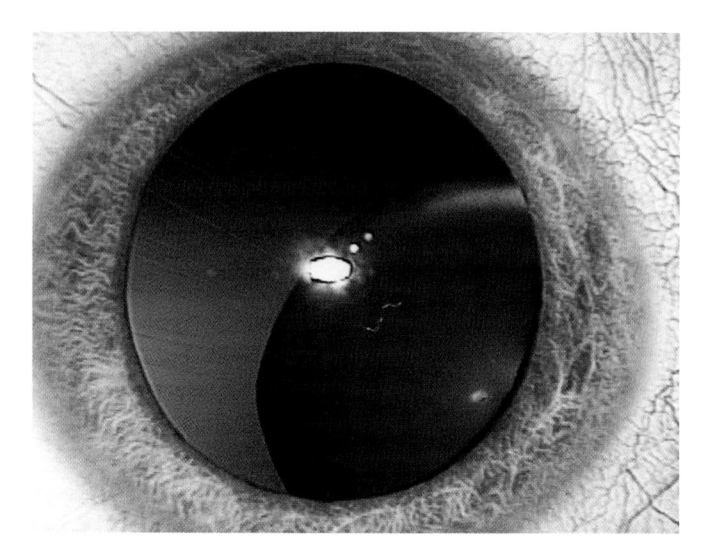

FIGURE 27-1 Subluxated lens in a young boy with Marfan syndrome.

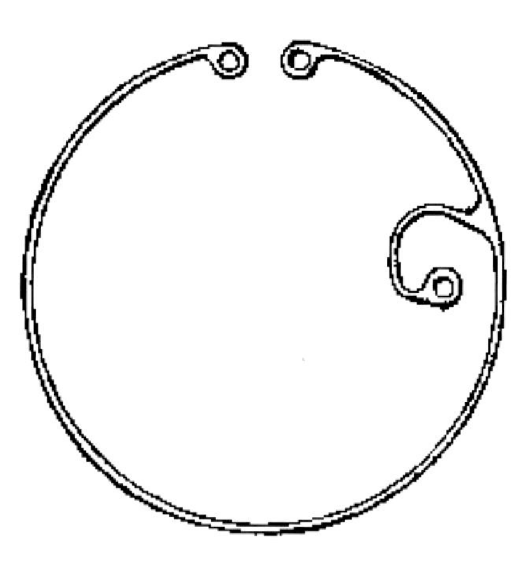

FIGURE 27-2 Diagram of the Cionni modified capsular tension ring (MCTR) (Model 1-L).

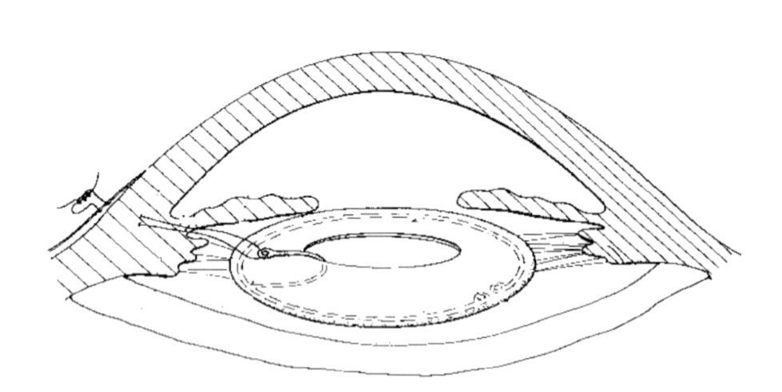

FIGURE 27-3 Diagram showing how the MCTR can be sutured through the ciliary sulcus and to the scleral wall to induce bag centration and stabilization.

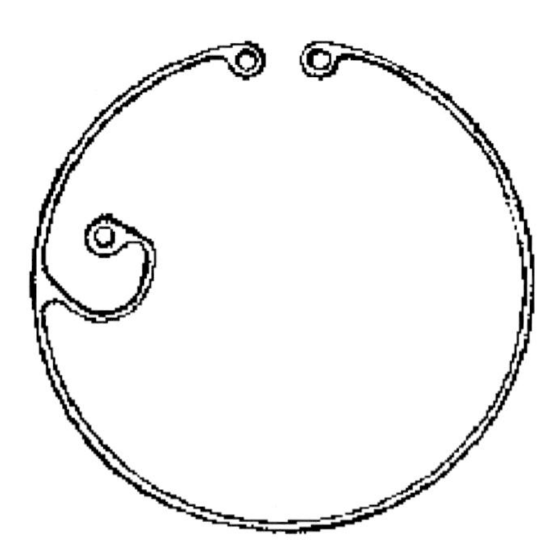

FIGURE 27-4 MCTR (Model 2-C) can be used with the Geuder shooter.

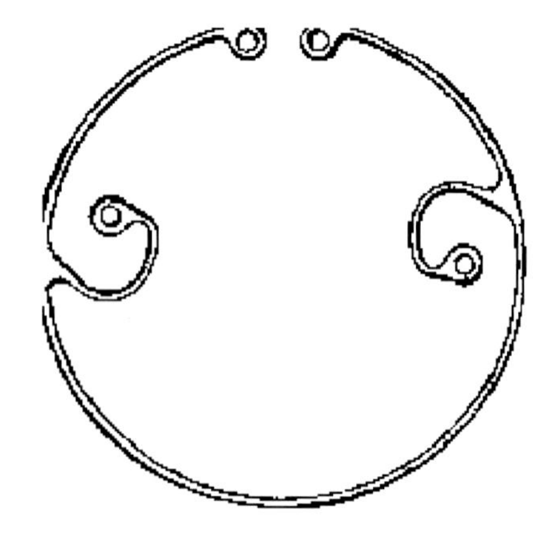

FIGURE 27-5 MCTR (Model 2-L) has two fixation hooks for maximal stabilization of the most significantly loose lenses.

through which a suture can be passed to allow scleral fixation (Figure 27-3). Currently, there are three MCTR models. Model 1-L has a single fixation hook distant from the insertion end of the ring. Model 2-C has a single fixation hook near the insertion end of the ring, allowing it to be implanted with the Geuder shooter (Figure 27-4). Model 2-L has two fixation hooks (Figure 27-5). This model is useful in patients with very significant generalized zonular weakness.

Preoperative Evaluation

An initial assessment of the best-corrected visual acuity for near and distance should be established, keeping in mind that the patient may see best with an aphakic correction if the lens is markedly subluxed. In young children, if the lens is not threatening to dislocate posteriorly or anteriorly and an accurate refraction can be obtained, observation is warranted and amblyopia treatment begun. Surgery should be considered when there is progressive subluxation of the lens with bisection of the pupil or if dislocation is imminent. In addition, if amblyopia cannot be effectively treated with conventional means, such as glasses, contact lenses, or patching, lens extraction may be the best option. For older children and adults, lens extraction should be considered if poor visual acuity is attributed to the subluxated lens or if the lens is threatening to dislocate anteriorly or posteriorly.

Before surgery, the surgeon should characterize the areas of zonular weakness in terms of degrees of loss, location of the defect, presence or absence of vitreous prolapse, and the presence or absence of phacodonesis. Phacodonesis is more noticeable and dramatic before dilation because dilation often stabilizes the ciliary body and iris, dampening any iris or lens movement. The surgeon should be wary of the inferiorly subluxated lens because inferior subluxation indicates 360 degrees of very significant zonular weakness combined with the effect of gravity. Such significant generalized zonular weakness makes it unlikely that the surgeon will be able to remove the lens while maintaining the capsular bag for PC IOL support. Pars plana lensectomy should be considered in these eyes. The presence or absence of additional ocular pathologic conditions that might affect the visual outcome must be considered and the patient counseled accordingly. Many patients with Marfan syndrome have significant systemic problems, which increase the risk of death or morbidity. These patients need to be evaluated by their primary medical doctor or cardiologist before surgery. Patients taking anticoagulant medicine for heart, vessel, and or valvular abnormalities need to be counseled in detail concerning the implications of discontinuing anticoagulants versus undergoing surgery while anticoagulated.

Surgical Technique

The surgeon should attempt to make the incision away from the area of zonular weakness. This will help reduce the stress placed on the existing zonules during phacoemulsification. Unfortunately, many of these patients have generalized zonular weakness. The surgeon should then try to place the incision over the quadrant of subluxation because the zonules in the opposite quadrant have proven to be the weakest. However, the surgeon should not compromise his or her surgical abilities by operating at a meridian that is uncomfortable. The surgeon should always work through the smallest incision possible without compromising his or her ability to perform the necessary maneuvers. Doing so will minimize fluid egress through the incision and therefore will help to limit anterior chamber collapses. The initial anterior chamber entry should be made just large enough to insert the viscoelastic cannula and place a generous amount of a highly retentive viscoelastic over the area of zonular dialysis to tamponade vitreous and to maintain a deep, noncollapsing anterior chamber.

The surgeon should start the capsulorhexis in an area remote from the dialysis and use the countertraction provided by the remaining healthy zonules (Figure 27-6). A second blunt instrument, such as the Osher Nucleus Manipulator (Duckworth and Kent, St. Louis, Mo.), may be used for countertraction or to push the lens into view if it is significantly decentered under the iris. With extensive zonular loss or weakness, it may be necessary to begin the tear by cutting the anterior capsule with a sharp-tipped 15-degree blade or a diamond blade. A 5.5- to 6-mm capsulorhexis should allow the surgeon to more easily manipulate the nucleus. The capsulorhexis must be made "off-center" because bag recentration with the MCTR will change what appears to be the center of the anterior capsule. Although the MCTR could be placed into the capsular bag after capsulorhexis, the bulk of the nucleus can make placement of the MCTR difficult. In addition, visualization during insertion is better if the nucleus is removed first. Instead, I prefer to stabilize the capsular bag by grasping the capsulorhexis edge with one to three titanium or disposable nylon iris retractors placed through limbal stab incisions[11] (Figure 27-7). Hydrodissection is then performed carefully, yet thoroughly, to maximally free the nucleus and thereby decrease zonular stress during manipulation of the nucleus. If the nucleus is soft, hydrodissection of the nucleus completely into the anterior chamber is preferred. Doing so will greatly simplify its removal via automated aspiration or phacoemulsification and will virtually eliminate zonular stress during phacoemulsification.[12]

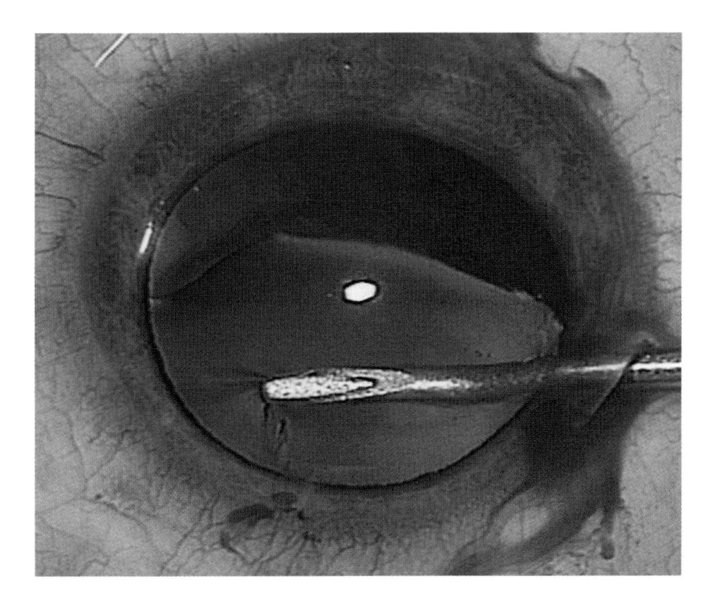

FIGURE 27-6 Remaining "strong zonules" provide the necessary countertraction to begin capsulorhexis with a 22-gauge bent needle.

Phacoemulsification should be performed using low vacuum and aspiration settings to keep the bottle height at a minimum.[13] High bottle heights cause higher inflow rates, which can force fluid through the areas of zonular weakness and lead to vitreous hydration. This in turn can lead to positive pressure, anterior chamber shallowing, and vitreous prolapse. However, it is important to not lower the bottle so much as to allow outflow to outpace inflow, for this can also lead to vitreous prolapse because the anterior segment would be less pressurized than the posterior segment.

For the denser nucleus, divide or chop techniques are preferred. These techniques will minimize zonular stress during

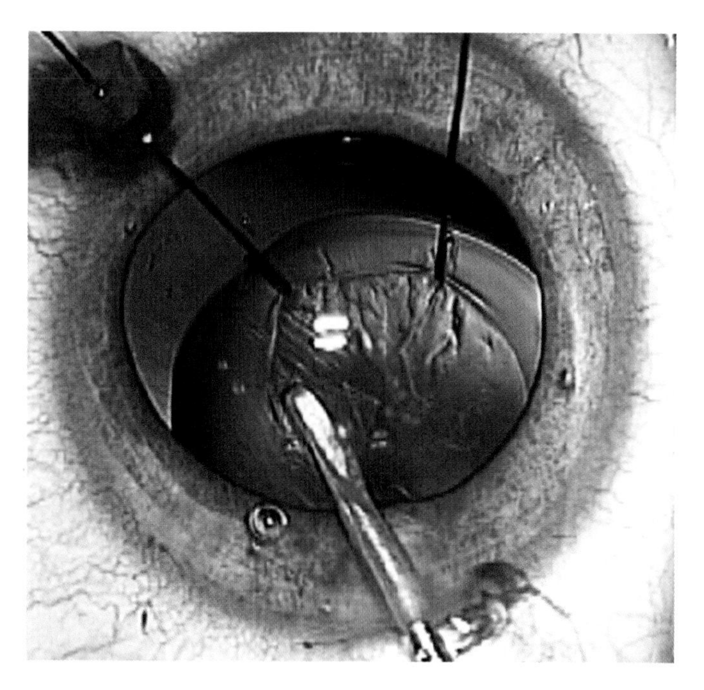

FIGURE 27-7 Two iris hooks are used to grasp the capsulorhexis edge for stabilization.

phacoemulsification if the surgeon is careful to apply equal forces in opposing directions to avoid displacing the nucleus. It is very helpful to "viscodissect" the nuclear halves or quadrants free from the cortex in areas of zonular weakness.[14] Viscoelastic injected between the nuclear quadrants and peripheral capsular bag will lift the nuclear fragments while expanding and stabilizing the bag.

Before inserting the MCTR, the surgeon should place viscoelastic just under the surface of the residual anterior capsular rim to create a space for the MCTR and to dissect residual cortex away from the peripheral capsule, making cortical entrapment by the MCTR less likely (Figure 27-8). Insertion of the ring begins by preplacing a 9-0 Prolene suture, double-armed with CIF-4 needles, through the eyelet of the fixation hook. Alternatively, the suture can be single-armed and the free end of the Prolene tied to the fixation hook eyelet. The MCTR is inserted with smooth forceps through the main incision and dialed into the capsular bag with a Y-hook (Figure 27-9). The fixation hook will often "capture" anterior to the capsulorhexis edge. If it does not do so, the hook is easily manipulated anteriorly with a Y-hook (Osher Y-Hook, Duckworth and Kent, St. Louis, Mo.) and a second dull instrument to retract the capsulorhexis edge. The Y-hook is used to "dial" the MCTR until the eyelet is centered at the site of zonular dehiscence or zonular weakness. A Y-hook can then be used to push the fixation hook to the scleral wall to be certain that the chosen location will result in bag centration (Figure 27-10). A scleral flap is fashioned at this site so that, once the Prolene suture is tied, the knot can be covered. Viscoelastic is then used to create space between the undersurface of the iris and the anterior capsule in preparation for needle passage. The needles are placed through the incision, into the pupil, and behind the iris. The needle and suture should remain anterior to the anterior capsule at all times (Figure 27-11). This needle pass is then continued out through the scleral wall at the site of the fixation hook. The needles should exit the scleral wall approximately 1.5 mm posterior to the corneal-scleral junction. This will position the fixation hook posterior enough to prevent postoperative iris chaffing. The sutures are cinched-up until centration is obtained and a temporary knot tied (Figure 27-12). If a single-armed suture is used, the needle is passed partial thickness through scleral bed beneath the scleral flap, and the suture is then tied to itself. After suture fixation of the MCTR, any remaining cortex can be aspirated

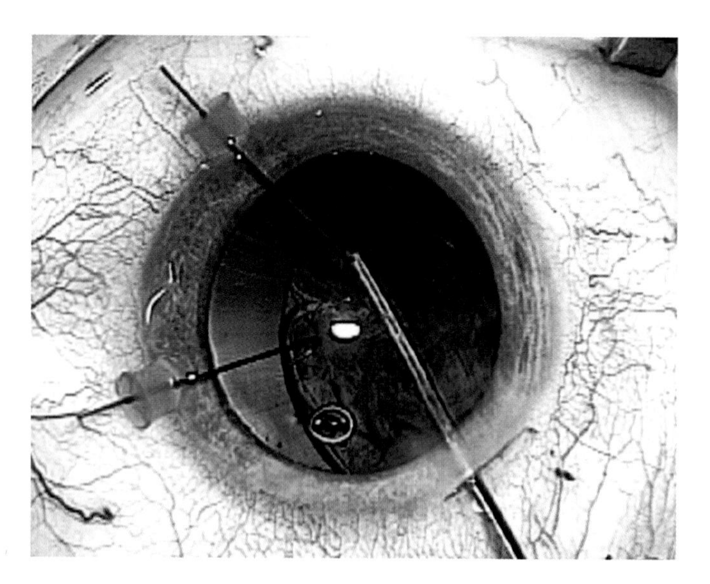

FIGURE 27-8 Viscodissection of anterior and peripheral cortex before placing MCTR.

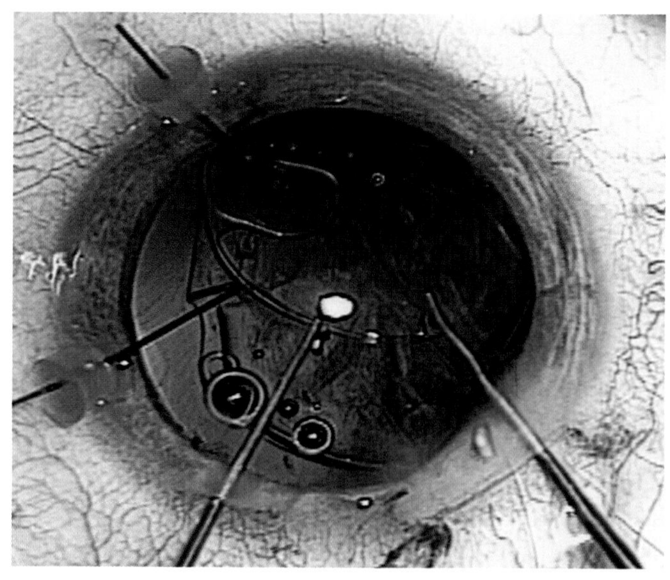

FIGURE 27-9 MCTR Model 1-L is dialed into the capsular bag with an Osher Y-hook and an Osher nucleus manipulator.

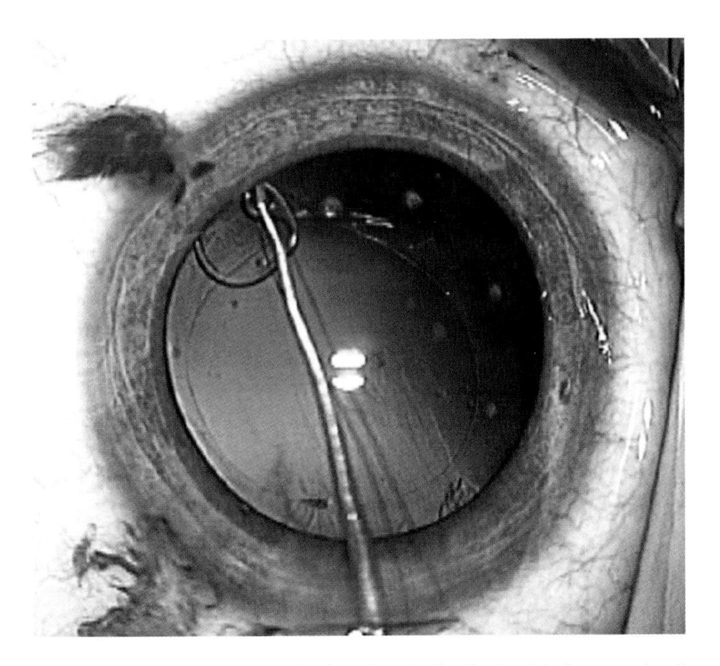

FIGURE 27-10 Osher Y-hook pushes the fixation hook to the scleral wall to determine the correct meridian of hook fixation to achieve bag centration before needle passage.

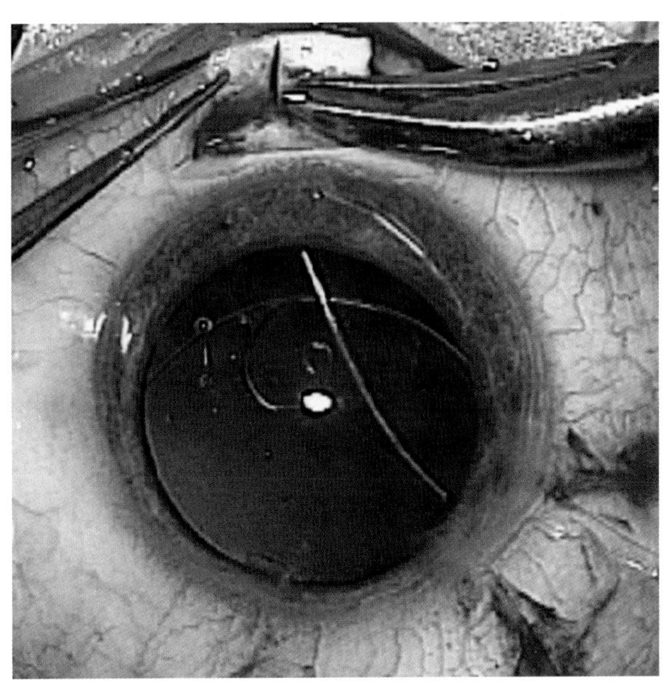

FIGURE 27-11 Needle is placed through the incision, between the anterior capsule and the undersurface of the iris and out through the ciliary sulcus and scleral wall.

manually with a 24- to 27-gauge cannula. Alternatively, one can use an automated irrigation-aspiration device, but vitreous hydration and prolapse may be more likely. The capsular bag is then reinflated with viscoelastic before PC IOL insertion.

I have found it easiest to insert a foldable-style PC IOL into the capsular bag in these cases. In addition, the ability to place a PC IOL with a 6-mm optic through a small, "near-clear" corneal incision makes wound closure easier in these young patients with more scleral elasticity. I currently favor the AcrySof SA60 in these younger patients because of the low level of inflammatory response and the low posterior capsule opacification rate found with this IOL material and design.[15-18] This single-piece foldable acrylic IOL can be injected completely into the capsular bag through a 3-mm incision (Figure 27-13) (Alcon AcrySof SA 60AT and Monarch II delivery system, Alcon Labs, Fort Worth, Tex.).

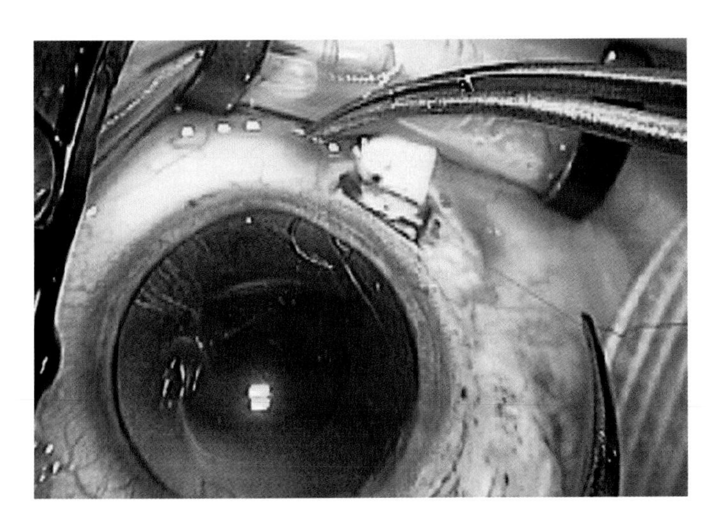

FIGURE 27-12 The 9-0 Prolene suture is tightened, and a temporary knot is tied to recenter and stabilize the capsular bag.

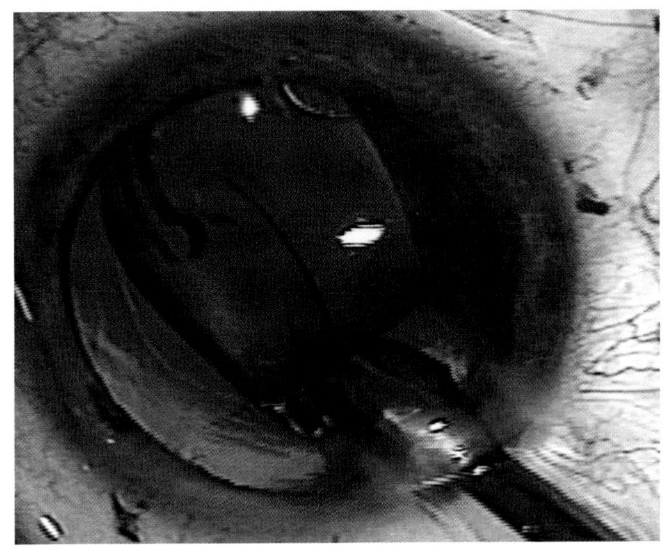

FIGURE 27-13 AcrySof SA 60AT is injected into the capsular bag using a so that both haptics unfold into the capsular bag without dialing the IOL.

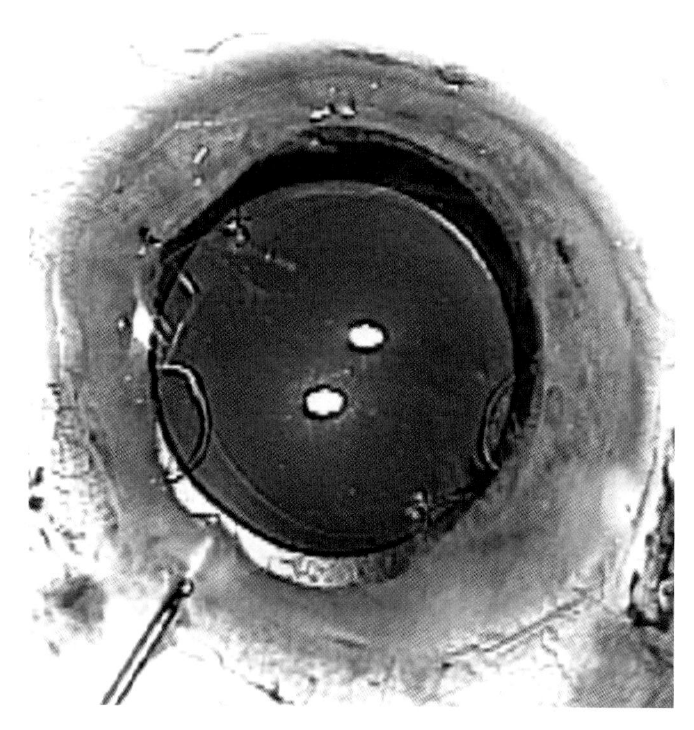

FIGURE 27-14 MCTR Model 2-L with a nicely centered AcrySof MA60 in a young boy with Marfan syndrome.

Once the PC IOL is in place, the temporary knot is released, and a permanent knot is tied with just enough tension to effect IOL centration. The knot can then be rotated beneath the sclera or simply buried beneath the scleral flap. If the two-hook model (2-L) is used, the fixation site for each hook must be ascertained by displacing each hook to the scleral wall before suturing. Depending on the size of the capsular bag, the best centration may be obtained with the hooks less than 180 degrees apart (Figure 27-14). Viscoelastic is removed manually through the side-port incision or with an automated irrigation-aspiration handpiece. Acetylcholine (Miochol) is instilled to ensure that the pupil rounds and that the anterior chamber is free of vitreous. Conjunctiva is reapproximated over the scleral flap and the near-clear corneal incision is hydrated and checked to be certain that it is watertight.

If vitreous presents at any time during the procedure, it should be carefully and completely removed from the anterior chamber. Small amounts of vitreous can be removed by using a "dry" vitrectomy technique with an automated vitrector and an anterior chamber filled with viscoelastic.[19] For significant vitreous prolapse, a bimanual vitrectomy should be performed. This is best accomplished by using a side-port incision for irrigation with a 25- or 27-gauge cannula. The vitrectomy handpiece can be inserted through the initial incision or through a pars plana sclerotomy.[20]

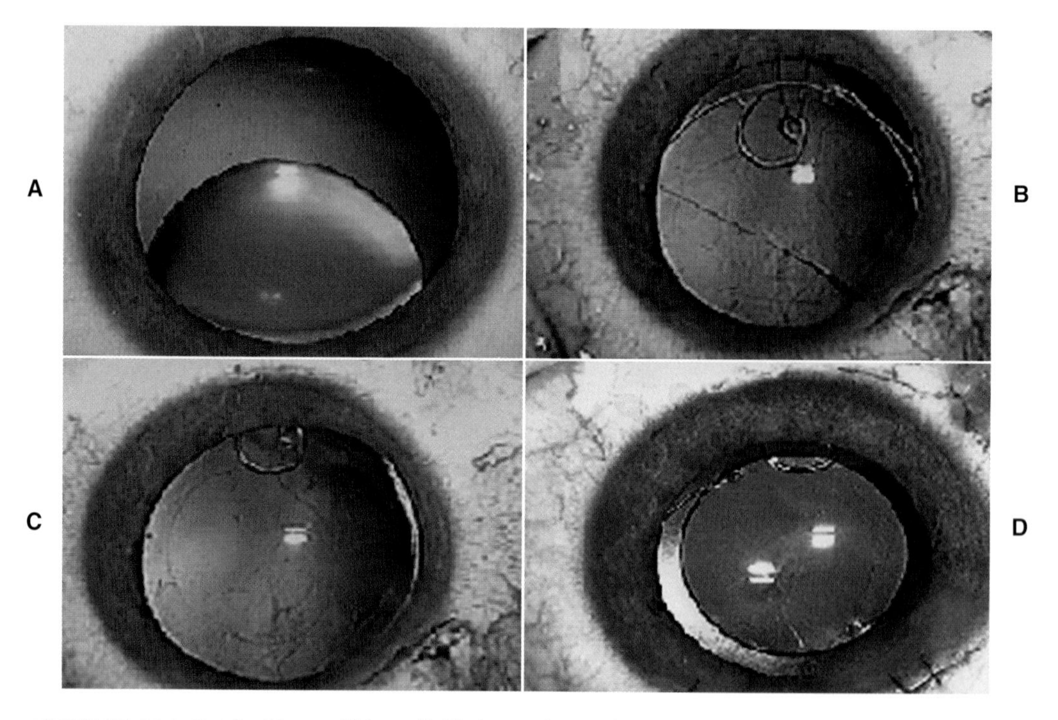

FIGURE 27-15 An 11-year-old boy with Marfan syndrome. **A,** Preoperative photo showing tremendous lens subluxation. **B,** After placement of the MCTR Model 2-C and before tightening the Prolene sutures, the bag is expanded yet remains decentered. **C,** Tightening the MCTR's Prolene sutures centers the expanded capsular bag. **D,** With the MCTR secured in place, the capsular bag and PC IOL are well centered and stable at the end of the case. The patient's vision after 24 hours measured 20/25 without glasses.

As of this writing, I have performed the procedure described previously in over 90 eyes with congenitally subluxed lenses, ranging in age from 2 to 65 years. The results have been phenomenal, with all patients thus far showing a marked improvement in vision. However, nine patients in whom I had used 10-0 Prolene for MCTR fixation presented more than a year after surgery with the fixation suture broken. In five of these patients, lens decentration was not symptomatic. One of these patients had significant pseudophacodonesis, and I therefore resutured the MCTR using 8-0 Gortex suture.

Surgical management of the congenitally subluxed lens is still somewhat challenging, and one should not expect successful placement of a MCTR in every case. A learning curve is to be expected. Accordingly, the majority of failed MCTR placements were early in my experience and occurred before learning to use iris hooks to stabilize the lens for phacoemulsification and MCTR insertion. Since incorporating iris hook stabilization, I have had only two failed MCTR attempts. These failures were due to a tear that developed in the capsulorhexis edge during phacoemulsification or with removal of the iris hooks. Without an intact capsulorhexis, or should a tear develop in the edge of the capsulorhexis or in the posterior capsule later in the procedure, the expansile forces of any MCTR or CTR will likely cause the capsular bag to rupture, necessitating MCTR removal.

The management of the congenitally subluxated lens remains challenging. However, newer surgical techniques now afford us the possibility of saving the capsular bag, recentering the capsular bag, and even placing a PC IOL within the capsular bag (Figure 27-15). This allows the surgery to be performed through a 3-mm incision, giving the patient a rapid visual recovery. This is most important in young children because prolonged visual deprivation could result in dense amblyopia.

REFERENCES

1. Jensen AD, Cross HE: Surgical treatment of dislocated lenses in Marfan's syndrome and homocystinuria, *Trans Am Acad Ophthalmol Otolaryngol* 76:1491-1499, 1972.
2. Varga B: The results of my operations improving visual acuity of ectopia lentis, *Ophthalmologica* 162:98-110, 1971.
3. Maumenee IH: The eye in Marfan's syndrome, *Trans Am Acad Ophthalmol Soc* 79:684-733, 1981.
4. Straatsma BR, Allen RA, Pettit TH et al: Subluxation of the lens with iris photocoagulation, *Am J Ophthalmol* 61:1312-1324, 1966.
5. Zetterstrom C, Lundvall A, Weeber Jr H et al: Sulcus fixation without capsular support in children, *J Cataract Refract Surg* 25:776-781, 1999.
6. Cionni RJ, Osher RH: Endocapsular ring approach to the subluxated cataractous lens, *J Cataract Refract Surg* 21:245-249, 1995.
7. Legler U, Witschel B et al: The capsular tension ring, a new device for complicated cataract surgery. Presented at the American Society of Cataract and Refractive Surgery, Seattle, Wash, May 1993.
8. Osher RH: Synthetic zonules, *J Cataract Refract Surg* 8(1), 1997 (video).
9. Pfeifer V: Video presentation at the American Society of Cataract and Refractive Surgery, San Diego, Calif, April 1998.
10. Cionni RJ, Osher RH: Management of profound zonular dialysis or weakness with a new endocapsular ring designed for scleral fixation, *J Cataract Refract Surg* 24:1299-1306, 1998.
11. Merriam J, Zheng L: Iris hooks for phacoemulsification of the subluxated lens, *J Cataract Refract Surg* 23:1295, 1997.
12. Maloney WF: Supracapsular phaco: achieving greater efficiency with phaco outside of the capsular bag—a 3-year experience. Presented at the American Society of Cataract and Refractive Surgery, Seattle, Wash, April, 1999.
13. Osher RH: Slow motion phacoemulsification approach, *J Cataract Refract Surg* 19:667, 1993 (letter).
14. Cionni RJ, Osher RH: Complications of phacoemulsification. In Weinstock FJ, editor: *Management and care of the cataract patient,* Cambridge, Mass, 1992, Blackwell Scientific, pp 209-210.
15. Hollick EJ, Spalton DJ, Ursell PG et al: Biocompatibility of poly(methylmethacrylate), silicone, and AcrySof intraocular lenses: randomized comparison of the cellular reaction on the anterior lens surface, *J Cataract Refract Surg* 24:361-366, 1998.
16. Ursell PG, Spalton DJ, Pande MV et al: Relationship between intraocular lens biomaterials and posterior capsule opacification, *J Cataract Refract Surg* 24:352-360, 1998.
17. Linnola RJ, Werner L, Pandey SK et al, Adhesion of fibronectin, vitronectin, laminin, and collagen type IV to intraocular lens materials in pseudophakic human autopsy eyes. Part 1: Histological sections, *J Cataract Refract Surg* 26:1792-1806, 2000.
18. Linnola RJ Werner L, Pandey SK et al: Adhesion of fibronectin, vitronectin, laminin, and collagen type IV to intraocular lens materials in pseudophakic human autopsy eyes. Part 2: Explanted intraocular lenses, *J Cataract Refract Surg* 26:1807-1818, 2000.
19. Osher RH: Dry vitrectomy, *J Cataract Refr Surg* 8(4), 1992 (video).
20. Snyder ME, Cionni RJ, Osher RH: Management of intraoperative complications. In Gills JP, editor: *Cataract surgery: the state of the art,* Thorofare, NJ, 1998, Slack, pp 149-152.

Techniques and Principles of Surgical Management for the Traumatic Cataract

28

Michael E. Snyder, MD
Robert H. Osher, MD

Management of the patient with a traumatized anterior segment often poses challenges both at initial evaluation and in the operating room. Traumatic cataract commonly occurs with severe penetrating ocular trauma, but it may also result from blunt injury by snowballs, water balloons,[1] and airbags.[2] Athletic events and other seemingly harmless everyday activities may also give rise to traumatic cataracts. For example, in a peculiar case, a golfer sustained a large corneal laceration while teeing off when a bird flew into his eye! Thus traumatic injuries are, by their very nature, highly variable, and the extent of damage can be difficult to determine at the initial presentation. The anterior segment injury may appear either much less or much greater than it actually is. Furthermore, concurrent posterior segment damage may require vitreoretinal intervention that may precede, follow, or be concurrent with the cataract operation, necessitating communication and coordination with the vitreoretinal surgeon. Traumatic cataracts are among the most technically demanding cases that the anterior segment surgeon may face. As with all surgeries, preparation and planning for any anticipated or unanticipated intraoperative events will serve to maximize both the patient's outcome and the surgeon's comfort with the operative procedure.

In acute, severe injuries, preparation may include appropriately counseling the injured patient, emphasizing the unpredictable nature of these cases and reasonable short-term and long-term expectations. The patient began with "normal vision" may anticipate returning to preinjury status; however, this may or may not be possible in any given case. Although it is important to offer reasonable hopes, we advocate the "underpromise and overdeliver" philosophy.

The goal of this chapter is to outline a careful, systematic approach to surgery for traumatic cataract and to describe several surgical techniques that may be helpful in these challenging settings.

Clinical Evaluation

Careful preoperative evaluation of the patient with a traumatic cataract is ideal to gaining a complete understanding of the disrupted ocular anatomy and anticipating events that may occur in the operating room. The goals of the preoperative evaluation are to assess the degree of ocular damage; formulate an operative plan; and determine all potentially needed instruments, equipment, sutures, and implants in advance. Careful preoperative planning should reduce the number and degree of intraoperative surprises, thereby enhancing the surgeon's comfort level with the operation and maximizing the patient's visual outcome.

History of the Injury

In the acute setting, the preoperative evaluation should include a careful history about how the injury occurred. The force and mechanism of the injury may give clues about whether an occult perforation or intraocular foreign body may exist or whether coexisting posterior segment damage should be anticipated. Metal-on-metal injuries should raise the suspicion of an iron-containing intraocular foreign body. In cases of an open globe, inquiry about the environment where the injury occurred may provide clues about the presence of potentially infectious or inflammatory material. Keep in mind that the history of events surrounding the injury may be notably unreliable when provided by children. In our experience, children and adolescents may not be entirely forthright initially, and often the real story is not disclosed for weeks or months. The implication for the clinician is to maintain a high degree of vigilance and refrain from eliminating any possibilities based on the history provided by a youth.

Some cases of traumatic cataract will present months, years, or even decades after the injury; the patient may have long forgotten the details or even the occurrence of the injury and may remember only after the surgeon poses several probing questions.

Examination

This section reviews those components of the ophthalmic examination that are particularly relevant to cases of traumatic cataract.

Assessing Visual Function

The examination should always begin with an assessment of visual acuity. Ideally, this will be a best-corrected Snellen visual acuity tested in the controlled setting of the office environment. Of course, in acute trauma, this ideal situation may not exist. When testing reveals hand motions or light perception vision, the ability to identify colored light gives some prognostic information about macular function. Confrontational visual fields give very helpful information but are not possible in eyes with mature cataracts. The patient's response to the Purkinje phenomenon may provide indirect evidence about whether the retina is attached or detached or if glaucomatous or visual field loss may be present. Recently, a patient with mature cataract noted the Purkinje phenomenon only in the nasal visual field. Magnetic resonance imaging (MRI) disclosed an otherwise asymptomatic pituitary tumor. Similarly, Karp and Fazio[3] reported a patient who presented 3 months after an ocular injury with a monocular nasal hemianopia confirmed by Humphrey 24-2 testing. The hemianopia resolved completely following extraction of a posterior subcapsular cataract. Purkinje testing is contraindicated in the presence of an open penetrating wound.

For evaluations performed in the emergency room, formal Snellen assessments may not be possible. We can, however, still document light perception, hand motions, and count fingers—all the way up to "recognizes faces" or even "reads 14-point print on hospital consent form." Although visual acuity measurements can underestimate visual potential in the setting of acute penetrating trauma, proper documentation and patient and family counseling may protect the surgeon from inaccuracies in a patient's or family's subsequent recollections of the severity of the initial injury.

As the only objective measure of visual function, assessment for an afferent pupillary defect should always be ascertained. Although assessment of the pupillary response can be extremely helpful in predicting prognosis, it is not always easily performed in the acute setting of an anxious patient with an open globe. Because traumatic mydriasis, miosis, and frank iris tears or incarceration may limit the function of the involved pupil, the ophthalmologist should always remember that visualization of only one pupil is required to determine the presence or absence of an afferent pupillary defect. Significant efforts to simultaneously open both lids should be avoided if that is likely to result in the patient squeezing them closed.

Biomicroscopy

Slit lamp biomicroscopy provides extremely helpful information for the operative intervention. First, the anterior chamber may be studied for possible vitreous prolapse or retained intraocular foreign body. The presence and degree of iris damage or loss can be assessed, and the crystalline lens can be scrutinized. In fact, the traumatic origin of cataract is sometimes revealed by noting the subtle findings of a gap between the iris margin and lens surface or decentration of the Y sutures relative to the pupil center. Phacodonesis, frank decentration, and zonular loss should be carefully documented in both location and degree. When the lens capsule is visibly damaged, the extent of a tear should be carefully delineated and recorded. A corrugated appearance to the lens capsule may indicate compromised capsular or zonular integrity. The anterior lens capsule can be ruptured even in cases of blunt (nonpenetrating) trauma.[4] The surgeon should already be thinking about how a capsulorhexis might be able to incorporate the defect. An anterior capsule tear will typically enlarge as the lens material swells. Therefore, if a defect is near the margin to which it could be incorporated into a capsulorhexis, intervention might be expedited. Posterior capsular breaks can, similarly, occur with either penetrating or blunt trauma,[5] although this may not be apparent on clinical examination because cataract formation may limit the examiner's view.

Some biomicroscopic findings may be fairly obvious in some cases. Netland et al.[6] describe a case of dislocation of the crystalline lens into the anterior chamber following blunt injury.

In the setting of an open corneoscleral laceration, careful preoperative evaluation at the slit lamp examination may be either impractical or impossible, making surgical planning much more challenging.

Ophthalmoscopy

Funduscopic evaluation (when view permits) should include an evaluation for retinal holes or tears or commotio retinae. Subretinal or suprachoroidal hemorrhage may portend a more guarded prognosis. When any suprachoroidal hemorrhage is present, the surgeon should expect positive posterior pressure in surgery.

Special Testing

When a mature cataract is present, B-scan ultrasonography is instrumental in surgical planning. First, the B-scan can provide crucial information about the status of the posterior lens capsule. In one case of mature cataract following penetrating injury, B-scan ultrasonography confirmed a displaced rupture of the posterior lens capsule (Figure 28-1). In addition to confirming the posterior segment status, B-scan information may alter the surgeon's approach to removing the cataract. When a suprachoroidal hemorrhage is detected, for example, the anterior segment surgeon should exercise caution in considering a pars plana approach for anterior vitrectomy. If possible, intervention should be delayed until the hemorrhage has resolved. If a large suprachoroidal hemorrhage is present, vitreoretinal consultation is recommended because drainage may be required. Although the drainage procedure is not particularly difficult, subsequent retinal detachment may occur as the choroidal mounds flatten. Ultrasound testing can also demonstrate vital features in the anterior segment. Sathish, Chakrabarti, and Prajna[7] reported a patient who sustained an anterior scleral rupture with ultrasound-documented dislocation of the crystalline lens into the subconjunctival space.

If the surgeon suspects an intraocular or intraorbital foreign body, computed tomography (CT) scan imaging of the orbits with thin slices is indicated. CT scanning may have some role in diagnosing traumatic cataract in the setting of acute trauma. One study reports that a low attenuation of the lens is diagnostic of current or near-term development of visually significant cataract.[8] In that study, no patients with normal attenuation developed cataract within 1 year. The ophthalmologist should

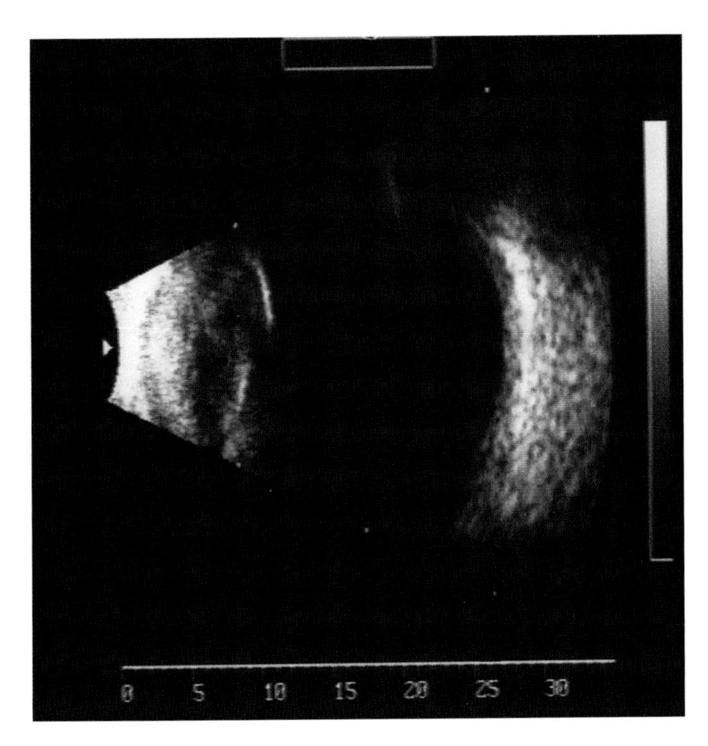

FIGURE 28-1 B-scan ultrasound demonstrates a full-thickness laceration of the lens with discontinuity of the two hemispheres. (This case is described in detail in Case One at the end of the chapter.)

be aware of another study demonstrating that an intumescent cataract may appear invisible on CT scan, giving a false impression of traumatic aphakia.[9] MRI scanning is not particularly helpful in the management of a traumatic cataract and could cause serious damage if a ferromagnetic foreign body is present in the eye or orbit.

Cataract Surgery in the Acutely Traumatized Globe

Although some articles advocate primary cataract extraction at the time of an open globe repair,[10] there are advantages to a staged approach. First, in many instances, corneal clarity, anterior chamber hyphema, clot or disorganization of the anatomy may obscure the view of anterior segment structures and may lead to unanticipated complications. Further examination and testing after repair of the primary laceration can lead to more accurate surgical planning. Second, at the time of an open globe injury, keratometry and biometry of the affected eye are virtually impossible, and usually the patient cannot cooperate maximally for accurate A-scan and keratometry measurements of the contralateral eye. This may lead to a greater likelihood of significant ametropia or anisometropia in what might be an otherwise optimal visual result.

Occasionally, the degree of injury to the lens may appear greater at the initial presentation, but, in fact, it may not require cataract extraction. One patient presented emergently with a full-thickness central corneal laceration that penetrated the anterior capsule of the lens. The cornea was closed primarily, and cataract extraction was not performed. The lens capsule sealed over and developed only a small, focal cataract. The patient retained 20/20 vision and was asymptomatic. Pieramici et al.[11] reported five cases in which a peripheral lens perforation occurred and lens clarity was maintained using a lens-sparing approach for intraocular foreign body removal. They noted that some inert (glass) foreign bodies were well tolerated without removal. Conversely, any potentially iron-containing foreign body should be removed because an iron-containing intralenticular foreign body may result in ocular siderosis with potentially devastating visual consequences.[12]

Cataract Surgery and the Acute Operative Intervention

Of course, in certain occasions, cataract surgery at the time of primary open globe repair is absolutely indicated. First, when traumatic cataract obscures the view for removal of a known intraocular foreign body, cataract extraction should be immediate, particularly when the foreign body may carry vegetable or other contaminated material. Delayed treatment of an intraocular foreign body significantly reduces the chances of a favorable outcome.[13] If the foreign body is in the posterior segment, the anterior segment surgeon should work in combination with a vitreoretinal surgeon. Preferably, the traumatic cataract should be removed using an anterior approach. Pars plana lensectomy leads to more capsular damage and may unnecessarily commit the patient to aphakia or the need for a sutured posterior chamber intraocular lens (PC IOL). If the posterior segment surgeon believes strongly that a pars plana lensectomy is required for vitreoretinal reasons, efforts should be made to retain as much capsular support as possible.

Also, some patients may have medical conditions that may significantly increase their anesthetic risks, making a single general anesthetic episode more desirable. In these instances an expeditious primary extraction is appropriate, although the surgeon should remember that the alternative of a secondary procedure may often be performed under regional anesthesia with a lesser anesthetic risk.

Preoperative patient counseling should be directed at setting realistic expectations based on the available prognostic information.

Surgical Planning and Technique

Ideally, the surgeon should be able to plan the case well in advance so that the operative procedure is a performance that has been mentally rehearsed. This means anticipating each surgical step to the best degree possible preoperatively. The first decision in any operative plan is the selection of the anesthetic approach. In traumatic cataract cases, the surgeon will usually be choosing between general and local anesthesia. For open globe situations, general anesthesia usually provides greater safety. In the setting of a secure globe, the decision about regional or general anesthesia may be based on factors relating to the patient's ability to cooperate and the anticipated length of the procedure. Topical anesthesia should be reserved for only the most straightforward traumatic cataract cases. If significant posterior pressure is anticipated, intravenous mannitol administered in the holding room may be helpful. Although some informal, anecdotal teachings suggested a link between intravenous mannitol and suprachoroidal hemorrhage, formal studies have not identified mannitol as an independent risk factor. Traumatic eye injury, however, is a well-documented risk for suprachoroidal hemorrhage.[14,15]

Selection of Wound Location

Once anesthetic concerns have been addressed, the surgeon must select the planned location of the scleral or corneal wound. The wound should preferably be positioned in the area of the most normal anterior segment anatomy. A cataract incision placed over a zonular dialysis will make scleral suturing of a modified Cionni capsular tension ring or sutured posterior chamber implant unnecessarily more difficult. Furthermore, the surgeon will be working directly over an exposed hyaloid face, increasing the chances of disturbing the vitreous. Sometimes a steep orbital rim will mandate a temporal approach, although if the traumatic wound crosses the temporal limbus, this area should be strictly avoided for the cataract incision. In such a case, an inferior incision may be considered. If the factors described previously do not limit the surgeon's choices of wound location, then astigmatic considerations may be taken into account. The planned wound location will usually dictate the most appropriate orientation for the surgeon to sit.

Managing the Conjunctiva

Often in traumatic cases, the additional strength of a scleral tunnel wound is preferable because a larger incision may be required if the surgeon has selected a polymethylmethacrylate (PMMA) implant. Although the conjunctival incision is not the most glamorous part of the procedure, careful consideration should be given to the location and extent of the peritomy. The conjunctival openings should allow ample access to the planned scleral tunnel wound sites and also should include access for a pars plana sclerotomy or a site for scleral suturing of a PC IOL or modified Cionni capsular tension ring. Although adequate access is of vital importance, uninvolved conjunctiva should be respected because several traumatic cataract cases may be referred to a glaucoma specialist at some point in the future.

Viscoelastic Options

Selection of the viscoelastic agent for a traumatic cataract case depends on several factors. In some cases more than one agent may be appropriate. When the intact hyaloid face is partly exposed, a highly retentive viscoelastic agent such as Viscoat (Alcon, Fort Worth, Tex.) or Vitrax (Allergan, Irvine, Calif.) may tamponade the vitreous and keep it back[16] (Figure 28-2). The highly retentive agents are also excellent endothelial protectants. This may be particularly relevant to cases in which the endothelial cell density has been reduced by the trauma.[17] The space-retaining qualities and ease of removal typical of highly cohesive viscoelastic agents, such as Healon GV and Healon 5 (Pharmacia, Monrovia, Calif.), make these agents more appropriate for the lens implantation stage of a procedure. In some cases one may choose the "soft shell" technique,[18] which combines the added endothelial protection of a highly dispersive agent with the space-maintaining abilities, ease of removal, and clarity of the cohesive agents. The soft shell is created by loosely filling the corneal dome with a dispersive viscoelastic and then instilling a cohesive viscoelastic just in front of the crystalline lens. This presses the dispersive agent against the corneal endothelium, creating a thin protective layer. The soft shell approach should be used cautiously when vitreous tamponade is desired because the cohesive agent may thin or displace the protective "plug" in front of the vitreous.

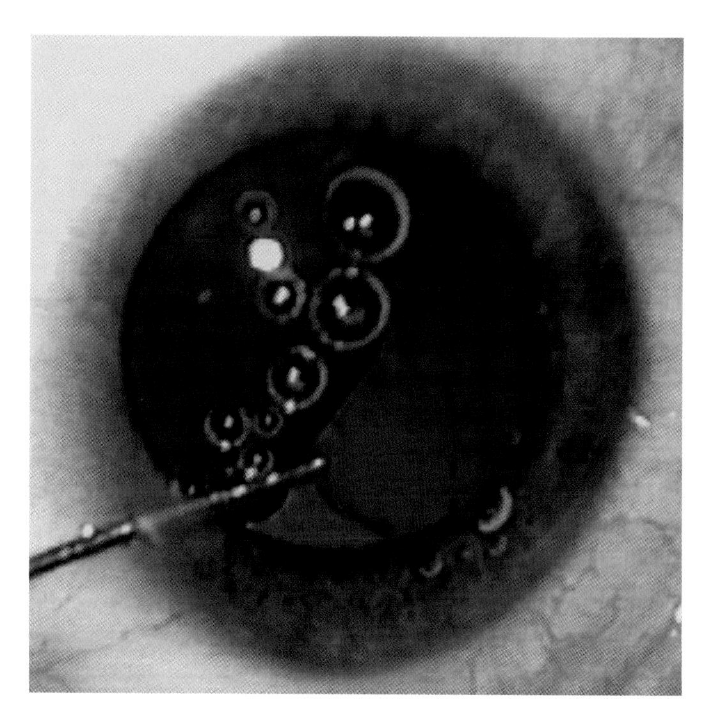

FIGURE 28-2 Dispersive viscoelastic can create a "plug" to protect an exposed hyaloid face.

Another option may offer both protection and space maintenance with a single agent. Healon 5 is a "pseudoplastic" agent with outstanding space maintenance properties. At higher aspiration flow rates, the cohesive agent sheers, providing properties similar to the dispersive materials. Healon 5 holds promise for use in traumatic cataracts; however, our experience in this setting is still early, and the surgeon should be alerted to the possibility of greater intraocular pressure elevation if any agent remains in the globe at the completion of the procedure.

When "dry" lens material aspiration under viscoelastic is anticipated,[19] a moderately cohesive agent such as Healon or ProVisc (Alcon, Fort Worth, Tex.) should be selected. Highly retentive viscoelastics tend to clog the cannula for manual aspiration techniques, and Healon GV tends to follow into the tip of the cannula, preferentially to the lens material, and, in fact, can inhibit aspiration of cortex.

The Capsulotomy

The anterior capsulotomy often determines the ease or difficulty of the cataract removal. Sometimes, the traumatic injury may have caused an anterior capsular defect either from a blunt rupture or from a sharp laceration. The opening may provide direct access to the lens material, yet every effort should be made to convert the capsular tear into an intact capsulorhexis. A complete capsulorhexis has far superior mechanical integrity to either a can-opener capsulotomy or a partial capsulorhexis[20] and will improve the safety of each subsequent step of the operative procedure. Occasionally, a vitrector may be useful in creating an anterior capsular opening. This type of capsulotomy has a greater structural integrity than a can-opener capsulotomy but is not as desirable as a complete capsulorhexis.[21] The vitrectorhexis technique can be less facile in practice than in theory because the lens capsule is not always easily aspirated to the cutting port. Moreover, when the capsule is engaged in the port, marginal zonules may be compromised.

Visualization for the capsulorhexis may be particularly difficult in cases of traumatic cataract, particularly when the capsule is torn or the cortex is opaque. Several dyes have been recommended to aid in visualization of the anterior capsule, including fluorescein,[22] methylene blue, gentian violet,[23] crystal violet, trypan blue,[24] and indocyanine green (ICG).[25] Clinically, ICG (IC-Green, Akorn, NJ) and trypan blue (Vision Blue, Dutch Ophthalmic Research Corporation, Netherlands) are extremely helpful and have acceptable safety profiles[26] (Figure 28-3). The initial descriptions of ICG recommended instillation under air. We have found that when the capsule is intact, gently painting a drop across the anterior capsule under viscoelastic is equally effective. The stain may even delineate the edges of a torn capsule. Trypan blue has some potential advantages, particularly its low cost, but is not currently available in the United States. Fluorescein has a high index of safety, but it stains the capsule only weakly and tends to cause a diffuse yellow appearance of the operative field, which may limit visualization of subsequent steps. Methylene blue and gentian violet have a known cytotoxicity.[27]

Tangential illumination of the anterior capsule using a sterile endoilluminator probe may also facilitate visualization for capsulotomy with a white lens. Metz[28] and, subsequently, Gimbel and Willerscheidt[29] reported aspirating liquefied, white cortical material through a tiny, central capsular opening to decompress the capsular bag in cases of intumescent white cataract. This may decrease the tendency for peripheral extension by lowering the endocapsular pressure.

The surgeon should exercise meticulous technique in creating a capsular tear in traumatized lenses. Zonular countertraction may not be uniform, so the physics of creating the tear are slightly different than the usual case. The surgeon should make special efforts to have the leading edge of the capsular flap *folded over* to control the path of the tear more predictably (Figure 28-4). If significant zonular instability is present, the surgeon may use a side port instrument to stabilize the lens nucleus during capsulorhexis. The anterior capsulorhexis in children with traumatic cataract may be even more challenging than their adult counterparts because the pediatric lens capsule has a stronger and more elastic consistency. For these younger patients, it may be easier to plan to make the capsulorhexis smaller initially and enlarge it later if necessary because these capsules have a greater tendency toward peripheral extension of the circular tear.

Nucleus Removal

Removal of the lens nucleus can be addressed by a number of different techniques, each of which have potential advantages

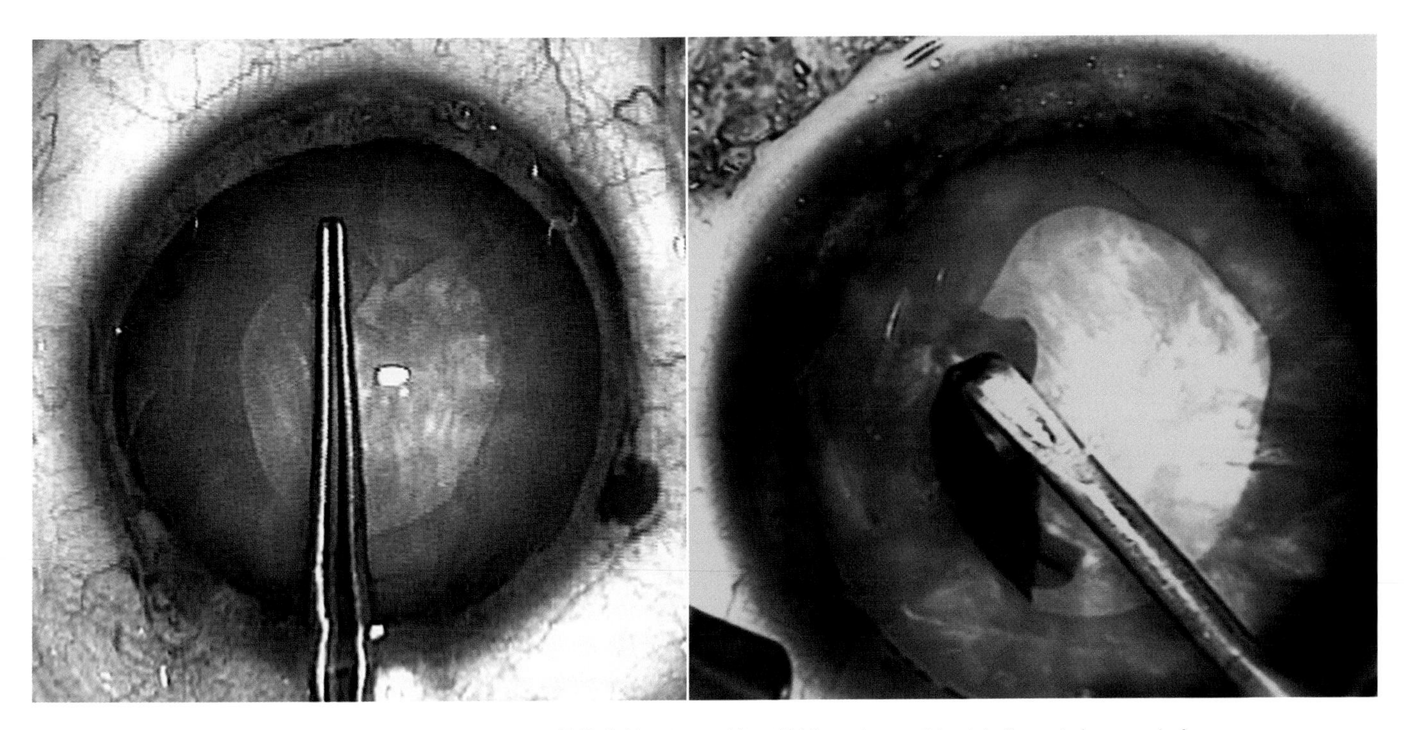

FIGURE 28-3 Indocyanine green (ICG) *(left)* or trypan blue *(right)* can be used to stain the anterior capsule for greater visibility in the white cataract.

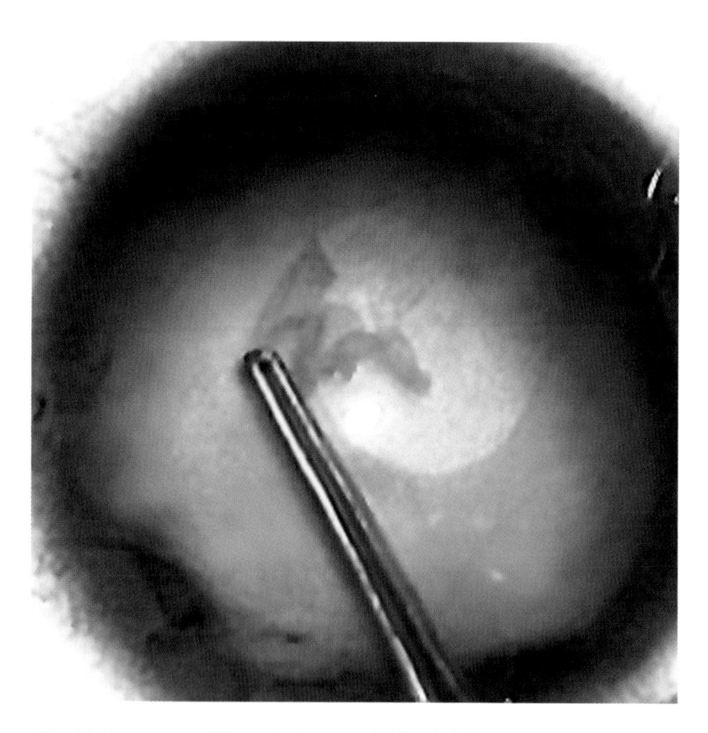

FIGURE 28-4 If the anterior capsular flap is folded over, the surgeon will have greater control over the direction of the capsular tear. ICG was used in this case to better demonstrate the capsular flap. In this case, ICG was administered under viscoelastic, and some residual dye is visible within the viscoelastic material.

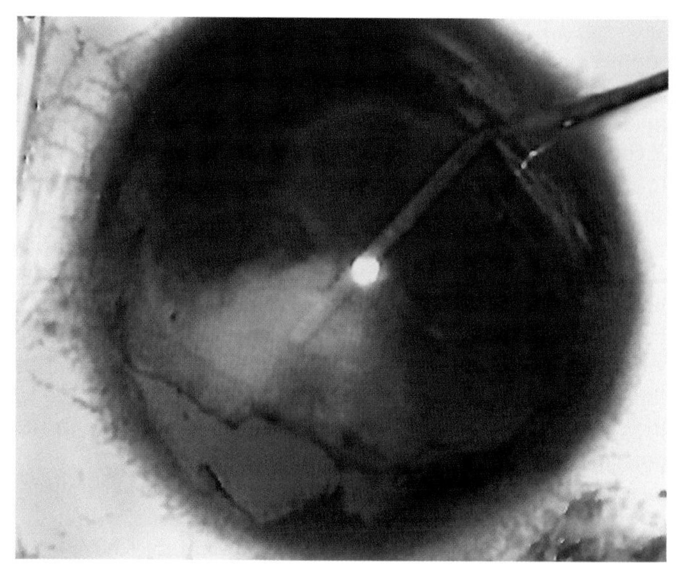

FIGURE 28-5 Remaining white cortical material within the capsular bag is aspirated manually with a 27-gauge cannula in a "dry" fashion. Viscoelastic material protects the exposed hyaloid face in an area of preexisting posterior capsular tear seen just up and to the left of the cannula tip.

and disadvantages, depending on the setting. In a young patient the nucleus is usually very soft and is amenable to many different options. For a patient with an intact capsulorhexis, phaco aspiration of the nucleus is typically safe and expeditious. If an anterior or posterior capsular tear is present, then manual aspiration with a Simcoe-style cannula affords greater control (Figure 28-5). "Dry" aspiration of the soft nucleus under viscoelastic material offers exquisite control, especially in the most complicated cases.[15]

Because the nucleus is more dense in older patients, its removal requires a more challenging disassembly. The superior control of a small-incision, closed system approach to nucleus removal shines particularly brightly in cases with distorted anatomy and potentially weakened zonules. Traumatized eyes are at greater risk for suprachoroidal hemorrhage, so maintaining a closed system reduces the chances of the catastrophic expulsive consequences. Furthermore, a closed system allows compartmentalization within the anterior segment. If the posterior capsule is broken or if a zonular dehiscence is present, viscoelastic tamponade of the vitreous can be best maintained in the setting of a closed system. Manual extracapsular cataract extraction and manual phacosection techniques require an open wound and thereby compromise an important degree of control over the intraocular environment.

The technique of phacoemulsification may vary somewhat depending on the surgeon's usual approach, although some important principles should be incorporated into these special traumatic cases. A cautious respect for the zonular support in the traumatic cataract should guide the surgeon away from choosing a "phaco-flip," "chip-and-flip," or other techniques that may exert trampoline-like pressure to the zonular apparatus, even when no frank zonular dialysis is detected preoperatively. Many variations of gentle, divide and conquer techniques or phaco-chop techniques can be modified to incorporate the principles of "slow motion phaco."[30]

Phacoemulsification in the Presence of Zonular Compromise

In some patients with very weak zonules, grooving for a divide and conquer and other endocapsular manipulations may stress the already compromised capsular support. A relatively large capsulorhexis will facilitate viscoexpression of the nucleus into the anterior chamber. Alternatively, a very gentle chopping procedure is protective to the remaining intact zonules because all applied forces are borne by the chopper instrument, the nucleus, and the countertraction of the phacoemulsification handpiece.

When severe zonular damage is present, the surgeon can use a capsular tension ring to help stabilize the lens nucleus before phacoemulsification begins. To facilitate endocapsular ring placement, cortical cleaving viscodissection will create the potential space for the ring to pass into the capsular bag. When more than four clock hours of zonular damage are present, the modified Cionni capsular tension ring (Morcher, Germany) adds suture fixation to the area of greatest zonular weakness[31] (Figure 28-6). We have found that it is easiest to load the suture through the fixation eyelet before ring implantation and then pass the transscleral sutures in an ab interno fashion once the fixation element has been guided into the proper meridian. Suture fixation improves the lens stability for the remainder of the case. If the lens nucleus is particularly large and dense, it may be difficult or impossible to place the endocapsular ring before

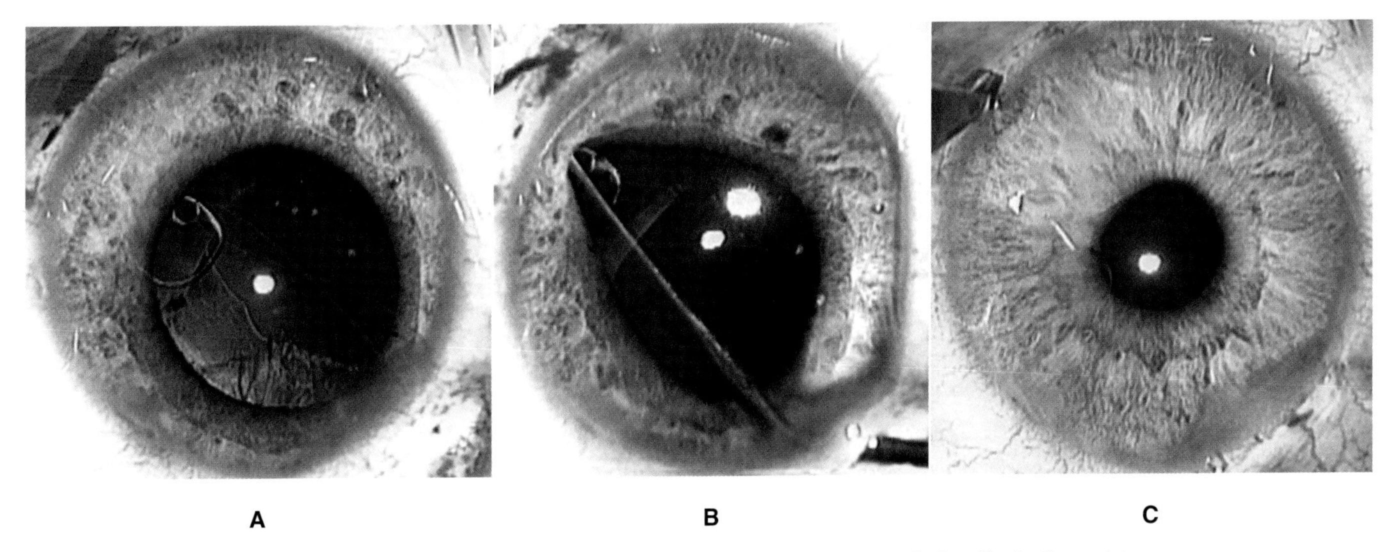

FIGURE 28-6 **A,** Modified (Cionni) capsular tension ring in situ within the capsular bag. The fixation eyelet courses in front of the capsulorhexis margin. The sutures have not yet been passed through the sclera. **B,** Position of the fixation element is seen after the fixation sutures have been tightened. The second light reflex is the second Purkinje-Sanson image from the front surface of the well-centered IOL. **C,** Appearance of the eye at the end of the procedure.

phacoemulsification. In such cases the surgeon can temporarily augment the native zonular support with flexible nylon "iris" retractors placed through a limbal incision to engage the capsulorhexis margin (Figure 28-7). The retractor can be placed through a paracentesis tract, although a pathway may be created with a curved S-14 spatula needle placed perpendicular at the conjunctival insertion, entering the anterior chamber just above the iris insertion. This method of placement creates less anterior movement of the lens-capsular complex, thereby providing a deeper anterior chamber to work in. The tract of an S-14 needle is self-sealing. Once the nucleus is emulsified, the endocapsular ring may be placed with greater ease.

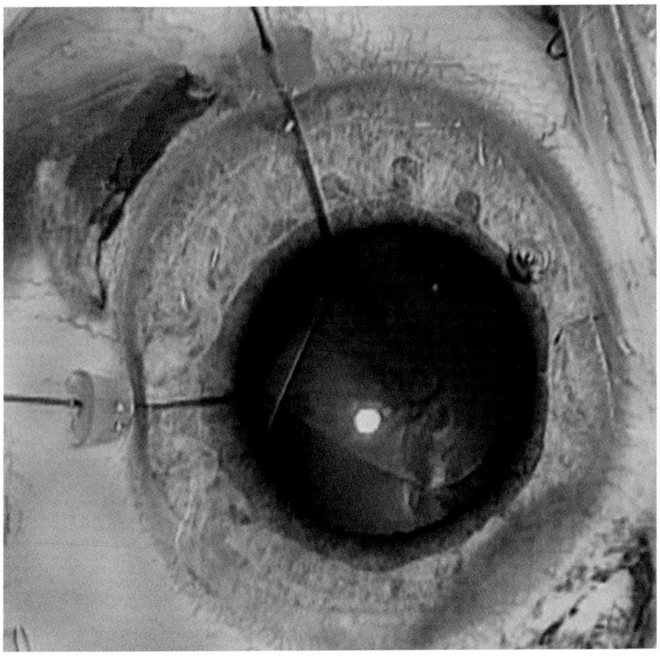

FIGURE 28-7 Flexible "iris" retractors can be placed to stabilize the capsular bag for phacoemulsification when zonular support is compromised. After phacoemulsification, the capsular tension ring can be more easily inserted.

Theoretically, the capsular tension ring could be inserted after a posterior capsular break if both an intact anterior and posterior capsulorhexis were present. Capsular tension ring placement should *not* be considered with any other setting of anterior or posterior capsular break. If a capsular tear or break were to occur with the endocapsular ring in situ, the device should be promptly retrieved from the anterior segment because its stability is no longer guaranteed.

Cortical Removal

Once the lens nucleus has been successfully removed, the capsular bag should be carefully inspected for integrity. Isolated posterior capsule rupture has been reported as a result of blunt injury.[32-35] When the capsular bag and zonular apparatus are intact, cortical removal can be routine, but when zonular damage is present, the cortex is best removed by a very gentle, controlled technique. Some of the principles discussed previously for soft nuclei apply particularly well to cortical removal and are reviewed in more detail here. If cortical cleaving hydrodissection was performed at the beginning of the case, this step may be much easier. If hydrodissection was incomplete or not performed, viscodissection can gently separate cortical material from the capsular bag[36] (Figure 28-8). When an automated irrigation and aspiration method is used, teasing the cortical strands parallel to the zonular dialysis will be less likely to cause the intact zonules to unzip. The same principle applies to manual aspiration with a Simcoe-type cannula, which offers a greater degree of control within a stable chamber. If a posterior capsular break is present, a viscoelastic tamponade of the intact hyaloid face, combined with a manual dry aspiration with a 25-

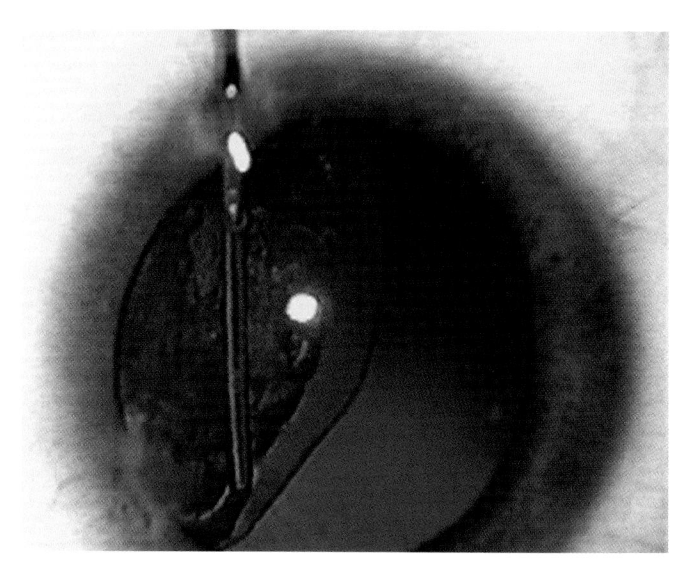

FIGURE 28-8 Cortical cleaving viscodissection can separate the lens material from the capsular bag, making the cortex easier to remove.

or 27-gauge cannula on a 3-cc syringe in a chamber filled with viscoelastic material, can facilitate complete cortical removal without vitreous loss. The exquisite control of the dry aspiration technique offsets the more tedious and time-consuming nature of this approach.[23]

Removal of Lens Material with Vitreous Prolapse

Vitreous in the anterior segment alone or admixed within the lens material increases the risks of posterior segment complications. It is not uncommon for penetrating injuries to go through the lens and into the vitreous. If the penetrating object is withdrawn, vitreous may be pulled into or through the lacerated crystalline lens. The surgeon should always try to avoid aspirating any vitreous material. Any traction on the firm attachments of the anterior vitreous to the vitreous base can create a retinal break and subsequent retinal detachment. If there is extensive loss of zonular support and the capsular remnants are severely lacerated, a pars plana lensectomy with vitrectomy may be the most appropriate course.

When vitreous is identified within the lens material but the lens support and peripheral lens anatomy are relatively intact, some special anterior segment approaches are indicated. First, any vitreous that has prolapsed through the laceration or surgical wound should be removed with an automated vitreous cutter. A dry vitrectomy can be performed at the wound site by placing the cutting port against the scleral or corneal opening. This will effectively remove any external vitreous without creating traction. The machine settings should have relatively low flow and low vacuum.

Next, the vitreous cutter can be placed into the anterior chamber, and a gentle anterior vitrectomy can be performed to remove the vitreous material from the anterior segment and sever any incarcerations or attachments to the anterior segment wounds. Coaxial irrigation on the vitrector handpiece can blow the vitreous away from the cutting port and thus cause unnecessary flow through the anterior chamber. Bimanual or split infusion via a separate paracentesis site is preferable using a 21-gauge butterfly or blunt cannula to allow control of the direction of the irrigation stream.

When the anterior chamber is clear of vitreous, attention is turned to the removal of the lens material. When the lens material is soft, it may be aspirated via the vitrector handpiece on "I/A cutter" settings so that the instrument behaves as an I/A device until foot position 3, in which cutting action is engaged. Use of the vitrector handpiece adds additional safety when vitreous may be admixed with lens material because if an errant strand of vitreous finds its way to the aspiration port, cutting may be immediately initiated, thereby releasing vitreous traction.

Dry Cortical Aspiration

If zonular damage is present and exquisite control is required, a dry aspiration technique under a chamber filled with viscoelastic can be carefully performed. A moderately cohesive viscoelastic agent can be injected to deepen the chamber. Special caution should be used to place the viscoelastic agent at the wound first and not to overfill the chamber. If too much viscoelastic material is injected, the increase in the intraocular pressure may cause vitreous to prolapse through the wound during instillation. The aspiration is most effective when introducing a 25- or 27-gauge cannula *into* the soft lens material with the cannula tip placed as far from the capsular break as possible. The lens material can be carefully stripped and aspirated, working from the area most distal to the capsular break. If vitreous is engaged at any point, it must be immediately released, and additional vitrectomy is performed.

Dense Capsular Plaques

Not infrequently, capsular plaques may line either the posterior capsule or, occasionally, the entire internal circumference of the capsular bag. Once an edge of the plaque is elevated, viscodissection, blunt dissection, and peeling of the plaque may result in a clear posterior capsule and clean capsular bag (Figure 28-9). Other times, a posterior capsulorhexis may be created, or alternatively, YAG laser capsulotomy may be performed after surgery.

Dense Nucleus and an Open Posterior Capsule

In the presence of dense cataractous lens material, phacoemulsification may be required. If the anterior segment has been entirely cleared of vitreous, an anterior chamber phaco over a bed of dispersive viscoelastic or a Sheets glide may be cautiously considered. In this setting, a side port instrument should be used to support the lens material. Sheets glide placement technique should be meticulous because inaccurate insertion can engage or tear remaining capsular support. The surgeon should consider that a Sheets glide can be very difficult to place from a clear corneal wound.

Preferentially, if a complete anterior capsulorhexis can be achieved, slightly smaller than the intraocular lens (IOL) optic,

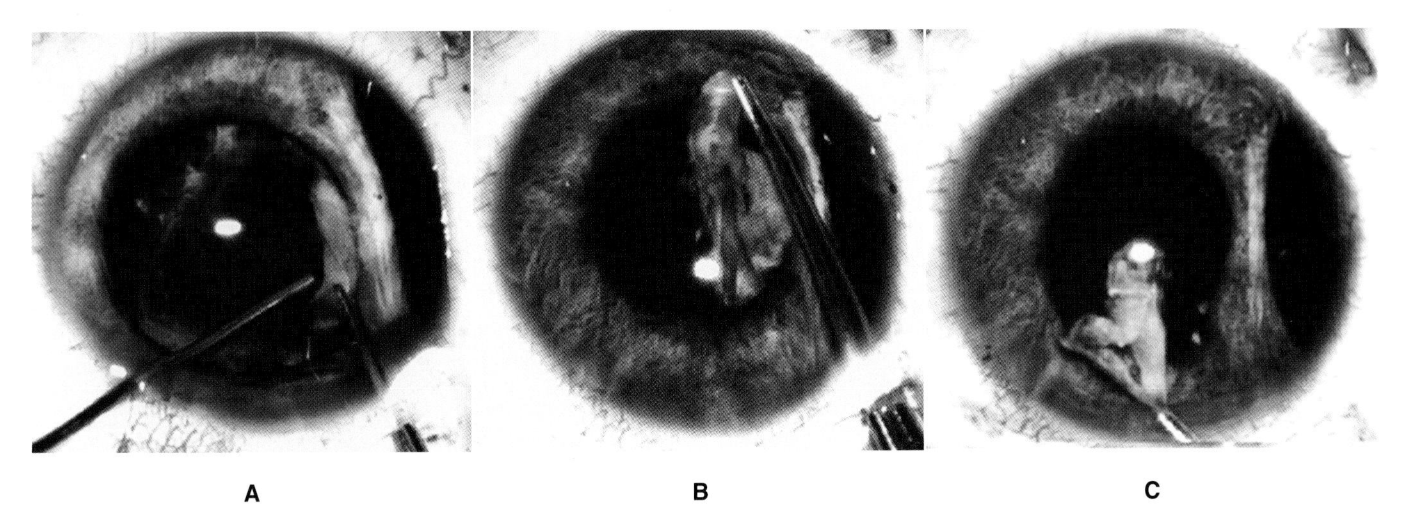

FIGURE 28-9 A, Dense capsular plaque is viscodissected from the capsular bag. Plaque encompasses the entire internal lining of the intact bag. **B,** Once the tightest adhesions have been lysed, the plaque can be peeled away from the capsule. **C,** Plaque is removed en bloc, leaving an intact and clear capsular bag.

then the nuclear fragments can be placed on the iris leaflet anteriorly, the cortex can be manually aspirated in a dry fashion, and the IOL can be placed in the ciliary sulcus. With posterior capture of the implant optic through the capsulorhexis, the barrier between the anterior and posterior segments has been reestablished, and anterior chamber phaco can be performed without concern for posterior dislocation of lens fragments (Figure 28-10).

Kelman[37] has proposed a technique that he calls "posterior assisted levitation" in which nuclear material is supported from behind via a second instrument placed through the pars plana. With this technique the surgeon should be vigilant in watching for vitreous at the port of the phacoemulsification handpiece. The surgeon should always avoid manual manipulation of the vitreous gel because traction on the anterior vitreous base may lead to serious retinal sequelae.

Anterior Segment Cleanup

Once the lens material is removed, the anterior segment is carefully reevaluated for any anteriorly displaced vitreous. If vitreous is identified, further vitrectomy should be performed. Once the anterior segment media permit a view through the pupillary space, vitrectomy through a pars plana incision, again with a split, anterior infusion, can be used. The vitrector handpiece is placed through a sclerotomy created 3 mm posterior to the limbus by a 20-gauge V-lance blade (Figure 28-11). The pars plana approach has several advantages over limbal vitrectomy. First, the vitreous material is aspirated posteriorly away from the anterior segment wounds. With anterior irrigation and posteriorly placed vitrector aspiration a localized pressure gradient occurs, creating a flow from anterior to posterior, as desired. Pulling the vitreous back into the vitreous cavity creates less traction on the vitreous base and allows better access to subincisional vitreous that may be coursing around the iris margin.[38] Furthermore, when the vitrector handpiece is placed through the cataract incision, the corneal dome is more likely to be distorted, leading to suboptimal visualization. With the pars plana approach, the view through the cornea is excellent. Once an adequate vitrectomy has been completed, the sclerotomy should be cleaned externally (as described earlier) and then closed with a suture, for example, a figure-of-eight, 7-0 Vicryl suture.

Managing the Compromised Capsule

When all lens material and any offending vitreous have been safely removed, the surgeon can breathe only a brief sigh of relief; he or she must then assess the degree of zonular and capsular support that remain. After filling the anterior segment with viscoelastic, the surgeon may gently retract the iris to directly visualize the underlying anatomy. When the anterior capsulorhexis is intact but a posterior capsular break is present, a few different options exist. Ideally, if the posterior capsular tear is small, some viscoelastic can be placed through the opening to retroplace the vitreous, and the posterior tear may be converted into a posterior capsulorhexis. This can preserve the capsular strength for endocapsular placement of a posterior chamber implant (Figure 28-12).

The experienced surgeon may be able to implant the IOL into the torn capsular bag even when the posterior tear cannot be safely converted to a capsulorhexis, yet it may be safer to place the haptics of a posterior chamber implant into the ciliary sulcus. If the anterior capsulorhexis is intact and measures 5 mm or less, the lens optic can be prolapsed into the capsular bag, providing additional support and centration. In this setting, the implant power would be chosen as usually calculated. If both the optic and the haptics are in the plane of the ciliary sulcus, one-half diopter should be subtracted from the calculated implant power.[39]

If significant capsular damage exists, a determination should be made as to whether there is enough support for the placement of a posterior chamber implant in the ciliary sulcus. The torn posterior capsular bag will often provide long-term fixation

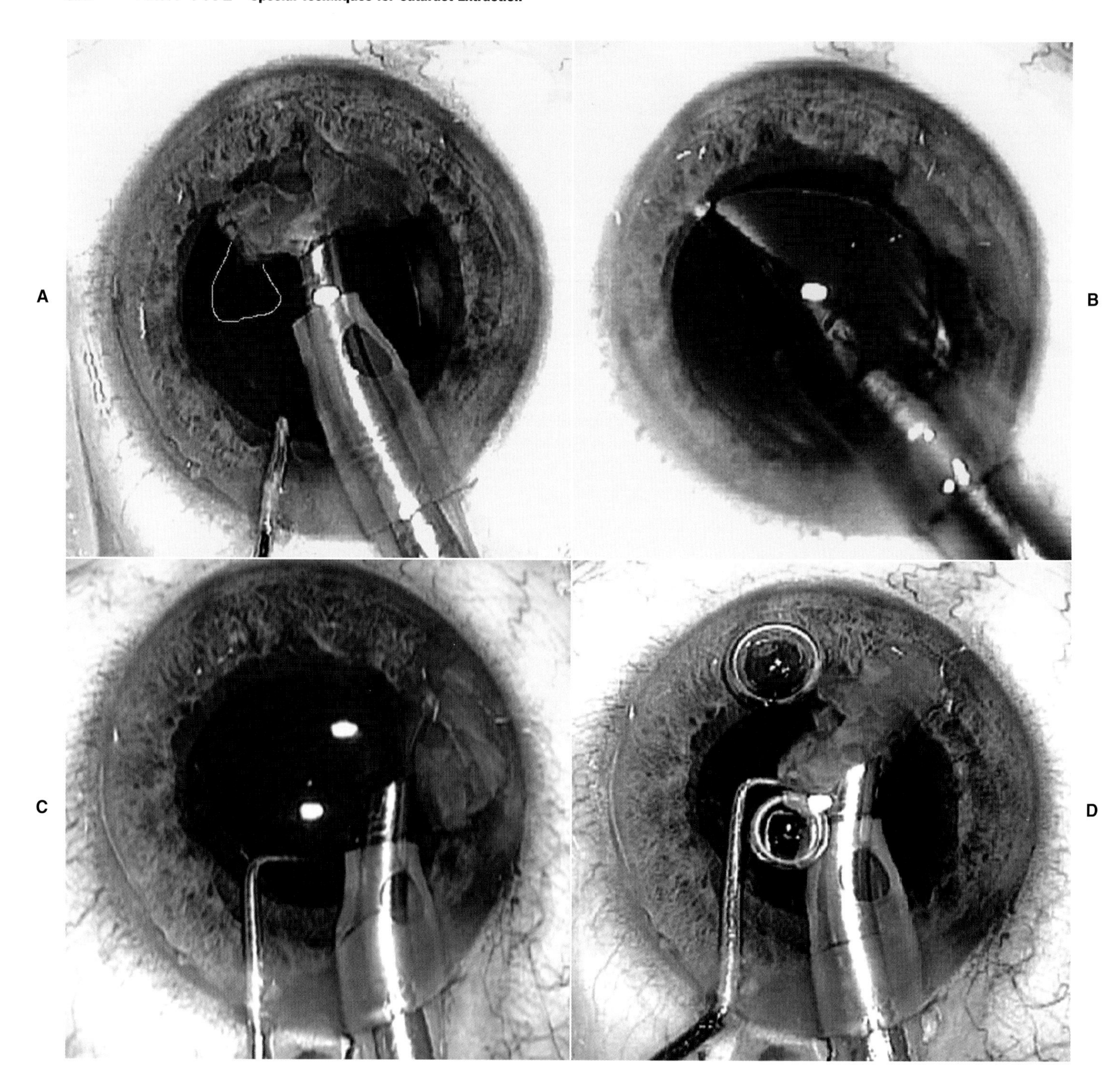

FIGURE 28-10 A, Posterior capsular break *(outlined in yellow)* becomes evident as the last large nuclear fragment is held at the phaco tip. The anterior chamber and bag were filled with viscoelastic material, tamponading the hyaloid face. The fragment was placed on the iris leaflet. **B,** PC IOL was inserted into the ciliary sulcus. **C,** Optic was captured into the capsulorrhexis, reestablishing a barrier between the anterior segment and the vitreous. **D,** Nuclear fragment is safely emulsified without risk of posterior dislocation.

of an IOL, yet the surgeon must be capable of modifying the implantation technique to safely insert the lens without further damaging the capsular remnants. Special attention should be given to the inferior support because gravity may gradually rotate a horizontally oriented implant. When the lens is placed and found to be centered, the "Osher bounce test" can confirm stability. The optic is gently decentered toward each haptic, then released; the implant should spontaneously recenter. If capsular support is absent or deemed to be inadequate, the surgeon should consider scleral suture fixation of one or both haptics of the posterior chamber implant. These techniques are covered in detail in Chapter 16.

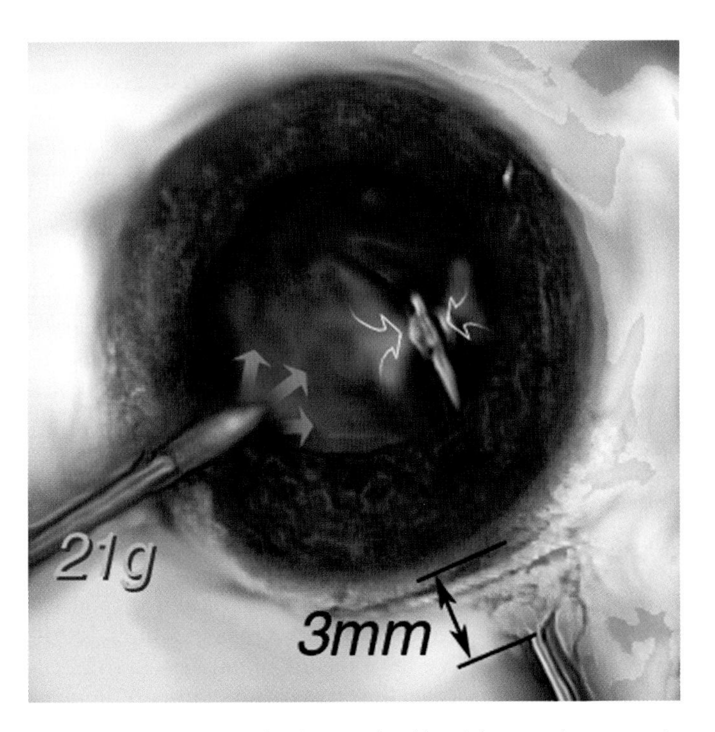

FIGURE 28-11 Anterior vitrectomy is achieved via a pars plana approach. The automated vitrector is placed through a 20-gauge opening 3 mm posterior to the limbus. Irrigation fluid is infused *(blue arrows)* through a 21-gauge butterfly needle placed through a corneal paracentesis tract. The prolapsed vitreous material is pulled back into the vitreous cavity and removed with the automated cutting device *(open white arrows)*.

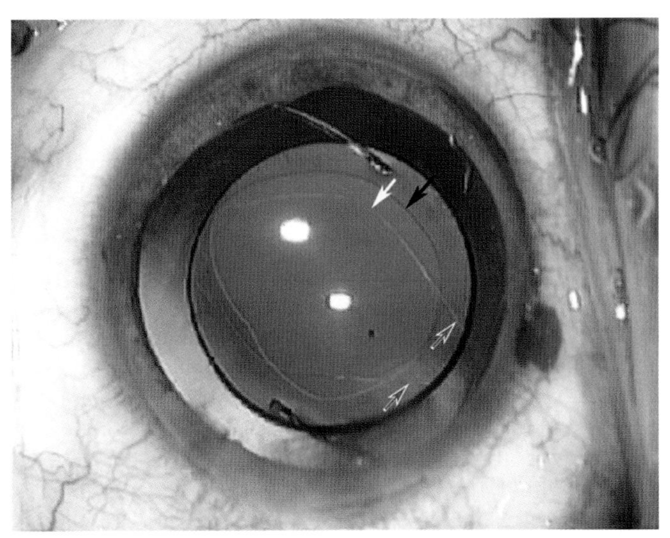

FIGURE 28-12 Three-piece acrylic PC IOL is placed within the capsular bag following posterior capsulorhexis. The anterior capsulorhexis *(black arrow)* maintains its usual round appearance, while the posterior capsulorhexis *(white arrow)* becomes ovoid from the tension of the haptic on the fornices of the bag, inducing some striae *(open white arrows)* in the posterior capsule.

Intraocular Lens Options

Once the cataract has been safely removed from the eye, the surgeon should consider some guidelines in the selection of an appropriate implant lens design and material. First, silicone-based lenses may increase the difficulty of future vitrectomy surgeries; therefore they are a suboptimal choice if the injury has included the posterior segment.[40,41] Both PMMA and acrylic lenses are well tolerated by the eye and preferred by vitreoretinal surgeons.

Because traumatic cataracts are not uncommonly associated with some degree of traumatic mydriasis, a 6-mm or larger diameter IOL optic seems prudent. Large optic diameters are also more forgiving of implant decentrations, which may be more likely in traumatic cataract cases.

When a sutured implant is required, a rigid, one-piece PMMA implant may provide additional stability and can be attached to the sclera with two- or four-point fixation, the latter decreasing the likelihood of tilt. A rigid implant, however, requires a larger incision. An implant with a fixation element on the apex of each haptic is preferable. Foldable acrylic lenses can be sutured to the ciliary sulcus as well, although with currently available implants only one suture can be affixed to each haptic, achieving just two points of fixation. A new implant haptic and suture guard (proprietary design by Michael E. Snyder, MD, Cincinnati, Ohio, patent pending) will facilitate four-point fixation of a foldable PC IOL.

One-piece acrylic lenses are suitable only for in-the-bag fixation. The surgeon should always consider the overall length of the IOL because sulcus support cannot be predictably achieved using IOLs with shorter overall lengths designed for endocapsular fixation.

In cases where glaucoma is present and preservation of conjunctiva for an existing or future filtering bleb is paramount, the surgeon may consider an acrylic lens with a clear corneal incision.

Some experts discourage the use of anterior chamber implants, especially in the setting of a traumatized eye, because "modern" angle-fixated implants, even when perfectly positioned, will have some contact with the delicate uveal tissue of the ciliary body band and may induce a low-grade chronic cyclitis and, perhaps, cystoid macular edema. Moreover, the relationship to the trabecular meshwork is of concern when traumatic glaucoma is present. A recent study reported *delayed onset* pupil deformity in 58% of patients with a Kelman-style anterior chamber implant.[42] This may represent a chronic inflammatory or ischemic response. Furthermore, the anterior chamber implant lens optics may be smaller than the preferred 6-mm or larger diameter. These angle-fixated lenses vault anteriorly in front of the iris plane, making the effective coverage of the entrance pupil even smaller yet, thereby accentuating the possibility of unwanted visual phenomena (such as halos, arcs, and edge glare). In some countries outside of the United States, anterior chamber iris-fixated "claw" lenses are popular (Artisan, Ophtec, Groningen, Netherlands). These lenses are not yet available in the United States.

Plate haptic silicone implants should not be used in traumatic cataract patients. They are unforgiving to capsular and zonular asymmetry, which may not be known at the time of surgery, and should YAG capsulotomy be required, the small size of the posterior capsule opening desired to prevent posterior dislocation[43] may afford an inadequate view of the retinal periphery.

Intraocular Lens Placement

If the capsular bag retains its integrity, intracapsular placement of the implant is desirable. Even in the face of zonular damage, a few options exist for capsular fixation of the implant lens. As described previously, the capsular tension rings can be inserted at any stage of the procedure, providing that an anterior capsulorhexis is intact and the capsular bag is intact. If the ring is placed before complete cortical removal, special effort should be taken to avoid trapping cortical fibers in the fornix of the bag because they can be extremely difficult to remove. If an endocapsular ring is not available and only a small area of zonular dehiscence is present, the haptics of the implant can be oriented along the axis of the weakness, unless it is obvious that the best centration is achieved in a different axis. Slowly unfolding the implant or gently placing a rigid lens will minimize the stress on the intact zonules.

Ciliary sulcus placement of a posterior chamber implant is still possible in the setting of a posterior capsular tear or zonular dialysis. If the anterior capsulorhexis is intact, yet a severe posterior capsule break exists, the haptics should be placed in the sulcus, and it may be possible to capture the lens optic posteriorly into the capsulorhexis. This will provide adequate support and will prevent the lens from subsequently dislocating. If the capsulorhexis is incompetent or larger than the implant optic, then simple sulcus fixation with a large diameter implant can be used. If an inferior zonulolysis is present and capture within the rhexis is not possible, then suture fixation can add additional safety because gravity may induce inferior lens migration over time (Figure 28-13).

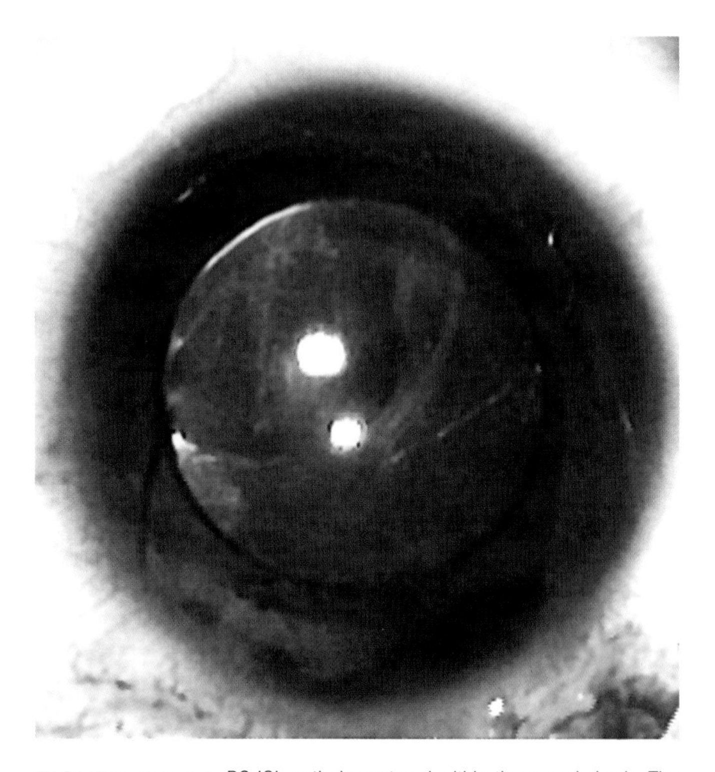

FIGURE 28-13 PC IOL optic is captured within the capsulorhexis. The capsule was stained with ICG. The lower haptic is fixated to the sclera by a suture. With this double-fixation method the implant was well centered and secure.

Intraocular Lenses and Children

Although many surgeons now commonly place IOLs in children, the correction of aphakia in children remains somewhat controversial. Traumatic injuries typically affect only one eye, and in uniocular aphakia, contact lens compliance may be even more poorly tolerated than in bilateral aphakia. IOLs can be safely tolerated in most children, even following trauma.[44] IOL implantation may be significantly easier at the time of cataract extraction than at a later date because iridocapsular adhesions and fusion of the anterior and posterior capsular flaps make a subsequent secondary implant procedure more challenging. In cases where the posterior capsule remains intact, the presence of an implant may reduce the risk of posterior capsular opacity,[45] and should YAG laser capsulotomy be required, the implant will also prevent vitreous prolapse into the anterior segment. Furthermore, as inferred from the literature addressing implants in uveitic patients, an IOL may decrease the chances of significant posterior synechiae.[46] Scleral-sutured posterior chamber implant lenses have been used successfully in children, although the long-term integrity of Prolene sutures is still unknown.[47] Although we favor the use of implants in children, each surgeon must evaluate the merits of any particular implant option for each case. The informed consent discussion with the parent or guardian should include the fact that most IOLs are still not approved by the Food and Drug Administration for use in children.

Some investigators in China have recently advocated the use of epikeratophakia for correction of pediatric aphakia following surgery for traumatic cataract. While they have had some promising successes, worldwide experience with this approach is still limited. Epikeratophakia lenticules are currently not available in the United States.[48] We feel that, currently, IOLs remain the best option in pediatric aphakia.

Iris Repair and Replacement

Unless the iris damage is extensive, preventing access to the lens or interfering with the operative procedure, the repair of iris defects can follow cataract extraction and lens implantation steps. The pseudophakos is significantly thinner than the intumescent cataract, and therefore the anterior chamber is deeper, allowing more working space. Also, the long needles used for iris repair may inadvertently engage lens capsule, cortex, or vitreous if the passes are placed early in the operative procedure. Gentle lysis of iridocapsular adhesions can be performed early; however, when the zonules are damaged, the iridocapsular adhesions may provide extra support during the capsulorhexis and phacoemulsification.

Five types of iris injury can be present with trauma: (1) holes, (2) sphincter tears, (3) iridodialyses, (4) traumatic mydriasis, and (5) partial or total loss of iris tissue. Repair of iris defects can be accomplished with transcameral 10-0 Prolene sutures. A paracentesis location and orientation are selected so that passage of a long, curved needle can be easily directed toward the iris defect. The needle is gently wiggled into the paracentesis, taking care not to catch any stromal fibers. The tip of the needle engages one edge of the iris at the proximal margin of the tear. The tip then engages the distal iris leaflet (from the underside), and the needle is passed through the peripheral cornea. For iris

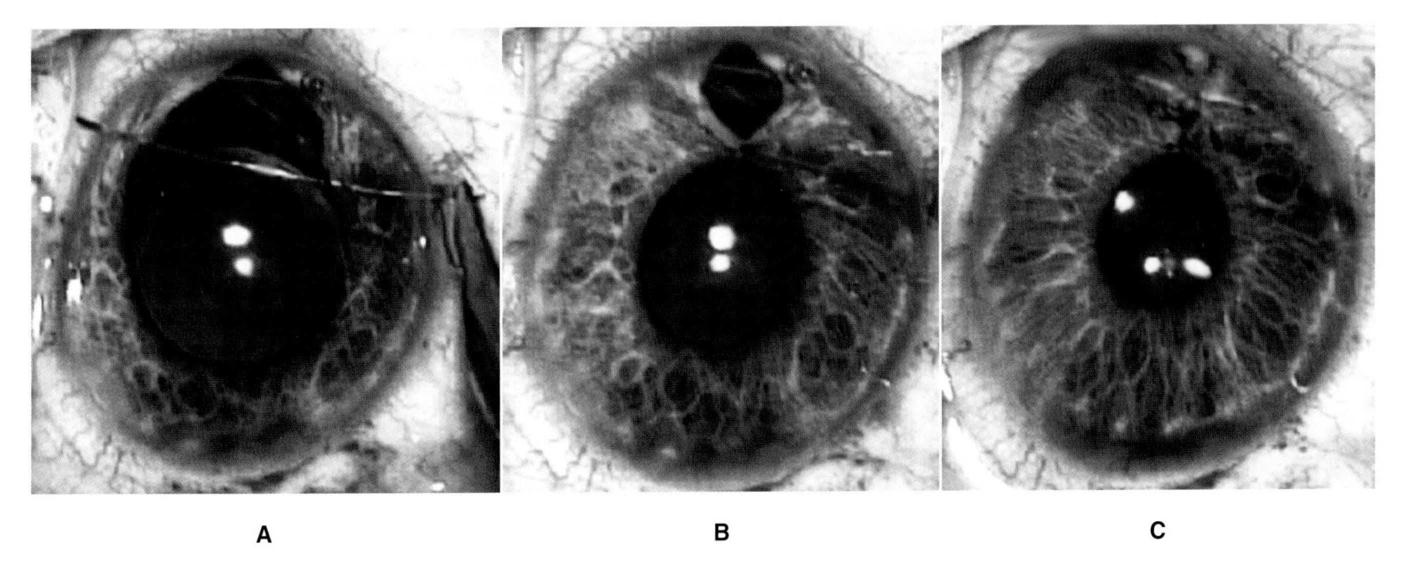

FIGURE 28-14 Cut margin of the iris sphincter is identified. **A,** A 10-0 Prolene suture on a long, curved needle is passed through the iris margin of each iris leaflet and then passed out the distal limbus. **B,** As the suture knot is secured, the pupil begins to return to a more normal shape. **C,** Appearance after closure of the remaining peripheral iris defect.

sphincter tears, it is best to identify the cut margin at each side and to take a healthy bite of iris tissue (Figure 28-14). The suture can be tied within the anterior chamber with the sliding knot technique, as described by Siepser.[49] Orientation of the suture ends is particularly important so that the suture will create a knot and not just a twist as the two ends are drawn together (Figure 28-15). We typically will use a double throw followed by a single throw. An iris defect also can be closed via a limbal incision using the basic technique described by McCannel.[50]

Iridodialysis can be repaired by passing each needle of a double-armed 10-0 Prolene suture through the disinserted peripheral iris and then out the scleral wall at the iris root.[51,52] The knot can be tied externally and rotated internally (Figure 28-16).

Traumatic mydriasis may result in postoperative glare from edge-related symptoms. A cerclage type of procedure can be performed to reduced the pupillary aperture.[53,54] Although different techniques may be used to pass the suture through the iris tissue, each approach attempts to create either a segmental or circumferential purse-string of the iris margin.

When significant iris tissue has been lost, implantation of a diaphragm IOL (Morcher and Ophtec), intracapsular iris rings (Morcher), occluding ring segments (Morcher), or the multi-piece iris prosthetic system of Hermeking (Ophtec) should be considered. Details of iris supplements are beyond the scope of this chapter.

Membranous Cataract and Long-standing Changes

Occasionally, a patient may present for evaluation of a white or brunescent cataract many years after a penetrating injury. In some of these cases, a significant portion of the lens material may have been resorbed, thus leaving little separation between the anterior and posterior capsules. Special caution will prevent inadvertent entry into the vitreous cavity. The surgeon may occasionally encounter a fibrotic or calcified capsule or lens remnant requiring sharp incision and scissors dissection and removal of the tough capsular material with the vitrector handpiece. Of benefit to the surgeon is the knowledge that long-standing traumatic capsular tears do not readily extend, as acute capsular tears tend to do.

Demonstrative Cases

Case One

A 14-year-old boy accidentally struck his right eye while cutting a piece of rubber with a carpet knife. He had a corneoscleral laceration extending from the superior limbus through cornea, iris, and lens. The laceration deviated paracentrally 1.5 mm around the corneal apex, severed the inferior limbus and ciliary body, and extended to just before the inferior rectus insertion. Vitreous was present at the limbus. The laceration was repaired primarily with automated vitrectomy performed at the scleral opening. Primary cataract extraction was not performed.

His clinical evaluation the next day revealed light perception vision with brisk identification of colored lights. The Purkinje phenomenon was present, and no afferent defect was noted. The corneal wound was secure, and the superior and inferior iris leaflets were bisected. A small amount of vitreous prolapse was noted at the inferior iris break. The anterior lens capsule was torn from the superior to inferior equatorial regions. B-scan ultrasonography showed a displaced rupture of the posterior crystalline lens (see Figure 28-1).

Problem list:
Intumescent traumatic cataract
Ruptured anterior capsule
Ruptured posterior capsule
Vitreous prolapse
Lacerated iris
Corneoscleral and ciliary body laceration (repaired)

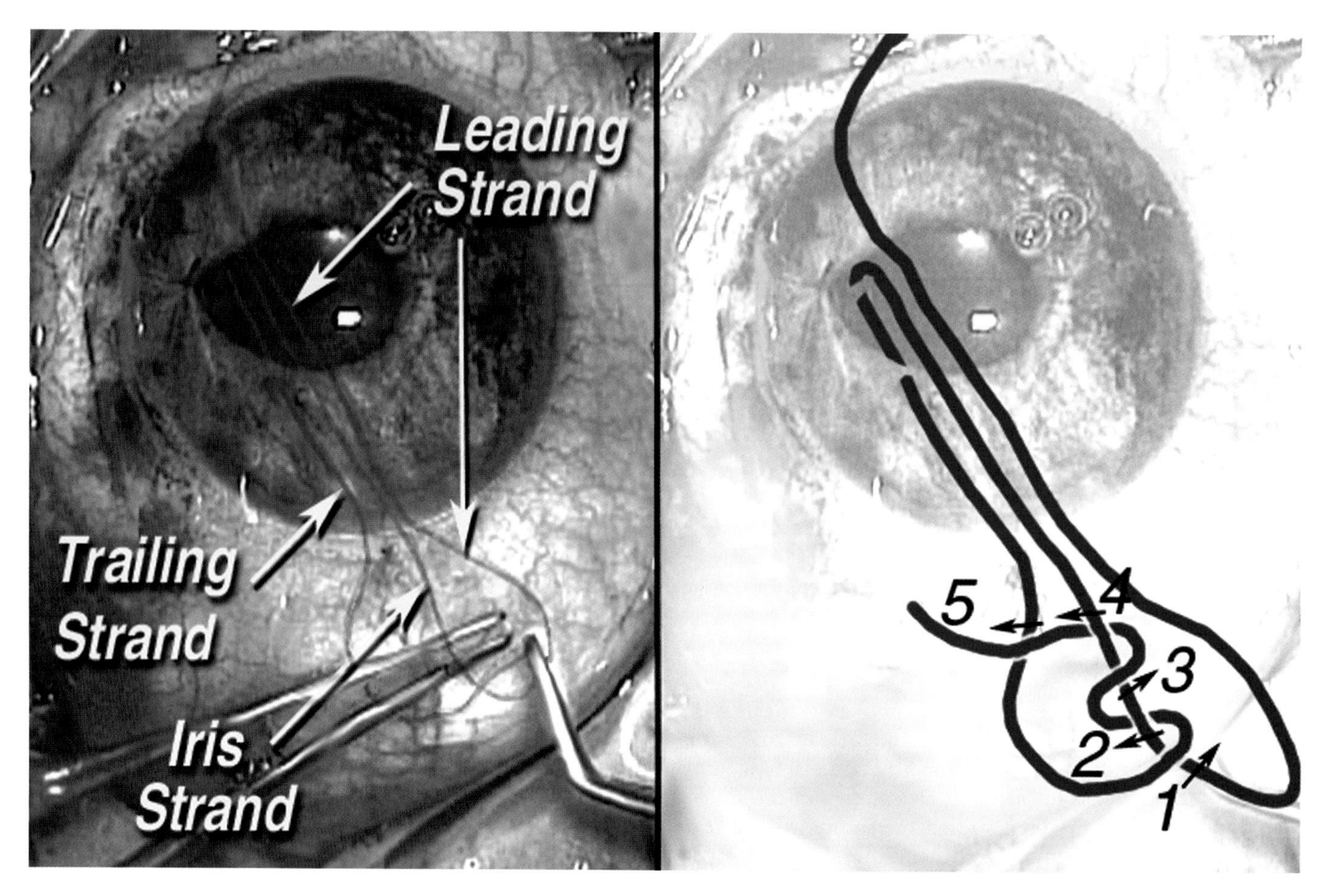

FIGURE 28-15 Tying the sliding suture knot requires meticulous attention to suture orientation. First, the suture loops should be laid out on the globe as shown with the strand coming from the iris margin (iris strand) adjacent to the free (trailing strand) end. The free end of the trailing strand is passed down through the retrieved loop *(1)*, under the iris strand *(2)*, down through the loop again *(3)*, under the strand again *(4)*, then over the trailing strand *(5)*. The distal and proximal ends are pulled, and the knot slides into the anterior chamber without causing any tension on the iris tissue. The knot is secured by a second retrieval and single or double throw.

The patient was brought back to the operating room 5 days later. A temporal wound site was chosen (the area of most normal anatomy). The corneal dome was filled with Viscoat (Alcon, Fort Worth, Tex.), and the anterior chamber was gently deepened with Healon (Pharmacia, Monrovia, Calif.) in the soft shell technique. A 19-gauge cannula was placed via the superotemporal paracentesis site, and the tip was placed into the peripheral lens material nasally where the lens anatomy was not damaged. Manual aspiration of lens material was undertaken in a dry fashion. Additional Healon was added serially to maintain the anterior chamber. The peripheral lens material was similarly removed from the temporal area via a nasal paracentesis. Viscoat was used to tamponade the anterior hyaloid centrally, allowing aspiration of the remaining central lens material. In this young boy, the soft lens nucleus was easily aspirated with a cannula alone. The area inferiorly around the prolapsed vitreous was carefully avoided. An inferotemporal pars plana sclerotomy was created, and an automated vitrectomy was performed locally using irrigation via the superior paracentesis site. The small knuckle of vitreous was pulled back posteriorly and removed with the cutter device. The small bit of lens material in this region was removed with the vitrector handpiece. An acrylic foldable lens (MA60BM AcrySof [Alcon, Fort Worth, Tex.]) was placed into the ciliary sulcus, oriented horizontally, with excellent support. The iris was then repaired in a closed-chamber sliding knot technique. The viscoelastic was removed with the vitrector handpiece. Postoperative uncorrected visual acuity improved to 20/40.

Case Two

A 25-year-old man presented with light perception vision in his left eye after hammering a nail that hit his left eye. Examination showed vague light perception vision and a questionable afferent pupillary defect. Testing was limited by poor cooperation. Brief glimpses during the slit lamp examination showed a central corneal full-thickness laceration. The anterior chamber was deep with an admixture of fibrin, heme, and, possibly, vitreous. The pupillary outline was irregular, but central. The status of the lens could not be ascertained.

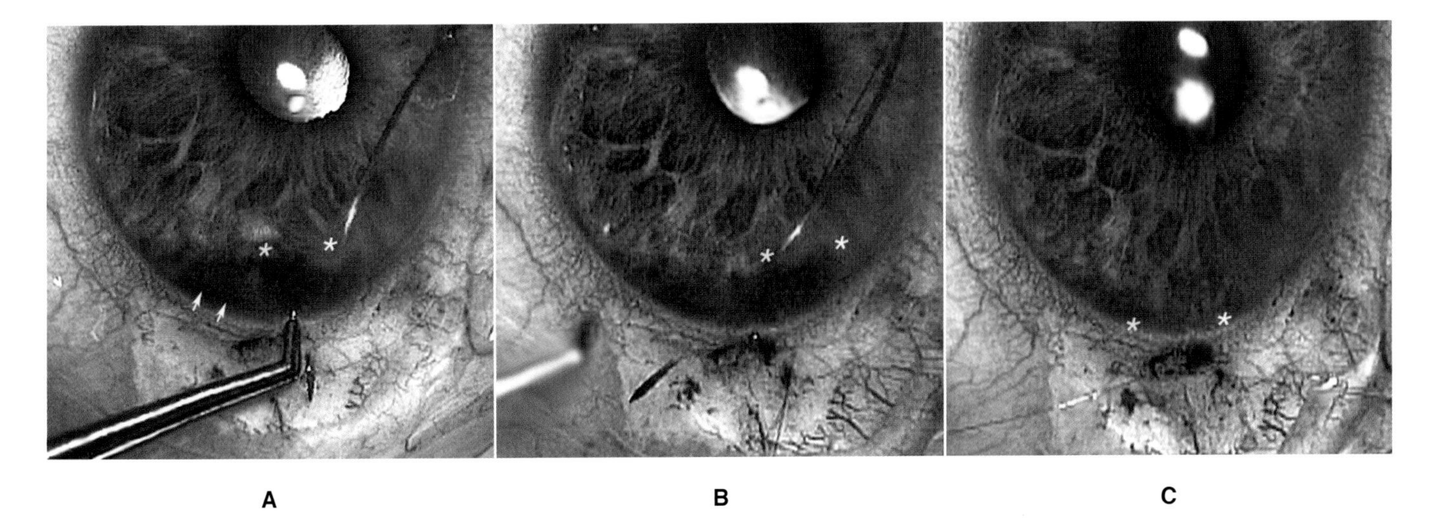

A B C

FIGURE 28-16 A, Double-armed 10-0 Prolene suture on a long, curved needle is passed via a corneal paracentesis through the disinserted peripheral iris at the junction between the middle and outer thirds and then out at the level of the iris insertion at the scleral wall. The white asterisk identifies the site of the first suture pass, and the yellow asterisk identifies the intended site of the second pass. Note that the peripheral iris anatomy is distorted by the needle during the suture pass. **B,** Second arm of the suture is similarly passed a few millimeters from the first. **C,** Suture is tied, achieving closure of the iridodialysis.

Problem list:
Central corneal laceration
Vitreous prolapse?
Lens status?
Status of anterior choroid/pars plana?

The patient was brought to the operating room, and the corneal wound was closed under general anesthesia. Vitreous was present outside the corneal wound and was carefully removed at the level of the laceration with the automated cutter. The lens was not removed.

The following day, vision was counting fingers, and the corneal wound was secure. Vitreous streamed through the inferior portion of the lens to the back of the cornea. Condensing fibrin filled the anterior chamber. The crystalline lens was obviously lacerated and was starting to turn white. B-scan showed a clear vitreous, an attached retina, and no suprachoroidal hemorrhage. Steroids, cycloplegics, and antibiotics were administered. A-scan ultrasonography was performed on each eye, and keratometry readings were obtained.

Problem list:
Repaired central corneal laceration
Vitreous through lens to posterior cornea
Traumatic, lacerated cataract

On postinjury day 4, the patient was brought to the operating room for cataract extraction, PC IOL implantation, and vitrectomy. A superotemporal wound site was selected. The anterior segment anatomy was most normal superiorly; in addition, a superotemporal incision would best offset the likely future induced astigmatism from the corneal wound. (Typically, the steep axis will be perpendicular to the sutured laceration.) Two paracenteses were created, one superonasally and the other temporally. A bimanual (split irrigation) anterior vitrectomy was performed via these two sites to sever the bands of vitreous going to the corneal wound and to clear the vitreous from the anterior chamber. Healon GV was used to maintain the anterior chamber and for endothelial protection. The cataract material in the area of the lens laceration was removed with the vitrector handpiece on "I/A cutter" mode. This successfully cleared a view through the pupillary space. A pars plana sclerotomy was then created 3 mm posterior to the limbus, and the remaining vitreous material was cleared form the pupillary and retropupillary space. The remaining lens material was removed with the vitrector on I/A cutter mode. Examination of the capsular remains showed no support inferiorly and inferonasally. It was elected to suture a 6-mm optic, single-piece, PMMA posterior chamber implant to the ciliary sulcus. Miochol was instilled. The vitrector was used to remove the viscoelastic material from the anterior chamber.

The postoperative course was unremarkable, and the patient achieved a suture-out 20/25 result with a –3.25 + 3.25 ± 090 correction, despite the central, apical corneal laceration. Topographic astigmatism was regular. Neither corneal transplant nor contact lens was required.

Case Three

A 66-year-old man sustained a blunt injury when a softball struck his right eye 2 years before evaluation. At his initial presentation, his right eye vision was counting fingers at 6 feet, and intraocular pressure was elevated to 36 mm Hg. An afferent pupillary defect was present. Slit lamp finding showed a subluxated dense nuclear, cortical, and posterior subcapsular cataract with obvious phacodonesis. Zonules were absent from the 10 o'clock to 4 o'clock position. Vitreous was prolapsed anteriorly around the lens equator and into the anterior chamber. Fundus exam showed a pale optic nerve head with no posterior segment details. Gonioscopy revealed seven clock hours of angle recession.

Problem list:
Subluxated, dense traumatic cataract
Vitreous prolapse
Angle recession glaucoma

The patient chose to undergo cataract extraction with endocapsular ring placement, IOL implantation, pars plana approach anterior vitrectomy, and trabeculectomy. First, the trabeculectomy site was prepared with a fornix-based flap. A superonasal paracentesis was created for anterior irrigation. A pars plana sclerotomy was performed 3 mm posterior to the 10:30 limbus. The prolapsed vitreous material was removed with the automated vitrector, pulling the vitreous back into the vitreous cavity (Figure 28-17). Viscoat (Alcon, Fort Worth, Tex.) was placed to tamponade the remaining vitreous posterior to the lens. A capsulorhexis was then performed, and the lens nucleus was meticulously emulsified with a phaco-chop technique. The cortical material was aspirated with a Simcoe cannula, and dry cortical stripping was performed. An endocapsular ring was placed. This resulted in nice recentration of the capsular bag. An acrylic implant (AcrySof MA60BM, Alcon, Fort Worth, Tex.) was placed intracapsularly. The scleral tunnel was then pedunculated to create a scleral flap, and several punches were taken from the posterior scleral rim. The flap was secured with releasable sutures, and conjunctiva was closed. The final postoperative vision was 20/20, and intraocular pressure was 16 mm Hg. The patient retained this result at 2-year follow-up.

Conclusion

Traumatic cataracts vary widely in nature, presentation, and degree of ocular comorbidity. With careful clinical evaluation and meticulous attention to surgical technique, these cases can often yield excellent visual, functional, and cosmetic results. In fact, rehabilitation of these challenging cases can often be among the most gratifying services that we can provides for our patients.

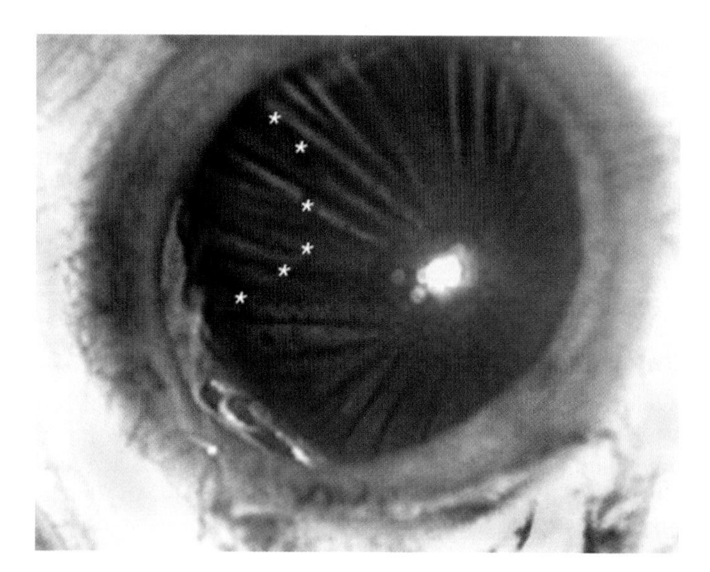

FIGURE 28-17 In this case of traumatic cataract, vitreous is prolapsed around the lens equator and into the anterior chamber. Asterisks outline pigment clumps along the edge of the prolapse knuckle of vitreous *anterior* to the crystalline lens. The vitrector is placed behind the lens, and the vitreous is pulled posteriorly out of the anterior chamber and removed with the cutter device. Folds in the lens capsule are not uncommon in cases of traumatic cataract.

REFERENCES

1. Bulluck JD, Ballal DR, Johnson DA et al: Ocular and orbital trauma from water balloon slingshots: a clinical, epidemiological, and experimental study, *Ophthalmology* 104:878-887, 1997.
2. McDermott ML, Shin DH, Hughes BH et al: Anterior segment trauma and air bags, *Arch Ophthalmol* 113:1567-1568, 1995.
3. Karp CL, Fazio JR: Traumatic cataract presenting with unilateral nasal hemianopsia, *J Cataract Refract Surg* 25:1302-1303, 1999.
4. Zabriskie NA, Hwang IP, Ramsey JF et al: Anterior lens capsule rupture caused by air bag trauma. *Am J Ophthalmol* 123:832-833, 1997.
5. Angra SK, Vajpayee RB, Titiyal JS et al: Types of posterior capsular breaks and their implications. *Opthalmic Surg* 22:388-391, 1991.
6. Netland KE, Martinez J, LaCour OJ III et al: Traumatic anterior lens dislocation: a case report, *J Emerg Med* 19:73-74, 2000.
7. Sathish S, Chakrabarti A, Prajna V: Traumatic subconjunctival dislocation of the crystalline lens and its surgical management, *Ophthalmic Surg Lasers* 30:684-686, 1999.
8. Boorstein JM, Titelbaum DS, Patel Y et al: CT diagnosis of unsuspected traumatic cataract in patients with complicated eye injuries: significance of attenuation value of the lens, *Am J Roentgenol* 164:181-184, 1995.
9. Almog Y, Reider-Groswasser I, Goldstein M et al: "The disappearing lens": failure of CT to image the lens in traumatic intumescent cataract, *J Comput Assist Tomogr* 23:354-356, 1999.
10. Rubsanen PE, Irvine WD, McCuen BW et al: Primary intraocular lens implantation in the setting of penetrating ocular trauma, *Ophthalmology* 102(1):101-107, 1995.
11. Pieramici DJ, Capone A, Rubsame PE et al: Lens preservation after intraocular foreign body injuries, *Ophthalomology* 103:1563-1567, 1996.
12. O'Duffy D, Salmon JF: Siderosis bulbi resulting from an intralenticular foreign body, *Am J Opthalmol* 127:218-219, 1999.
13. Jonas JB, Budde WM: Early versus late removal of retained intraocular foreign bodies. *Retina* 19:193-197, 1999.
14. Speaker MG, Guerriero PN, Met JA et al: A case-control study of risk factors for intraoperative suprachoroidal expulsive hemorrhage, *Ophthalmology* 98:202-209, 1991.
15. Arnold PN: Study of acute intraoperative suprachoroidal hemorrhage, *J Cataract Refract Surg* 18:489-494, 1992.
16. Osher RH: Complications: The torn posterior capsule: management principles, *J Cataract Refract Surg* 8(1), 1991 (video).
17. Fukagawa K, Tsubota K, Kimura C et al: Corneal endothelial cell loss induced by air bags, *Ophthalmology* 100:1819-1823, 1993.
18. Arshinoff SA: Dispersive-cohesive viscoelastic soft shell technique, *J Cataract Refract Surg* 25:167-173, 1999.
19. Osher RH, Cionni RJ: The torn posterior capsule: its intraoperative behavior, surgical management, and long-term consequences, *J Cataract Refract Surg* 16:490-494, 1990.
20. Krag S, Thim K, Corydon L et al: Biomechanical aspects of the anterior capsulotomy, *J Cataract Refract Surg* 20:410-416, 1994.
21. Andreo LK, Wilson ME, Apple DJ: Elastic properties and scanning electron microscopic appearance of manual continuous curvilinear capsulorhexis and vitrectorhexis in an animal model of pediatric cataract, *J Cataract Refract Surg* 25:534-539, 1999.
22. Fenzl R: Avoiding the complication cascade, In Gills JP, editor: *Cataract surgery: the state of the art,* Thorofare, NJ, 1998, Slack, pp 130-131.
23. Prieto I, Cabral I, Rogue J: Capsular staining—Gentian violet, *Vid J Catarct Refract Surg* XV(2), 1999.
24. Melles GR, de Waard PW, Pameyer JH et al: Trypan blue capsule staining to visualize capsulorhexis in cataract surgery, *J Cataract Refract Surg* 25:7-9, 1999.
25. Horiguchi M, Miyake K, Ohta Y et al: Staining of the lens capsule for continuous circular capsulorhexis in eyes with white cataract, *Arch Ophthalmol* 116:535-537, 1998.
26. Newsom TH, Oetting TA: Indocyanine green staining in traumatic cataract, *J Cataract Refract Surg* 26:1691-1693, 2000.
27. Wainwright M, Phoenix DA, Rice L et al: Increased cytotoxicity and phototoxicity in the methylene blue series via chromophore methylation, *J Photochem Photobiol B* 40:233-239, 1997.

28. Metz G: Lens induced glaucoma, *J Catract Refract Surg* 2(3), 1986 (audiovisual).
29. Gimbel HV, Willerscheidt AB: What to do with limited view: the intumescent cataract, *J Cataract Refract Surg* 19:657-661, 1993.
30. Osher RH: Slow motion phacoemulsification approach, *J Cataract Refract Surg* 19:667, 1993 (letter; comment).
31. Cionni RJ, Osher RH, Solomon K: The Cionni ring, *J Cataract Refract Surg* 14(4), 1998 (video).
32. Camponella PC, Aminlari A, DeMaio R: Traumatic cataract and Weigert's ligament, *Ophthalmic Surg Lasers* 28:422-423, 1997.
33. Yasukawa T, Kita M, Honda Y: Traumatic cataract with a ruptured posterior capsule from a nonpenetrating ocular injury, *J Cataract Refract Surg* 24: 868-869, 1998.
34. Thomas R: Posterior capsular rupture after blunt trauma, *J Cataract Refract Surg* 24:283-284, 1998.
35. Rao SK, Parikh S, Padhmanabhan P: Isolated posterior capsule rupture in blunt trauma: pathogenesis and management, *Ophthalmic Surg Lasers* 29:338-342, 1998.
36. Osher RH: Surgery of the loose cataract, *J Cataract Refract Surg* 5(3), 1989 (video).
37. Kelman C: Posterior capsular rupture: PAL technique, *J Cataract Refract Surg* 12(2), 1996 (video).
38. Eller AW, Barad RF: Miyake analysis of anterior vitrectomy techniques, *J Cataract Refract Surg* 22:213-217, 1996.
39. Oscher H: Unpublished data presented at American Society of Cataract and Refractive Surgeons Annual Meeting, 1984.
40. Khawly JA, Lambert RJ, Jaffe GJ: Intraocular lens changes after short- and long-term exposure to intraocular silicone oil: an in vivo study, *Ophthalmology* 105:1227-1233, 1998.
41. Bartz-Schmidt KU, Kirchhof B, Heimann K: Condensation on IOL's during fluid-air exchange, *Ophthalmology* 103:199, 1996 (letter).
42. Sawada T, Kimura W et al: Long-term follow-up of primary anterior chamber intraocular lens implantation, *J Cataract Refract Surg* 24:1515-1520, 1998.
43. Dick B, Schwenn O, Stoffelns B et al: [Late dislocation of a plate haptic silicone lens into the vitreous body after Nd:YAG capsulotomy: a case report], *Ophthalmologe* 95:181-185, 1998.
44. Churchill AJ, Noble BA, et al: Factors affecting visual outcome following uniocular traumatic cataract, *Eye* 9:285-291, 1995.
45. Ram J, Apple DJ, et al: Update on fixation of rigid and foldable posterior chamber intraocular lenses. Part II: choosing the correct haptic fixation and intraocular lens design to help eradicate posterior capsule opacification, *Ophthalmology* 106:891-900, 1999.
46. Holland GN, Van Horn SD, Margolis TP: Cataract surgery with ciliary sulcus fixation of intraocular lenses in patients with uveitis, *Am J Ophthalmol* 128:21-30, 1999.
47. Lam SC, Joan SK et al: Short-term results of scleral sutured intraocular lens fixation in children, *J Cataract Refract Surg* 24:1474-1479, 1998.
48. Feng C, Chen J, Liu H et al: The preliminary report of epikeratophakia in the treatment of pediatric aphakia after traumatic cataract extraction, *Yan Ke Xue Bao* 13:38-40, 1997.
49. Seipser SP: The closed chamber slipping suture technique for iris repair, *Ann Ophthalmology* 26:71-72, 1994.
50. McCannel M: A retrievable suture idea for anterior uveal problems, *Ophthalmic Surg* 7:98-103, 1976.
51. Wachler BB, Krueger RR: Double-armed McCannel suture for repair of traumatic iridodialysis, *Am J Ophthalmol* 122:109-110, 1996.
52. Kaufman SC, Insler MS: Surgical repair of traumatic iridodialysis, *Ophthalmic Surg Lasers* 27:963-966, 1996.
53. Osher RH: Consultation section, *J Cataract Refract Surg* 20:665-669, 1994.
54. Ogawa GS: The iris cerclage suture for permanent mydriasis: a running suture technique, *Ophthalmic Surg Lasers* 29:1001-1009, 1998.

Iris Repair

29

Roger F. Steinert, MD
Scott E. Burk, MD, PhD

Iris abnormalities that present in conjunction with cataract or intraocular lens (IOL) surgery are usually the result of accidental or surgical trauma. Less commonly, the iris abnormalities may be congenital, such as an iris coloboma or corectopia, or the abnormality may be the result of a later-onset degenerative process.

Penetrating injuries of the cornea or anterior sclera may result in iris injury from direct laceration or as a consequence of iris prolapse through the wound. Blunt, nonpenetrating trauma to the anterior segment may also injure the iris.[1-3] The most common patterns of iris injury after severe blunt trauma are localized sphincter tears, generalized sphincter paralysis, and dialysis of the iris root.[4]

Preservation of iris tissue and restoration of normal iris architecture are important for two principal reasons. Most importantly, the optical performance of the eye is highly dependent on the pupillary aperture.

A large and nonreactive pupil results in photophobia and glare. In addition, aberrations from the peripheral cornea, as well as the peripheral IOL and/or exposed capsule, can be highly disturbing to the functional vision of a patient. Pupillary distortions are better tolerated by a patient with a clear crystalline lens than a pseudophakic patient because the IOL has a substantially smaller optical diameter than the crystalline lens.

The first step in management of traumatic iris abnormalities is therefore to minimize damage to the iris and to preserve as much iris tissue as possible. Prolapsed iris tissue does not necessarily need to be excised; the surgeon performing the primary repair must judge the likelihood of microbial contamination of the iris before sacrificing a prolapsed iris.

Iris Reconstruction

Surgical Principles of Iris Suturing

Although iris deformities have an infinite number of possible configurations, the basic principles of surgical repair can be summarized in a few basic techniques.

PRINCIPLE 1: MOBILIZATION

The first principle is to free up and mobilize as much iris tissue as possible. Synechia to the cataract or capsule should be bluntly dissected. Most iridocapsular adhesions are strongly attached only at the sphincter edge. Often there is some proliferation of iris pigment epithelium from the posterior iris surface to the capsule involving the more peripheral iris, but these adhesions are weak and can be easily separated with an instrument such as a cyclodialysis spatula or a cannula with viscoelastic agent. If iridocapsular adhesions cannot be bluntly dissected, then careful excision with a scissors or blade should be performed, preserving as much iris tissue as possible by taking care not to excise any iris tissue that is avoidable.

After freeing up all iridocapsular adhesions, the surgeon should then release any peripheral adhesions. Peripheral anterior synechia usually can be released with traction using forceps or a pointed hook such as a Sinskey hook or Osher Y hook or by sweeping maneuvers with a spatula. In addition, inflammation sometimes causes the iris stroma to form adhesions internally, causing contraction of the iris in a manner similar to accordion pleats. Again, gentle traction can release many of these adhesions and produce a surprising amount of iris tissue necessary for the subsequent repair. Mobilization of iris tissue from peripheral synechiae is illustrated later in Case Studies 1, 2, and 5.

PRINCIPLE 2: INTRAOCULAR SUTURING AND KNOT TYING

The second fundamental principle is the method for suturing iris and tying knots within the eye. Often the knot is central, and traction to bring the iris with the knot to a limbal wound will damage the iris repair. Figure 29-1 illustrates the basic technique for passing the suture into the anterior chamber via a paracentesis, through a radially oriented iris defect, and then out through the peripheral cornea on the opposite side of the paracentesis. In all cases, a nonbiodegradable suture material should be used. The most common suture employed is 10-0 polypropylene (Prolene). A long, gently curved needle is typically used. The Ethicon CIF-4 needle is strong and relatively easy to control. Although it has a noncutting needle tip, the bulk of the needle has the disadvantage of leaving a small new iris puncture defect in its path. Finer needles that create less of an iris defect but are correspondingly more difficult to handle are the Ethicon CTC-6 (curved) and STC-6 (straight).

A flaccid iris and a knot close to a wound may allow the surgeon to tie the knot at the limbus without undue iris damage. Successful completion of many cases of iris reconstruction

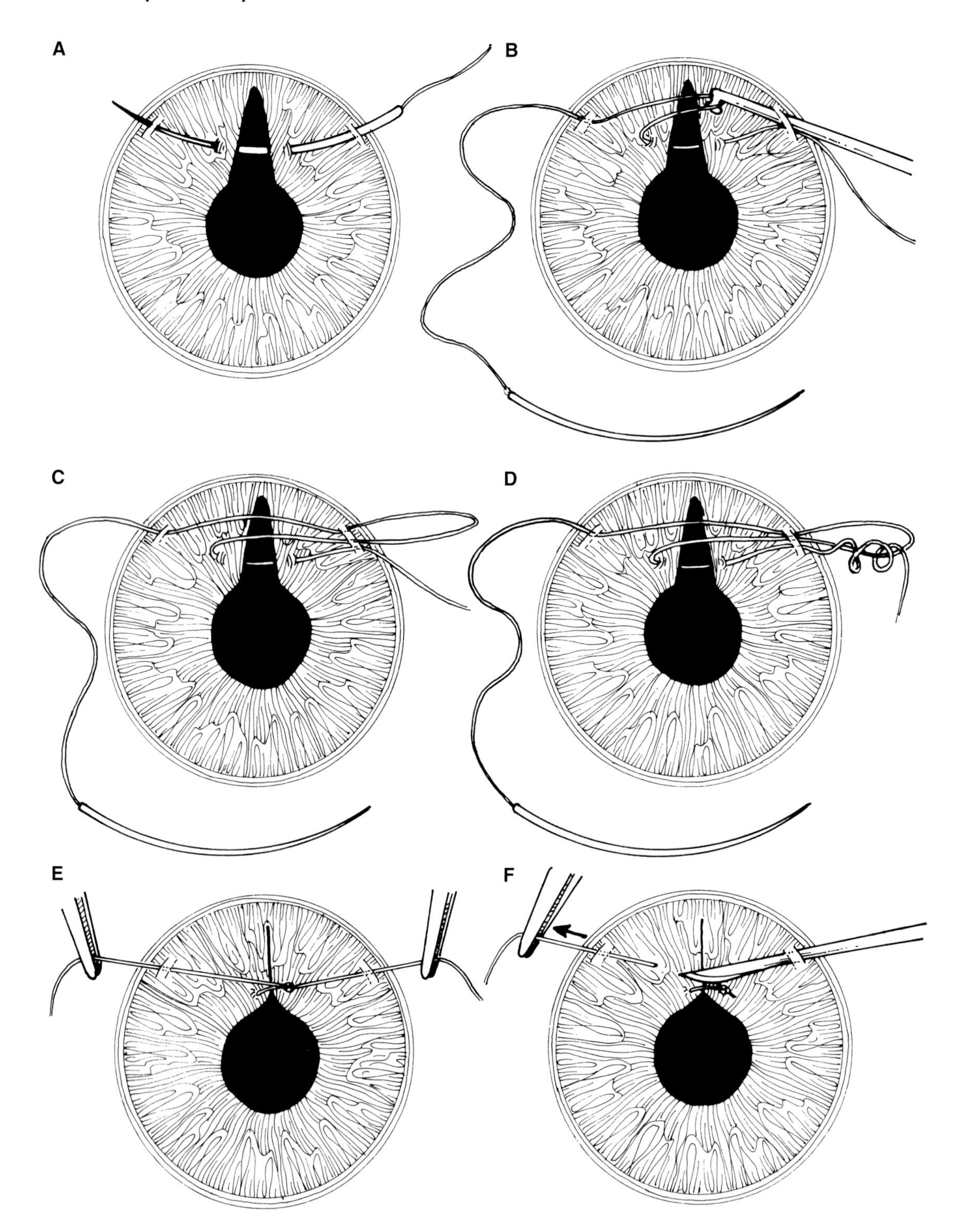

FIGURE 29-1 A, Long needle enters through a paracentesis, across the iris defect, and exits by puncturing through the peripheral cornea. **B,** Hook such as a Kuglen hook retrieves a loop of the distal arm of the suture, making sure that the needle end of the suture remains external to the eye. **C,** Loop is now external through the paracentesis. **D,** Proximal end of the suture is wrapped around the suture loop twice, creating one throw of what will become the knot. **E,** Tension on each end of the suture draws the knot into the eye and tightens it. **F,** After four throws, the suture ends are cut with a thin sharp knife such as a Wheeler blade.

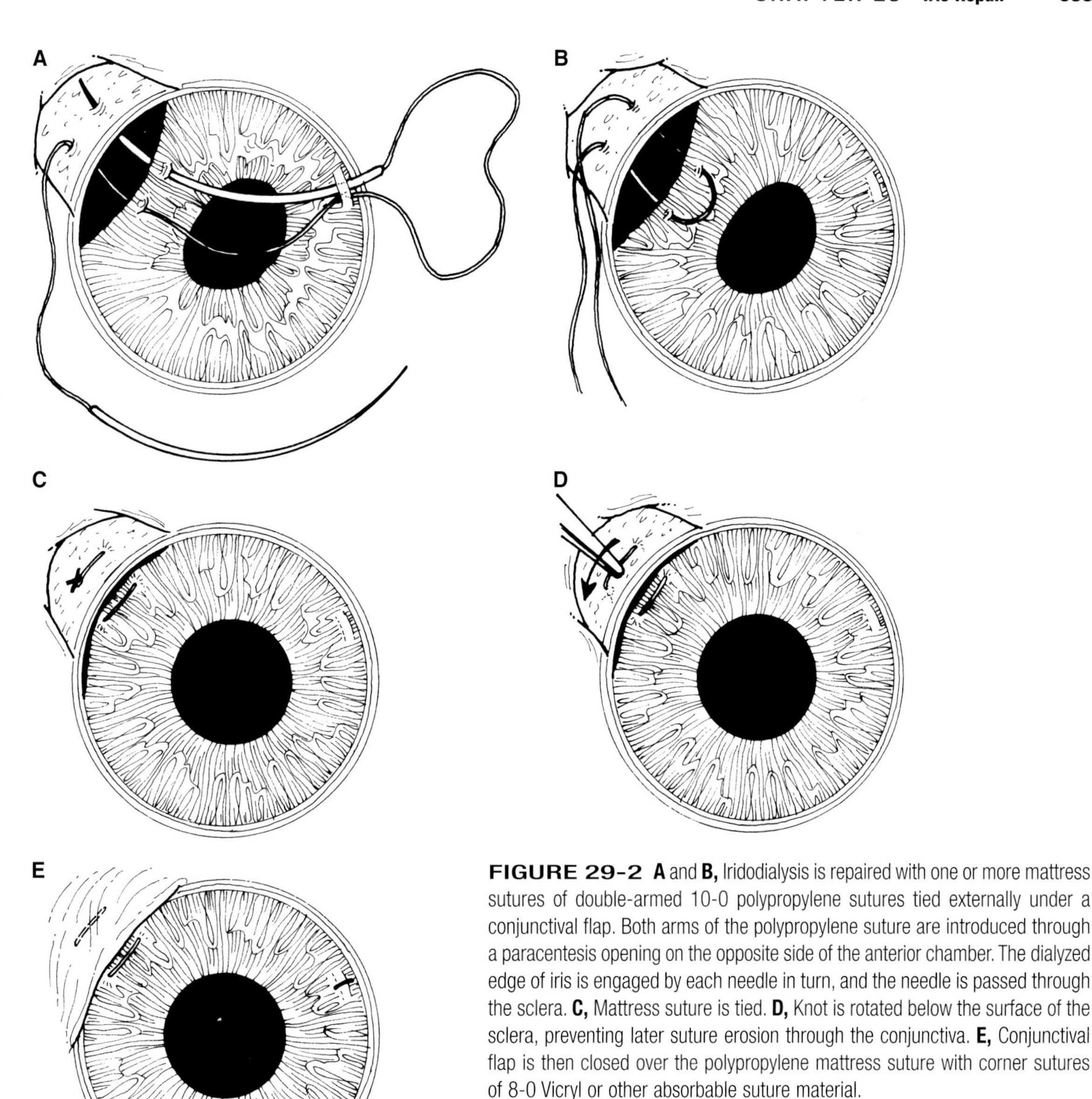

FIGURE 29-2 **A** and **B,** Iridodialysis is repaired with one or more mattress sutures of double-armed 10-0 polypropylene sutures tied externally under a conjunctival flap. Both arms of the polypropylene suture are introduced through a paracentesis opening on the opposite side of the anterior chamber. The dialyzed edge of iris is engaged by each needle in turn, and the needle is passed through the sclera. **C,** Mattress suture is tied. **D,** Knot is rotated below the surface of the sclera, preventing later suture erosion through the conjunctiva. **E,** Conjunctival flap is then closed over the polypropylene mattress suture with corner sutures of 8-0 Vicryl or other absorbable suture material.

requires that no additional traction be placed on the iris, however. The knot must be advanced into the eye and tied internally. One method to accomplish a knot deep inside the anterior chamber is to form the knot loop externally and then use a hook such as a Kuglen hook to advance the loop into the eye and make it snug. The procedure is repeated three or four times, achieving a secure knot at completion. The disadvantage of this technique is that it requires a skilled assistant, as it is necessary to maintain gentle traction on each of the suture ends while simultaneously advancing the knot with the hook. Three skilled hands are therefore needed.

Figure 29-1 illustrates an alternative two-handed technique popularized by Stephen Siepser, MD. In this variation, the knot is tied by passing loops externally, but the two ends of the suture can then be tightened, which draw the knot internally into the eye. This technique is elegant and does not require the third hand of a skilled assistant.

PRINCIPLE 3: REATTACHMENT OF IRIS TO SCLERA

The third principle is the technique for repair of a peripheral iris defect with the use of horizontal mattress sutures. A double-armed suture is employed. The mattress suture brings the iris back to its origin, if possible (Figure 29-2), or closes a peripheral defect using available adjacent iris tissue (Figure 29-3, *A* and *B*). The knot is tied externally but then rotated below the surface so that only a smooth loop of external suture remains. By using this technique of suture rotation and burying the knot, identical to the concept used in transscleral suturing of secondary posterior chamber (PC) IOLs (see Chapter 25, Figure 25-1), only a smooth loop of suture material remains. A scleral flap does not need to be dissected, and conjunctiva alone provides adequate coverage of the suture material. A large iridodialysis will require several adjacent horizontal mattress sutures.

A large defect may require a combination of these techniques (see Figure 29-3). Typically the repair begins by using horizontal

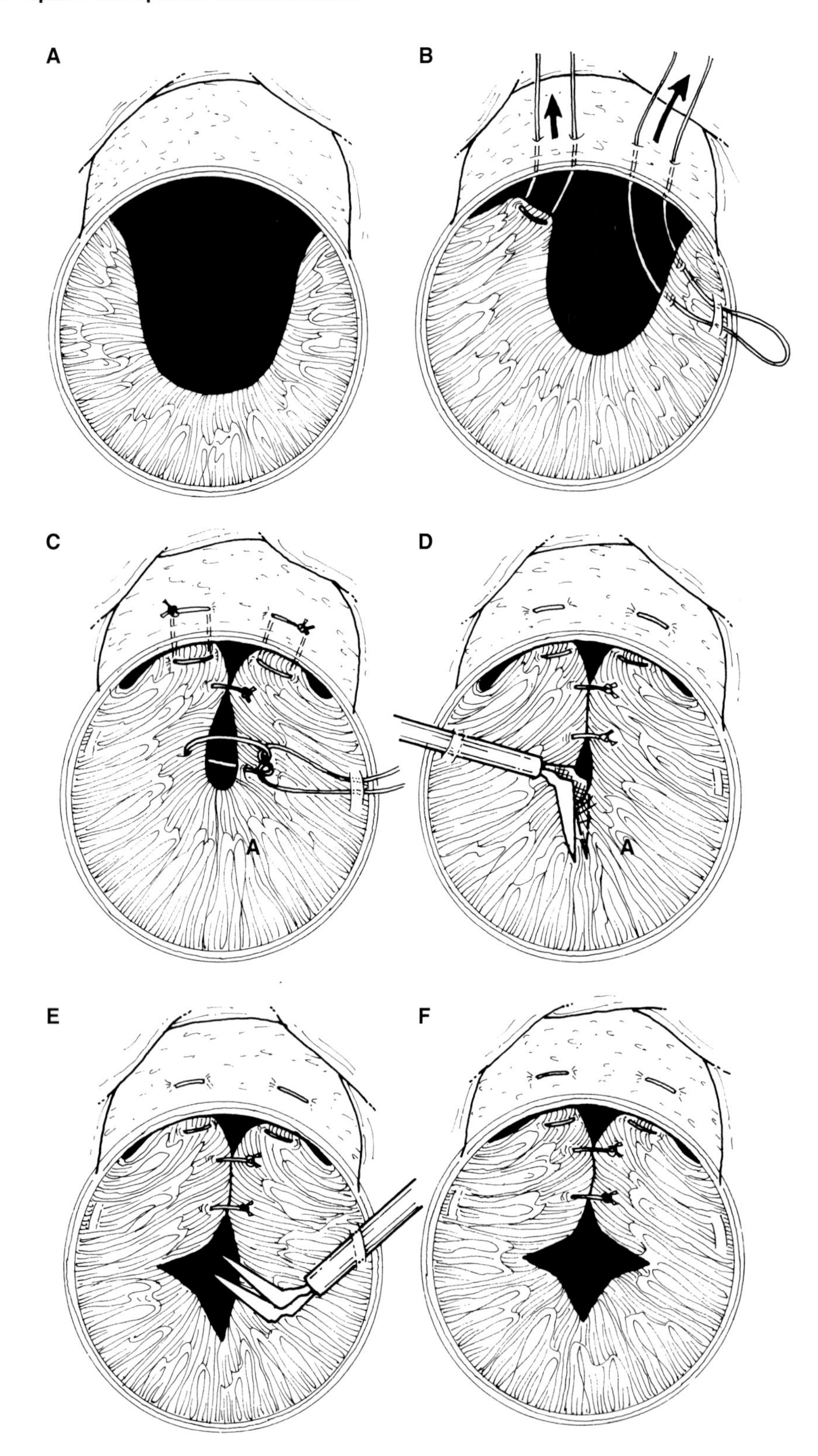

FIGURE 29-3 **A,** Conjunctival flap is recessed in the area of a sector iris defect. **B,** Horizontal mattress sutures bring midperipheral iris tissue into the basal area without iris. **C,** Interrupted sutures close the midperipheral space. **D to F,** "Sphincterotomies" in the central zone create a new pupillary aperture.

mattress sutures to create as much coverage of the peripheral and midperipheral cornea as possible (see Figure 29-3, *A* and *B*). Often this results in a distortion of the pupil itself (see Figure 29-3, *C*). A new pupil is constructed by judicious incisions in the iris and placement of additional sutures (see Figures 29-3, *C* to *F*). Case Studies 3 and 4 particularly illustrate these techniques. Second, the iris is highly visible and often important to the patient cosmetically.

In general, the surgeon should err on the side of leaving a pupil too small rather than too big. Postoperatively, a surgeon can use the neodymium: yttrium-aluminum-garnet (Nd:YAG) laser to expand the pupil by performing sphincterotomies with Nd:YAG laser pulses. The technique is similar to peripheral iridectomies with the Nd:YAG laser. A focusing contact lens is helpful. The laser setting is typically 6 mJ.

PRINCIPLE 4: PUPIL REPAIR

Blunt trauma often causes injury to the iris sphincter. An isolated rupture of the sphincter muscle is repaired with single interrupted sutures, similar to the technique illustrated in Figures 29-1 and 29-2. Case Study 1 illustrates the repair of local sphincter damage with interrupted sutures. When there is more generalized damage to the iris sphincter, caused by either multiple ruptures or ischemia, a different technique is needed. The surgeon can generally determine by careful preoperative inspection whether generalized iris sphincter injury has occurred. At the slit lamp examination, while varying the illumination through the pupil, the surgeon can inspect whether there is reactivity of the iris sphincter. In addition, the iris sphincter architecture is carefully inspected. When the iris sphincter architecture is not preserved and there is little to no reactivity, then a larger-scale repair of the pupil is needed.

The surgeon has two choices. The simpler choice is to place multiple interrupted sutures. This will typically result in a square or diamond-shaped pupil (Figure 29-4). Although cosmetically suboptimal, the optical benefit to the patient is substantial.

Alternatively, the surgeon can perform a 360-degree purse-string suture. This procedure was originally demonstrated by Dr. Pius Bucher of Austria and is illustrated in Case Study 6. The placement of the suture occurs after the completion of any cataract removal and IOL placement, of course. In the iris cerclage purse-string suture technique, a 10-0 Prolene suture on a CTC-6 needle (Ethicon) is recommended. In addition to the larger principal incision used for the cataract and IOL surgery, the surgeon should place two or three paracentesis openings at approximately equally spaced intervals. The needle is introduced through the principal incision and is passed in and out of the midperipheral iris stroma, typically for three or four passes. The needle is then passed out of the paracentesis by "docking" the needle tip into the end of a blunt 27-gauge irrigating cannula that has been passed through the paracentesis into the anterior chamber. In this manner, the pointed needle can be externalized without engaging the corneal tissue around the paracentesis. The needle is then regrasped with the needle holder and reintroduced into the eye, repeating the process for another quadrant or third of the iris. In reintroducing the needle through the paracentesis, great care must be taken not to inadvertently engage the lip of Descemet's membrane or any of the stroma. If the surgeon encounters difficulty passing the tip of the needle through the paracentesis cleanly, placement of some viscoelastic in the paracentesis can be a great aid in opening the passageway.

It is important that the bites of the cerclage suture be in the midperipheral iris, not close to the pupillary margin. The reason is that, once the suture is tightened, the suture between each of the bites will tighten and constrict. If the suture bites are near the pupillary edge, the suture material will be pulled into the pupillary opening. In contrast, if the suture material is kept in the midperiphery, the suture material itself will not be able to cross over the pupillary zone itself.

After completing the 360-degree passage of the suture, the knot is carefully tied through the principal limbal incision. The pupil is drawn down to a size of 3 to 4 mm. The postoperative appearance of the pupil is usually only slightly irregular.

If a major retinal problem occurs subsequently, such as retinal detachment, the iris cerclage suture can be released with either laser spots or intraoperatively by cutting the suture.

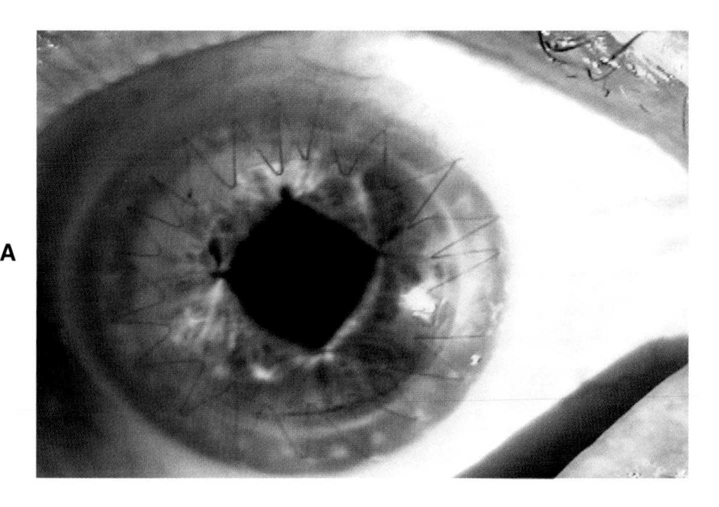

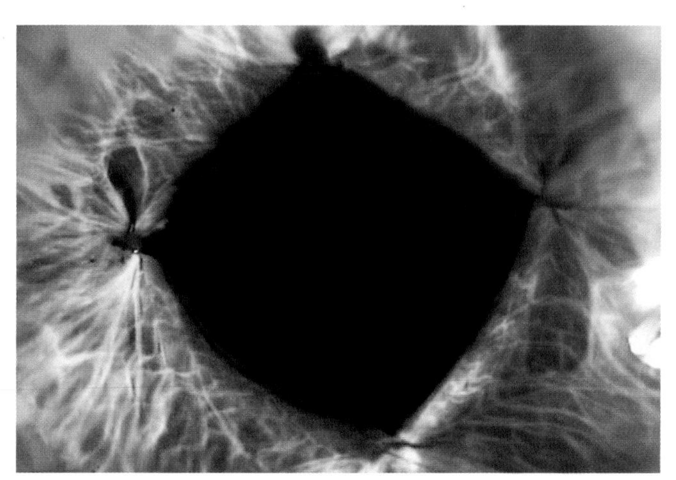

FIGURE 29-4 **A,** Diamond-shaped appearance of the pupil after four interrupted sutures reduced a large atonic pupil at the time of penetrating keratoplasty. **B,** High magnification shows the four polypropylene suture knots.

Case Studies in Iris Reconstruction

Case 1: Traumatic mydriasis caused by localized sphincter rupture

This patient had blunt trauma from a paintball gun injury, resulting in cataract and traumatic mydriasis (Figure C1-1). Preoperative slit lamp examination showed that the sphincter muscle had ruptured temporally with atrophy of the sphincter in that region and that the remainder of the sphincter muscle reacted normally to light. After cataract surgery and IOL implantation, a Y-hook was used to bring the iris tissue out of the angle (Figure C1-2). Repair of the temporal iris consisted of placing two interrupted 10-0 polypropylene sutures (Figures C1-3 through C1-6, surgeon's view temporally). One day after surgery, a reasonably well-centered pupil was present, centered over the IOL (Figure C1-7, slit lamp view).

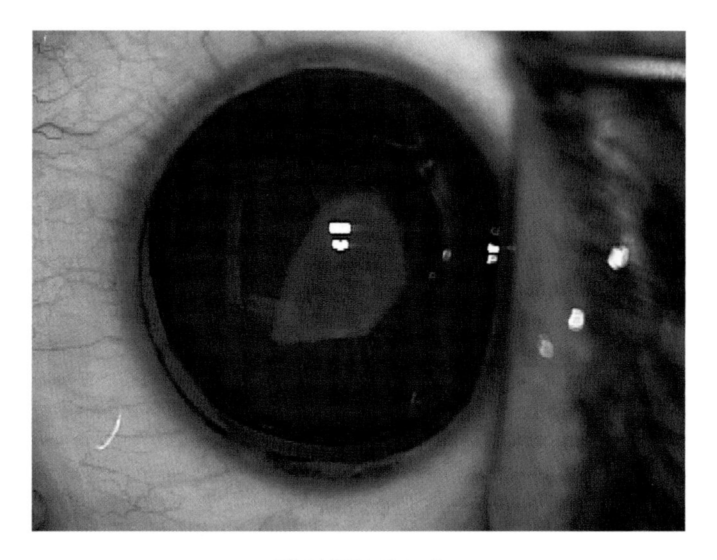

FIGURE C1-1

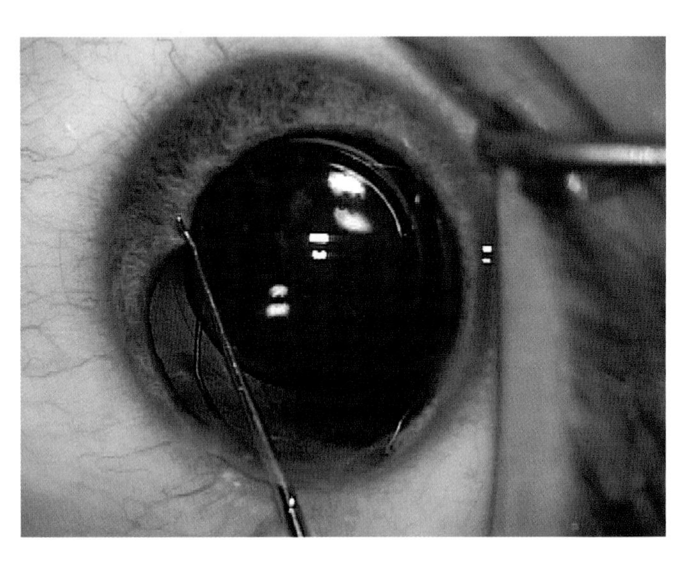

FIGURE C1-2

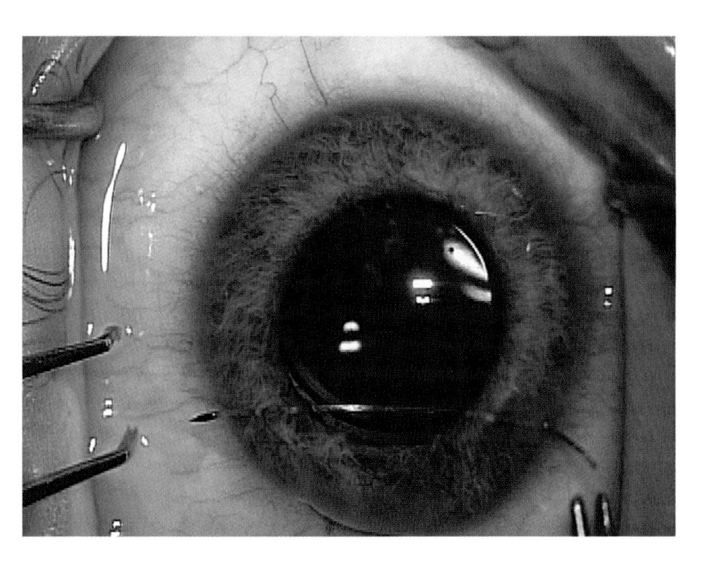

FIGURE C1-3

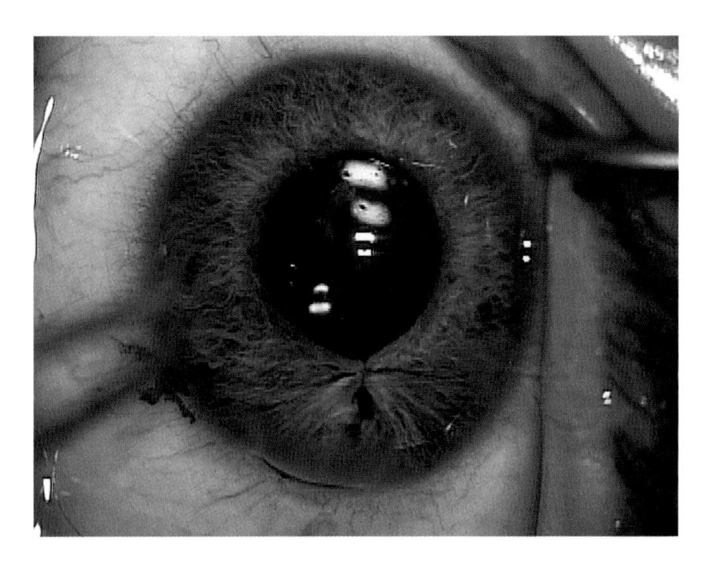

FIGURE C1-4

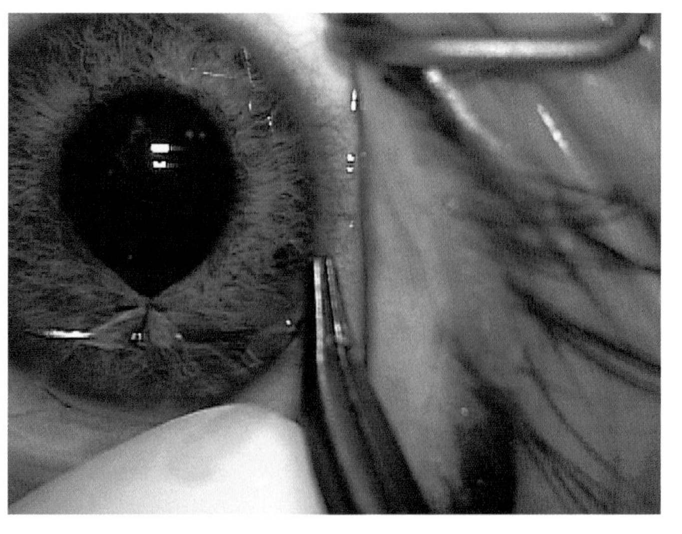

FIGURE C1-5

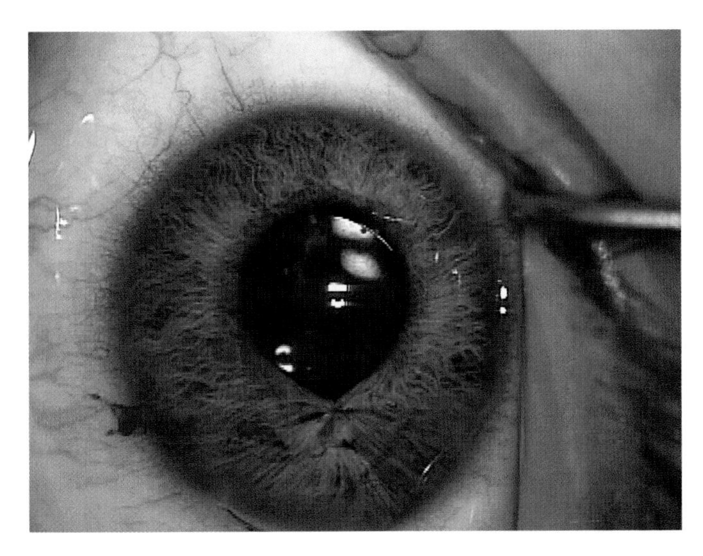

FIGURE C1-6

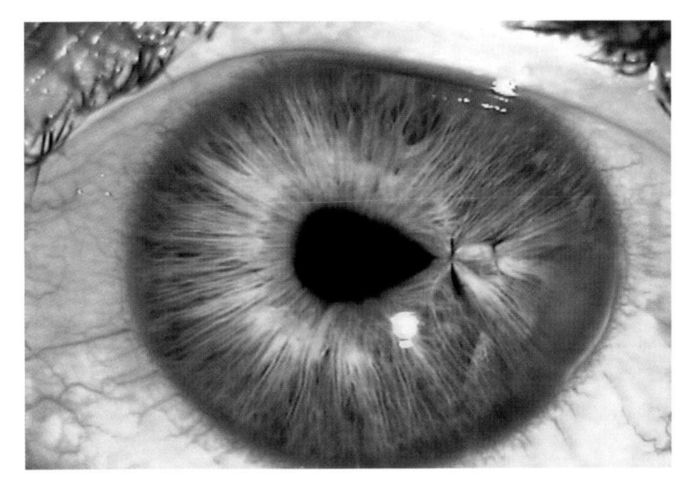

FIGURE C1-7

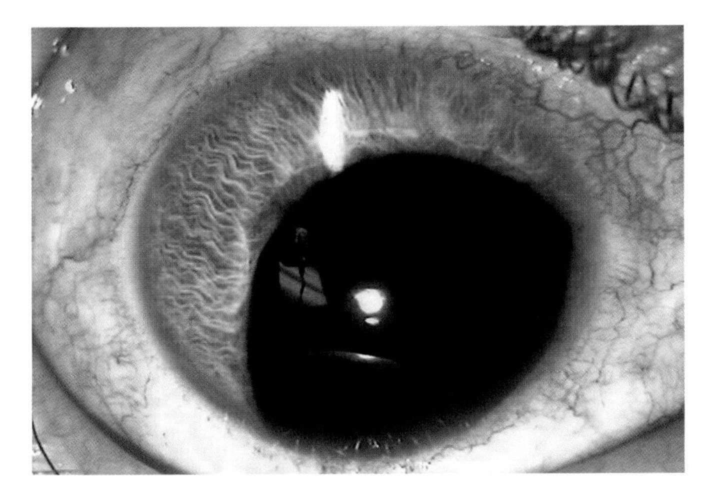

FIGURE C2-1

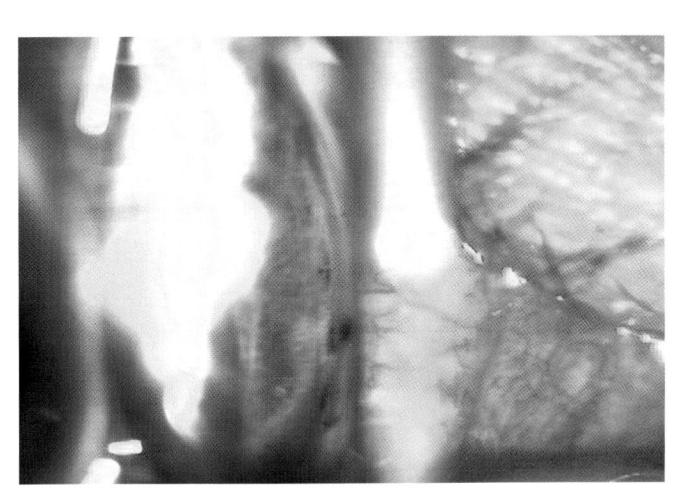

FIGURE C2-2

Case 2: Airbag injury

A severely eccentric pupil and cataract resulted from an airbag injury in a motor vehicle accident. The iris appeared absent inferotemporally (Figure C2-1). Preoperative gonioscopy showed that the iris appeared bunched up into the angle of the area corresponding to the pupil abnormality (Figure C2-2). The surgical photos are from the surgeon's perspective, sitting superiorly. At surgery, the severely subluxated lens had been removed by pars plana lensectomy and vitrectomy (Figure C2-3). A posterior chamber IOL with a 7-mm optic was secured through transscleral sutures, deliberately decentered in the direction of the pupil deformity in case the pupil cannot be fully shifted centrally (Figure C2-4). Repair of the iris began with traction on the peripheral iris to release adhesions, taking care to avoid dialysis of the iris root (Figures C2-5 through C2-7), markedly improving the amount of peripheral iris tissue but leaving a nonreactive pupil that was still large enough to cause glare (Figure C2-8). A single interrupted suture across the inferotemporal pupil (Figure C2-9) reduced the pupil to an acceptable size and shape (Figure C2-10).

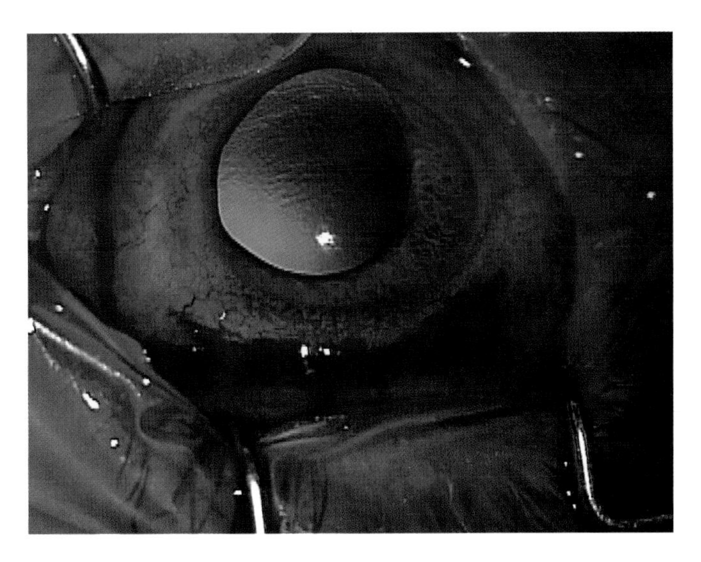

FIGURE C2-3

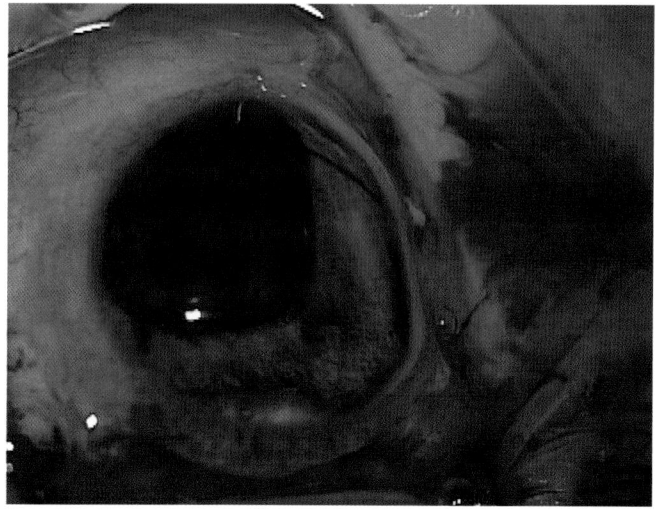

FIGURE C2-4

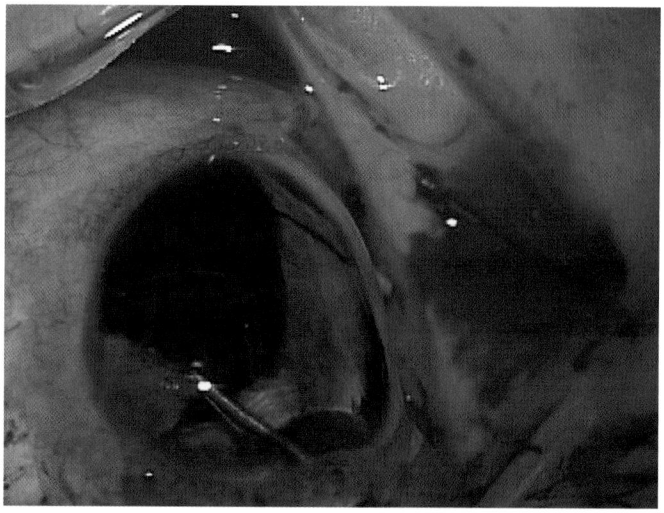

FIGURE C2-5

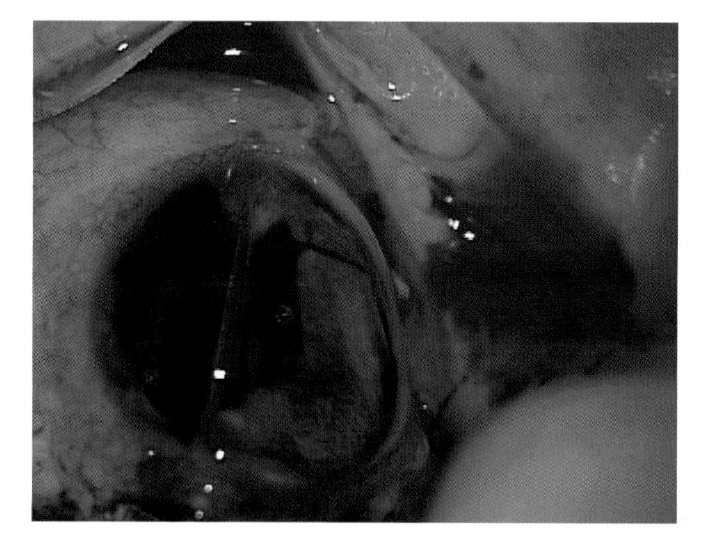

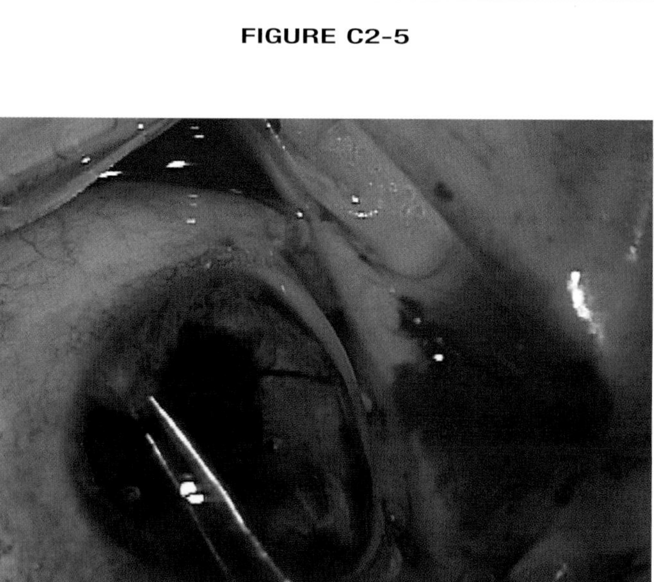

FIGURE C2-6

FIGURE C2-7

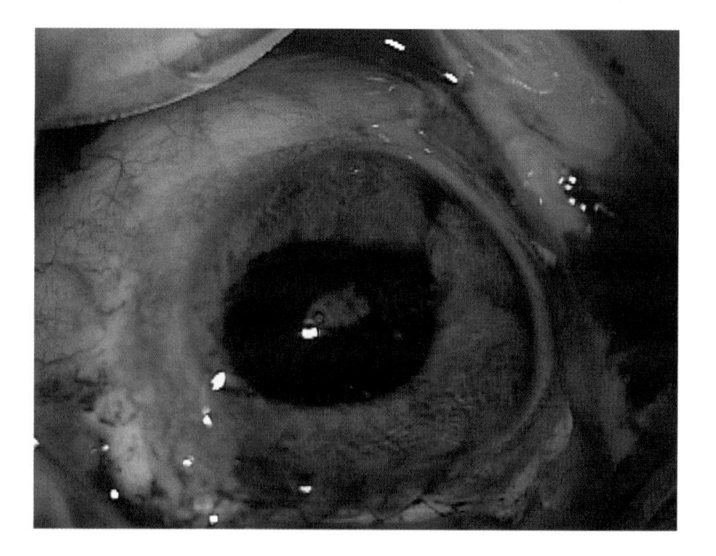

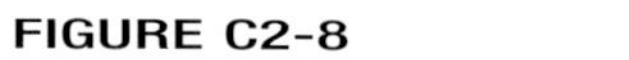

FIGURE C2-8

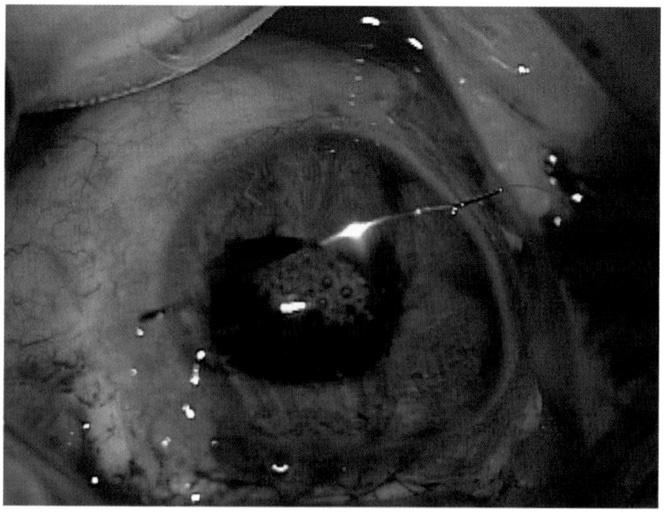

FIGURE C2-9

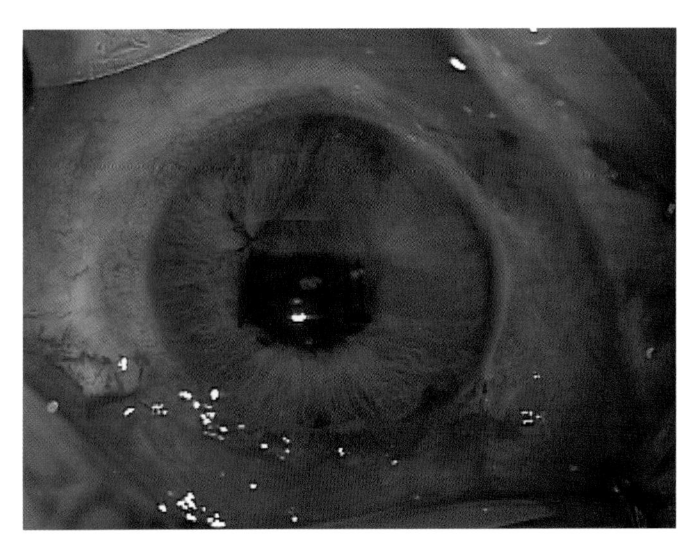

FIGURE C2-10

Case 3: Sector iris defect after melanoma excision

A slowly expanding iris melanoma, observed and documented for over a decade, threatened to invade the angle in a patient with developing cataract (Figures C3-1 and C3-2). The surgeon sat superiorly (Figure C3-3) to have a better angle of access for excising the tumor after phacoemulsification cataract extraction and capsular bag placement of a PC IOL in this right eye.

The melanoma was isolated first with radial incisions by a Gills-Vannas scissors, with a small margin of normal iris (Figures C3-4 and C3-5). The basal iris was excised as close as possible to the angle using horizontal vitreous scissors (Figures C3-6 and C3-7) and the tumor placed on a sterile tongue blade (Figure C3-8) to maintain a flat orientation for pathologic examination.

The reconstruction began with a 10-0 polypropylene suture reapproximating the sphincter edges (Figures C3-9 and C3-10). Note how much larger the defect became because of relaxations of the iris, compared with the original area of excision (Figure C3-4). A second

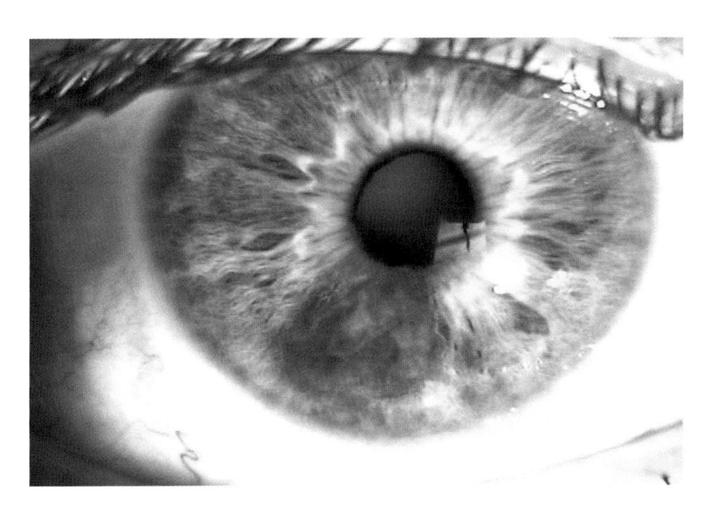

FIGURE C3-1

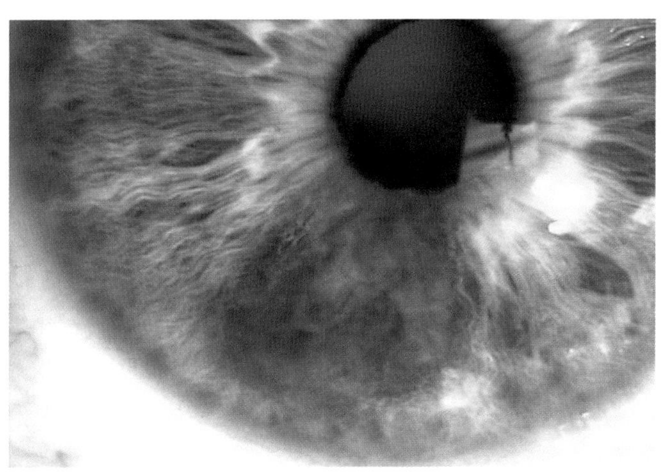

FIGURE C3-2

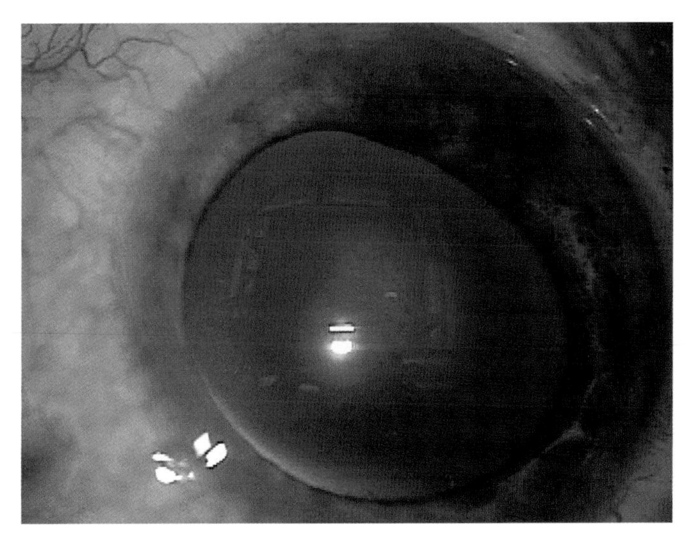

FIGURE C3-3

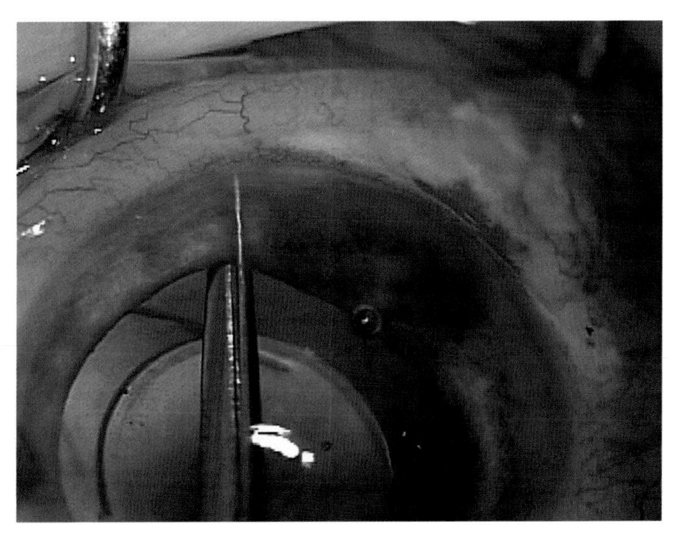

FIGURE C3-4

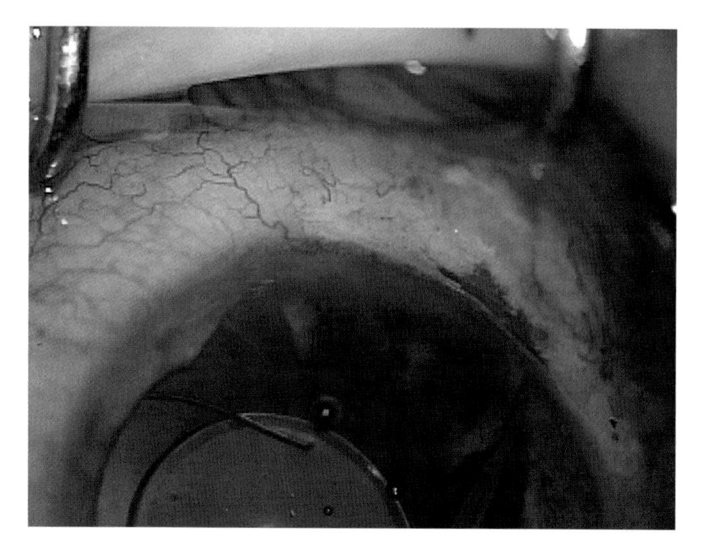
FIGURE C3-5

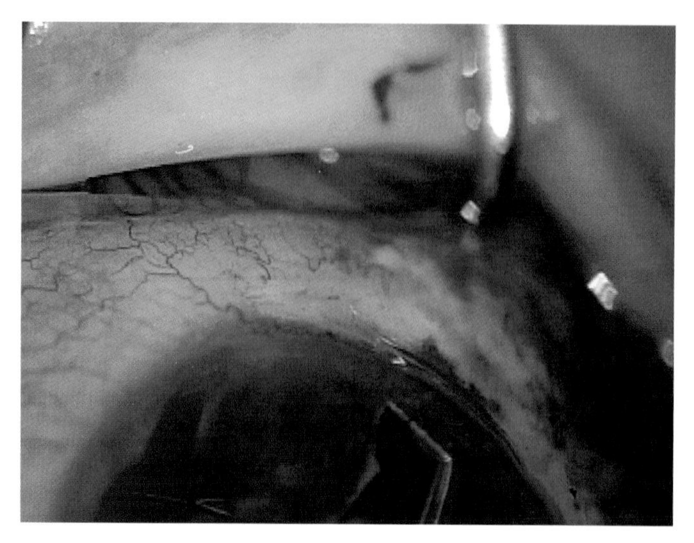
FIGURE C3-6

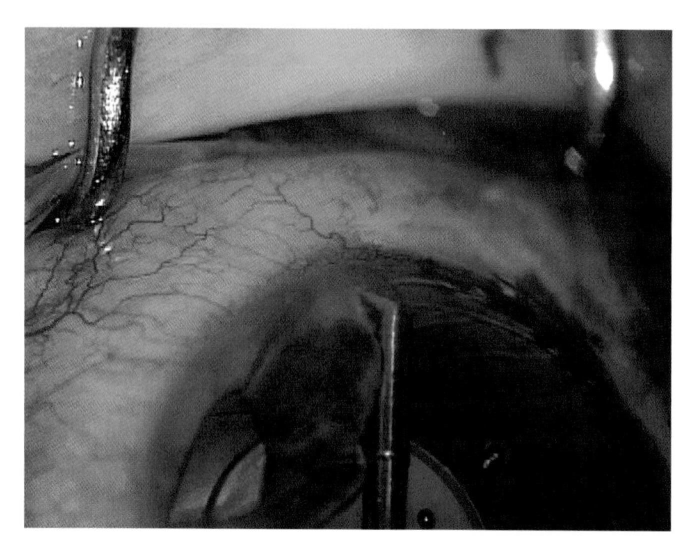
FIGURE C3-7

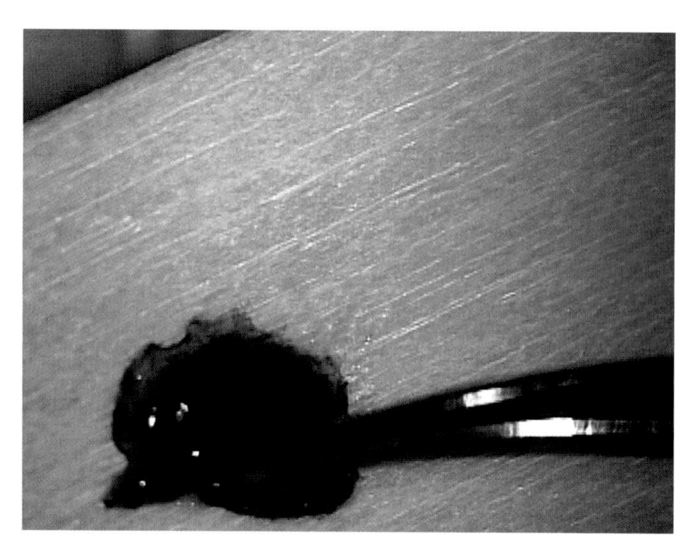
FIGURE C3-8

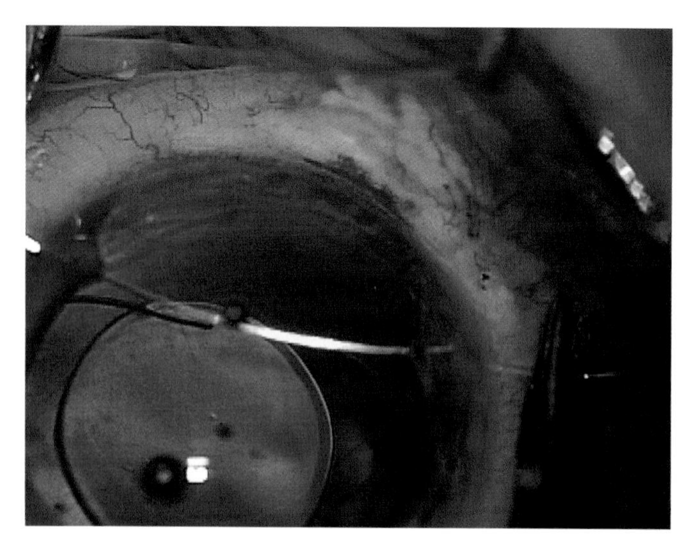
FIGURE C3-9

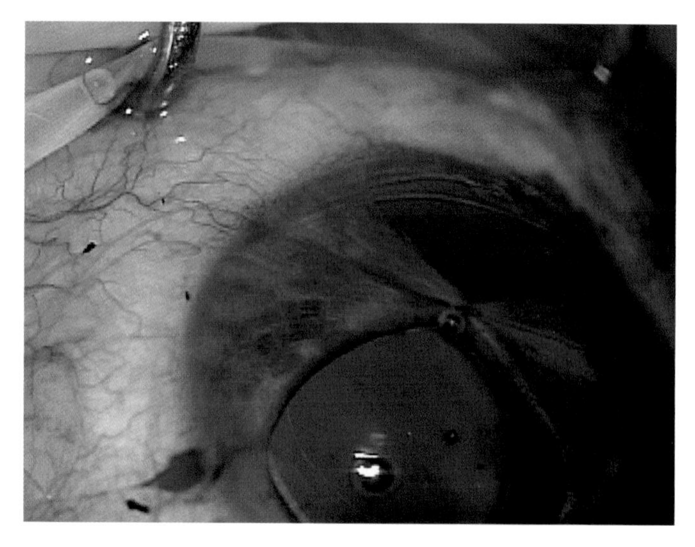
FIGURE C3-10

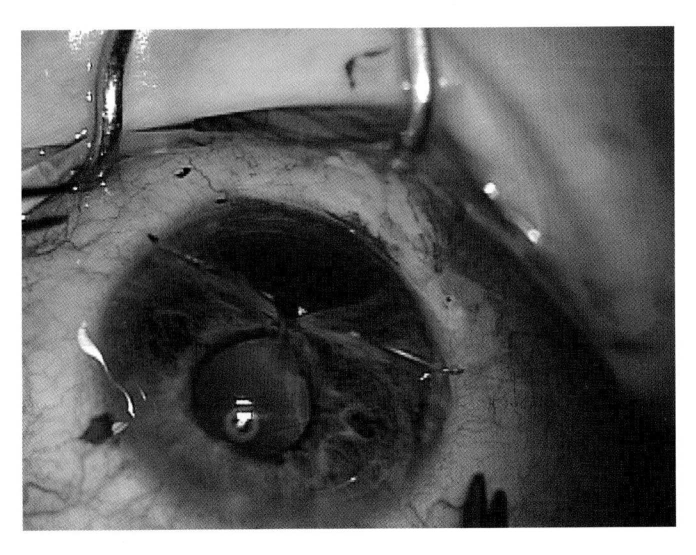

FIGURE C3-11

suture added reinforcement (Figures C3-11 and C3-12), but it became apparent that a large basal defect would persist that, given the exposed inferior location, would be a source of glare.

To close the basal defect, a double-armed 10-0 polypropylene suture was passed in a horizontal mattress orientation (Figures C3-13 and C3-14) through the iris and the limbus, which closed the basal defect when tied (Figure C3-15). The knot was rotated beneath the scleral surface to prevent later erosion through the conjunctiva (Figure C3-16).

As a consequence, the pupil was shifted eccentrically. Two additional sutures closed the eccentric opening (Figures C3-17 and C3-18), restoring a nearly round and well-centered pupil (Figure C3-19). The appearance on the first postoperative day showed a somewhat small pupil (Figure C3-20), but the patient had no complaints of dark vision. It is better to err on the side of leaving the pupil too small at the time of the surgical repair, as later expansion of the pupil can be achieved easily with laser sphincterotomies (see Chapter 45) and/or lysis of a suture.

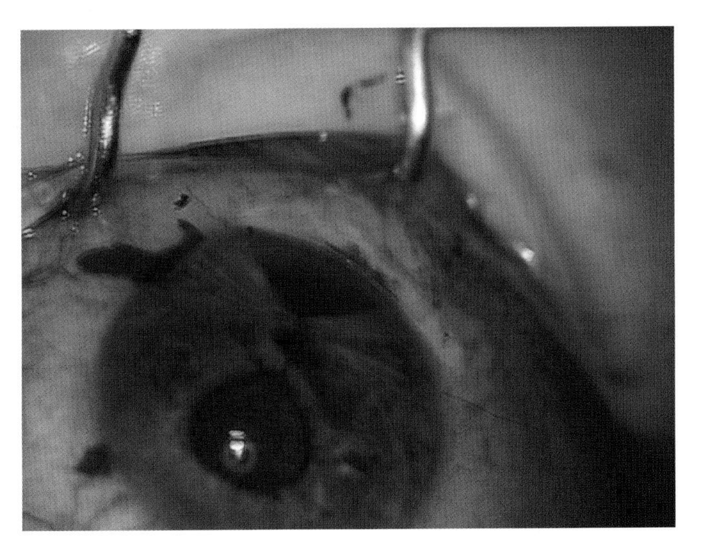

FIGURE C3-12

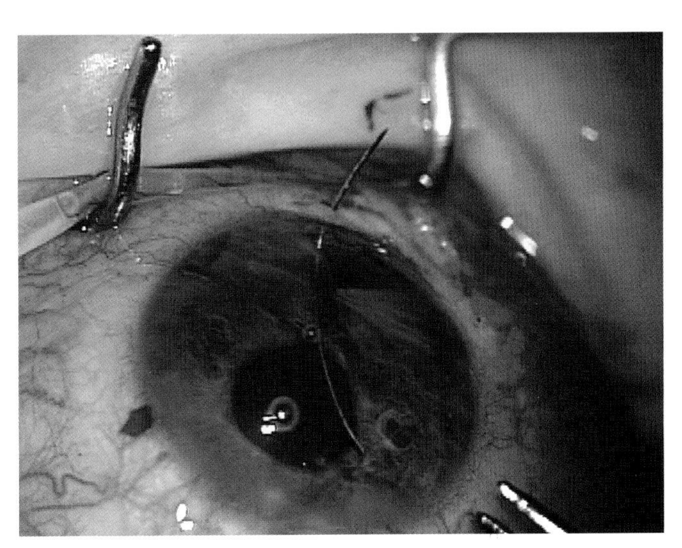

FIGURE C3-13

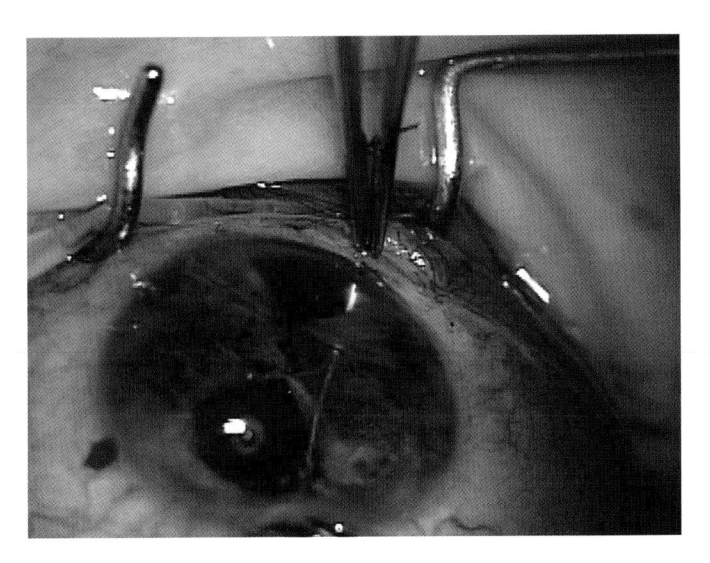

FIGURE C3-14

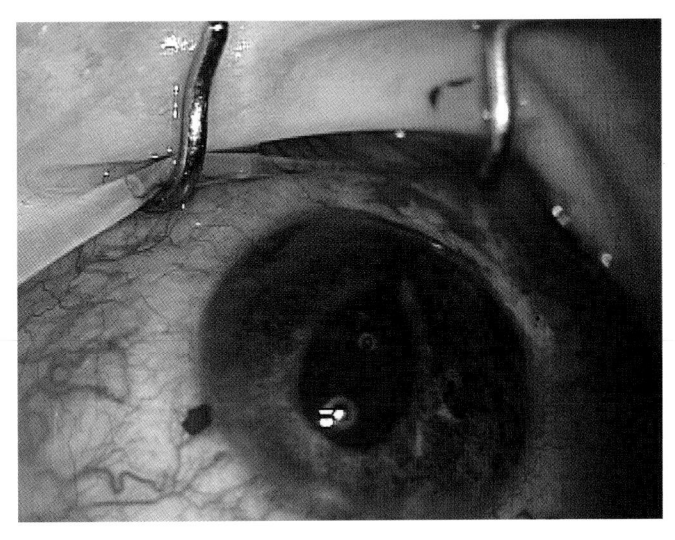

FIGURE C3-15

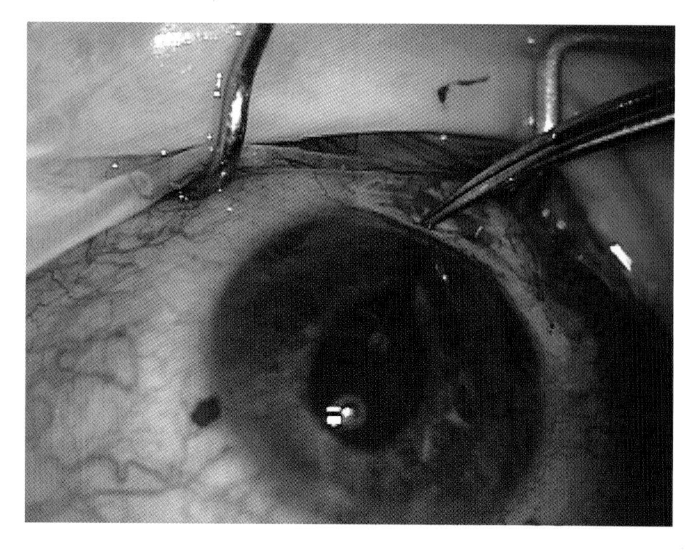

FIGURE C3-16

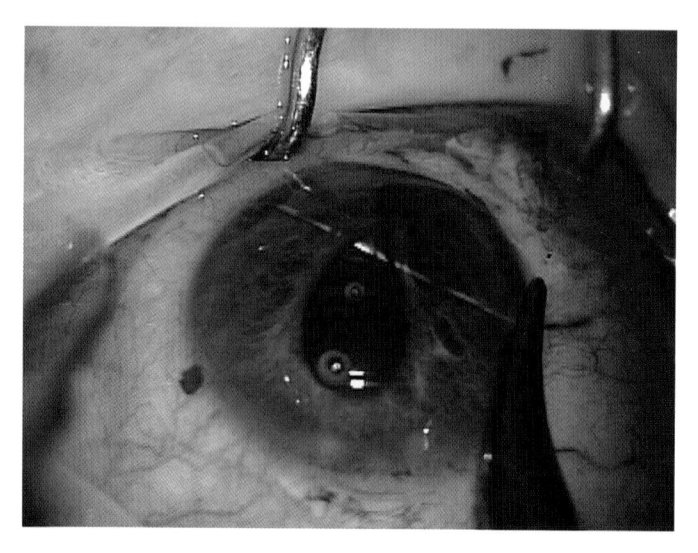

FIGURE C3-17

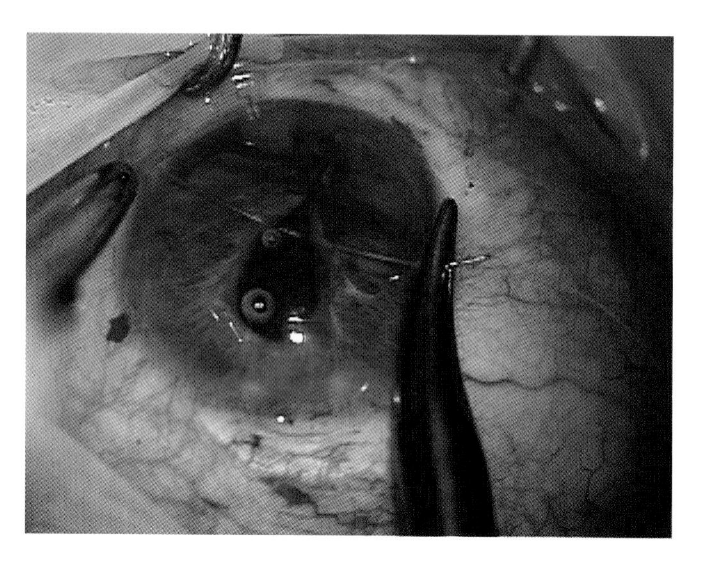

FIGURE C3-18

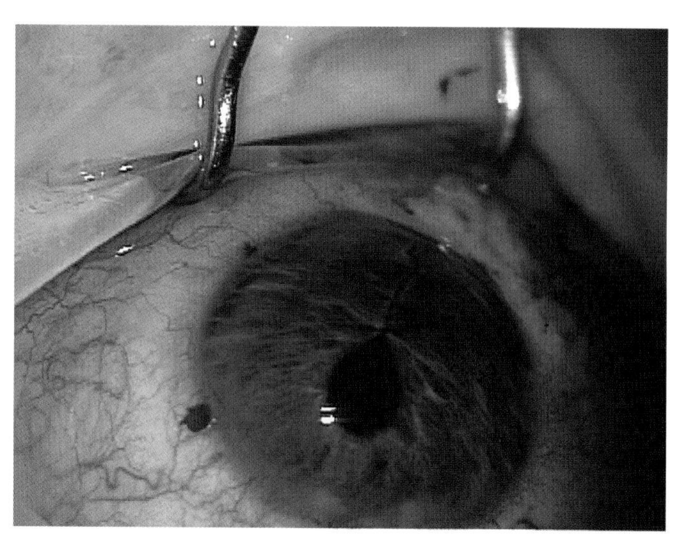

FIGURE C3-19

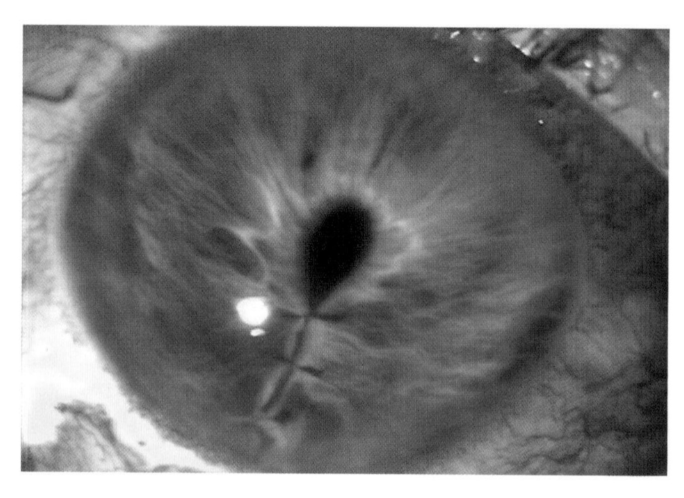

FIGURE C3-20

Case 4: Iris loss at cataract surgery

This patient experienced iris prolapse and subsequent bleeding from the iris root during attempted implantation of a phakic IOL for correction of high hyperopia. A secondary cataract developed, and uncomplicated cataract surgery with PC IOL implantation was performed. The patient complained about severe glare postoperatively resulting from exposure of the IOL edge (Figure C4-1). An artificial prosthetic iris was recommended, but the patient was unhappy with the prospect of implantation of an investigational device and sought other surgical remedies.

From the surgeon's perspective seated superiorly (Figure C4-2), the first area to be addressed was the loose stub of iris tissue. A double-armed 10-0 polypropylene suture was passed as a horizontal mattress closure (Figures C4-3 and C4-4) that provided partial coverage when the suture was tightened (Figure C4-5).

The inferior pupil appeared to be too superior after the horizontal mattress suture, and an inferior sphincterotomy was performed with Gills-Vannas scissors (Figure C4-6). The superior gape was closed with two interrupted sutures (Figures C4-7 through C4-9). The pupil appeared too small, with a vertical slit configuration. Small sphincterotomies were then placed horizontally to the left and right (Figure C4-10).

At this point, the original inferior sphincterotomy shown in Figure C4-6 appeared excessive, with exposure of the inferior edge of the capsulorrhexis margin (Figure C4-11). The exposure was remedied with an interrupted suture (Figure C4-12). Postoperatively, the patient reported elimination of the glare and was pleased by the improvement in the appearance of her highly visible iris (Figure C4-13). The upper lid in its natural position covered the remaining superior peripheral iris defect.

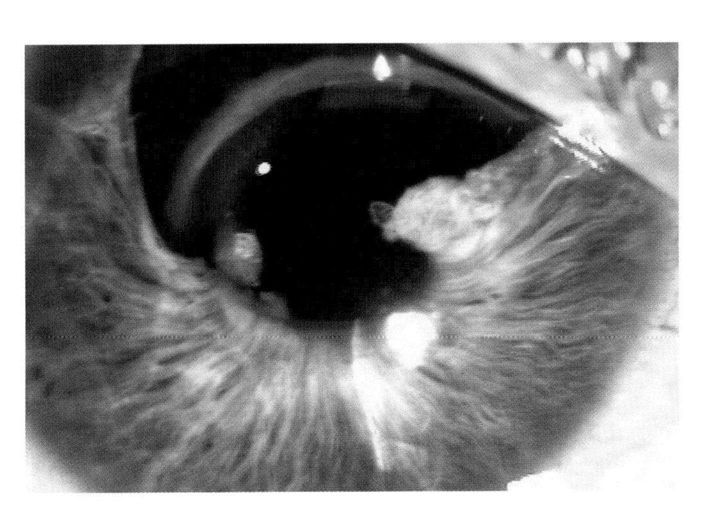

FIGURE C4-1

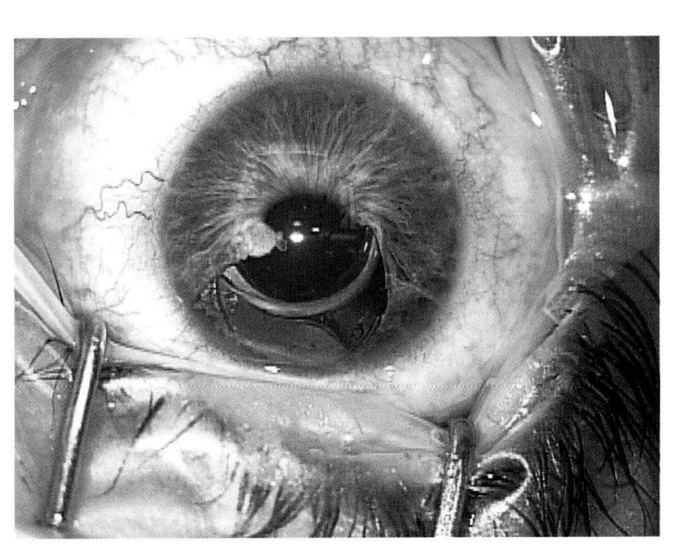

FIGURE C4-2

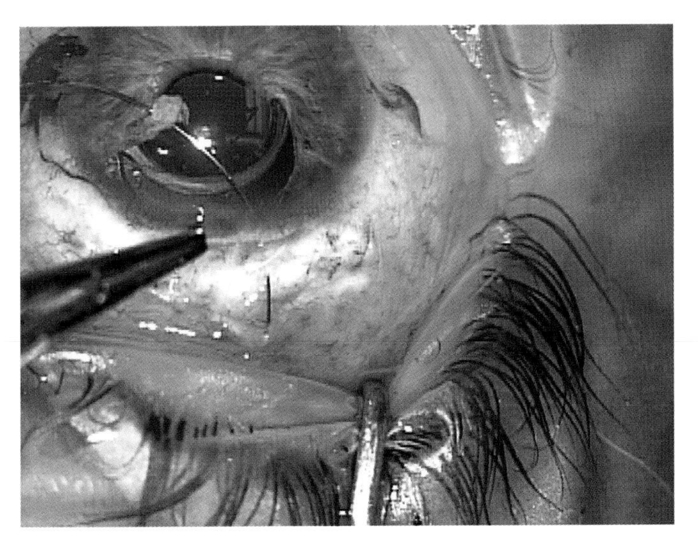

FIGURE C4-3

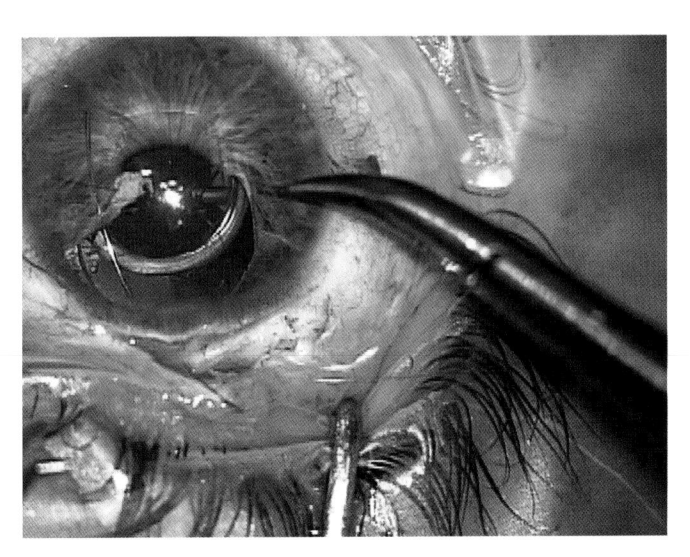

FIGURE C4-4

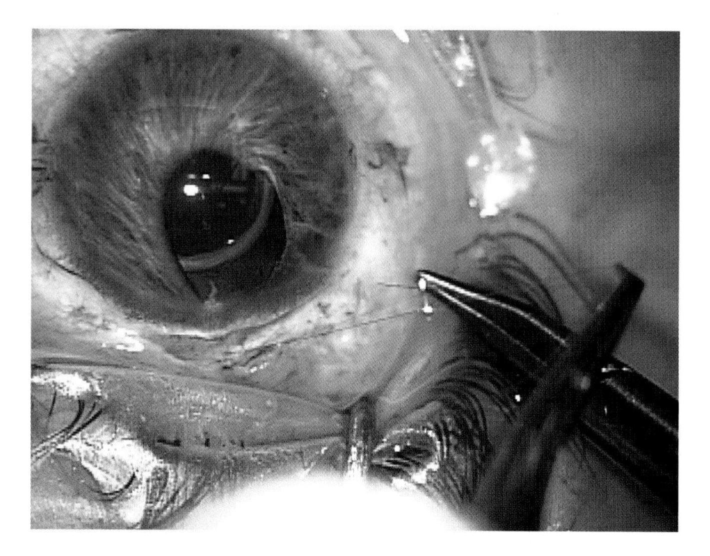

FIGURE C4-5

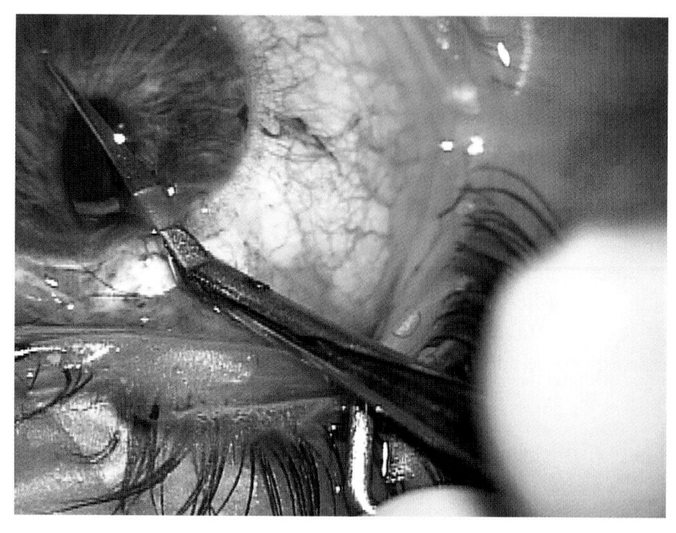

FIGURE C4-6

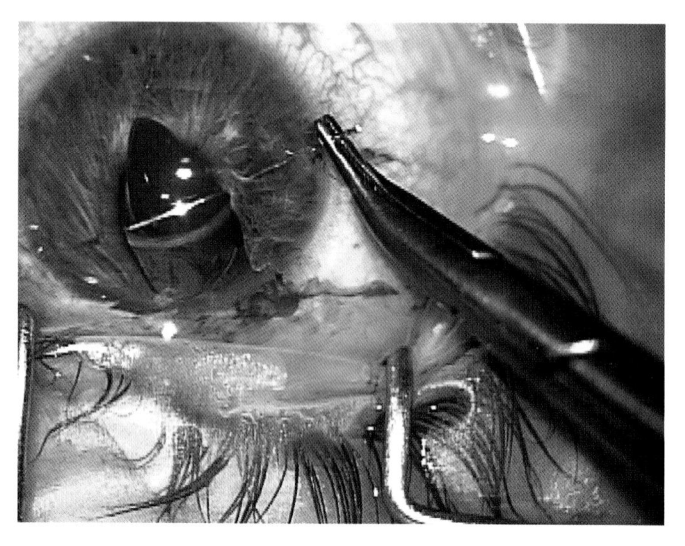

FIGURE C4-7

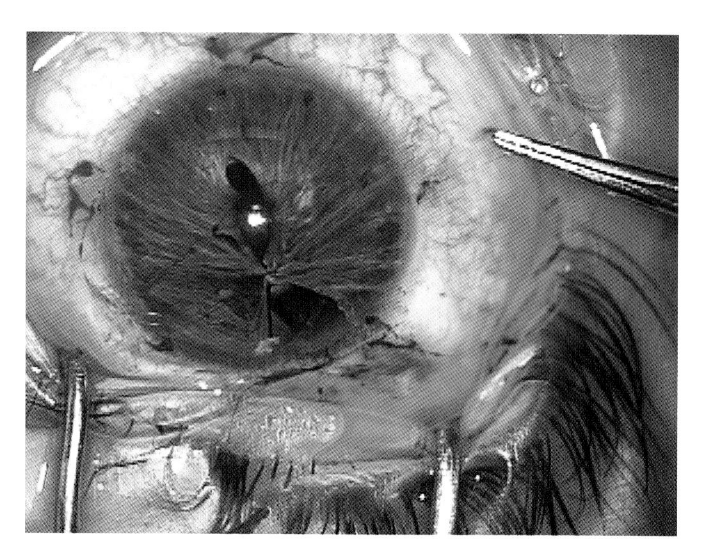

FIGURE C4-8

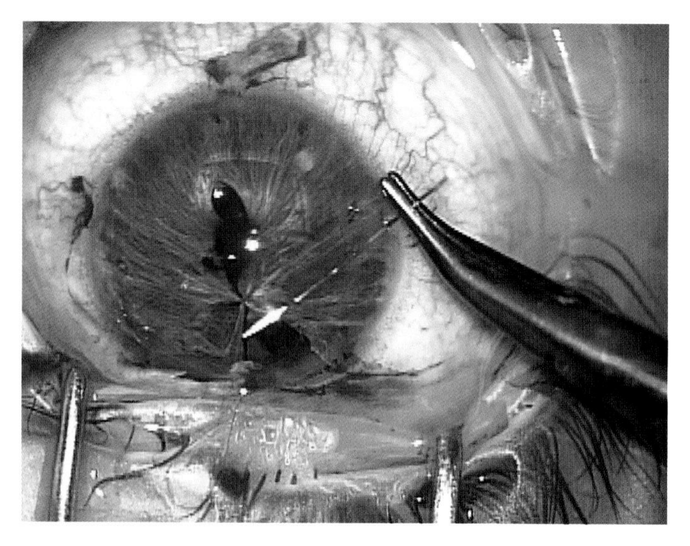

FIGURE C4-9

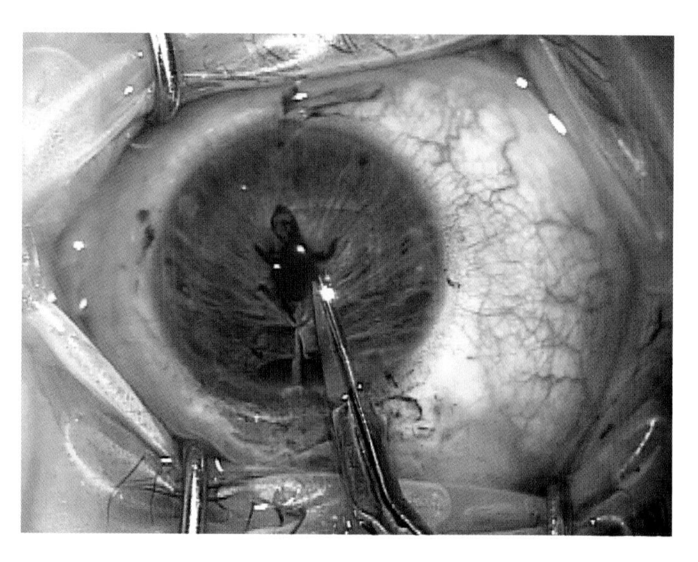

FIGURE C4-10

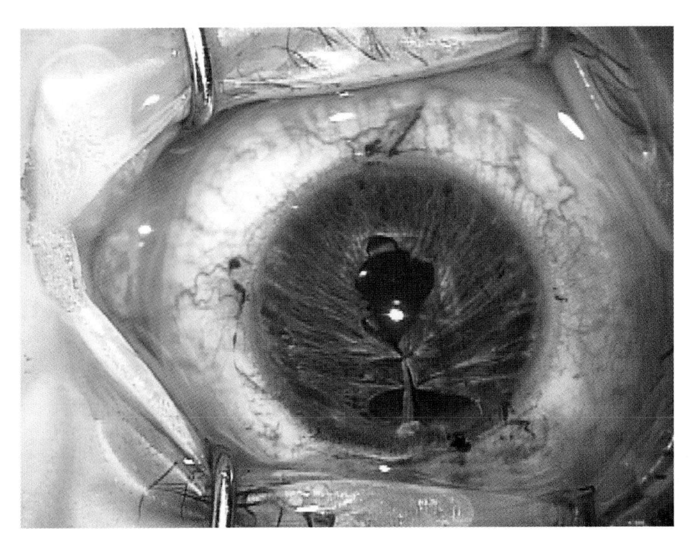

FIGURE C4-11

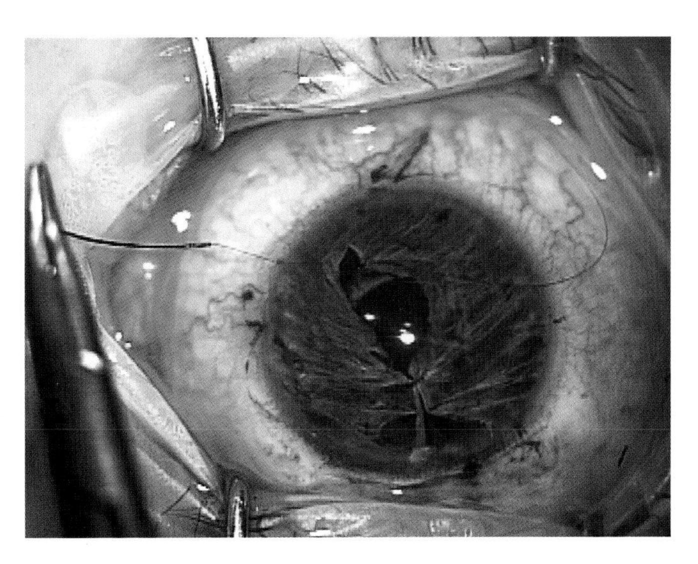

FIGURE C4-12

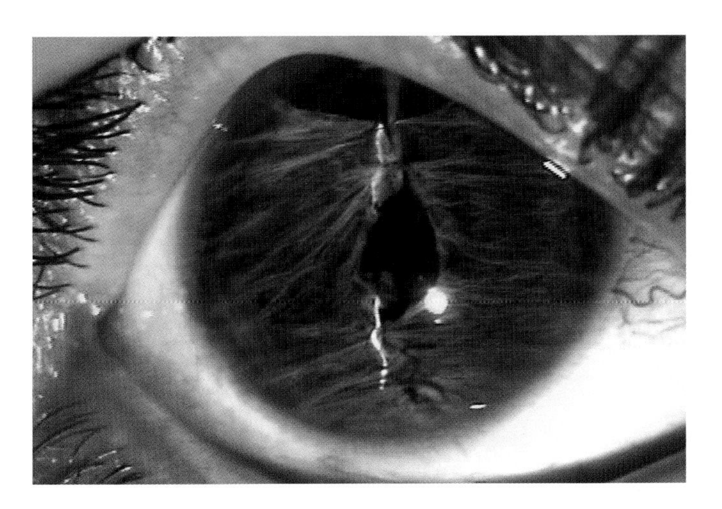

FIGURE C4-13

Case 5: Anterior chamber IOL–Induced pupillary distortion

The patient was experiencing both severe glare and loss of vision caused by cystoid macular edema associated with iris tuck 6 months after secondary implantation of flexible open-loop anterior chamber IOL. The view of the surgeon sitting superiorly is shown in Figure C5-1. Simple removal of the misplaced haptics that caused the iris tuck did not relieve the pupillary distortion (Figure C5-2).

After thorough vitrectomy and placement of a transscleral suture–fixated PC IOL, traction on the peripheral iris released some peripheral synechiae (Figure C5-3) Next, the large iridectomy was closed with a single interrupted suture (Figure C5-4).

The pupillary aperture was then reduced with interrupted sutures nasally and temporally (Figures C5-5 and C5-6). To create a rounder pupil, small sphincterotomies were added inferiorly (Figure C5-7) and superiorly (Figure C5-8). On the first postoperative day, the view was mildly hazy because of the inflammatory reaction, but the slit lamp appearance showed a reasonably sized central pupil (Figure C5-9). Over

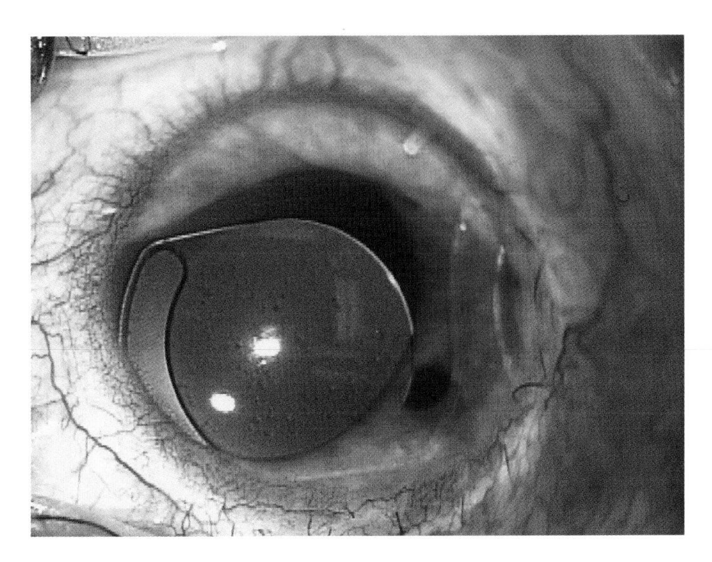

FIGURE C5-1

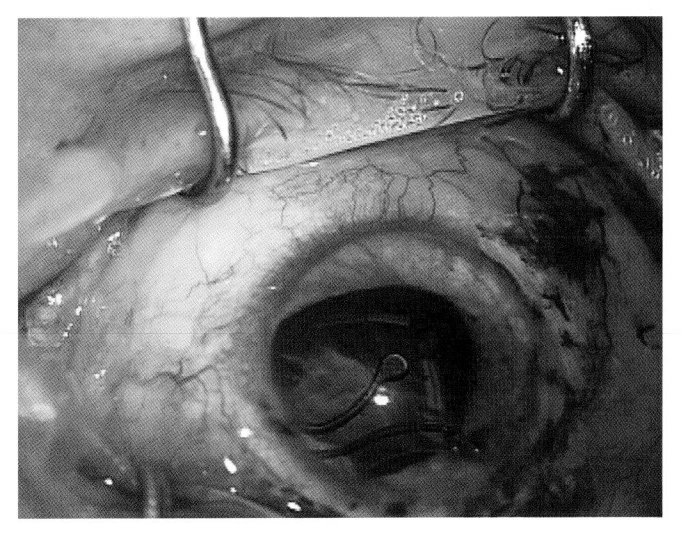

FIGURE C5-2

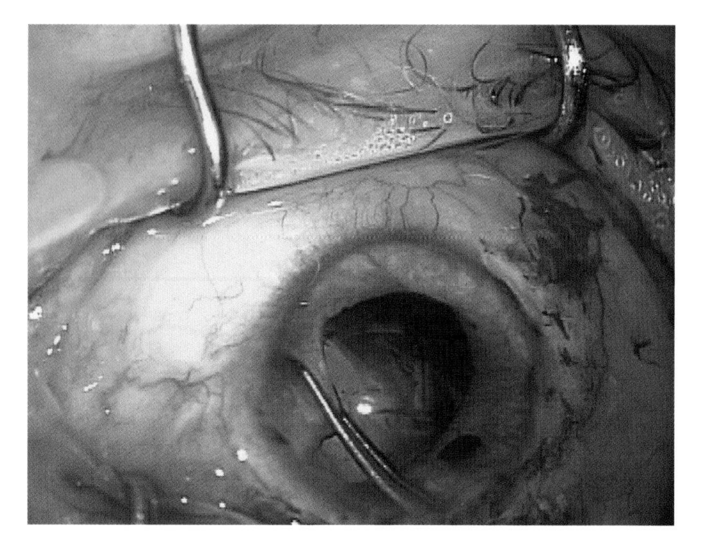

FIGURE C5-3

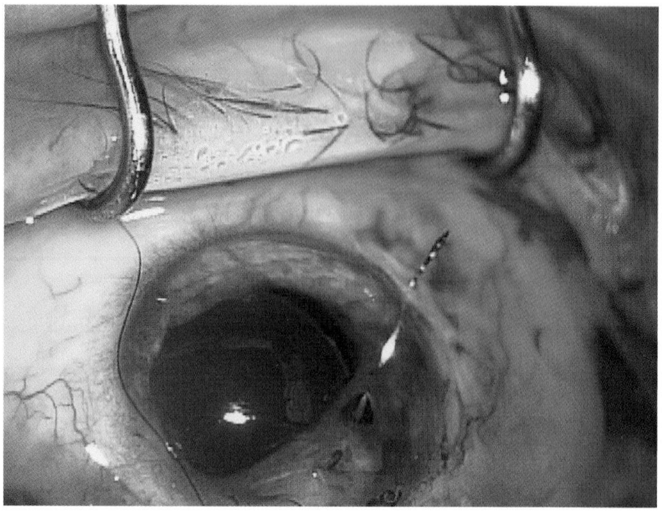

FIGURE C5-4

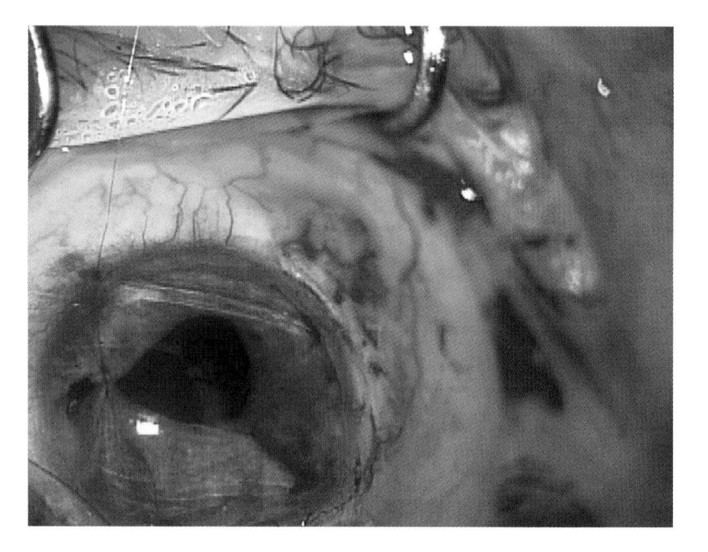

FIGURE C5-5

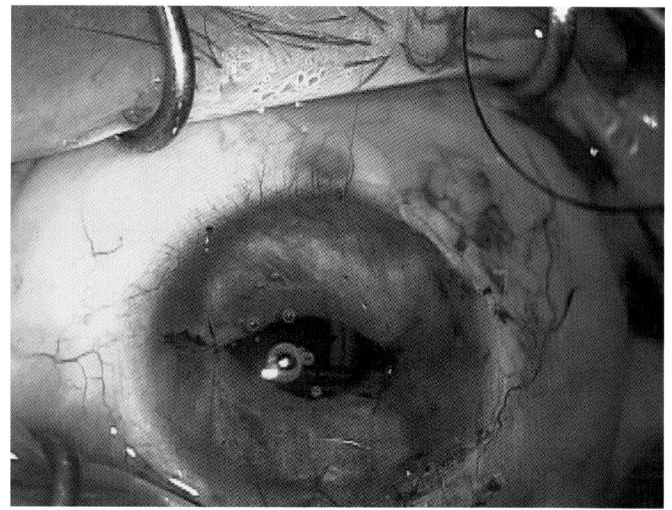

FIGURE C5-6

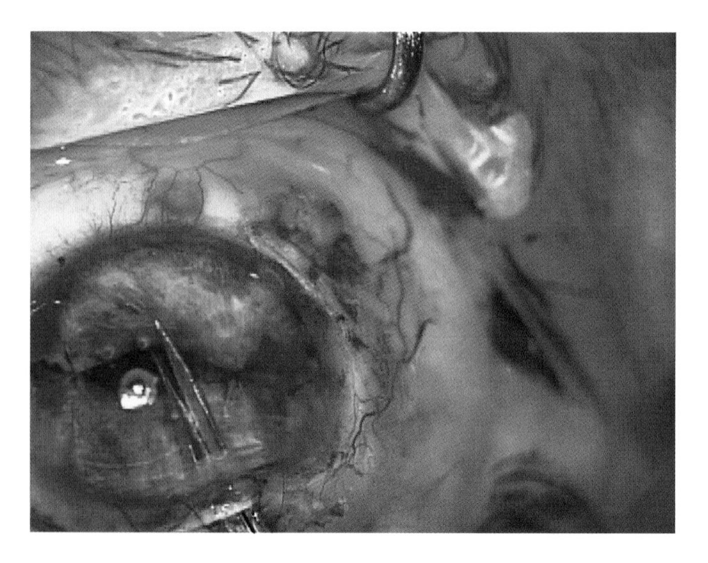

FIGURE C5-7

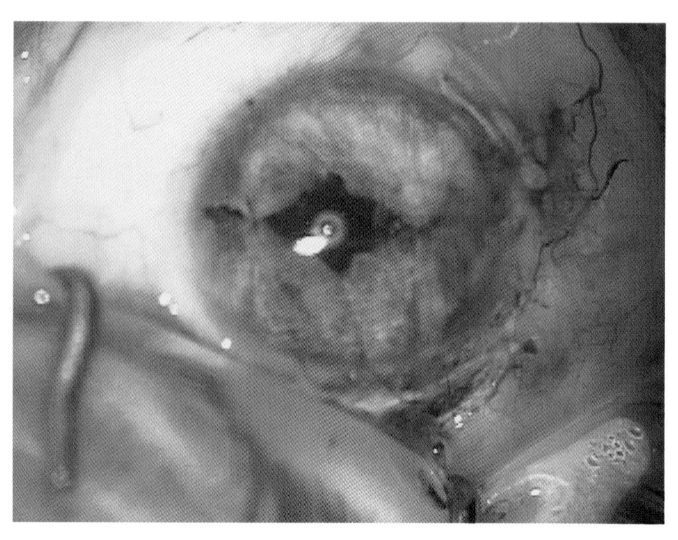

FIGURE C5-8

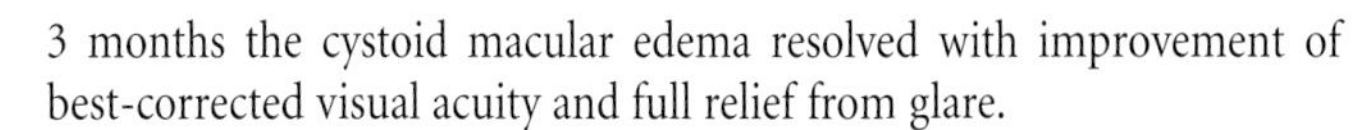

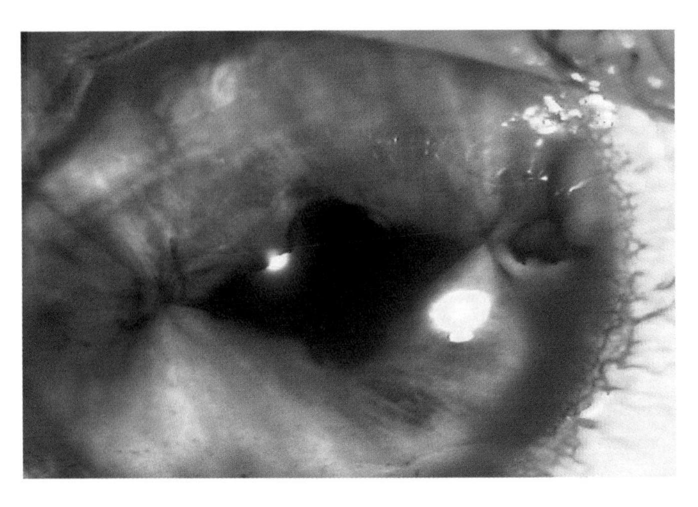

FIGURE C5-9

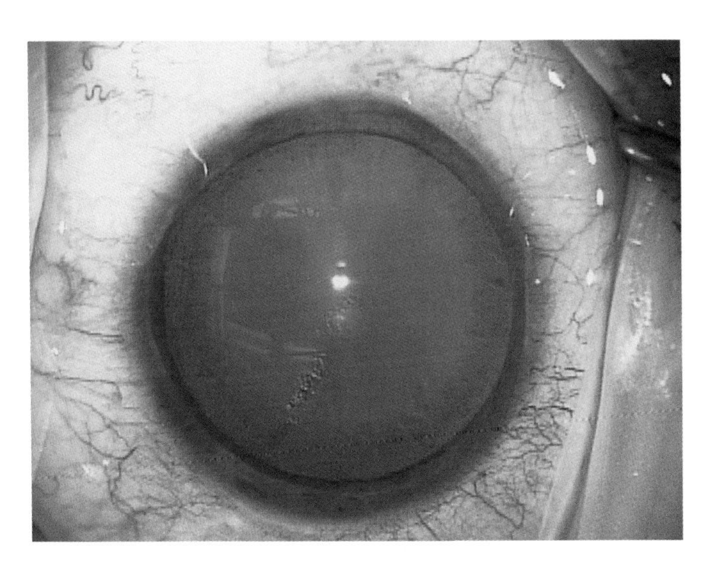

FIGURE C6-1

3 months the cystoid macular edema resolved with improvement of best-corrected visual acuity and full relief from glare.

Case 6: Atonic pupil corrected with iris circlage purse-string suture

This patient requiring cataract surgery had a lifelong history of isolated bilateral atonic pupils that measured 8 mm without dilation and non-reactive to light. His clinical presentation is more commonly seen after blunt trauma leading to generalized atrophy of the sphincter muscle. Glare symptoms will be worsened after cataract surgery because the IOL optic edge will not be covered by iris.

The appearance of the pupil at the start of surgery is shown in Figure C6-1. The appearance after completion of phacoemulsification and PC IOL implantation through a temporal clear corneal incision is shown in Figure C6-2. Two additional paracentesis openings were made at 4 o'clock and 8 o'clock positions relative to the principal incision (120-degree spacing).

A 10-0 polypropylene suture on a CTC-6 (Ethicon) needle initially made three full-thickness bites in the midperipheral iris (Figure C6-3), moving from the principal incision toward the first paracentesis. For the needle tip to exit the paracentesis without engaging any corneal tissue, a blunt-tip 27-gauge cannula was inserted into the anterior chamber, and the needle tip "docked" inside the cannula (Figure C6-4). The needle and cannula were then externalized as a unit (Figure C6-5). The needle was reinserted through the paracentesis, taking care to make sure that no corneal tissue was engaged, and the purse-string iris suture technique was repeated in each remaining sector, ending at the original incision (Figures C6-6 and C6-7).

The suture ends were then tied externally, and the knot was advanced into the eye with a Kuglen hook while the surgeon and assistant maintained gentle tension on each suture end (Figures C6-8). After four throws, the suture ends were cut with a Gills-Vannas scissors, leaving a central, normal-sized pupil (Figure C6-9).

Postoperatively, the appearance of the pupil was grossly normal, for the first time in the patient's life (Figure C6-10). High-magnification inspection revealed two barely visible strands of the polypropylene suture across small gaps in the gathered-up iris (Figure C6-11). Although this is of no optical consequence, it illustrates the importance of placing

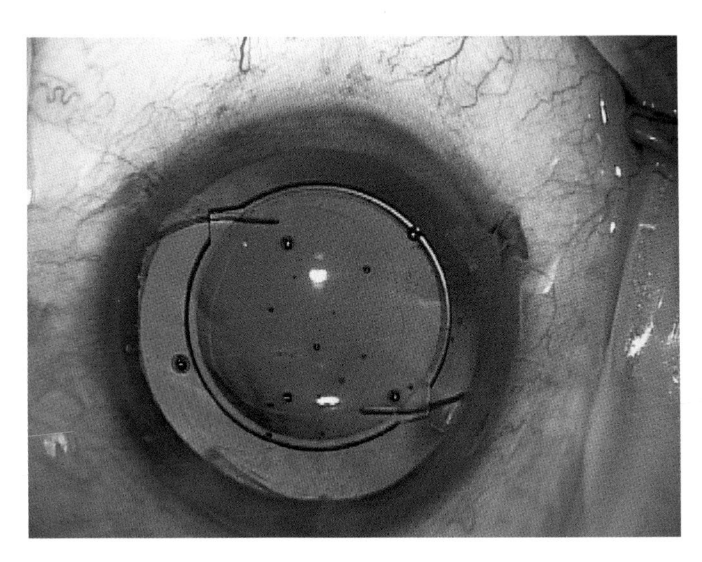

FIGURE C6-2

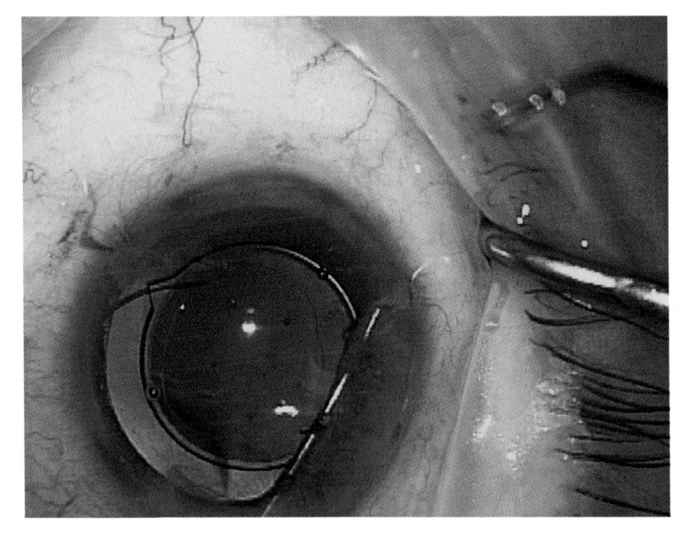

FIGURE C6-3

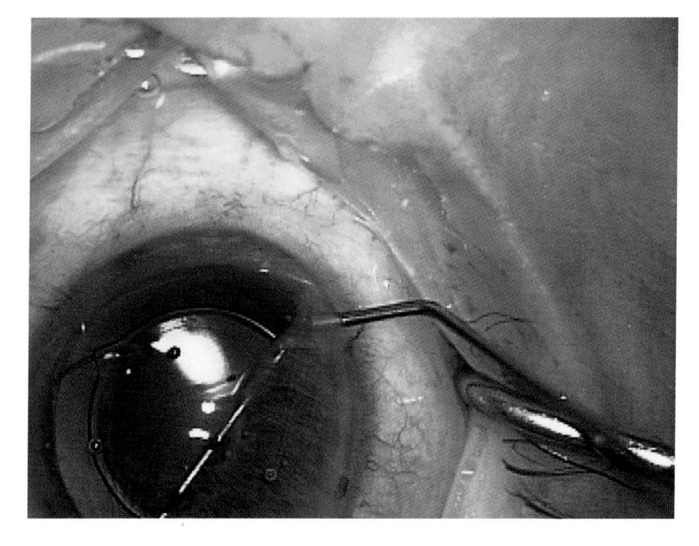

FIGURE C6-4

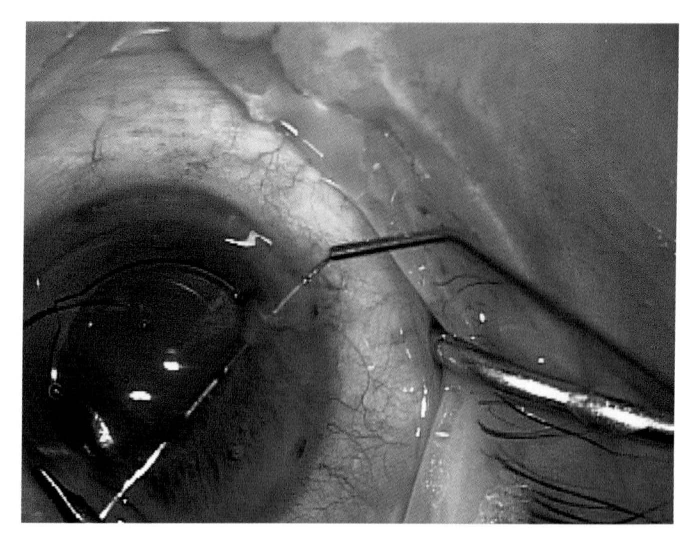

FIGURE C6-5

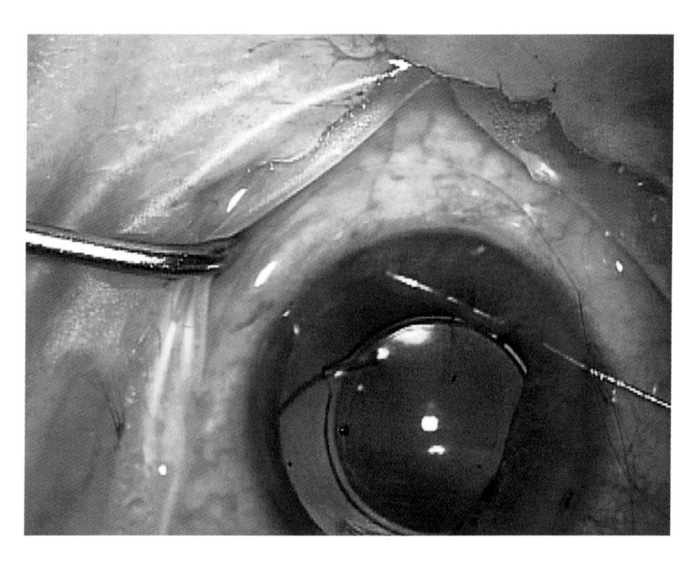

FIGURE C6-6

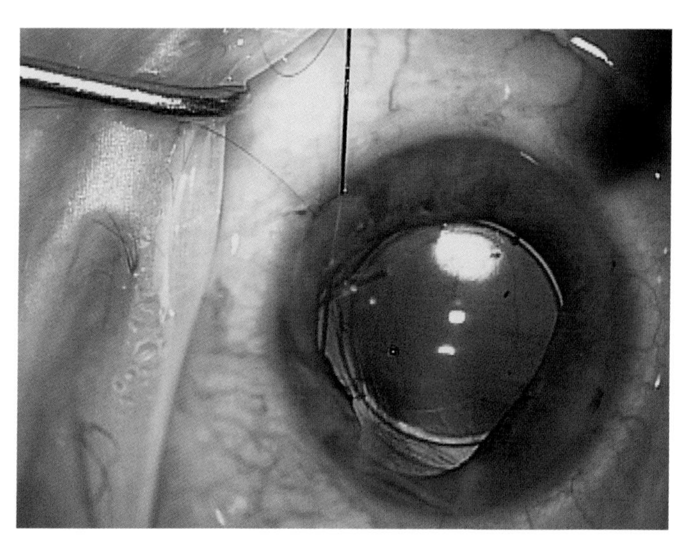

FIGURE C6-7

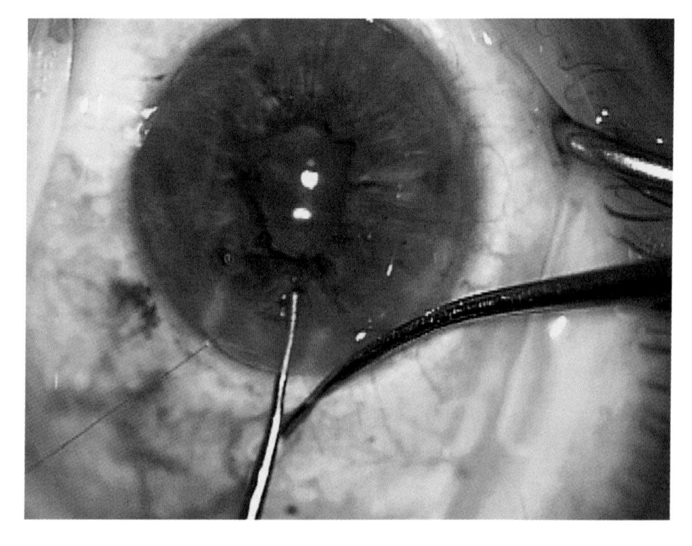

FIGURE C6-8

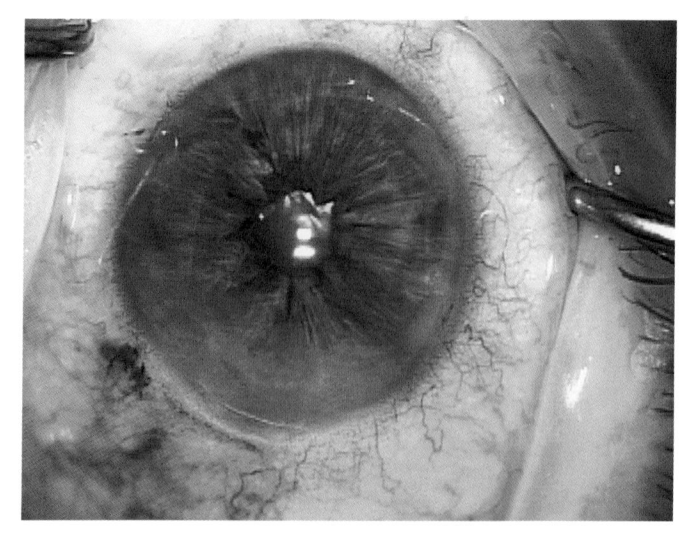

FIGURE C6-9

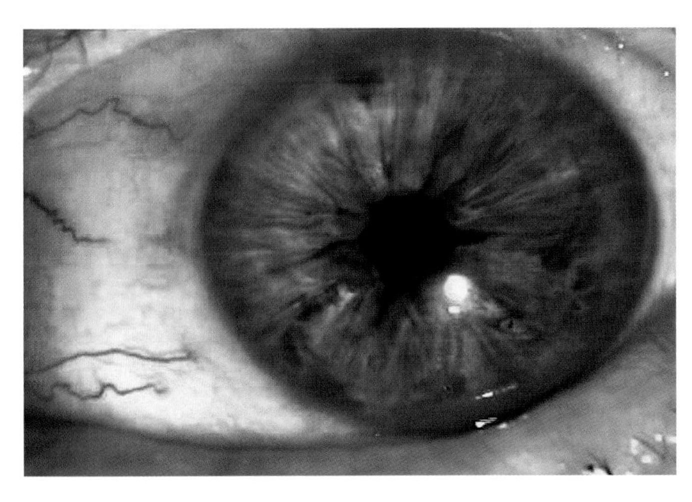

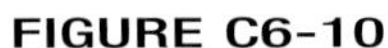

FIGURE C6-10

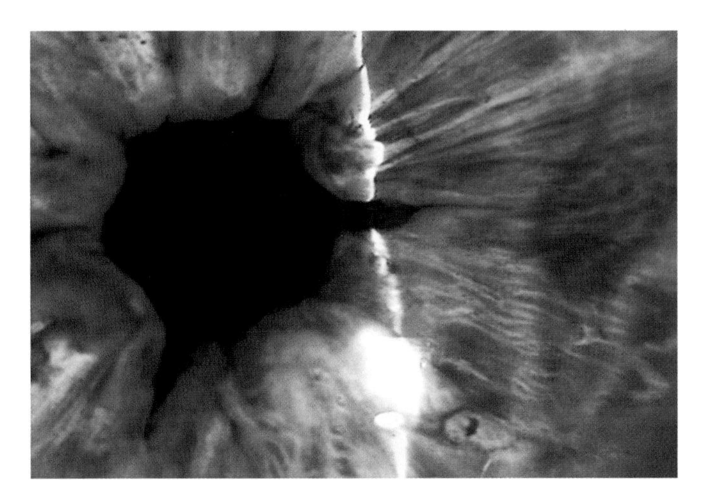

FIGURE C6-11

the suture bites in the midperipheral iris rather than near the sphincter edge. Suture bites near the sphincter margin will result in more gaps with exposed suture and a more irregularly bordered pupil.

Case 7: Preservation of iris

This complex multistep case is presented in summary form to illustrate the critical importance of never sacrificing iris tissue that may be salvaged for reconstruction. This 37-year-old man suffered massive accidental blunt trauma that ruptured the superior limbus and dialyzed all iris attachments except two to three clock hours inferiorly. Emergency repair closed the superior wound with iris prolapse covered by conjunctiva and no visible pupil (Figure C7-1). The patient was referred for repair.

At surgery, a conjunctival flap was dissected back, exposing a large amount of prolapsed iris tissue (Figure C7-2). Viscoelastic agent infusion separated the iris pillars, revealing the original pupillary space (Figure C7-3). The iris pillars were reattached to the sclera with multiple horizontal mattress double-armed sutures (Figures C7-4 and C7-5).

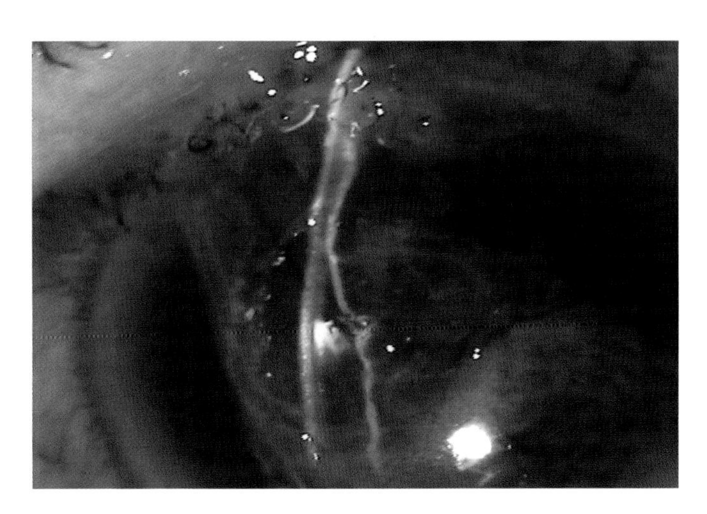

FIGURE C7-1

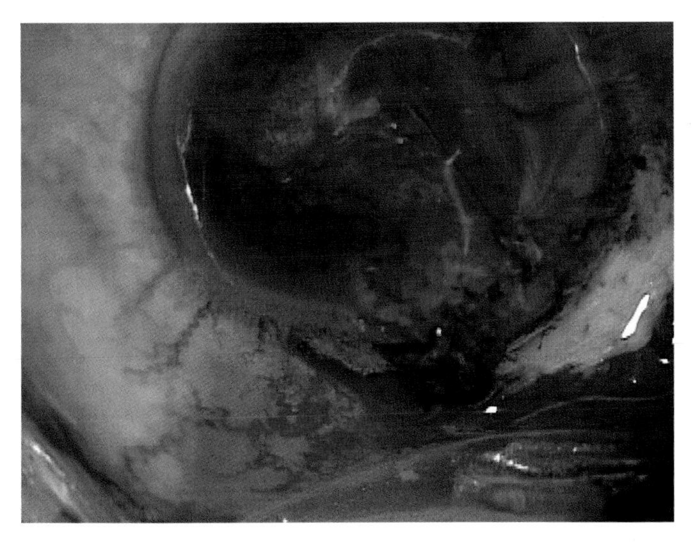

FIGURE C7-2

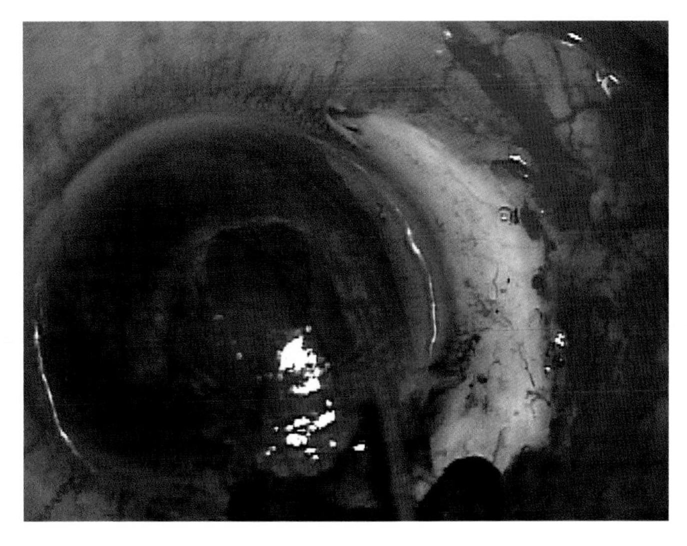

FIGURE C7-3

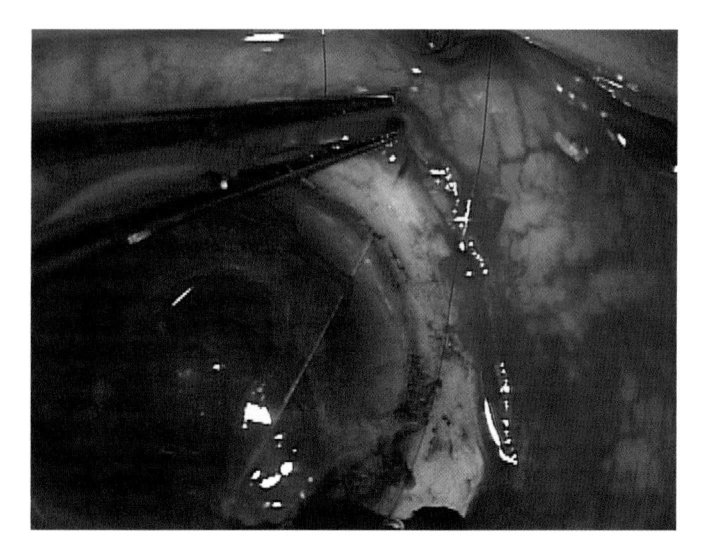

FIGURE C7-4

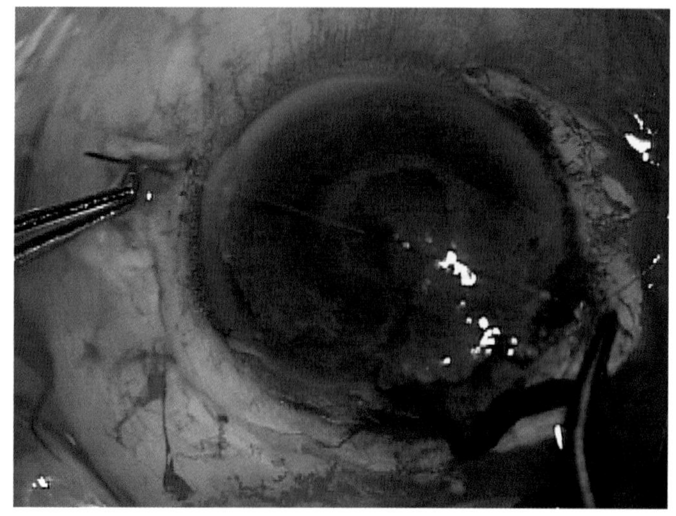

FIGURE C7-5

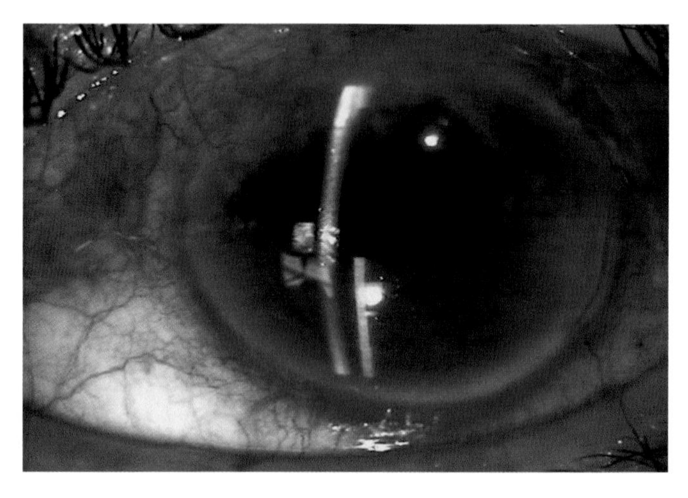

FIGURE C7-6

The result was a marked improvement, particularly in the critical areas inferiorly, nasally, and temporally where most glare originates (Figure C7-6). If glare proves to be a problem, despite maximal reconstruction of available iris, then subsequent implantation of a prosthetic iris device can be considered.

Iris Prostheses

Every effort should be made to reconstruct the natural iris. However, some patients do not have adequate residual iris tissue to prevent glare and other optical aberrations. Under these circumstances, the surgeon has two principal options. The first is to attempt to fit the patient with a contact lens with an "artificial iris" peripheral pigmentation. Some patients have been greatly helped by these devices, but these lenses are expensive and need periodic replacement. In the absence of the contact lens, the patient has a return of the visual impairment.

Alternatively, IOL and polymer technology have permitted the development of pigmented materials that can be permanently implanted as iris prostheses within the eye.

The artificial iris implant was first introduced and published in Europe by Sundmacher, Reihnhard, and Althaus[5-7] in 1994. They reported using a single-piece black diaphragm IOL in traumatic and congenital aniridia. The first use of small-incision artificial iris ring implants was reported at the Welch Cataract Congress by Kenneth Rosenthal in 1996. Subsequently, two independent series of cases have been reported, demonstrating the safety and efficacy of both the single-piece black diaphragm IOL and the endocapsular prosthetic iris rings.[8,9]

When contemplating use of a prosthetic iris device, the surgeon must first define the clinical situation and choose the appropriate device based on the relevant anatomy. Currently there are two main categories of prosthetic iris implant available, each with specific indications.

The single-piece black diaphragm IOL (Figure 29-5) provides a full iris diaphragm and IOL that can be placed in the ciliary sulcus on capsular support or transsclerally sutured. However, a significant drawback of the single-piece diaphragm IOL is that it requires a relatively large incision size, which is associated with delayed visual rehabilitation, increased astigmatism, and increased risk of intraoperative suprachoroidal hemorrhage. Nonetheless, this is the implant of choice when capsular support is weak or absent. When implanting the single-piece iris diaphragm IOL, care must be taken while manipulating the haptics because they are brittle and easily broken.

The other main category of iris prosthetic devices currently available is the Morcher endocapsular ring with iris diaphragm developed by Volker Rasch of Potsdam, Germany. The aniridia rings do not have an optical portion and therefore can be inserted through the same small incision as the foldable IOL. This approach offers the advantages of a full iris diaphragm and separate optical system, both of which may be inserted through a sutureless small incision.

There are two styles of endocapsular ring used as iris prostheses. One ring with a single fin (Type 96G) is used for sectoral iris loss (Figure 29-6). Two rings with multiple fins that interdigitate (Type 50C) are used to create a full iris diaphragm (Figure 29-7). The Type 50C rings produce an iris diaphragm with a pupil size of approximately 6 mm, which reduces the

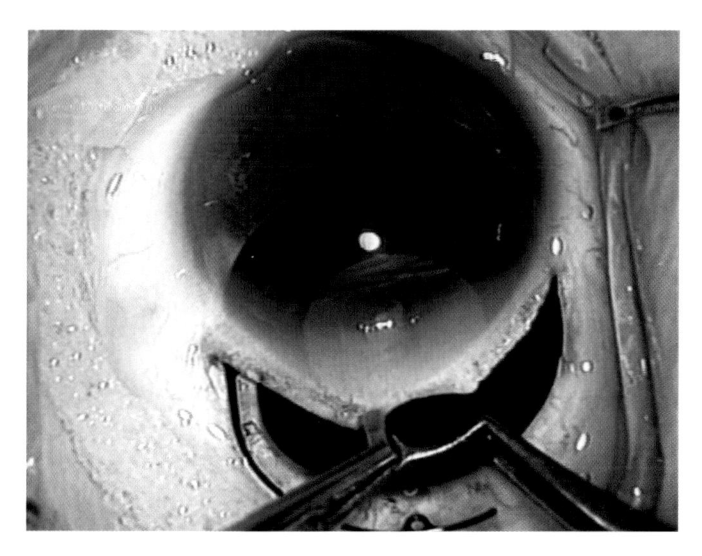

FIGURE 29-5 IOL with a peripheral pigment skirt for cases of aniridia or other generalized absence of iris tissue. Implantation of this large IOL requires an incision of at least 10 mm.

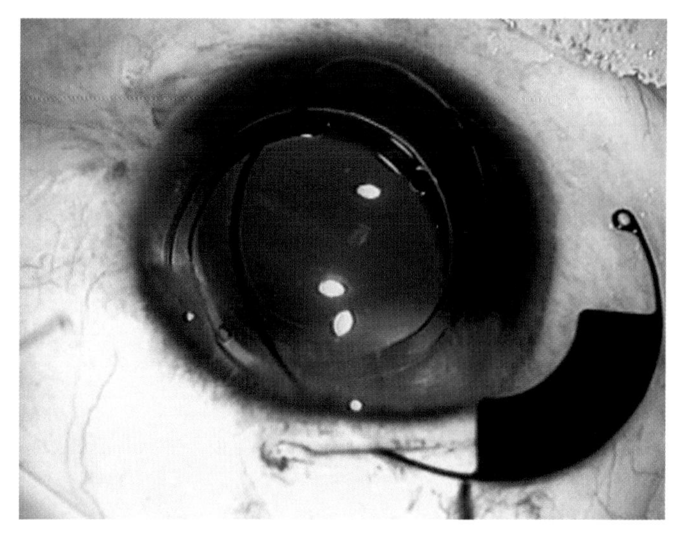

FIGURE 29-6 Segment of single-fin opaque implant for blocking a sector defect.

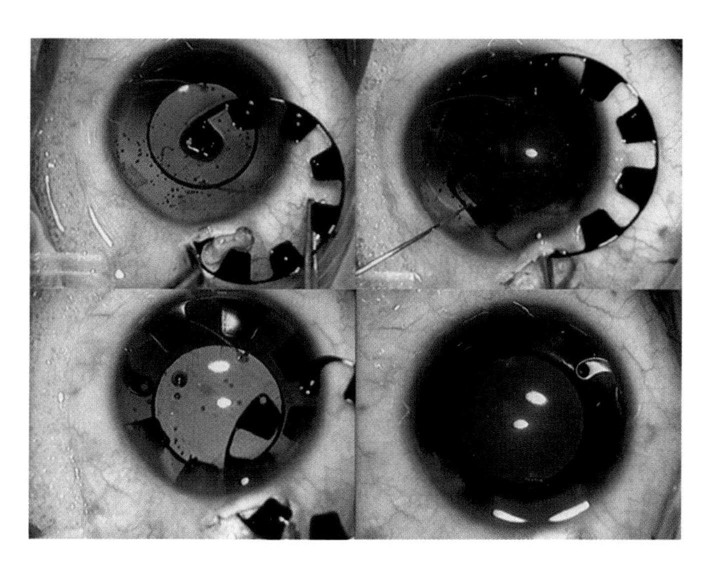

FIGURE 29-7 Implantation of two multiple-fin segments that are aligned to obtain 360-degree artificial iris coverage through a small incision.

stray light entering the eye by 75% yet provides an aperture compatible with excellent fundus viewing postoperatively.

The foldable optic chosen should have a diameter of 6.5 mm to eliminate edge glare, and the ideal optic position is posterior to both rings.

After implantation, the artificial iris rings remain quite stable and can lend support to the capsule by distributing zonular tension evenly around the equator of the capsular bag.

Caution should be exercised when implanting these devices because they are brittle and susceptible to fracture. Furthermore, the capsular bag can become somewhat crowded after three devices have been inserted. Finally, great care must be taken not to damage the fragile capsule of patients with congenital aniridia.

The technology for iris reconstruction will continue to improve as several groups are working on other prosthetic iris devices. In the future we can expect refinements in the structure, flexibility, implantation techniques, and even the ability to choose the color. The black coloration of the Morcher devices provides excellent reduction of glare but is not helpful cosmetically, particularly in a patient with a lighter color iris.

REFERENCES

1. Britten MJA: Follow-up of 54 cases of ocular contusion with hyphaema, with special reference to the appearance and function of the filtration angle, *Br J Ophthalmol* 49:120-127, 1965.
2. Weidenthal DT: Experimental ocular contusion. *Arch Ophthalmol* 71:77-81, 1964.
3. Wolff SM, Zimmerman LE: Chronic secondary glaucoma associated with retrodisplacement of iris root and deepening of the anterior chamber angle secondary to contusion, *Am J Ophthalmol* 54:547-563, 1962.
4. Paton D, Craig J: Management of iridodialysis, *Ophthalmic Surg* 4:38-39, 1973.
5. Reihnhard T, Sundmacher R, Althaus C: Irisblenden-IOL bei traumatischer aniridie, *Klin Monatsbl Augenheilkd* 205:196-200, 1994.
6. Sundmacher R, Reihnhard T, Althaus C: Black diaphragm intraocular lens for correction of aniridia, *Ophthalmic Surg* 25:180-185, 1994.
7. Sundmacher R, Reihnhard T, Althaus C: Black diaphragm intraocular lens in congenital aniridia, *Ger J Ophthalmol* 1994;3:197-201, 1994.
8. Thompson CG, Fawzy K, Bryce IG et al: Implantation of a black diaphragm intraocular lens for traumatic aniridia, *J Cataract Refract Surg* 25:808-813, 1999.
9. Osher RH, Burk SE: Cataract surgery combined with implantation of an artificial iris, *J Cataract Refract Surg* 25:1540-1547, 1999.

High Myopia

30

Roger F. Steinert, MD

Cataract surgery in the presence of high axial myopia poses a number of challenges for the surgeon. Special consideration must be given to these patients at each stage of the preoperative, operative, and postoperative periods. Table 30-1 summarizes these key considerations in high myopia.

Preoperative Evaluation

A comprehensive preoperative evaluation is performed on all cataract patients. In the case of high axial myopia, however, the surgeon must pay particular attention to the fundus exam. High myopia is associated with a higher risk of both peripheral and macular retinal pathologic conditions. Measurement of macular visual potential is important if there is disturbance of the pigment epithelium or evidence of atrophy or neovascularization from the choroid. Preoperative evaluation of potential visual acuity is covered in Chapter 3.

The peripheral retina in high axial myopia is more vulnerable to pathologic conditions that increase the risks of retinal detachment. A careful preoperative peripheral retinal examination is mandatory. However, visualization of the peripheral retina, even with aggressive scleral depression, may not reveal preexisting peripheral retinal pathologic conditions because of impaired visualization caused by the cataract.

The other primary challenge facing the cataract surgeon preoperatively, in the presence of high myopia, is determination of the intraocular lens (IOL) power. First, the accuracy of the A-scan biometry and the subsequent calculation of the IOL power are subject to more variability in high myopia than in patients with a normal-sized eye. If the axial myopia is accompanied by a posterior staphyloma, the precise determination of the axial length at the fovea is often imprecise.

Even with an accurate determination of the axial length, the IOL power formulas have less accuracy in the more extreme ranges. Studies have indicated that the SRK-T formula is more accurate in high axial myopia than other formulas (see Hoffer KJ [1993] and Holladay JT [1998] in Suggested Readings and Chapter 4). Even then, however, there is considerably more variability in the IOL power accuracy in these cases.

The surgeon must discuss with the patient the intended postoperative IOL power goal. While some myopes value excellent distance uncorrected vision, other myopes have enjoyed the ability to read with spectacles. Determining the desired postoperative refractive goal is a key step in the preoperative surgical planning.

Intraoperative Considerations

High axial myopia poses a high risk of complication with retrobulbar or peribulbar anesthesia. The larger and longer globe fills more of the orbit, and the passage of a needle posteriorly is more prone to inadvertently penetrating the sclera. Moreover, the sclera in high axial myopia is thinner, resulting in less resistance to penetration by an anesthetic injection needle (see Chapter 8).

High myopes typically have deeper anterior chambers and less residual formed vitreous than the average patient. Therefore the surgeon may face excessive anterior chamber deepening on introducing the phacoemulsification tip and irrigation. If so, the height of the infusion bottle should be lowered. There may also be more mobility of the nucleus, related both to zonular laxity and the lack of vitreous support. The vitreous body is frequently more liquefied than in a similar-aged emmetrope. As a result, the surgeon should expect to face a deeper anterior chamber and more anteroposterior movement of the crystalline lens and capsule in the course of the phacoemulsification. Moreover, there is less vitreous support for the posterior capsule, and many surgeons have observed that the posterior capsule has the potential for rupturing during surgery at a higher rate in high axial myopia. Furthermore, if the posterior capsule does rupture, the liquefied vitreous will not provide normal resistance to posterior migration of nuclear fragments. The patient is therefore at higher risk for loss of nuclear fragments into the deep vitreous and against the retina. Should this complication occur, the anterior segment surgeon should obtain the assistance of a skilled vitreoretinal surgeon to remove the nuclear fragments safely. If a vitreoretinal surgeon is available, this can be done immediately in the course of the cataract surgery. If not, then the cataract surgeon should complete the anterior cleanup and obtain an immediate postoperative consultation to schedule the patient for an expeditious removal of the posterior lens fragments by the vitreoretinal surgeon. Chapter 18 explores these issues in more detail.

In the presence of this complication, a frequently debated issue is whether the cataract surgeon should place the IOL

TABLE 30-1

Special Elements in Cataract Surgery for High Myopia

PREOPERATIVE
Peripheral retina exam
Macular exam
Potential acuity testing
Biometry, postoperative refractive goal determination, and IOL power calculation
INTRAOPERATIVE
Risk of retrobulbar/peribulbar anesthetic injection
Increased anterior chamber depth
Reduced nuclear support
POSTOPERATIVE
Preservation of a clear posterior capsule/capsulotomy complications minimized
Surveillance for peripheral retinal breaks/early detection of retinal detachments

primarily or whether the patient should be left in an aphakic state. If the nuclear fragments that remain are quite large and dense, a vitreoretinal surgeon may choose to bring the fragments up through the pupil and deliver them through a limbal incision, rather than attempt a posterior ultrasonic fragmentation of a very large and dense nucleus. If the nuclear fragments are reasonably small, however, the vitreoretinal surgeon will usually feel comfortable with posterior ultrasonic fragmentation of the remaining nucleus. In that case, the presence of an IOL will not impede the vitreoretinal surgeon's maneuvers. Ideally, a cataract surgeon should develop a good working relationship with a vitreoretinal surgeon and explore the vitreoretinal surgeon's preferences regarding IOL placement under these circumstances.

High axial myopia presents one other challenge for a surgeon who wishes to perform surgery through a corneal scleral incision rather than a limbal or fully clear corneal incision. In true high axial myopia, the sclera may be markedly thinned. The surgeon needs to anticipate that dissection should be more shallow than usual to avoid inadvertent penetration through the sclera onto the ciliary body while attempting to dissect a scleral tunnel incision.

Postoperative Care

Maintaining the integrity and clarity of the posterior capsule is generally regarded as important in reducing the frequency of vitreoretinal complications. In addition, a broad area of clear posterior capsule and a large optic assist in the examination of the patient's retina postoperatively. A pupil that is not traumatized during surgery and does not have postoperative synechia inhibiting dilation also contributes to good postoperative care. Therefore the cataract surgeon should use a meticulous technique with a centered capsulorhexis, thorough cortical cleanup, and great care to maintain the integrity and clarity of the posterior capsule. The choice of IOL should be influenced by these considerations.

A large optic, either 6 or 6.5 mm, is preferable to a smaller optic. Using an IOL optic material that will least interfere with subsequent vitreoretinal surgery, if needed, and an IOL optic edge that is configured to inhibit posterior capsule opacification is recommended. Currently, the lens of choice in this circumstance has a square or modified square edge (see Chapter 35).

Because the high axial myopic patient is at higher risk for retinal detachment, it is advisable to carefully examine the peripheral retina with wide dilation and scleral depression with indirect ophthalmoscopy early postoperatively, such as several weeks, but also to perform such an examination at more frequent intervals. Many postoperative detachments do not occur for many months or years after the surgery. If there is difficulty in visualization of the peripheral retina or question about the advisability of "prophylactic" laser treatment of suspicious peripheral lesions, consultation with a vitreoretinal surgeon is recommended (see Chapter 49).

If the posterior capsule opacifies to the point of functional visual impairment, then Nd:YAG laser posterior capsulotomy may be indicated. To minimize the disturbance to any residual formed vitreous and to maintain as much integrity of the barrier function of the capsule-IOL complex, the surgeon is advised to use the lowest amount of energy necessary to open the posterior capsule and to keep the size of the capsular opening smaller than the optic (see Chapter 44).

SUGGESTED READINGS

Alldredge CD, Elkins B, Alldredge OC: Retinal detachment following phacoemulsification in highly myopic cataract patients, *J Cataract Refract Surg* 24:777-780, 1988.

Apple DJ, Solomon KD, Tetz MR et al: Posterior capsular opacification, *Surv Ophthalmol,* 37:73-115, 1992.

Buratto L, editor: *Phacoemulsification: principles and techniques.* Thorofare, NJ, 1988, Slack.

Buratto L, Buratto LE, editors: *Cataract surgery in axial myopia,* Milano, 1994, Ghedini.

Coonan P, Fung WE, Webster RG et al: The incidence of retinal detachment following extracapsular cataract extraction: a ten year study, *Ophthalmology* 92:106, 1985.

Curtin BJ: *The myopias: basic science and clinical management,* Hagerstown, 1985, Harper and Row.

Duke-Elder S, Abrams D: *System of ophthalmology,* St Louis, 1976, Mosby.

Francois JG, Goes F: Comparative study of ultrasonic biometry of emmetropes and myopes, with special heredity of myopia, *Biometrie Oculaire Clinique* Parigi, Masson, 1976.

Hoffer KJ: The Hoffer Q formula: a comparison of theoretic and regression formulas, *J Cataract Refract Surg* 19:700-712, 1993.

Hoffman P, Pollock A, Oliver M: Limited choroidal hemorrhage associated with intracapsular cataract extraction, *Arch Ophthalmol* 102:1761-1765, 1984.

Holladay JT: IOL power calculation for the unusual eye. In Gills, JP, Fenzyl R, Martin RG, editors: *Cataract surgery: the state of the art,* Thorofare, NJ, 1998, Slack, pp 197-205.

Hollick EJ, Spalton DJ: The effect of capsulorhexis size on posterior capsule opacification. Presentation at ASCRS Meeting, Boston, 1997.

Hollick EJ, Spalton DJ, Ursel PG et al: Lens epithelial cell regression on the posterior capsule with different intraocular lens material, *Br J Ophthalmol* 82:1182-1188, 1998.

Hymans SW, Bialik M, Neumann E: Myopia-aphakia. *Br J Ophthalmol* 59:480, 1975.

Jaffe NS, Clayman HM, Jaffe MS: Retinal detachment in myopic eye after intracapsular and extracapsular cataract extraction, *Am J Ophthalmol* 97:48-52, 1984.

Koch PS: Phacoemulsification in patients with high myopia. In *Phacoemulsification in difficult and challenging cases,* New York, 1999, Thieme Medical Publishers.

Osterlin S: Vitreous changes after cataract extraction. In Freeman HM, Hirose T, Schepens CL, editors: *Vitreous surgery and advances in fundus diagnosis and treatment,* New York, 1977, Appleton-Century Crofts, pp 15-21.

Percival SPB: Long term complications from extracapsular cataract surgery, *Trans Ophthalmol. Soc U K* 104: 915-918, 1985.

Praeger DL: Five years' follow-up in the surgical management of cataracts in high myopia treated with the Kelman phacoemulsification technique, *Ophthalmology* 86:2024-2033, 1979.

Retzlaff J: A new intraocular lens calculation formula, *J Am Intraocul Implant Soc* 6:148-152, 1980.

Retzlaff JA, Sanders DR, Kraff MC: Development of the SRK/T intraocular lens implant power calculation formula, *J Cataract Refract Surg* 16:333-340, 1990.

Rickman-Barger L, Florine CW, Larson RS et al: Retinal detachment after neodymium YAG laser capsulotomy, *Am J Ophthalmol* 107:531-536, 1989.

Sanders DR, Retzlaff J, Kraff MC: Comparison of empirically derived and theoretical aphakic refraction formulas, *Arch Ophthalmol* 101:956-967, 1983.

Selley LF, Barraquer J: Surgery of the ectopic lens, *Ann Ophthalmol* 35:1127, 1973.

Shah GR, Gills JP, Durham DG et al: Three thousand YAG laser posterior capsulotomies: an analysis of complications and comparison to polishing and surgical discission, *Ophthalmic Surg* 17:473-477, 1986.

Ursell PG, Spalton DJ, Pande MV et al: The relationship between intraocular lens biomaterials and posterior capsule opacification, *J Cataract Refract Surg* 24:352-360, 1998.

Nanophthalmos, Relative Anterior Microphthalmos, and Axial Hyperopia

31

Ruthanne B. Simmons, MD
Marianne B. Mellem Kairala, MD
Richard J. Simmons, MD
Charles D. Belcher III, MD

Ophthalmic surgeons have been aware for years that surgery in small eyes can be difficult and challenging. Not all small eyes are the same, and some present far more serious potential problems than others. Thanks to the work of Robert Brockhurst, Donald Gass, and others, we now have a better understanding of which short eyes are the most precarious and ways to try to lessen the risk.

The literature is often confusing on this subject. No classification is perfect, and categories usually overlap. We have tried to clarify the different types of small eyes based on anatomic differences in order to give surgeons a framework for surgical planning in these problematic cases.

Classification and Terminology

Microphthalmos is a developmental arrest of ocular growth during gestation. Most cases of microphthalmos are sporadic, but the condition can be inherited in an autosomal dominant or recessive pattern. Often it is associated with one of many different systemic diseases, including genetic or environmental disorders, or those of unknown causes.[1,2] Therefore the evaluation of microphthalmic patients should be interdisciplinary, with special attention given to the history of the disease and examination of other family members. This is especially true for pediatric patients, and the ophthalmologist and the pediatrician should evaluate together the risks and benefits of performing any kind of surgery in such eyes.

Because microphthalmos is a heterogeneous disease, with different pathophysiologies and many possible and overlapping presentations, we prefer to use an anatomic classification for these eyes, based on anterior chamber depth and total axial length (Tables 31-1 and 31-2).[3,4]

Short Anterior Chamber Depth with Short Axial Length: Nanophthalmos, Colobomatous, and Complex Microphthalmos

Duke-Elder[5] in 1964 described three categories of microphthalmos: simple microphthalmos, or nanophthalmos, which is essentially a short eye with no other associated morphologic anomalies; colobomatous microphthalmos, related to incomplete closure of embryonic fissure; and complex microphthalmos, not related to closure of the fissure but associated with systemic anomalies and other anterior and posterior malformations of the eye.

NANOPHTHALMOS (SIMPLE MICROPHTHALMOS)

Nanophthalmos is a rare condition characterized by a short eye. The total axial length is at least two standard deviations below the mean for age or less than 20.5 mm.[6] There is an absence of systemic or other ocular morphologic abnormalities.[5,7] Many authors, including Duke-Elder and Naumann, have synonymously used the terms *simple microphthalmos* and *nanophthalmos* to refer to such eyes.[5,6,8,9]

Although microphthalmos in general is a fairly common ocular malformation in all races,[1] nanophthalmos is a rare form of it. Most cases of nanophthalmos described in the literature are sporadic, but recently genetic studies of several nanophthalmic pedigrees showed autosomal recessive inheritance.[10] In 1998, the first human gene locus associated with autosomal dominant nanophthalmos was identified on chromosome 11 and named *NNO1*.[11] In our experience, a family history of nanophthalmos is often unknown, but patients sometimes report relatives who were blind from unknown cause consistent with angle closure glaucoma. There appears to be no gender predilection in this condition.

Younger patients are usually first brought to the attention of an ophthalmologist because of a high refractive error, which

TABLE 31-1

Relationship Between Axial Length and Anterior Chamber Depth

Anterior chamber depth ↓	Axial length → Shorter	Axial length → Longer
Shallower	Simple microphthalmos = Nanophthalmos Colobomatous microphthalmos Complex microphthalmos	Relative anterior microphthalmos
Deeper	Axial hyperopia	Normal

Modified from Holladay J: Achieving emmetropia in extremely short eyes with two piggyback posterior chamber intraocular lenses, *Ophthalmology* 1996;103:1118-1123, 1996; Auffarth GU, Blum M, Faller U et al: Relative anterior microphthalmos: morphometric analysis and its implications for cataract surgery, *Ophthalmology* 107:1555-1560, 2000.

TABLE 31-2

Anatomic Classification of Short Eyes

2.1 Short anterior chamber (AC) depth with short axial length
- 2.1.1. Nanophthalmos (simple microphthalmos)
- 2.1.2. Colobomatous microphthalmos
- 2.1.3 Complex microphthalmos

2.2 Short AC depth with normal axial length
- Relative anterior microphthalmos

2.3 Normal AC depth with short axial length
- Axial hyperopia

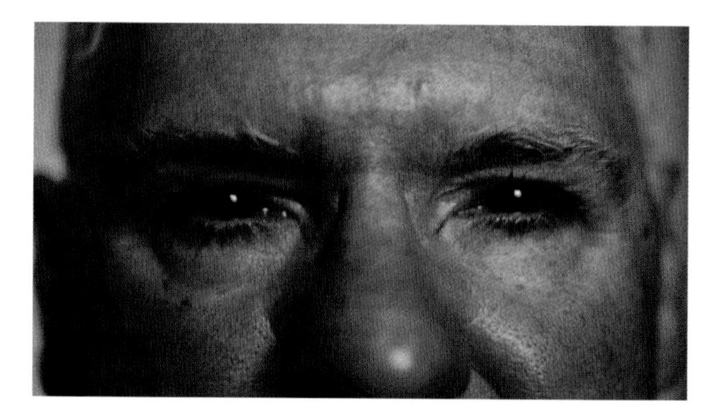

FIGURE 31-1 Nanophthalmos. Eyes deeply set with narrow palpebral fissures.

usually is fully correctable with corrective lenses. Consequently, these patients often remain undiagnosed until middle age, when complications most commonly develop. If one or more clinical features (to be discussed next) are present, the diagnosis of nanophthalmos should be considered. If left untreated, this condition often results in blindness.

Clinical features. The most prominent clinical features seen in nanophthalmos are described here and are summarized in Table 31-3.

Nanophthalmos is a bilateral disease in which the eyes are deeply set with narrow palpebral fissures (Figure 31-1).

The eyes are uniformly small, usually about two thirds of the normal volume, but have an increased lens/eye volume ratio. The crystalline lens can be normal or can have a slightly increased anteroposterior length (Figure 31-2). Nanophthalmos is typically associated with microcornea, with corneal diameters between 9.5 and 11 mm. The anterior chamber is also shallow, with depths from less than 1 mm to 2.7 mm.[6] Pupils usually dilate poorly, even without prolonged miotic therapy, and there often is a wide amplitude of intraocular pulse pressure, which is still present after cataract extraction. The mechanism of both features is unknown.

The disproportion between lens and ocular volume contributes to the shallowing of the anterior chamber and to the marked convexity of the iris, which sometimes shows the appearance of "Vesuvio iris" with central shallowing of the chamber (Figure 31-3). Early, the angle can remain wide open despite the central shallowing of the anterior chamber, but later in the course of nanophthalmos the peripheral anterior chamber becomes shallow, followed by closure of the angle.

TABLE 31-3

Nanophthalmic Clinical Features

Short axial length	Moderate to high axial hyperopia
Small cornea	Thick sclera
Shallow anterior chamber	Thickened choroid
Marked iris convexity	Angle closure glaucoma*
Normal or increased lens thickness	Uveal effusions*
High lens/eye volume ratio	Exudative retinal detachment*

*May develop these features in the late course of the disease.

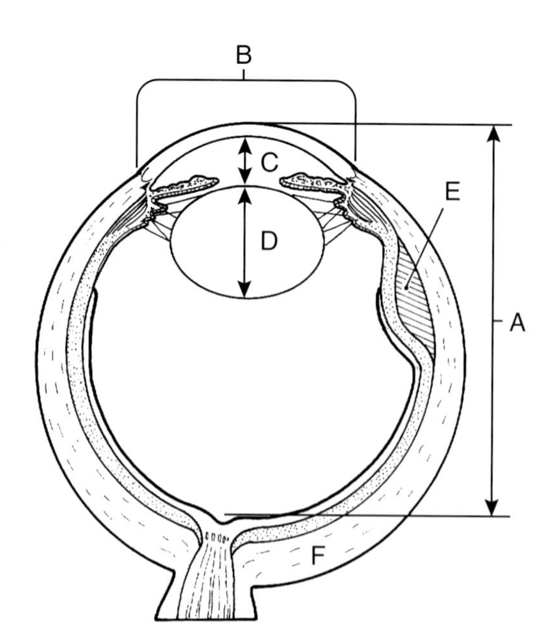

FIGURE 31-2 Schematic drawing of nanophthalmic eye showing the main ocular findings: **A,** short axial length; **B,** reduced corneal diameter; **C,** shallow anterior chamber; **D,** normal or increased lens thickness and high lens/eye volume ratio; **E,** thickened uveal tract with intrachoroidal or suprachoroidal peripheral uveal effusions; **F,** thickened scleral wall.

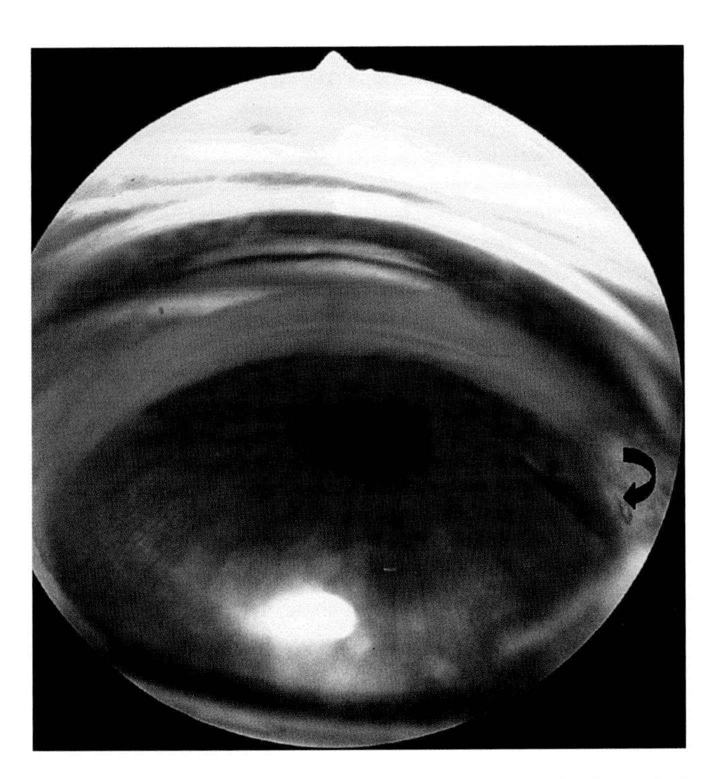

FIGURE 31-3 Gonioscopic view of a nanophthalmic eye showing marked iris convexity, "Vesuvio iris." Note the patent surgical iridectomy *(arrow)*.

Marked hypermetropia is characteristic with a range between +7.25 and +20.00.[6] Depending on the corneal and lens refractive power, nanophthalmic patients can have lower degrees of hyperopia or, very rarely, myopia.[2,5-8,12-14]

Nanophthalmic eyes also present increased thickness of the choroid and sclera. Although normal eyes present mean combined sclerochoroidal thickness of 1.01 mm, nanophthalmic patients have values between 0.75 and 4 mm (mean of 2.78 mm), as we found in a series of 32 eyes of 16 patients with nanophthalmos.[6]

Retinal findings reported in nanophthalmic patients include chorioretinal folds, macular hypoplasia, cystic macular degeneration, retinal pigmentary degeneration, retinitis pigmentosa, and disc drusen.[15-18] The retinal findings are not prominent or important criteria for diagnosing nanophthalmos.

The most distinctive feature in nanophthalmic eyes is the abnormality of the sclera, which is thicker[8,19,20] and more inelastic than normal sclera. Ultrastructural and histochemical studies demonstrated abnormal scleral collagen fibers (Table 31-4) and an alteration in the metabolism of glycosaminoglycans and fibronectin production by scleral cells.[21-28] By restricting normal eye growth, it is speculated that this finding is related to the pathophysiology of nanophthalmos.

Untreated nanophthalmic patients are likely to undergo gradual progressive narrowing of the angle, angle closure, formation of peripheral synechiae, and elevation of intraocular pressure. Nanophthalmic patients characteristically develop spontaneous uveal effusion in the late course of the disease. These are often followed by exudative retinal detachment (Figure 31-4).

The association of nanophthalmos and uveal effusion was described by Brockhurst in 1974.[8] The pathophysiology of nanophthalmic uveal effusion has been explained by compression of vortex veins, as postulated by Brockhurst, or by reduced scleral permeability to proteins, as postulated by Gass. In both cases, the primary cause is the abnormal sclera found in nanophthalmic eyes.[13,19,27,30-32]

TABLE 31-4
Scleral Abnormalities in Nanophthalmic Eyes

COLLAGEN FIBERS
Variations in the size of collagen fibers[23,27,28]
Increased fraying and splitting of collagen fibers[23]
Disordered lamellar arrangement of collagen bundles[22,29]
EXTRACELLULAR MATRIX
Glycosaminoglycan deposits[22-24]
Increased fibronectin content[28]

Nanophthalmic uveal effusion can be intrachoroidal, suprachoroidal, or both.[33] It can occur spontaneously, usually becoming clinically apparent between the fourth and seventh decades, or acutely after any kind of surgical intervention. When spontaneous, it is typically noninflammatory, often annular, and anteriorly located.

Uveal effusion can lead to choroidal and exudative retinal detachment spontaneously or after surgical intervention. The choroidal detachment causes retinal pigment epithelium dysfunction, which promotes leakage of serous fluid into the subretinal space and an exudative retinal detachment that can be localized or total.

The progressive accumulation of fluid in the choroid leads to an increase in the sclerochoroidal[34] thickness and can be noted by ultrasound or magnetic resonance imaging.

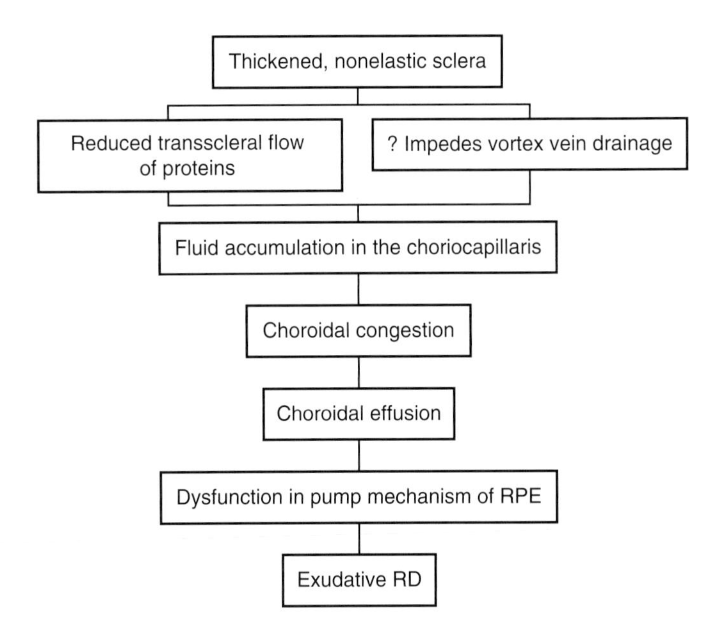

FIGURE 31-4 Proposed pathogenesis of uveal effusion and retinal detachment in nanophthalmic eyes. *RD*, Retinal detachment; *RPE*, retinal pigment epithelium.

The onset of angle-closure glaucoma usually occurs in middle age and is characteristically chronic and painless, with progressive elevation of intraocular pressure. As the lens enlarges with age, there is an increase in the relative pupillary block, with progressive crowding and shallowing of the anterior chamber, narrowing, and gradually closing of the angle.[33] Angle closure is usually precipitated by gradual peripheral uveal effusion and/or exudative retinal detachment, which causes a forward rotation of the ciliary body, forward movement of the peripheral iris, and consequent increase in the relative pupillary block.[9,33] Pupillary block is an early component of this angle closure but is not the entire mechanism because in the presence of iridotomy, which eliminates pupillary block, progressive choroidal effusion usually results in further angle closure.

COLOBOMATOUS MICROPHTHALMOS

Colobomatous microphthalmos results from involution of the primary optic disc or incomplete closure of the embryonic fissure,[5] which is usually closed by the sixth week of gestation. The typical colobomatous defect is located inferonasally. This condition is typically characterized by the presence of other ocular anomalies. According to the grade of disorganization of ocular and surrounding tissues, these anomalies can vary from a small iris coloboma or choroidal coloboma to clinical orbital cysts, with extrusion of intraocular tissues through the sclera.[1,4] The visual pathways and the occipital cortex may be also hypoplasic.[5]

COMPLEX MICROPHTHALMOS

Complex microphthalmos is associated with other syndromes (Table 31-5)[35] and further anatomic malformations of the anterior or posterior segment of the eye, but it is not related to the incomplete closure of the embryonic fissure. This is a heterogeneous group of conditions in which the microphthalmia is secondary to the other ocular abnormalities.[4,5]

The presence of congenital cataracts is common[1] and is usually associated with poorly developed or defective retinal and optic nerve structures, which further compromise the visual prognosis.

Short Anterior Chamber Depth with Normal Axial Length: Relative Anterior Microphthalmos

In 1980, Naumann coined the term *relative anterior microphthalmos* (RAM) to describe those eyes that did not fit into any of the existing classifications. He described eyes with an axial length of more than 20 mm and horizontal corneal diameter between 9 and 11 mm, but with disproportionately smaller anterior segment.

The terminology and classification between RAM and microcornea can be confusing, mostly because of the misinterpretation of the latter. Microcornea is a classification based exclusively on the size of the cornea (smaller than 10 mm), and it can occur as part of the simple, colobomatous, and/or complex microphthalmos.

RAM refers to those eyes that present a normal axial length and a disproportionate smaller anterior segment, despite the corneal diameters, which can be on the microcornea or in the lower normal range. These eyes show no other morphologic macroscopic malformations and can easily be overlooked at slit lamp examination. RAM is more common than nanophthalmos and high hyperopia (Table 31-6).

Like nanophthalmic patients, RAM patients also have a high incidence of chronic angle closure glaucoma, which appears to be related to the crowded anterior segment. There is no evidence for scleral abnormalities or uveal effusion in this group of patients. If untreated, the angle closure glaucoma is progressive and difficult to control.

Normal Anterior Chamber Depth with Short Axial Length: Axial High Hyperopia

There is a third group of microphthalmic eyes that are severely hyperopic but present a normal anterior chamber depth, despite the short axial length. These eyes usually do not have the same complications as the two previous groups because of the normal morphology of the anterior chamber. The main issue in this group of patients is the high refractive error.

TABLE 31-5

Syndromes Associated with Microphthalmia

Trisomy 13 (Patau's syndrome)
Chromosome 18 deletion syndrome
Congenital rubella
Hallermann-Streiff syndrome
LSD (lysergic acid diethylamide) embryopathy
Goldenhar's syndrome
Oculodentodigital syndrome
Pierre Robin syndrome
Oculocerebrorenal syndrome
Focal dermal hypoplasia
Francois' syndrome
Ullrich's syndrome

Modified from Ritch R: Glaucoma related to other ocular disorders. In Richt R, Shields M, editors: *The secondary glaucomas,* St Louis, 1982, Mosby, pp 55-57.

TABLE 31-6

Anatomic Parameters in Relative Anterior Microphthalmos vs. Nanophthalmos

Ocular Parameters	Relative Anterior Microphthalmos	Nanophthalmos
Corneal diameter	Average: 10.7 mm Range: 9-11 mm	Average: 10.3 mm Range: 9.5-11 mm
Anterior chamber depth	Average: 2.2 mm Range: 0.98-3.70 mm	Average: 1.46 mm Range: 1-2.7 mm
Anteroposterior lens thickness	Average: 5.05 mm Range: 3.49-6.46 mm	Average: 5.18 mm Range: 4.20-7.26 mm
Total axial length	Average: 21.92 mm Range: 20.29-23.89 mm	Average: 17 mm Range: 14.5-20.5 mm
Refractive error	Average: –0.13 diopters Range: –6.0-+7.5 diopters	Average: +13.60 diopters Range: +7.25-+20.00 diopters

Modified from Auffarth GU, Blum M, Faller U et al: Relative anterior microphthalmos: morphometric analysis and its implications for cataract surgery, *Ophthalmology* 107:1555-1560, 2000.

Preoperative Assessment

Because of the potential hazards of cataract surgery or glaucoma surgery in eyes with nanophthalmos and, to a lesser extent, RAM, it is important to identify these conditions preoperatively in order to take the necessary prophylactic measures to avoid serious complications during cataract surgery and in the postoperative period.

Nanophthalmos

EVALUATION FOR POTENTIAL NANOPHTHALMIC GLAUCOMA

Any eye with a small corneal diameter and more than 8 diopters of hypermetropia, as well as an axial length of less than 20.5 mm, should be evaluated for other features of nanophthalmos before intraocular surgery is undertaken, and special attention should be given to evaluation of potential nanophthalmic glaucoma.

Gonioscopy can be performed with a mirrored goniolens, such as Zeiss, Goldmann, or Sussman. This procedure can be challenging because of the extreme convexity of the iris in these microphthalmic eyes and because indentation of the small cornea can cause Descemet's folds, which obscure visualization of the angle. A child's 12-mm Koeppe lens, bilaterally inserted, offers a clear view with simultaneous comparison of both eyes and allows examination by multiple observers without moving the lens.[33] We find this technique of great value.

Ultrasound biomicroscopy (UBM) can help document the relationship between the anterior chamber's structures and the anatomy of the angle. In addition, it can identify peripheral choroidal effusions (Figure 31-5).

B-scan ultrasonography may be used to verify the thickness of the sclera and choroid, as well as the presence of uveal effusions that can be difficult to detect by clinical exam.

Given the high incidence of narrow angles and angle-closure glaucoma, it is important to evaluate and document the optic disc even in eyes with normal intraocular pressure. Disc visualization and photography may not be possible because in nanophthalmic eyes, pupils dilate poorly. If the angle is dangerously narrow, laser iridotomy should be performed before attempting pharmacologic mydriasis. In these cases, documentation of the disc may have to be done by drawings or imaging techniques that do not require dilation (e.g., nerve fiber analyzers, laser confocal disc topographers, and others).

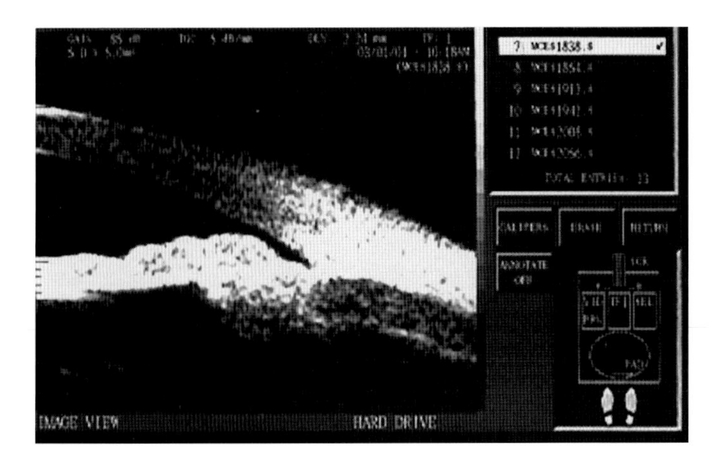

FIGURE 31-5 UBM of nanophthalmic eye showing the anatomy of the angle. Note the thickened choroidal layer.

TABLE 31-7
Stages of Nanophthalmic Glaucoma

Stage 1	Narrow angles; nanophthalmos recognized/no elevation of intraocular pressure
Stage 2	Progressive narrowing of the angle/angle closure threatened but not present
Stage 3	Progressive narrowing of the angle/angle partially closed
Stage 4	Extensive angle closure/increased intraocular pressure controlled with medical therapy
Stage 5	Angle closed by synechiae/intraocular pressure uncontrolled by medical therapy

In nanophthalmic patients, our prophylactic and therapeutic approach depends on the status of this condition, which may be divided into five stages (Table 31-7).[33]

THERAPY OF NANOPHTHALMOS

In 1980, Brockhurst[30] described the successful use of vortex vein decompression by dissection of a large partial-thickness sclerectomy around the vortex veins for treatment of nanophthalmic uveal effusions. In 1983, based on his hypothesis that the primary cause of the idiopathic uveal effusion syndrome was the impairment of transscleral outflow of proteins by the abnormal sclera, Gass[19] proposed a new surgical technique—a quadrantic equatorial partial-thickness sclerectomy. The successful use of this scleral thinning procedure without vortex vein decompression in patients with nanophthalmic uveal effusion supports the hypothesis that the barrier effect of sclera is more important than the vortex vein obstructing effect.[31,36-38]

Uveal effusion usually resolves within several months after surgical intervention[19,31,38]; however, recurrence of uveal effusion several months or years after the first scleral thinning procedure has been reported, in which case, repetition of the surgery proved to be successful.[31,36] This can be explained by the regeneration of the sclera over the sclerectomy, with the scar tissue blocking the bypass created surgically.[39] Recently, new techniques have been proposed to minimize the scarring of the sclerectomy sites and to promote long-term control of uveal effusion. Akduman, Adelberg, and Del Priore[40] described the successful use of topical mitomycin-C (0.3 mg/ml for $2\frac{1}{2}$ minutes) over the sclerectomy sites, and Krohn and Seland[41] reported the use of absorbable gelatin film to cover the scleral bed after the procedure in order to maintain a low resistance to transscleral outflow and prevent massive scarring of the area.

In stage 1 and 2 nanophthalmic eyes in which gonioscopy reveals narrow, occludable angles, prophylactic laser iridotomy is indicated. Even so, uveal effusions following prophylactic laser trabeculoplasty and retinal photocoagulation in nanophthalmic patients have been reported in the literature.[36,42]

Because of the thicker iris present in nanophthalmic eyes, penetration of the stroma with neodymium: yttrium-aluminum-garnet (Nd:YAG) laser is usually more difficult than in normal

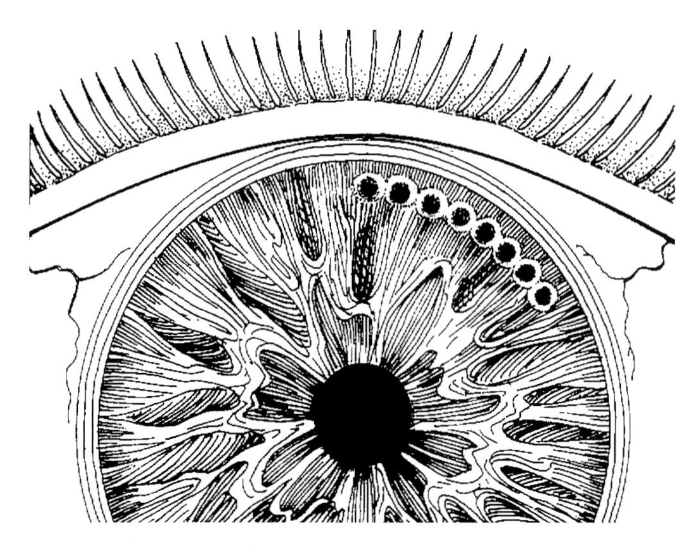

FIGURE 31-6 Gonioplasty burns from one to two clock hours.

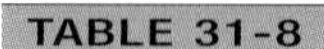

TABLE 31-8
Laser Settings for Gonioplasty in Nanophthalmos

Power	200-500 mW
Spot size	250-500 μm
Time	0.2-0.5 seconds
Applications	Three to five burns per clock hour
Each session	Three to four clock hours

eyes, and therefore we recommend that argon laser be applied to thin the proposed iridotomy site before final penetration with the Nd:YAG laser.[43]

Even after successful iridotomies eliminating pupillary block, the peripheral iris can remain convex, and the angle often remains narrow in these eyes. Eventually, despite the patent iridotomy, the angle progressively narrows (stage 3). Laser gonioplasty, also called iridoplasty, can flatten the peripheral iris, widen the angle, and prevent angle closure before the occurrence of peripheral anterior synechiae. Gonioplasty in some cases will cause separation of early synechiae.

To perform gonioplasty, after miosis with 2% pilocarpine, we use a mirrored contact gonioscopic lens and apply argon laser to the periphery of the iris. We start with a spot size of 250 to 500 μm and a laser power of 200 mW, slowly increasing it until we achieve a localized burn with contraction and not an explosion with perforation of the iris. Gonioplasty is applied to three to four clock hours at a time (Figures 31-6 and 31-7, Table 31-8), with caution taken not to overtreat, otherwise causing iatrogenic mydriasis.

Widening of the angle achieved by gonioplasty may gradually disappear over months, in which case we recommend repeating the procedure multiple times until it is no longer beneficial. In many cases, one is thus able to keep the anterior chamber angle from closing for a period of years (Figure 31-8).

If and when gonioplasty fails to keep the angle open, as ultimately usually occurs, but before intraocular pressure is out of control, sclerectomies alone should be employed to widen the angle. The technique we have been using since the 1980s is illustrated in Figure 31-9, *A* to *E*.

At stage 4, when angle closure is extensive and there is an increase in the intraocular pressure, we opt to treat glaucoma with topical medicines until they become ineffective. Stage 5 occurs when there is extensive synechial closure of the angle and further laser iridotomy, laser gonioplasty, and medical therapy are ineffective. At this point, two choices are available: filtering surgery and a ciliary destructive procedure.

In stage 5, when glaucoma is such that trabeculectomy can be temporarily deferred, we prefer to perform prophylactic anterior sclerectomies (as shown in Figure 31-9, *A* to *E*) in the two lower quadrants 4 to 6 weeks before the filtering procedure to allow full recovery before trabeculectomy. However, if the glaucoma is so severe that immediate surgery is necessary, we

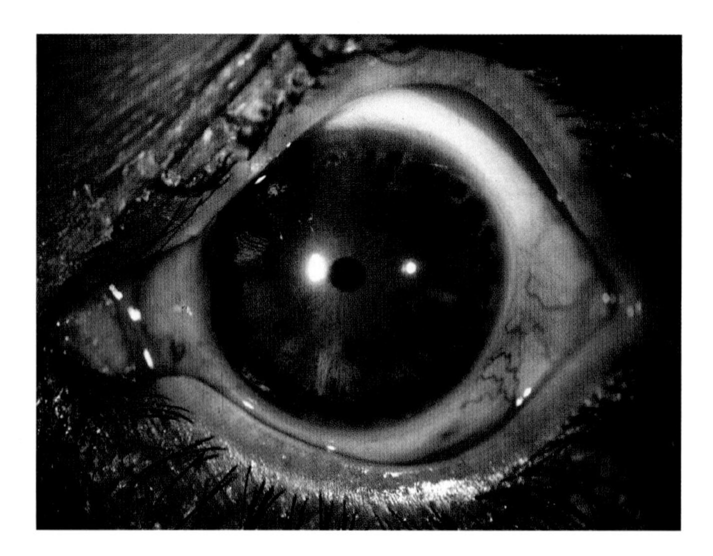

FIGURE 31-7 Appearance of nanophthalmic eye following successful opening of the entire angle with argon laser gonioplasty, done in multiple sessions.

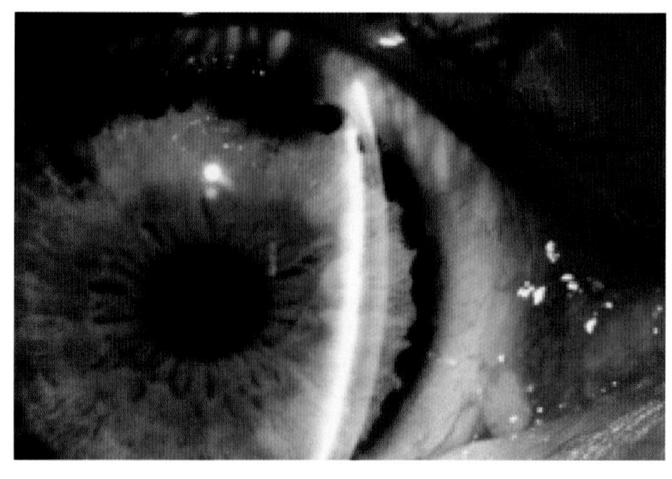

FIGURE 31-8 Nanophthalmic eye showing the narrow but open angle maintained with multiple sessions of argon laser gonioplasty.

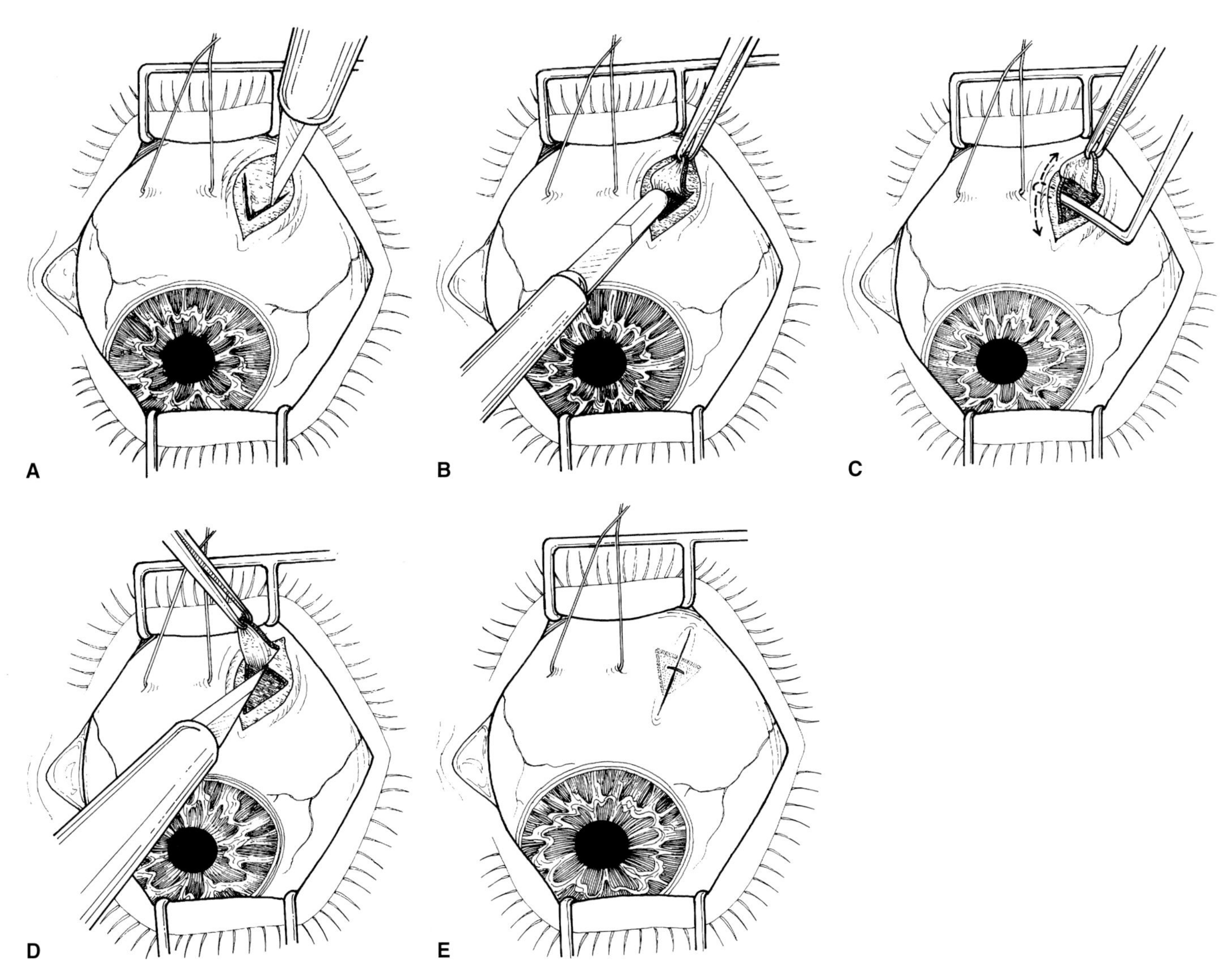

FIGURE 31-9 A, After a radial incision is created in both lower quadrants, a full-thickness triangular scleral flap 4 × 4 × 4 mm is created, with its apex at 3.5 mm from the limbus, over the pars plana. **B,** Flap is dissected posteriorly to expose the underlying choroid. **C,** Cyclodialysis spatula is then advanced to both sides of the sclerectomy, tangentially to the sclera, to drain any existing fluid from the suprachoroidal spaces. **D,** Full-thickness scleral flaps are excised completely, leaving two full-thickness triangular sclerectomies in each lower quadrant. **E,** Conjunctival incisions are closed with one or two 10-0 interrupted nylon sutures.

recommend that anterior sclerectomies be done at the time of the trabeculectomy. We modified our trabeculectomy procedure to minimize hypotony in nanophthalmic eyes, using high-viscosity viscoelastic in the anterior chamber to prevent sudden decompression of the anterior chamber, preplacing sutures in the flap to allow rapid closure and making scleral flap closure tighter than usual.

Cyclodestructive procedures are used as a last resort when all other attempts to control intraocular pressure are unsuccessful.

Phacoemulsification in nanophthalmic patients is done when intraocular pressure is under control and should be performed after or simultaneously with prophylactic sclerectomies. The use of early phacoemulsification as a therapy for narrow angles and as a prophylaxis of angle-closure glaucoma in nanophthalmos is hypothetical and controversial. It can be considered in the face of progressive narrowing of the angle despite other treatments, before extensive synechiae is formed.

Colobomatous and Complex Microphthalmos

Despite different pathophysiologies, colobomatous and complex microphthalmos can be assessed in the same manner because the common and more important feature is the presence of associated ocular or systemic pathologic conditions. In both cases, the final visual acuity is extremely variable and depends on the grade of disorganization of ocular tissues and integrity of visual pathway. The presence of congenital cataracts is common in both diseases[1] and is usually associated with poorly developed or defective retinal and optic nerve structures that will further compromise the visual prognosis.

For these reasons, cataract surgery is not always indicated in these patients. In children, the health and potential of the child should be carefully considered, and the pediatrician should perform a thorough comprehensive evaluation before the decision to perform cataract surgery is made.

In viable eyes with some expectation of visual acuity improvement, some surgeons[44] recommend using corneal diameter measurements to determine surgical planning as follows:

- Eyes with corneal diameters of less than 5 mm probably should not have cataract surgery unless the cataracts are bilateral. In such cases, surgery without an intraocular lens (IOL) is indicated. Surgery should be performed in the eye with the largest cornea and longest axial length or the one presenting the most normal ocular structures. The correction of aphakia in these cases should be done with spectacles.
- If the corneal diameter is between 6 and 9 mm, rigid gas-permeable contact lens with a reduced diameter could be adapted.
- In complex microphthalmic eyes with corneal diameters greater than 9 mm, a posterior chamber IOL should be considered.

Patients with choroidal colobomas are at a higher risk for retinal detachment and should be warned of the symptoms.[1] Therefore any retinal area susceptible to retinal detachment should be treated prophylactically before surgery.

Relative Anterior Microphthalmos

Indications for cataract extraction in eyes with relative anterior microphthalmos are the same as normal eyes. Auffarth et al.[4] found that lens removal alone leads to a significant intraocular pressure reduction and a decrease in the number of glaucoma medicines in eyes with RAM. The main complication after cataract surgery in these eyes is iridovitreal block. Because of the increased incidence of cornea guttata, transitory or permanent corneal edema can occur following cataract surgery. Another risk factor for cataract surgery in this group is the increased incidence of the pseudoexfoliation syndrome.[4]

Axial Hyperopia

Phacoemulsification surgery in high hyperopic patients is done using the surgeon's standard techniques. In addiction to cataract extraction, clear lensectomy for refractive correction in the absence of significant opacity of the lens is another indication for phacoemulsification. Other techniques for refractive correction in low to moderate hyperopic patients include laser in situ keratomileusis (LASIK), photorefractive keratectomy, and laser thermal keratoplasty.[45]

Clear lens extraction in high hyperopic eyes was first described by Lyle and Jin[46] in 1994, in six patients with refraction errors between +4.25 and +7.87, all of them with axial length greater than 20.5 mm. They did not report any complications during surgery or in the postoperative period. Refractive lensectomy for high hyperopia offers many advantages when compared with other refractive techniques. It has the capability to correct higher refractive errors, offers a higher predictability of refractive outcome, does not cause irregular astigmatism, and has no regression.[47] However, besides the potential of retinal detachment, loss of accommodation, and risk of endophthalmitis encountered in any cataract surgery, it is difficult to obtain an optimal IOL selection, and a piggyback IOL implantation may be necessary. For these reasons, this procedure remains controversial in these high hyperopic patients.

Regardless of the indication for phacoemulsification, either cataract extraction or refractive correction, there may be difficulties in the calculation of the implant power[48,49] because of the disproportion between anterior and posterior segments. In addition, extremely high hyperopic eyes require high-power IOLs that are often not available. Piggyback implantation of two IOLs has been used in these with mixed results.

Intraocular Lens Assessment in Eyes with Extremely Short Axial Length

Axial Length Measurement

The measurement of axial length is a critical determinant of the IOL power and final refractive results in any patient. This is particularly true in extremely short eyes, where a minor error in axial length measurement can lead to a large and unexpected refractive error.[3] An accurate axial length determination can be a challenge in these eyes because most ultrasound biometry devices are calibrated with average velocities of normal-sized eyes, and some still have limitations of axial length range, not measuring values of less than 21.5 mm.[49] Because of the short axial length, the posterior wall echo can be of great intensity, sometimes making it necessary to reduce the gain to obtain a clear echo (Figure 31-10).[48] Any flattening of the corneal surface can also account for significant IOL calculation errors, and immersion biometry may be used.

Lens Power Calculation

IOL power calculations for extremely short eyes remain a problem for the cataract surgeon. This can be attributed to the poor predictability of the older formulas. Current third-generation formulas (SRK/T, Holladay II, Hoffer Q, and Haigis)

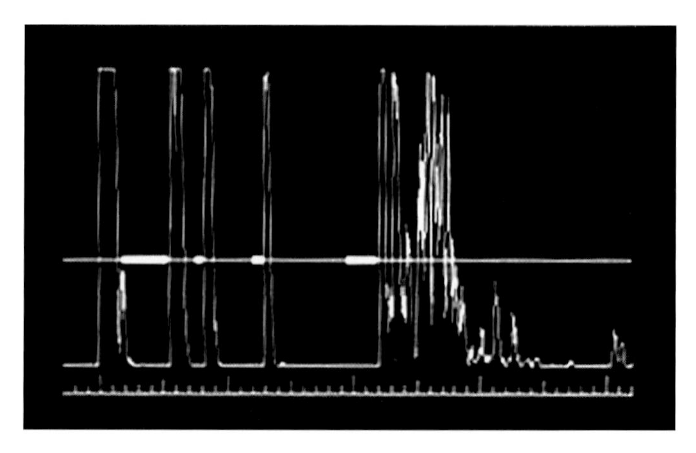

FIGURE 31-10 Biometry of a nanophthalmic eye. Total axial length is 16.98 mm, lens thickness is 5.05 mm, and anterior chamber depth is 2.77 mm.

that take into account variables such as anterior chamber depth, corneal diameter, and lens thickness have improved refractive predictability.[3,49-51] Theoretical formulas proved to be more accurate than empirical ones in microphthalmic eyes.[52,53] In a study of IOL calculation, Inatomi et al.[52] demonstrated that although the SRK/T produced the best results for these short eyes, all the formulas tested still showed a tendency for residual hypermetropia. Therefore calculations for eyes with less than 22 mm in axial length should be made with more than one formula for comparison, until newer and more accurate formulas are available.

Implant Choice

Implant choice is another challenge for the surgeon because rigid polymethylmethacrylate (PMMA) IOLs with a power greater than +45.0 diopters (D) and foldable lenses greater than +30.0 D are not available.[54] Implanting two PMMA posterior chamber lenses to achieve the desired total lens power was proposed by Gayton[55] in 1993, when +35.0 D was the maximum power available. These "piggyback" implantations later proved to offer better optical quality and cause less spherical aberration than a single lens with such a high dioptric power.[3] In 1996, Shugar[56] implanted two acrylic foldable lenses in six patients. He combined the advantages of small-incision surgery and the increased biocompatibility of the acrylic material. Acrylic lenses are also highly suitable for the piggyback procedure because the high refractive index allows acrylic lenses to be thinner and flatter than PMMA or silicone. Since then, polypseudophakia has become a frequently used procedure to achieve emmetropia in severely hyperopic eyes.

Gills and Cherchio[57] calculate the lens power by dividing the total power equally between the two lenses, whereas others prefer to place two thirds of the lens power in the more posterior lens and one third anteriorly.[49] This last option offers more advantages. By placing the more powerful lens posteriorly and in the bag, spherical aberrations can be reduced, and by inserting the least powerful lens in the sulcus, the access to the lens is also facilitated in case an exchange for a different power lens is needed.

Modifications in Cataract Surgery Technique in Microphthalmic Eyes

Standard large-incision extracapsular cataract extraction in eyes with increased intraocular pressure results in a sudden drop in pressure to atmospheric value, which can lead to dilation of the choroidal vascular bed and increases the risk of intrachoroidal effusion, suprachoroidal or intrachoroidal hemorrhage, or expulsive hemorrhage. This technique is dangerous in eyes with short anterior chamber depth and specifically in nanophthalmic eyes, in which the inelasticity of the sclera makes these complications likely.

Phacoemulsification allows avoidance of intraocular hypotony during surgery. When performing phaco surgery, these eyes should be carefully prepared and the intraocular pressure lowered to normal levels. If topical medications and mechanical pressure-lowering device (e.g., Honan's balloon) are not enough to lower the pressure to less than 25 mm Hg, 20% mannitol IV, 1 to 2 ml/kg body weight, should be employed 15 to 30 minutes before surgery. If needed, the surgery can be performed under general anesthesia with controlled hypotension, which will cause a reduction in arterial pressure.[48]

Topical/intracameral anesthesia may have some advantage because local infiltration can provoke increased orbital pressure and lead to an increase in the posterior pressure and vortex vein congestion. Clear corneal incisions in eyes with shallow anterior chamber offer the surgeon an anatomically better approach to the lens and allow the employment of smaller and safer incisions.[49] A shorter and more anterior corneal tunnel will help to prevent iris prolapse and facilitate manipulation of the nucleus.[48] A temporal approach is especially useful in these microphthalmic eyes, typically deeply set in the normal-sized orbit.

Maximal control over intraocular fluid dynamics is critical, and the new technology phaco machines offer great advantages over older ones. Paracentesis should be done carefully and gradually, avoiding the iris and anterior capsule. Intraoperative hypotony should be avoided as much as possible.

In severely hyperopic eyes, RAM, and nanophthalmic eyes with shallow anterior chamber, besides the proximity of the cataract from the cornea, there is often a low endothelial cell count. The Arshinoff soft-shell technique using a cohesive viscoelastic in the center of the anterior chamber and a dispersive viscoelastic above it may better stabilize the eye, decrease iris prolapse, and protect the endothelium.[49,58]

Posterior synechiae and pupillary membranes, if present, can be initially lysed with an iris spatula, and if viscoelastic substance and pharmacologic agents (we use 8 drops of 10% phenyl diluted in 2 ml of balanced salt solution [BSS]) fail to increase the pupil size, mechanical dilation of the pupil or sphincterotomies may be needed.

The size of capsulorhexis should be selected in accordance with the IOL plan. For a single implant, 5 to 6 mm is a good diameter. Because of the posterior vitreous pressure, the use of as much viscoelastic as necessary to hyperinflate and maintain the anterior chamber depth will help depress and flatten the anterior capsule, thus preventing radial extension of the capsulorhexis. For piggyback implantation of two lenses, a larger (6.5 to 7 mm) capsulorhexis is preferred so that the border of the anterior capsule does not cover the edge of the IOL.[59]

The use of a Kelman-Mackool phaco tip may facilitate surgical manipulation because its tip is bent down toward the position of the cataract.[49,54] It is important to remember to enter the eye with the phacoemulsification handpiece in the irrigation position. Chilled BSS may help prevent incision burns in these shallow anterior chambers.[59]

Before starting with emulsification of the nucleus, removal of the anterior epinucleus offers more space to work in the anterior chamber. During nucleus removal, a chopping technique[48,49,58] with high vacuum and short pulses of ultrasound may be helpful. The surgeon should start with a lower phaco power and increase it as dictated by nuclear density up to an efficient rate. Working in the nucleus at the level of the iris plane or in the posterior chamber avoids the endothelium and helps the integrity of the incision.

The risk of a posterior capsule rupture is increased in these eyes because of the frequent presence of significant posterior pressure, weakened zonules, and floppy capsules.[60] To reduce the incidence of this complication, low vacuum is used, and a second instrument is positioned between the posterior capsule and the phaco tip during the removal of the last pieces of nucleus.

Automated irrigation-aspiration should be done thoroughly to prevent interlenticular opacification in the case of piggyback implantation.

If a single IOL is planned, there are no changes in the technique. In the case of piggyback implantation, the first lens should be placed in the bag, with the haptics oriented vertically. The second lens is then inserted in the sulcus vertically with forceps, while maintaining downward pressure on the optic through the side port with the second instrument. The haptics of the two lenses should remain perpendicular to each other, increasing the separation between the optics and perhaps decreasing the incidence of interlenticular opacification.[54] Special attention should be given to viscoelastic removal from behind and between the two lenses.

It is safer to close the incision with a 10-0 nylon suture to protect against wound leakage and hypotony in the postoperative period, which could lead to a disastrous outcome, especially in nanophthalmic eyes.

Postoperative Monitoring

Careful observation is required following any anterior segment surgery in microphthalmic eyes. Some surgeons see the patient 4 to 6 hours after surgery for intraocular pressure and anterior chamber depth evaluation.

Cataract extraction can dramatically improve some cases with narrow angles (e.g., RAM), lowering intraocular pressure in most of the cases. After surgery, eyes with persistent intraocular pressure elevation can often be treated with laser trabeculoplasty because their angles are now accessible.[48]

In patients who received piggyback IOL implantation, follow-up should be done every 4 to 6 months, when a full dilation is indicated and the lenses are checked for interlenticular opacification.[48]

Complications of Surgery

Many complications that may arise during and after surgery in microphthalmic eyes are for the most part the same as those observed in phacoemulsification of normal-sized eyes, but they occur with much more frequency, depending on the disproportion between anterior and posterior chambers.[48] Microphthalmic eyes are predisposed to positive vitreous pressure and iris prolapse.[59]

Corneal Burns

Microphthalmic eyes with shallow anterior chambers are at greater risk of corneal wound burns given the proximity of the endothelium and the phacoemulsification tip. To prevent this, using chilled BSS and carefully inserting the phaco handpiece in the irrigating position along with careful positioning of the tip in the anterior chamber before starting to use phacoemulsification have been advocated.

Rupture or Disinsertion of Posterior Capsule

The posterior capsule is thin in microphthalmic eyes and very susceptible to ruptures that can extend dramatically because of the positive vitreous pressure present in small eyes. Surgery may lead to partial or total zonular dialysis. There is no consensus on the best course of action when a posterior chamber IOL is not feasible. An anterior chamber IOL is almost impossible in the majority of cases of microphthalmia, whereas immediate or later scleral fixation of the implant is an extremely risky maneuver.[48] This is especially true for the very susceptible nanophthalmic eyes.

Uveal Effusions/Hemorrhages

As emphasized earlier, nanophthalmos is a special group of microphthalmic eyes distinguished by its abnormal sclera. Uveal effusions in this group of patients can occur spontaneously or be precipitated by cataract extraction, glaucoma surgery, argon laser trabeculoplasty, and even prophylactic laser iridotomy.[42,61] Any eye surgery can precipitate or worsen a previous effusion by inflammatory increase of protein leakage or by reduction of transscleral hydrostatic pressure during intraoperative and/or postoperative hypotony. The effusions can be intrachoroidal, suprachoroidal, or both.

Suprachoroidal hemorrhage is more common in nanophthalmic patients. The sudden decompression of the eye during surgery may lead to choroidal engorgement that cannot be handled because of the inelastic sclera.

In case of sudden uveal effusion or hemorrhage, surgery must be interrupted, and tight closure of wounds should be performed. If sclerectomies have not been done preoperatively, they should be performed now. No further intervention is advised until the complication is resolved.

Retinal Detachments

Exudative retinal detachment can occur isolated after surgery or following postoperative uveal effusion if treatment of the latter is delayed or fails. Treatment of exudative retinal detachment consists of performing multiple sclerectomies as described previously in this chapter (see Figure 31-9, *A* to *E*).[37,41,42,61,62]

Angle Closure Glaucoma

Because crowding of the anterior chamber and narrow angles occurs in many nanophthalmic and RAM eyes, the surgeon should consider the possibility that a strong preoperative dilation may induce a primary angle closure attack in the most susceptible eyes.[59] Secondary angle closure can be caused by sudden peripheral uveal effusion and/or exudative retinal detachment, which causes a forward rotation of the ciliary body, forward movement of the peripheral iris, and pseudophakic pupillary block.[9,33]

If the aqueous is misdirected to the vitreous instead of the posterior chamber, malignant glaucoma can occur. Cycloplegic and mydriatic therapy should be initiated, together with steroids, and Nd:YAG laser to the anterior hyaloid face through a patent iridectomy may be attempted. If suprachoroidal effusion is also present, surgical drainage of fluid may be required. Posterior vitrectomy should be kept as a last resort for treatment of this complication.[48]

Interlenticular Opacification

Also known as interpseudophakos opacification or interpseudophakos Elschnig pearls, this late complication of piggyback IOL implantation recently became the subject of diverse studies and research.[56,63,64] It is characterized by the ingrowth of lens epithelial cells in the space between the two IOLs and is related to the hyperopic shift seen in these patients. It has been reported to occur 1 to 3 years following the piggyback IOL implantation.

This complication seems to be related to the border apposition of the anterior capsule toward the surface of the anterior lens. Attempts to avoid this problem use a larger capsulorhexis and insertion of the two lenses in the bag, or insertion of one lens in the bag and the other in the sulcus. Both strategies should follow a thorough cleaning of epithelial cells of the remaining anterior and posterior capsule. The first strategy seems to work better in patients with microphthalmos and narrow angles because it maximizes the anterior chamber depth and angle dimensions.[56]

There is insufficient data regarding the influence of the IOL material in this matter. If an interlenticular opacity develops, treatment varies from the use of Nd:YAG in the borders of anterior capsulorhexis to a new surgical intervention to clean the space between the lenses or exchange them.

If a lens exchange is necessary, the surgeon should base the calculation of IOL on previous measurements because a hyperopic shift may have occurred.

REFERENCES

1. Bateman J: Microphthalmos in development abnormalities of the eye, *Int Ophthalmol Clin* 24:87-106, 1984.
2. Warburg M: Genetics of microphthalmos, *Int Ophthalmol* 4:45-65, 1981.
3. Holladay J: Achieving emmetropia in extremely short eyes with two piggyback posterior chamber intraocular lenses, *Ophthalmology* 103:1118-1123, 1996.
4. Auffarth GU, Blum M, Faller U et al: Relative anterior microphthalmos: morphometric analysis and its implications for cataract surgery, *Ophthalmology* 107:1555-1560, 2000.
5. Duke-Elder S: Normal and abnormal development: congenital deformities. In Duke-Elder S, editor: *System of ophthalmology,* St Louis, 1964, Mosby, pp 488-495.
6. Singh O: Nanophthalmos: a perspective on identification and therapy, *Ophthalmology* 89:1006, 1982.
7. Weiss A: Simple microphthalmos, *Arch Ophthalmol* 107:1625-1630, 1989.
8. Brockhurst R: Nanophthalmos with uveal effusion: a new clinical entity, *Trans Am Ophthalmol Soc* LXXII:371-404, 1974.
9. Ryan E: Nanophthalmos with uveal effusion, *Ophthalmology* 89:1013-1017, 1982.
10. Altintas A, Acar MA, Yalvac IS et al: Autosomal recessive nanophthalmos, *Acta Ophthalmol Scand* 75:325-328, 1997.
11. Othman MI, Sullivan SA, Skuta GL et al: Autosomal dominant nanophthalmos (NNO1) with high hyperopia and angle-closure glaucoma maps to chromosome 11, *Am J Hum Genet* 63:1411-1418, 1998.
12. O'Grady R: Nanophthalmos, AJO 71:1251-1253, 1971.
13. Calhoun F: The management of glaucoma in nanophthalmos, *Trans Am Ophthalmol Soc* 73:97, 1975.
14. Cross H: Familial nanophthalmos, *AJO* 81:300-306, 1976.
15. Ghose S: Bilateral nanophthalmos, pigmentary retinal dystrophy, and angle closure glaucoma: a new syndrome? *Br J Ophthalmol* 69:624, 1985.
16. MacKay C: Retinal degeneration with nanophthalmos, cystic macular degeneration, and angle closure glaucoma, *Arch Ophthalmol* 105(366), 1987.
17. Buys YM, Pavlin CJ: Retinitis pigmentosa, nanophthalmos, and optic disc drusen: a case report, *Ophthalmology* 106:619-622, 1999.
18. Serrano JC, Hodgkins PR, Taylor DS et al: The nanophthalmic macula, *Br J Ophthalmol* 82:276-279, 1998.
19. Gass J: Uveal effusion syndrome: a new hypothesis concerning pathogenesis and technique of surgical treatment, *Retina* 3:159-163, 1983.
20. Gass J: Idiopathic serous detachment of the choroid, ciliary body, and retina (uveal effusion syndrome), *Ophthalmology* 89:1018-1032, 1982.
21. Yamani A, Wood I, Sugino I et al: Abnormal collagen fibrils in nanophthalmos: a clinical and histologic study [published erratum appears in *Am J Ophthalmol* 127:635, May 1999], *Am J Ophthalmol* 127:106-108, 1999.
22. Trelstad R: Nanophthalmic sclera: ultrastructural, histochemical, and biochemical observations, *Arch Ophthalmol* 100:1935, 1982.
23. Stewart D: Abnormal scleral collagen in nanophthalmos, *Arch Ophthalmol* 109:1017-1025, 1991.
24. Shiono T: Abnormal sclerocytes in nanophthalmos, *Graefes Arch Clin Exp Ophthalmol* 230:348-351, 1992.
25. Kawamura M: Biochemical studies of glycosaminoglycans in nanophthalmic sclera, *Graefes Arch Clin Exp Ophthalmol* 233:58-62, 1995.
26. Kawamura M: Immunohistochemical studies of glycosaminoglycans in nanophthalmic sclera, *Graefes Arch Clin Exp Ophthalmol* 234:19-24, 1996.
27. Yue B: Nanophthalmic sclera: morphologic and tissue culture studies, *Ophthalmology* 93:534, 1986.
28. Yue B: Nanophthalmic sclera: fibronectin studies, *Ophthalmology* 95:56-60, 1988.
29. Ward RC, Gragoudas ES, Pon DM et al: Abnormal scleral findings in uveal effusion syndrome, *Am J Ophthalmol* 106:139-146, 1988.
30. Brockhurst R: Vortex vein decompression for nanophthalmic uveal effusion, *Arch Ophthalmol* 98:1987-1990, 1980.
31. Johnson M: Surgical management of the idiopathic uveal effusion syndrome, *Ophthalmology* 97:778-785, 1990.
32. Shaffer R: Discussion of Calhoun FP Jr: The management of glaucoma in nanophthalmos, *Trans Am Ophthalmol Soc* 73:119-120, 1975.
33. Simmons R: Nanophthalmos: diagnosis and treatment. In Epstein D, editor: *Chandler and Grant's glaucoma,* Philadelphia, 1986, Lea & Febiger, pp 251-259.
34. Jalkh A: Diffuse choroidal thickening detected by ultrasonography in various ocular disorders, *Retina* 3:277-283, 1983.
35. Ritch R: Glaucoma related to other ocular disorders. In Ritch R, Shields M, editors: *The secondary glaucomas,* St Louis, 1982, Mosby, pp 55-57.
36. Good W: Recurrent nanophthalmic uveal effusion syndrome following laser trabeculoplasty, *Am J Ophthalmol* 106:234-235, 1988.
37. Casswell AG, Gregor ZJ, Bird AC: The surgical management of uveal effusion syndrome, *Eye* 1(pt 1):115-119, 1987.
38. Allen KM, Meyers SM, Zegarra H: Nanophthalmic uveal effusion, *Retina* 8:145-147, 1988.
39. Morita H: Recurrence of nanophthalmic uveal effusion, *Ophthalmologica* 207:30-36, 1993.
40. Akduman L, Adelberg DA, Del Priore LV: Nanophthalmic uveal effusion managed with scleral windows and topical mitomycin-C, *Ophthalmic Surg Lasers* 28:325-327, 1997.
41. Krohn J, Seland JH: Exudative retinal detachment in nanophthalmos, *Acta Ophthalmol Scand* 76:499-502, 1998.
42. Lesnoni G, Rossi T, Nistri A et al: Nanophthalmic uveal effusion syndrome after prophylactic laser treatment, *Eur J Ophthalmol* 9:315-318, 1999.
43. Belcher CD, Greff LJ: *Laser therapy of angle-closure glaucoma.* In Albert DM, Jakobiec FA, editors: *Principles and practice of ophthalmology,* Philadelphia, 2000, WB Saunders.
44. Biglan AW: Pediatric cataract surgery. In Albert DM, editor: *Ophthalmic surgery: principles and techniques,* Cambridge, 1999, Blackwell Science, pp 970-1014.
45. Fink A: Refractive lensectomy for hyperopia, *Ophthalmology* 107:1540-1548, 2000.
46. Lyle W, Jin GJ: Clear lens extraction for the correction of high refractive error, *J Cataract Refract Surg* 20:273-276, 1994.
47. Vicary D: Refractive lensectomy to correct ametropia, *J Cataract Refract Surg* 25:943-948, 1999.

48. Buratto L, Bellucci R: Cataract surgery and intraocular lens implantation in severe hyperopia. In Buratto L, Osher RH, Masket S, editors: *Cataract surgery in complicated cases,* Milano, Italy, 2000, Slack Inc, pp 73-85.
49. Fine IH, Hoffman RS: Phacoemulsification in high hyperopia. In Buratto L, Osher RH, Masket S, editors: *Cataract surgery in complicated cases,* Milano, Italy, 2000, pp 67-72.
50. Fenzl R: Refractive and visual outcome of hyperopic cataract cases operated on before and after implementation of the Holladay II formula, *Ophthalmology* 105:1759-1764, 1998.
51. Bartke TU, Auffarth GU, Uhl JC et al: Reliability of intraocular lens power calculation after cataract surgery in patients with relative anterior microphthalmos, *Graefes Arch Clin Exp Ophthalmol* 238:138-142, 2000.
52. Inatomi M, Ishii K, Koide R et al: Intraocular lens power calculation for microphthalmos, *J Cataract Refract Surg* 3:1208-1212, 1997.
53. Huber C: Effectiveness of intraocular lens calculation in high ametropia, *J Cataract Refract Surg* 15:667-672, 1989.
54. Shugar JK: Cataract surgery in microphthalmos. In Buratto L, Osher RH, Masket S, editors: *Cataract surgery in complicated cases,* Milano, Italy, 2000, Slack Inc, pp 90-93.
55. Gayton J: Implanting two posterior chamber intraocular lenses in a case of microphthalmos, *J Cataract Refract Surg* 19:776-777, 1993.
56. Shugar J: Implantation of multiple foldable acrylic posterior chamber lenses in the capsular bag for high hyperopia, *J Cataract Refract Surg* 22:1368-1372, 1996.
57. Gills JP, Cherchio M: Phacoemulsification in high hyperopic cataract patients. In Lu LW, Fine IH, editors: *Phacoemulsification in difficult and challenging cases,* New York, 1999, Thieme Medical Publishers, pp 21-31.
58. Dodick JM, Hsu J: Personal technique for cataract removal in high hyperopia. In Buratto L, Osher RH, Masket S, editors: *Cataract surgery in complicated cases,* Milano, Italy, 2000, Slack Inc, p 86.
59. Gayton J: Cataract surgery and hyperopia. In Buratto, L, Osher RH, Masket S, editors: *Cataract surgery in complicated cases,* Milano, Italy, 2000, Slack Inc, pp 87-88.
60. Buratto L, Osher RH, Masket S: *Cataract surgery in complicated cases,* Milano, Italy, 2000, Slack Inc, p 466.
61. Bellows A: Choroidal effusion during glaucoma surgery in patients with prominent episcleral vessels, *Arch Ophthalmol* 97:493-497, 1979.
62. Faulborn J, Kolli H: Sclerotomy in uveal effusion syndrome, *Retina* 19: 504-507, 1999.
63. Stasiuk R: Interface Elschnig pearl formation with piggyback implantation, *J Cataract Refract Surg* 26:157-158, 2000.
64. Gayton J: Interlenticular opacification: clinicopathological correlation of a complication of posterior chamber piggyback intraocular lenses, *JCRS* 26:330-336, 2000.

Cataract Surgery in the Presence of Other Ocular Comorbidities

32

Hiroko Bissen-Miyajima, MD

The indication and technique of cataract surgery in the presence of other ocular morbidities have dramatically changed with the development of modern technique, such as phacoemulsification and intraocular lens (IOL) implantation, and the introduction of ophthalmic viscosurgical devices (OVDs). When phacoemulsification or IOL was first introduced, the indication was limited to cataractous eyes without any other ocular pathologic condition. For these eyes, extracapsular extraction was the first choice, and IOL was implanted in limited cases. Recent advances in techniques of phacoemulsification and IOL have changed the indication completely; that is, we hardly ever encounter contraindications.

However, for eyes with other ocular morbidities, special caution should be paid before, during, and after surgery.

Ocular Surface Problems

Dry Eye

Research on the effect of cataract surgery on the cornea mostly focused on the endothelium. However, the effects on epithelium such as superficial punctate keratitis (SPK) and epithelial defect seem to be more common. Often patients complain of ocular discomfort with dry eye sensation after surgery. Dry eye following cataract surgery is divided into two groups. One is the worsening of preexisting dry eye symptoms, and the other is surgically induced dry eye. The possible effects of cataract surgery on ocular surface are shown in Table 32-1.

PREOPERATIVE MANAGEMENT

Dry eye should be diagnosed before surgery because the condition of preexisting dry eye can be easily worsened by cataract surgery. Epithelial defect following cataract surgery often happens to the patients with decreased tear production. If dry eye is suspected, fluorescein staining of the corneal epithelium, Rose-Bengal staining, and tear film break-up time (BUT) should be examined before surgery. If SPK exists, artificial tears or eyedrops containing hyaluronic acid should be prescribed to improve their corneal condition. If SPK is resistant to this treatment, intracanalicular plug should be considered. Any eyedrops that contain preservative such as benzalkonium chloride should be avoided.[1]

Another important point is to inform patients with dry eye that their symptoms may worsen for a couple of months after cataract surgery.

SURGICAL PROCEDURE

The side effect of topical anesthesia on the corneal epithelium is well known. Anesthetic eyedrop application should be kept to a minimum. The exposure to the light source of the operating microscope should be kept to a minimum as well. The incision technique of either sclerocorneal or corneal does not seem to be matter in these patients. Our study revealed that BUT (Figure 32-1) and the barrier function of corneal epithelium (Figure 32-2) were affected for a month postoperatively in both sclerocorneal and corneal incisions.

POSTOPERATIVE MANAGEMENT

Any eyedrops that contain preservative tend to cause an epithelial problem. Nonsteroidal antiinflammatory drugs such as diclofenac sodium are known to affect the corneal epithelium in certain cases. For patients already diagnosed with dry eye, only antibiotic and steroid regimens are used. Additional eyedrops such as artificial tears are important to increase the stability of the precorneal tear film. If SPK is severe in the early stage, the treatment plan may have to be changed to avoid resistant keratitis. Sometimes severe SPK is observed 1 week after surgery (Figure 32-3). In cases like this, all the eyedrops, except artificial tears, may have to be stopped. If no recovery is seen with this procedure, serum eyedrops may be prescribed.[2] The procedure to make this type of eyedrops is shown in Table 32-2. Another method is to use an eye protector or goggles to avoid evaporation from the tear film.

Intracanalicular plugs are useful when the patient still has dry eye sensation. Absorbable plugs developed for the dry eye following laser in situ keratomileusis (LASIK) can also be used.

Stevens-Johnson Syndrome and Ocular Pemphigoid

Cataract surgery for patient with severe cicatricial keratoconjunctivitis such as Stevens-Johnson syndrome or ocular pemphigoid is a challenge. The choice of surgery was limited to penetrating keratoplasty and open-sky cataract extraction. The new technique of surgical reconstruction of the ocular surface

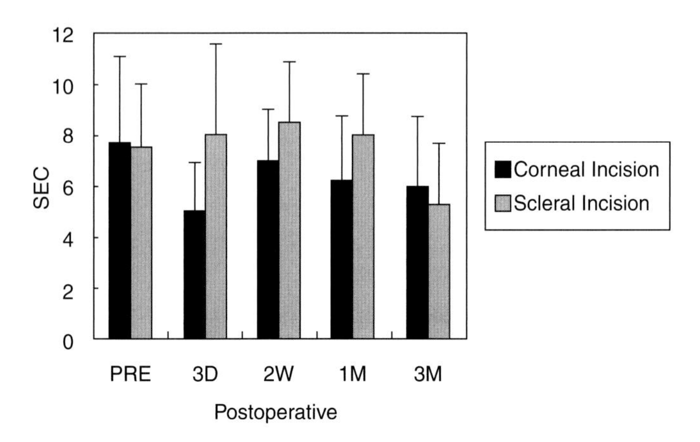

FIGURE 32-1 Tear film break-up time (BUT) decreased 3 days after surgery in the group with corneal incision.

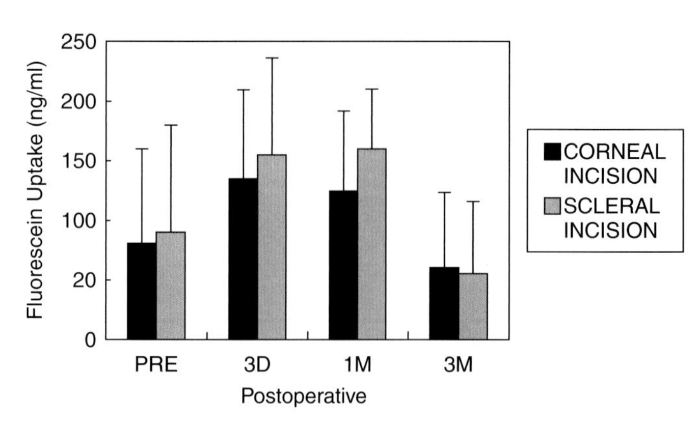

FIGURE 32-2 Barrier function of corneal epithelium. Barrier function of corneal epithelium recovered to preoperative level at 3 months after surgery.

using amniotic membrane and allograft limbal tissue at the time of cataract surgery has extended the surgical indication. Possible problems are shown in Table 32-3.

PREOPERATIVE MANAGEMENT

Not very much can be done before surgery. The surgical plan should be precisely considered.

SURGICAL PROCEDURE

Anesthesia. In most cases, need either peribulbar or retrobulbar anesthesia is used. An extra procedure such as removal of dermal tissue, dissection of palpebral-bulbar conjunctiva, and excessive coagulation may be applied. Also the rotation of the eye is limited, and bridal suture may be necessary to control the eye position.

Incision. The conjunctiva or dermal tissue that covers the cornea usually must be removed (Figure 32-4). Thus a scleral

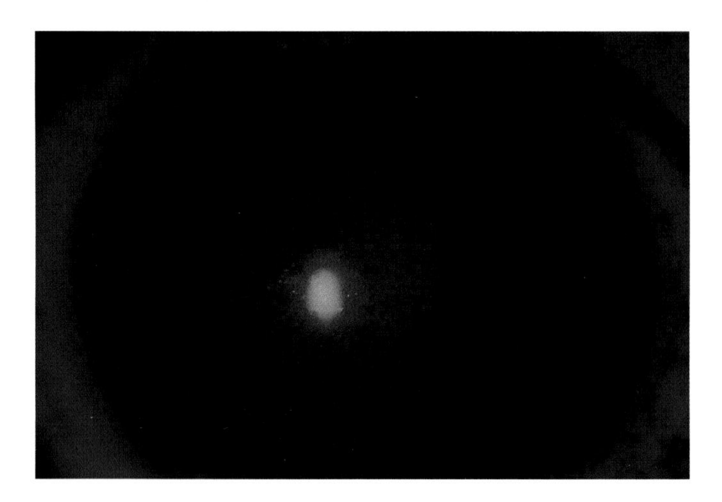

FIGURE 32-3 Severe superficial punctate keratitis. Fluorescein staining over the whole cornea is observed.

TABLE 32-1

Effects of Cataract Surgery on the Ocular Surface

PREOPERATIVE
Dry eye
DURING SURGERY
Dryness of cornea and conjunctiva because of their exposure
Drying from the light source of operating microscope
Topical anesthesia
INCISION
Transient ischemia resulting from the disconnect of conjunctival and episcleral vessels
Denervation of cornea
POSTOPERATIVE
Incomplete lid closure
Eyedrops (steroid, diclophenac natrium, preservative)

TABLE 32-2

Preparation of Autologous Serum Application

1. Obtain 40 ml of blood
2. Centrifuge for 5 minutes at 1500 revolutions/min
3. Separate the serum
4. Put into a bottle with ultraviolet light cut coating
5. Dilute the serum to 20% with physiologic saline

TABLE 32-3

Problems in Cataract Surgery with Cicatricial Keratoconjunctivitis

Eyelid	Adhesion of palpebral and bulbar conjunctiva
Cornea	Dermal tissue over the cornea
	Irregular surface
	Delayed epithelization
Wound closure	

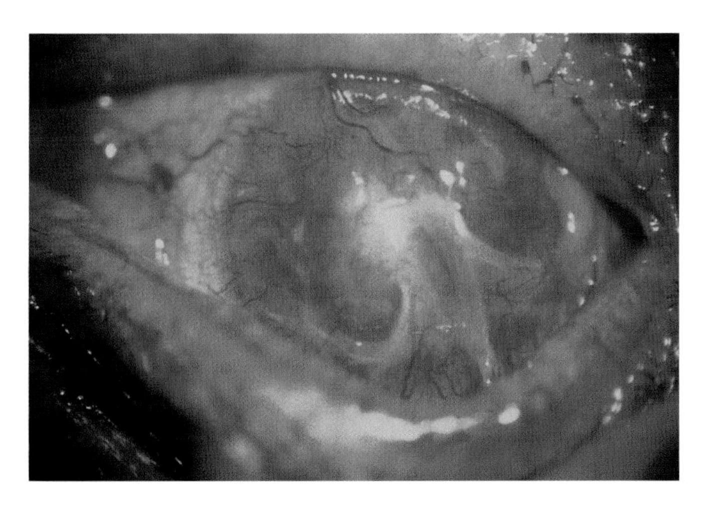

FIGURE 32-4 Ocular pemphigoid. Conjunctival tissue covers the cornea.

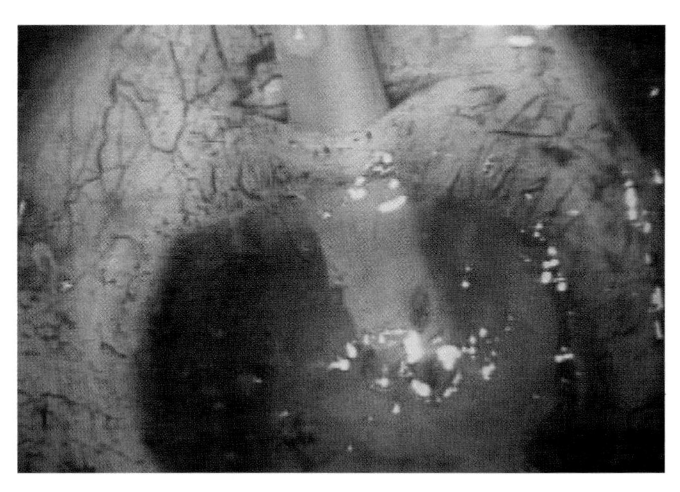

FIGURE 32-5 Phacoemulsification is carefully done under poor visibility.

incision is the first choice. If the surgeon feels more confident with a corneal incision, suturing the incision is mandatory. Epithelization is critical in such a case, and a smaller incision is preferable. However, if the transparency of the cornea is poor, phacoemulsification may not be possible, and an extracapsular or intracapsular extraction may have to be performed.

Removal of the lens. Capsulorhexis is critical in this surgery. Even if some transparency could be obtained after the removal of conjunctival or dermal tissue over the cornea, the surface is still irregular. Focusing on the anterior capsule is sometimes impossible, and the surgeon may need to choose the can-opener technique. Even following this technique, phacoemulsification can be performed (Figure 32-5). If the existence of the posterior capsule is uncertain because of poor corneal condition, viscodelineation may be helpful. Similar to hydrodissection, ophthalmic viscoelastic substance is injected between the capsule and cortex. If the cortex or epinucleus is separated from the capsule, it is not very difficult to continue phacoemulsification. The aim of cataract surgery in this particular case is to improve vision. Unlike usual cataract cases, perfect lens removal is not required.

Intraocular lens implantation. If the lens is safely removed, an IOL is implanted in the usual manner. If the surgeon is familiar with a polymethylmethacrylate IOL, the incision is enlarged and the IOL is implanted from a 6- to 7-mm incision. As mentioned earlier, a smaller incision is preferable. A foldable IOL is also indicated.

Wound closure. The corneal or scleral tissue is usually very thin. Suture is necessary.

Amniotic membrane implantation. Amniotic membrane is an ideal material for the bulbar conjunctiva because there is no immunogenicity.[3] Frozen amniotic membrane obtained from a Cesarean section is defrosted and manually dissected from the chorion. The amniotic membrane is placed on the eye and sutured to the eye with 9-0 silk (Figure 32-6).

Allograft limbal tissue implantation. Allograft limbal tissue is used to grow corneal epithelium. After trephination of the central cornea from eyes obtained from an eye bank, the scleral and the stromal portions of the limbal tissue are manually dissected to obtain a thin, ring-shaped section of limbal tissue (Figure 32-7). The limbal tissue is sutured to the peripheral cornea with 10-0 nylon.[4]

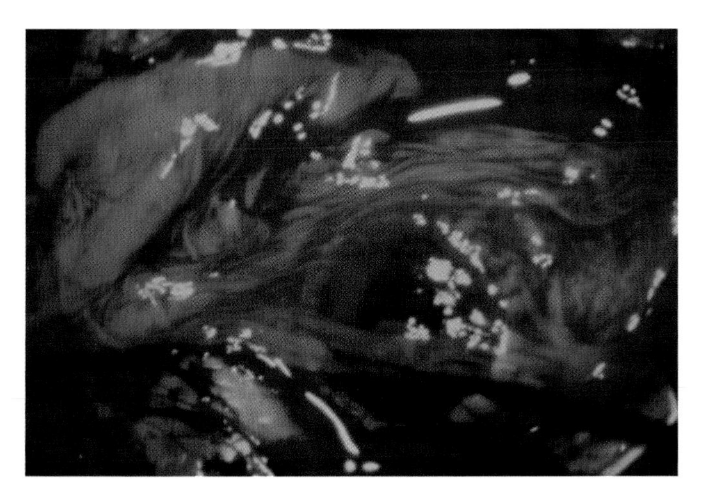

FIGURE 32-6 Implantation of amniotic membrane. Amniotic membrane is covered over cornea and sclera.

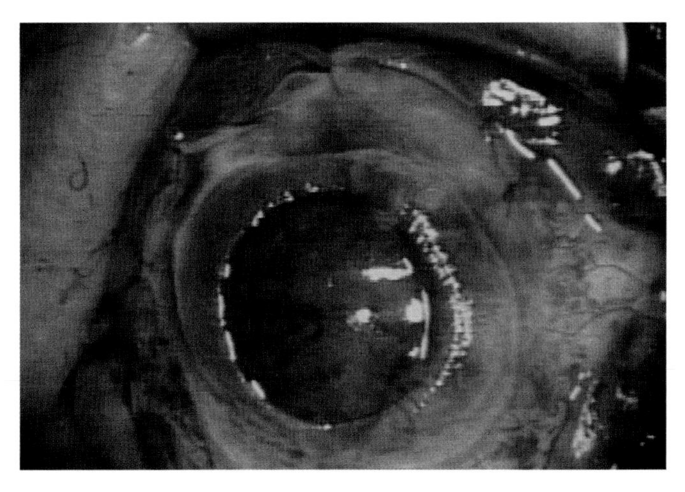

FIGURE 32-7 Allograft limbal transplantation. Ring-shaped limbal tissue is prepared.

POSTSURGICAL MANAGEMENT

In addition to the eyedrops used routinely after cataract surgery, cyclosporine eyedrops and autoserum eyedrops should be considered. Preservative-free artificial tears also were frequently administered. Systemic steroid (dexamethasone) and cyclosporine A are usually helpful.

Diabetes

In patients with diabetes, several complications seem to happen more often compared with otherwise healthy patients (Table 32-4).

PREOPERATIVE MANAGEMENT

The control of diabetes is necessary. With the help of primary doctor or internist, a hemoglobin A1c (HbA1c) test should be the best way to measure the condition.

SURGICAL PROCEDURE

Minimum invasion should be considered. Surgery sometimes becomes complicated from poor dilation. Phacoemulsification can be done in the same manner as with as small pupil. Excessive contact with iris will increase the postoperative inflammation in the anterior chamber and may cause unexpected bleeding. If vitrectomy for diabetic retinopathy has been performed, the surgeon should be prepared for unstable anterior chamber and preexisting rupture in the posterior capsule. If laser coagulation for diabetic retinopathy is planned following cataract surgery, the larger size of anterior capsulotomy and optic diameter of IOL should be considered. Difficulty is also experienced in controlling intraocular pressure in patients undergoing hemodialysis. For these patients, OVD in the anterior chamber should be removed completely.

POSTOPERATIVE MANAGEMENT

The control of anterior chamber inflammation should be more carefully done than in usual cases. Some reports show a higher incidence of cystoid macular edema in diabetic patients. Synechia is more common, and mydriatic eyedrops may be used if there is a possibility of posterior synechia developing. Epithelial problems are also common. Artificial tears may be added for a while.

TABLE 32-4
Possible Complications of Cataract Surgery in Patient with Diabetes

Bleeding
Poor dilation
Delayed epithelization
Iritis
Possible effect on diabetic retinopathy
Insufficient would closure
Infection
Increased blood sugar level caused by the topical or general steroid

Retinitis Pigmentosa

PREOPERATIVE MANAGEMENT

Anterior subcapsular opacification is common in patients with retinitis pigmentosa. Such a small opacity in the center of the lens may diminish visual acuities because the visual field is concentric in such patients. Some may complain about glare as the first symptom of cataract.

SURGICAL PROCEDURE

The capsule is thin, and handling of the capsule is rather complicated. The size of capsulorhexis has a tendency to become smaller after the surgery.[5] If the capsulorhexis happened to be rather small, it should be enlarged at the end of surgery. Phacoemulsification is usually not difficult because the type of cataract is an anterior subcapsular opacification and the nucleus is not very hard. IOL with ultraviolet cut is preferable.

POSTOPERATIVE MANAGEMENT

If the capsulotomy has become too small and affects visual acuity, YAG laser capsulotomy is performed. In general, sunglasses are recommended when patients are under sunlight.

Eyelid Abnormalities

PREOPERATIVE MANAGEMENT

The surgical problem of the patient with eyelid abnormality is how to get enough exposure of the eye. For most of these cases, a lid speculum cannot be used, and suture may be necessary to open both upper and lower lids (Figure 32-8). Cases with symblepharon are especially a challenge. The surgeon should plan how to open the eyelid and be ready to perform cataract surgery under poor exposure of the eye.

SURGICAL PROCEDURE

With any difficult case, the usual technique, with which the surgeon is most confident, should be performed. If the eye can

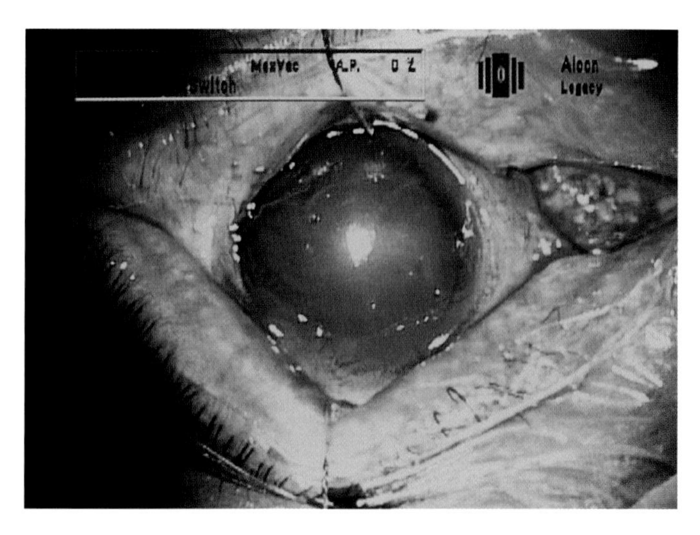

FIGURE 32-8 Lid opening. Suture was used to open upper and lower lids.

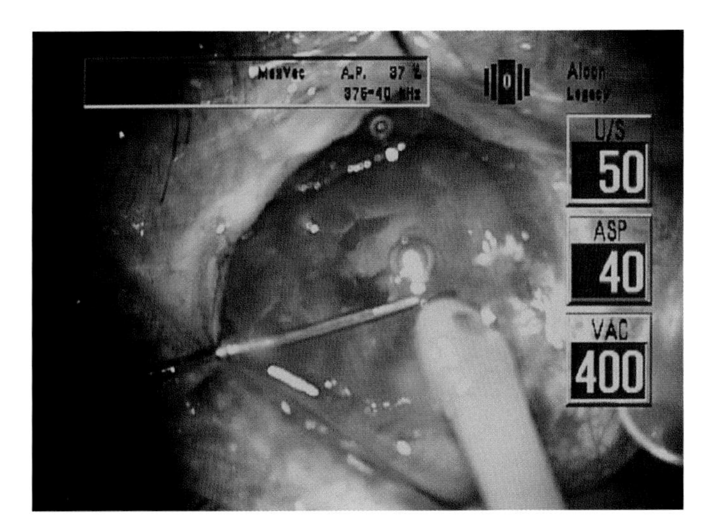

FIGURE 32-9 Phacoemulsification. The site of incision is carefully chosen, and two-handed phacoemulsification is performed.

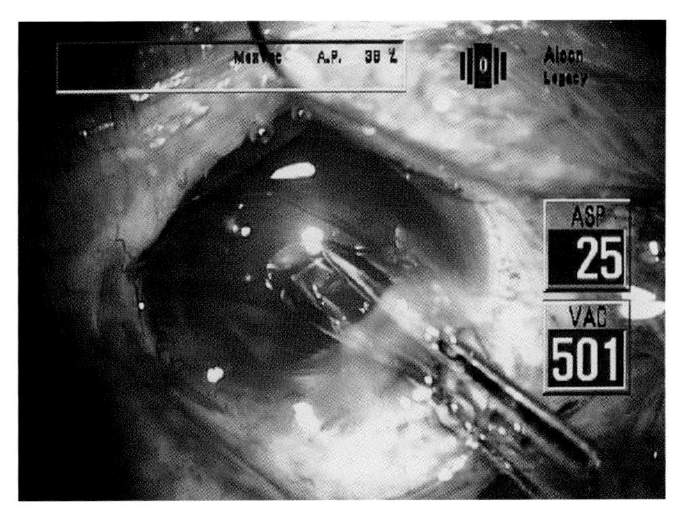

FIGURE 32-10 Intraocular lens (IOL) implantation. Foldable IOL is inserted in the usual manner.

be opened, the entrance of the incision should be considered. In cases with symblepharon, pannus is also common. As for the incision, the site should be planned to avoid unnecessary hemorrhage (Figure 32-9). If phacoemulsification is completed, IOL implantation can be done in the usual manner (Figure 32-10). Another problem is visibility during surgery. If the eye is opened with a suture or lid speculum, the irrigating water will stay and disturb the visibility of the anterior capsule. The water will stay and pool between upper and lower lids. Any cannula that absorbs the water should be used.

Bleeding Disorders

Most common in this category is the use of anticoagulant therapy. With the introduction of topical anesthesia and clear corneal incisions, routine cataract surgery can be performed for patients with bleeding disorders.

PREOPERATIVE MANAGEMENT

If the surgery is planned with peribulbar or retrobulbar anesthesia, there is a risk of hemorrhage during injection. The risk of stopping the anticoagulants, in patients with a general condition such as thrombosis or embolism should be considered. The doctor who prescribed anticoagulants for this matter should be consulted if the general condition seems to be critical. If cataract surgery is performed through a clear corneal incision with topical anesthesia, the patient does not have to stop anticoagulant therapy.[6]

SURGICAL PROCEDURE

The technique chosen should be the one that has less risk of encountering vessels. If the surgeon is performing a clear corneal incision with topical anesthesia, the patient can continue to take the anticoagulant medicine.

POSTOPERATIVE MANAGEMENT

If no extra hemorrhage is seen on the first postoperative day, the patient may start taking anticoagulants.

REFERENCES

1. Gasset AR: Benzalkonium chloride toxicity to the human cornea, *Am J Ophthalmol* 84:169-171, 1977.
2. Tsubota K, Goto E, Shimmura S et al: Treatment of persistent corneal epithelial defect by autologous serum application, *Ophthalmology* 106:1984-1989, 1999.
3. Shimazaki J, Tsubota K: Amniotic membrane transplantation for ocular surface reconstruction in patients with chemical and thermal burns, *Ophthalmology* 104:2068-2076, 1997.
4. Tsubota K, Satake Y, Ohyama M et al.: Surgical reconstruction of the ocular surface in advanced ocular cicatricial pemphigoid and Stevens-Johnson syndrome, *Am J Ophthalmol* 52:38-52, 1996.
5. Hayashi K, Hayashi H, Matsuo K et al: Anterior capsule contraction and intraocular lens dislocation after implant surgery in eye with retinitis, *Ophthalmology* 105:1239-1243, 1998.
6. Shuler JD, Paschal JF, Holland GN: Antiplatelet therapy and cataract surgery, *J Cataract Refract Surg* 18:567-569, 1992.

The Evolution of the Intraocular Lens

33

Kenneth J. Hoffer, MD, FACS

In a short book chapter, it would be impossible to cover every aspect and personality in the history of the intraocular lens (IOL). Therefore this synopsis is limited by the historical materials at my disposal and my personal recollections.

Prehistory

The history of implanting a lens in the human eye to eliminate the "first complication of cataract surgery"—aphakia—dates back to Casanova[1-3] (1725-1798.) In his memoirs he related that in 1764 the Italian oculist Tadini had mentioned to him the idea of implanting a lens after cataract surgery. Casanova passed the idea to Casaamata[2] of Dresden in 1795, and he attempted to introduce a glass lens into the eye after removing a cataract and watched it immediately slide back toward the fundus. Choyce[4] stated that in 1939, John Foster of Leeds, England, made a jocular reference to the possibility of artificial lens implantation in an after-dinner speech at the Leeds Medical Society. Strampelli[5] told of the unpublished fruitless attempts of Marchi to fixate quartz lenses with platinum wires in the anterior chambers of animals in 1940.

Ridley Era

In the autumn of 1948, a medical student was observing Harold Ridley extract a cataract at St. Thomas's Hospital in London. The student asked him why he was not going to replace the lens he had just removed. This simple question was the direct stimulus for Ridley to consider implanting an IOL. Ridley was born in Leicestershire, the eldest son of a Navy eye surgeon, and attended Cambridge. He was the head of his surgical division and a well-respected eye surgeon of his time. Fortunately (before his death on May 25, 2001), I had the opportunity to visit him and his charming wife Elizabeth at their home in August of 1999 (Figure 33-1). I asked him if this story of the medical student was apocryphal, and he told me it was absolutely true. In addition, he told me what few have known: the medical student was a woman, and she corresponded with him yearly to that day. Therefore it was a woman who had sparked the idea for IOLs. He had then asked John Pike of Rayners (Rayner & Keeler, Choleywood, England) to fashion a lens of polymethylmethacrylate (PMMA [from International Chemical Industries]) because he had noted no ill effects from stationary particles of PMMA in the eyes of Royal Air Force pilots (especially Gordon Cleaver, a Battle of Britain pilot) who had sustained injuries from shattered Spitfire canopies during World War II. The lens (Figure 33-2, *B*) that they made was shaped like the human lens with a diameter of 8.35 mm weighing 112 mg, and it was sterilized using 1% cetrimide solution.

History was made on November 29, 1949, when Ridley implanted the first lens in a 42-year-old woman after extracapsular cataract extraction. The surgery went well, but unfortunately, lens power calculation prediction became of utmost importance when her postoperative refractive error was $-18.00-6.00 \times 120°$ (a -21.0 diopter [D] overcorrection). I had assumed that Sir Harold (see Figure 33-2, *A*) had removed the lens and replaced it with a proper power, but he told me that he was not able to do anything to correct the situation. The second lens was implanted 9 months later with the same result. Needless to say, they changed their method of predicting the correct power. After Ridley's first public report at Oxford in 1951, many others followed his example, such as Arruga, Barraquer, Epstein, and Pafique, as well as Warren Reese of Philadelphia (the first American to implant an IOL on St. Patrick's Day in 1952). The first paper published on IOLs was by Ridley in 1951.[6-7] The major complications were severe hyphema, downward decentration, iris atrophy, glaucoma, and anterior and posterior (6%) dislocation and inflammation. The cetrimide molecule was found to cling to the IOL and later release, causing the inflammation. In 1956, Cornelius Binkhorst[8] of Terneuzen, Holland suggested sterilizing the IOLs using ultraviolet (UV) (253.7 nm) radiation (later used by some [Cox-Uphoff] in America in the 1970s). In 1958, Strampelli placed IOLs into the patient's earlobes for 3 to 4 months to "humanize" them before implanting them into the eye. Precipitates on the implants did not occur. In 1957, Frederick Ridley[9] of England (no relation) introduced the sodium hydroxide sterilization method (Figure 33-3, *A*) (soak in 10% NaOH for 1 hour at 30° C, store in 0.1% NaOH, neutralize on use with 0.5% $NaHCO_3$, rinse with saline). This method was embraced and used by all until 1978 when the U.S. Food and Drug Administration (FDA) mandated ethylene oxide sterilization, which had been introduced by American manufacturers.

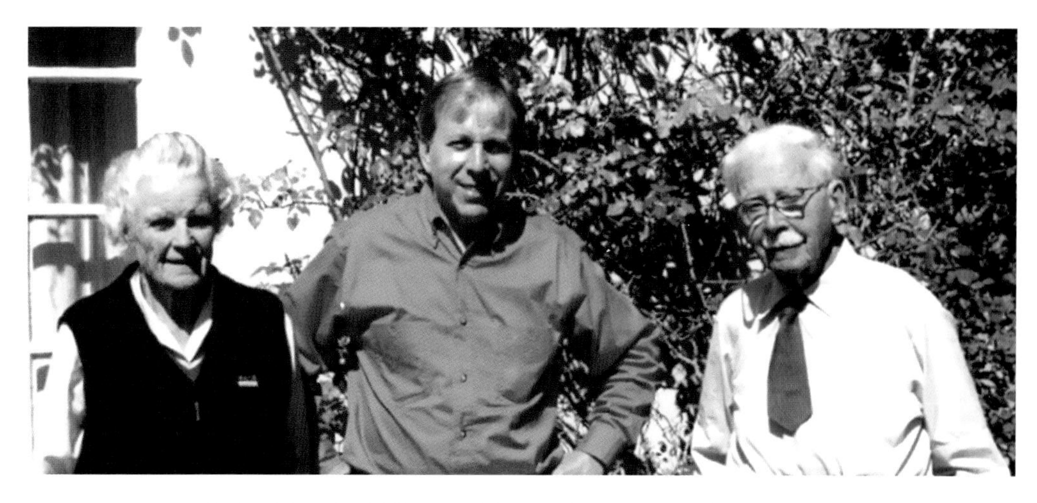

FIGURE 33-1 Sir Harold and Lady Elizabeth Ridley with the author at their home near Salisbury, England, on August 30, 1999. (Photo by Marcia Hoffer.)

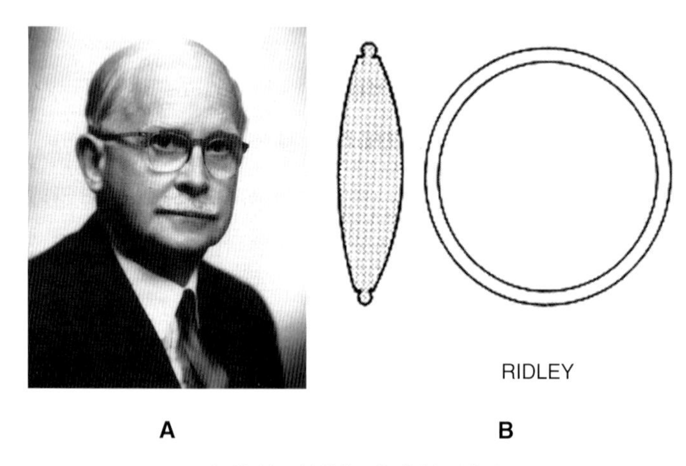

FIGURE 33-2 A, Sir Harold Ridley. **B,** Original Ridley posterior chamber lens implant circa 1949.

Overall, Ridley implanted about a thousand of these lenses. I had the opportunity to examine one of his patients [see Figure 33-3, *B*) in Santa Monica in 1979. The 85-year-old woman had received the implant in 1951 (at age 57) and had an uncorrected visual acuity of 20/20 with a perfectly placed lens for over a quarter of a century. These lenses weren't all bad; however, because of complications, 15% of the Ridley designs were removed, and the implant was beginning to lose favor with those who were using it. Because of this, the pioneers looked for a better place to put Ridley's invention.

Strampelli Era

The next site considered for IOL placement was the anterior chamber so as to prevent posterior dislocation and to be able to

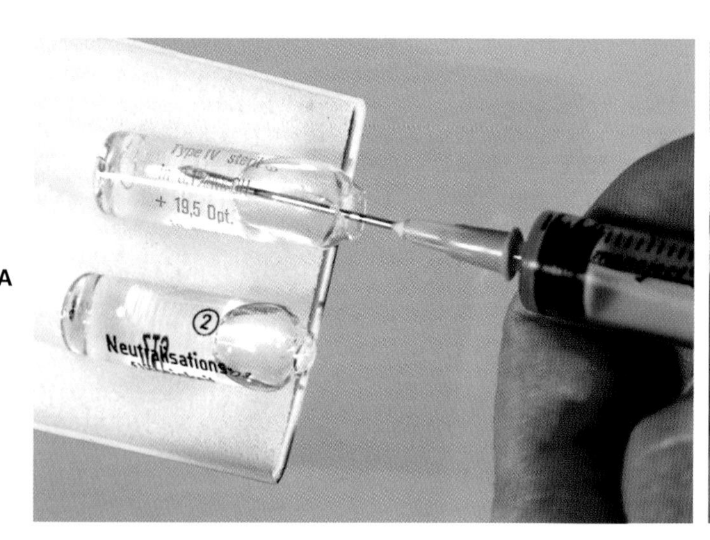

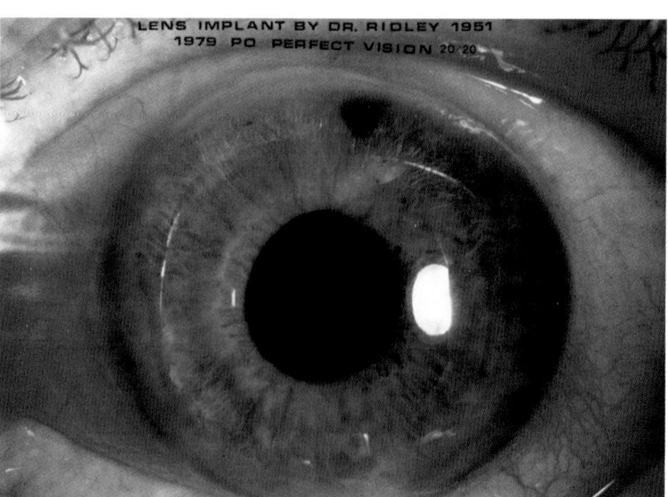

FIGURE 33-3 A, Sodium hydroxide/bicarbonate sterilization method. **B,** An eye with a Ridley posterior chamber IOL (implanted by Sir Harold Ridley in 1951) with uncorrected 20/20 vision in 1979. (Photo by Kenneth J. Hoffer, in 1979.)

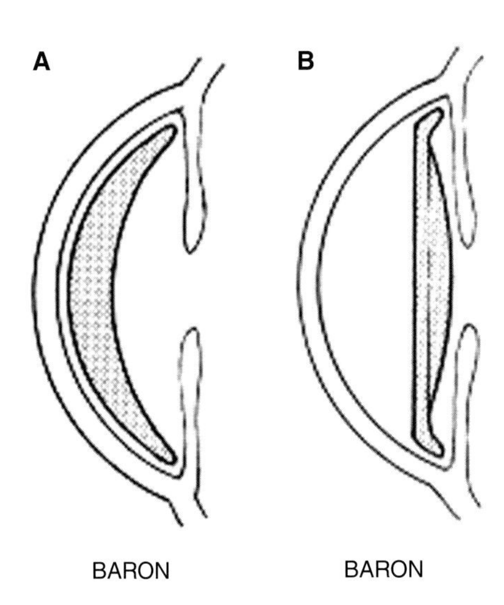

FIGURE 33-4 A, Original Baron anterior chamber lens, the very first anterior chamber lens. **B,** Baron plano-convex anterior chamber lens design.

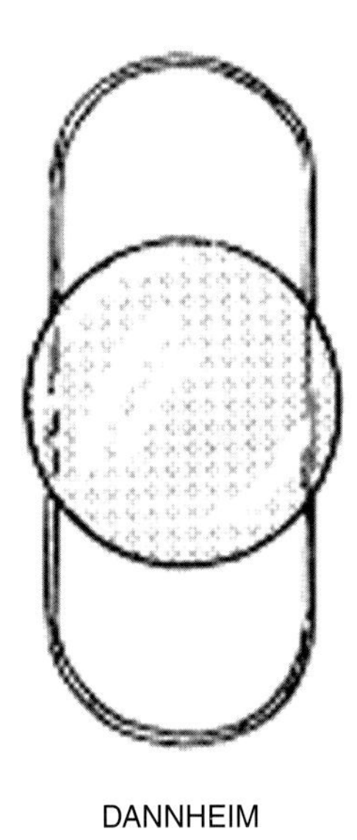

FIGURE 33-6 Original Dannheim closed-loop anterior chamber lens design.

use the lens in intracapsular and extracapsular surgery. The first to do this was Baron[10] of France on May 13, 1952. He designed a huge convexo-concave piece of plastic (Figure 33-4, *A*) that was 1-mm thick centrally and rested in (filled) the angle. It came into contact with the corneal endothelium with the expected results. He changed it to a plano-convex design (Figure 33-4, *B*) to no avail. Scharf[11] of Germany was next with his quadripodal design, which he first implanted on September 26, 1953. Then 2 days later, Strampelli[12] of Rome implanted the first of his designs (Figure 33-5), which looked like an Iolab Azar lens (B&L, San Dimas, Calif.) but was of solid plastic. Because of his early success and Choyce's later modifications of his original design, Strampelli has been credited with originating the anterior chamber IOL. Many got into the act after this. Schrek, Bietti and even Sir Harold with his own tripod design. It was Dannheim[13] of Germany who came up with the idea of a closed-loop haptic (Figure 33-6) using elastic-supporting loops made of supramide (similar to the Leiske lens [Surgidev] of the late 1970s and 1980s). Over 650 of these IOLs were implanted. Lieb and Guerry followed with a lens using three closed loops. Barraquer[14] of Barcelona removed half of each loop (Figure 33-7) of the Dannheim lens (giving it an S shape), creating the first open-loop lens, which was later used by Shearing of Las Vegas to create the first flexible-loop posterior chamber lens in the late 1970s. However, I'm jumping ahead. The primary result of all these early forays into the anterior chamber was bullous keratopathy, dissolving of supramide loops, and chronic inflammation, but the lenses did not dislocate into the vitreous.

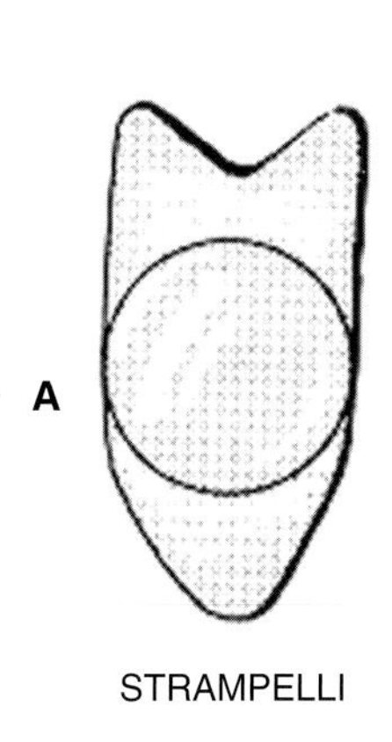

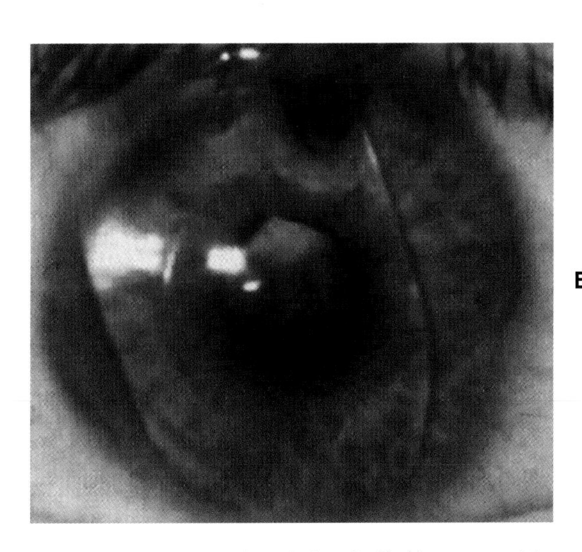

FIGURE 33-5 A, Original Strampelli tripod anterior chamber lens design. **B,** Phakic eye containing an original Strampelli anterior chamber lens.

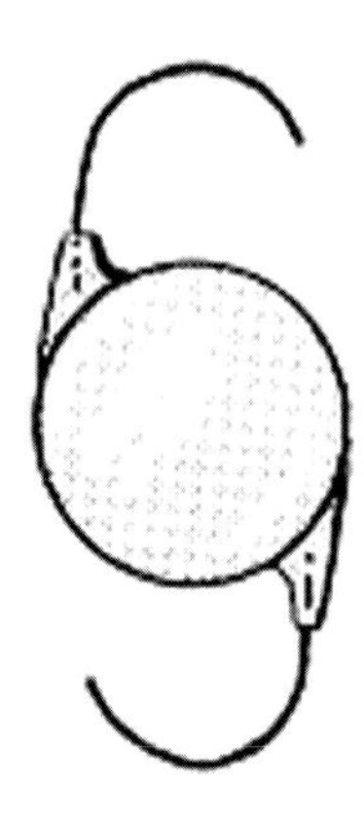

FIGURE 33-7 Original Barraquer open-loop anterior chamber lens design.

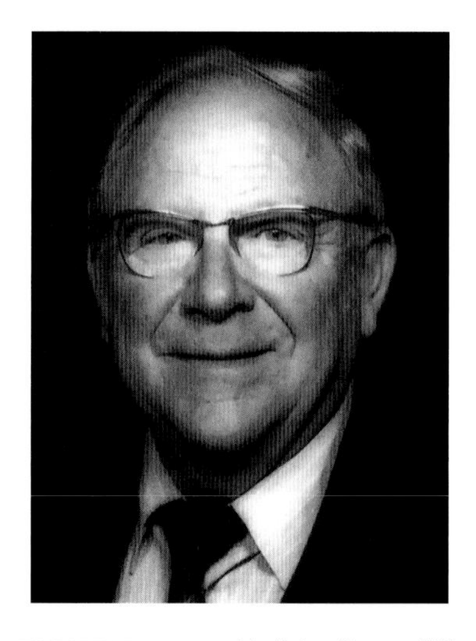

FIGURE 33-8 Mr. Peter Choyce, MD.

Choyce Era

D. Peter Choyce (Figure 33-8) (died August 8, 2001), who assisted Sir Harold in London, took up the Strampelli concept and implanted his first Choyce Mark I anterior chamber lens (Rayner) in 1956 (Figure 33-9, *A*). The Mark II to VIII (Figure 33-9, *B*) (including the final Mark IX) (Figure 33-9, *C*) designs modified the optic curvature and the form of the haptic feet and tips. He perfected the Strampelli design such that it became the very first IOL (Coburn Optical, Ind.) to receive FDA approval in the United States, for which he was justifiably proud. Jerrold Tennant of Dallas, Texas, patented the Choyce Mark VIII design in the United States and helped popularize the lens in America as an alternative to the American-made metal-looped prepupillary lenses (Figure 33-10), which were causing so many problems for intracapsular surgeons. Choyce never benefited financially from the success of his IOL designs. In the early 1980s, Charles Kelman took the Choyce design a step further to the designs we use today.

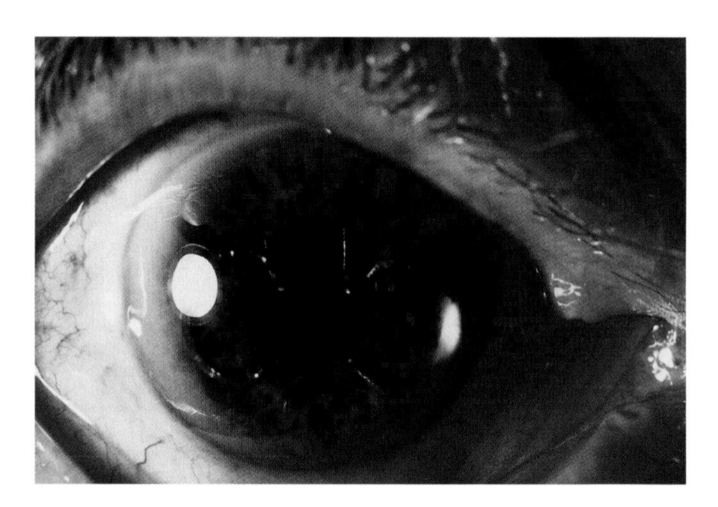

FIGURE 33-10 First patient ever to receive an American-made (McGhan) metal-loop intracapsular iris clip lens design by Dennis Shepard in 1976. The eye ultimately became blind after several years.

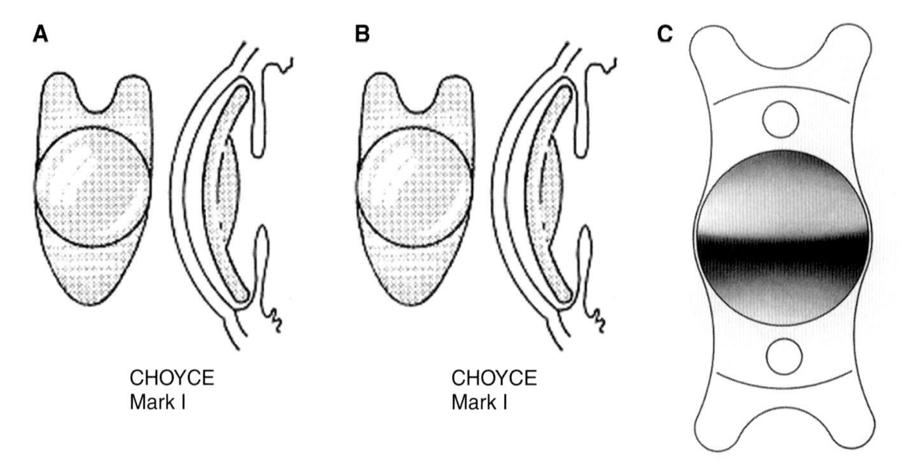

FIGURE 33-9 **A,** Choyce Mark I tripod anterior chamber lens design. **B,** Choyce Mark VIII quadripod anterior chamber lens design. **C,** Final Choyce Mark IX anterior chamber lens design.

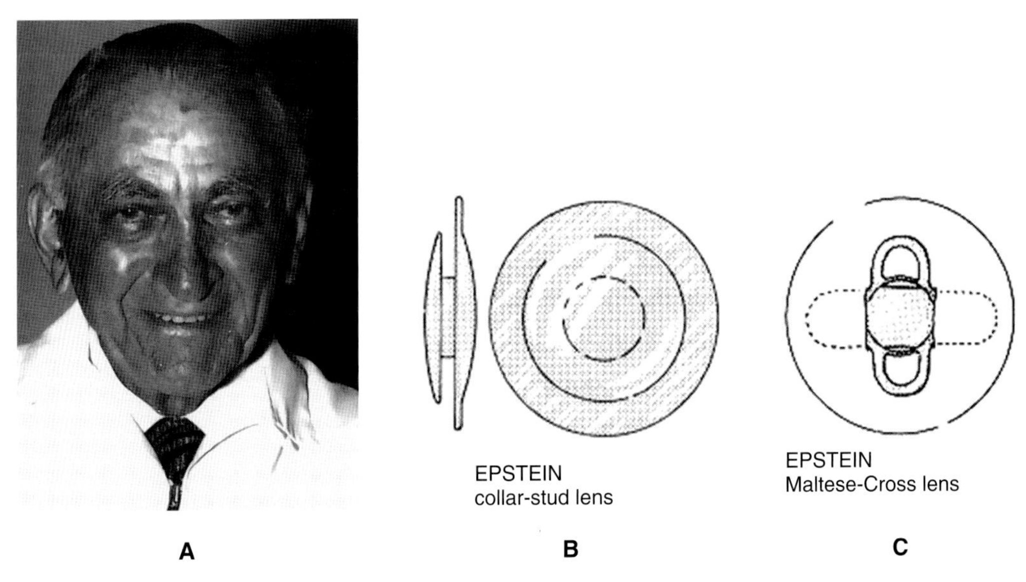

FIGURE 33-11 A, Dr. Edward Epstein. **B,** Epstein Collar-Stud pupil-fixated lens design. **C,** Epstein Maltese-Cross pupil-fixated lens design.

Edward Epstein (Figure 33-11, *A*) of Johannesburg, South Africa, had fairly good success with the original Ridley implant, but because of dislocations, he changed the design to fixate the lens using the pupil. He called this the Collar-Stud lens (see Figure 33-11, *B*) and implanted the first one in June 1953. After noting pigmentary glaucoma in a high percentage of the 40 eyes he had given implants, he switched to some anterior chamber designs and then developed the Maltese-Cross lens (see Figure 33-11, *C*). This lens had four plates (blades) extending from the optic. The anterior two were fenestrated, and the posterior two were solid. The pupil was woven around the plates such that the lens was held in the pupil. In America, at the instigation of Richard Troutman and Cornelius Binkhorst's brother Richard, the same design with four solid plates was produced by an optician named Michael Copeland and became known as the Copeland-Binkhorst lens. This lens was used prominently by many American surgeons such as Jaffe, Galin, Osher, and Hamdi. Epstein was never given credit for his design by his American copiers.

Binkhorst Era

Things were not looking good for lens implants in the late 1950s and 1960s, and many of the pioneers were abandoning their designs. The bad results led prominent ophthalmologists, especially in America, to deride and ridicule the entire concept. Statements such as "implanting such a foreign body is malpractice," "recklessness," "viciousness" (Derrick Vail, publicly to Ridley on the podium at the American Academy of Ophthalmology (AAO) after Ridley gave his invited lecture [Vail's remarks are published in the *Transactions of the American Academy of Ophthalmology and Otolaryngology,* January/February 1953]) and "intraocular time bomb" (Richard Troutman) caused many who might have been interested to be wary of joining this merry band. Sir Stewart Duke-Elder of London hated Ridley for what he had done, and he and Vail were very close friends. This public ridicule for his new idea caused much psychologic pain to Ridley, which led to depression for some time.

It was the integrity, pioneering perseverance, and intellectual and surgical acumen of one man that kept this subject alive to herald in the modern era. Cornelius Binkhorst (Figure 33-12, *A*), of Terneuzen, Holland, had learned lens implantation from Sir Harold in London and gradually believed there had to be a better way. He came up with a totally different design that he thought would prevent corneal decompensation, as well as posterior dislocation. He designed the prepupillary iris clip lens (see Figure 33-12, *B*) in 1957 and implanted the first one on August 11, 1958. They were manufactured by both Rayner and Kurt Morcher (Bad Cannstatt, Ebitzweg, Germany). He first presented this lens publicly in Middelburg on the Isle of Walcheren on October 3, 1958. The term "pseudophakia" to indicate the presence of an IOL was inaugurated by Binkhorst at Oxford in 1959. The 5 × 0.6 mm biconvex lens had two pairs of flexible supramide wire loops. The posterior pair was drilled into the posterior surface of the optic and bent at right angles to extend peripherally. They were inserted through the pupil and came to lie against the posterior surface of the iris, but they did not touch the ciliary body. The distance, loop tip to loop tip, was 7 mm, and they prevented the lens from moving forward. After being constricted, the pupil took the shape of a square with a diagonal length of 4 mm. The anterior loops were parallel to the posterior but 0.75 mm anterior to them. They were mounted on the equator of the optic and were adjacent to the anterior surface of the iris with a safe distance from the anterior chamber angle. The lens weighed 6 mg, compared with the Ridley lens at 112 mg.

In 1963, Fyodorov[15] (Figure 33-13) of Russia changed the relationship of the anterior and posterior loops from parallel to perpendicular, and it was known as the Binkhorst-Fyodorov lens, which became quite popular in America. He also published the first IOL power formula in 1967.

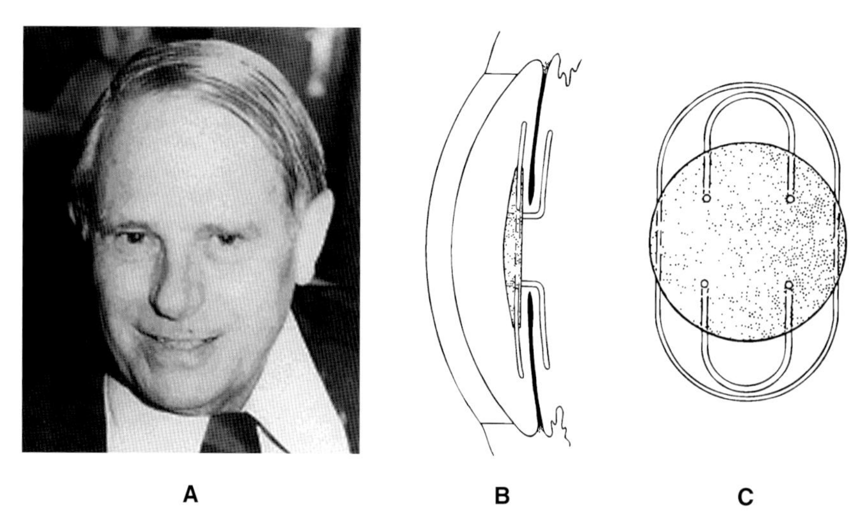

FIGURE 33-12 A, Dr. Cornelius D. Binkhorst. **B,** Binkhorst Iris Clip pupil-fixated lens design (side view). **C,** Iris-clip lens (front view).

Few realize that in 1967 the biconvex lens shape for IOLs was changed by Binkhorst to a simple convexo-plano shape at the suggestion of his brother Richard (New York) for the purpose of decreasing obstruction of aqueous flow through the pupil, increasing the accuracy of IOL power calculation, and theoretically lessening spherical aberration. By the 1970s, this became the shape of all IOLs until the American manufacturer Coburn Optical (later Storz, now Bausch & Lomb) came out with their first PMMA biconvex lens designs in the late 1980s. Although there were really no accounts of optical aberrations with the convexo-plano design, Holladay championed the biconvex design for the company, based on theoretical grounds, and it soon became the shape of all IOLs by all manufacturers today. Later, several published reports (including Atchison[16]) establishing that for PMMA lenses, the convexo-plano was the best optically and that biconvex was only superior in lenses made of silicone. Nothing changed, the die had been cast. In 1968 Fyodorov,[17] working with Zakharov, replaced the anterior loops with three equidistant small prongs (pintles) and changed the posterior loops from two to three. Because of its "antennae" appearance, it was called the Fyodorov Sputnik lens (see Figure 33-13, *B*). With the increase of posts in the pupil from four to six, the pupil took on a rounder shape when constricted. The lens only weighed 0.9 mg in aqueous and the design was quite successful for intracapsular and extracapsular implantation, but it was difficult to obtain them in America during the Cold War years.

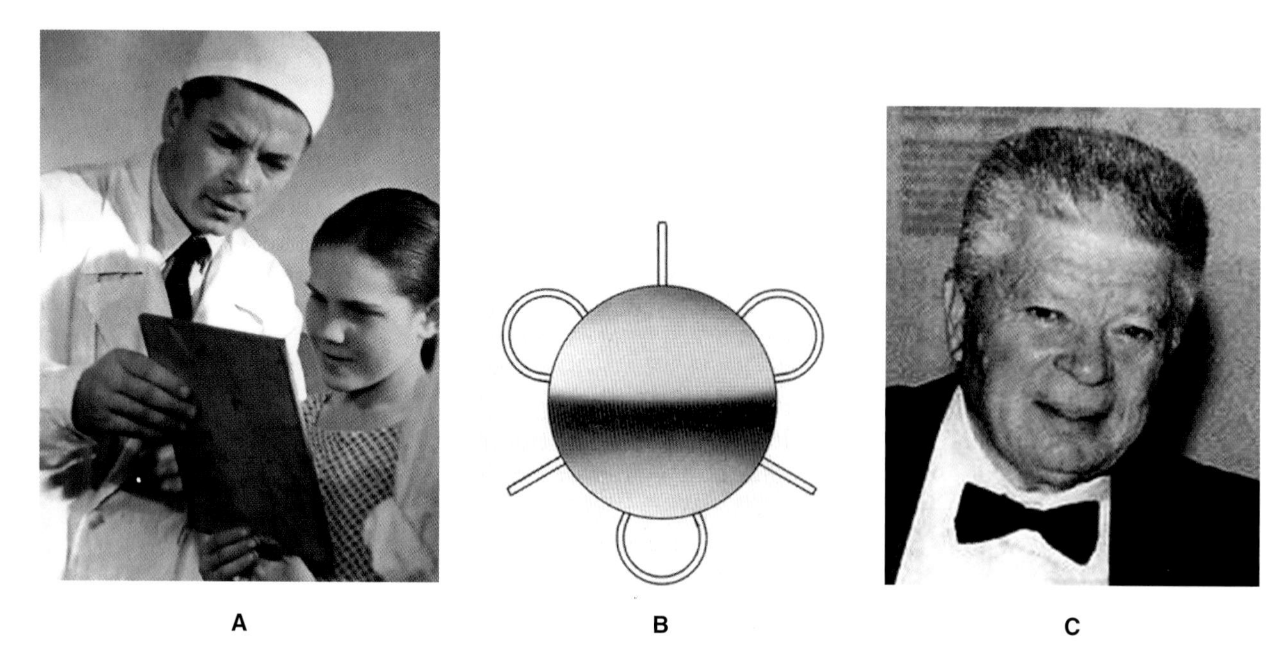

FIGURE 33-13 A, Dr. Syvataslav Fyodorov as a young surgeon in Archangel, Russia. **B,** Fyodorov-Zakharov pupil-fixated Sputnik lens design. **C,** Fyodorov in later life.

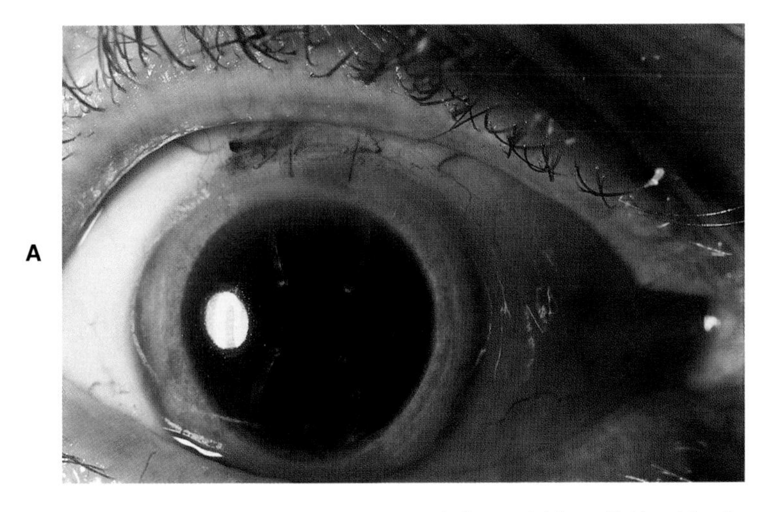

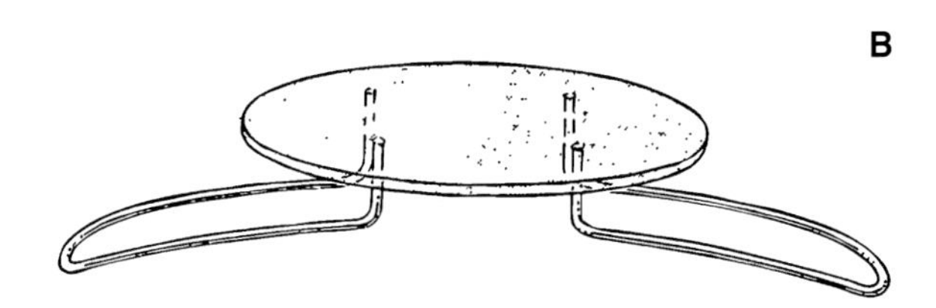

FIGURE 33-14 A, Eye containing a Binkhorst two-loop iridocapsular lens implant circa 1976. **B,** Binkhorst two-loop iridocapsular lens design.

To meet the demand, American manufacturers copied it, but they used heavier metal posterior loops and pintles that, because of their weight, caused tearing of the iris sphincter, chronic cystoid macular edema (CME), and dislocation, and the lens fell in popularity.

Various other changes were made in the iris clip lens from 1961 to 1971, but what really created the IOL revolution in the early 1970s was the change by Binkhorst[18] to his iridocapsular design (Figure 33-14) and the change by Jan Worst, his Dutch protégé, to his Medallion sutured lens (Figure 33-15, *A*).

Binkhorst originally designed the iridocapsular lens for use in children in 1965 but soon realized that it was the lens of choice for all eyes. The anterior loops of the iris clip lens were removed, and the posterior loops were changed to 0.15-mm platinum-iridium wire because they would be imbedded in iris and capsule tissue (he feared supramide could biodegrade over time like Dannheim lenses.) This increased the lens weight to 15.1 mg. He implanted the first style with supramide loops on September 16, 1965, and with metal loops on October 27, 1965. The two-loop lens became his lens of choice for all cataract cases by 1973. What is most interesting in the evolution of IOLs is that from the 1974 American Revolution of IOL surgery, Binkhorst advocated extracapsular surgery and the use of the two-loop lens. His successes were the basis for the rapid interest in IOLs in America, but Americans ignored Binkhorst's advice and proceeded with intracapsular designs such as the iris clip and Copeland lenses. Phacoemulsification was completely ignored by most IOL surgeons because the "incision had to be extended to get the lens in."

Jan Worst, of Groningen, Holland attempted to eliminate the anterior loops and replaced them with a flat, thin superior plate extension of the optic with two holes to allow the lens to be sutured to the superior iris. It was called the Worst Medallion lens (Medical Workshop, Groningen, Holland) (see Figure 33-15, *A*), and he implanted the first one on December 18, 1970. His success added to the enthusiasm and excitement in America in 1974. Worst made several other designs with iridectomy clipping devices (Platina, 1973) (see Figure 33-15, *B*) and recommended stainless steel sutures for fixation. These ideas were not as popular in America.

So far I have liberally relied on the first textbook on IOLs by Marcel Nordlohne[19] (Figure 33-16) in 1975 for many of these

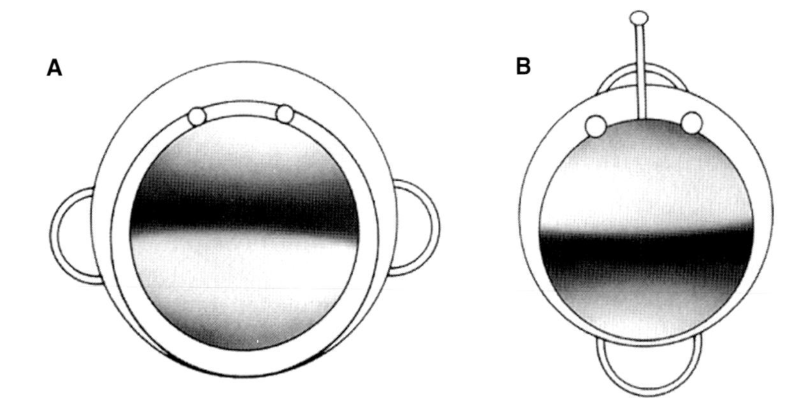

FIGURE 33-15 A, Worst Medallion sutured pupil-fixated lens design. **B,** Worst Platina iridectomy clip pupil-fixated lens design.

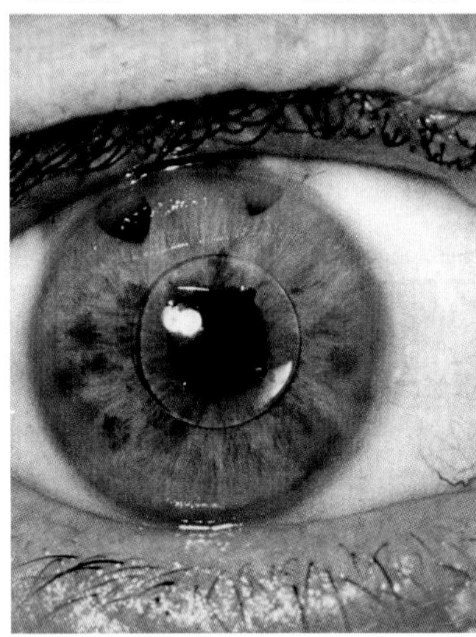

FIGURE 33-16 The cover of the first IOL textbook by Nordlohne (Junk Publishers) in 1975.

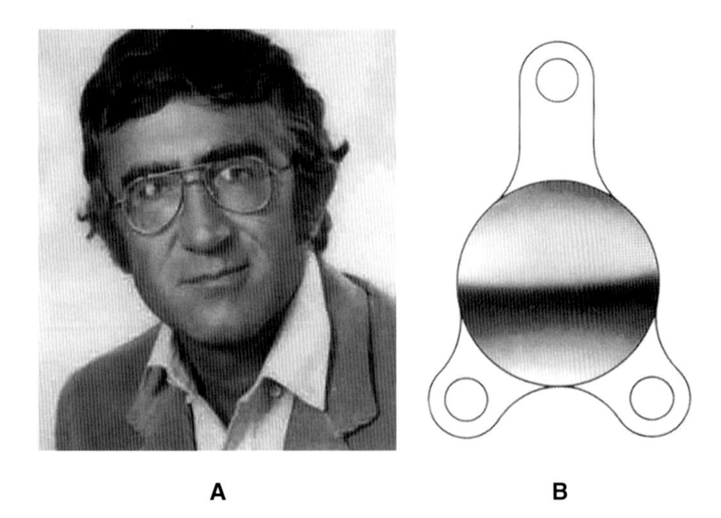

FIGURE 33-17 **A,** Mr. John L. Pearce, MD. **B,** Original Pearce tripod posterior chamber lens design.

historical facts and subsequently relied on the excellent textbook on IOLs by David Apple.[20]

The Revolution: 1970s

The 1970s were the decade of revolution and change in IOL surgery. It began with the use of the lenses such as the Copeland, Binkhorst iris clip, Sputnik, iridocapsular, and Choyce Mark VIII and ended with the Simcoe and Shearing posterior chamber lenses.

Posterior Chamber Era

Through most of the 1970s, two camps of lens implanters developed: those performing intracapsular surgery and using their favorite IOL design (90%) and those (including myself) using phacoemulsification and implanting the iridocapsular lens (10%). In 1975, John Pearce[21] (Figure 33-17, *A*) of England took the lead back into the posterior chamber with his one-piece PMMA tripod lens (see Figure 33-17, *B*). James Little of Oklahoma City and Eric Arnott of London followed suit with their design and later so did William Harris of Dallas in 1977. Things were rather quiet until 1977, when Shearing[22] of Las Vegas advocated implanting a flexible-loop Barraquer anterior chamber lens into the posterior chamber and called it "ciliary body" (later ciliary sulcus) fixation. Several prominent phacoemulsification trainers in California, such as Richard Kratz and Robert Sinskey, began using the Shearing lens (Model 101, Iolab Corp.) (Figure 33-18, *A*) and teaching it in their courses. The loops were stiff and in the shape of the letter J. Often the lens would become trapped in the pupil, so at the suggestion of Kratz (Iolab ignored Shearing's previous request to do this[23]), the loops were angulated 10 degrees anteriorly to keep the optic posterior to the pupil. This was the very first modification of this posterior chamber IOL and was given the name Model 101K because Kratz refused to attach his name to it. What many will find surprising is that the next modification ever made to this posterior chamber IOL was the addition of the Hoffer[24] ridge to the optic, and for the same reason it was called the Model 101H (see Figure 33-29, *C*).

Through the early and mid-1980s, it became increasing evident that the posterior chamber lens should be implanted completely in the capsular bag to eliminate all contact with uveal tissue. The stiffness of the loops and the jagged "can opener" capsulotomy made this technically difficult. In the same year as Shearing (1977) (or perhaps earlier), William Simcoe of Tulsa designed long sweeping loops (Figure 33-19, *A*) that came off the lens optic at a very low angle rather than perpendicular so that they were very flexible and could be "dialed" into the capsular bag. Simcoe and others later recommended shortening the loops so that they took on the shape of the letter C (see Figure 33-19, *B* and *C*).

Shearing had obtained a method patent for his design and, in attempting to protect his intellectual property, filed legal actions against all the manufacturers making a posterior chamber lens that were not licensed. In their defense, these manufacturers used Simcoe's story of having really been the first to implant a posterior chamber lens when he cut off the posterior loops and snipped the anterior loops of an iris clip lens and implanted them into the capsular bag before Shearing's patent. These court battles were notorious and contentious and even led to a podium fistfight, as well as the exhumation of the body of a patient in whom Simcoe claimed to have inserted such an implant (the family was paid to exhume the body).[23] The claimed lens was not found, but Simcoe states that the hospital records were in disarray and that it would be impossible to know which patients had received these initial lenses. Perhaps we will never know who was first.

All posterior chamber lenses had loops of supramide and latter Prolene. In the mid-1980s, Wayne Callahan* used computer

Presently of ThinOptX, Abington, Virginia.

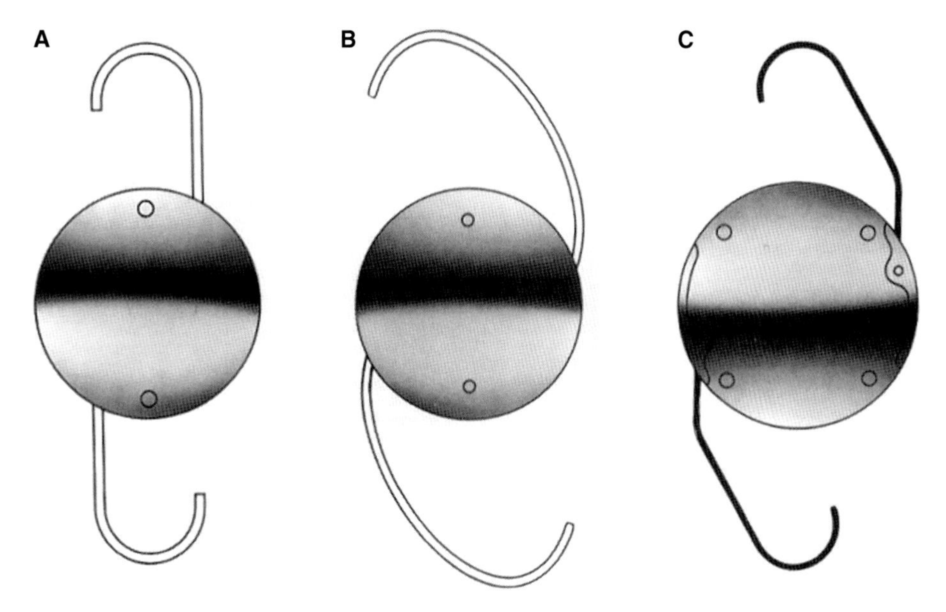

FIGURE 33-18 Shearing flexible-loop posterior chamber lens designs. **A,** Original Shearing stiff J loop. **B,** "Sinskey" soft J loop. **C,** Kratz-Johnson crimped J loop.

lathes (Cilco, Huntington, WVa.; now Alcon Surgical, Ft. Worth, Tex.) to fashion the first all-PMMA one-piece posterior chamber lenses. They were stiff and thick in the early models, but as development proceeded, they became thin and flexible. The Jaffe, Arnott,[25] and Bechert designs (with Hoffer ridges) became popular throughout the 1980s (Figure 33-20).

In 1980, Kratz asked Iolab to make a crimp in the J loop (to decrease its stiffness) but refused to allow his name to be used on the lens model, so Iolab called it the Sinskey lens[23] (see Figure 33-18, *B*). Later, other manufacturers copied this "soft-J" design, and they were called the Kratz and Kratz-Johnson lenses (see Figure 33-18, *C*). Other posterior chamber designs such as the Anis lens (Figure 33-21, *A*) and the Galand disc lens (Figure 33-21, *B*) were defining the future direction of lens design until the foldable lenses caused their demise.

The 1980s Anterior Chamber Lens Disaster

The use of anterior chamber lenses continued throughout the 1980s and became extremely popular with intracapsular surgeons, especially when problems with American-manufactured iris-supported lenses (with metal loops [see Figure 33-10]) became an issue. Choyce slimmed down the Mark VIII to the Mark IX in 1978. American manufacturers copied the Mark VIII lens, and most were poorly made and poorly polished, leading

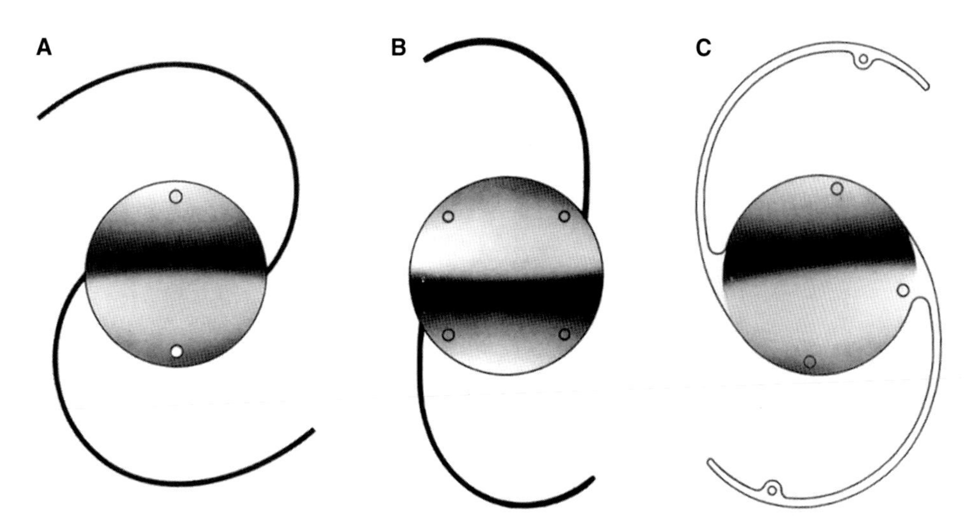

FIGURE 33-19 Simcoe flexible-loop posterior chamber lens designs. **A,** Original Simcoe wide C loop. **B,** Modified short C loop. **C,** One-piece PMMA C-loop lens.

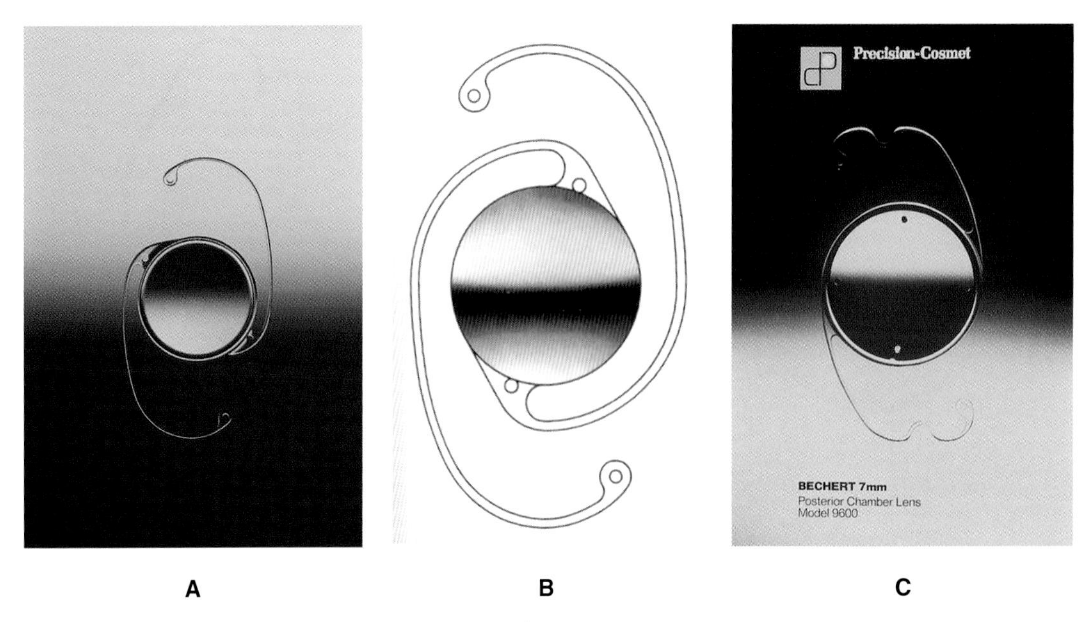

FIGURE 33-20 **A,** Jaffe short, encircling loop, all-PMMA one-piece lens with Hoffer ridge. **B,** Arnott large, encircling loop, all-PMMA one-piece lens. **C,** Bechert all-PMMA one-piece 7-mm lens design with Hoffer ridge.

to the Ellingson uveitis-glaucoma-hyphema syndrome.[26] In 1977, Robert Azar of New Orleans came out first with a copy of the Strampelli lens with the letters of his last name embossed as molded projections on the surface of the optic, lest someone forget who designed it. He later (1982) changed the design to one with closed loops, called the Azar 91Z (Iolab) (Figure 33-22, *A*), to compete with the Leiske closed-loop lens (Figure 33-22, *B*), both of which became extremely popular in the United States.

Other surgeons designed closed-loop designs (see Figure 33-22) fashioned after the original Dannheim lens. History was repeating itself by those unfamiliar with it or totally willing to ignore its lessons. Lens designs such as the Leiske (1978, Surgidev), Shepard (1979), Hessberg (1981, Intermedics), Dubroff (1981), Optiflex (1981), Feaster (1982), Stableflex (1983, Optical Radiation Corp.), and the Copeland anterior chamber lens (see Figure 33-22, *B* through *G*) were being implanted in great numbers throughout the United States. Many of these lenses ultimately led to multiple complications and had to be removed, often during a corneal transplantation for bullous keratopathy. These designers were all committed to the concept that a one-size anterior chamber lens could fit eyes of all sizes, to the detriment of many patients.

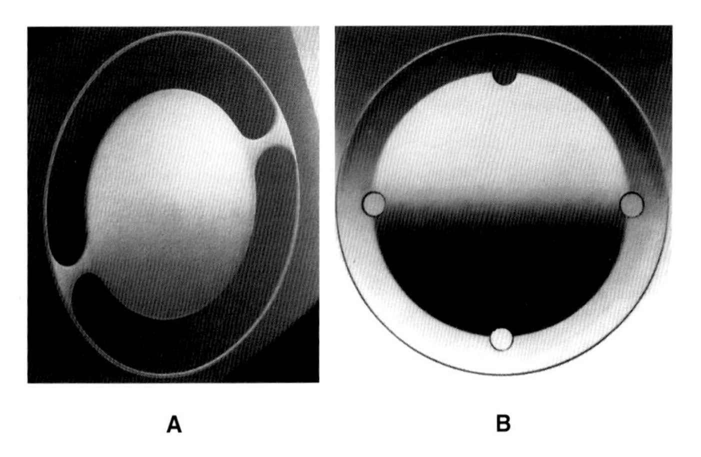

FIGURE 33-21 Later "Ridleyesque" posterior chamber lens designs. **A,** Anis large closed-circle lens. **B,** Galland disc lens design.

During the same period, Charles Kelman[27] of New York (Figure 33-23, *H*), the inventor of phacoemulsification, refrained from implanting IOLs. He finally gave in and designed an anterior chamber lens tripod (by "cutting the plastic out of it" [similar to the attempt by Boberg-Ans in 1961]). It was made of solid PMMA lathe-cut in the shape of a "pregnant 7," with an optic of 4.5 mm and special foot plates to impinge in the angle that he first implanted in 1978. The first to make this lens was Precision-Cosmet of Minnesota (Figure 33-23, *A*). A slight modification was later made by Heyer-Schulte (Irvine, Calif. [later AMO]), and they improved it to the Omnifit in 1981 (see Figures 33-23, *B* and *C*). Collaborating with Wayne Callahan at Cilco, Kelman designed the extremely flexible Quadriflex (1981) quadripodal design, which later was modified to the Multiflex I (1982) (see Figures 33-23, *D* and *E*). Both had four-point angle fixation with the haptics coming off the same side of the lens optic. The former looked like a "pregnant E," but the haptics of the Multiflex were unique in that their design allowed internal flexion in the same plane as the haptics without forward movement of the optic. This was the answer and is now the basis for all safe anterior chamber lenses used today. When a high incidence of optic entrapment by the pupil was noted, Kelman directed that the haptics should exit the lens optic from opposite sides, and these became the S-flex and the Multiflex II (see Figure 33-23, *F*). The most unique attribute of the Multiflex II was that Cilco originally made the lens in seven different sizes (see Figure 33-23, *G*), from 11.5 to 14.5 mm (in 0.5-mm steps), so that any size eye could be fitted safely without making the eye

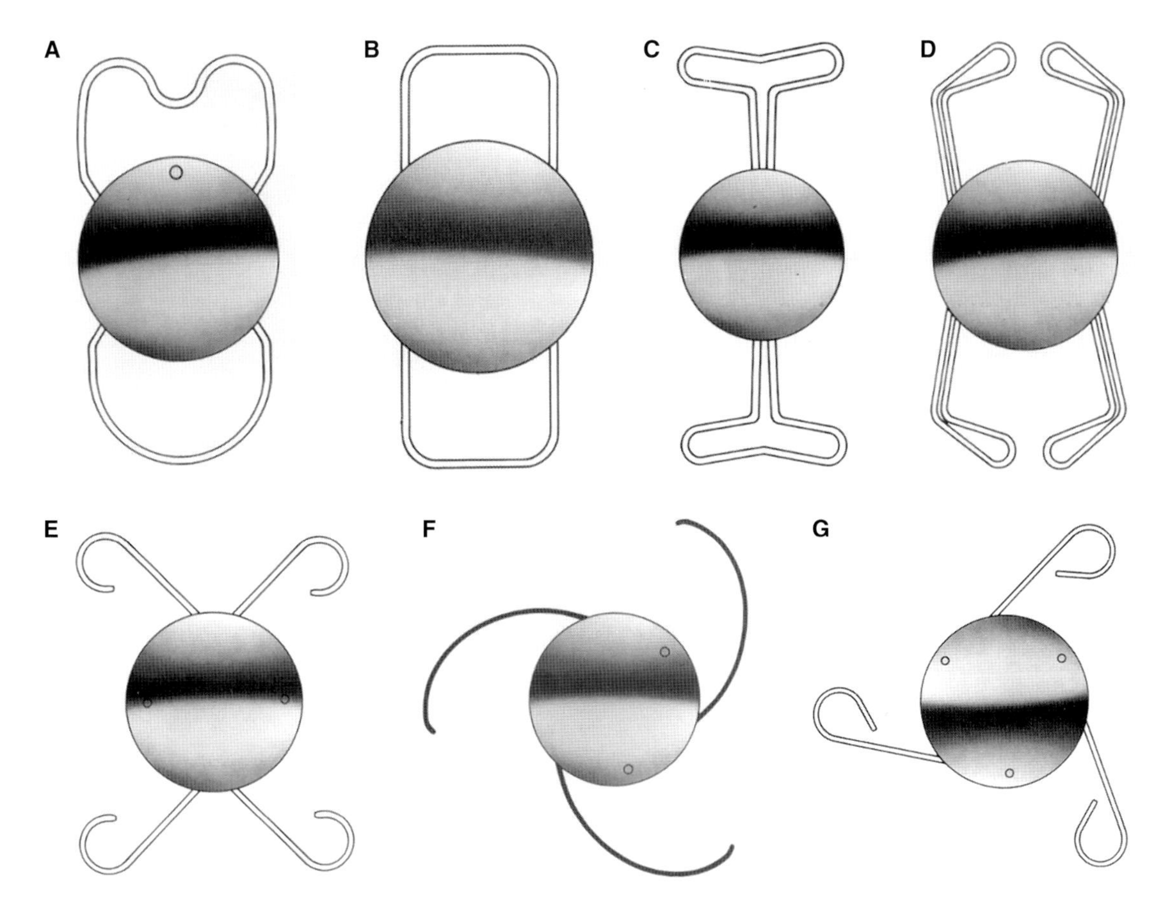

FIGURE 33-22 The troublesome closed-loop anterior chamber lenses. **A,** Azar 91Z lens (1982). **B,** Leiske lens (1978). **C,** Hessberg lens (1981). **D,** Stableflex lens (1983). **E,** Shepard lens (1979). **F,** Dubroff lens (1981). **G,** Copeland anterior chamber lens (1982).

withstand the constant pressure of an oversized lens. This was never repeated by any other company. It has always been my theory that if this had been done with all the closed-loop anterior chamber lenses, the disasters they caused might have been prevented. The "one-size-fits-all" anterior chamber lens goal was a cause of untold loss of sight by the surgeons who experimented with it.

Kelman always strongly advocated precise horizontal corneal diameter measurement and intraoperative gonioscopy to ensure proper sizing during the procedure. This advice was ignored by most implanting surgeons to their peril. For intracapsular cataract extraction (ICCE), secondary and backup implantations, I switched from the Rayner Choyce Mark VIII to the Cilco Kelman Multiflex II in 1983 and, following Kelman's teachings, have not had to remove a Multiflex II that was personally implanted for any reason.

Phakic Intraocular Lenses to Correct Ametropia

Jan Worst designed his iris plane Lobster Claw lens for aphakia in 1976, which sat on the surface of the iris and was fixated by two haptic claws that imbricated the anterior stroma of the iris in the nondilating midperiphery portion. This lens was used extensively in Europe, India, and Pakistan for aphakia and today is being used in a different version as a phakic IOL for the correction of refractive errors (Artisan Lens, Ophtec, Fla.) (Figure 33-24, *A*). Undeterred by the failures of Strampelli, Barraquer, and many other early pioneers who attempted to use anterior chamber lenses in phakic eyes, Georges Baikoff of Marseilles, France, modified the Multiflex II lens for the same purpose, beginning with the Domilens ZB lens (see Figure 33-24, *B*). This was later changed to the B&L Nuvita lens (see Figure 33-24, *C*) and ultimately the CIBA Vision Vivere lens, which has PMMA haptics but an acrylic foldable optic that is multifocal (see Figure 33-24, *D*). In the 1980s, Fyodorov and Zuev were working on phakic IOLs for the posterior chamber, starting with the Mushroom pupillary centering lens, which ultimately led to the Staar ICL (Collamer) (see Figure 33-25, *A*), and the Medennium PRL (Silicone) (Figure 33-25, *B* and *C*), which was developed by Dr. Dimitrii Dementiev (see Figure 33-25, *D*) of Milano, Italy.

Small Incision Era

Phacoemulsifiers always disliked enlarging their small, 3.5-mm incision to implant a 6 to 7-mm solid PMMA optic IOL. What was needed was a lens optic that could be folded and enter the 3.5-mm incision.

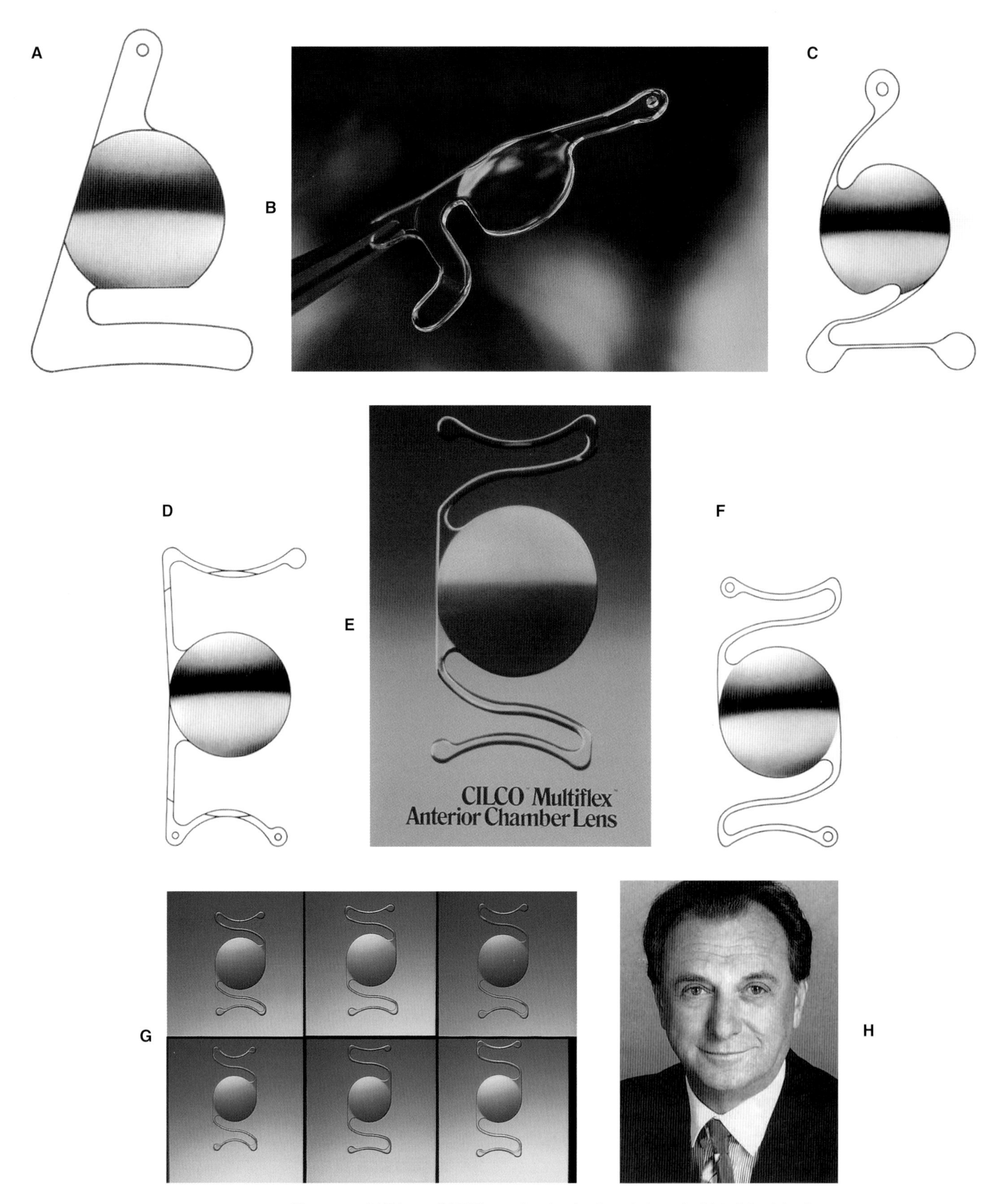

FIGURE 33-23 The successful Kelman all-PMMA anterior chamber lens designs. **A,** Original Precision-Cosmet "pregnant-7" tripod lens (1978). **B,** Heyer-Schulte tripod design. **C,** AMO Omnifit tripod lens. **D,** Cilco Quadriflex lens (1981). **E,** Cilco Multiflex I lens. **F,** Cilco Multiflex II lens (1982). **G,** Six (of seven) different sizes of the Cilco Multiflex II lens (note difference in design between the shortest and the longest). **H,** Charles D. Kelman, MD.

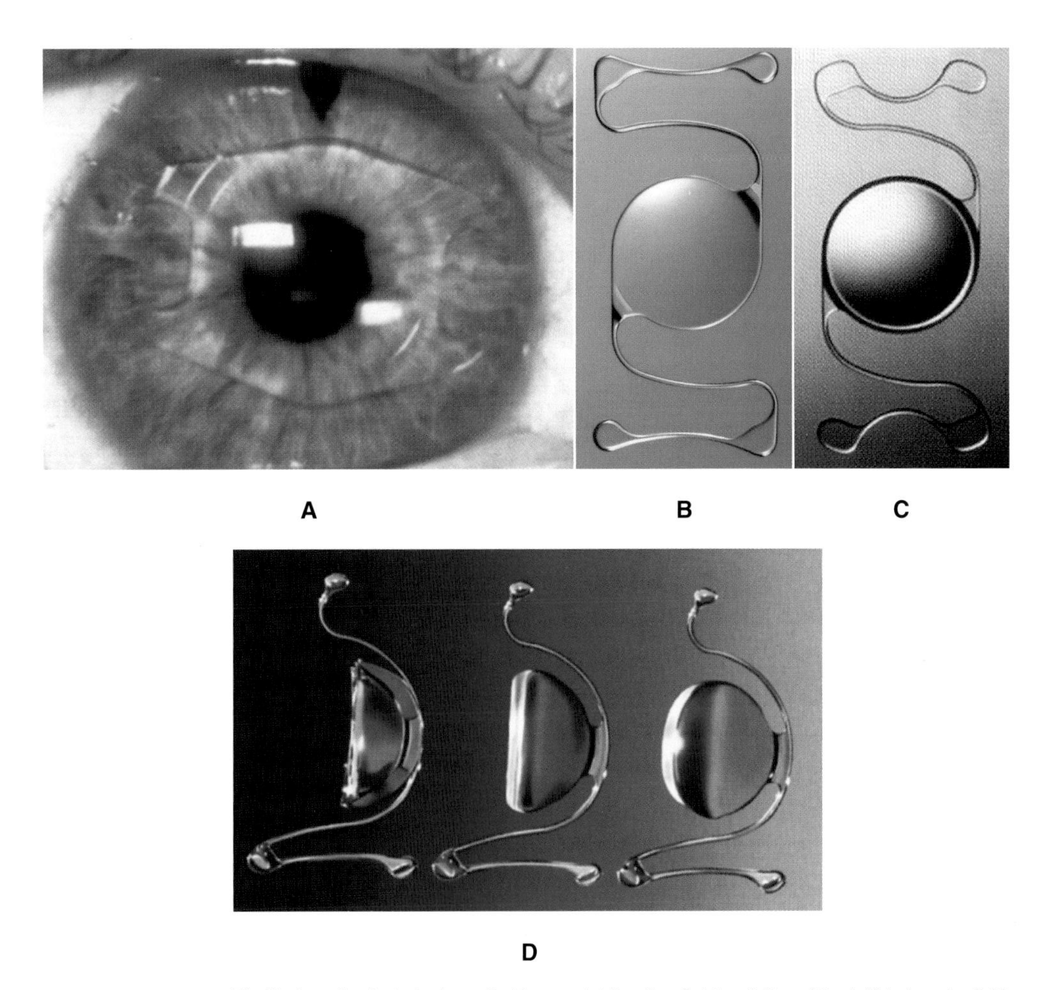

FIGURE 33-24 Phakic lens implant designs. **A,** Eye containing the Ophtec Artisan Worst "lobster claw" iris-supported lens. **B,** Original Baikoff Domilens ZB anterior chamber lens. **C,** Baikoff B&L Nuvita anterior chamber lens. **D,** Latest Baikoff foldable-optic acrylic/PMMA CIBA Vision Vivere anterior chamber lens.

In the mid-1970s, Keiki Mehta[28] (Figure 33-26) of Bombay, India, fabricated iris clip lenses using silicone for the optic with no intention of folding them. He told me what he was doing at the time and 10 years later told how they all turned yellow with time and he abandoned their use. In the early 1980s, Edward Epstein started making posterior chamber IOLs of silicone with the intention of folding them. But when Thomas Mazzacco (Van Nys, Calif.) (see Figure 33-26) began folding and implanting plate haptic silicone IOLs (Staar Surgical, Covina, Calif.) through a 3.5-mm phaco incision, the world of lens implantation was about to change forever. From this point on, the popularity of phacoemulsification went from 40% to 95%. At first, they didn't ensure that the lenses were entirely in the capsular bag, and complications ensued. Around 1981, Calvin Fercho[29] of Fargo, ND (see Figure 33-27, *A*), invented the complete circular capsulorhexis (later to be popularized by Thomas Neuhann [Munich, Germany] and Howard Gimble [Calgary, Canada] while Fercho was undergoing prostate cancer treatment) (see Figure 33-27, *B*). It soon became apparent that the plate haptic silicone lens worked best if placed entirely in the capsular bag with an intact, round central capsulorhexis of adequate size. The FDA only approved it with this stipulation.

Viscoelastics

Endre Balazs[30] began the research on using hyaluronic acid as a replacement for vitreous. Soon David Miller (Boston) and Roger Stegman (South Africa) began talking about its use for anterior segment surgery. Balazs presented his work at the 1979 AAO meeting in San Francisco. It just so happened that the AAO had asked me to be the discussant for that paper. After giving my presentation, in which I cautiously lauded the idea, I recommended that it be supplied in a preset syringe ready for use in all cataract surgery. I also warned of antigenicity and intraocular pressure rise. After sitting down, I was approached by two gentlemen from Pharmacia (of Sweden) who asked if I would be interested in doing some research with their new product called Healon. When I agreed, I soon received vials of Healon and performed the first phacoemulsification/IOL viscosurgery in America in late 1979. I was soon using it for every cataract surgery I performed. After 6 months of excellent results (except for temporary rises in intraocular pressure), I warned the company that they had better be well prepared with a huge supply before they bring it to the market because I

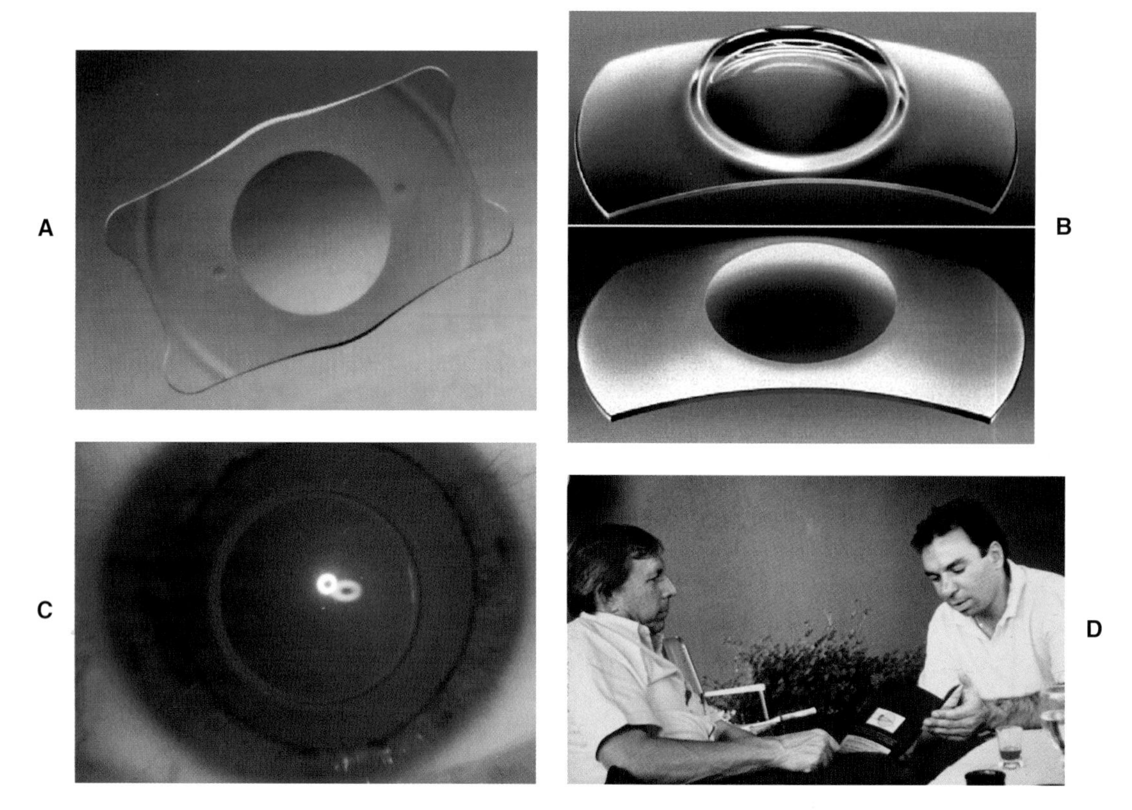

FIGURE 33-25 Phakic posterior chamber lens implant designs. **A,** Staar ICL. **B,** Medennium myopic (upper) and hyperopic (lower) PRL lenses. **C,** Eye containing myopic Medennium PRL. **D,** The author (Dr. Kenneth Hoffer) with Dr. Dimitrii D. Dementiev (designer of PRL) in Milano, Italy.

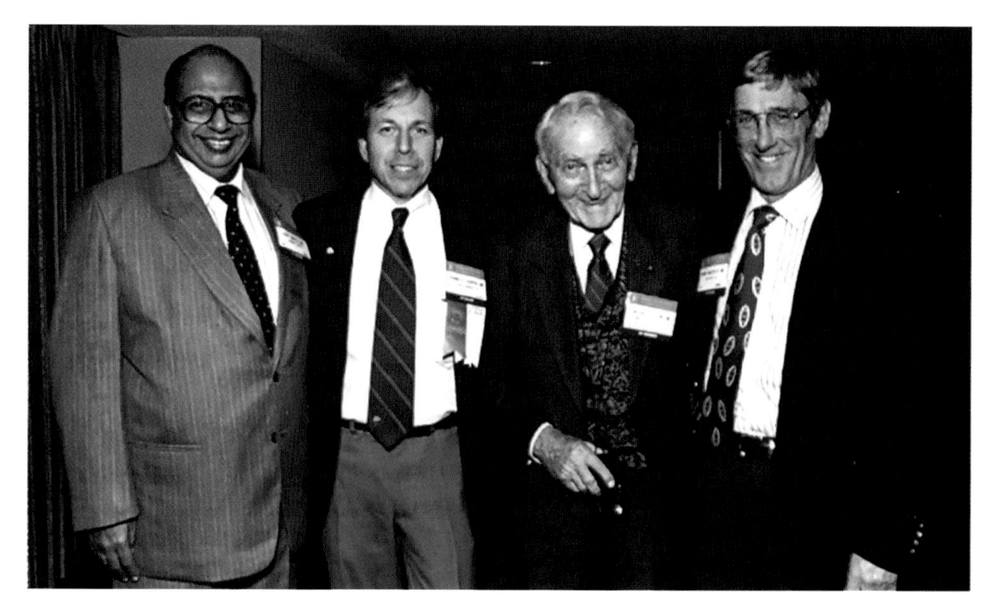

FIGURE 33-26 The silicone pioneers. *Left to right:* Drs. Keiki Mehta, Kenneth Hoffer (the author), Edward Epstein, and Thomas Mazzacco.

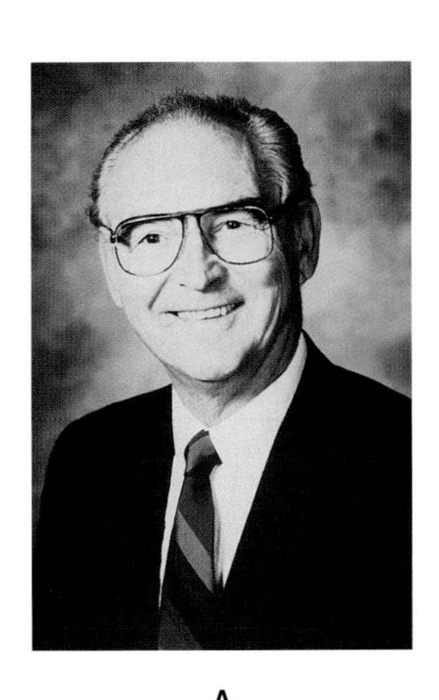

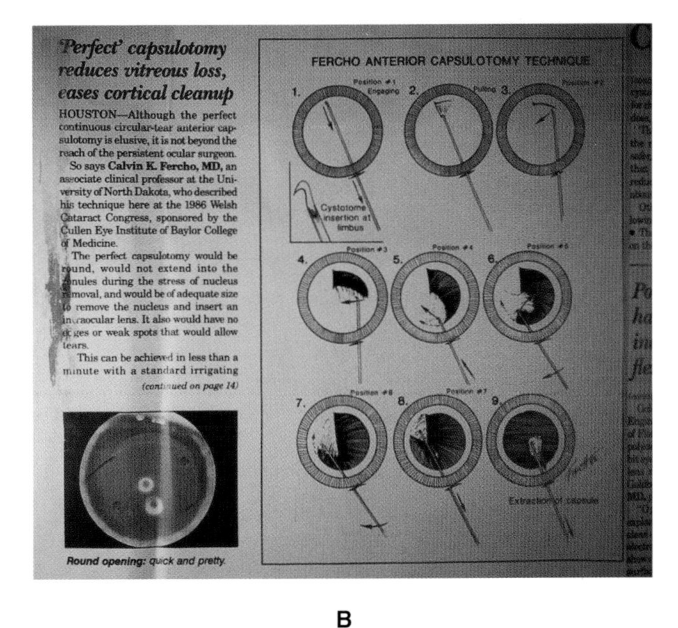

'Perfect' capsulotomy reduces vitreous loss, eases cortical cleanup

HOUSTON—Although the perfect continuous circular-tear anterior capsulotomy is elusive, it is not beyond the reach of the persistent ocular surgeon.

So says **Calvin K. Fercho, MD,** an associate clinical professor at the University of North Dakota, who described his technique here at the 1986 Welsh Cataract Congress, sponsored by the Cullen Eye Institute of Baylor College of Medicine.

The perfect capsulotomy would be round, would not extend into the zonules during the stress of nucleus removal, and would be of adequate size to remove the nucleus and insert an intraocular lens. It also would have no edges or weak spots that would allow tears.

This can be achieved in less than a minute with a standard irrigating

(continued on page 14)

Round opening: quick and pretty.

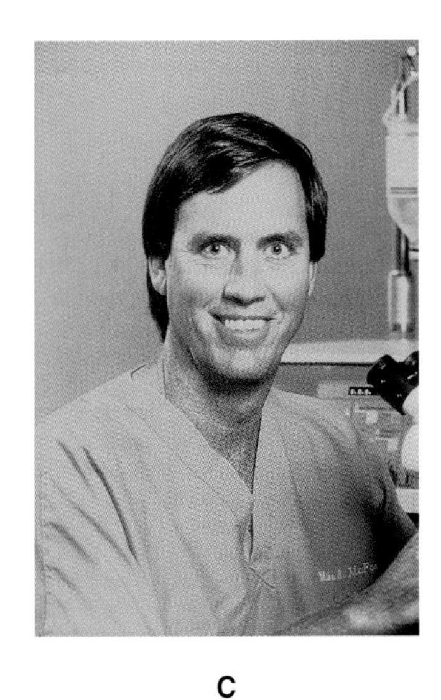

A B C

FIGURE 33-27 Cataract surgery innovators. **A,** Dr. Calvin Fercho. **B,** *Ocular Surgery News* article (November 15, 1986) first to describe *circular capsulotomy.* **C,** Dr. Michael McFarland.

believed that it would become the standard in cataract surgery immediately. They did not follow my advice, and 6 months after its introduction, they were back-ordered on the product for almost a year. In that intervening period, many surgeons looked for ways to bring about the same result without the expense of Healon. Needless to say, everyone is aware of the profound effect Healon and subsequent viscoelastics have had on the safety and ease of lens implant surgery.

Chronic Developments

Probably the most important development for cataract and lens implant surgery was the introduction of the Zeiss motorized zoom microscope in 1965 to allow surgeons to see the red reflex while operating. The first motorized zoom, focus, and X-Y controls were introduced in 1970. This had a great effect on the increasing use of extracapsular surgery.

Based on the experience of James Gills of Tarpon Springs, Florida, many surgeons abandoned the routine use of a peripheral iridectomy with posterior chamber lenses during the 1980s. Michael McFarland (see Figure 33-27,*C*) of Pinebluff, Arkansas, first proposed the concept of self-sealing sutureless incisions, and Howard Fine popularized making the incision in clear corneal surgery. In 1990, John Shepherd[31] of Las Vegas invented the in-the-bag fracturing, hydration, and quartering of the nucleus for phacoemulsification, later popularized by Gimble and others. All these advances made the surgery simpler and safer, as well as shortened the recovery time for the eye dramatically.

One of the most interesting developments was the elimination of retrobulbar injections. R.M. Redmond[32] of Belfast, Northern Ireland, had written a paper in April 1990 about performing extracapsular cataract surgery using local anesthesia without a retrobulbar injection (Figure 33-28, *A*). After reading the paper, I invited him to present his experience at my IOL Course[33] at the AAO Meeting in October 1991 (Figure 33-28, *B*). Many prominent cataract surgeons were also lecturing at or attending this course, and Redmond's presentation drew excited interest. Soon there followed many surgeons attempting topical anesthetics for IOL surgery, especially with clear corneal incisions. Redmond Smith of London had also eliminated retrobulbar injections since April of 1985. He also eliminated O'Brien lid akinesia as well in June 1987 and used a locking speculum to prevent the patient from blinking. Gills recommended intraocular Xylocaine in addition to the topical anesthetic.

In 1979 Barasch and Poler[34] tried making IOL optics out of glass. This was done by Lynell, Inc., and they used a new polymer, Elastimide, to fashion haptics to hold the glass optic. Because of the increased index of refraction of glass, the lenses were very thin. When the yttrium-aluminum-garnet (YAG) laser caused several of these lenses to crack inside the eye, the FDA recalled them. Staar Surgical used the Elastimide material for the haptics of their three-piece silicone posterior chamber lenses.

Acrylic lenses were the next logical offshoot from research into optical-quality materials that could be folded like silicone. The edge architecture of the original popular models caused persistent haloes (because of acrylic's higher index of refraction) in a sporadic but persistent number of extremely unhappy patients. After many years of ignoring the issue, Alcon finally made changes in the edge design in the newer acrylic lens styles, but there are still reports of this nagging phenomenon.

YAG Laser and Lens Design

The annoying surgical posterior capsulotomy became outdated when Aron-Rosa[35] of Paris and Fankhauser[36] of Switzerland

A

Extracapsular cataract extraction under local anaesthesia without retrobulbar injection

R M Redmond, N L Dallas

Abstract
Day-case cataract surgery and the need for local anaesthesia are likely to increase. Retrobulbar (and peribulbar) anaesthetic injection is a common technique in cataract surgery, but serious complications are persistently reported. Subconjunctival injection is an alternative that avoids these risks. This retrospective study compares two groups of patients that underwent extracapsular cataract surgery under local anaesthetic. One group (retrobulbar) had uncomplicated retrobulbar injection with bupivicaine and hyaluronidase. The other group (non-retrobulbar) had superior bulbar, subconjunctival infiltration

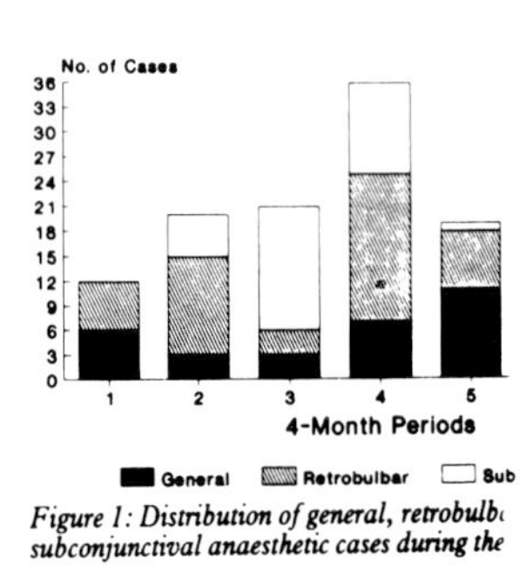

Figure 1: Distribution of general, retrobulb… subconjunctival anaesthetic cases during the

Patients and methods

ACADEMY Instruction Courses — Tue OCT 15, 1991

Course 261 **Room: CTR – B2**
Periods 2 through 5 *9:45 AM – 4:15 PM*
Modern Phaco/ECCE Implant Surgery: 1991 †
Kenneth J Hoffer, MD, Santa Monica, CA; Bradley R Straatsma, MD, Los Angeles, CA; David B Davis II, MD, Hayward, CA; R D Redmond, MD, Belfast, Northern Ireland; William F Maloney, MD, Vista, CA; Thomas V Cravy, MD, Santa Maria, CA; Stephen A Obstbaum, MD, New York, NY; Calvin K Fercho, MD, Fargo, SD; Howard V Gimbel, MD, Calgary, AB, Canada; Thomas Neuhann, MD, Munich, West Germany; David J Apple, MD, Charleston, SC; Aziz Y Anis, MD, Lincoln, NE; R M Redmond, MD, London, England

This course will cover, step-by-step, the latest techniques and options available to achieve 100% in-the-bag IOL placement using either ECCE or Phaco and any size incision and lens style. Due to its rise in popularity, there will be an emphasis on phacoemulsification. Preop and postop considerations will be covered as well as IOL designs, preventing power errors, incision control, and newer ideas in handling vitreous encounters. Practical clinical information will be stressed in areas such as anesthesia, incisions, capsulorrhexis, hydrodissection, nuclear cracking, lens insertion techniques, and incision closure. Novice and experienced phaco surgeons should gain useful tips. (Bas, Int, Adv)

B

FIGURE 33-28 A, Article by Mr. R.M. Redmond, MD, on topical anesthesia in the *British Journal of Ophthalmology* in April 1990. **B,** Academy course where Redmond first presented topical anesthesia in America.

independently introduced the YAG laser in the early 1980s. Aron-Rosa began clinical trials in October 1978 and did 5000 eyes over a period of 4 years. Fankhauser did his first YAG capsulotomy in November 1980. Soon reports of IOL damage from the laser began to appear. Contrary to common belief, the Hoffer ridge optic[37] was designed in 1978 for two equally important purposes. The first was to increase the pressure at the edge of the optic to create an increased barrier to the migration of lens epithelial cells onto the posterior capsule (Figure 33-29, *B* and *C*) The second was to create a space between the back surface of the IOL and the posterior capsule to prevent damage to the IOL during the performance of a posterior capsulotomy. Iolab made the first ridge lenses (Figure 33-29, *A*), but they were soon followed by Cilco, CooperVision (Bellevue, Wash.) and then most other companies. The stimulus for its popularity was the increased use of the YAG laser, which was causing severe pitting in lens optics without the spacing. Other ideas for spacing ensued, such as a meniscus optic (William Myers, CooperVision), Prolene riders (Lawrence Castleman, MD, Ioptex, San Leandro, Calif.), and partial ridges (Kratz-Johnson, AMO). For the Hoffer ridge to block Elschnig pearl formation and prevent posterior capsule opacification (PCO), the haptics had to be angled anteriorly (to increase posterior pressure) and the lens had to be placed entirely in the capsular bag (uniform pressure on entire ridge). Because neither of these rules was adhered to during the lenses popular period from 1983 to 1989, reports of the effects of the ridge on PCO were conflicting, although several studies showed a definite positive effect.[38] No adverse effects of this lens modification have been reported after 18 years of use. After the disastrous recall of the Azar 91Z, Iolab

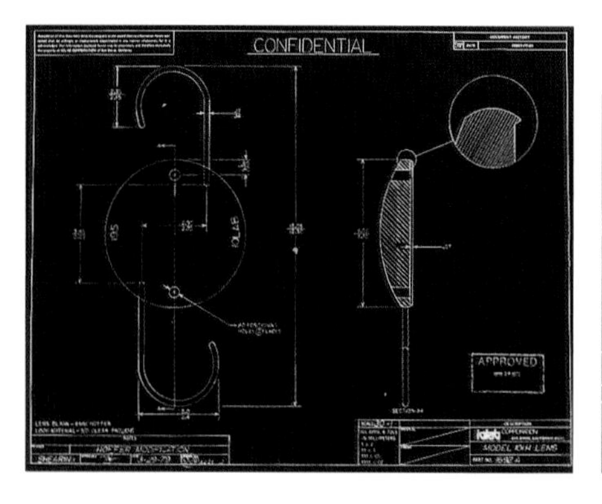

A

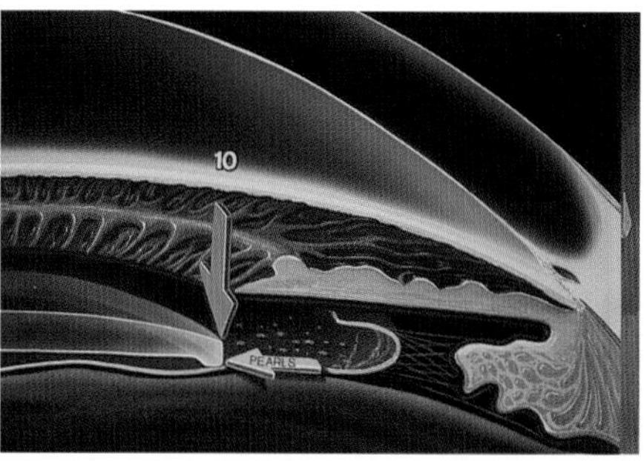

B

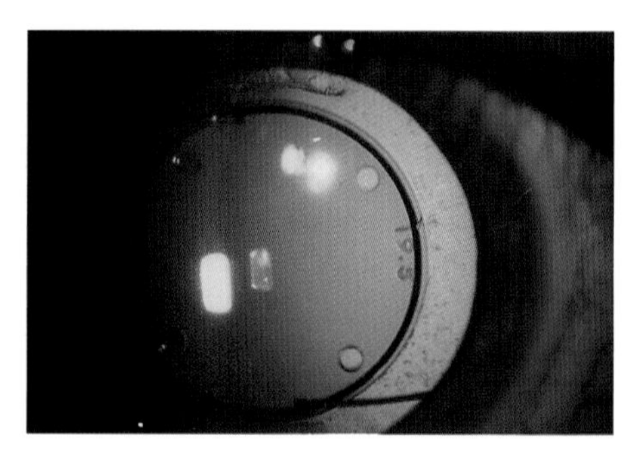

C

FIGURE 33-29 A, First mechanical drawing by Iolab of the Hoffer ridge Lens. **B,** Graphic depiction of the increased pressure caused at the edge of the lens by the ridge. **C,** An eye with an Iolab ridge lens demonstrating the blockage of Elschnig pearls at the edge of the lens optic.

claimed that it was the Hoffer ridge lenses that kept them afloat. As studies began to show that convex-surface-posterior lenses decreased PCO, and with the increased production of more-accurate lasers, most surgeons turned toward biconvex IOLs without the ridge in the 1990s. The Hoffer ridge optic was successfully made on biconvex PMMA IOLs (Coburn Optical) and with silicone (AMO), but never brought on the market.

UV protection was also an issue strongly advocated by Diana Langley in the 1980s and soon it became a standard in IOL fabrication.

Multifocal IOLS

In 1982, after seeing a patient referred with severely decentered Shearing lenses bilaterally (Figure 33-30, *B*), I postulated a concept[39] of multifocality for IOLs. The patient had 20/20 vision without correction but was also correctable to 20/20 with an aphakic spectacle correction. I concluded that the only way this could be possible would be if her brain were selecting the clearest image of the two being presented by the pseudophakic and aphakic zones of her pupil. I immediately attempted to patent the concept, but Jack Hartstein had already applied in 1975 (Figure 33-30, *A*). I pressured Iolab into fabricating a 50/50 split bifocal IOL for research purposes. After they made five such lenses (see Figure 33-30, *C*) for me in their research and development division, they lost interest in the idea while they turned their attention to research with partial-depth positioning holes. Frustrated, I was able to get Ioptex to clean, polish, verify the powers, and sterilize these lenses. With thorough informed consent, I implanted them in three patients uniocularly. They worked, but I had to remove one because of annoying images. Three years later, I learned that John Pearce, working with Iolab, was implanting central bullet bifocal IOLs by Iolab in England. This was soon followed by the diffractive multifocal (3M) and the various other manufacturer designs, including the Array lens by Allergan (AMO). After Alcon purchased the 3M IOL division, they abandoned the multifocal because of the strict FDA testing asked of them. Allergan persisted, and they ultimately received FDA approval. All the other designs gradually faded away. Ironically, I do not implant multifocal IOLs.

Lens Implant Societies

It is impossible to relate the history of IOLs without touching on the societies that sprang up to deal with them. Choyce[4] came up with the idea of setting up an organization for the study of lens implants in 1964. It took several years for him to convince Ridley, but they did it in 1966 and held their first meeting as the Intraocular Implant Club (IIC) on Wednesday, July 14, 1966, in Oxford, England. Ridley was the first president, followed by Strampelli in 1970. It was the Paris meeting on Saturday, June 1, 1974, at the Meridien Hotel adjoining the Palais des Congres after the close of the Twenty-second International Congress of Ophthalmology, that saw the tremendous surge of interest in IOLs. Forty-four members and 88 nonmembers attended, most from America. After the formation of the American society and other national implant societies, they changed the name to the International IIC (IIIC).

In March 1974, I conceived of the idea of an American society for lens implantation to bring together the disparate factions then present in the implant world here in the United States. I had not yet heard of the IIC. I wanted the society to hold educational meetings and publish a scientific journal because at that time there was no forum for presenting or publishing reports on the subject. I persuaded three colleagues to help me (Drs. John Darin, Jeremy Levenson, and Stephen Cooperman). Together we organized and incorporated the society as the American Intra-Ocular Implant Society (AIOIS) in August 1974, whose name was changed to the American Society of Cataract & Refractive Surgery (ASCRS) in 1983 (Figure 33-31).

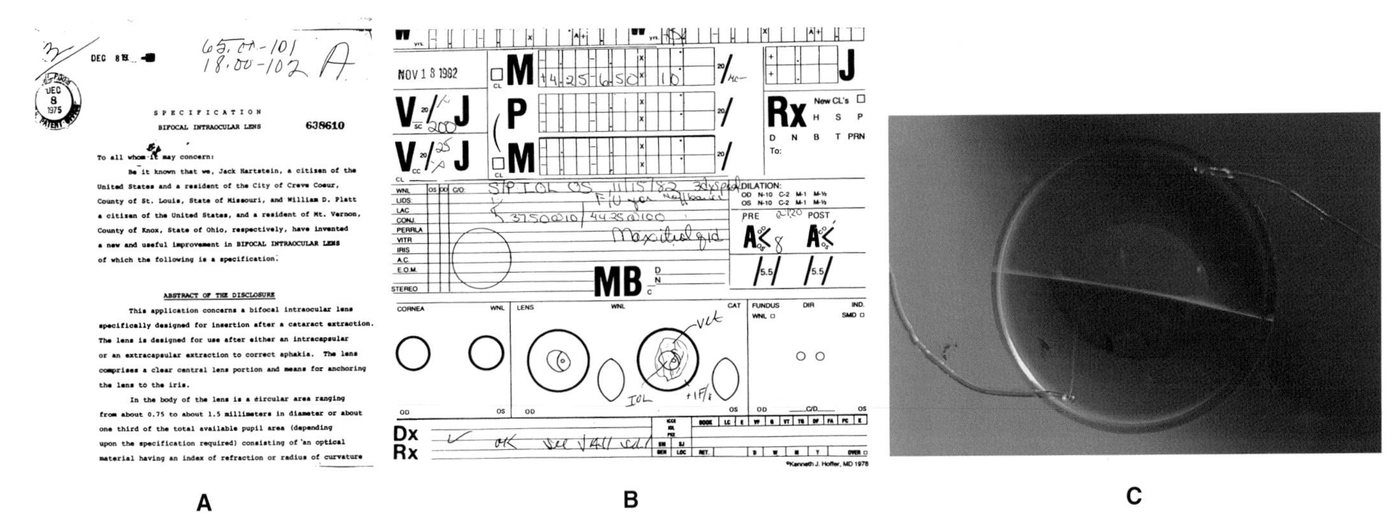

DEC 8 1975

SPECIFICATION

BIFOCAL INTRAOCULAR LENS 638610

To all whom it may concern:

Be it known that we, Jack Hartstein, a citizen of the United States and a resident of the City of Creve Coeur, County of St. Louis, State of Missouri, and William D. Platt a citizen of the United States, and a resident of Mt. Vernon, County of Knox, State of Ohio, respectively, have invented a new and useful improvement in BIFOCAL INTRAOCULAR LENS of which the following is a specification.

ABSTRACT OF THE DISCLOSURE

This application concerns a bifocal intraocular lens specifically designed for insertion after a cataract extraction. The lens is designed for use after either an intracapsular or an extracapsular extraction to correct aphakia. The lens comprises a clear central lens portion and means for anchoring the lens to the iris.

In the body of the lens is a circular area ranging from about 0.75 to about 1.5 millimeters in diameter or about one third of the total available pupil area (depending upon the specification required) consisting of an optical material having an index of refraction or radius of curvature

FIGURE 33-30 **A,** Harstein bifocal IOL patent application, December 8, 1975. **B,** Chart of patient with bilateral dislocated posterior chamber lenses, November 18, 1982. **C,** Original 1983 Hoffer split bifocal intraocular lens.

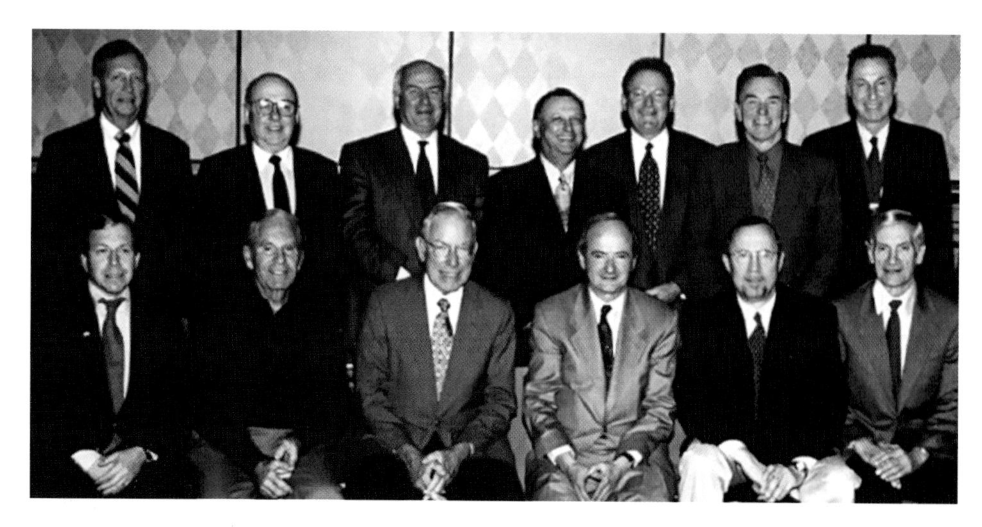

FIGURE 33-31 Past presidents of the American Society of Cataract & Refractive Surgery (ASCRS) (in chronological order of holding office). *Bottom row:* Kenneth J. Hoffer (1974-1975), Norman S. Jaffe (1975-1977), Robert C. Drews (1977-1979), Miles A. Galin (1979-1980), Henry M. Clayman (1980-1983), Manuc C. Kraff (1983-1985). *Top row:* Guy E. Knolle (1989-1991), Jack M. Dodick (1991-1993), John D. Hunkeler (1993-1995), Charles D. Kelman (1995-1997), David Karcher (Executive Vice President 1981-present), Spencer P. Thornton (1997-1999), Robert M. Sinsky (1999-2000).

When I visited Cornelius Binkhorst in Terneuzen, Holland, in November 1974, he was very kind to me but expressed his great concern about this "American Implant Society" he had heard I had founded. I reassured him that we had no intention of overshadowing the IIC, of which he was then president.

I don't think he completely believed me, but he finally dropped the subject. Needless to say I was disconcerted because I never thought of the little society I had started as trying to take over for the IIC, but looking back on it now, he was right; it did. A year later, to quell his continued fears about AIOIS, I urged him to create a European Implant Lens Council, which would be an amalgamation of European national implant societies over which he could preside. As president, he ultimately did just that, and the European Council later became the European Society of Cataract & Refractive Surgery (ESCRS).

First Intraocular Lens Power Calculations

As proven by Sir Harold's first two cases, correct calculation of the IOL power is essential and a vital part of the history of IOLs. When I learned in 1974 that Jan Worst was using A-scan ultra-

A

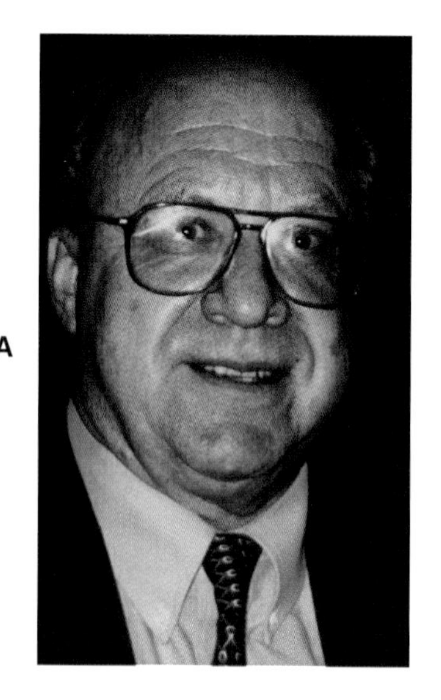

B

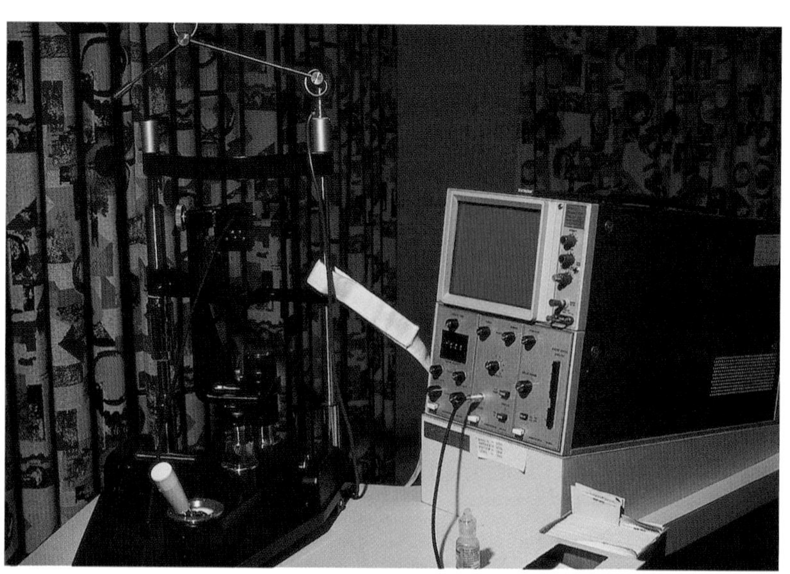

FIGURE 33-32 **A,** Karl C. Ossoinig, MD, of Iowa City. **B,** The first IOL power specific A-scan ultrasound unit in 1975 (Sonometrics DBR-100).

sound axial length for IOL power calculation, I had remembered Karl Ossoinig's (Figure 33-32, *A*) (Iowa City) A-scan lectures[40] (1972) and called him regarding the instrument to be used. Santa Monica Hospital agreed to purchase the recommended Kretz 7200-MA unit from Austria and a keratometer and provide a facility where I could perform the tests. I called the new facility the "Eye Lab."

Before inserting my first IOL (Medallion ICCE) on April 22, 1974, I performed the first A-scan IOL power calculation in the Western Hemisphere.[41] Dr. Ossoinig was on the telephone from Iowa talking me through the calibration of the Kretz unit and the measurement of the photographs. For his willingness to help me, I will be eternally grateful. It worked!

Before this time, American lens implanters used a standard 18.0-D prepupillary lens for all eyes, expecting the patient to be as myopic or hyperopic as he or she was before surgery. In the mid-1970s, Dennis Shepard (Santa Maria, Calif.) devised a nomogram based on the patient's preoperative refractive error. After the word spread about our Eye Lab, many other ophthalmologists sent their patients to the Eye Lab for IOL power calculation, including Dr. Henry Hirschman, who limousined his patients to Santa Monica from Long Beach. After months of performing the exam myself, I finally decided I had to train a technician to do it. Our photographer, Don Allen, was the closest at hand, and after 2 months he picked it up easily and became the first IOL power calculation technician in America. Don died several years ago, and I honor him here.

Working with Lou Katz of Sonometrics, I designed the first A-scan ultrasound unit (see Figure 33-32, *B*) specific for IOL power calculation (DBR-100).[41] It ushered in the era of automatic measuring gates and the applanation technique, of which the latter turned out to be less accurate then the Ossoinig immersion technique but became the standard to this day. In 1974, I programmed the Colenbrander and Hoffer IOL formulas on a Hewlitt-Packard programmable calculator. It took hundreds of presentations at the AAO and ASCRS meetings, as well as numbers of "9-diopter surprises" to make A-scan the standard of care nationwide. The efforts of formula developers such as Tom Lloyd, Don Sanders, John Retzlaff, Manus Kraff, Thomas Olsen, Jack Holladay, and Wolfgang Haigis cannot be left unmentioned.

Conclusion

One thread runs clear through this history of IOLs. Since Jaques Daviel[42] (Paris) performed the first intentional intracapsular cataract extraction on April 8, 1747, most, if not all, the steps of innovation (and mistakes) leading to what we do today were devised and carried out by individual private practitioner cataract surgeons throughout the world without university or government research funding. To all of them, we owe a debt of gratitude.

Ridley lived long enough (94 years) to have his invention implanted into his own eyes, realize the benefit to humanity he provided, and be knighted by his Queen (Figure 33-33). For that we can all be grateful; what a unique and lucky man he was.

With the passing of four giants, Ridley, Choyce, Binkhorst, and Fyodorov, I dedicate this chapter to their memory.

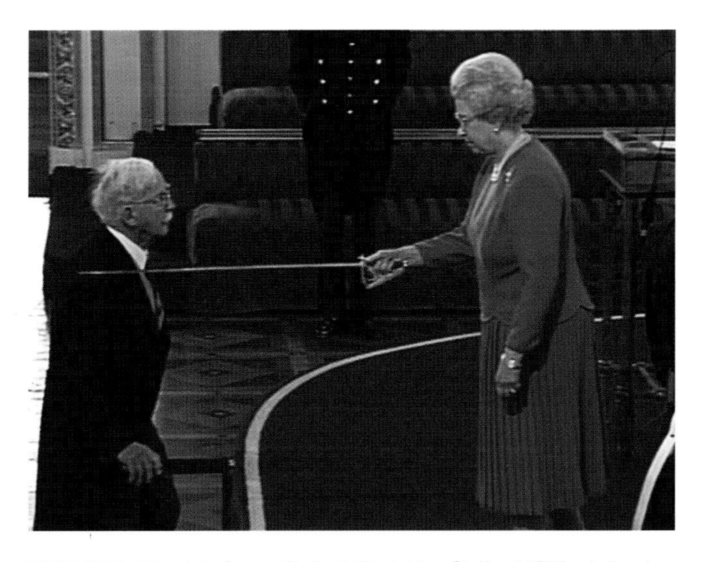

FIGURE 33-33 Queen Elizabeth II knighting Sir Harold Ridley in London, March 2000.

REFERENCES

1. Taieb A: Des mèmoires di Casanova á l'operation di Ridley, *Arch Ophtalmol (Paris)* 15:501-503, 1955.
2. Münchow W: Zur Geschichte der intraokularen Korrektur der Aphakie, *Klin Monatsbl Augenheilkd* 145:771-777, 1964.
3. Ascher KW: Prosthetophakia two hundred years ago, *Am J Ophthalmol* 1965; 59:445-446.
4. Choyce DP: Recollections of the early days of intraocular lens implantation, *J Cataract Refract Surg* 16:505-508, 1990.
5. Strampelli B: L' évolution des lentilles plastiques de chambre antérieuri: derniéres acquisitions techniques, *An Inst Barraquer* III-4:519-530, 1962.
6. Ridley H: Intra-ocular acrylic lenses, *Trans Ophthalmol Soc U K* 71:617-621, 1951.
7. Ridley H: Intra-ocular acrylic lenses after cataract surgery, *Lancet* I:118-121, 1952.
8. Binkhorst CD, Flu FP: Sterilization of intra-ocular acrylic lens prostheses with ultra-violet rays, *Br J Ophthalmol* 40:665-668, 1956.
9. Ridley F: Safety requirements for acrylic implants, *Br J Ophthalmol* 41:359-367, 1957.
10. Baron A: Tolérance di l'oeil à matiére plastique: prosthéses optiques cornéennes, *Bull Soc Ophtalmol Paris* 9:982-988, 1953.
11. Scharf J: Demonstration eiener neuartigen Kunststofflinse zur Korrecttur der Aphakie, mit Vorstellung operierter Patienten, *Klin Monatsbl Augenheilkd* 128:233-235, 1956.
12. Strampelli B: Sopportabilità di lenti acriliche in camera anteriore nella afachia e nei vizi di refrazione, *Ann Otall* 80:75-82, 1954.
13. Dannheim H: Vorderkammerlinse mit elastischen Halteschlingen, *Ber Dtsch Ophthal Ges Heidelberg* 60:267-268, 1956.
14. Barraquer J: Complicaciones de la inclusion segun los diversos tipos de lentes, *An Inst Barraquer* III-4:588-592, 1962.
15. Fyodorov SN: Application of intraocular pupillary lenses for aphakia correction (translation), *Vestn Oftal (Mosk)* 78:76-83, 1965.
16. Atchison DA. Optical design of poly(methyl methacrylate) intraocular lenses, *J Cataract Refract Surg* 16:178-188, 1990.
17. Fyodorov SN: Scientific research in behalf of the medical practice (translation), *Nauka I Zjiznj (Science Life)* 8:93-95, 1972.
18. Binkhorst CD, Gobin MHMA: Pseudophakia after lens injury in children, *Ophthalmologica (Basel)* 154:81-87, 1967.
19. Nordlohne ME: History of intraocular lens implants. In *The intraocular implant lens: development and results with special reference to the Binkhorst lens*, The Hague, 1975, Dr W Junk BV, pp 14-36.
20. Apple DJ, Kincaid MC, Mamalis N et al: *Intraocular lenses: evolution, designs, complications and pathology*, Baltimore, 1989, Williams & Wilkins, pp 11-41.
21. Pearce JL: New lightweight sutured posterior chamber lens implant, *Trans Ophthalmol Soc U K* 96:6-10, 1976.
22. Shearing SP: Mechanism of fixation of the Shearing posterior chamber intra-ocular lens, *Contact Intraocul Lens Med J* 5:74-77, 1979.

23. Shearing SP: The genesis of the posterior chamber lens. In Kwitko ML, Kelman CD, editors: *The history of modern cataract surgery,* The Hague, Netherlands, 1998, Kuglen Publications, 1998 pp 139-146.
24. Hoffer KJ: Five Year's Experience with the ridged laser lens implant. In Emery, JM, Jacobson AC, editors: *Current concepts in cataract surgery (eighth congress),* New York, 1983, Appleton-Century Crofts, pp 296-299.
25. Arnott EJ, Condon R: The totally encircling loop lens-followup of 1,800 cases, *Cataract* 2:13-18, 1985.
26. Ellingson FT: Complications with the Choyce Mark VIII anterior chamber implant (uveitis-glaucoma-hyphema), *J Am Intraocul Implant Soc* 3:199-201, 1977.
27. Kelman CD: Anterior chamber lens design concepts. In Rosen ES, Haining WM, Arnott EJ, editors: *Intraocular lens implantation,* St Louis, 1984, Mosby, pp 239-245.
28. Mehta KR, Sathe SN, Karyekar SD: The new soft intraocular lens implant, *J Am Intraocul Implant Soc* 4:201-205, 1978.
29. Fercho C: "Perfect" capsulotomy reduces vitreous loss, eases cortical cleanup, *Ocular Surgery News* November 15, 1986.
30. Pape LG, Balazs EA: The uses of sodium hyaluronate (Healon) in human anterior segment surgery, *Ophthalmology* 87:699-705, 1980.
31. Shepherd JR: In situ fracture, *J Cataract Refract Surg* 16:436-438, 1990.
32. Redmond RM, Dallas NL: Extracapsular cataract extraction under local anesthesia without retrobulbar injection, *Br J Ophthalmol* 74:203-204, 1990.
33. Modern Phaco/ECCE Implant Surgery: 1991 AAO Course #261, Anaheim, Calif, October 1991.
34. Barasch KR, Poler S: Intraocular lens weights and the vitreous, *Ophthalmic Surg* 10:65, 1979.
35. Aron-Rosa D, Aron JJ, Griesemann M et al: Use of the neodymium YAG laser to open the posterior capsule after lens implant surgery: a preliminary report, *J Am Intraocul Implant Soc* 6:352-354, 1980.
36. Fankhauser F, Roussel P, Steffen J et al: Clinical studies on the efficacy of high power laser radiation upon some structures of the anterior segment of the eye, *Int Ophthalmol* 3:129-139, 1981.
37. Hoffer Ridge Patent; US Patent #4,244,060, issued January 13, 1981, US Patent #RE 31,626, reissued July 10, 1984.
38. Westliing AK, Calissendorff BM: Factors influencing the formation of posterior capsular opacities after extracapsular cataract extraction with posterior chamber lens implant, *Acta Ophthalmol* 69:315-320, 1991.
39. Hoffer KJ: Personal history in bifocal intraocular lenses. In Maxwell A, Nordan LT, editors: *Current concepts of multifocal intraocular lenses,* Thorofare, NJ, 1991, Slack, Inc, pp 127-132.
40. Ossoinig KC: Standardized echography: basic principles, clinical applications, and results, *Int Ophthalmol Clin* 19:127, 1979.
41. Hoffer KJ: The history of IOL power calculation in North America. In: Kwitko ML, Kelman CD, editors: *The history of modern cataract surgery,* The Hague, Netherlands, 1998, Kuglen Publications, pp 193-208.
42. Daviel J: A new method of curing cataracts by extraction of the lens, *Mem Royal Acad Surg (Paris)* 2:337, 1753.

Polymethylmethacrylate Intraocular Lenses

34

Richard L. Lindstrom, MD
Elizabeth A. Davis, MD

This chapter reviews the historical evolution and current status of intraocular lenses (IOLs) with an optic manufactured of polymethylmethacrylate (PMMA). Although a comprehensive review of the literature has been performed and selected references provided, the perspectives presented are those of the authors. In the following chapters, the historical evolution and current status of IOLs with an optic manufactured from foldable materials and those with a multifocal optic also are reviewed.

The earliest reference to lens implantation is credited to Tadini, an eighteenth-century oculist.[1-3] According to his memoirs, Casanova met him in 1766 in Warsaw, where Tadini showed him a box with small spheres that were well polished and suggested that such globes might be placed under the cornea in the place of the crystalline lens. No confirmation is available that Tadini ever actually did perform such an implant operation.

Approximately 30 years later, in 1795, a Dresden ophthalmologist, Casaamata, performed a cataract operation and implanted an artificial lens.[1-3] Apparently, Casaamata performed the procedure by inserting the glass lens through a wound in the cornea. He immediately realized the procedure would not be successful as the glass lens fell deeply into the vitreous. Thus the first implantation of an IOL and the first severe complication, total lens dislocation into the vitreous, appear to belong to Casaamata.

The modern era of lens implantation begins with Harold Ridley of London.[4-6] At the end of a cataract operation in the fall of 1949, Ridley reported he was asked by a medical student why he did not replace the cataractous lens he was removing with a new one. Apparently this gave Ridley the impetus to explore the possibility of lens implantation. During World War II, many ophthalmologists had noted that perforating eye injuries from airplane canopies made from acrylic Perspex plastic often resulted in minimal intraocular irritation secondary to the material itself. It therefore became accepted that acrylic was relatively inert in the eye. This, and the fact that acrylic has a relatively high refractive index of 1.49 and a low specific gravity of 1.19, prompted Harold Ridley to select this material for his initial investigations into lens implantation.

Ridley originally designed his lens to imitate the natural lens. Its diameter was 8.35 mm, and its weight was 112 mg in air and 70.4 mg in water, as compared with a modern IOL, which weighs less than 4 mg in water. On November 29, 1949, at St. Thomas Hospital in London, Harold Ridley implanted the first posterior chamber lens into the capsular bag after an extracapsular cataract extraction. It is amazing that his original choice of material, method of cataract extraction, and selection of in-the-bag implantation have been affirmed after more than 40 years of trial-and-error investigation in this field.

The second lens was implanted almost 1 year later, on August 23, 1950. Unfortunately, the initial two patients' postoperative refractive results were significantly myopic, one refracting at –20.0 and one at –15 diopters (D). Ridley then recalculated the basic optics for the lens and began a series of about 750 implants, which extended to approximately 1959. These early lens implant patients had a significant rate of complications, including severe postoperative inflammation and lens dislocation. Lens dislocation occurred in approximately 13% of the cases, usually into the vitreous. Many patients also developed late secondary glaucoma. Nonetheless, many of these implants performed well for many years (Figure 34-1).

Ridley's work stimulated several other surgeons to become interested in the idea of lens implantation. In an attempt to reduce the high incidence of dislocation, most of these surgeons abandoned the posterior chamber and began to design anterior chamber angle-fixated lenses. The first published reports of such lenses came from Strampelli.[7] His lens can be considered the precursor of the rigid, one-piece anterior chamber lenses. Of particular interest is the original work by Dahnheim, whose closed-loop anterior chamber lens most closely resembles the closed-loop anterior chamber lenses that gained great popularity in the United States in the 1980s before being withdrawn from the market for an unexpectedly high incidence of uveitis, glaucoma, hyphema, cystoid macular edema, and corneal decompensation.[8] Of equal interest is the open-loop anterior chamber lens of Barraquer, which was later modified successfully as a posterior chamber lens by Shearing.[9,10] It remains today one of the most popular IOL designs in the world.

Unfortunately, the early anterior chamber angle-fixated lenses resulted in a very high incidence of secondary corneal decompensation. Barraquer actually reported a 67% incidence of late corneal decompensation, and he had to remove 50% of his lens implants, many of which were implanted for the correction of myopia in phakic eyes.[9]

These anterior chamber angle-fixated lenses were the first lenses that suggested to ophthalmologists that long-term

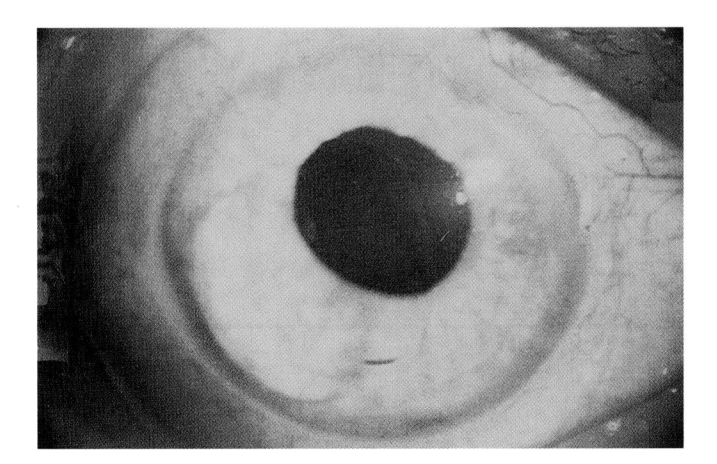

FIGURE 34-1 Ridley posterior chamber lens implant in an eye, nearly 40 years after implantation.

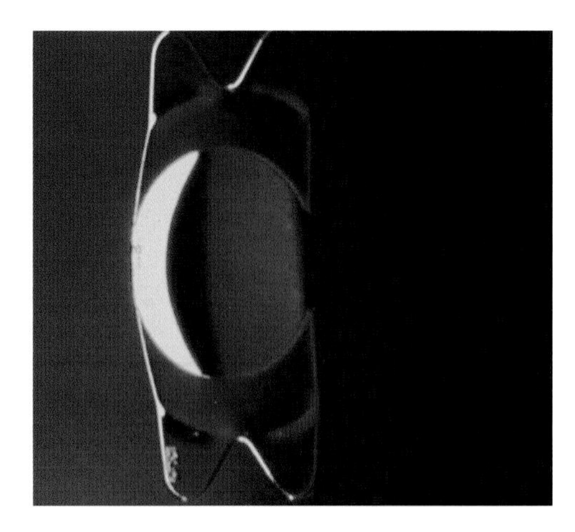

FIGURE 34-2 Choyce-Tennant rigid anterior chamber intraocular lens.

follow-up might be required to confirm the level and severity of complications. For example, Strampelli did not notice a high incidence of bullous keratopathy until almost 5 years postoperatively, with most of his patients doing well in the initial postoperative period.

In 1964, Peter Choyce designed a lens, named the Mark VIII, based on his continuing work in anterior chamber angle fixation (Figure 34-2).[8] This was the first lens implant to perform in a reasonable fashion over an extended period in many surgeons' hands. This lens was implanted without any major change in design between 1964 and 1978. One of the major factors in the improved success of the Mark VIII lens of Choyce was a significant improvement in the quality of manufacturing, which was quite crude in many of the early implant designs.

A continuing significant complication rate with the anterior chamber angle-fixated lens caused many ophthalmologists to turn to the pupil or iris for fixation of a lens implant. Pioneers of iris-fixated lenses included Epstein of South Africa,[11] Binkhorst[12-14] and Worst[15] in the Netherlands, and Fyodorov[8] in the Soviet Union.

The original work of Edward Epstein led to a lens shaped like a Maltese cross, with four wings extending from a central optical part. Epstein abandoned this design because of secondary complications, especially inflammation. A similar lens under the name of Copeland was widely used in the United States in the 1970s (Figure 34-3). Unfortunately, a high incidence of chronic iris irritation, secondary cystoid macular edema, and bullous keratopathy caused this lens also to fall into disuse.

A major contributor to the generation of iris support and later iridocapsular lenses was Cornelius Binkhorst, who developed the concept of the iris clip implant. Modifications of this lens, especially the Binkhorst four-loop iris clip lens, gave results superior to those that had been obtained with the early posterior chamber and anterior chamber angle-fixated implants.

Jan Worst, also working in Holland, had the concept of improved fixation through the use of a suture or metal clip. This led to a series of lenses called the Medallion lens implants, which also showed improved results over the previous generation of implants.

At the same time, working in the Soviet Union, Syvataslav Fyodorov developed a group of lenses commonly called the Sputnik lenses, which also became popular. However, there continued to be a significant rate of dislocation, cystoid macular edema, and secondary corneal decompensation with these lens implants. Unsatisfied with the results himself, Binkhorst recognized the benefits of extracapsular cataract extraction. He went on to develop a series of iridocapsular lenses, which achieve their primary fixation from the capsular bag after extracapsular cataract extraction and a secondary fixation and centration through pupil support.[13] It was soon discovered that the frequency and severity of cystoid macular edema, dislocation, and corneal decompensation were significantly lower with the capsular-fixated lenses.

The concept of iridocapsular fixation gained increasing support and led to a renewed interest in extracapsular cataract extraction. This set the stage for a return to the posterior chamber.

In 1977, John Pearce, working in England, reevaluated the concept of capsular fixation of a posterior chamber lens.[16-17] Beginning with a small, 4-mm optic, tripod-shaped lens, which he sutured to the iris to obtain secondary fixation, he showed that posterior chamber lenses could be safely and effectively implanted without a high complication rate. The work of Pearce stimulated the imagination of several other ophthalmologists, including Shearing[10] and Simcoe,[18] who modified the Barraquer flexible, open-loop anterior chamber lens for use in the posterior chamber. Shearing developed the J-loop posterior chamber lens; with semiflexible loops for implantation either into the

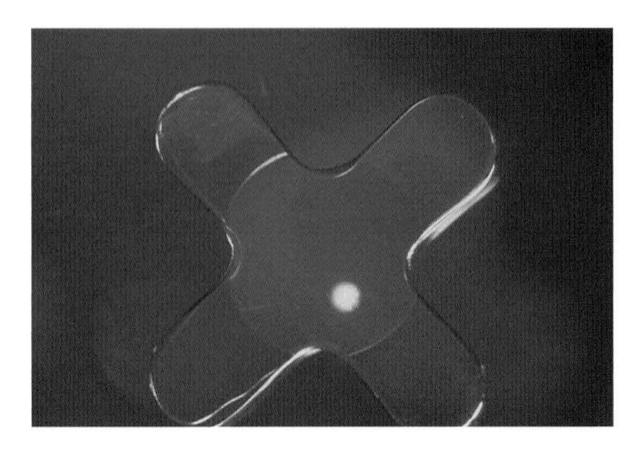

FIGURE 34-3 Copeland pupil-supported lens.

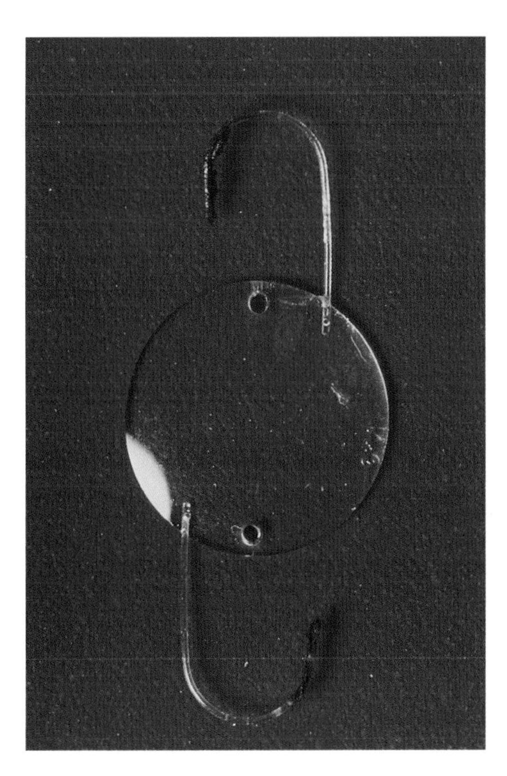

FIGURE 34-4 Original Shearing J-loop posterior chamber lens used a 5-mm optic and polypropylene loops.

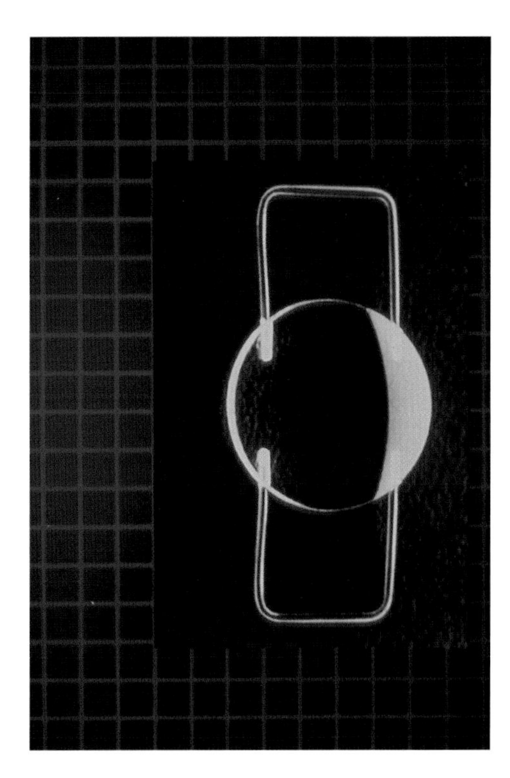

FIGURE 34-5 The popularity of the Leiske closed-loop anterior chamber lens peaked between 1982 and 1983.

ciliary sulcus or the capsular bag[10] (Figure 34-4).This lens proved almost immediately to be successful and demonstrated a relative ease of implantation with a lower complication rate than had been noted with any other implant design. Many brilliant and innovative surgeons then dedicated themselves to improving on the open-loop posterior chamber lens implant.[19-50] The end result of the evolution is discussed later in this chapter.

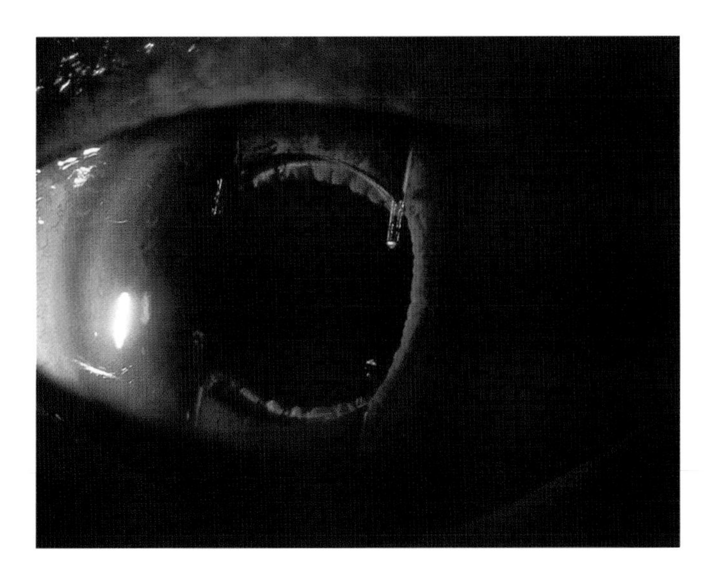

FIGURE 34-6 Pupil-blocked glaucoma associated with uveitis and recurrent microhyphema in a patient who received a Leiske closed-loop anterior chamber lens implant.

About the same time that one group of pioneers was returning to the posterior chamber with good success, there was a rebirth in interest in the closed-loop anterior chamber lens (Figure 34-5). The attractiveness of this concept was clear in that most surgeons were accomplished at intracapsular cataract extraction and did not wish to learn the skill of extracapsular extraction required for posterior chamber lens implantation. The popularity of the closed-loop anterior chamber lenses peaked in approximately 1982, followed by a total withdrawal from the market by 1988 because of an intolerable incidence of secondary complications, including cystoid macular edema, secondary glaucoma, uveitis, hyphema, and corneal decompensation[51-55] (Figure 34-6).

About the same time, Charles Kelman introduced his flexible, three-point and four-point fixation, one-piece PMMA open-loop anterior chamber lenses, which have continued to perform successfully to this day (Figure 34-7).

Optic Materials

The optic material for an IOL is required to meet several challenges. It must be able to be lathed or molded and polished to a high optical quality, it must be biocompatible and durable with minimal induction of inflammation, it must be non-antigenic and noncarcinogenic, and it must be sterilizable. To meet the requirement for a light weight, it requires a high index of refraction. It is remarkable that Harold Ridley, in his first work, selected a material that has continued to stand the test of time, PMMA.

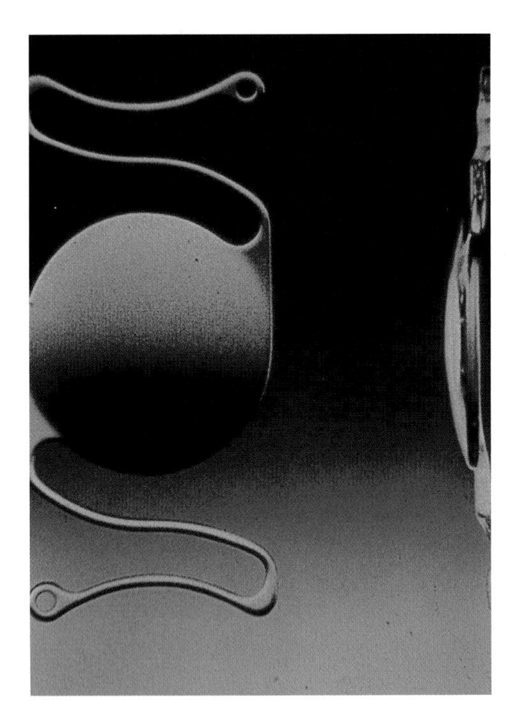

FIGURE 34-7 Kelman flexible, open-loop, one-piece anterior chamber lens.

PMMA is a polymer of methylmethacrylate monomer (Figure 34-8). PMMA is manufactured through addition polymerization of methylacrylic acid methyl ester, which is itself derived from acrylic acid.[56] Additional agents such as ultraviolet light absorbers may be added to the plastic to enhance its capabilities.[57-59] Various forms of PMMA are available commercially. PMMA used in lathe-cut or compression-molded IOLs is a high-molecular-weight type, such as the Perspex CQ, manufactured by Imperial Chemical Industries. Another form of manufacturing, injection molding, uses a lower-molecular-weight PMMA, such as that manufactured by Rohm & Haas.

PMMA is a light, durable material with a specific gravity of 1.19. It has a refractive index of 1.49. The average molecular weight of Perspex CQ is in the range of 2.5 to 3 million Daltons. At temperatures lower than 100° C it is hard, but the material can melt at temperatures of 140° C or higher.

Although the monomer is toxic, the polymer is inert and is well tolerated in the eye with minimal inflammatory reaction.[60-62] Release of monomer from PMMA was not a concern until the development of the neodymium:yttrium-aluminum-garnet (Nd:YAG) laser for capsulotomy, which has the potential to damage the PMMA optic.[63-67] It has been shown that substances toxic to cultures of various ocular cell lines can be released from PMMA IOLs that are directly hit with Nd:YAG laser bursts in the range of 5 mJ. Fortunately, this has not resulted in significant problems because much lower energy levels are used, and direct blows to the lens are rare. The higher-molecular-weight lathe-cut, compression-molded, and cast-molded IOLs are more resistant to Nd:YAG laser damage than the injection molded lenses.

$$\left[-\overset{H}{\underset{H}{C}} - \overset{CH_3}{\underset{CO\,OCH_3}{C}} - \right]_n$$

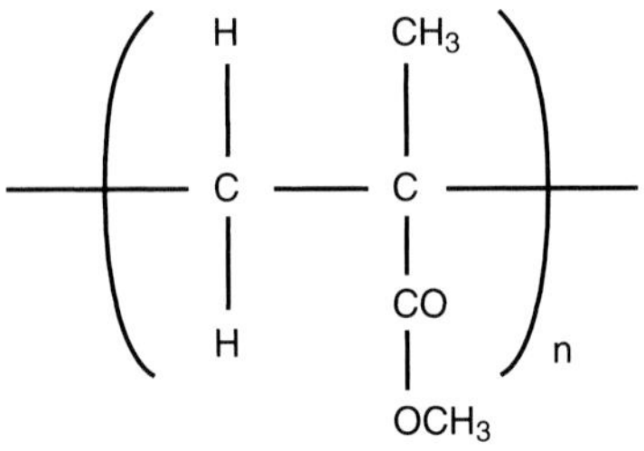

FIGURE 34-8 Chemical structure of PMMA.

Although PMMA is relatively inert, it is not totally inert in the eye. It does not appear to activate complement or induce chemotaxis of leukocytes, but a cellular reaction does occur on its surface, even in clinically well-tolerated implants.[68-70]

PMMA transmits a broad spectrum of light, including near-ultraviolet light, a possible source of retinal damage.[71] Therefore ultraviolet-absorbing materials have been added to PMMA optics to reduce this potential toxicity.[57-59] The ultraviolet absorber may be added through covalent bonding or by simply mixing the chromophores with the PMMA. Although it has not been confirmed that ultraviolet absorption has a clinical value, most current PMMA lenses contain ultraviolet light absorbers, usually a benzophenone or benzotriazole.

Loop and Haptic Materials

Most PMMA optic lenses are supported by one or more loops or haptic configurations. These may be broadly divided onto one-piece and multipiece IOLs. In the one-piece lenses, the entire lens is manufactured of the same PMMA. In the multipiece lenses, the loop or haptic is composed of a second material. These alternative materials are discussed in the following paragraphs.

An initial material selected for support loops was polyamide, a synthetic material consisting of long molecular chains that contain the amido group at regular intervals. The polyamides include materials such as Nylon 6, Supramid, and Perlon. In the American literature, nylon is basically synonymous with polyamide. These materials retain a high degree of breakage resistance and are quite flexible. They can be manufactured in various diameters, and the manufacturing technology to create various shapes is readily available. Unfortunately, nylon undergoes hydrolysis, resulting in fragmentation over time after implantation into tissue.[15,72] For this reason, polyamide materials were abandoned for use as loops to support optics.

Another suture material, polyethyleneglycolterephthalate, commonly known as Dacron or Mersilene, is also a potential material for IOL loops.[73] Unlike nylon, it is hydrophobic rather than hydrophilic and does not appear to undergo biodegradation. However, it is less elastic and stiffer than the favored polypropylene. Although it is not currently popular for use in IOL loops, Mersilene suture is often used for wound closure and can be used for iris fixation or transscleral fixation of posterior chamber or iris-supported IOLs.

The most popular material for three-piece posterior chamber lenses other than PMMA has been polypropylene (Prolene).[74] Polypropylene has a high tensile strength and, in contrast to nylon, has no hydrolysable binding sites. In a vascular tissue, it is biologically inert and relatively stable, although it is subject to oxidative biodegradation, especially when exposed to light.[72] Elongation of polypropylene is significantly greater than that of Mersilene. It also appears to have a relatively short structural memory, making it possible to implant lenses with compressible polypropylene loops in a space smaller than the diameter of the lens without the loops causing continuous pressure on the tissues.

Polypropylene continues to be a widely employed material for loops of posterior chamber lenses. However, it has two potential problems.

In vitro, polypropylene materials have demonstrated increased levels of complement fragments, which attract circulating inflammatory cells.[70] The clinical importance of this finding is not clear. To date, only one study by Tuberville and Wood[75] has measured complement levels in pseudophakic eyes. This study found that complement levels in posterior chamber IOL pseudophakic eyes were not different than in phakic eyes. The type of haptic material in the patients studied was not differentiated, however.

One in vitro assay indicated that more bacteria adhere to polypropylene than to PMMA haptics.[76] In a retrospective case-control clinical comparison of endophthalmitis, Menikoff et al.[77] reported that 87% of their cases involved polypropylene-looped lenses. Because of the low incidence of endophthalmitis and the time frame of this study, it is not clear if the more frequent involvement of polypropylene-looped lenses is a function of other confounding factors or represents a clinically significant phenomenon.

Nonetheless, polypropylene has stood the test of time as a support loop in posterior chamber lenses. Yet most surgeons have come to favor PMMA. Metal-looped, iris-supported lenses had a short period of popularity, particularly platinum-iridium and titanium. Today, all metal-looped lenses have been removed from the market because of a high rate of complications.[78]

Another potential haptic material put to use more recently is polyimide. This is a synthetic material of variable construction that contains an imino (NH) group and benzoyl ring. This material is capable of withstanding high temperatures and high-energy radiation and may be heat sterilized. At this time, polyimide is used as a support loop in some three-piece silicone IOLs, and it is performing in a satisfactory fashion.

In summary, the most popular materials to provide haptic support for a lens implant continue to be PMMA itself, polypropylene, and polyimide. All three appear to perform in a satisfactory fashion, especially if placed inside the capsular bag. The possible oxidative biodegradation of polypropylene and its ability to induce inflammation have reduced its popularity, especially when sulcus fixation or anterior chamber angle fixation is selected. The dominant trend is toward one-piece, all-PMMA posterior chamber lenses.

Manufacturing Techniques

There are at least five different ways to manufacture IOLs today from PMMA material.[78] Although the exact details of the manufacturing process are often proprietary, a brief review follows.

The most popular method is lathe cutting, in which lenses are cut out of a PMMA blank, usually of a high-molecular-weight acrylic such as Perspex CQ. Initially, PMMA cast sheets are received as raw material. PMMA cast sheets are preformed and then, using a computer-aided microlathe, lens blanks are cut to the appropriate specific spherical radius for the optic power. The lens blanks are polished. In three-piece lenses, the loops are then formed and attached. In one-piece lenses, the lens optic is lathe cut with a diamond-tip tool to the radius of curvature, and the haptic shape is milled to size and shape. A modern lathe can be programmed to produce a variety of lens shapes and powers. After formation, most lenses are tumble polished, using a drum filled with small spheres that rotate slowly for hours to days. This results in very smooth edges. As an alternative, polishing pads may be used to buff the surface and edges.

In a second manufacturing technique, compression molding is added to the lathe cutting. After creating the lens with a lathe, the implant is placed into a mold, and heat and pressure are applied to shape the lens into its final form. The lens is then carefully polished. This manufacturing technique produces a lens that requires less polishing than a lens produced solely by lathe cutting.

A third method is compression polymerization, in which well-aged and dried base material is poured into a hard stainless steel mold and slowly warmed under high pressure until polymerization occurs. High pressure is maintained as the material is cooled by blowing.

Fourth, the lenses may be cast molded. Cast molding requires the use of resin in a distilled and purified form. PMMA monomer is crystallized into a pregel or prepolymer residue. The pregel is vacuum processed, filtered, and poured into molds of the desired optical configuration. Lens blanks are cast in a curing cycle similar to that used to prepare cast sheet PMMA.

Finally, lenses may be injection molded. In injection molding, the plastic is heated and then injected into a steel mold. As it softens, it takes the shape of the PMMA mold. After the PMMA cools, the blank is removed from the mold and the edges are polished.

It is clear that manufacture of IOLs by any of these techniques is sophisticated and requires highly skilled technical capability. For an IOL to be suitable for implantation, it must be within 0.25 D of stated power; have the proper shape and configuration within 0.25 mm; have a uniform, smooth surface and edges; be chemically pure without any residual monomer, ethylene oxide, or contaminants; be clean of surface debris; and be sterile. Although all manufacturers incorporate careful practices and all IOLs are inspected, it is the surgeon's responsibility to perform a final inspection as well. This may be done under high power with the operating microscope. If the lens shows any imperfection, it should be rejected for implantation and returned to the manufacturer.

Sterilization

PMMA lenses cannot be heat sterilized because the material will melt. Most PMMA lenses are sterilized by ethylene oxide, which is the only technique that is approved by the United States Food and Drug Administration. Ethylene oxide is a cyclic ether that can be toxic to tissue and adheres only to plastic. Although it is an effective sterilizer, all IOLs must be quarantined after sterilization until excess ethylene oxide evaporates and reaches a nontoxic level. Ethylene oxide residual continues to be a concern as a possible cause of postoperative inflammation after implantation of IOLs. The alternative technique of sodium hydroxide sterilization is not used in the United States but is potentially effective.

General Design Characteristics, Optic Size, and Shape

IOL optics range in size from 4.5 to 7.5 mm. The potential advantage of a larger optic is a lens that is more forgiving of decentration and one that is less likely to produce unwanted optical aberration as a result of light deflecting off the edge of the optic.[79,80] In addition, there is a reduced likelihood of complications such as pupillary capture. An optic size of 6.5 to 7 mm is appropriately popular with surgeons using planned extracapsular cataract extraction in which a large incision is made (Figure 34-9).

As more surgeons convert to phacoemulsification and use of continuous-tear anterior capsulectomy, smaller optic lenses are becoming more popular.[81-83] In particular, lenses with a round optic of 5 to 5.5 mm are currently favored by many phacoemulsification surgeons (Figure 34-10). Because lens implants placed inside the bag after capsulorhexis show minimal decentration, this optic size seems satisfactory for most older patients.[79] However, these lenses have the potential for increased optical aberration as a result of edge light deflection. Several manufacturers are working on edge treatments to reduce the unwanted visual images created when a lens implant edge is exposed in the pupil.

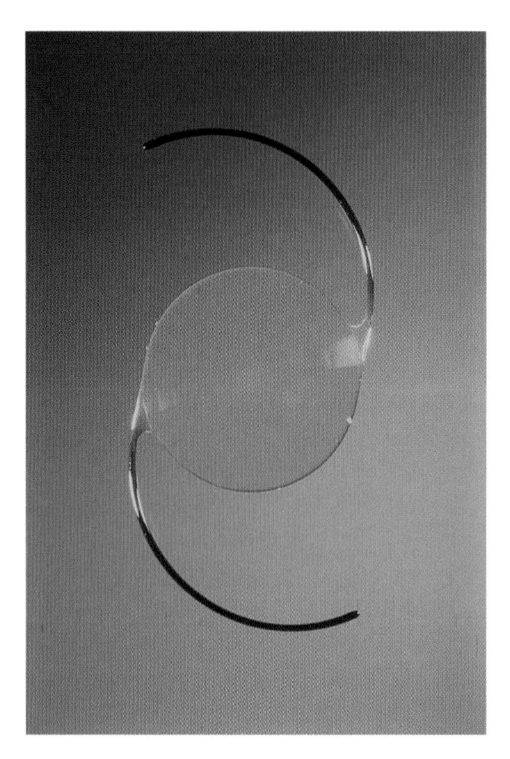

FIGURE 34-9 Modern one-piece, all-PMMA, open-loop posterior chamber lens with a 6.5-mm optic. (Courtesy IOLAB Corporation, Claremont, Calif.)

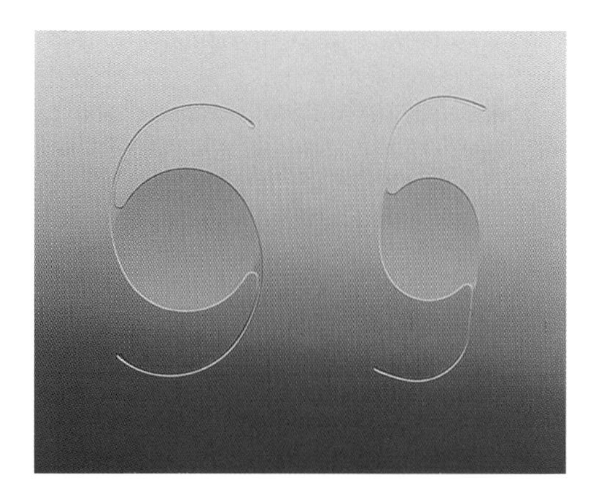

FIGURE 34-10 A 7-mm round optic, one-piece, all-PMMA posterior chamber lens side by side with a 5- × 6-mm oval lens. (Courtesy Storz Corporation, St. Louis, Mo.)

Oval optics, especially those 5 by 6 mm in diameter, are available and also allow implantation through a relatively small incision. Unfortunately, inside a continuous-tear circular anterior capsulectomy, some lenses decenter in the axis perpendicular to the loops, rendering the extra optical diameter in the opposite meridian less helpful. In addition, the oval lenses appear to induce a higher incidence of unwanted glare or reflection off the edge of the 5-mm portion of the optic, which is usually somewhat thicker. Currently, oval lenses are rarely used as most surgeons favor round optic lenses.

In regard to shape, biconvex lenses appear to be the soundest design. In addition to simulating the natural lens and providing a good optical quality, the posterior convex portion of the optic in close apposition to the posterior capsule appears capable of retarding opacification from Elschnig pearls.[84-86] A biconvex implant design also presents a relatively low profile, which enhances implant-to-iris clearance.

Other design shapes, including meniscus, planoconvex, and those with laser spacing ridges, are still preferred by some surgeons but are significantly less popular. Many lenses have one or more small holes placed in the optic or adjacent to the optic-haptic junction to aid the surgeon in positioning the lens within the eye. Although some surgeons find these useful, with modern flexible-loop capsular bag lenses, positioning holes are probably unnecessary and in some cases can produce unwanted optical aberrations.[37] Use of the optic-haptic junction for manipulation as an alternative to positioning holes in the optic is currently favored by most surgeons because this configuration reduces the chance of postoperative unwanted visual aberrations.

Loop Size, Shape, and Configuration

Loop materials currently used in most posterior chamber lenses include PMMA, polypropylene, and polyamide. One-piece and three-piece PMMA lenses, three-piece polypropylene lenses, and polyamide haptic lenses have excellent track records with no strong scientific evidence to support one or the other. However, there is an increasing trend toward use of one-piece, all PMMA lenses among experienced surgeons. Theoretically, the absence of a junction between two materials reduces the chance for a discontinuity at which inflammatory cells and debris could accumulate. Several studies have shown that the capsular bag stretches only from approximately 9.5 to approximately 11 mm after cataract extraction and that the diameter of the ciliary sulcus is only 11.5 to 12.5 mm.[46] This has led to a trend toward shortening the overall tip-to-tip diameter of posterior chamber IOLs. These so-called capsular bag lenses are usually 11.5 to 12.5 mm from tip to tip. These lenses provide a relative ease of implantation without excess capsular stretch and striae in the postoperative period. Nonetheless, the longer tip-to-tip diameter lenses have achieved an excellent track record over the past 10 years.

Multiple-loop configurations—beginning with the J-loop lens, followed by the Y-loop configurations popularized by Kratz and Sinskey, through the longer and more gradual C-loop, and on to the modified C loop, which is most popular today—are available without any strong scientific proof favoring one over the other. The choice of loop configuration is usually made by the preference of the individual surgeon and influenced by ease of implantation. The majority of surgeons use a modified or short C configuration. Loops are usually angled to a small degree, in the belief that this will reduce pupil capture and iris chafe and place the optic more directly in contact with the posterior capsule.[87] An angulation of 3 to 10 degrees is usually preferred. Some loops also contain holes or notches for specialized implantation forceps or for use in scleral fixation. Some loops are colored to provide easier visualization during and after implantation into the eye. Increased visibility of the loops can assist in ensuring that the implant is inside the capsular bag (Figure 34-11).

The most popular lenses of today appear to be those manufactured with biconvex optics, which are round and between 5 and 6.5 mm in diameter. In most cases, these lenses are one-piece or three-piece tumble-polished biconvex optics with haptics of PMMA. The preferred overall diameter is 12 to 12.5 mm, with a modified short C loop and an angulation of approximately 5 degrees. Results with these lenses are superb, and surgeons can use them with confidence. Other alternative lens designs continue to attract small but loyal followings, including various closed-loop designs such as those advocated by Sheets and Anis for capsular bag fixation.[29,88] In addition, disc or plate lenses have been investigated, especially in Europe.[6]

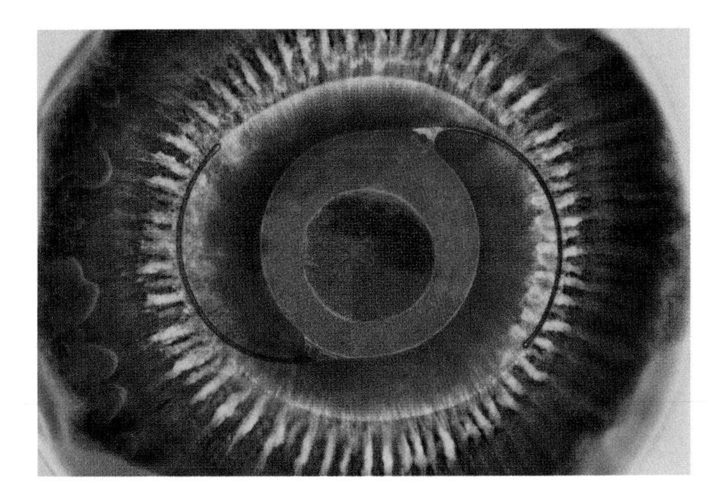

FIGURE 34-11 A colored-loop, one-piece, all-PMMA posterior chamber lens inside the capsular bag, as viewed by a Miyake eye model posterior photograph. (Courtesy IOLAB Corporation, Claremont, Calif.)

Surface Modification of PMMA Lenses

With improvements in surgical technique and equipment, the incidence of postoperative inflammation following cataract surgery has decreased dramatically. Nevertheless, evidence has shown that a low-grade inflammatory response occurs to the IOL implant.[89-91] Clinical and histologic studies have demonstrated that a foreign body reaction likely occurs in all eyes following IOL implantation.[92-94] This inflammatory reaction may result in synechiae, cellular and pigmented deposits on the IOL, and uveitis. Certain conditions, such as preexisting uveitis, diabetes, glaucoma, or a young age may predispose a patient to this event.

Despite PMMA being a relatively inert material in the human eye, its biocompatibility is compromised in one respect, that of surface molecular structure. The ends of the long polymer chains of PMMA, when exposed to the surface of the IOL, can induce inflammatory responses. Knowledge of this interaction potential has stimulated much research into methods of modifying the surface of PMMA lenses such that the exposed polymer ends are either chemically modified or coated with another material.[42,43]

In particular, the use of a heparin coating on the IOL has been investigated and has been shown to reduce early postoperative inflammation in high-risk eyes.[44,45] This IOL is created by inducing electrostatic adsorption of heparin onto the surface of the PMMA IOL. In vitro experiments have demonstrated a reduced activation of human granulocytes with heparin coating of PMMA. Furthermore, platelet adhesion and growth of human fibroblasts are reduced.[95]

A coating of heparin has been shown to decrease the number and severity of lens deposits. In addition, the likelihood of formation of adhesions to the IOL is decreased.[96-98] Some have found heparin-coated IOLs to be free of cellular deposits and to reduce the incidence of inflammatory complications, compared with unmodified PMMA lenses.[99] In addition, fewer lens deposits lead to a clearer implant and better visual acuity.[100] These benefits have been found not only for high-risk eyes but for routine cases as well.[101] Care must be taken in implanting heparin-coated IOLs because the heparin can be mechanically destroyed in the areas where the lens is grasped.[102] The clinical consequences of this occurrence are not currently known.

Another modification of PMMA IOL surfaces has been introduced by Bausch & Lomb Surgical. This innovation, known as fluorine surface modification, is unique in that it produces a permanent, irreversible change in the molecular structure and composition of the IOL surface. Again, this results in enhanced biocompatibility with decreased cellular adsorption and adhesions.[103] Fluorine-surface modified lenses have been used in the correction of pediatric aphakia, a procedure in which the postoperative inflammatory response can be significant. These lenses have demonstrated a reduced cicatricial response compared with unmodified PMMA lenses.[104]

Conclusions

Although IOLs have historically been placed in the anterior chamber angle, pupillary space, or posterior chamber, the posterior chamber has been confirmed to be the safest and most effective for primary implantation.

Surgeons have the opportunity to select from a large variety of IOL designs. Most of the differences are small modifications based on individual preference, but some design features have been shown to be advantageous through clinical experience and scientific study. PMMA is clearly a superior material for lens implant. Biconvex optics appear to be preferred over other shapes. In addition, a round optic appears to be superior to an oval optic. The trend is therefore toward one-piece, biconvex PMMA lenses, which may have a slight advantage over three-piece lenses.

The short modified C-loop haptic appears to be a good compromise between ease of implantation and solid fixation and centration. Reduction in the overall tip-to-tip loop diameter to 12 to 12.5 mm is consistent with ocular anatomy, and loops that angle forward 3 to 10 degrees reduce contact between the lens and the iris and thereby the chance for pupillary capture. In addition, implantation within the capsular bag appears to be superior to sulcus fixation because the lens is sequestered from contact with vascular tissue.

Positioning holes and notches on the lens loops are unnecessary for most surgeons for routine implantation and may result in secondary complications, such as optical aberration or difficulty in IOL removal. Most lenses incorporate an ultraviolet light absorber in spite of the absence of strong evidence in its favor. Loop coloration may ease implantation for the beginning surgeon but is not required for most experienced surgeons. Surface modification may be useful to reduce the postoperative inflammatory response, particularly in high-risk cases.

The evolution to the current state of the art in posterior chamber lenses over a period of more than 40 years represents a marvel of collaboration among manufacturers, ophthalmic surgeons, and patients throughout the world.

REFERENCES

1. Jaffe NS, Clayman HM, Hirschman H et al: *Pseudophakos,* St Louis, 1978, Mosby.
2. Alpar JJ, Fechner PU: *Fechner's intraocular lenses,* New York, 1986, Thieme-Stratton.
3. Gorin G: *History of ophthalmology,* Wilmington, Del, 1982, Publish or Perish Inc.
4. Ridley H: Intraocular acrylic lenses, *Trans Ophthalmol Soc U K* 71:617-621, 1951.
5. Ridley H: Intraocular acrylic lenses: 10 years' development, *Br J Ophthalmol* 44:705-712, 1960.
6. Ridley H: Safety requirements for acrylic implants, *Br J Ophthalmol* 41:359-367, 1957.
7. Strampelli B: Les lentilles camerules après six annees d'experience, *Acta Ophthalmol Belgica* 2:1692-1698, 1958.
8. Nordlohne ME: *The intraocular implant lens: development and results with special reference to the Binkhorst lens,* The Hague, 1975, Dr W Junk Publishers.
9. Drews RC: The Barraquer experience with intraocular lenses: 20 years later, *Ophthalmology* 89:386-393, 1982.
10. Shearing S: A practical posterior chamber lens, *Contact: IOL Med J* 4:114-117, 1978.
11. Epstein E: Modified Ridley lenses, *Br J Ophthalmol* 43:29-33, 1959.
12. Binkhorst CD, Leonard PAM: Results in 208 iris-clip pseudophakos implantations, *AM J Ophthalmol* 64:947-956, 1967.
13. Binkhorst CD, Kats A, Leonard PAM: Extracapsular pseudophakia, *Am J Ophthalmol* 73:625-636, 1972.
14. Binkhorst CD: Iris-clip and irido-capsular lens implants (pseudophakia): personal techniques of pseudophakia, *Br J Ophthalmol* 51:761-771, 1967.
15. Worst JGF: Iris sutures for artificial lens fixation: Perlon vs. stainless steel, *Trans Am Acad Ophthalmol Otolaryngol* 88:102-104, 1976.
16. Pearce JL: Pearce-style posterior chamber lenses, *J Am Intraocul Implant Soc* 6:33-36, 1980.
17. Pearce JL: Intraocular lenses, *Curr Opin Ophthalmol* 3:29-38, 1992.
18. Baikoff F: L'insertion capsulaire des implants de Simcoe, *J Fr Ophtalmol* 4:14-23, 1981.
19. Clayman HM: Ultraviolet-absorbing intraocular lenses, *J Am Intraocul Implant Soc* 10:429-432, 1984.
20. Olson RJ, Kolodner H, Kaufman HE: The optical quality of currently manufactured intraocular lenses, *Am J Ophthalmol* 88:548-555, 1979.
21. Simpson MJ: Optical quality of intraocular lenses, *J Cataract Refract Surg* 18:86-90, 1992.
22. Drews RC, Smith ME, Okun N: Scanning electron microscopy of intraocular lenses, *Ophthalmology* 85:415-424, 1978.
23. Yamanaka A, Matsumoto T, Nakama K et al: Physical and chemical analysis of intraocular materials, *J Am Intraocul Implant Soc* 5:131-136, 1979.
24. Apple DJ, Mamalis N, Olson RJ et al: *Intraocular lenses: evolution, designs, complications and pathology,* Baltimore, 1989, Williams & Wilkins, pp 405-426.
25. Shepard DD: The dangers of metal-loop intraocular lenses, *J Am Intraocul Implant Soc* 3:42-45, 1977.
26. Drews RC: Quality control and changing indications for lens implantation. Seventh Binkhorst Medical Lecture, 1982. *Ophthalmology* 90:301-310, 1983.
27. Clayman HM: Intraocular lenses. In Duane TD, Jaeger EAD, editors: *Clinical ophthalmology,* Philadelphia, 1991, JB Lippincott.
28. Galin MA, Turkish L: Studies of intraocular lens sterilization: the effect of NaOH on *B. subtillis* spores, *J Am Intraocul Implant Soc* 6:18-20, 1980.
29. Maida JW, Sheets JH: Intraocular lenses: a review of 1,000 consecutive cases, *Contacts: IOL Med J* 4:95-101, 1978.
30. Olmos EZ, Roy FH: Results of over 1,000 intraocular lens implants in the last five years, *Contact: IOL Med J* 6:162-170, 1980.
31. Jaffe NS: Results of intraocular lens implant surgery, *Am J Ophthalmol* 85:13-23, 1978.
32. Kaufman HE, Katz JI: Endothelial damage from intraocular lens insertion, *Invest Ophthalmol* 15:996-1000, 1976.
33. Miller D, Doane MG: High-speed photographic evaluation of intraocular lens movements, *Am J Ophthalmol* 97:752-759, 1984.
34. Severin SL: The Severin posterior chamber lens for intracapsular surgery, *Contact: IOL Med J* 6:291-293, 1980.
35. Kratz RP, Mazzocco TR, Davidson B et al: A comparative analysis of anterior chamber, iris-supported, capsule-fixated, and posterior chamber intraocular lenses following cataract extraction by phacoemulsification, *Ophthalmology* 88:56-58, 1981.
36. Stark WJ, Worthen DM, Holladay JT et al: The FDA report on intraocular lenses, *Ophthalmology* 90:311-317, 1983.
37. Brems RN, Apple DJ, Pfeffer BR, et al: Posterior chamber intraocular lenses in a series of 75 autopsy eyes. Part III: Correlation of positioning holes and optic edges with the pupillary aperture and visual axis, *J Cataract Refract Surg* 12:367-371, 1986.
38. Kratz RP: Intraocular lenses: complications associated with intraocular lenses, *Ophthalmology* 86:659-661, 1979.
39. Crawford JB: A histopathological study of the position of the Shearing intraocular lens in the posterior chamber, *Am J Ophthalmol* 91:458-461, 1981.
40. Hoffer KJ: Five years' experience with the ridges laser lens implant. In Emery JM, Jacobson AC, editors: *Current concepts in cataract surgery,* Norwalk, Conn, 1984, Appleton & Lange, pp 296-299.
41. Maltzman B, Haupt E, Cucci P: Effect of laser ridge on posterior capsular opacification, *J Cataract Refract Surg* 15:644-647, 1989.
42. Ratner BD, Mateo NB: Surface modification of intraocular lenses, *Ophthalmol Clin North Am* 4:277-293, 1991.

43. Hofmeister FM, Yalon MS, Iida S et al: In vitro evaluation of iris chafe protection afforded by hydrophilic surface modification of polymethylmethacrylate intraocular lenses, *J Cataract Refract Surg* 14:514-519, 1988.
44. Larson R, Selen G, Bjorklund H et al: Intraocular PMMA lenses modified with surface-immobilized heparin: evaluation of bio-compatibility in vitro and in vivo, *Biomaterials* 10:511-516, 1989.
45. Phillipson B, Fagerholm P, Calel B et al: Heparin surface modified intraocular lenses: three month follow-up of a randomized, double-masked clinical trial, *J Cataract Refract Surg* 18:71-77, 1992.
46. Assia El, Legler UFC, Libby CC et al: Size and configuration of the capsular bag after short and long-term fixation of PC-IOL's in-the-bag. Presented at the American Society of Cataract and Refractive Surgery Annual Meeting, Boston, 1992.
47. Masket S: Pseudophakic posterior iris chafing syndrome, *J Cataract Refract Surg* 12:252-256, 1986.
48. Van-Oye R, Budo C, Galand A et al: Two year postoperative results of Galand lens implantation, *J Cataract Refract Surg* 12:135-139, 1986.
49. Gunning FP, Greve EL: Intracapsular cataract extraction with implantation of the Galand disc lens: a retrospective analysis in patients with and without glaucoma, *Ophthalmic Surg* 22:531-538, 1991.
50. Kratz RP: Intracapsular versus extracapsular cataract extraction for intraocular lens implantation, *Int Ophthalmol Clin* 19:179-194, 1979.
51. Keates RH, Ehrlich DR: "Lenses of chance": complications of anterior chamber implants, *Ophthalmology* 85:408-414, 1978.
52. Reidy JJ, Apple DJ, Googe JM et al: An analysis of semi-flexible, closed loop anterior chamber intraocular lenses, *J Am Intraocul Implant Soc* 11:344-352, 1985.
53. Lim ES, Apple DJ, Tsai JC et al: An analysis of flexible anterior chamber lenses with special references to the normalized rate of explantation, *Ophthalmology* 98:243-246, 1991.
54. Beehler CC: A review of 100 cases of flexible anterior chamber lens implantation, *J Am Intraocul Implant Soc* 10:188-190, 1984.
55. Smith PW, Wong SK, Start WJ et al: Complications of semi-flexible closed loop anterior chamber intraocular lenses, *Arch Ophthalmol* 105:52-57, 1987.
56. Saunders JJ: *Organic polymer chemistry,* New York, 1973, Chapman and Hall.
57. Mainster MA: Spectral transmittance of intraocular lenses and retinal damage from intense light sources, *Am J Ophthalmol* 85:167-170, 1978.
58. Gupta A: Long-term aging behavior of ultraviolet absorbing intraocular lenses, *J Am Intraocul Implant Soc* 10:309-314, 1984.
59. Kraff MC, Sanders DR, Jampol LM et al: Effect of an ultraviolet filtering intraocular lens on cystoid macular edema, *Ophthalmology* 92:366-369, 1985.
60. Holyk PR, Eifrig DE: Effects of monomeric methylmethacrylate on ocular tissues, *Am J Ophthalmol* 88:385-395, 1979.
61. Galin MA, Chowchuvech E, Turkishfd L: Uveitis and intraocular lenses, *Trans Ophthalmol Soc UK* 96:16-167, 1976.
62. Turkish L, Galin MA: Methylmethacrylate monomer in intraocular lenses of polymethylmethacrylate, *Arch Ophthalmol* 98:120-121, 1980.
63. Terry AC, Stark WJ, Newsome DA et al: Tissue toxicity of laser-damaged intraocular lens implants, *Ophthalmology* 92:414-418, 1985.
64. Mellerio J, Capon MMRC, Docchio F et al: A new form of damage to PMMA intraocular lenses by Nd: YAG laser photodisruptors, *Eye* 2:376-381, 1988.
65. Bath PR, Romberger AB, Brown P: A comparison of Nd:YAG-laser damage thresholds for PMMA and silicone intraocular lenses, *Invest Ophthalmol Vis Sci* 27:795-798, 1986.
66. Loertscher H: Laser-induced breakdown for ophthalmic applications. In Troken SL, editor: *YAG Laser ophthalmic microsurgery,* Norwalk, Conn, 1983, Appleton & Lange, pp 40-67.
67. O'Connell RM, Deaton TF, Saito TT: Single and multiple shot laser damage properties of commercial grade PMMA, *Appl Optics* 23:682-688, 1984.
68. Wolter JR: Foreign body giant cells on intraocular lens implants, *Graefes Arch Clin Exp Ophthalmol* 1219:103-111, 1982.
69. Sievers H, Von Domarus D: Foreign-body reaction against intraocular lenses, *Am J Ophthalmol* 97:743-751, 1984.
70. Tuberville AW, Galin MA, Perez HD et al: Complement activation by nylon and polypropylene-looped prosthetic intraocular lenses, *Invest Ophthalmol Vis Sci* 22:727-733, 1982.
71. Grossman LW, Knight WB: Resolution testing of intraocular lenses, *J Cataract Refract Surg* 71:84-90, 1991.
72. Kronenthal FL: Intraocular degradation of non-absorbable sutures, *J Am Intraocul Implant Soc* 3:222-238, 1977.
73. Jaffe NS: Polyethylene terephthalate (Dacron) in intraocular surgery, *Ophthalmology* 88:955-958, 1981.
74. Clayman HM: Polypropylene, *Ophthalmology* 88:959-964, 1981.
75. Tuberville AW, Wood TO: Aqueous humor protein and complement in pseudophakic eyes, *Cornea* 9:249-253, 1990.
76. Dilly PN, Sellors PJ: Bacterial adhesion to intraocular lenses, *J Cataract Refract Surg* 15:317-320, 1989.
77. Menikoff JA, Speaker MG, Marmor M et al: A case-control study of risk factors for postoperative endophthalmitis, *Ophthalmology* 98:761-1768, 1991.
78. Olson RJ: Intraocular lens quality: update 1979, *J Am Intraocul Implant* Soc 6:16-17, 1980.
79. Hansen SO, Tetz MR, Solomon KD et al: Decentration of flexible loop posterior chamber intraocular lenses in a series of 222 postmortem eyes, *Ophthalmology* 95:344-349, 1988.
80. Assia El, Castanada VE, Legler UF et al: Studies on cataract surgery and intraocular lenses at the Center for Intraocular Lens Research, *Ophthalmol Clin North Am* 4:251-266, 1991.
81. Gimbal HV, Neuhann T: Development, advantages and methods of the continuous tear capsulorhexis technique, *J Cataract Refract Surg* 16:33-37, 1990.
82. Apple DJ, Assia EI, Wasserman D et al: Evidence in support of the continuous tear anterior capsulotomy (capsulorhexis technique). In Cangelosi GC, editor: *Advances in cataract surgery: transaction of the New Orleans Academy of Ophthalmology,* Thorofare, NJ, 1991, Slack, pp 21-47.
83. Armstrong TA: Refractive effect of capsular bag lens placement with the capsulorhexis technique, *J Cataract Refract Surg* 18:121-124, 1992.
84. Hansen SO, Solomon KD, McKnight GT et al: Posterior capsule opacification and intraocular lens decentration. Part I: Comparison of various posterior chamber lens designs implanted in the rabbit model, *J Cataract Refract Surg* 14:605-613, 1988.
85. Born CF, Ryan DK: Effect of intraocular lens optic design on posterior capsule opacification, *J Cataract Refract Surg* 16:188-192, 1990.
86. Setty S, Percival S: Intraocular lens design and inhibition of epithelium, *Br J Ophthalmol* 73:918-921, 1989.
87. Johnson SH, Kratz RP, Olson PF: Transillumination defect and microhyphema syndrome, *J Am Intraocul Implant Soc* 10:425-428, 1984.
88. Galand A, Van Oye R, Budo C et al: Results of implantation in the capsular bag: a short-term review of 1588 cases, *Trans Ophthalmol Soc U K* 105: 562-566, 1985.
89. Jennette JC, Eifrig DE, Paranjape YB: The inflammatory response to secondary methylmethacrylate challenge in lens-implanted rabbits, *J Am Intraocul Lens Implant Soc* 8:35-37, 1982.
90. Mondino BJ, Nagata S, Glovsky MM: Activation of the alternative complement pathway by intraocular lenses, *Invest Ophthalmol Vis Sci* 26:905-908, 1985.
91. Mondino BJ, Rao H: Effect of intraocular lenses on complement levels in human serum, *Acta Ophthalmol* 61:76-84, 1983.
92. Ohara K: Biomicroscopy of surface deposits resembling foreign body giant cells on implanted intraocular lenses, *Am J Ophthalmol* 11:260-267, 1985.
93. Wolter JR: Cytopathology of intraocular lens implantation, *Ophthalmology* 92:135-142, 1985.
94. Bryan JA III, Peiffer RL Jr, Brown DT et al: Morphology of pseudophakic precipitates on intraocular lenses removed from human patients, *J Am Intraocul Lens Implant Soc* 11:260-267, 1985.
95. Larsson R, Selen G, Bjorklund H, et al: Intraocular PMMA lenses modified with surface-immobilized heparin: evaluation of biocompatibility in vitro and in vivo, *Biomaterials* 10:511-516, 1989.
96. Ygge J, Wenzel M, Philipson B: Cellular reactions on heparin surface-modified versus regular PMMA lenses during the first postoperative month, *Ophthalmology* 97:1216-1223, 1990.
97. Miyake K, Maekubo K: Comparison of heparin surface modified and ordinary PCLS: a Japanese study, *Eur J Implant Refract Surg* 3:95-97, 1991.
98. Borgioli M, Coster DJ, Fan RFT: Effect of heparin surface modification on polymethylmethacrylate intraocular lenses on signs of postoperative inflammation after extracapsular cataract extraction, *Ophthalmology* 99:1248-1255, 1992.
99. Percival SPB, Pai V: Heparin-modified lenses for eyes at risk for breakdown of the blood-aqueous barrier during cataract surgery, *J Cataract Refract Surg* 19:760-765, 1993.
100. Jones NP: Extracapsular cataract surgery with and without intraocular lens implantation in Fuchs' heterochromic uveitis, *Am J Ophthalmol* 108: 310-314, 1989.
101. Trocme SD, Hung-ir L: Effect of heparin-surface-modified intraocular

lenses on postoperative inflammation after phacoemulsification: a randomized trial in a United States patient population, *Ophthalmology* 107:1031-1037, 2000.

102. Dick B, Kohnen T, Jacobi KW: Alteration of heparin coating on intraocular lenses caused by implantation instruments, *Klin Moatsbl Augenheilkd* 206:460-466, 1995.

103. Eloy R, Parrat D, Tran Min Duc CE et al: In vitro evaluation of inflammatory cell response after CF4 plasma surface modification of poly(methyl methacrylate) intraocular lenses, *J Cataract Refract Surg* 19:364-370, 1993.

104. Thouvenin D, Arne JL, Lesueur L: Comparison of fluorine-surface-modified and unmodified lenses for implantation in pediatric aphakia, *J Cataract Refract Surg* 22:1226-1231, 1996.

Foldable Intraocular Lenses

35

Roger F. Steinert, MD

Foldable Intraocular Lenses and Small-Incision Surgery

The soft implant material that makes up a foldable intraocular lens (IOL) enables a 6-mm IOL to be inserted through a 3-mm incision with minimal trauma. For forceps insertion, the surgeon grasps the IOL, bends it in half with folding forceps, grasps the folded IOL with insertion forceps, then maneuvers the lens through the incision until the IOL and haptics are appropriately situated. For insertion with an implantation device, the surgeon grasps the IOL with holding forceps, positions the IOL in the device, inserts the tip of the device through the incision, and implants the IOL. Some lenses are available for insertion without the need for folding forceps or inserters.

As the IOL slides into position inside the capsular bag or within the ciliary sulcus, the optic unfurls to resume its original shape. Visual recovery from the aphakic state is almost immediate. Visual acuity after cataract surgery and IOL implantation is nearly always an improvement over vision through a crystalline lens with a cataract, especially with small foldable IOLs and small-incision surgical techniques.

A major advantage of small-incision cataract surgery is that it minimizes corneal shape changes that induce astigmatism and delay visual recovery.[1-3] Rigid polymethylmethacrylate (PMMA) lenses require a wound size of at least the size of the optic diameter, 6 mm for example, to be able to insert the lens. Foldable IOLs can be inserted through incisions of 3.5 mm, 3 mm, or less, depending on the IOL and insertion system used.

The scope of this chapter is the restoration of lenticular refraction and correction of refractive errors at the time of cataract surgery. Most of the literature cited is from 1995 to 2001 because the IOL technologies, surgical techniques, and systems of analysis have more in common than in the early years of foldable IOL development. Some earlier reports are included to show trends over time.

The major foldable IOLs and their manufacturers are listed in Table 35-1. The physical properties of these IOLs are listed in Table 35-2.

Small-Incision Surgery

Effect of Incision Size on Astigmatism

Surgically induced changes in the structural stability of the cornea may produce or aggravate corneal astigmatism that may not be amenable to correction postoperatively with a spherocylindrical lens. Surgically induced astigmatism can adversely affect postoperative refraction and the stability of the patient's vision over time. Incision length, location, shape, orientation, and suture technique and material are factors. The following investigators compared the effect of incision length on astigmatism following implantation of a foldable IOL through a small incision or a rigid PMMA IOL through a larger incision. Incision sizes and their impact on astigmatism are summarized in Table 35-3.

Hayashi et al.[2] conducted a prospective, randomized study of the correlation between incision size and corneal shape changes in sutureless surgery in 200 eyes at 1 week and 1, 3, and 6 months after surgery. Group A had 64 eyes implanted with a high-refractive-index silicone IOL through a 3.2-mm incision. Group B had 65 eyes implanted with a lower-refractive-index silicone IOL through a 4-mm incision. Group C had 71 eyes implanted with a PMMA lens through a 5-mm incision. According to corneal topography measurements, eyes implanted with the high-refractive-index lens through a 3.2-mm incision had wound-related flattening in the peripheral cornea at 1 week that disappeared by 1 month and did not reoccur. Eyes in the 4-mm incision group had less wound-related peripheral flattening but developed an irregular steepening in the lower central cornea at 6 months. Eyes in the 5-mm incision group experienced a similar steepening in the lower cornea that persisted and extended to the upper central cornea at 3 and 6 months. Based on these findings, the authors recommended incision sizes of 3 mm or less to improve uncorrected postoperative visual acuity.

Pfleger et al.[4] observed 103 consecutive patients with postoperative astigmatism for 1 year to determine if there was a correlation between surgically induced astigmatism and incision sizes. A foldable silicone IOL was implanted through incision

TABLE 35-1

Manufacturers of IOLs and IOL Trade Names

Company	Location	Product
Alcon Laboratories	Fort Worth, TX	AcrySof
Advanced Medical Optics (AMO)	Santa Ana, CA	Array Multifocal ClariFlex PhacoFlex II Sensar with OptiEdge
Bausch & Lomb Surgical	Rochester, NY	ChiroFlex EasAcryl HydroView SoFlex
CIBA Vision/Novatris	Duluth, GA	MemoryLens
IOLTech	La Rochelle, France	MF4 Multifocal Lens Haptibag Tripode XL Stabi XL Octo Stabibag Bigbag FZ60
Medical Developmental Research	Clearwater, FL	HydroFlex II
Rayner Intraocular Lenses	East Sussex, UK	Centerflex Raysoft
Pharmacia	Peapack, NJ	CeeOn CeeOn Edge
STAAR Surgical	Monrovia, CA	AA-4203TF and TL (toric) AA-4203, 4204, 4207 Collamer Elastic Elastimide

IOL, Intraocular lens.

sizes of 3.2 mm (n = 35) and 4 mm (n = 37), and a PMMA lens was implanted through an incision size of 5.2 mm (n = 31). The smaller incisions were self-sealing, and the 5.2-mm incisions were closed with a suture as needed. Mean preoperative cylinder was similar in all three groups. Immediately after surgery there was a small with-the-rule astigmatic shift in all groups that resolved by the 1-year follow-up. The smallest incision was associated with the least surgically induced astigmatism and axial change.

Olson and Crandall[5] conducted a prospective, randomized, masked clinical comparison of 3.2-mm and 5.5-mm incision sizes to determine if foldable lenses had long-term benefits over rigid lenses. In all 55 eyes (55 patients) in the 3.2-mm incision group, a foldable silicone three-piece IOL was implanted, whereas in the 56 eyes (56 patients) in the 5.5-mm incision group, a one-piece PMMA IOL was implanted. All incisions were in the superior vertical meridian, commenced 1.5 mm posterior to the limbus, and extended into the cornea for a total length of 2.5 to 3 mm. All incision sizes were determined before the IOL was implanted. Keratometry was performed in a masked fashion and not by the surgeon. A general change to against-the-wound astigmatism and a significant difference in the astigmatic shift between the two incision sizes were seen over the 3-year follow-up. Eyes in the 3.2-mm incision group had significantly less astigmatic shift (–0.18 vs. –0.88 D; $P < .001$) and better visual acuity (logMAR, 0.14 vs. 0.26; $P = .04$) than eyes in the 5.5-mm incision group. The depth and length of the incision (forces that relax the wound) were the major factors in against-the-wound shifts, and wound healing (forces that tighten the wound) was the major factor in with-the-wound shifts. Based on the findings of their 3-year evaluation, the authors concluded that smaller-incision surgery with a foldable IOL has statistical and clinical advantages over a 5.5-mm incision.

Oshika et al.[6] came to the same conclusion in their 3-year prospective, randomized study of foldable silicone IOLs (n = 99) implanted through a 3.2-mm incision and PMMA IOLs (n = 98) implanted through a 5.5-mm incision. Eyes implanted with foldable lenses had significantly better uncorrected and corrected visual acuity in the immediate postoperative period and less surgically induced astigmatism throughout the study than eyes implanted with rigid lenses.

Müller-Jensen and Barlinn[7] looked at corneal refractive changes after implantation with a foldable acrylic (AcrySof) or PMMA IOL. All of the 147 patients in the study had spherical corneas (n = 47) or preoperative astigmatism of 0.5 to 2.5 D (n = 100). Corneal topography was measured preoperatively and at 3 days and 6 months postoperatively. Analyses were performed using the subtractive method, Jaffe's vector analysis, Naeser's polar value method, and the formula by Holladay. Patients with spherical corneas (no preoperative astigmatism) had significantly less induced astigmatism with the 3.2-mm incision than the 4.1-mm incision. The 4.1-mm incision was associated with 0.8 D and the 3.2-mm incision with 0.4 D of induced astigmatism. For patients with preoperative astigmatism, there was more postoperative astigmatism in the 4.1-mm than the 3.2-mm incision group, but the differences were less clear. For those having with-the-wound changes in astigmatism, the differences were significant with the subtraction and Holladay methods (both $P = .02$) than for those with against-the-wound astigmatism. The postoperative polar value of Naeser showed significant differences ($P = .01$) between the two incisions.

Hayashi et al.[8] conducted a prospective study of 224 eyes randomly assigned for implantation with a silicone IOL (SI40NB, AMO) through a 3.5-mm incision, acrylic IOL (MA60BM, Alcon) through a 4.1-mm incision, or a PMMA IOL (MZ60BD, Alcon) through a 6.5-mm incision. The silicone group had 77 eyes; foldable acrylic group, 75 eyes; and PMMA group, 72 eyes. All incisions were scleral tunnel, and patients were observed for 3 months. Fourier analysis was used to quantify irregular astigmatism. The Fourier system captures videokeratographic data points and translates them into spherical equivalent, regular astigmatism, and irregular astigmatism components. The PMMA group had a significant increase in regular astigmatism over preoperative levels ($P < .0001$) and significantly greater regular astigmatism than the foldable IOLs at 2 days, 4 days, 10 days, and 1 month ($P \leq .017$). Induced regular astigmatism increased slightly with the 3.5-mm and 4.1-mm incisions and increased significantly with the 6.5-mm arch-shaped incision. Higher-order irregularities of the anterior corneal surface increased significantly in all three groups but declined to preoperative levels by 4 days in the foldable IOL groups and 1 month in the PMMA group ($P \leq .0016$). Best spectacle-corrected visual acuity

TABLE 35-2

Physical Properties of Intraocular Lenses

Material	Trade Name	Model	Optic (mm)	Length (mm)	Configuration	Haptics	Other
HYDROPHOBIC ACRYLIC							
	AcrySof	SA60AT	6.0	13.0	Asymmetric biconvex	Acrylic, 0° angulation	1-piece
	AcrySof	SA30AL	5.5	12.5	Biconvex	Modified L, 0° angulation	1-piece
	AcrySof	MA30BA	5.5	12.5	Biconvex	PMMA, modified-C, 5° angulation	3-piece
	AcrySof	MA60BM	6.0	13.0	Biconvex	PMMA, modified C, 10° angulation	3-piece
	Sensar	AR40	6.0	13.0	Biconvex	PMMA, modified C, 5° angulation	3-piece
	Sensar OptiEdge	AR40e	6.0	13.0	Biconvex	PMMA, modified C, 5° angulation	Square edge
HYDROPHILIC ACRYLIC							
	Bigbag	—	6.5	10.35	Concave Convex	Loop angle 0°	For myopia
	Centerflex	570H	5.75	12.0	Biconvex (Equiconvex)	—	1-piece
	EasAcryl	—	6.0	11.0	Biconvex	Plate haptic, no angulation	—
	FZ60	—	6.0	12.5	Biconvex	Angulation 10°	1-piece
	Haptibag Angulé	—	6.0	12.0	Biconvex	Loop angle 10°	1-piece
	HydroFlex II	SC-25B-OUV	6.0	12.5	Co-convex	Modified C, 5° angulation	1-piece
		SP-60S-4UV	6.0	11.0	Co-convex	Variable angulation	1-piece
	HydroView	H60M	6.0	13.0	Biconvex	PMMA, modified C, 10° angulation	—
	MemoryLens	CV232	6.0	13.0	Equiconvex	Prolene, modified C, 10° angulation	Prefolded
	MF4 Multifocal	—	6.0	10.5	Biconvex	Monobloc, 1-piece	1-piece
	Raysoft	574H	5.75	10.5	Biconvex (Equiconvex)	—	1-piece
	STAAR Collamer	CC4204BF	6.0	10.8	Biconvex	0.9-mm fenestrations, 0° angulation	Plate foldable
	Stabibag	—	5.5	10.5	Biconvex	Angulation 10°	1-piece
	Tripode	—	6.0	10.5	Biconvex	Loop angle 0°	1-piece
	XL Octo	—	6.0	10.75	Biconvex	Loop angle 0°	1-piece
	XL Stabi	—	6.0	10.5	Biconvex	—	1-piece
SILICONE							
	Array Multifocal	—	6.0	13.0	Biconvex	PMMA, modified C, 10° angulation	3-piece
	CeeOn	920	6.0	12.5	Equi-biconvex	Blue modified C, 5° angulation	3-piece
	CeeOn	912	5.5	12.0	Equi-biconvex	PMMA, Cap C, 6° angulation	3-piece
	CeeOn Edge	911A	6.0	12.0	Equi-biconvex	Polyvinylidene fluoride, Cap C, 6° angulation	Square edge
	ChiroFlex	C11UB	6.0	10.5	Equiconvex	Plate haptic, 0° angulation	1-piece
	ClariFlex	—	6.0	13.0	Biconvex	PMMA, modified C, 10° angulation	3-piece
	Elastic	AA-4207VF	5.5	10.8	Biconvex	Plate haptic 1.15-mm fenestrations	—
	Elastimide	AQ-1016V	6.3	13.5	Biconvex	Polyimide, modified J loop	—
		AQ-2003V	6.3	12.5	Biconvex	Polyimide, modified C loop, 0° angulation	—
		AQ2010V	6.3	13.5	Biconvex	Polyimide, modified C loop, 10° angulation	3-piece
		AQ-2017V	5.5	12.5	Biconvex	Polyimide, modified C loop, 10° angulation	—
		AQ-5010V	6.3	14.0	Concave/Plano	Polyimide, modified C loop, 10° angulation	For myopia
	PhacoFlex II	SI40NB	6.0	13.0	Biconvex	PMMA, modified C, 10° angulation	3-piece
	PhacoFlex II	SI30NB	6.0	13.0	Biconvex	Polypropylene, modified C, 10° angulation	3-piece
	PhacoFlex II	SI55NB	5.5	13.0	Biconvex	PMMA, modified C, 10° angulation	3-piece
	SoFlex	LI61U	6.0	13.0	Equiconvex (biconvex)	PMMA, modified C, 5° angulation	3-piece
		C31UB	6.3	12.5	Equiconvex	Polyamide haptics	—
	STAAR	AA-4203TL	6.0	11.2	Biconvex	Plate haptic 1.15-mm fenestrations	Toric
		AA-4203TF	6.0	10.8	Biconvex	Plate haptic 1.15-mm fenestrations	Toric
		AA-4203VF	6.0	10.8	Biconvex	Plate haptic 1.15-mm fenestrations	—

PMMA, Polymethylmethacrylate.

TABLE 35-3
Incision Sizes and Impact on Surgically Induced Astigmatism (SIA)

	Foldable IOLs			
	Silicone (mm)	Acrylic (mm)	PMMA IOL (mm)	Incision size with least SIA (mm)
Hayashi et al, 1995[2]	3.2 or 4.0	—	5.0	3.2
Pfleger et al, 1996[4]	3.2 or 4.0	—	5.2	3.2
Olson and Crandall, 1998[5]	3.2	—	5.5	3.2
Oshika et al, 1998[6]	3.2	—	5.5	3.2
Müller-Jensen and Barlinn, 2000[7]	—	3.2	4.1	3.2
Hayashi et al, 2000[8]	3.5	4.1	6.5	3.5 or 4.1

was significantly worse at 2 days after surgery than at later examinations for all IOLs ($P <.001$).

Shimizu[9] examined induced astigmatism at 1 month in eyes with 4-, 3.2-, 3-, or 2.8-mm temporal corneal incisions. Using regression analysis, Shimizu determined that surgically induced astigmatism should approach zero at an incision size of 2.64 mm or less.

Effect of IOL Implantation on Incision Size

Surgically induced astigmatism may correlate with small incision sizes, but forcible insertion of the folded IOL through the wound may widen the wound, and the final incision may not be as small as the initial keratome incision. Steinert and Deacon[10] developed a set of incision-size gauges to study the dimensional stability of incisions during cataract extraction and IOL implantation. Steinert-Deacon gauges (Capital Instruments, Ltd., Wan Chai, Hong Kong) are the equivalent thickness of conventional metal keratomes and are manufactured in 0.2-mm increments (Figure 35-1). The gauges were initially tested in 51 consecutive patients undergoing phacoemulsification.

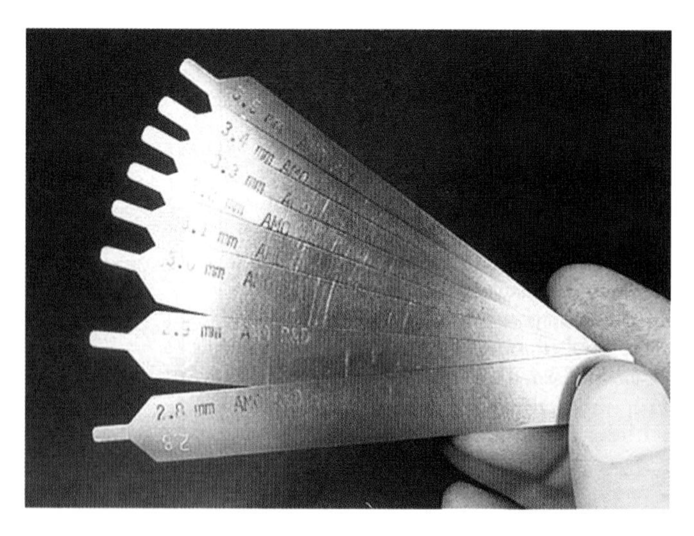

FIGURE 35-1 Steinert-Deacon incision-size gauges. (From Steinert R, Deacon J: Enlargement of incision width during phacoemulsification and folded intraocular lens implant surgery, *Ophthalmology* 103:220-225, 1996.)

In the 46 cases of temporal clear corneal incisions performed with diamond keratomes, the initial incision was significantly wider than the keratome blade (0.16 ± 0.08-mm; $P <.0001$). After phacoemulsification and irrigation-aspiration, the incision was again significantly wider (0.09 ± 0.06 mm; $P <.0001$). If the incision was not widened before insertion of the folded silicone IOL, significant enlargement occurred once more (0.26 ± 0.05-mm; $P <.0001$). The final insertion size after forceps insertion of a three-piece silicone foldable IOL was not statistically different than injector insertion of a plate haptic silicone IOL ($P = .56$). The investigators concluded that the incision has limited capacity for elastic deformation and may be vulnerable to tearing or irreversible stretching.

Implantation Devices for Small-Incision Surgery

Implantation devices were developed to provide uniform folding of the IOL and to allow the IOL to be inserted through smaller incisions than are possible with forceps. Unlike forceps, inserters isolate the IOL from the external environment, reducing the risk of introducing surface pathogens into the eye at the time of implantation. For most inserters, the surgeon or technician fills the cartridge with viscoelastic, grasps the IOL with holding forceps, loads the IOL in the cartridge, closes the cartridge, and places it in the handpiece. The surgeon enters the incision with the insertion tip of the handpiece and delivers the IOL into the capsular bag or ciliary sulcus. Not all inserters are appropriate for inserting the IOL into the sulcus.

The primary insertion devices in use in the United States are the Monarch II IOL delivery system from Alcon, the Unfolder implantation systems (Silver, Gold, and Sapphire) from AMO, and the M-Port and Passport II injector delivery systems from Bausch & Lomb.

MONARCH II DELIVERY SYSTEM

The Monarch II delivery system is designed to insert the three-piece (MA30BA) and one-piece (SA30AL) AcrySof acrylic IOLs into the capsular bag. The Monarch II has a reusable, titanium handpiece and single-use insertion cartridge. Hagan[11] evaluated the first 100 cases of the Monarch I delivery system for implantation of the 5.5-mm AcrySof MA30BA IOL into the capsular bag. He found the Monarch system to require less manipulation and provide better control of the IOL than folding and insertion with forceps. The Monarch II is designed to implant AcrySof IOLs through a 3- to 3.2-mm incision.

THE UNFOLDER IMPLANTATION SYSTEM

The Unfolder Silver Series implantation system is designed to implant AMO's SI30NB, SI40NB, ClariFlex, and Array multifocal lenses through a 3-mm incision. The Unfolder Gold is designed to implant the SI55NB silicone IOL through a 2.8-mm incision, and the Unfolder Sapphire is designed to implant the Sensar (AR40) and Sensar with OptiEdge (AR40e) acrylic IOLs through a 3.2-mm incision. All three systems have a reusable handpiece with disposable cartridges. The Silver and Gold Series have an additional sheath and tip, both of which are disposable.

Olson et al.[12] conducted an open-label evaluation of the original Unfolder by six investigators at six sites. Investigators compared the clinical performance of the device with other insertion systems they had used and measured the internal incision size with Steinert-Deacon incision gauges. All investigators reported that the Unfolder allowed slow, controlled delivery of the IOL into the capsular bag. Mean incision size before IOL implantation was 3 ± 0.1 mm (range 2.7 to 3.2 mm) and after implantation was 3.1 ± 0.1 mm (range 2.9 to 3.3 mm).

M-PORT AND PASSPORT II INJECTOR SYSTEMS

Bausch & Lomb's M-Port is a disposable injector system designed to implant the SoFlex LI61U, C31UB, and Silens 6 multipiece silicone IOLs. It provides uniform folding of the IOL into an M-fold and allows the IOL to be inserted through a 3- to 3.3-mm incision. The Passport II injector is a syringe-type system designed to propel the ChiroFlex C11UB single-piece silicone IOL into the capsular bag.

Summary

Evidence in the clinical literature to date supports a correlation between incision size and postoperative astigmatism, with foldable acrylic and silicone IOLs inserted through small incisions generally resulting in less induced astigmatism than PMMA IOLs inserted through larger incisions. Implantation and injector systems have been developed to insert a folded IOL through a smaller incision than is generally possible with insertion forceps. There is no consensus on the appropriate incision length because other wound construction variables have to be considered.

Materials and Optics

In the early 1950s, Scales[13] suggested that an ideal material for implantation into human tissues should be chemically inert, stable, not physically modified by contact with tissues, and acceptable to the body, with no inflammation, foreign body response, or tissue chafe. The desired material would not be carcinogenic or allergenic and would be capable of fabrication into the desired form, able to resist mechanical strains, and easy to sterilize.

For ophthalmic applications, the material should be optically transparent and able to remain so for long periods, capable of being manufactured into a high resolving power, able to block ultraviolet (UV) radiation in the 330- to 400-nm wavelengths, and implantable through a small incision.

Acrylic Polymers

The history of acrylic materials used in foldable IOLs begins with PMMA, an acrylic material with excellent tissue tolerance that has been used successfully in ophthalmology, oral and dental surgery, orthopedics, and plastic and reconstructive surgery. Acrylic materials are polymers synthesized from esters (monomers) of acrylic acid or methacrylic acid. The methyl ester of methacrylic acid, methylmethacrylate, readily polymerizes to polymethylmethacrylate. PMMA is a hard, rigid, strong thermoplastic material with excellent optical clarity. It has low water and gas diffusion constants and is highly resistant to the effects of light, oxygen, and hydrolysis. The pure polymer readily transmits UV light but can be manufactured with UV-absorbing chromophores to block ultraviolet energy from reaching the retina.

HYDROPHOBIC ACRYLIC POLYMERS

IOLs made of hydrophobic acrylic polymers include the AcrySof (Alcon) and Sensar (AMO). These polymers are members of the same family as rigid PMMA, but they are tailored for specific optical and mechanical properties by altering the side groups of a standard methacrylate backbone. PMMA and hydrophobic acrylic polymers are similar in their negligible water content and high refractive indices (1.55 for AcrySof, 1.49 for PMMA, and 1.47 for Sensar). Unlike PMMA, hydrophobic acrylic materials have a relatively long hydrocarbon side chain for increased flexibility at typical operating room temperatures of 18° to 22° C. The glass transition temperature (T_g) for PMMA is 105° C, approximately 15.5° to 21.5° C for AcrySof,[14] and 13° C for Sensar. The T_g is the temperature at which the polymer chains soften from their low-temperature rigid state to their flexible high-temperature form. Thus the lower the T_g, the easier the IOL material is to fold at standard room temperatures.

The AcrySof lens optic is molded from a phenylethyl acrylate and phenylethyl methacrylate polymer (US Patent 5,290,892; 1994). The Sensar lens optic is cut from a sheet of ethyl acrylate, ethyl methacrylate, and trifluoroethyl methacrylate polymer, then cryolathed into its final shape (US Patent 4,834,750; 1989).

HYDROPHILIC ACRYLIC POLYMERS

IOLs made with hydrophilic acrylic (hydrogel) polymers include the Hydroview and EasAcryl (Bausch & Lomb), HydroFlex II (Medical Developmental Research; Clearwater, Fla.), MemoryLens (Novartis Ophthalmics), Collamer (STAAR), Haptibag and Stabibag (IOLTech), and CenterFlex and Raysoft (Rayner).

HydroView IOLs are lathe cut and polished from a composite material. The foldable optic is cut from the central hydrogel portion, which contains a bonded UV absorber; the haptics appear blue and are formed from the outer PMMA portion (product labeling). The HydroView IOL has been associated with deposits of calcium phosphate on the IOL, some of which necessitated IOL explantation.[15,16] The cause of the calcification is currently under investigation.

MemoryLens IOLs come prerolled. They are produced from a hydrophilic polymer made of methylmethacrylate and

2-hydroxyethyl methacrylate (HEMA) and a UV-protector.[17] The polymer is rigid below temperatures of 25° C. During manufacturing, the lens is warmed above its Tg, then tightly rolled and cooled. The prerolled lens is kept cool until it is inserted through the phaco incision. As the lens warms to body temperature, it slowly unrolls.

The Collamer IOL (STAAR) is a plate haptic design. Collamer is a hydrogel-collagen copolymer consisting of a HEMA-based acrylic copolymer into which about 0.01% porcine collagen and a UV-absorbing chromophore have been bonded.[18] Because of its high water content, it is wet packed in a glass vial containing the sterile lens in balanced salt solution and placed in a pouch for shipping. The lens is removed from the vial with blunt forceps and loaded into a disposable plastic cartridge. The cartridge is inserted into a disposable plastic injector.

Silicone Elastomers

Silicone is used in medicine for prosthetic devices, estradiol-releasing vaginal rings, intracoronary stents, subdermal and transdermal implants, intrauterine contraceptive devices, catheters, nasolacrimal intubation tubes, finger joints, and a variety of other clinical situations. In ophthalmology, silicone is used for contact lenses, scleral buckles, keratoprostheses, glaucoma shunts, and IOLs. Silicone is inert, stable at high temperatures, flexible and elastic at a wide range of temperatures, and nonadhesive to tissues. Silicone IOLs are optically clear and have refractive indices ranging from 1.42 to 1.46.

The Array multifocal and PhacoFlex II monofocal IOLs (AMO), CeeOn (Pharmacia), SoFlex and ChiroFlex IOLs (Bausch & Lomb), and Elastimide (STAAR) are among the lenses made of silicone elastomers. The Array and PhacoFlex II IOLs are composed of high-refractive polydimethylsiloxane, a second-generation silicone material that has been covalently bonded to UV-light absorbing benzotriazole (product labeling). The silicone material is called SLM-2/UV. The CeeOn, SoFlex three-piece, ChiroFlex plate haptic, and Elastimide IOLs are silicone copolymers.

Silicone elastomers are safe, stable, and inert over the long term. Silicone IOLs showed no change in optical performance or surface quality in UV and hydrolytic stress tests designed to mimic 20 years of aging.[19-20] Questions have been raised about the advisability of implanting silicone IOLs in patients at risk for vitreoretinal surgery because silicone oil used as an intravitreal tamponade may adhere to the silicone lens and obstruct the surgeon's view.[21-23] Acrylic IOLs have frequently been the lenses of choice for patients with a history of ocular inflammation, pseudoexfoliation, and diabetic retinopathy or for patients at risk of future vitreoretinal surgery; however, McLoone et al.[24] showed silicone oil adherence to acrylic lenses in vitro. The mean percentage coating of silicone oil on PMMA IOLs was 20.8% and that on foldable hydrophobic acrylic IOLs was from 17.1% to 21.5% (P = NS). One hydrogel IOL (Aqua-Sense, Ophthalmic Innovations International; Ontario, Calif.) had 17.8%, and another (Raysoft, Rayner Intraocular Lenses, UK) had 5.2% ($P < .001$ vs. the other lenses).

Vacuoles within the IOL have been reported in several studies of patients with AcrySof IOL implants.[25-29] Christiansen et al.[26] reported that 42 eyes implanted with AcrySof IOLs all exhibited some degree of vacuole formation that appeared as glistenings under slit lamp observation. Laboratory studies suggest that temperature elevations increase the level of glistenings[30] as does the addition of serum to AcrySof IOLs in aqueous humor.[31] The presence of vacuoles in the IOL at mild to moderate levels does not appear to affect visual function. However, high levels of vacuole formation can decrease visual acuity,[26,28] decrease contrast sensitivity,[25,28,29] and interfere with the ability to target a neodymium: yttrium-aluminum-garnet (Nd:YAG) laser for posterior capsulotomy.[28]

Optic Edge Designs

Until recently, most PMMA and foldable IOLs had rounded edges. Manufacturers have been developing optics with sharp or squared edges to inhibit the growth of lens epithelial cells over the posterior capsule. Nishi, Nishi, and Sakanishi[32] reported that an AcrySof IOL with a sharp optic edge had a significantly greater effect in inhibiting posterior capsule opacification (PCO) than a PMMA IOL with rounded edges. Later, Nishi, Nishi, and Wickstrom[33] looked at the influence of IOL design and materials, implanting an AcrySof acrylic IOL in one eye and a CeeOn silicone IOL in the other eye of seven rabbits. Both IOLs had a sharp, rectangular optic edge. Miyake-Apple views showed that migrating lens epithelial cells were inhibited at the optic edge of five of the six rabbits available for evaluation. Overall, there was no apparent difference in PCO development between the two IOLs for the first 3 to 4 weeks. The study suggests that IOL design is an important factor in preventing PCO.

Schmack and Gerstmeyer[34] conducted a study in 42 eyes of 36 patients to look at the long-term efficacy and safety of the recently introduced CeeOn Edge silicone IOL. They found no signs of haze or discoloration of the IOL and no inflammatory cell deposits on the IOL surface. PCO was found at 3 years, but it did not cause clinically relevant restrictions on the patients' vision.

With the square-edge hydrophobic acrylic IOL, some patients have reported bothersome edge glare and negative dysphotopsias.[35-38] Holladay, Lang, and Portney[39] conducted ray tracings of biconvex IOLs that were identical except that the edge was either round or square. The sharp-edge design formed an arclike pattern of reflected light on the retina, and the round-edge design formed a diffuse image (Figure 35-2).

Rounding the biconvex lens reduced the peak intensity of the reflected glare image by 90%. The authors concluded that the glare images from the sharp edge appeared like a thin crescent or partial ring in the periphery of the retina opposite the image of the glare source and that rounding the edges significantly reduced the peak intensity of the reflected glare image.

An alternative explanation for the photic phenomena reported by patients with the square-edge AcrySof IOL comes from a study comparing equiconvex silicone (LI16U) and PMMA (P359UV) IOLs with an unequal biconvex acrylic (MA60BM) IOL.[40] The refractive indices for the three IOLs were 1.43, 1.49, and 1.55, respectively. This study suggested that the unequal biconvex design produced greater postoperative glare and external reflections than the equiconvex IOLs. Further, an increase in the refractive index from 1.43 to 1.55 increased the amount of reflected light fivefold.

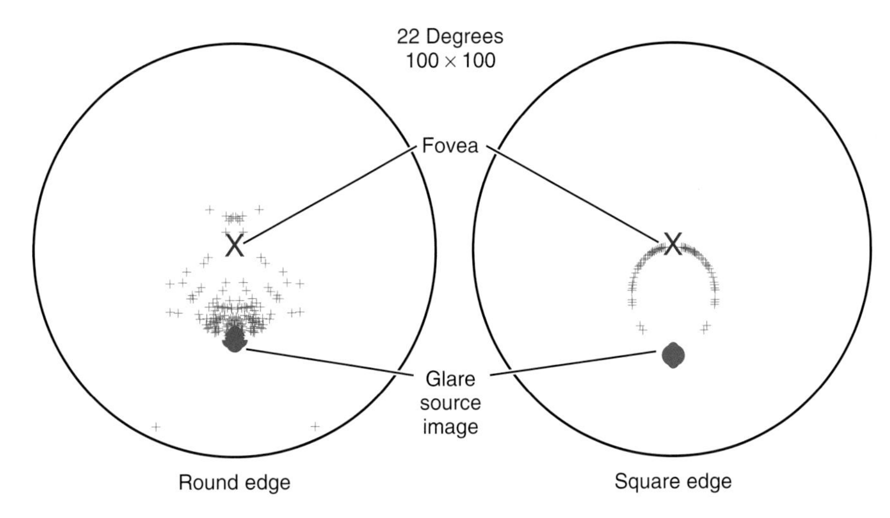

FIGURE 35-2 Distribution of internally reflected light on the retina. (From Holladay J, Lang A, Portney V: Analysis of edge glare phenomena in intraocular lens edge designs, *J Cataract Refract Surg* 27:614-621, 2001.)

There have been no published reports of high levels of photic phenomena with the square-edge silicone CeeOn Edge IOL. However, the IOL has only recently been released.

Another approach to edge design was taken by the Sensar (acrylic) and ClariFlex (silicone) lenses. The Sensar IOL has a standard rounded edge. The Sensar with OptiEdge and ClariFlex have a sharp vertical edge on the posterior surface, a sloped edge along the side of the IOL, and a rounded anterior edge (Figure 35-3).

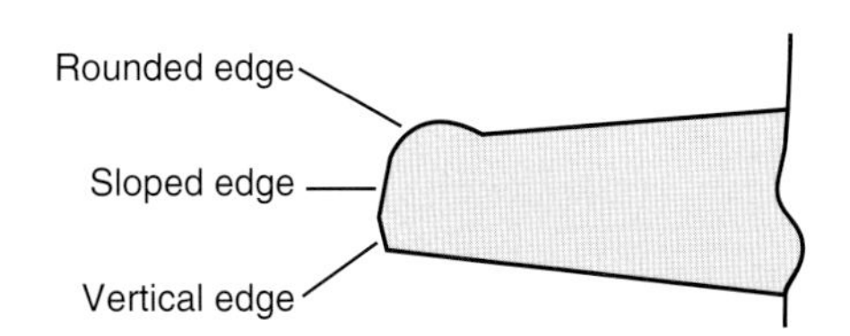

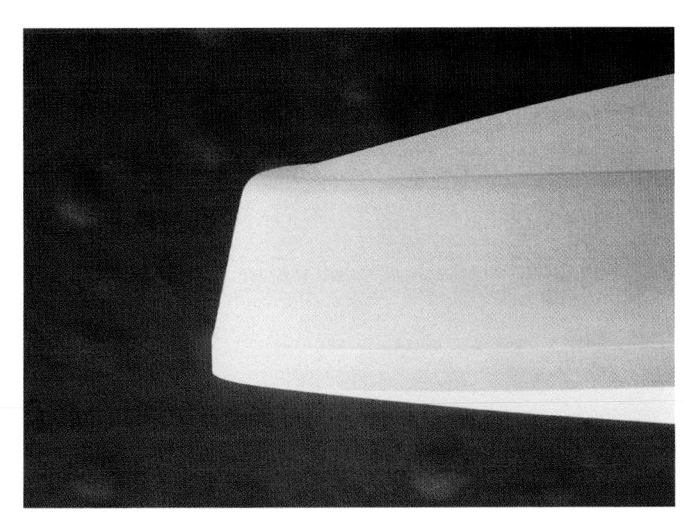

FIGURE 35-3 Edge design of the Sensar with OptiEdge and ClariFlex IOLs. (Courtesy AMO Surgical.)

The ray tracings of this new design show less reflection off the posterior surface than a conventional square-edge design and dispersion of light rays through the anterior surface (Figure 35-4; AMO Surgical Data on File). The IOLs are newly released, so information is not yet available as to the effect on PCO or photic phenomena.

Haptics

Haptic design is important in keeping the IOL centered and stable within the capsular bag or ciliary sulcus. IOL decentration or tilt may result in decreased visual acuity and increased photic phenomena such as glare and halos. Anterior-posterior shifts of the IOL can cause a shift in dioptric power, requiring further visual correction or IOL explantation. IOLs with fairly rigid

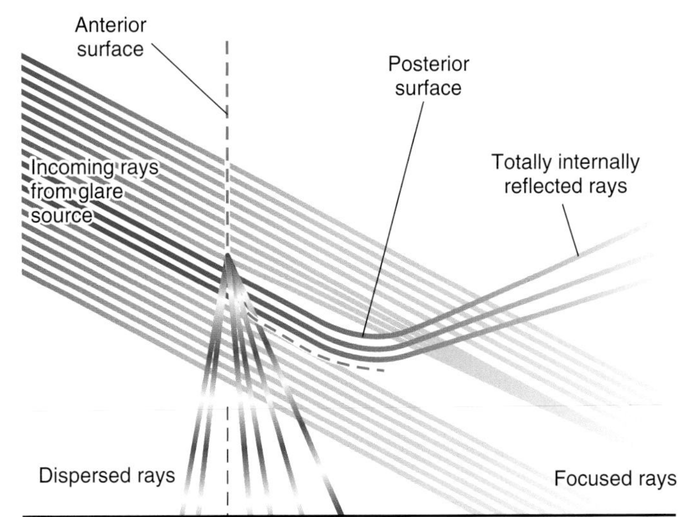

FIGURE 35-4 Ray tracings of the Sensar with OptiEdge. (Courtesy AMO Surgical.)

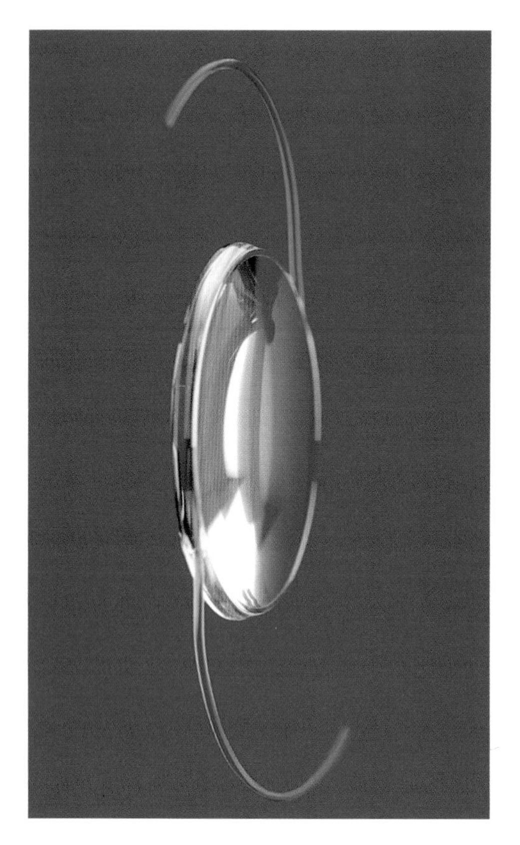

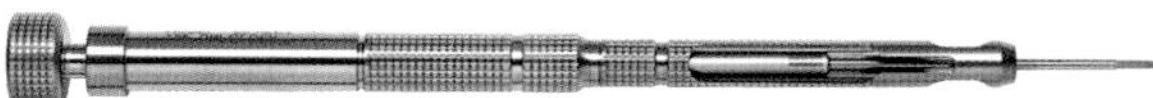

FIGURE 35-5 AMO ClariFlex silicone IOL with OptiEdge design *(top)* and Unfolder Injector *(bottom)*.

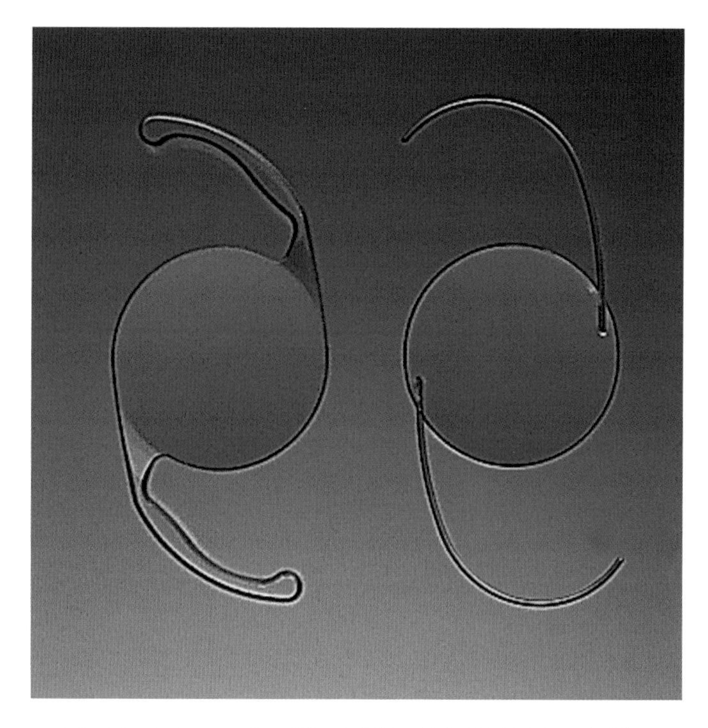

FIGURE 35-6 Alcon SA-30 *(left)* and MA-30 *(right)* acrylic IOLs.

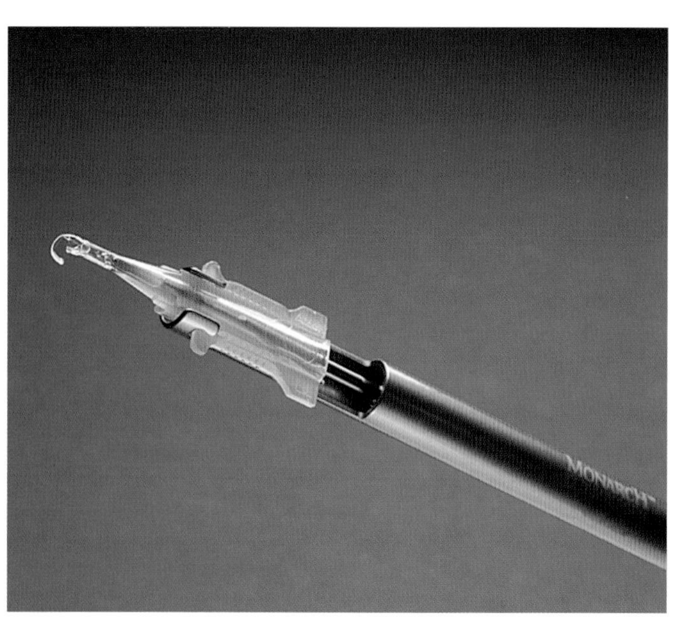

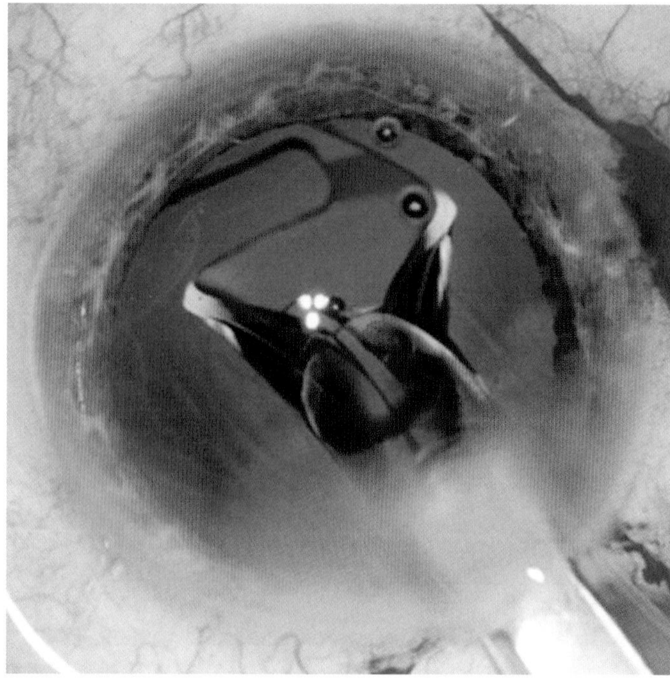

FIGURE 35-7 Monarch II injector *(left)* placing an SA-60 single-piece PC IOL *(right)*.

haptics, such as PMMA or polyimide, provide good in-the-bag fixation and IOL stability.[41,42] C-haptics do not deform the capsular bag and offer good contact between the haptic arc and the capsular equator.[42,43] Posterior angulation of the haptics increases the area of contact between the IOL optic and the posterior capsule, stabilizing the IOL in the bag.[42] This angulation may also serve to inhibit the migration of lens epithelial cells across the posterior capsule.[41] Most nonplate design foldable IOLs have C-shaped optics that come off the optic at an angle, a design that was the gold standard for PMMA IOLs.

Summary

The hydrophobic acrylic and silicone foldable IOLs have garnered the largest share of the overall IOL market in the United States. Figures 35-5 to 35-9 illustrate several of the most commonly implanted foldable IOLs. Hydrogel IOLs have been available for almost two decades, but the literature does not yet demonstrate significant advantages of this material over the nonhydrogel IOLs.

Optic designs have been undergoing changes in an effort to inhibit the growth of lens epithelial cells over the posterior capsule without producing glare, streaks of light, or dark shadows (negative dysphotopsia). Biocompatibility issues are discussed later in this chapter.

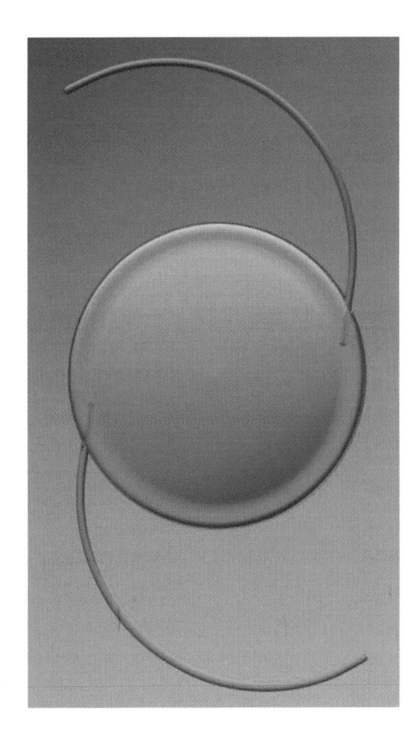

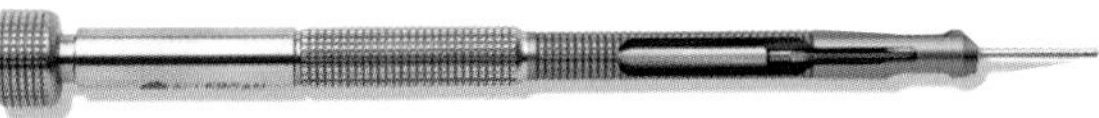

FIGURE 35-8 AMO Sensar Acrylic IOL *(top)* with OptiEdge and Unfolder injector *(bottom)*.

Efficacy of Foldable IOLs

Visual acuity at distance and near, spectacle corrected or uncorrected, is the primary efficacy variable for judging IOLs. Monofocal IOLs focus distant images on the retina; reading glasses or bifocals are generally required to provide adequate vision for near activities, such as reading, gardening, and playing cards. Multifocal IOLs provide both distance and near vision simultaneously. Spectacle dependence is minimized and may only be needed for reading very small print or for precision tasks such as watch repair.

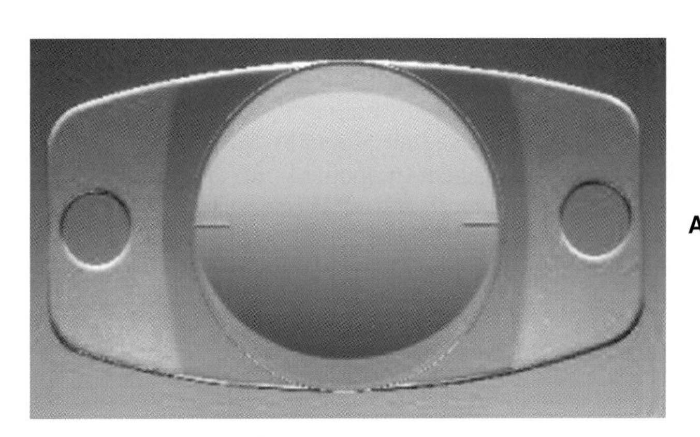

A

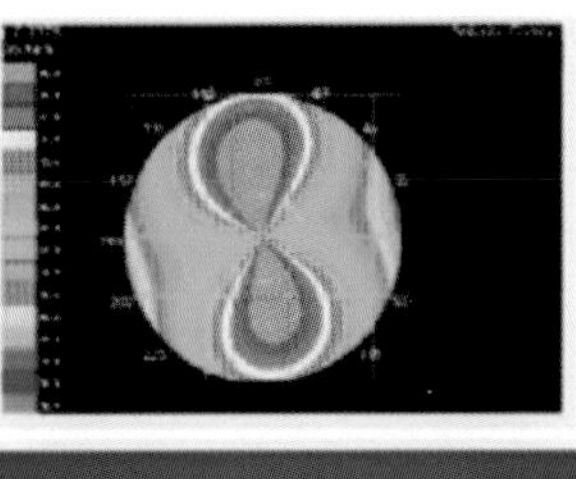

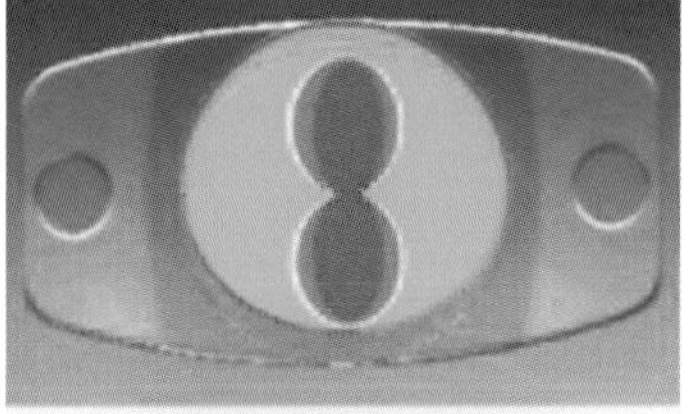

B

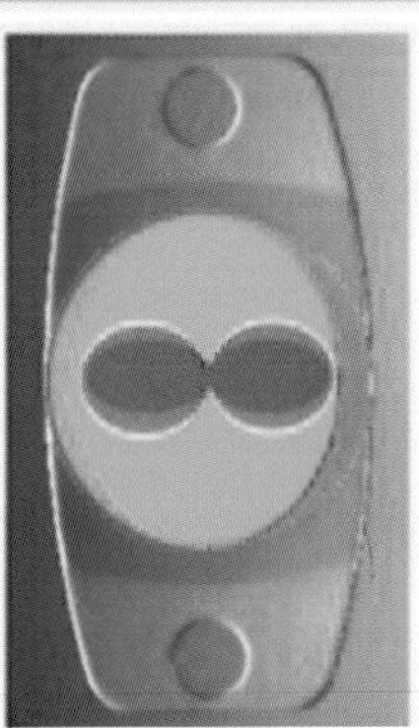

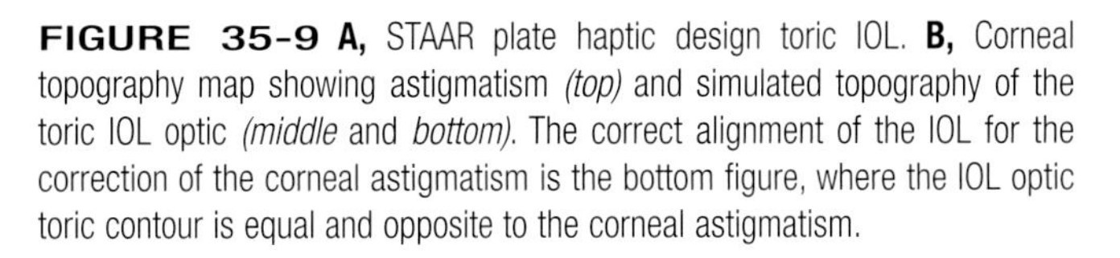

FIGURE 35-9 A, STAAR plate haptic design toric IOL. **B,** Corneal topography map showing astigmatism *(top)* and simulated topography of the toric IOL optic *(middle* and *bottom)*. The correct alignment of the IOL for the correction of the corneal astigmatism is the bottom figure, where the IOL optic toric contour is equal and opposite to the corneal astigmatism.

Distance Visual Acuity

Cataracts adversely affect visual acuity and cause glare and contrast sensitivity. Uncomplicated cataract surgery can resolve or improve these symptoms, with new symptoms or worsened symptoms occurring in only a few patients.[44] Overall, clinical studies of foldable IOLs demonstrate excellent best corrected distance visual acuity (BCVA) after cataract surgery (Table 35-4).

Prospective clinical trials comparing the Array multifocal IOL with a similar silicone monofocal IOL showed the Array to have uncorrected and best corrected distance visual acuity comparable to the monofocal IOL. Vaquero-Ruano et al.[45] reported mean uncorrected distance visual acuities of 20/40 (Snellen equivalent) for both IOLs in 50 patients, each observed for 18 months. Steinert et al.[46] reported Snellen equivalent values of 20/32 (multifocal) and 20/30 (monofocal) in 102 patients observed for 1 year. Javitt and Steinert[47] found Snellen equivalent values of 20/21 (multifocal) and 20/22 (monofocal) in 123 patients observed for 3 months. Mean BCVA was 20/25 (multifocal) and 20/23 (monofocal) in the Vaquero-Ruano study, 20/25 (multifocal) and 20/23 (monofocal) in the Steinert study, and 20/18 (multifocal) and 20/18 (monofocal) in the Javitt and Steinert study.

Near Visual Acuity

The Array multifocal IOL provides better uncorrected near visual acuity than an equivalent monofocal IOL. Mean uncorrected near visual acuity was Jaeger 3 (multifocal) and Jaeger 7 (monofocal) in the Vaquero-Ruano study, 20/33 (multifocal) and 20/54 (monofocal) in the Steinert study, and 20/26 (multifocal) and 20/40 (monofocal) in the Javitt and Steinert study.

Patients in the studies who wore corrective lenses for distance also had better near visual acuity if they received the multifocal lens implant. Mean distance-corrected near visual acuity was Jaeger 2 (multifocal) and Jaeger 5 (monofocal) in the Vaquero-Ruano study, 20/33 (multifocal) and 20/53 (monofocal) in the Steinert study, and 20/26 (multifocal) and 20/45 (monofocal) in the Javitt and Steinert study.

Summary

Foldable IOLs provide aphakic patients with visual acuity that is equivalent or superior to that achieved with rigid PMMA IOLs. Multifocal lenses studied to date provide distance visual acuity equivalent to monofocal IOLs and near visual acuity superior to monofocal IOLs. An optimal result with multifocal IOLs, and to a slightly lesser degree with monofocal IOLs, requires accurate biometry and control of astigmatism. Multifocal IOLs are discussed in greater detail in Chapter 36.

Biocompatibility

Foreign-Body Reaction

Clinical measures of biocompatibility include cellular deposits on the capsule, capsule opacification, postoperative blood-aqueous barrier breakdown, cellular reaction at the anterior capsule–IOL interface, and postoperative inflammation. Amon[48] calls *biocompatibility* one of the most important prerequisites of an intraocular implant and raises concerns about the use of the term in the medical literature. He quotes the definition from the International Dictionary of Medicine and Biology, "Biocompatibility is the capability of a prosthesis implanted in the body to exist in harmony with tissue without causing deleterious changes."[49]

Ideally, the IOL should remain an inert refractive element within the intraocular structures, but it does react with different tissues in the eye, specifically the uvea and the capsular bag. Capsular biocompatibility, according to Amon, occurs when there is minimal or no lens epithelial cell proliferation over the posterior or anterior capsule. Similarly, uveal biocompatibility exists when the IOL causes only a very mild foreign-body

TABLE 35-4
Studies of Foldable IOLs and Best Corrected Distance Visual Acuity*

Study	Material	IOL	Number of Patients	Follow-up	BCVA 20/40 or better (Snellen or Snellen equivalent)
Steinert, Giamporcaro, and Tasso, 1997[69]	SLM-2/UV	Phacoflex II	501	3 yr	95.2%
Menapace, 1995[70]	SLM-2/UV	Phacoflex II	35	3 to 17 mo	100%
Colin, 1996[71]	Silicone	ChiroFlex	125	3 to 18 mo	100%
Oshika et al, 1996[72]	Hydrophobic acrylic	AcrySof	64	2 yr	100%
Mengual et al, 1998[73]	Hydrophobic acrylic	AcrySof	81	9 mo	100%
Vaquero-Ruano et al, 1998[45]	Silicone	Array	100	18 mo	100%
Brown et al, 1998[18]	Hydrophilic acrylic	Collamer	125	4 to 6 mo	97.1%
Afsar et al, 1999[74]	Hydrophobic acrylic	AcrySof	67	2 mo	100% (20/30 or better)
Steinert et al, 1999[46]	Silicone	Array	123	1 year	100%
Kobayashi et al, 2000[75]	Hydrophobic acrylic	AcrySof	279	3 yr	96.4% of best case patients
Jirásková et al, 2000[17]	Hydrophilic acrylic	MemoryLens	150	1 yr	90.6% (20/30 or better)
Javitt and Steinert, 2000[47]	Silicone	Array	245	3 mo	20/18 or better

*Note: Because of differences in study design, direct comparisons among studies are inappropriate.
BCVA, Best corrected distance visual acuity; *IOL,* intraocular lens.

reaction despite the close proximity or direct contact between the IOL and uveal tissue.

Posterior Capsule Opacification

PCO is a common postoperative complication of cataract surgery that occurs when lens epithelial cells proliferate and migrate across the posterior capsule. Lens epithelial cells are generally clear or translucent, and migration is minimal and transparent. When they are confluent, persistent, fibrotic, and cover the optic, the patient may have complaints of loss of visual acuity, contrast sensitivity, and dysphotopsias such as disabling glare. Currently, PCO is treated by Nd:YAG laser, which cuts an opening in the opacified, fibrotic posterior capsule to clear the visual axis.

Schaumberg et al.[50] conducted a meta-analysis of the incidence of PCO reported in published articles in the literature. PCO occurred in 11.8%, 20.7%, and 28.4% of cases at 1, 3, and 5 years, respectively. They concluded that visually significant PCO develops in more than 25% of patients with posterior chamber IOL implantation over the first 5 postoperative years.

Nd:YAG capsulotomy rates are frequently used as a surrogate measure of PCO. Studies comparing Nd:YAG capsulotomy rates of foldable IOLs with their PMMA predecessors are summarized in Table 35-5. Overall, with the exception of the HydroView IOL in the study by Hollick et al.,[51] foldable IOLs had lower Nd:YAG capsulotomy rates than PMMA IOLs.

Other measures of PCO, such as digital photography and capsular light scatter, have shown the decrease in PCO with the advent of foldable IOLs. In the Olson and Crandall study,[52] the lens opacity meter scores showed less PCO in the silicone IOL group than the PMMA IOL group (8.6% vs. 10.4%; P = .02). This was consistent with the subjective slit lamp scoring (0.88 vs. 1.79; P = .0001).

Hollick et al.[53] studied the influence of IOL material on the process of lens epithelial cell migration. They randomly assigned 90 eyes of 91 patients for implantation with a PMMA (MC60BM), first-generation silicone (LI41U), or foldable acrylic (AcrySof) IOL after extracapsular cataract extraction.

TABLE 35-6

LEC Ongrowth on PMMA, First-Generation Silicone, and Foldable Acrylic IOLs at 90 Days and 2 Years After ECCE

	Number of Patients (%)	
IOL Type	**No LEC Ongrowth**	**LEC Ongrowth**
PMMA		
Day 90, n = 28	1 (4%)	27 (96%)
Year 2, n = 25	0 (0%)	25 (100%)
FIRST-GENERATION SILICONE		
Day 90, n = 27	2 (7%)	25 (93%)
Year 2, n = 21	0 (0%)	21 (100%)
FOLDABLE ACRYLIC		
Day 90, n = 26	14 (54%)	12 (46%)
Year 2, n = 16	6 (38%)	10 (62%)

From Hollick EJ, Spalton DJ, Ursell PG et al: Lens epithelial cell regression on the posterior capsule with different intraocular lens materials, *Br J Ophthalmol* 82:1182-1188, 1998.
ECCE, Extracapsular cataract extraction; *IOL,* intraocular lens; *LEC,* lens epithelial cell; *PMMA,* polymethylmethacrylate.

They observed the patients at 7, 30, 90, and 180 days and at 1 and 2 years with digital retroillumination imaging through dilated eyes. Table 35-6 shows the findings at 90 days and 2 years. Patients with foldable acrylic IOLs had significantly fewer lens epithelial cells on the posterior capsule than those with first-generation silicone or PMMA IOLs (P = .001) despite the small numbers of patients available at 2 years in the foldable acrylic IOL group.

Ursell et al.[54] reported on the same patient population as Hollick et al.[53] using digital retroillumination imaging and dedicated image processing software. They reported their findings as the median percentage of PCO at each follow-up. The findings support those of Hollick, showing significantly

TABLE 35-5

Nd:YAG Capsulotomy Rates of Different Studies by Type of IOL*

		Nd:YAG Capsulotomy % (Number of Patients)				
			Acrylic		Silicone	
Study	**Years postsurgery**	**PMMA**	**Hydrophobic**	**Hydrophilic**	**First generation**	**Second generation**
Oner, Gunenc, and Ferliel, 2000[76]	1.5	6.5% (77)	1.3% (80)	— —	— —	— —
Hollick et al, 2000[51]	2	14% (28)	— —	28% (25)	— —	0% (25)
Hayashi et al, 1998[55]	2	30.4% (69)	2.7% (73)	— —	— —	5.7% (70)
Ursell et al, 1998[54]	2	0% (25)	0% (16)	— —	0% (21)	— —
Hollick et al, 1999[77]	3	26% (23)	0% (19)	— —	14% (22)	— —
Olson and Crandall, 1998[52]	3	33% (59)	— —	— —	— —	24% (60)
Brown and Ziémba, 2001[78]	1	— —	— —	8% (40)	— —	— —
Hayashi et al, 200158	2	29% (26)	4.2% (4)	— —	— —	14.4% (12)

*Note: Because of differences in study design, direct comparisons among studies are inappropriate.
Nd:YAG, Neodymium: yttrium-aluminum-garnet; *PMMA,* polymethylmethacrylate.

TABLE 35-7

LEC Ongrowth on PMMA, First-Generation Silicone, and Foldable Acrylic IOLs at 90 Days, 1 Year, and 2 Years After ECCE

	6 Months Median (%)	1 Year Median (%)	2 Years Median (%)
	n = 25*	n = 21*	n = 24*
PMMA	19.9	26.1	43.7
	n = 24*	n = 23*	n = 21*
LI41U†	20.0	22.2	33.5
	n = 21*	n = 25*	n = 16*
AcrySof	8.2	10.7	11.8

From Ursell PG, Spalton DJ, Pande MV et al: Relationship between intraocular lens biomaterials and posterior capsule opacification, *J Cataract Refract Surg* 24:352-360, 1998.
*Images analyzed.
†First-generation silicone.
ECCE, Extracapsular cataract extraction; *IOL,* intraocular lens; *LEC,* lens epithelial cell; *PMMA,* polymethylmethacrylate.

TABLE 35-8

Mean PCO Value and Nd:YAG Capsulotomy Rates

	PMMA (MZ60BD) N = 69	Silicone (SI30NB) N = 70	Acrylic (MA60BM) N = 73	P
ND:YAG CAPSULOTOMY				
Number of eyes	21	4	2	
Rate	30.4%	5.7%	2.7%	<.001
PCO VALUE				
Number of eyes	48	66	71	
Postoperative exam (month ± SD)	25.7 ± 2.5	25.6 ± 2.2	25.7 ± 2.8	
PCO density measure	26.3 ± 12.2	12.0 ± 8.3	16.0 ± 10.3	<.001

From Hayashi H, Hayashi K, Nakao F et al: Quantitative comparison of posterior capsule opacification after polymethylmethacrylate, silicone, and soft acrylic intraocular lens implantation, *Arch Ophthalmol* 116:1579-1582, 1998.
Nd:YAG, Neodymium: yttrium-aluminum-garnet; *PCO,* posterior capsule opacification; *PMMA,* polymethylmethacrylate.

less PCO with the AcrySof IOL than with the first-generation silicone and PMMA IOLs, which were not significantly different (Table 35-7).

Hayashi et al.[55] quantified the density of PCO after implantation of PMMA (MZ60BD, Alcon), second-generation silicone (SI30NB), and soft acrylic (MA60BM) IOLs in 212 eyes of 212 patients. Patients were evaluated at 2 years. The examiner took Scheimpflug slit images of the implanted IOL at four meridians of the lens. The highest quality image of each meridian was captured as a computer image for axial densitometry measurements. The average measure for each meridian was the PCO value for that meridian. Mean PCO values and Nd:YAG rates were significantly higher in the PMMA group than in the silicone or foldable acrylic group (Table 35-8).

These values correlated with a loss of visual acuity among the three lenses. Patients with the PMMA IOL implant had a significantly greater loss of best corrected visual acuity than either of the foldable IOLs (P <.001; Table 35-9).

The findings of this sizeable study using an objective measurement to evaluate PCO in foldable and rigid lenses, as well as the loss of visual acuity among the three lenses, favor the use of foldable IOLs.

Wang and Woung[56] conducted a prospective, randomized study of 40 eyes, 20 with a PMMA IOL and 20 with an SI30NB second-generation silicone IOL. At 1 year, digital retroillumination images were taken with the EAS-1000 anterior segment analysis system (Nidek). The images were analyzed for transparency and opacity over the central 3- and 5-mm optic zones. The central posterior capsule was significantly more transparent in the silicone group than in the PMMA group at 1 year. Mean transparency over the central 3-mm optic zone was 97.17% (± 5.96% SD) in the silicone group and 86.32% (± 19.60%) in the PMMA Group (P = .048).

Postmortem studies by Apple, Werner, and Pandey[57] identified the Nd:YAG rates for eight foldable IOL styles in 5416 pseudophakic human eyes with posterior chamber IOLs obtained between January 1988 and January 2000. Foldable IOLs were present in 814 (15%) of the cadaver eyes. These included designs manufactured by STAAR, Bausch & Lomb, Alcon, and AMO. Only U.S.-marketed lenses were included in the analysis. The overall laser capsulotomy rate was 14.1% (115 of 814) for the foldable IOLs in this group and 31.1% (1430 of 4602) for the PMMA IOLs. All of the newer models had lower rates of Nd:YAG laser capsulotomy than older models, suggesting that improvements in lens design and surgical technique played a role in reducing the incidence of PCO and the need for laser intervention to restore visual acuity. The study does not give clear clinical direction as to IOL choice. Autopsy globe analysis,

TABLE 35-9

Loss of Best Corrected Visual Acuity

	PMMA (MZ60BD) N = 69		Silicone (SI30NB) N = 70		Acrylic (MA60BM) N = 73	
	n	(%)	n	(%)	n	(%)
No loss	25	(1.4)	51	(72.9)	53	(72.6)
1 line	4	(5.8)	5	(7.1)	8	(11.0)
2 lines	13	(18.8)	6	(8.6)	3	(4.1)
3 lines	5	(7.2)	4	(5.7)	5	(6.8)
4 lines	7	(10.1)	1	(1.4)	0	(0.0)
5 lines	4	(5.8)	2	(2.9)	0	(0.0)
6 lines	6	(8.6)	1	(1.4)	1	(1.4)
7 lines	3	(4.3)	0	(0.0)	1	(1.4)
8 lines	2	(2.9)	0	(0.0)	0	(0.0)

From Hayashi H, Hayashi K, Nakao F et al: Quantitative comparison of posterior capsule opacification after polymethylmethacrylate, silicone, and soft acrylic intraocular lens implantation, *Arch Ophthalmol* 116:1579-1582, 1998.
PMMA, Polymethylmethacrylate.

TABLE 35-10

Mean PCO Value and Nd:YAG Capsulotomy Rates at 24 Months

	PMMA (MZ60BD) N = 90	Silicone (SI30NB) N = 83	Acrylic (MA60BM) N = 96	P
ND:YAG CAPSULOTOMY				
Number of eyes	26	12	4	
Rate	28.9%	14.4%	4.2%	
PCO VALUE				
Mean PCO values (±SD)	23.2 ± 13.8	14.1 ± 9.2	11.7 ± 7.6	<.001

From Hayashi K, Hayashi H, Nakao F et al: Changes in posterior capsule opacification after poly(methylmethacrylate), silicone, and acrylic intraocular lens implantation, *J Cataract Refract Surg* 27:817-824, 2001.
Nd:YAG, Neodymium: yttrium-aluminum-garnet; *PCO,* posterior capsule opacification; *PMMA,* polymethylmethacrylate.

to date, does not include time variables, such as the interval between implantation and death, which can provide important clues about the development of PCO. Nevertheless, this is a valuable, ongoing study into one of the leading causes of loss of visual acuity after cataract surgery.

Hayashi et al.[58] reported on their 2-year study of the changes in PCO after implantation of PMMA (MZ60BD, Alcon), second-generation silicone (SI30NB), and soft acrylic (MA60BM) IOLs in 269 eyes of 269 patients. As with their previous study in 1998 (reported earlier), Scheimpflug images were analyzed by computer to give PCO values. Mean PCO values and Nd:YAG rates were significantly higher in the PMMA group than in the silicone or foldable acrylic group (Table 35-10).

Anterior Capsule Opacification

Lens epithelial cells can also migrate onto the anterior surface of the IOL. Hollick, Spalton, and Ursell[59] looked at surface cytologic features of PMMA, silicone, and hydrogel IOLs and their effect on the blood-aqueous barrier as an indicator of biocompatibility. They found that patients who had hydrogel IOLs implanted were significantly more likely to have lens epithelial cells on the anterior surface of the IOL for a longer period than those with PMMA or silicone IOLs ($P < .001$). The investigators commented that lens epithelial cells grew over the anterior surface to a much greater extent and in a completely different pattern on the hydrogel IOLs than the PMMA or silicone IOLs.

Müllner-Eidenböck et al.[60] conducted a prospective, randomized clinical study of lens epithelial cell migration onto the anterior capsule in 15 eyes, each implanted with one of four IOLs: the HydroView, MemoryLens, AcrySof, or CeeOn 920. The greatest ongrowth was seen with the hydrophilic acrylic IOLs, HydroView and MemoryLens, which had 86.7% and 73.4%, respectively, at 30 days and 86.7% and 22%, respectively, at 180 days. The lowest rates were seen with the hydrophobic acrylic AcrySof IOL (86.7% at 30 days and 0% at 180 days) and CeeOn 920 silicone IOL (26.7% at 30 days and 19.9% at 180 days).

Lenis and Philipson[61] observed 25 cataract patients with HydroView hydrogel IOL implants for up to 12 months. Lens epithelial cells were detected on the anterior IOL surface in 13 patients (52%). Most of these were within 1 mm of the capsulorhexis border, with 4 cases of cell proliferation centrally. Overall, this migration and proliferation did not affect visual acuity.

House et al.[62] evaluated 41 cases of AcrySof IOL implantation in 31 patients. They found granular deposits of what they classified as lens epithelial cell proliferation on the anterior surface of the IOL in 18 cases (44%) at 3 to 5 weeks after surgery. The deposits did not have an effect on visual acuity.

Koch, Kalicharan, and van der Want[63] reported on 62 (of 196; 33.2%) eyes implanted with a HydroView IOL that developed a layer of lens epithelial cells on the anterior surface of the IOL optic between 8 and 98 weeks after surgery. The presence of the lens epithelial cell membrane produced visual symptoms varying from low vision to hazy vision or light scatter. Removal of the membrane by Nd:YAG laser treatment or surgical membranectomy alleviated the visual symptoms.

Schauersberger et al.[64] found significantly higher levels of anterior ongrowth of lens epithelial cells on the round-edge HydroView hydrophilic acrylic IOL than the square-edge AcrySof or round-edge Sensar hydrophobic acrylic IOLs from 30 days to 1 year after surgery ($P \leq .015$). They concluded that, unlike in PCO, IOL material plays a greater role than edge design in anterior lens epithelial cell ongrowth.

Inflammatory Reaction

The trauma of cataract surgery and IOL implantation can trigger a breakdown in the blood-aqueous barrier, with an outpouring of proteins and macrophages to repair tissue and isolate the foreign body from the ocular tissues. The foreign body reaction depends on the IOL material and the preexisting status of the ocular tissues, such as diabetic retinopathy. The inflammatory response is measured subjectively by slit lamp grading of cells and flare or objectively by a laser flare photometer.

Hollick, Spalton, and Ursell[59] measured the effect of PMMA, silicone (SI30NB), and hydrogel (HydroView) IOL implantation on the blood-aqueous barrier by laser flare and cell meter (Kowa, Osaka, Japan). At 1 month after surgery, small cells were present on 4 of 30 hydrogel, 11 of 30 PMMA, and 15 of 30 silicone IOLs ($P = .01$). The hydrogel lenses showed a significantly shorter duration and lower grades of small cells than the silicone or PMMA IOLs ($P < .001$ for both). At the same visit, epithelioid cells were most pronounced on the PMMA (11 of 30), present in only 1 of 30 silicone IOLs, and not present on the hydrogel IOLs ($P < .001$). Lens epithelial cells, on the other hand, were present at 1 month on 20 of 30 hydrogel IOLs, 12 of 30 PMMA IOLs, and 0 of 30 silicone IOLs. Lens epithelial cells reached a peak between 1 week and 1 month after surgery and then regressed. The hydrogel IOLs had significantly greater numbers that did not regress, and in half the patients the lens epithelial cells formed a confluent sheet along the entire 360 degrees of the capsulorhexis rim, probably because of migration from the capsulorhexis.

In a study by Samuelson, Chu, and Kreiger[65] the levels of postoperative inflammatory giant-cell deposits were measured in patients 6 months after combined cataract and glaucoma surgery. The level of inflammatory giant-cell deposits was slightly higher in patients with an acrylic IOL (AcrySof) than in patients with a silicone IOL (PhacoFlex II); however, the difference was not statistically or clinically significant.

Summary

Nd:YAG capsulotomy rates are not an accurate measure of PCO. Surgeons vary considerably in the criteria they use, and patients vary in the amount of opacification that compromises their vision. Objective measures of PCO, anterior capsule opacification, and ocular inflammation show greater biocompatibility with foldable lenses than PMMA, and greater biocompatibility with newer IOL designs and materials than older ones.

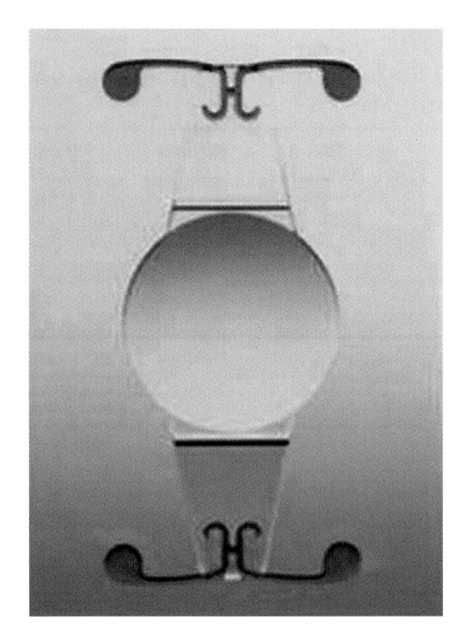

FIGURE 35-10 AT-45 accommodating IOL from C&C Vision.

The Future

The purpose of cataract surgery and IOL implantation has been to remove the barriers to vision caused by the loss of transparency at the lenticular plane. The current state of the surgical art is to remove the cloudy lens contents through a small incision and restore lenticular function with a prosthesis with one or more focal lengths. We can expect the near future to produce improvements in surgical technique, surgical equipment, and foldable IOLs. A greater knowledge of how IOL materials interact with ocular tissues will lead to improvements in biocompatibility. Continued improvements in both IOL and inserter designs will improve the ease of use for surgeons.

At the time of this writing, an area of intense research is focused on restoring accommodative function and lenticular refractive function to the aging eye. Other areas include correcting refractive errors—hyperopia, myopia, ametropia, and presbyopia—at the time of cataract surgery or even before the cataract has fully developed.

C&C Vision (Aliso Viejo, Calif.) is developing a third-generation silicone lens, the AT-45 CrystaLens, that can be injected through a 2-mm incision into the bag. The lens has a small optic on two long hinges, with the theory that the hinges take advantage of residual accommodative function to move the optic forward and back to give approximately 2.5 D of accommodation (Figure 35-10).

Calhoun Vision, Inc. (Pasadena, Calif.), is developing a laser-light sensitive lens that can be implanted in the capsular bag and adjusted by laser to correct up to 2 D of myopia, hyperopia, and astigmatism.

Other investigators are looking at removing the precataractous crystalline lens and implanting a multifocal IOL to solve the problem of presbyopia.[66-68] This is referred to as refractive lensectomy, presbyopic lens exchange (Prelex), or clear lens extraction.

Improvements in IOL technology and surgical technique have moved cataract surgery into the refractive realm. The future holds great promise for cataract refractive surgery.

REFERENCES

1. Steinert RF, Brint SF, White SM et al: Astigmatism after small incision cataract surgery: a prospective, randomized, multicenter comparison of 4- and 6.5-mm incisions, *Ophthalmology* 98:417-423, 1991; discussion 423-424.
2. Hayashi K, Hayashi H, Nakao F et al: The correlation between incision size and corneal shape changes in sutureless cataract surgery, *Ophthalmology* 102:550-556, 1995 (see comments).
3. Brint S, Ostrick D, Bryan J: Keratometric cylinder and visual performance following phacoemulsification and implantation with silicone small-incision or poly(methyl methacrylate) intraocular lenses, *J Cataract Refract Surg* 17:32-36, 1991.
4. Pfleger T, Skorpik C, Menapace R et al: Long-term course of induced astigmatism after clear corneal incision cataract surgery, *J Cataract Refract Surg* 22:72-77, 1996.
5. Olson R, Crandall A: Prospective randomized comparison of phacoemulsification cataract surgery with a 3.2-mm vs a 5.5-mm sutureless incision, *Am J Ophthalmol* 125:612-620, 1998.
6. Oshika T, Nagahara K, Yaguchi S et al: Three year prospective, randomized evaluation of intraocular lens implantation through 3.2 and 5.5 mm incisions, *J Cataract Refract Surg* 24:509-514, 1998.
7. Müller-Jensen K, Barlinn B: Corneal refractive changes after AcrySof lens versus PMMA lens implantation, *Ophthalmologica* 214:320-323, 2000.
8. Hayashi K, Hayashi H, Oshika T et al: Fourier analysis of irregular astigmatism after implantation of 3 types of intraocular lenses, *J Cataract Refract Surg* 26:1510-1516, 2000.
9. Shimizu K: Clear-cornea cataract incision: astigmatic consequences. In Masket S, Crandall AS, editors: *Atlas of cataract surgery,* London, 1999, Martin Dunitz Ltd, pp 129-139.
10. Steinert R, Deacon J: Enlargement of incision width during phacoemulsification and folded intraocular lens implant surgery, *Ophthalmology* 103: 220-225, 1996.
11. Hagan Jr: Initial experience with the MONARCH IOL delivery system for insertion of the 5.5 mm: ACRYSOF intraocular lens, *Mo Med* 6:555, 561-562, 1999.
12. Olson R, Cameron R, Hovis T et al: Clinical evaluation of the Unfolder, *J Cataract Refract Surg* 23:1384-1389, 1997.
13. Scales J: Discussion on metals and synthetic materials in relation to tissues: tissue reactions to synthetic materials, *Proc R Soc Med* 46:647-652, 1953.
14. Anderson C, Koch DD, Green G et al: Alcon AcrySof Acrylic Intraocular Lens. In Martin RG, Gills JP, Sanders DR, editors: *Foldable intraocular lenses,* Thorofare, NJ, 1993, Slack, Inc, pp 161-177.
15. Fernando GT, Crayford BB: Visually significant calcification of hydrogel intraocular lenses necessitating explantation, *Clin Experiment Ophthalmol* 28:280-286, 2000.

16. Werner L, Apple D, Escobar-Gomez M et al: Postoperative deposition of calcium on the surfaces of a hydrogel intraocular lens, *Ophthalmology* 107:2179-2185, 2000.
17. Jirásková N, Rozsíval P, Liláková D et al: Evaluation of 150 MemoryLens implantations, *InterNet J Ophthalmol* 5:7-11, 2000; www.unich.it/injo/200.htm.
18. Brown D, Grabow H, Martin R et al: Staar Collamer intraocular lens: clinical results from the phase I FDA core study, *J Cataract Refract Surg* 24:1032-1038, 1998.
19. Francese JE, Pham L, Christ FR: Accelerated hydrolytic and ultraviolet aging studies on SI-18NB and SI-20NB silicone lenses, *J Cataract Refract Surg* 18:402-405, 1992.
20. Christ FR, Fencil DA, Van Gent S et al: Evaluation of the chemical, optical, and mechanical properties of elastomeric intraocular lens materials and their clinical significance, *J Cataract Refract Surg* 15:176-184, 1989.
21. Khawly J, Lambert R, Jaffe G: Intraocular lens changes after short- and long-term exposure to intraocular silicone oil: an in vivo study, *Ophthalmology* 105:1227-1233, 1998.
22. Apple D, Federman J, Krolicki T et al: Irreversible silicone oil adhesion to silicone intraocular lenses: a clinicopathologic analysis, *Ophthalmology* 103:1555-1561, 1996; discussion 1561-1562.
23. Apple DJ, Isaacs RT, Kent DG et al: Silicone oil adhesion to intraocular lenses: an experimental study comparing various biomaterials, *J Cataract Refract Surg* 23:536-544, 1997.
24. McLoone E, Mahon G, Archer D et al: Silicone oil-intraocular lens interaction: which lens to use? *Br J Ophthalmol* 85:543-545, 2001.
25. Dhaliwal DK, Mamalis N, Olson RJ et al: Visual significance of glistenings seen in the AcrySof intraocular lens, *J Cataract Refract Surg* 22:452-457, 1996.
26. Christiansen G, Durcan FJ, Olson RJ et al: Glistenings in the AcrySof intraocular lens: pilot study, *J Cataract Refract Surg* 27:728-733, 2001.
27. Dogru M, Tetsumoto K, Tagami Y: Optical and atomic force microscopy of an explanted AcrySof intraocular lens with glistenings, *J Cataract Refract Surg* 26:571-575, 2000.
28. Mitooka K, Shiba T, Tsuneoka H et al: [A case of intraocular lens eye with decrease in visual function by glistening], *Ganka* 40:1501-1504, 1998.
29. Mitooka K, Tsuneoka H: [Glistening], *Practical Ophthalmol* 52:66-67, 1999.
30. Shiba T, Mitooka K, Tsuneoka H: [Study of causal mechanism of glistening occurring in AcrySof intraocular lens], *IOL & RS* 14:2000.
31. Dick HB, Olson RJ, Augustin AJ et al: Vacuoles in the Acrysof intraocular lens as factor of the presence of serum in aqueous humor, *Ophthalmic Res* 33:61-67, 2001.
32. Nishi O, Nishi K, Sakanishi K: Inhibition of migrating lens epithelial cells at the capsular bend created by the rectangular optic edge of a posterior chamber intraocular lens, *Ophthalmic Surg Lasers* 9:587-594, 1998.
33. Nishi O, Nishi K, Wickstrom K: Preventing lens epithelial cell migration using intraocular lenses with sharp rectangular edges, *J Cataract Refract Surg* 26:1543-1549, 2000.
34. Schmack W, Gerstmeyer K: Long-term results of the foldable CeeOn Edge intraocular lens, *J Cataract Refract Surg* 26:1172-1175, 2000.
35. Davison JA: Positive and negative dysphotopsia in patients with acrylic intraocular lenses, *J Cataract Refract Surg* 26:1346-1355, 2000.
36. Farbowitz MA, Zabriskie NA, Crandall AS et al: Visual complaints associated with the AcrySof acrylic intraocular lens (1), *J Cataract Refract Surg* 26:1339-1345, 2000.
37. Mamalis N: Complications of foldable intraocular lenses requiring explanation or secondary intervention: 1998 survey, *J Cataract Refract Surg* 26:766-772, 2000.
38. Masket S: Truncated edge design, dysphotopsia, and inhibition of posterior capsule opacification, *J Cataract Refract Surg* 26:145-147, 2000.
39. Holladay J, Lang A, Portney V: Analysis of edge glare phenomena in intraocular lens edge designs, *J Cataract Refract Surg* 25:748-752, 1999.
40. Erie JC, Bandhauer MH, McLaren JW: Analysis of postoperative glare and intraocular lens design, *J Cataract Refract Surg* 27:614-621, 2001.
41. Apple D, Auffarth G, Peng Q et al: Foldable intraocular lenses: evolution, clinicopathologic correlation, and complications, Thorofare, NJ, 2000, Slack Inc.
42. Tana P, Belmonte J: Experimental study of different intraocular lens designs implanted in the bag after capsulorhexis, *J Cataract Refract Surg* 22:1211-1221, 1996.
43. Assia EI, Legler UF, Apple DJ: The capsular bag after short- and long-term fixation of intraocular lenses, *Ophthalmology* 102:1151-1157, 1995.
44. Adamsons I, Vitale S, Stark W et al: The association of postoperative subjective visual function with acuity, glare, and contrast sensitivity in patients with early cataract, *Arch Ophthalmol* 114:529-536, 1996.
45. Vaquero-Ruano M, Encinas J, Millan I et al: AMO array multifocal versus monofocal intraocular lenses: long-term follow-up, *J Cataract Refract Surg* 24:118-123, 1998.
46. Steinert R, Aker B, Trentacost D et al: A prospective comparative study of the AMO ARRAY zonal-progressive multifocal silicone intraocular lens and a monofocal intraocular lens, *Ophthalmology* 106:1243-1255, 1999.
47. Javitt J, Steinert R: Cataract extraction with multifocal intraocular lens implantation: a multinational clinical trial evaluating clinical, functional, and quality-of-life outcomes, *Ophthalmology* 107:2040-2048, 2000.
48. Amon M: Biocompatibility of intraocular lenses, *J Cataract Refract Surg* 27:178-179, 2001.
49. *International dictionary of medicine and biology,* New York, 1986, Churchill Livingstone.
50. Schaumberg D, Dana M, Christen W et al: A systematic overview of the incidence of posterior capsule opacification, *Ophthalmology* 105:1213-1221, 1998.
51. Hollick EJ, Spalton DJ, Ursell PG et al: Posterior capsular opacification with hydrogel, polymethylmethacrylate, and silicone intraocular lenses: two-year results of a randomized prospective trial, *Am J Ophthalmol* 129:577-584, 2000.
52. Olson R, Crandall A: Silicone versus polymethylmethacrylate intraocular lenses with regard to capsular opacification, *Ophthalmic Surg Lasers* 29:55-58, 1998.
53. Hollick E, Spalton D, Ursell P et al: Lens epithelial cell regression on the posterior capsule with different intraocular lens materials, *Br J Ophthalmol* 82:1182-1188, 1998.
54. Ursell P, Spalton D, Pande M et al: Relationship between intraocular lens biomaterials and posterior capsule opacification, *J Cataract Refract Surg* 24:352-360, 1998.
55. Hayashi H, Hayashi K, Nakao F et al: Quantitative comparison of posterior capsule opacification after polymethylmethacrylate, silicone, and soft acrylic intraocular lens implantation, *Arch Ophthalmol* 116:1579-1582, 1998.
56. Wang M, Woung L: Digital retroilluminated photography to analyze posterior capsule opacification in eyes with intraocular lenses, *J Cataract Refract Surg* 26:56-61, 2000.
57. Apple D, Werner L, Pandey S: Newly recognized complications of posterior chamber intraocular lenses, *Arch Ophthalmol* 119:581-582, 2001.
58. Hayashi K, Hayashi H, Nakao F et al: Changes in posterior capsule opacification after poly(methyl methacrylate), silicone, and acrylic intraocular lens implantation (1), *J Cataract Refract Surg* 27:817-824, 2001.
59. Hollick E, Spalton D, Ursell P: Surface cytologic features on intraocular lenses: can increased biocompatibility have disadvantages? *Arch Ophthalmol* 117:872-878, 1999.
60. Müllner-Eidenböck A, Schauersberger J, Kruger A et al: [Cellular reactions on anterior surfaces of four different types of foldable lenses], *Spektrum der Augenheilkunde* 12:218-223, 1998.
61. Lenis K, Philipson B: Lens epithelial growth on the anterior surface of hydrogel IOLs: an in vivo study, *Acta Ophthalmol Scand* 76:184-187, 1998.
62. House P, Barry C, Morgan W et al: Postoperative deposits on the AcrySof intraocular lens, *Aust N Z J Ophthalmol* 27:301-305, 1999.
63. Koch MU, Kalicharan D, van der Want JJ: Lens epithelial cell layer formation related to hydrogel foldable intraocular lenses, *J Cataract Refract Surg* 25:1637-1640, 1999.
64. Schauersberger J, Amon M, Kruger A et al: Lens epithelial cell outgrowth on 3 types of intraocular lenses, *J Cataract Refract Surg* 27:850-854, 2001.
65. Samuelson TW, Chu YR, Kreiger RA: Evaluation of giant-cell deposits on foldable intraocular lenses after combined cataract and glaucoma surgery, *J Cataract Refract Surg* 26:817-823, 2000.
66. Fine I, Hoffman R, Packer M: Clear-lens extraction with multifocal lens implantation, *Int Ophthalmol Clin* 41:113-121, 2001.
67. Auffarth G, Dick H: [Multifocal intraocular lenses: a review], *Ophthalmologe* 98:127-137, 2001.
68. Ge J, Arellano A, Salz J: Surgical correction of hyperopia: clear lens extraction and laser correction, *Ophthalmol Clin North Am* 14:301-313, 2001.
69. Steinert RF, Giamporcaro JE, Tasso VA: Clinical assessment of long-term safety and efficacy of a widely implanted silicone intraocular lens material, *Am J Ophthalmol* 123:17-23, 1997.
70. Menapace R: Evaluation of 35 consecutive SI-30 PhacoFlex lenses with high-refractive silicone optic implanted in the capsulorhexis bag, *J Cataract Refract Surg* 21:339-347, 1995.
71. Colin J: Clinical results of implanting a silicone haptic-anchor-plate intraocular lens, *J Cataract Refract Surg* 22:1286-1290, 1996.
72. Oshika T, Suzuki Y, Kizaki H et al: Two year clinical study of a soft acrylic intraocular lens, *J Cataract Refract Surg* 22:104-109, 1996.
73. Mengual E, Garcia J, Elvira JC et al: Clinical results of AcrySof intraocular lens implantation, *J Cataract Refract Surg* 24:114-117, 1998.

74. Afsar AJ, Patel S, Woods RL et al: A comparison of visual performance between a rigid PMMA and a foldable acrylic intraocular lens, *Eye* 13:329-335, 1999.
75. Kobayashi H, Ikeda H, Imamura S et al: Clinical assessment of long-term safety and efficacy of a widely implanted polyacrylic intraocular lens material, *Am J Ophthalmol* 130:310-321, 2000.
76. Oner FH, Gunenc U, Ferliel ST: Posterior capsule opacification after phacoemulsification: foldable acrylic versus poly(methyl methacrylate) intraocular lenses, *J Cataract Refract Surg* 26:722-726, 2000.
77. Hollick E, Spalton D, Ursell P et al: The effect of polymethylmethacrylate, silicone, and polyacrylic intraocular lenses on posterior capsular opacification 3 years after cataract surgery, *Ophthalmology* 106:49-54, 1999; discussion 54-55.
78. Brown D, Ziemba S: Collamer intraocular lens: clinical results from the US FDA core study, *J Cataract Refract Surg* 27:833-840, 2001.

Multifocal Intraocular Lenses

36

Roger F. Steinert, MD
Richard L. Lindstrom, MD

The normal eye is constructed to allow the various refracting surfaces and ocular media to focus parallel rays of light coming from a distant object onto the retina. The eye can also adjust its refractive power through the accommodative process to bring near objects into focus. The cortex of the young lens is a soft, easily molded material contained in an elastic capsule. The traction of the zonular fibers opposes the natural tendency of the lens to assume a spherical shape. Contraction of the ciliary muscles relaxes the zonular attachment sites inward toward the lens equator, reducing the tension on the zonules and allowing the lens to move anteriorly and the highly elastic capsule to increase the convexity of the lens.[1] The resultant steepening of the anterior and posterior poles and anterior movement of the lens change the focal plane, resulting in accommodation.

For the cataract patient, intraocular lens (IOL) implantation surgery has overcome the loss of visual function associated with the removal of cataracts. However, because most IOLs are monofocal, the loss of accommodation becomes significant with surgery. Although the loss of accommodation is not absolute because increased depth of field secondary to small pupillary diameter[2,3] or mild astigmatism[4-7] provides a degree of apparent accommodation (pseudoaccommodation), the need to correct the resultant loss of accommodation (presbyopia) is clinically apparent.

The most common treatment methods for presbyopia are reading glasses or, in cases of ametropia, bifocal spectacles. The difficulties in adapting to bifocal lenses can be considerable. As the add power is increased in strength, trifocal or multifocal reading segments may be required to enable a greater range of focus.

In what may be considered an evolutionary step, bifocal and multifocal IOLs of several different designs have been introduced.[1,8] They differ from conventional monofocal IOLs by potentially providing both distance and near vision without additional bifocal or reading spectacle correction. This chapter describes the multifocal IOL and bifocal designs available in the United States and Europe and those under investigation at this time.

Intraocular Lens Design

Bifocal and multifocal spectacles and some contact lenses are designed for alternating vision. The individual's gaze is directed through the portion of the lens containing the appropriate dioptric power for the target plane of focus. Usually the majority of the lens provides distance vision, and an inset dioptric add at the bottom of the lens is used for near vision. Such a design is not feasible for a multifocal IOL. An individual cannot "look through" different areas of an IOL.

Multifocal IOLs use the principle of simultaneous vision. Different areas of the IOL are designed with different focal planes, usually for near and distance vision. At any given time, one image is in focus at the retina, and the second image is highly defocused with very little structure. Distant objects are focused by the distance power of the lens and defocused by the near power. For near objects, the reverse is true; near objects are focused by the near power of the lens and defocused by the distance power.

Optics

Multifocal IOLs produce simultaneous images using either diffractive or refractive optics (Table 36-1). Although we have used the term *multifocal IOLs,* most designs are actually bifocal.

All diffractive IOLs, such as the CeeOn 811E/808X and the 3M 825X/815LE, are bifocal (see Table 36-1). These IOLs consist of an anterior spherical surface with multiple, concentric, microslope rings on the posterior surface (Figure 36-1). The microslope rings diffract the incoming light, creating a diffraction pattern. Distance and near foci are formed by the combination of the anterior refractive surface with the zero and first orders of diffraction, respectively, created by the posterior surface.

Refractive IOLs (see Table 36-1) achieve more than one plane of focus by alternating zonular rings of different refracting power. IOLs such as the True Vista or MF4 are bifocal (Figure 36-2). Each zone is powered for either distance or near vision. The

TABLE 36-1
Multifocal and Bifocal Intraocular Lenses

Design and Model	Material	Optics and Features
REFRACTIVE MULTIFOCAL		
Array (Advanced Medical Optics [AMO], Santa Ana, Calif.)	Three-piece silicone	Zonal-progressive with repeatable, continual power distributions on anterior surface; aspheric; biconvex; distance dominant, 3.5 D add
Domilens Progress 1 (Bausch & Lomb, Claremont, Calif.)	One-piece PMMA	Optic diameter of 7 mm; central 4.7 mm anterior surface of progressively increasing power to a final add of +5 D surrounded by an annular distance ring; aspheric; biconvex; near dominant
Domilens Progress 3 (Bausch & Lomb, Claremont, Calif.)	One-piece PMMA	Same as Progress 1 with 6.5-mm optic diameter and 4.75 D add
REFRACTIVE BIFOCAL		
True Vista (Bausch & Lomb, Claremont, Calif.)	PMMA	Three-zone (central distance, near annulus with 4 D add, peripheral distance); biconvex; distance dominant
MF4 (IOLTECH, La Rochelle, France)	One-piece hydrophilic acrylic	Four-zone (central near with 4.0 D add, alternating zones of near and distance vision from center); biconvex; near dominant
DIFFRACTIVE BIFOCAL		
CeeOn 811E (Pharmacia Upjohn, Kalamazoo, Mich.)	One-piece PMMA	Bifocal; UV absorbing; concentric diffractive microstructure superimposed on posterior surface of conventional refractive lens; 6-mm biconvex optic; 4.0 D add
CeeOn 808X (Pharmacia Upjohn, Kalamazoo, Mich.)	One-piece PMMA	Same as above with a diameter of 6.5 mm
3M 825X (Alcon, Fort Worth, Tex.)	Three-piece PMMA	Meniscus-shaped optic; anterior spherical surface with multiple diffraction zones on posterior surface; 4.0 D add
3M 815LE (Alcon, Fort Worth, Tex.)	One-piece PMMA	Twenty-seven concentric microslope rings on posterior surface; 3.5 D add

D, Diopter; *PMMA*, polymethylmethacrylate; *UV*, ultraviolet.

True Vista is distance dominant, with the central zone powered for distance vision. The MF4 is near dominant, and the central zone contains the dioptric add for near vision.

True multifocality has been attempted with the designs of the Array and the Domilens Progress IOLs (see Table 36-1). The Array is a distance-dominant, simultaneous-vision, zonal-progressive lens (Figure 36-3). It combines a posterior refractive surface with multiple anterior aspheric refractive zones of continuously varying power (Figure 36-4). Beginning with the central zone, distance power is placed centrally in each odd ring (1, 3, and 5). The power increases toward the periphery of the odd-numbered rings to form a smooth transition with the even

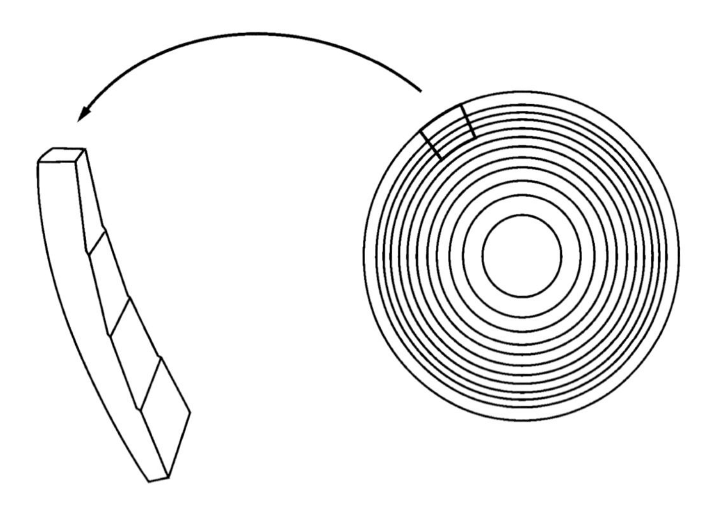

FIGURE 36-1 Alcon 3M Microslope diffractive bifocal intraocular lens. The anterior surface is a spherical refractive surface. The posterior surface is a diffractive surface creating two focal points, near and distance, which can be captured by the retina.

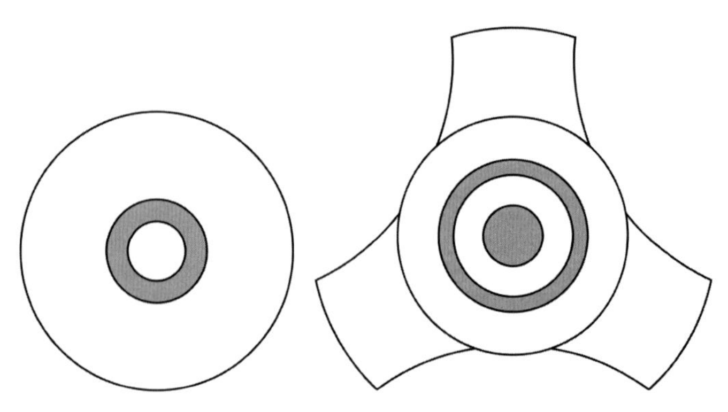

FIGURE 36-2 *Left:* Bausch & Lomb True Vista bifocal IOL optic. The inner and outer zones are powered for distance. The middle zone *(shaded area)* has a 4-D add for near vision. *Right:* IOLTECH MF4 autofocus IOL. Zones 1 and 3 *(shaded areas)* have a 4-D add for near vision. Zones 2 and 4 *(unshaded)* are powered for distance vision.

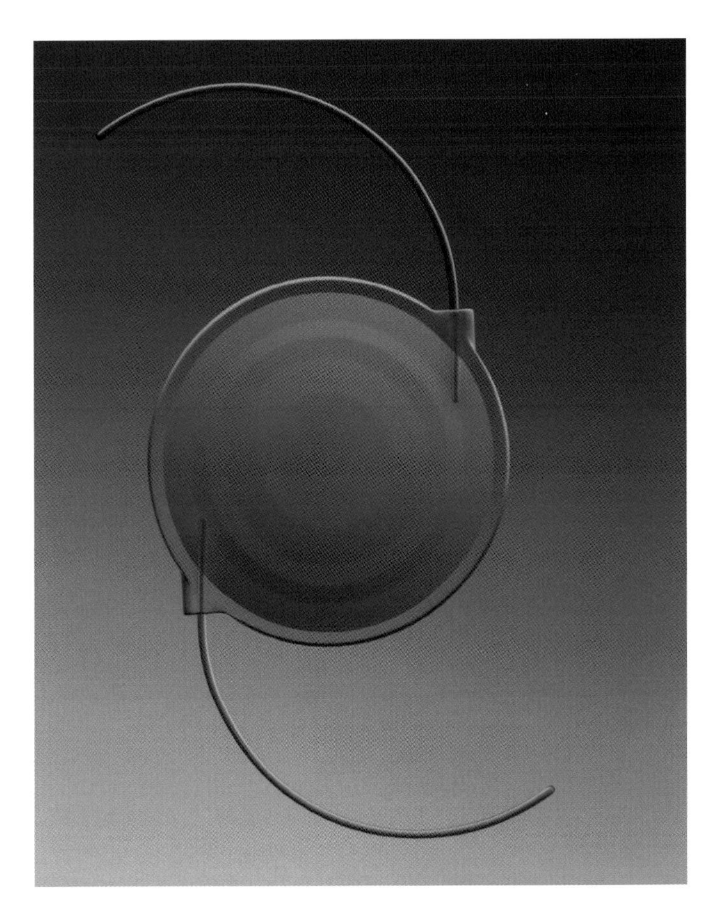

FIGURE 36-3 AMO Array multifocal intraocular lens is a distance-dominant, simultaneous-vision, zonal-progressive lens.

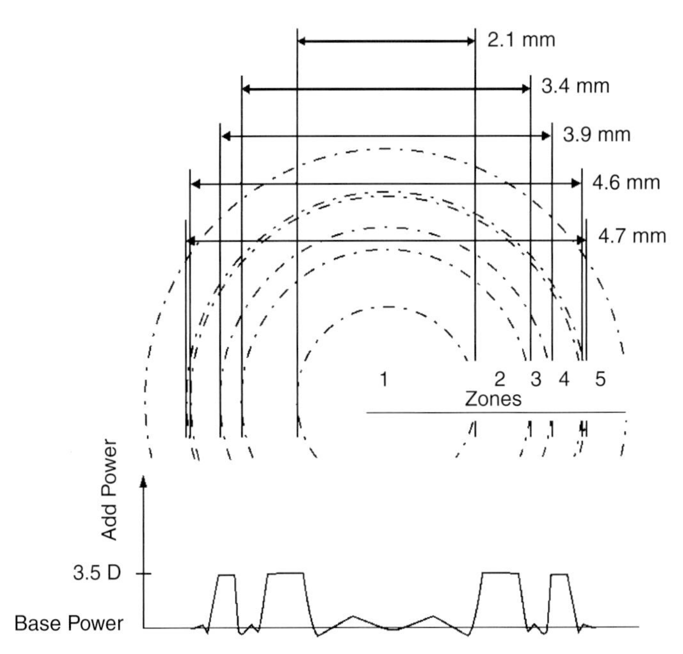

FIGURE 36-4 Frontal view of the AMO Array zonal-progressive IOL showing the add power in diopters associated with each zone.

zones (2 and 4) that emphasize near vision with a 3.5 diopter (D) add. This provides continuous refractive power across the lens to minimize dependence on pupil size.

The Domilens Progress series are near-dominant refractive IOLs with a central aspheric zone of progressive power that provides near vision through the central portion of the lens, distance vision through the periphery of the aspheric portion, and intermediate vision in between.

Each IOL design has different strengths. The diffractive optical effect is simultaneously located throughout the central and paracentral regions of the lens. Thus relative power distribution tends to be little affected by pupil size or IOL centration. Conversely, because of the localized nature of the dioptric power in alternating zones, pupil size and lens centration can affect the refractive zones available in refractive bifocal IOLs.[2] This is less of a problem with the Array multifocal IOL (MIOL) because of the gradation of power across each distance zone.[9,10]

The amount of light transmitted to the retina for image formation also differs among IOL designs. With diffractive IOLs, approximately 41% of the transmitted light is allocated to the distance focus and 41% to the near focus. The remaining 18% of the transmitted light is lost to higher orders of diffraction that are not focused at the retina.[11] In contrast, refractive IOLs transmit all of the available light to the retina. For bifocal refractive IOLs, the transmitted light is divided between near and distance foci. Multifocal IOLs focus the transmitted light for intermediate vision in addition to near and distance vision. For example, the Array MIOL allocates 50% of transmitted light to distance focus, 37% to near focus, and 13% to intermediate focus (based on a 4-mm pupil). The decrease in the percentage of light transmitted through diffractive bifocal IOLs compared with the Array MIOL may result in decreased contrast acuity for patients' distance and intermediate vision.[12]

Clinical Studies

Array Multifocal

The Array MIOL has undergone more studies than any other multifocal IOL and is the only multifocal IOL approved for marketing in the United States. As can be seen in Table 36-2, the Array MIOL provided excellent distance vision.[13-21] Studies comparing the performance of the Array MIOL with monofocal IOL controls found no significant difference in distance uncorrected visual acuity (UCVA).[14,15,17,21]

The advantage of a multifocal IOL is the added ability to focus on near targets. In studies comparing near vision in the Array MIOL and monofocal IOLs, the Array MIOL consistently produced significantly improved levels of near vision.[14,17,21] In a large, prospective, randomized, masked clinical trial, 97% (119 of 123) of Array MIOL patients achieved J3 (20/40) or better uncorrected near visual acuity compared with 66% (72 of 109) of monofocal IOL patients ($P <0.0001$). Further, 73% (90 of 123) of Array MIOL patients achieved J1 (20/20) or better uncorrected near visual acuity compared with 28% (30 of 109) of monofocal IOL patients ($P <0.0001$).[14] Steinert and et al.[17] reported similar results; uncorrected near visual acuity of 20/40 or better and 20/20 or better was achieved by 86% (87 of 101) and 47% (47 of 101) of Array MIOL eyes, respectively. For monofocal eyes, 49% (49 of 101) achieved 20/40 or better and

TABLE 36-2
Visual Acuity with the Array Multifocal IOL

Study	Design	Lens Model	N*	Time Postsurgery	Mean Distance UCVA	Mean Distance BCVA
Steinert et al, 1992	P, DM	MPC-25NB	32 (M)	3-6 months	20/30	88% 20/25 or better
Vaquero et al, 1996	P	MPC-25NB	42 (M)	9.9 months (mean)	—	20/25
Weghaupt et al, 1996	P	SSM 26-NB	14 (M)	6.5 months (mean)	0.79 (20/25)	0.94 (20/21)
Walkow et al, 1997	R	PA154N	40 (M)	1 month	82% 20/30 or better	100% 20/30 or better
Arens et al, 1999	RT	N/A	21 (M)	≥2 years	0.53 (~20/40)	0.82 (20/25)
Steinert et al, 1999	P, C	SSM-26NB	400 (M)	1 year	20/26	20/20
Brydon et al, 2000	RT	SA-40N	15 (B)	≥1 month	93% 20/40 or better	100% 20/30 or better
Javitt and Steinert, 2000	P, R, M	SA-40N	64 (B)	3 months	20/21	20/18
Javitt et al, 2000	P, R, DM	SA-40N	127 (M)	3 months	20/21	20/22

*Number of patients receiving the Array multifocal IOL, not the total number of the study; *B,* binocular implant; *M,* monocular implant.
BCVA, Best corrected visual acuity; *C,* comparative; *DM,* double masked; *M,* masked; *N/A,* not available; *P,* prospective; *R,* randomized; *RT,* retrospective; *UCVA,* uncorrected visual acuity.

12% (12 of 101) achieved 20/20 or better uncorrected near visual acuity. Seventy-seven percent of Array MIOL patients and 57% of monofocal IOL patients achieved a UCVA of J3 (20/40) or better in a study by Brydon et al.[15] In a group of 62 patients, the mean uncorrected near visual acuity was J3+ (20/36) for the Array MIOL group and J7 (20/74) for the monofocal IOL group.[21] A similar mean uncorrected near visual acuity of J2.75 for patients with the Array MIOL was reported by Weghaupt, Pieh, and Skorpik.[20]

Similar near uncorrected visual acuities were found for Array MIOL patients (0.68 [20/29]) and monofocal IOL patients (0.53 [20/38]) who were targeted for slight myopia (–0.5 D or –0.75 D). However, when best distance correction was added to both groups, the Array MIOL patients (0.91 [20/22]) had significantly better ($P < 0.05$) near visual acuity than the monofocal IOL patients (0.52 [20/38]).[16]

A prospective study of patients with cataract and concurrent disease such as macular degeneration, glaucoma, or diabetic retinopathy found that even in compromised eyes, the Array MIOL (n = 81) still produced distance visual acuity comparable to or better than a monofocal IOL (SI-40NB, Advanced Medical Optics [AMO], Santa Ana, Calif.).[22]

Patients with bifocal/multifocal IOLs gain the ability to see at near but may lose some contrast sensitivity in low light conditions. Contrast sensitivity is typically examined using the contrast acuity charts of 96%, 50%, 25%, and 11% thresholds. Studies (n = 291 patients total) consistently reported no significant difference in contrast sensitivity at high thresholds (96% and 50%) between the Array MIOL and monofocal IOLs.[16-18,21] These same studies found that at 11% contrast, contrast sensitivity was significantly lower (approximately 1 line) with the Array MIOL than with a monofocal IOL. However when comparing binocular vision, contrast sensitivity at 11% did not differ significantly between the Array MIOL and the monofocal IOL.[16-18,21] The findings at 25% were mixed; some studies found a significant decrease in contrast sensitivity with the Array MIOL (n = 193 total patients),[17,18] whereas other studies did not (n = 98 total patients).[16,21] The reduction in low-contrast acuity had little effect on everyday visual tasks.[17] Bilateral implantation of the Array MIOL may alleviate reduced contrast sensitivity at low contrast levels.[16]

Driving simulation studies can help define any potential for functional visual performance loss associated with a reduction in low-contrast acuity. At night, car headlights can decrease contrast sensitivity and increase glare. A prospective, masked, parallel-group comparison of 33 bilateral Array MIOL patients and 33 bilateral monofocal IOL patients assessed driving performance during night, night with glare, and fog conditions.[23] There was no significant difference between the groups for 26 of the 30 driving performance measurements. The four measures that were different were in favor of the monofocal subjects. These were the percentage of correctly recognized warning signs at night in clear weather, sign recognition distances for guide and warning signs in fog, and detection distance for one of four hazards (suitcase). The multifocal patients performed, on average, within safety guidelines (American Association of State Highway and Transportation Officials).[23] Schmitz and et al.[24] compared the effect of glare from halogen lights (which are similar to oncoming automobile headlights) on contrast sensitivity in patients with an Array MIOL or a monofocal IOL. There were no significant differences in contrast sensitivity between the two groups in the presence of moderate or strong glare. A significant difference between the two groups was found only at the lowest spatial frequency (3 cpd) without halogen glare. Together, these studies suggest that driving vision with an Array MIOL is similar to that with a monofocal IOL. Nevertheless, patients with multifocal IOLs should exercise caution when driving at night or under poor visibility conditions.

Photic phenomena such as glare and halos occasionally occur in patients with bifocal, multifocal, and monofocal IOL implants.* Haring and et al.[26] queried cataract patients from four study centers who had received an Array MIOL or a monofocal IOL implant. Nine percent (8 of 93) of patients in the monofocal group reported some form of photic phenomena (halo, flare, flash, glare or streak) compared with 41% (57 of 138) of the Array MIOL group. Ninety percent (124 of 138) of the Array MIOL group and 97% (90 of 93) of the monofocal group rated their disturbance by the photic phenomena as none or slight. The degree of disturbance was moderate or severe for 10% (14 of 138) of the Array MIOL group and 3% (3 of 93) of

*References 13, 14, 16, 17, 20, 24-26.

the monofocal group. The grade of patient complaints in the Array MIOL group varied significantly across the four study sites, suggesting that surgical technique or patient selection criteria may affect postoperative reports of photic phenomena.

Even though some patients experienced halos or glare with the Array multifocal IOL, they would choose to have the Array MIOL implanted again.[13,14,17] Further, overall quality of life and satisfaction were higher in multifocal patients than monofocal patients.[13,14]

Overwhelmingly, studies demonstrated that patients with the Array MIOL implant wear spectacles less frequently than patients with monocular IOLs.[13-15,21,27] Patients with the Array MIOL rated their distance, intermediate, near, and overall vision without glasses better than patients with monofocal IOLs.[13,14,27] This finding was true irrespective of the implant combination: bilateral Array MIOL, monofocal-Array MIOL combination, or unilateral Array MIOL with a phakic fellow eye.[17] A significantly higher proportion of patients with bilateral Array MIOLs reported that they could function comfortably at near distance.[17]

CeeOn 811E and 808X

The CeeOn 811E and CeeOn 808X diffractive bifocal IOLs (Pharmacia Upjohn, Kalamazoo, Mich.) are marketed in Europe. They are the same diffractive bifocal design, with a near add of +4.0 D. The CeeOn 811E has a 6-mm optic, and the CeeOn 808X has a 6.5-mm optic. The CeeOn 811E provides good visual performance for distance and near vision (uncorrected distance = 0.79 [20/25], best-corrected distance = 1.0 [20/20], uncorrected near = J1.6 [between 20/25 and 20/30], near with best distance correction = J1.19 [~20/20]).[28] When comparing the 811E bifocal diffractive IOL and the Array refractive MIOL, there was no significant difference in contrast sensitivity,[19] glare visual acuity,[19] or distance visual acuity.[29]

A study of 149 patients found that the Pharmacia 808X IOL produced similar distance visual acuity as a monofocal lens (all achieved best-corrected visual acuity of 0.5 [20/40] or better), but the 808X was significantly better for near vision (uncorrected near acuity of J3 [20/40] or better: 93% of 79 808X patients, 9% of 70 monofocal patients).[30] Contrast sensitivity was slightly lower for patients with the 808X IOL than a monofocal IOL.[30,31] However, contrast sensitivity was better in patients with bilateral 808X IOLs.[31]

Domilens Progress

Domilens Progress 1 and 3 IOLs (Laboratories Domilens division of Bausch & Lomb Surgical, Claremont, Calif.) are marketed in Europe. The design is the same for both IOLs. The Progress 1 has a final add of +5.0 D for near vision and a 7-mm optic. The Progress 3 has a +4.75 D add for near vision and a 6.5-mm optic diameter.

The first clinical results with the Domilens Progress 1 showed that 65% of the patients (n = 20) had an uncorrected distance acuity of 8/10 (20/25) or better and uncorrected near visual acuity of J2 (20/30) or better.[32] In medium and bright light, visual acuity was decreased by 0.01 and 0.05 Snellen lines, respectively.[32] The quality of vision at various focal distances can be determined by assessing the spatial resolution threshold. The mean spatial resolution threshold was not significantly different between the Domilens Progress 1 IOL and either the CeeOn 811X bifocal IOL or the Array MIOL for distance vision. The Domilens Progress 1 IOL performed significantly less well than the Array MIOL for intermediate vision and significantly less well than the Array MIOL or CeeOn 811X bifocal IOL for near vision.[33] Contrast sensitivity was decreased in patients with the Domilens Progress 1 compared with a monofocal IOL.[32]

A study examining the Domilens Progress 3 IOL (n = 59) found a mean uncorrected distance visual acuity of 20/26 and mean corrected acuity of 20/21.[34] With this IOL, distance visual acuity was not influenced by pupillary diameter. Mean uncorrected near visual acuity was J4.75 (between 20/50 and 20/40) and distance corrected was J4 (between 20/50 and 20/40). Patient satisfaction was high when viewing objects under good light conditions or when viewing larger objects but decreased under poor lighting conditions.[34]

True Vista

The True Vista IOL (Bausch & Lomb Surgical, Claremont, Calif.) is also marketed in Europe. It has three zones: a central zone for distance focus, an annulus for near focus (add power of +4.0 D), and a peripheral zone for distance focus (Figure 36-5).

The True Vista multifocal IOL provides good visual acuity. A prospective study of 446 patients found that at 7 to 11 months after surgery, 70% and 98% (n = 145) had 20/40 or better uncorrected and best-corrected distance acuity, respectively. Uncorrected near acuity was 20/30 or better in 69% of the patients, and distance-corrected near acuity was 20/30 or better in 78% (n = 131) of the patients.[35] Near acuity was better with the True Vista than with monofocal IOLs.[35] Distance and near acuity decreased with increasing astigmatism or increasing age.[35]

In dim light, at the lowest contrast levels, patients with the True Vista IOL had significantly greater loss of visual acuity compared with patients with monofocal IOLs.[35,36] Compared with the 3M 815LE diffractive IOL, the True Vista IOL provides a good compromise because distance contrast acuity is good and near vision is sufficient.[37] Another study compared the True Vista with the 3M 815LE and 3M 825X diffractive IOLs and found that the True Vista IOL performed slightly but significantly better than the 3M IOLs in bright light (96% and 25% contrast Regan charts).[36]

Blurring and glare were reported 2 to 3 times more often in the True Vista eye than in the monofocal eye.[35] Quality of vision was generally rated to be lower in the True Vista eye compared with the monofocal fellow eye. Knorz[35] concluded that based on the clinical findings, True Vista IOLs should not be implanted in patients with a monofocal fellow eye. In contrast, Charman et al.[38] found that 48% (n = 27) of the patients preferred the True Vista, 26% preferred the monofocal fellow eye, and 11% could not distinguish between the True Vista and the monofocal fellow eye.[38]

3M

The 3M 825X and 3M 815LE (Alcon, Fort Worth, Tex.) are diffractive IOLs under investigation. The near add is +4.0 D for the 825X and 3.5 D for the 815LE.

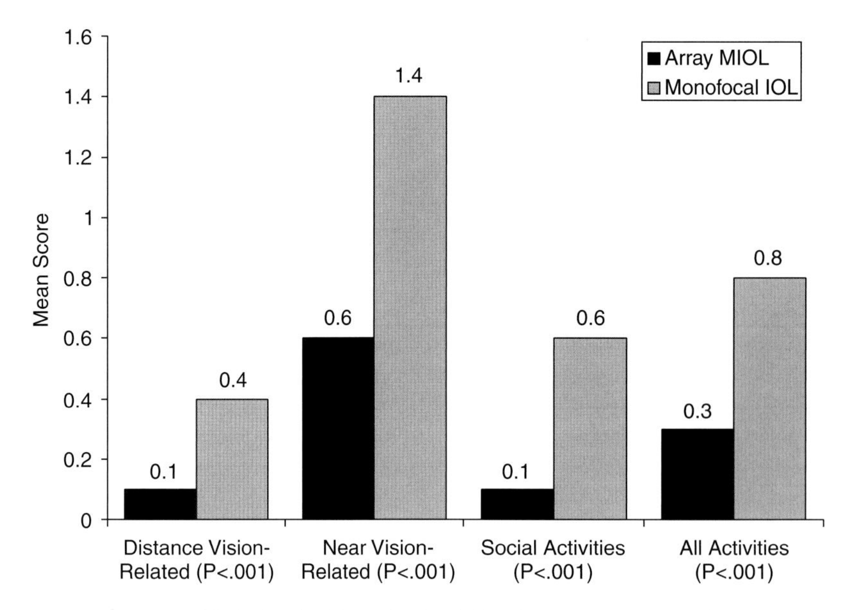

FIGURE 36-5 Summary of limitations in vision-related activities: 0 = no limitation, 1 = slight limitation, 2 = somewhat limited.

The 3M multifocal IOL provides good uncorrected distance visual acuity (Table 36-3).[39-42] In two studies that compared the 3M diffractive IOL to a monofocal IOL, slightly more monofocal IOL patients achieved 20/25 or better uncorrected distance visual acuity than 3M diffractive IOL patients; however, the differences were not statistically significant.[39,40]

Uncorrected near visual acuity was superior in the 3M diffractive IOL patients compared with monofocal IOL patients.[40] Thirty percent of 39 3M diffractive and 4% of 38 monofocal IOL patients achieved J1 (20/20) or better uncorrected near visual acuity.[40] An uncorrected near visual acuity of 20/40 or better was achieved by 93.9% of patients (n = 35) with the 3M diffractive IOL in a study by Auffarth et al.[42] and 66.7% of patients (60 of 90) in a study by Slagsvold.[41] Knorz et al.[37] reported a mean uncorrected near visual acuity of 20/35 for 10 patients implanted with a 3M815LE diffractive IOL.

Contrast sensitivity was lower in patients with 3M diffractive IOLs than in patients with monofocal IOLs.[36,39,43-45] The contrast sensitivities of the 3M diffractive IOL for distance and near focus were identical.[45,46] However, in a comparison with the refractive multifocal Array IOL, patients with the 3M diffractive bifocal IOL had contrast sensitivities 8% to 12% lower (at 3 to 11.4 cpd) than patients with the multifocal Array IOL. The decreased contrast sensitivity may be due to the smaller amount of transmitted light allocated to distance focus in the 3M diffractive compared with the Array MIOL.[12] Contrast acuity at near focus was better with 3M 815LE than True Vista IOLs.[37]

Patients (n = 149) with bilateral 3M diffractive IOLs had significantly more glare, flare, and halos than patients (n = 131) with bilateral monofocal IOLs.[39] Patients with 3M 815LE diffractive IOLs may also be more sensitive to glare than those with Array refractive MIOLs.[12]

Patients implanted with 3M diffractive IOLs wear spectacles less frequently than patients with monocular IOLs.[39] However, two long-term follow-up studies found that nearly half of the patients with 3M diffractive IOLs preferred to use spectacles for distance and/or near.[41,42] Bilaterally implanted 3M diffractive IOL patients needed spectacles less frequently than monocularly implanted patients.[41]

MF4

The MF4 (IOLTECH SA, La Rochelle, France) has four zones: a central zone (add power of +4.0 D) surrounded by alternating

TABLE 36-3
Visual Acuity with the 3M Lens

Study	Design	Lens Model	N*	Time Postsurgery	Mean Distance UCVA	Mean Distance BCVA
Slagsvold, 2000	F	815LE	76 (M)	8 years	90% 0.5 (20/40) or better	100% 0.5 (20/40) or better
Auffarth et al, 1993	F	815LE/825X	50 (M)	2.5 years	86% 20/40 or better	100% 20/40 or better
Knorz et al, 1993	C, P	815LE	10 (M)	4-6 months	20/33	20/25
El-Maghraby et al, 1992	P, R	815LE	39 (M)	2-4 months	79% 20/40 or better	96% 20/40 or better
Gimbel et al, 1991	RT	N/A	149 (B)	29 weeks, median	78% 20/40 or better	96% 20/40 or better

*Number of patients receiving the 3M bifocal IOL, not the total number of the study; *B*, binocular implant; *M*, monocular implant.
BCVA, Best corrected visual acuity; *C*, comparative; *F*, follow-up; *N/A*, not available; *P*, prospective; *R*, randomized; *RT*, retrospective; *UCVA*, uncorrected visual acuity.

annular zones for distance and near focus (see Figure 36-2). To date, no clinical studies of the MF4 have been published. A preliminary report at the 2001 meeting of the American Society of Cataract and Refractive Surgeons[47] compared the MF4 bifocal with the Array MIOL. Mean uncorrected distance visual acuity was 0.72 (20/25) with the Array MIOL (n = 20) and 0.63 (20/32) for the MF4 bifocal IOL (n = 20). Mean uncorrected near visual acuity was 0.72 with the Array MIOL and 0.78 with the MF4 bifocal IOL.

Optimizing Results

Patients with bifocal[30,41,42] or multifocal[14,17,21,27] IOLs depend less on spectacles than patients with monofocal IOLs. Patients with the Array MIOL reported significantly less limitation in vision-related function than patients with a monofocal IOL (see Figure 36-5).[27] A quality-of-life survey of patients with monofocal IOLs or the Array MIOLs indicated that patients would be willing to pay approximately $2.00 a day to avoid having to wear eyeglasses to read.[27] To maximize the benefits of bifocal/multifocal IOLs, patient selection, accurate preoperative evaluation, and astigmatic control are important.

Patient expectations must be realistic for bifocal or multifocal IOL implants to be successful. This may require more of the surgeon's time to educate the patient. Although all bifocal and multifocal IOLs lead to some loss of contrast sensitivity compared with monofocal IOLs, this loss may have little clinical impact. Human vision is designed to adapt to large changes in image contrast with small effects on performance. It would be expected that patients with multifocal IOLs would have contrast difficulties only under low-contrast viewing, in compromised eyes, or near the limit of visual acuity, where tolerance to contrast reduction breaks down. This is supported by a study demonstrating no impact of a multifocal IOL on reading speed unless the text had tiny letters or was of low contrast.[45]

Photic phenomena such as glare and halos occur with monofocal IOL implants, but their incidence is higher in bifocal and multifocal IOLs. Patients differ widely in their tolerance of photic phenomena and should be counseled accordingly before deciding on a bifocal or multifocal IOL. The trade-off for slightly greater glare disability and decreased contrast sensitivity is the increased depth of focus provided by multifocal IOLs.[42,45]

Lens selection, preoperative evaluation, astigmatism control, and postoperative care are important considerations when choosing a specific IOL. For example, a lens that provides constant vision regardless of pupil size may be best for patients with small or nonreactive pupils.[2,9,48] The status of the fellow eye should be considered to avoid conditions that may preclude an optimal result, such as extreme aniseikonia. How well the lens is centered and positioned along the axis of the eye will have direct bearing on how well the lens functions. Insight can be gained into the lens's likely optical performance by considering retinal point-spread functions (blur patches) according to the geometrical optics.[38]

Proper preoperative evaluation that includes accurate biometry is essential to obviate or minimize the use of spectacles with a multifocal IOL.[11,49,50] Small errors in lens power calculations may be well tolerated by patients, but larger errors may require spectacle correction for distance vision to fully use the properties of multifocal lenses.

Adequate surgical control of astigmatism contributes to an optimal result in patients with multifocal lenses, just as it does in those with monofocal lenses.[4,7,51] Both distance and near acuity decrease with increasing astigmatism.[37,52] The technique of wound closure used and final wound size can influence the induced astigmatism.[53] Astigmatism-induced deterioration of both distance and intermediate visual acuity was significantly worse with a multifocal lens (Array or True Vista) than with a monofocal lens.[52,54] However, near visual acuity was better with a multifocal lens in patients with astigmatism.[52] Therefore care should be taken to avoid or control the extent of surgically induced astigmatism at all times.

The Future

The future for bifocal and multifocal IOLs may be in refractive lensectomy. Presentations at the 2001 meeting of the American Society of Cataract and Refractive Surgery demonstrated the successful use of the Array MIOL to provide pseudoaccommodation to presbyopic patients.[55,56] A number of studies have reported replacing noncataractous lenses in high myopes[57,58] and hyperopes[57,59-63] with monofocal IOLs to achieve good distance visual acuity. The use of bifocal or multifocal IOLs in place of monofocal IOLs would provide the patient with both near and distance visual acuity.

An alternative to bifocal or multifocal IOLs is to produce an accommodating IOL. One approach is the CrystaLens AT-45 (C & C Vision, Aliso Viejo, Calif.), which is currently in development (see Figure 35-10). This IOL has two hinges positioned at the edges of the plate portion of the haptic.[64] The hinges allow the lens to flex anteriorly and posteriorly with contraction of the ciliary muscles. This may provide up to 2.5 D of accommodation.

Future development of multifocal optics that use an even smaller-incision lens design will allow improved control of astigmatism and rapid visual rehabilitation. In the future, many patients will be able to achieve visual acuities of 20/20 and J1 on the first postoperative day without spectacle correction. The pioneering work discussed here heralds the beginning of an exciting new era for cataract surgeons and their patients.

REFERENCES

1. Duffey RJ, Zabel RW, Lindstrom RL: Multifocal intraocular lenses, *J Cataract Refract Surg* 16:423-429, 1990.
2. Koch DD, Samuelson SW, Haft EA et al: Pupillary size and responsiveness: implications for selection of a bifocal intraocular lens, *Ophthalmology* 98:1030-1035, 1991.
3. Verzella F, Calossi A: Multifocal effect of against-the-rule myopic astigmatism in pseudophakic eyes, *Refract Corneal Surg* 9:58-61, 1993.
4. Bradbury JA, Hillman JS, Cassells-Brown A: Optimal postoperative refraction for good unaided near and distance vision with monofocal intraocular lenses, *Br J Ophthalmol* 76:300-302, 1992.
5. Percival P: An update on multifocal lens implants, *Doc Ophthalmol* 81: 285-292, 1992.
6. Sawusch MR, Guyton DL: Optimal astigmatism to enhance depth of focus after cataract surgery, *Ophthalmology* 98:1025-1029, 1991.
7. Datiles MB, Gancayco T: Low myopia with low astigmatic correction gives cataract surgery patients good depth of focus, *Ophthalmology* 97:922-926, 1990.

8. Holladay JT, Van Dijk H, Lang A et al: Optical performance of multifocal intraocular lenses, *J Cataract Refract Surg* 16:413-422, 1990.
9. Koch DD, Samuelson SW, Villarreal R, Haft EA et al: Changes in pupil size induced by phacoemulsification and posterior chamber lens implantation: consequences for multifocal lenses, *J Cataract Refract Surg* 22:579-584, 1996.
10. Knorz MC, Bedoya JH, Hsia TC et al: Comparison of modulation transfer function and through focus response with monofocal and bifocal IOLs, *Ger J Ophthalmol* 1:45-53, 1992.
11. Akutsu H, Legge GE, Luebker A, Lindstrom RL et al: Multifocal intraocular lenses and glare, *Optom Vis Sci* 70:487-495, 1993.
12. Pieh S, Weghaupt H, Skorpik C: Contrast sensitivity and glare disability with diffractive and refractive multifocal intraocular lenses, *J Cataract Refract Surg* 24:659-662, 1998.
13. Javitt J, Brauweiler HP, Jacobi KW et al: Cataract extraction with multifocal intraocular lens implantation: clinical, functional, and quality-of-life outcomes. Multicenter clinical trial in Germany and Austria, *J Cataract Refract Surg* 26:1356-1366, 2000.
14. Javitt JC, Steinert RF: Cataract extraction with multifocal intraocular lens implantation: a multinational clinical trial evaluating clinical, functional, and quality-of-life outcomes, *Ophthalmology* 107:2040-2048, 2000.
15. Brydon KW, Tokarewicz AC, Nichols BD: AMO array multifocal lens versus monofocal correction in cataract surgery, *J Cataract Refract Surg* 26:96-100, 2000.
16. Arens B, Freudenthaler N, Quentin CD: Binocular function after bilateral implantation of monofocal and refractive multifocal intraocular lenses, *J Cataract Refract Surg* 25:399-404, 1999.
17. Steinert RF, Aker BL, Trentacost DJ, Smith PJ et al: A prospective comparative study of the AMO ARRAY zonal-progressive multifocal silicone intraocular lens and a monofocal intraocular lens, *Ophthalmology* 106:1243-1255, 1999.
18. Vaquero M, Encinas JL, Jimenez F: Visual function with monofocal versus multifocal IOLs, *J Cataract Refract Surg* 22:1222-1225, 1996.
19. Walkow T, Liekfeld A, Anders N et al: A prospective evaluation of a diffractive versus a refractive designed multifocal intraocular lens, *Ophthalmology* 104:1380-1386, 1997.
20. Weghaupt H, Pieh S, Skorpik C: Visual properties of the foldable Array multifocal intraocular lens, *J Cataract Refract Surg* 22:1313-1317, 1996.
21. Steinert RF, Post CT Jr, Brint SF et al: A prospective, randomized, double-masked comparison of a zonal-progressive multifocal intraocular lens and a monofocal intraocular lens, *Ophthalmology* 99:853-860, 1992; discussion 860-861.
22. Kamath GG, Prasad S, Danson A et al: Visual outcome with the array multifocal intraocular lens in patients with concurrent eye disease, *J Cataract Refract Surg* 26:576-581, 2000.
23. Featherstone KA, Bloomfield JR, Lang AJ et al: Driving simulation study: bilateral array multifocal versus bilateral AMO monofocal intraocular lenses, *J Cataract Refract Surg* 25:1254-1262, 1999.
24. Schmitz S, Dick HB, Krummenauer F et al: Contrast sensitivity and glare disability by halogen light after monofocal and multifocal lens implantation, *Br J Ophthalmol* 84:1109-1112, 2000.
25. Dick HB, Krummenauer F, Schwenn O et al: Objective and subjective evaluation of photic phenomena after monofocal and multifocal intraocular lens implantation, *Ophthalmology* 106:1878-1886, 1999.
26. Haring G, Dick HB, Krummenauer F et al: Subjective photic phenomena with refractive multifocal and monofocal intraocular lenses: results of a multicenter questionnaire, *J Cataract Refract Surg* 27:245-249, 2001.
27. Javitt JC, Wang F, Trentacost DJ et al: Outcomes of cataract extraction with multifocal intraocular lens implantation: functional status and quality of life, *Ophthalmology* 104:589-599, 1997.
28. Avitabile T, Marano F, Canino EG et al: Long-term visual results of bifocal intraocular lens implantation, *J Cataract Refract Surg* 25:1263-1269, 1999.
29. Liekfeld A, Walkow T, Anders N et al: [Prospective comparison of 2 multi-focal lens models], *Ophthalmologe* 95:253-256, 1998.
30. Allen ED, Burton RL, Webber SK et al: Comparison of a diffractive bifocal and a monofocal intraocular lens, *J Cataract Refract Surg* 22:446-451, 1996.
31. Haaskjold E, Allen ED, Burton RL et al: Contrast sensitivity after implantation of diffractive bifocal and monofocal intraocular lenses, *J Cataract Refract Surg* 24:653-658, 1998.
32. Ravalico G, Baccara F, Isola V: [Functional evaluation of a new type of intraocular lens: Domilens type progress 1], *J Fr Ophtalmol* 17:175-181, 1994.
33. Ravalico G, Parentin F, Pastori G et al: Spatial resolution threshold in pseudophakic patients with monofocal and multifocal intraocular lenses, *J Cataract Refract Surg* 24:244-248, 1998.
34. Bleckmann H, Schmidt O, Sunde T et al: Visual results of progressive multifocal posterior chamber intraocular lens implantation, *J Cataract Refract Surg* 22:1102-1107, 1996.
35. Knorz MC: Results of a European multicenter study of the True Vista bifocal intraocular lens, *J Cataract Refract Surg* 19:626-634, 1993.
36. Boesten IE, Beekhuis WH, Hassmann E et al: Comparison of the Storz bifocal zonal and the 3M diffractive multifocal intraocular lenses, *J Cataract Refract Surg* 21:437-441, 1995.
37. Knorz MC, Claessens D, Schaefer RC et al: Evaluation of contrast acuity and defocus curve in bifocal and monofocal intraocular lenses, *J Cataract Refract Surg* 19:513-523, 1993.
38. Charman WN, Murray IJ, Nacer M et al: Theoretical and practical performance of a concentric bifocal intraocular implant lens, *Vision Res* 38:2841-2853, 1998.
39. Gimbel HV, Sanders DR, Raanan MG: Visual and refractive results of multifocal intraocular lenses, *Ophthalmology* 98:881-887, 1991; discussion 888.
40. el-Maghraby A, Marzouky A, Gazayerli E et al: Multifocal versus monofocal intraocular lenses: visual and refractive comparisons, *J Cataract Refract Surg* 18:147-152, 1992.
41. Slagsvold JE: 3M diffractive multifocal intraocular lens: eight year follow-up, *J Cataract Refract Surg* 26:402-407, 2000.
42. Auffarth GU, Hunold W, Wesendahl TA et al: Depth of focus and functional results in patients with multifocal intraocular lenses: a long-term follow-up, J Cataract Refract Surg 19:685-689, 1993.
43. Ravalico G, Baccara F, Rinaldi G: Contrast sensitivity in multifocal intraocular lenses, *J Cataract Refract Surg* 19:22-25, 1993.
44. Olsen T, Corydon L: Contrast sensitivity in patients with a new type of multifocal intraocular lens, *J Cataract Refract Surg* 16:42-46, 1990.
45. Akutsu H, Legge GE, Showalter M et al: Contrast sensitivity and reading through multifocal intraocular lenses, *Arch Ophthalmol* 110:1076-1080, 1992.
46. Ruther K, Eisenmann D, Zrenner E et al: [Effect of diffractive multi-focal lenses on contrast vision, glare sensitivity and color vision], *Klin Monatsbl Augenheilkd* 204:14-19, 1994.
47. Rau M: Visual acuity and contrast sensitivity after IOL implantation: array versus Autofocus MF-4. Annual Meeting of the American Society of Cataract and Refractive Surgery, San Diego, 2001.
48. Atebara NH, Miller D: An optical model to describe image contrast with bifocal intraocular lenses, *Am J Ophthalmol* 110:172-177, 1990.
49. Holladay JT, Hoffer KJ: Intraocular lens power calculations for multifocal intraocular lenses, *Am J Ophthalmol* 114:405-408, 1992.
50. Namiki M, Tagami Y: [Perimetric glare test and evaluation of intraocular lenses], *Nippon Ganka Gakkai Zasshi* 97:210-216, 1993.
51. Percival P: An update on multifocal lens implants, *Doc Ophthalmol* 81: 285-292, 1992.
52. Hayashi K, Hayashi H, Nakao F et al: Influence of astigmatism on multifocal and monofocal intraocular lenses, *Am J Ophthalmol.* 130:477-482, 2000.
53. Steinert RF, Brint SF, White SM et al: Astigmatism after small incision cataract surgery: a prospective, randomized, multicenter comparison of 4- and 6.5-mm incisions, *Ophthalmology* 98:417-423, 1991; discussion 423-424.
54. Knorz MC, Koch DD, Martinez-Franco C et al: Effect of pupil size and astigmatism on contrast acuity with monofocal and bifocal intraocular lenses, *J Cataract Refract Surg* 20:26-33, 1994.
55. Woodcock M: Predictability of refractive results after Array implantation versus LASIK. Annual Meeting of the American Society of Cataract and Refractive Surgery, San Diego, 2001.
56. Alexander A: Clear lens extraction with the Array multifocal IOL for hyperopia and presbyopia. Annual Meeting of the American Society of Cataract and Refractive Surgery. San Diego, 2001.
57. Vicary D, Sun X-Y, Montgomery P: Refractive lensectomy to correct ametropia, *J Cataract Refract Surg* 25:943-948, 1999.
58. Jimenez-Alfaro I, Miguelez S, Bueno J et al: Clear lens extraction and implantation of negative-power posterior chamber intraocular lenses to correct extreme myopia, *J Cataract Refract Surg* 24:1310-1316, 1998.
59. Siganos D, Pallidaris I, Siganos C: Clear lensectomy and intraocular lens implantation in normally sighted highly hyperopic eyes: three-year follow-up, *Eur J Implant Ref Surg* 7:128-133, 1995.
60. Siganos D, Pallikaris I: Clear lensectomy and intraocular lens implantation for hyperopia from +7 to +14 diopters, *J Refract Surg* 14:105-113, 1998.
61. Pop M, Payette Y, Amyot M: Clear lens extraction with intraocular lens followed by photorefractive keratectomy or laser in situ keratomileusis, *Ophthalmology* 108:106-109, 2001.
62. Lyle A, Jin G: Clear lens extraction to correct hyperopia, *J Cataract Refract Surg* 23:1051-1056, 1997.
63. Kolahdouz-Isfahani A, Rostmian K, Wallace D et al: Clear lens extraction with intraocular lens implantation for hyperopia, *J Refract Surg* 15:316-323, 1999.
64. Cumming JS, Kammann J: Experience with an accommodating IOL, *J Cataract Refract Surg* 22:1001, 1996.

Secondary Intraocular Lenses

37

Roger F. Steinert, MD
Martin S. Arkin, MD

The surgeon has four main alternatives for secondary intraocular lenses (IOLs): (1) standard capsular bag–fixated or sulcus-fixated posterior chamber (PC) lenses, (2) transscleral suture–fixated PC lenses, (3) peripheral iris suture–fixated PC IOLs, and (4) anterior chamber (AC) lenses.

If capsular support is available, standard PC lenses, placed in the ciliary sulcus or, preferably, in the capsular bag, are the standard of care. If capsular support is absent, the decision is more controversial. Sutured PC IOLs have become increasingly popular over the past decade, but most surgeons will select an open-loop flexible AC IOL in the absence of a specific contraindication. Extensive debate persists between these options because of the limited number of studies that are available and the lack of controlled studies with long-term follow-up.

IOLs have been widely used for less than 30 years. The first suture-fixated IOL was implanted a half century ago by Parry.[1] Worst was a pioneer in the use of iris pupil–fixated lenses in the mid-1970s.[1] McCannel reported the use of midperipheral iris fixation sutures to stabilize dislocated pupil-fixated IOLs in 1976.[1] Since then, numerous techniques using sutures to secure PC lenses to the iris or sclera have been described. Although many studies report on relatively small numbers of patients with short-term follow-up and fairly good results, few large prospective controlled studies exist. Most of the studies involve concomitant corneal transplantation to treat pseudophakic bullous keratopathy (PBK). This makes the analysis more difficult because these eyes often have a high degree of existing pathologic conditions, and corneal transplants have their own complications, including astigmatism, glaucoma, cystoid macular edema (CME), and graft rejection.

It is rare to find an aphakic patient with an intact posterior capsule. Most aphakic patients have had a complicated phacoemulsification or extracapsular cataract extraction. Aphakic patients with residual capsule often have synechiae between the anterior capsule and posterior iris or between the anterior capsule and posterior capsule. The surgeon has the option of placing a PC IOL in the ciliary sulcus after lysing iridocapsular adhesions or attempting capsular bag placement after reopening the bag. Stability and complication rates are thought to be similar to those of primary PC IOL placement in the sulcus.

Three primary options exist for IOL fixation in the absence of capsular support: transscleral-sutured PC IOLs, peripheral iris-sutured PC IOLs, and flexible open-loop AC IOLs. If both the posterior capsule and the iris are disrupted or absent, then sutured transscleral PC IOLs are the only IOL option. Tables 37-1 though 37-4 review the advantages and disadvantages of each of these IOL styles and those of nonsutured standard PC IOLs.[2-5]

Table 37-5 lists the principal indications for secondary IOL implantation. Clinical scenarios include rupture of the posterior capsule at the time of cataract surgery or a patient with a threatened expulsive hemorrhage in whom the cataract surgery was aborted without IOL placement. Some patients with closed-loop AC IOLs who have been followed closely and have not yet developed generalized corneal edema have been found to have decreasing endothelial cell counts, increasing corneal thickness, localized peripheral corneal edema, or CME. These patients may be candidates for IOL exchange. AC IOLs and sutured PC IOLs are also used to replace malpositioned lenses that are decentered, subluxated into the vitreous, or dislocated near the endothelium. Panton et al.[6] described the use of iris sutures and IOL exchange for scleral-sutured PC IOLs to manage subluxed primary PC IOLs. Price et al.[7] believe that capsulorhexis should help decrease the incidence of this complication. Finally, cataract surgery complications that can lead to IOL exchange include the uveitis-glaucoma-hyphema (UGH) syndrome or chronic pain from closed-loop AC lenses without corneal edema. Doren, Stern, and Driebe[8] found that the UGH syndrome was usually associated with a relatively poor outcome even with lens exchange. See Chapters 40 and 42 for further discussion of corneal decompensation and the technique of removing closed-loop AC IOLs.

Surgical Procedure

Few patients have an intact posterior capsule and no IOL present. Occasionally, PC IOLs dislocate without extensive capsular bag disruption, and an IOL exchange or repositioning is necessary. Some patients with old-style rigid AC IOL and PBK may have some capsular support evident at the time of penetrating keratoplasty and IOL exchange. For the few patients in whom secondary placement of a nonsutured standard PC IOL is possible, the two options are capsular bag or ciliary

TABLE 37-1

Theoretical Properties—Nonsutured Standard PC IOLs

Advantages	Disadvantages
Low incidence of CME, pupillary block, UGH, PBK	Requires intact posterior capsule and zonules
Less endothelial loss*	Increased risk of dislocation
Mechanical barrier against vitreous movement or diffusion of vasoactive substances that could lead to CME or retinal detachment	
Positioned at nodal point of the eye	
Distant from trabecular meshwork	

*Soong HK, Meyer RF, Sugar A: Techniques of posterior chamber lens implantation without capsular support during penetrating keratoplasty: a review, *J Refract Corneal Surg* 5:249-255, 1989.
CME, Cystoid macular edema; *UGH,* uveitis-glaucoma-hyphema; *PBK,* pseudophakic bullous keratopathy.

TABLE 37-2

Theoretical Properties—Scleral-Sutured Standard PC IOLs

Advantages	Disadvantages
? Share advantages of nonsutured PC IOLs	Technically difficult to insert
Can be used with limbal wound or penetrating keratoplasty	Increased operating time
Not dependent on presence of iris tissue	Often requires extensive vitrectomy
Vitreous supported by lens	Suture-related endophthalmitis
Limited pseudophacodonesis	? Risk of epithelial downgrowth from suture path
Minimizes uveal contact	Risk of retinal detachment from vitrectomy and manipulation near the vitreous base
	Risk of hemorrhage from suture passage through ciliary body
	Long-term dependence on fixation of IOL by a suture
	Ciliary body erosion from haptics*

*Duffey RJ, Holland EJ, Agapitos PJ et al: Anatomic study of transsclerally sutured intraocular lens implantation, *Am J Ophthalmol* 108:300-309, 1989.
PC IOL, Posterior chamber intraocular lens.

TABLE 37-3

Theoretical Properties—Iris-Sutured PC-IOLs

Advantages	Disadvantages
? Share advantages of nonsutured PC IOLs	? CME from uveal irritation
	Pigment dispersion
	Technically difficult to insert
	Technique limited to use with penetrating keratoplasty
	Limited pupillary dilation*
	Pseudophacodonesis
	Requires sufficient iris tissue

*Spigelman AV, Lindstrom RL, Nichols BD et al: Implantation of a posterior chamber lens without capsular support during penetrating keratoplasty or as a secondary lens implant, *Ophthalmic Surg* 19:396-398, 1988.
PC IOL, Posterior chamber intraocular lens.

TABLE 37-4

Theoretical Properties—Flexible Open-Loop AC IOLs

Advantages	Disadvantages
Easier insertion	Difficult to insert properly—iris tuck and sizing
Less operating time	? Risks of older-style AC IOLs, including uveitis, glaucoma, hyphema, CME, PBK

AC IOL, Anterior chamber intraocular lens; *CME,* cystoid macular edema; *PBK,* pseudophakic bullous keratopathy.

sulcus placement. In patients with an intact posterior capsule, a significant surgical obstacle is reopening the capsular bag. Nevertheless, in cases without extensive fibrosis, the anterior and posterior capsules can be separated. The key is to locate one area in which the anterior capsule edge is not strongly adherent to the posterior capsule. Using this entry point, viscoelastic agents can be very helpful in the separation of the capsular layers. If adhesions are very dense, blunt dissection with cannulas or other instruments can be attempted. In some cases, the adhesions can be left intact focally by creating an extension of an anterior capsulotomy peripheral to the adhesion, using either capsulorhexis-like tearing techniques or scissors cutting of the anterior capsule. A final alternative is sharp dissection between the anterior and posterior capsules, but this carries greater risk of penetrating the posterior capsule.

If reopening of the capsular bag is not feasible, ciliary sulcus fixation of the IOL is a reasonable alternative. This requires at least peripheral capsular support and intact zonular support. A frequent situation is a posterior capsular rent with an intact anterior capsulorhexis. It is often necessary to lyse adhesions between capsular remnants and the posterior iris to reconstruct the ciliary sulcus before IOL placement. It is important to visually confirm that the haptics are not inadvertently directed under the anterior capsule during insertion to ensure proper support and avoid vitreous entanglement. If capsular support is focally uncertain, suturing one of the IOL haptics to the iris or sclera is advisable.

It is commonly stated that AC IOLs are easy to insert but difficult to insert correctly. The three most common mistakes made during insertion are incorrect sizing, not taking sufficient steps to avoid iris tuck, and insufficient attention to location of iridectomies and the capacity of haptics to rotate through them. Table 37-6 lists the most important steps in AC IOL placement.

Peripheral Iris Suture Fixation

Peripheral iris suture fixation of the haptics of a PC IOL is commonly referred to as "McCannel suturing," in recognition

TABLE 37-5

Indications for Surgery—Secondary IOL or IOL Exchange

Corneal Edema
PBK (usually with IOL exchange)
Closed-loop AC IOLs
Iris-supported IOLs
Modern open-loop AC IOLs
ABK
Aphakia
Prior intracapsular cataract extraction
Contact lens intolerance
IOL Complications
Complications during planned extracapsular cataract extraction
IOL exchange of closed-loop AC IOL
Decreased endothelial cell counts
Cystoid macular edema
Malpositioned IOL
UGH syndrome
Pain
IOL Power error

ABK, Aphakic bullous keratopathy; *AC IOL*, anterior chamber intraocular lens; *PBK*, pseudophakic bullous keratopathy; *UGH;* uveitis-glaucoma-hyphema.

TABLE 37-6

Surgical Procedure for AC IOL Placement

Correct sizing—length 1 mm greater than horizontal white-white distance (limbal diameter)
If feasible, orient incision on steep meridian to reduce postoperative astigmatism
Orient incision to place haptics away from peripheral iridectomies, or rotate IOL away from iridectomies after insertion
Construct pupil preoperatively (e.g. pilocarpine 2% drops, 30 min before operation)
Use viscoelastic substance to maintain anterior chamber
Vitrectomy to clear anterior chamber and wound of vitreous if necessary
Avoid iris tuck, dialysis; some surgeons prefer the use of a Sheets guide
Haptics should rest securely at level of ciliary body band—perform "bounce" test to evaluate both stable fixation and absence of iris tuck

AC IOL, Anterior chamber intraocular lens.

of the contribution of Malcom McCannel, who first described the technique for passing sutures through the iris to stabilize an IOL that had dislocated postoperatively. McCannel's description was in the context of a pupil-fixated IOL, a style abandoned long ago. However, the basic maneuvers that McCannel described, using long needles to pass sutures through the iris and around elements of the IOL, remain highly useful for the stabilization or secondary implantation of a PC IOL in the absence of adequate capsular support.

Some surgeons advocate these techniques over transscleral suturing in all cases. Others reserve peripheral iris suture fixation for particular indications. These include glaucoma patients for whom an AC IOL is thought inadvisable or anatomically impossible and patients in whom the conjunctiva needs to be preserved for possible future filtration surgery or a filtering bleb is already present and must be protected. The technique is also attractive in the setting of phacoemulsification under topical anesthesia when capsular support is inadequate. Most patients can be comfortable with intracameral anesthetic, such as 1% nonpreserved lidocaine, while the surgeon places and sutures the IOL to the peripheral iris, whereas taking down conjunctival flaps and passing sutures through the ciliary sulcus and sclera may be unacceptably painful.

The fundamental technique for peripheral iris suturing of a PC IOL begins with constricting the pupil adequately to temporarily capture the PC IOL optic in the pupil anterior to the iris plane, while the haptics remain in the posterior chamber. The technique is illustrated in Figure 37-1. A key in obtaining a round central pupil is to keep the length of the iris suture pass as short as possible and as peripheral as possible. Long suture passes bunch up iris tissue. Nonperipheral suture passes inhibit free movement of the pupil. Both errors result in distorted, nonreactive pupils.

Transscleral Suturing

Many different alternatives have been presented in the literature for placement of transscleral-sutured PC lenses. Soong et al.[9] describe both two-point and four-point iris fixation for PC lenses. Scleral-sutured lenses can be sutured from the inside out (ab interno) or by passing the needles from the outside of the eye inward (ab externo). A combination of scleral and iris sutures has also been decribed.[10] Transscleral sutures can be oriented vertically, obliquely, or horizontally, except that direct 3 and 9 o'clock horizontal fixation is inadvisable because of the danger of suturing through the long ciliary arteries and nerves in these locations.[11] It is important to do an extensive anterior vitrectomy in most cases before placement of a sutured PC lens to avoid vitreous incarceration and subsequent retinal traction and detachment.[9,11,12]

Many of the early surgeries performed with scleral-sutured PC IOLs placed the haptics too far posteriorly. The goal is to have the haptics resting in the ciliary sulcus. Anatomic studies have shown that the ciliary sulcus is only 0.83 mm posterior to the limbus in the vertical meridian and only 0.46 mm posterior to the limbus in the horizontal meridian.[4] Duffey et al.[4] passed needles perpendicular to the sclera at 1, 2, and 3 mm posterior to the limbus and found that the needles exited internally at the ciliary sulcus, pars plicata, and pars plana, respectively. These anatomic studies emphasize the importance of keeping transscleral needle penetration sites anteriorly. The surgeon can detect that a needle is being passed too anteriorly by iris movement as the needle penetrates the peripheral iris stroma near the angle. In determining the correct location, the surgeon must be mindful that the anatomic studies are based on a strict perpendicularity of the needle relative to the scleral wall. If the surgeon passes the needle through the scleral wall at an oblique angle (usually tilted toward the iris plane), then the external scleral point will need to be more posterior for the interior scleral point to be at the level of the ciliary sulcus.[13]

The surgeon has the option of creating scleral flaps so that the polypropylene (Prolene) suture knot is buried, avoiding exposed suture ends. Cautery is recommended to retract exposed barbs, should they occur postoperatively, to avoid a possibly

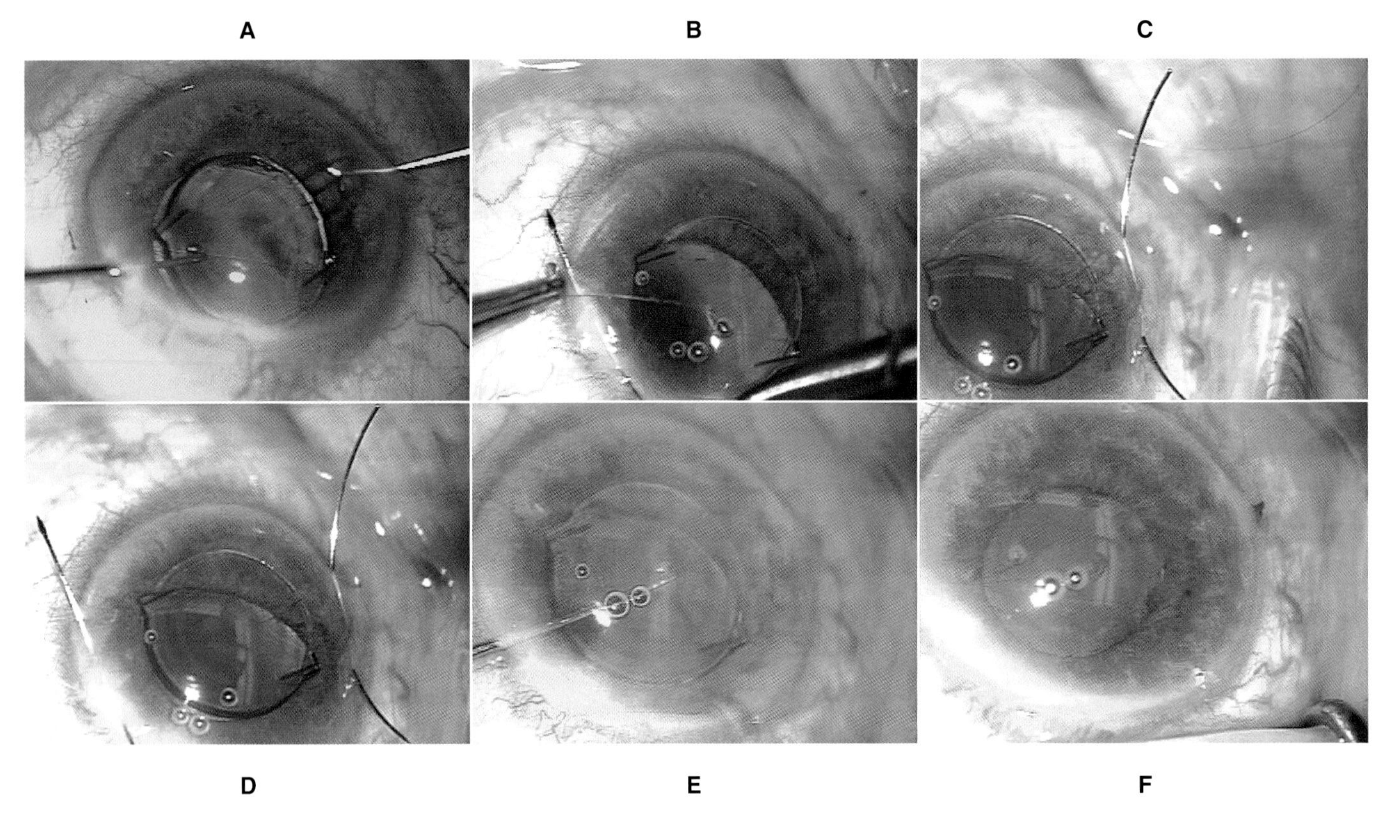

FIGURE 37-1 **A,** Kuglen hook in the surgeon's left hand and an Osher Y-hook in the surgeon's right hand are introduced through two paracentesis openings and used to elevate the optic above the iris plane, capturing the optic in the pupil while the haptics remain in the posterior chamber. **B,** A 10-0 polypropylene suture on a fine long needle (Ethicon CTC-6) is passed through the paracentesis, penetrates the iris in the periphery just in front of the haptic, which is indenting the iris stroma, exits the iris as soon as possible after the haptic, and then is driven up through the peripheral clear cornea. **C,** Same maneuver is performed under the opposite haptic. **D,** With both needles remaining in place behind the haptics, the successful capture of the haptics and acceptable location of the IOL in the pupil are verified. **E,** Sutures are tied and cut inside the eye using the "slip knot" technique illustrated for iris suturing in Figure 29-1. Kuglen hook presses the IOL optic posteriorly. **F,** Pupil is round, and the IOL is well centered.

entry tract for microorganisms or epithelium. If the suture knot is rotated, as in the technique of Stephen Lane shown in Figure 37-2, then no scleral flap is needed.

PC IOLs made specifically for suturing to the sclera have eyelets on the haptic to aid suture fixation and large-diameter optics (7 mm) to compensate for possible decentration. Some commonly used models of scleral-sutured IOLs include the Pharmacia 722Y,[14] Alcon CZ70BD,[15] and the CIBA C540MC.

The ab interno technique for transscleral suture fixation of a PC IOL typically uses polypropylene (Prolene) suture material. A long needle is required for the pass across the anterior chamber: the Ethicon CIF-4 and Ethicon STC-6 are commonly employed[16] (Figures 37-3 and 37-4). The needles are passed under the iris, aiming for the ciliary sulcus. A girth hitch can be used to attach the polypropylene suture loop to the IOL haptic (Figure 37-5). Alternatively, sutures can be tied to the haptic, to the haptic eyelets, or proximal to a haptic eyelet.[17] The needles exit the eye under the previously dissected scleral flaps, and the sutures are tied (Figure 37-6). Alternatively, to avoid dissecting scleral flaps and the potential for later erosion of the flap and conjunctiva, with exposure of the suture ends, the suture is passed through the positioning hole in the haptic, and the knot is rotated below the scleral surface (see Figure 37-2). The ab interno technique is adaptable to foldable IOL implantation as well, allowing suture fixation of the IOL while retaining a small incision, which is particularly important if capsule support is lost during primary cataract surgery through a small, clear corneal incision.[18]

The principal advantages of the ab interno (inside-to-outside) approach are that it is more straightforward and possibly faster than the ab externo (outside-to-inside) technique. It is also easier with penetrating keratoplasty. The disadvantages include the fact that the needle is passed under the iris without direct visualization, and the surgeon has to rely on indentation of the iris with the needle from behind to ensure correct placement in the ciliary sulcus.

Lewis[19] first described the ab externo technique of passing the scleral needles from the outside inward. The sutures used for the procedure are 10-0 polypropylene with a long straight needle, such as Ethicon STC-6. Alcon produces Pair Pack Fixation Suture, which is a hybrid combining an SC-5 straight needle on one end and an AUM-5 corneal needle on the other. This is specifically made for the outside-to-inside technique of scleral-sutured PC IOLs. The long straight needle is passed

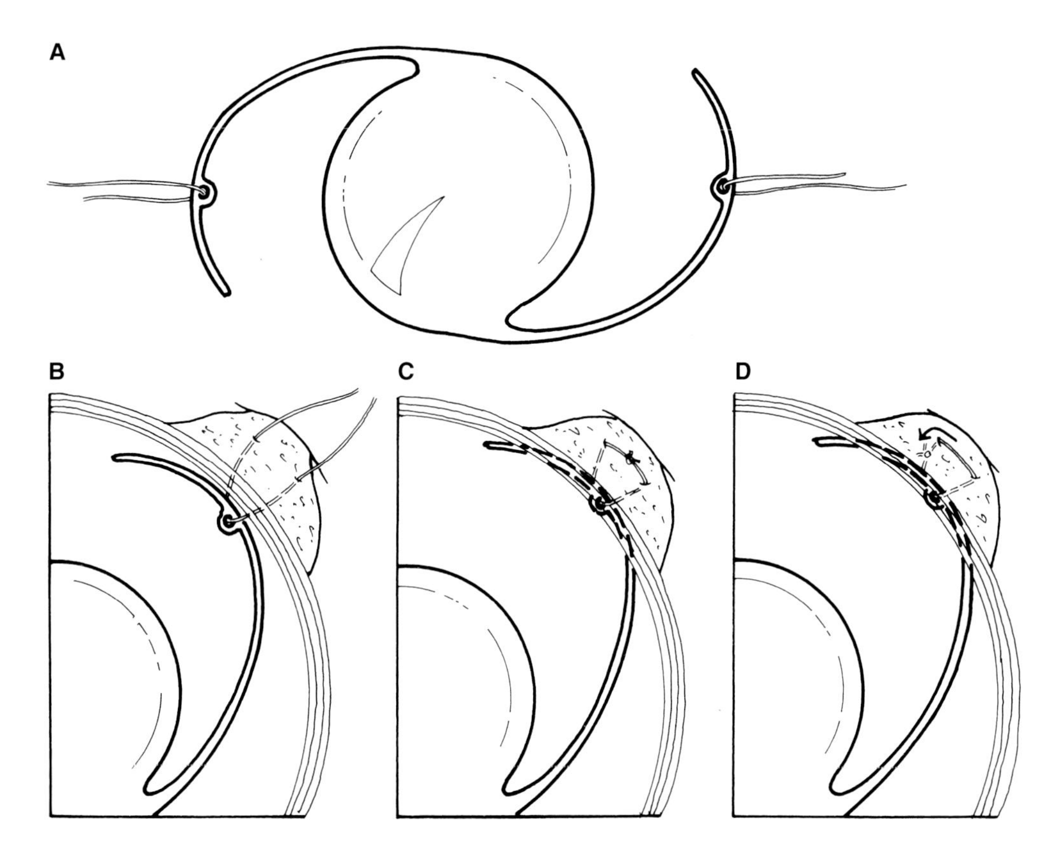

FIGURE 37-2 Lane technique to avoid scleral flaps. **A,** Double-armed polypropylene suture is passed through the haptic positioning hole. **B,** Suture is passed ab interno through the ciliary sulcus, as in Figures 37-3 and 37-4, except that no scleral flap is required. The sutures should be spaced 1.5 to 2 mm apart. **C,** Suture is tightened and tied with a small 1-1-1-1 knot. **D,** Knot is rotated internally. Conjunctiva is then closed over the smooth suture loop.

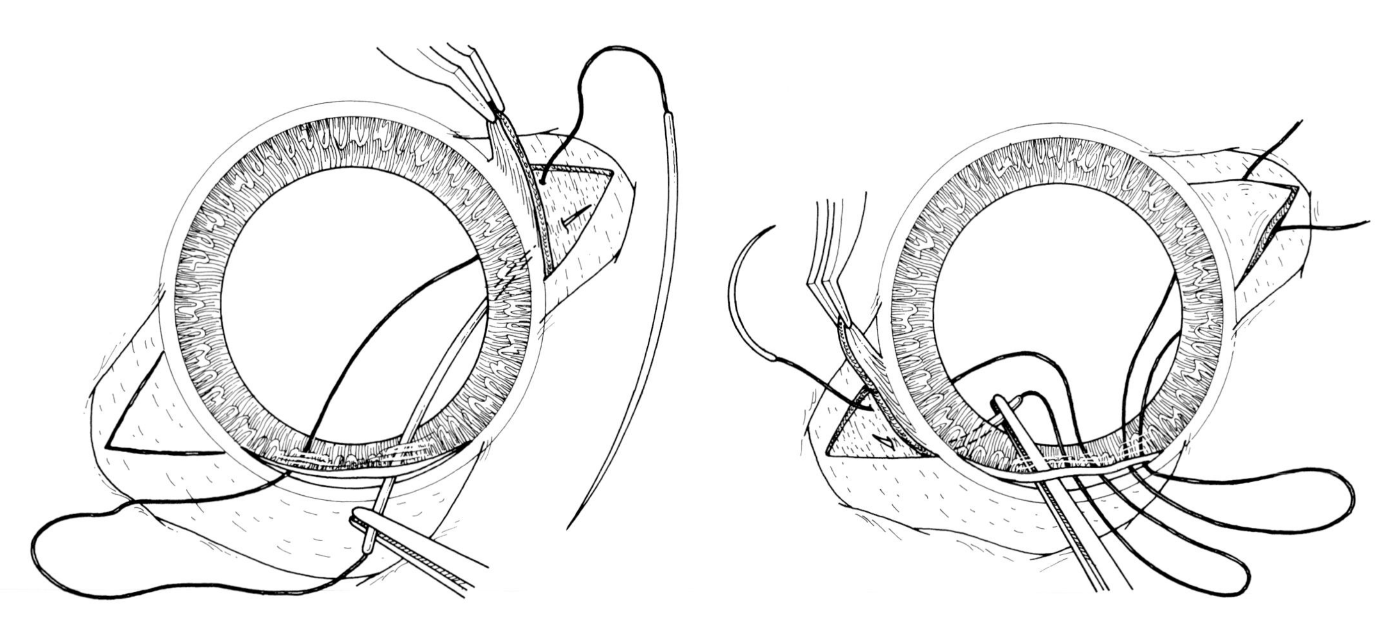

FIGURE 37-3 Technique for the ab interno approach (also see Figures 37-4 to 37-6). First the long needles are passed under the iris, aiming for the inferior ciliary sulcus. Two needle passes are made for each haptic if four-point fixation is desired. Needles exit under previously dissected scleral flaps.

FIGURE 37-4 A second pair of short needle passes is made under the superior iris for the suture to be tied to the second haptic.

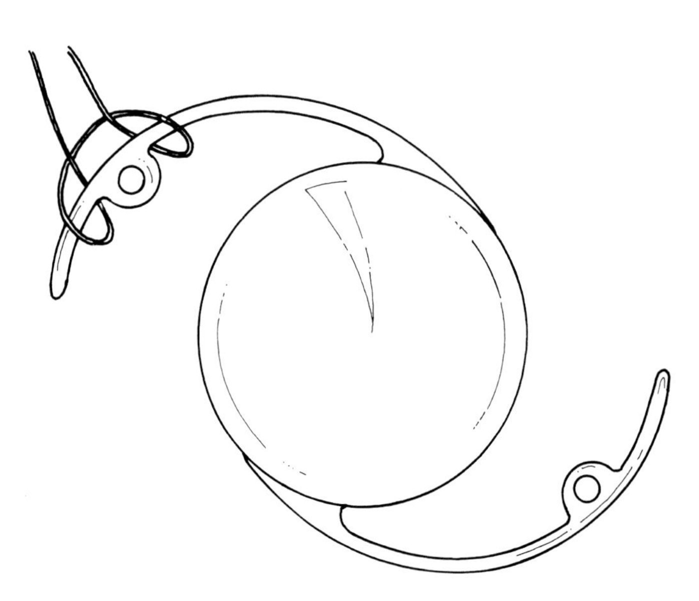

FIGURE 37-5 Girth hitch can be used to attach the polypropylene suture loop to the IOL haptic. This technique is more rapid than tying the suture to the haptic. Alternately, the suture can be attached to the IOL haptics before the transscleral needle passes, but the surgeon must avoid tangling the long sutures.

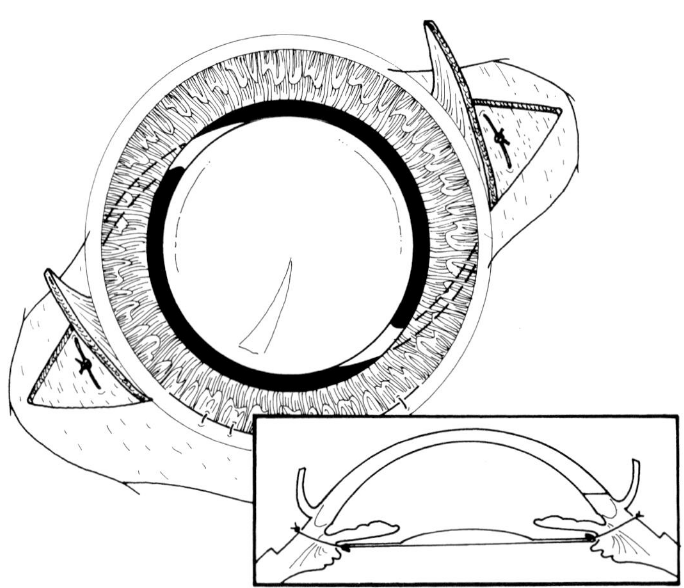

FIGURE 37-6 After exiting the eye under the previously dissected scleral flaps, the sutures are tied, securing the IOL into position. Appropriate suture tension is important to avoid lens decentration. The inset shows the cross-sectional view of the eye with the IOL correctly positioned in the ciliary sulcus.

perpendicularly through the sclera (usually under partial-thickness scleral flaps) approximately 0.75 mm posterior to the limbus (Figure 37-7). Inside the eye, the needle should penetrate at the ciliary sulcus. The needle is then "docked" inside the tip of a 25-, 27-, or 28-gauge hollow needle, which has been passed through the ciliary sulcus on the opposite side, also with an outside-to-inside technique (Figure 37-8). After the long straight needle with the 10-0 polypropylene is docked within the hollow needle, the hollow needle is withdrawn with the solid needle inside of it. In this way, the polypropylene suture is pulled across the eye. A hook is used to then pull the suture out through a superior limbal wound (Figure 37-9). The suture is cut, and each end is tied to a haptic of the IOL (Figure 37-10). After the IOL is placed into position, the scleral sutures are secured to the sclera.

This procedure can be performed with two sutures per haptic if the surgeon desires four-point fixation to ensure stability (Figure 37-11). The surgeon ties the sutures to the haptics and

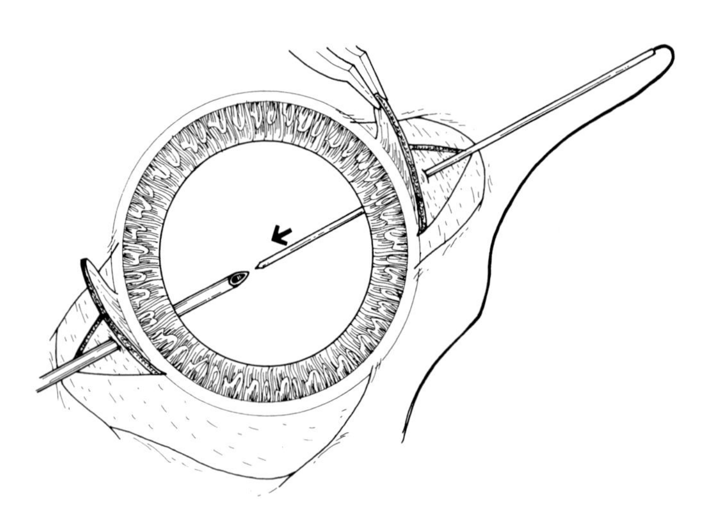

FIGURE 37-7 Technique for the ab externo approach (also see Figures 37-8 to 37-10). The long, straight solid needle is passed through the sclera (usually under partial-thickness scleral flaps) approximately 0.75 mm posterior to the limbus. Inside the eye, the needle should exit at the ciliary sulcus. A second hollow needle is passed from the opposite side of the eye. A pair of sutures can be used if four-point fixation is desired.

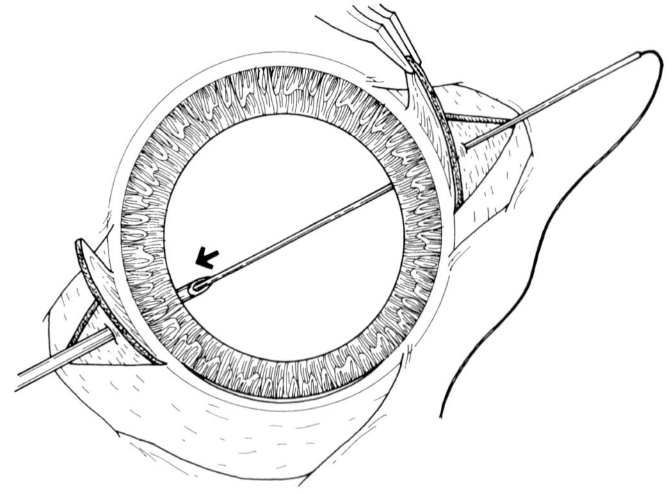

FIGURE 37-8 Solid needle is "docked" inside the tip of the hollow needle, which has been passed through ciliary sulcus on the opposite side. After docking, the pair of needles are withdrawn together from the eye, with the solid needle inside the hallow needle.

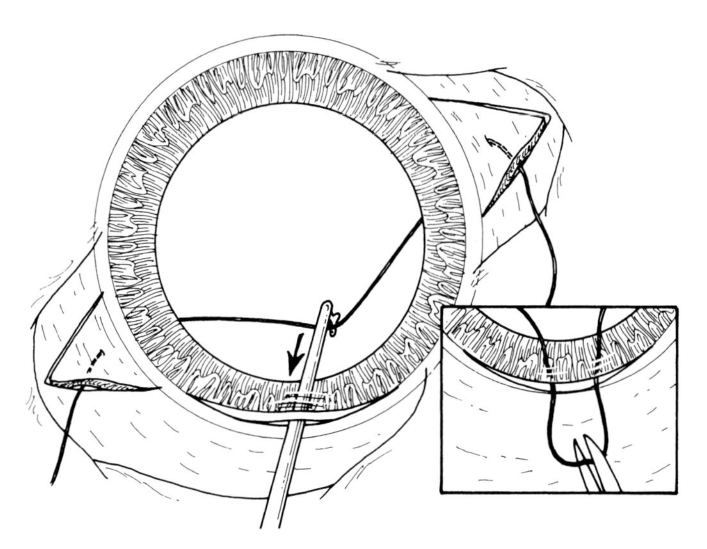

FIGURE 37-9 A hook is used to pull the suture out through a superior limbal wound so that it can be tied to the IOL.

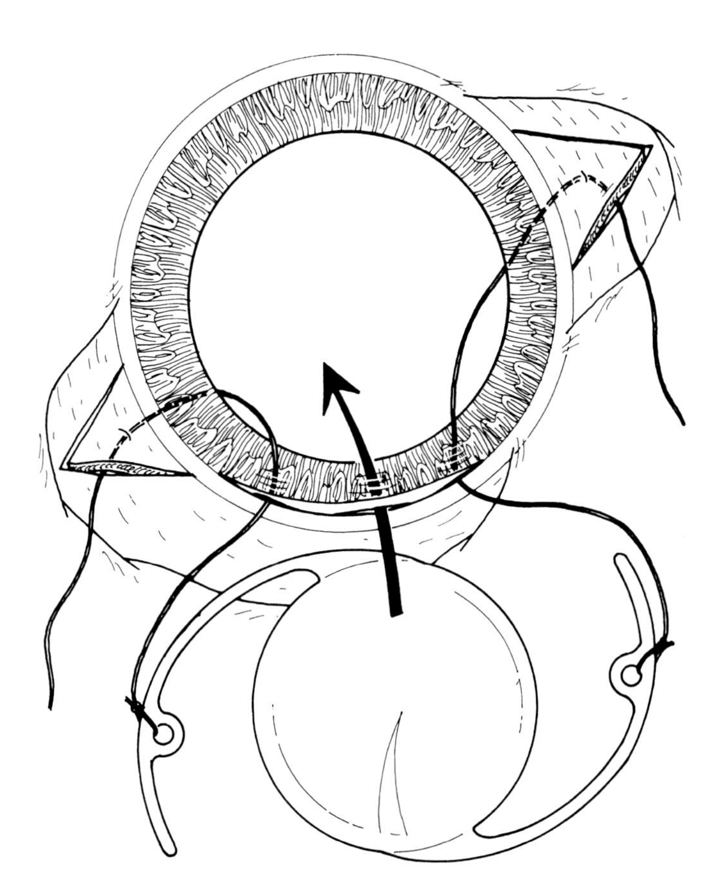

FIGURE 37-10 Suture is cut, and each end is tied to a haptic of the IOL. After the IOL is placed into position, the scleral sutures must be anchored to the sclera. Either a "blind pass" in the sclera is made so that the suture is tied to itself, or the transscleral suture is tied to a second suture that has been tied to the sclera with a short partial-thickness pass within the bed of the scleral flap.

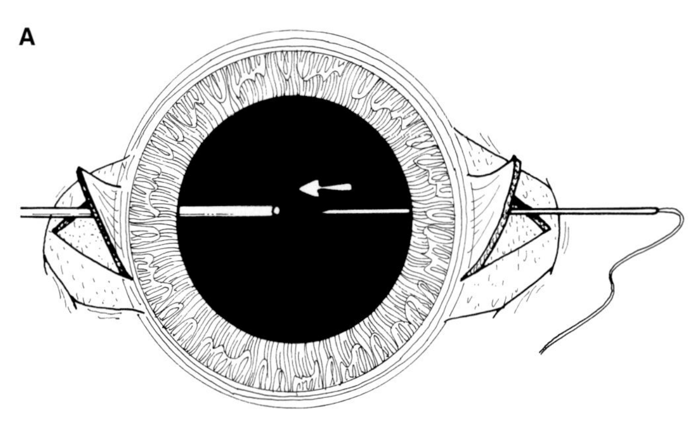

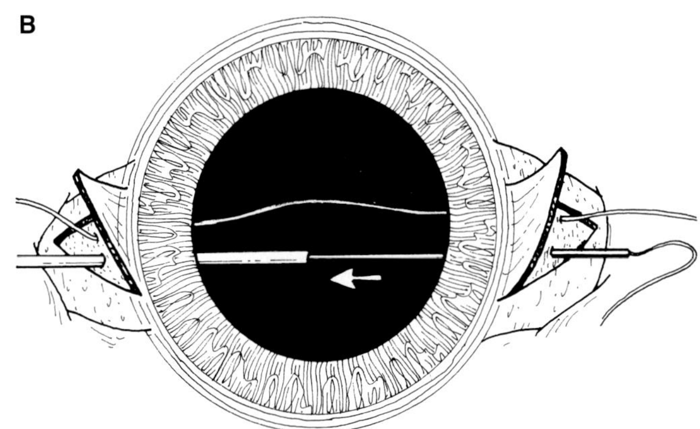

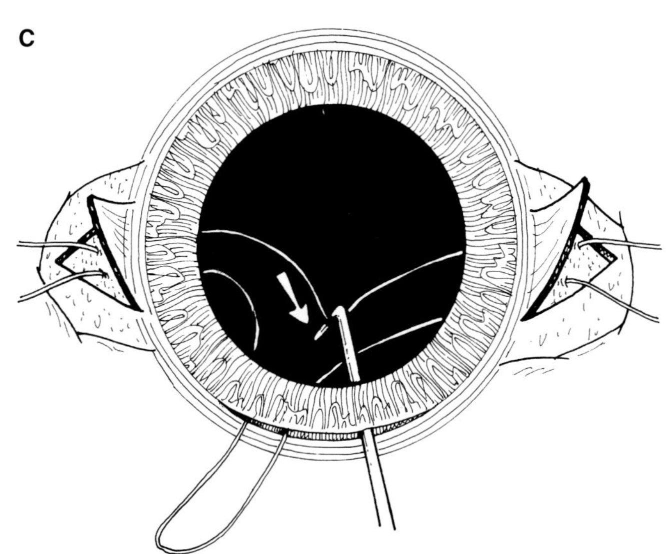

FIGURE 37-11 A, Double-suture variant of the Lewis ab externo technique begins similar to the single-suture technique, except that the suture entry point under the scleral flap is displaced to one side. **B,** Second suture is passed parallel to the first, with 1 to 1.5 mm between the two sutures. **C,** Care must be taken to keep the sutures taut to avoid crossing them or confusing which suture originates from each scleral site, while a Kuglen hook or similar instrument withdraws the suture loop through the previously prepared principal incision.

buries the external knot under a scleral flap (Figure 37-12). The alternative procedure, illustrated in Figure 37-13, allows rotation of the knot to avoid the necessity for scleral flaps and the potential of late exposure of the suture ends, but the antirotational stability of true four-point fixation is not achieved.[17-20]

The advantage of the outside-to-inside approach is greater assurance of the location of internal scleral penetration at the ciliary sulcus. Bleeding may be minimized by using precise measurements and avoiding the highly vascularized pars plicata. In addition, the anterior chamber remains closed during

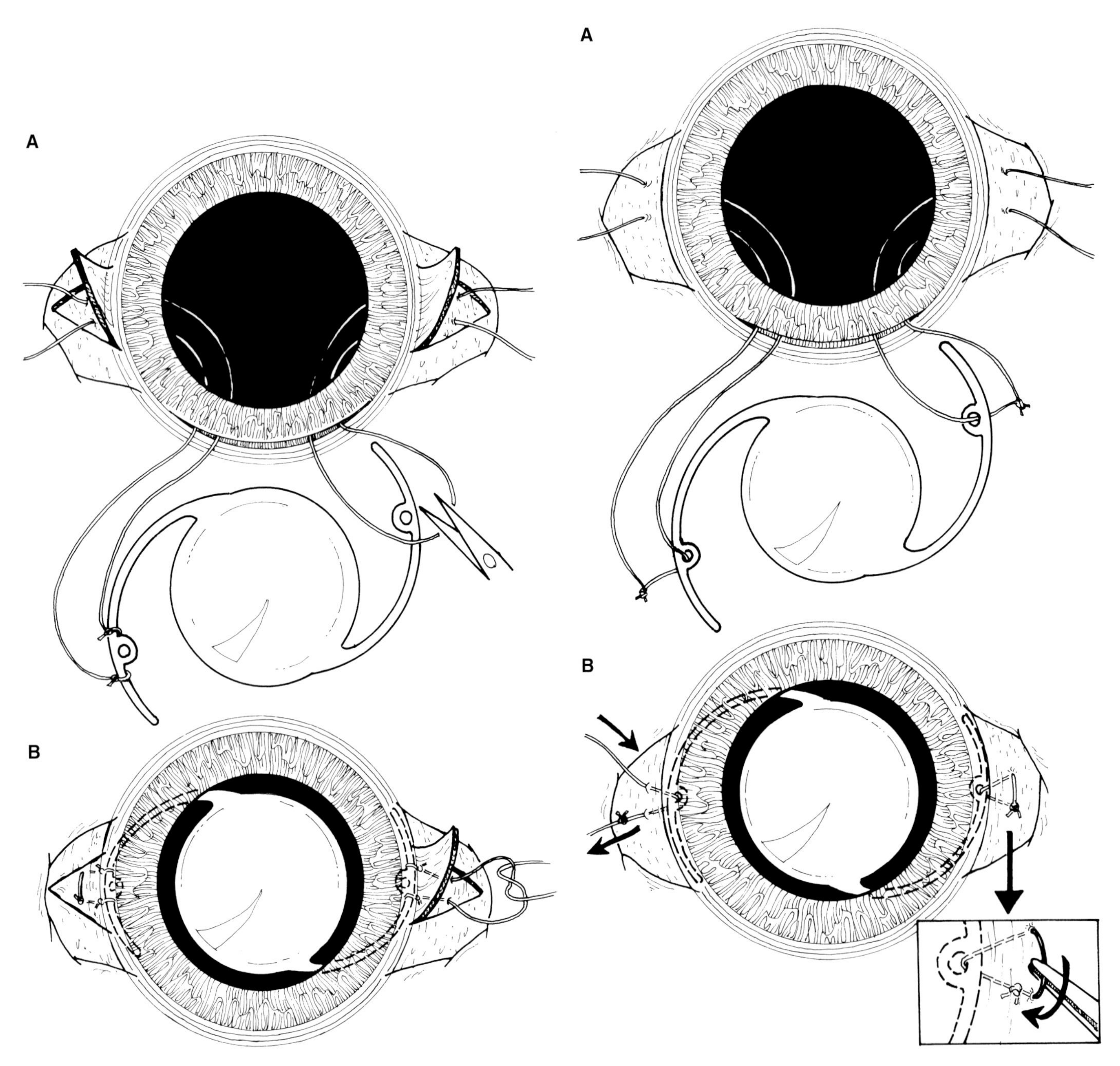

FIGURE 37-12 **A,** To achieve four-point stable fixation, the cut sutures are tied to the haptic on either side of the eyelet. **B,** IOL is then placed in the posterior chamber, keeping the sutures taut to avoid entanglement. The ends are then tied under the scleral flaps, and the conjunctiva closed over the flaps.

FIGURE 37-13 In this variant of the double-suture ab externo technique, the goal is to achieve a loop of suture where the knot can be rotated beneath the sclera, avoiding the necessity of a scleral flap and the potential for late erosion of the knot or suture ends. **A,** Cut ends of each suture are passed through the haptic positioning hole and tied. **B,** As the IOL is positioned in the posterior chamber, one end of the suture on each side is pulled so that the knot passes through the sclera to the external eye, where it is cut off. Remaining suture ends are then tied together, and the knot is rotated beneath the sclera *(inset),* achieving the same end result as illustrated in Figure 37-2.

the needle passes, decreasing the duration of ocular hypotony. The disadvantage of the ab externo approach is that it takes longer and it is not applicable with the open-sky situation of penetrating keratoplasty. In addition, if more than one suture pass is performed, it may be hard to keep track of the origin and course of the various suture ends.

If a double-suture technique with knot rotation is selected (see Figures 37-2 and 37-13), the surgeon must be meticulous in achieving a suture orientation that permits easy rotation of the knot (Figure 37-14, *A* and *B*) and avoiding suture configurations that will resist rotation of the knot (Figure 37-14, *C* through *H*). Furthermore, the surgeon should orient the suture pass through the opposite haptics in a direction that will resist rotation of the IOL out of the iris plane (Figure 37-14, *I*) rather than allow rotation (Figure 37-14, *J*).

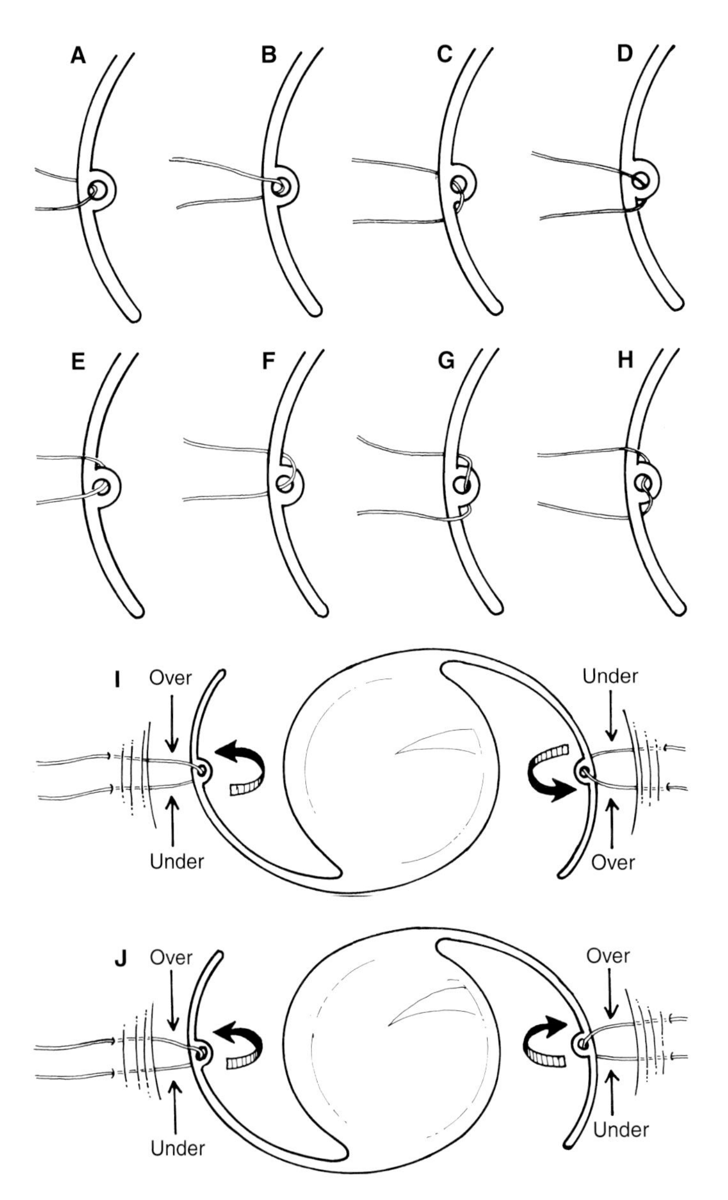

FIGURE 37-14 Suture passed through the positioning hole may wrap around the haptic in eight basic configurations. Only **A** and **B** illustrate appropriate pathways. In **C** through **H,** the ability to rotate the suture will be impaired or fully prevented by the circuitous route taken by the suture. Because there are two haptics, a total of 16 configurations are therefore possible. **I,** Surgeon should take care to use configuration A on one haptic and the opposite configuration B on the other haptic. In that manner, torque of the IOL is resisted; as one haptic starts to rotate in the direction not resisted by the suture loop, the other haptic meets more resistance *(arrows)*. **J,** When both suture loops have the same configuration, the suture does not resist torque of the IOL *(arrows)*.

Studies of Secondary IOLs

In studies in conjunction with penetrating keratoplasty, there does not appear to be a major difference in short-term overall results among scleral-sutured PC IOLs, iris-sutured PC IOLs, and modern AC IOLs. Kornmehl et al.[21] reported good results with flexible Kelman Omnifit AC IOLs compared with previous reports of sutured PC IOLs in penetrating keratoplasty. Lindquist et al.,[12] studying scleral-sutured PC IOLs without penetrating keratoplasty, also found results comparable to those in published reports using AC IOLs. Although the difference in complication rate is not striking in any series, some authors have found more complications with the scleral-sutured PC IOLs, compared with either iris-sutured PC IOLs or modern, flexible open-loop AC IOLs. Schein et al.[22] reported that iris-sutured PC IOLs had the lowest rate of early complications. This may have been a result of the increased complexity of the scleral-suturing techniques, which were relatively new at the time of that study.

Overall results of secondary IOL surgery are better if the initial cataract surgery had been uncomplicated.[8] Eyes with previous cataract surgery complicated by vitreous loss have worse results regardless of the type of IOL used at the second surgery. Vitrectomy at the time of placement of a scleral-sutured IOL does not seem to relate to the final visual acuity.[21,23,24] However, there is at least one report in the literature that contradicts this conclusion; Wong, Koch, and Emery[25] found a 28% incidence of retinal complications if vitrectomy was done at the time of secondary IOL placement.

Visual acuity results with scleral-sutured PC IOLs during penetrating keratoplasty have been similar, for the most part, to those achieved with other modern lens types.

Eighty-two percent of patients had better vision postoperatively compared with the preoperative vision if a combined corneal transplant and scleral-sutured PC IOL was performed.[26] Only 4% to 10% of patients had worse vision postoperatively, compared with preoperative vision, after scleral-sutured PC IOLs with or without corneal transplantation.[26,27] Several studies agree that approximately 30% of patients have vision of 20/40 or better after penetrating keratoplasty with scleral-sutured PC IOLs.[16,26,28,29] Lass et al.[28] included a control group of patients who had corneal transplants with modern AC IOLs and found that 25% of the AC IOL group had a final vision of 20/40 or better. Thirty-five percent of patients after penetrating keratoplasty with scleral-sutured PC IOLs had a vision of 20/200 or worse.[26] For iris-sutured PC IOLs with corneal transplantation, the final vision was 20/40 or better in approximately 45% of patients.[23] Most authors conclude that modern AC IOLs, scleral-sutured PC IOLs, and iris-sutured PC IOLs all achieve similar short-term results if used with penetrating keratoplasty. There are fewer studies of visual results of sutured lenses alone, without corneal transplantation, and they typically report on smaller numbers of patients. Nonetheless, visual results are reasonable. Patients with good preoperative corrected visual acuity and secondary sutured PC IOL placement usually maintained their preoperative vision.

Complications

Although overall visual acuity rates are similar among IOL groups, there may be a tendency toward an increased risk of unusual but serious complications with scleral-sutured PC IOLs. These serious complications include retinal detachment, hemorrhagic choroidal detachment, and later lens dislocation.[16] Sundmacher et al.[27] found that there was a 12% rate of severe complications with scleral-sutured PC IOLs. However, they pointed out that many of these eyes had preoperative disease, and half the complications were unrelated to the surgical method. These researchers believed that vascular risk factors predisposed patients to complications from scleral-sutured IOLs. Schein et al.[22] found a greater overall rate of complications with scleral-sutured PC IOLs compared with iris-sutured PC IOLs or modern AC IOLs. However, Heidemann and Dunn[16] reported that the incidences of glaucoma, CME, and graft failure with scleral-sutured PC IOLs were comparable to those with iris-sutured PC IOLs and modern AC IOLs used with penetrating keratoplasty. Table 37-7 compares the relative rates of various complications among the different lens options. This table extrapolates from data derived from initial studies and should be only considered a rough approximation of true relative complication rates.

The most common postoperative complication after scleral-sutured PC IOL implantation is persistent CME.[9] A range of 9% to 36% of patients with scleral-sutured lenses and penetrating keratoplasty had this complication.[9,30] Schein et al.[22] reported that slightly less macular edema was clinically observed if iris-sutured PC IOLs were used, compared with scleral-sutured PC IOLs or flexible open-loop AC IOLs. Although CME was a relatively frequent acute postoperative complication of scleral-sutured lenses, some patients who had a long-standing decrease in vision preoperatively because of CME improved greatly after AC IOL exchange for a scleral-sutured lens.[9,12] Thirty-two percent of patients with preoperative CME had a vision of 20/40 or better postoperatively with penetrating keratoplasty combined with a scleral-sutured PC IOL.[16]

Glaucoma is the second most common complication with scleral-sutured PC IOLs implanted at the same time as a penetrating keratoplasty.[16] It is difficult to determine the cause of this glaucoma because keratoplasty alone is associated with a 5% to 65% incidence of new onset of glaucoma.[3] Lass et al.[28] found that the mean intraocular pressure was significantly higher with scleral-sutured PC IOLs when compared with penetrating keratoplasty with flexible open-loop AC lenses. However, they admitted that their study may have been somewhat biased by case selection because patients with extensive peripheral synechiae preoperatively did not receive AC IOLs. Holland et al.[29] suspected that scleral-sutured lenses were associated with glaucoma; they found new-onset ocular hypertension in 30.3% of patients after a penetrating keratoplasty with a scleral-sutured PC IOL. Heidemann and Dunn[16] found that 59% of their patients with corneal transplant and scleral-sutured lenses required additional glaucoma medication postoperatively. Therefore, although sutured PC IOLs were not expected on theoretical grounds to be associated with glaucoma, initial studies suggest a possible correlation above that found with corneal transplant alone. Bias resulting from case selection may be responsible for most or all of this trend, however.

TABLE 37-7

Relative Frequency of Complications Associated with Secondary IOLs—Initial Studies*

Complication	Capsular-Supported PC IOL	AC IOL	Scleral-Sutured PC IOL	Iris-Sutured PC IOL
Acute CME	+	++	++	++
Chronic CME	–	+	+	+
Glaucoma	–	++	+	+
Lens tilt or decentration	–	+	++	++
Polypropylene knot erosion	NA	NA	++	NA
Suture-related endophthalmitis	NA	NA		NA
Endophthalmitis (unrelated to polypropylene suture)	+	+	+	+
Corneal edema	+	++	+	+
Intraoperative bleeding	+	+	++	++
Synechiae	–	++	–	+
Retinal detachment	–	+	++	+
Choroidal detachment	–	+	++	+
Uveitis/iritis	–	++	–	+
Long-term corneal graft failure	–	+	–	–
Risk of polypropylene suture failure	NA	NA	+	+

* –, not associated; +, mild association; ++, strong association; NA, not applicable.
AC, Anterior chamber; *CME,* cystoid macular edema; *IOL,* intraocular lens; *PC,* posterior chamber.

Lens tilt or decentration is found in 5% to 10% of patients after scleral-sutured PC lens implantation.[27,30] IOLs with large optics are recommended, so a small degree of decentration is not usually clinically significant. Proper polypropylene suture placement and tension are important in avoiding this complication.

Initially, scleral-sutured lenses were tied under conjunctival flaps alone. However, the high incidence of erosion of the sutures through the conjunctiva prompted surgeons to place these knots under scleral flaps. Solomon et al.[31] found that polypropylene suture erosion was the most common complication of scleral-sutured PC IOLs. Even with scleral flaps, up to 17% of patients have sutures that erode through the conjunctiva.[29,31] This rate greatly exceeds the experience of most surgeons, however. Without scleral flaps, 23.8% of patients have sutures erode through the conjunctiva. Because suture-related endophthalmitis has been reported,[32] it is recommended that all exposed sutures be treated either with cautery or with free scleral grafts.[18] Some have recommended leaving the polypropylene suture ends long so that they lie flatter on the globe, thus avoiding exposure.[12]

PBK has not been a frequently reported complication of scleral-sutured PC IOLs, perhaps partially because of the relatively short follow-up in these early studies of a new technique. If endothelial cell counts are measured after corneal transplantation with scleral-sutured lenses and compared with the results from corneal transplantation with modern AC IOLs, there is no significant difference in endothelial cell loss.[28] Soong et al.[9] found a 19% endothelial cell loss after 1 year with iris-sutured PC IOLs, compared with 28% with closed-loop AC IOLs. Sugar[33] points out that specular microscopy provides a good prognostic measure of later corneal decompensation.

Although bleeding in the form of vitreous hemorrhage or hyphema would be anticipated to be a frequent problem with scleral-sutured lenses because of the proximity of the needle path to the ciliary body, this has not turned out to be the case, and hemorrhages are relatively infrequent.[14,17]

Heidemann and Dunn[16] reported an 11% incidence of hyphema or vitreous hemorrhage in association with scleral-sutured PC IOLs. Holland et al.,[29] however, reported no hyphemas in 115 cases. The highest reported incidence of bleeding was 22%, reported by Kora, Fukado, and Yaguchi.[34] However, their experience was atypical. Proper passage of the needles through the ciliary sulcus rather than the pars plicata may help prevent this complication. Vitreous hemorrhage, if it occurs, is usually self-limited and spontaneously clears. Massive suprachoroidal hemorrhage is rare.

Although few studies address the question of synechial progression, at least one early report seems to contradict theoretical expectations. Schein et al.[22] found less synechial progression with modern AC IOLs compared with scleral- or iris-sutured PC IOLs. This may, however, result from the fact that AC lenses were oriented in the same meridian as the closed-loop AC lenses that they replaced. New synechiae formation may be limited by the synechiae already present from the older AC lens.

There appears to be a slightly greater risk of retinal detachment with sutured PC IOLs. Soong et al.[9] reported a 2.3% risk of retinal detachment with corneal transplant combined with iris-sutured PC IOL implantation. Three studies with corneal transplantation and scleral-sutured PC lenses reported a 2.7% to 5.4% risk of retinal detachment after this combined procedure.[16,26,29] Several retinal detachments have been reported with a retinal hole in the meridian of one of the transscleral sutures.[35] Not all studies have identified transscleral suture fixation of PC IOLs as a risk factor for retinal detachment, however.[36] Pathology studies examining eyes that have had sutured PC lenses implanted have found that haptics are usually posterior to the ciliary body adjacent to the pars plana rather than in the ciliary sulcus.[1,4,37] This may increase the risk of retinal detachment. The location of the haptics at the pars plana was found in pathology specimens from both iris- and scleral-sutured PC lenses. The authors explain this finding by the fact that the iris often sags when the globe is fluid filled, making the ciliary sulcus inaccessible internally.[4] They recommend the use of an air bubble to help pull the iris away from the ciliary sulcus. One surgeon used an endoscope to locate the ciliary sulcus intraoperatively.[34] A second explanation for the poor positioning of the haptics with sutured PC lenses is incorrect measurements used in placing the scleral sutures. A surgeon may easily overestimate the distance between the limbus and the ciliary sulcus.

Theoretically, the risk of choroidal detachment ought to increase with the length of operative hypotony. Also, transscleral sutures ought to increase the risk of choroidal hemorrhage or effusion.[16] Early studies seem to bear out this expectation to a small degree. Holland et al.[29] found that choroidal detachments, if they occurred, were often located alongside the site of a transscleral suture. Heidemann and Dunn[26] found that 3.6% of scleral-sutured PC IOLs were associated with a choroidal detachment, although these were nonexpulsive.

Uveitis does not seem to be frequently associated with sutured PC lenses. In a series of 105 penetrating keratoplasties with scleral-sutured PC lenses, there were no reported cases of chronic uveitis.[29] Theoretically, iris-sutured lenses may cause more inflammation as a result of irritation of uveal tissue because of suspension of the relatively heavy IOL from the iris. Pathology specimens from iris-sutured PC lenses show mild to moderate local inflammation, but this has not been shown to be clinically significant.

A disturbing late complication is the report of spontaneous polypropylene suture breakage leading to displaced PC IOLs. Price et al.[38] reported five such cases of late breakage of previously stable iris-supported PC IOLs. It appears that the polypropylene suture was cut by persistent rubbing at the optic hole of the IOL over time. This occurred an average of 9 years after the initial surgery. Pathology studies have shown that sutures are the primary fixation point for both iris- and scleral-sutured PC IOLs.[1,37] There is no postoperative fibrosis[16] and no inflammatory reaction around the polypropylene suture.[37]

Accidental cutting of the polypropylene suture is sometimes associated with dislocation of the IOL into the vitreous cavity.[37] This dislocation often is delayed after the cutting of the polypropylene suture, suggesting that the haptic may be embedded into tissue over time, but this fixation is not necessarily adequate to support the IOL long term in the absence of the suture.

Several visual complications are unrelated to the sutured PC IOL procedure. Often age-related macular degeneration was discovered after lens implantation. Vision was found to be limited by this condition in 5.7% of cases after penetrating keratoplasty with scleral-sutured PC IOL.[29] Maculopathy from other causes, such as vascular causes, was found in a minority of cases.

Comparison of Sutured PC IOLs with Open-Loop Flexible AC IOLs

In most cases of secondary IOLs, the management decision is between a scleral-sutured PC IOL and an AC IOL. There has been no convincing study implicating the modern, flexible open-loop AC IOLs with the many problems associated with the older, rigid closed-loop designs. Modern AC lenses have a greatly decreased incidence of postoperative pain and a decreased incidence of UGH syndrome.[39] Many studies have shown that there is a low rate of overall complications with these newer designs. Apple et al.[1] found that, although 75% of AC IOLs inserted now are of modern, flexible open-loop design, fewer than 15% of complicated AC IOL cases involved flexible open-loop AC IOLs. Mamalis et al.[40] found a favorable outcome in 86% of IOL exchanges to a flexible open-loop design, compared with 90% with exchanges to a standard, nonsutured, in-the-bag PC IOL. The similarity in the results between even standard nonsutured PC IOLs and AC IOLs supports the assertion that both are very stable in the eye. Uveitis is rare with the newer open-loop flexible AC IOLs.[40]

Soong et al.[9] found similar results after penetrating keratoplasty with IOL exchange whether the new lens was an iris-sutured PC lens or a modern AC IOL. Visual results showed that 57% to 63% of patients after penetrating keratoplasty and modern AC lens placement achieved 20/40 vision or better.[21,41] Endothelial cell counts were also similar with AC and PC lens types. Soong et al.[9] stated that not only were the endothelial cell counts as low with modern AC lenses as with unsutured standard PC IOLs, but they were lower than counts seen with iris-sutured PC lenses: 11.2% versus 19% loss. The rate of new glaucoma with AC lenses and penetrating keratoplasty is similar to that with penetrating keratoplasty alone.[41] Although persistent CME is a frequent postoperative problem after penetrating keratoplasty and IOL exchange with any lens type, modern AC lenses perform similarly to other lens types in terms of the incidence of CME. Synechiae are usually not formed with the modern AC lenses. Synechiae are commonly seen in the meridian of the haptics with older, rigid AC lens types.

If one accepts the premise that the behavior of an IOL that is retained at penetrating keratoplasty is an indication of the stability of the lens in the eye in general, then the study by Sugar[33] is illuminating. He found that the corneal transplant failure rate (as opposed to corneal rejection) was highest if closed-loop rigid AC lenses were left in the eye at the time of corneal transplantation and lowest for retained in-the-bag PC IOLs. Retained rigid closed-loop AC lenses were associated with a 33.6% rate of transplant failure. Iris pupillary-supported (not sutured) IOLs were associated with a 28.9% corneal transplant failure rate, and retained primary implanted PC IOLs (standard, unsutured) were associated with only a 6.4% rate of transplant failure. Endothelial cell counts confirmed this data for penetrating keratoplasty and retained IOLs.[33] The rigid closed-loop AC lenses were associated with a 34% drop in endothelial cell counts. Iris pupillary-supported IOLs were associated with a 31% drop in endothelial cell count. However, retained PC IOLs (unsutured) were associated with only a 17% drop in endothelial cell count.

The results with the modern AC lenses were assessed by Sugar[33] by studying IOL exchange at the time of penetrating keratoplasty. In a study of 469 patients over a 10-year period, he found that vision was best if the older lens was exchanged for a flexible open-loop AC IOL. The results were even better than if iris-sutured PC IOLs were used. Also, corneal transplant failure rates were lowest if flexible open-loop AC lenses were used at the time of penetrating keratoplasty. The rate of transplant failure was 24% with rigid closed-loop AC lenses but only 5% with flexible open-loop AC IOLs. If the new lens was a PC lens (not sutured, with an intact posterior capsule), there was an 8% rate of corneal failure. Endothelial cell counts in patients who had IOL exchange again confirmed the stability of flexible open-loop AC design. Rigid closed-loop AC lenses had a 28% loss of endothelial cells at 1 year. However, flexible open-loop AC lenses had only a 17% decline in endothelial cells. PC IOLs (not sutured, with an intact posterior capsule), had a 19% drop in endothelial cell counts 1 year after a penetrating keratoplasty with IOL exchange.[33] Thus flexible open-loop AC IOL lens designs appear to be relatively well tolerated in the eye.

Conclusions

Little debate exists that the placement of a standard PC IOL is the method of choice for a secondary IOL in the presence of sufficient capsular support. In the cases without capsular support, the decision is more difficult. It is impossible to reach firm conclusions regarding sutured PC lenses with present information. It seems clear that modern AC lenses have been disregarded prematurely by some surgeons and that they provide a valuable alternative to sutured PC lenses for many patients. The visual results for most patients with scleral-sutured lenses are comparable to those with other lens types. However, there is some reason to be concerned about the higher risk of some serious complications with scleral-sutured PC IOLs. These complications include a higher risk of retinal detachment, choroidal hemorrhage, lens dislocation, suture exposure and endophthalmitis, glaucoma, and persistent CME. On the other hand, scleral-sutured PC IOLs are an attractive alternative for patients with complications attributable to an AC IOL, such as chronic iritis and CME, and for patients where relative contraindications to an AC IOL are present, such as iris or angle abnormalities.

No large study has yet addressed long-term outcomes in patients randomized between modern, flexible open-loop AC IOLs and scleral-sutured PC IOLs, especially regarding endothelial cell loss.

REFERENCES

1. Apple DJ, Price FW, Gwin T et al: Sutured retropupillary posterior chamber intraocular lenses for exchange or secondary implantation, *Ophthalmology* 96:1241-1247, 1989.
2. Soong HK, Meyer RF, Sugar A: Techniques of posterior chamber lens implantation without capsular support during penetrating keratoplasty: a review, *J Refract Corneal Surg* 5:249-255, 1989.
3. Gaster RN, Ong HV: Results of penetrating keratoplasty with posterior chamber intraocular lens implantation in the absence of a lens capsule, *Cornea* 10:498-506, 1991.
4. Duffey RJ, Holland EJ, Agapitos PJ et al: Anatomic study of transsclerally sutured intraocular lens implantation, *Am J Ophthalmol* 108:300-309, 1989.
5. Spigelman AV, Lindstrom RL, Nichols BD et al: Implantation of a posterior chamber intraocular lens without capsular support during penetrating keratoplasty or as a secondary lens implant, *Ophthalmic Surg* 19:396-398, 1988.
6. Panton RW, Sulewski ME, Parker JS et al: Surgical management of subluxed posterior-chamber intraocular lenses, *Arch Ophthalmol* 111:919-926, 1983.
7. Price FW, Whitson WE, Collins K et al: Explantation of posterior chamber intraocular lenses, *J Cataract Refract Surg* 18:475-479, 1992.
8. Doren G, Stern G, Driebe WT: Indications for and results of intraocular lens explantation, *J Cataract Refract Surg* 18:79-85, 1992.
9. Soong HK, Musch DC, Kowal V et al: Implantation of posterior chamber intraocular lenses in the absence of lens capsule during penetrating keratoplasty, *Arch Ophthalmol* 107:660-665, 1989.
10. Stark WJ, Gottsch JD, Goodman DF et al: Posterior chamber intraocular lens implantation in the absence of capsular support, *Arch Ophthalmol* 107:1078-1083, 1989.
11. Smiddy WE, Sawusch MR, O'Brien TP et al: Implantation of scleral-fixated posterior chamber intraocular lenses, *J Cataract Refract Surg* 16:691-696, 1990.
12. Lindquist TD, Agapitos PJ, Lindstrom RL et al: Transscleral fixation of posterior chamber intraocular lenses in the absence of capsular support, *Ophthalmic Surg* 20:769-775, 1989.
13. Yasukawa T, Suga K, Akita J et al: Comparison of ciliary sulcus fixation techniques for posterior chamber intraocular lenses, *J Cataract Refract Surg* 24: 840-845, 1998.
14. Stark WJ, Goodman G, Goodman D et al: Posterior chamber intraocular lens implantation in the absence of posterior capsular support, *Ophthalmic Surg* 19:240-243, 1988.
15. Kershner RM: Vertical transscleral sulcus fixation of intraocular lenses in the absence of a posterior capsule, *J Cataract Refract Surg* 18:201-202, 1992.
16. Heidemann DG, Dunn SP: Transsclerally sutured intraocular lenses in penetrating keratoplasty, *Am J Ophthalmol* 113:619-625, 1992.
17. Hu BV, Shin DH, Gibbs KA et al: Implantation of posterior chamber intraocular lens in the absence of capsular and zonular support, *Arch Ophthalmol* 106: 416-420, 1988.
18. Oshima Y, Oida H, Emi K: Transscleral fixation of acrylic intraocular lenses in the absence of capsular support through 3.5 mm self-sealing incisions, *J Cataract Refract Surg* 24:1223-1229, 1998.
19. Lewis JS: Ab externo sulcus fixation, *Ophthalmic Surg* 22:692-695, 1991.
20. Lewis JS: Sulcus fixation without flaps, *Ophthalmology* 100:1346-1350, 1993.
21. Kornmehl EW, Steinert RF, Odrich MG et al: Penetrating keratoplasty for pseudophakic bullous keratopathy associated with closed-loop anterior chamber intraocular lenses, *Ophthalmology* 97:407-414, 1990.
22. Schein OD, Kenyon KR, Steinert RF et al: A randomized trial of intraocular lens fixation techniques with penetrating keratoplasty, *Invest Ophthalmology* 100:1437-1443, 1993.
23. Van Der Schaft TL, Van Riij G, Renardel De Lavalette JGC et al: Results of penetrating keratoplasty for pseudophakic bullous keratopathy with the exchange of an intraocular lens, *Br J Ophthalmol* 73:704-708, 1989.
24. Hayward JM, Noble BA, George N: Secondary intraocular lens implantation: eight year experience, *Eye* 4:548-556, 1990.
25. Wong SK, Koch DD, Emery JM: Secondary intraocular lens implantation, *J Cataract Refract Surg* 13:17-20, 1987.
26. Heidemann DG, Dunn SP: Visual results and complications of transsclerally-sutured intraocular lenses in penetrating keratoplasty, *Ophthalmic Surg* 21:609-614, 1990.
27. Sundmacher R, Althaus C, Webster R et al: Two years experience with transscleral fixation of posterior chamber lenses, *Dev Ophthalmol* 22:89-93, 1991.
28. Lass JH, DeSantis DM, Reinhart WJ et al: Clinical and morphometric results of penetrating keratoplasty with one-piece anterior-chamber or suture-fixated posterior-chamber lenses in the absence of lens capsule, *Arch Ophthalmol* 108:1427-1431, 1990.
29. Holland EJ, Daya SM, Evangelista A et al: Penetrating keratoplasty and transscleral fixation of posterior chamber lens, *Am J Ophthalmol* 114: 182-187, 1992.
30. Hayashi K, Hayashi H, Nakao F et al: Intraocular lens tilt and decentration, anterior chamber depth, and refractive error after trans-scleral suture fixation surgery, *Ophthalmology* 106:878-882, 1999.
31. Solomon K, Gussler JR, Gussler C et al: Incidence and management of complications of transsclerally sutured posterior chamber intraocular lenses, *J Cataract Refract Surg* 19:488-493, 1993.
32. Schechter RJ: Suture-wick endophthalmitis with sutured posterior chamber intraocular lenses, *J Cataract Refract Surg* 16:755-756, 1990.
33. Sugar A: An analysis of corneal endothelial and graft survival in for pseudophakic bullous keratopathy, *Trans Am Ophthalmol Soc* 87:762-801, 1990.
34. Kora Y, Fukado Y, Yaguchi S: Sulcus fixations of posterior chamber intraocular lenses by transscleral sutures, *J Cataract Refract Surg* 17:636-639, 1991.
35. Rajpal RK, Carney MD, Weinberg RS et al: Complications of transscleral sutured posterior chamber lenses, *Ophthalmology* 98:98, 1991.
36. Lee J, Lee J, Chung H: Factors contributing to retinal detachment after transscleral fixation of posterior chamber intraocular lenses, *J Cataract Refract Surg* 24: 697-702, 1998.
37. Lubniewski AJ, Holland EJ, Van Meter WS et al: Histologic study of eyes with transsclerally sutured posterior chamber intraocular lenses, *Am J Ophthalmol* 110:237-243, 1990.
38. Price FW, Whitson WE, Collins K et al: Changing trends in explanting intraocular lenses: a single center study, *J Cataract Refract Surg* 18:470-474, 1992.
39. Hahn TW, Kim MS, Kim JH: Secondary intraocular lens implantation in aphakia, *J Cataract Refract Surg* 18:174-179, 1992.
40. Mamalis N, Crandall AS, Pulsipher MV et al: Intraocular lens explantation and exchange: a review of lens styles, clinical indications, clinical results, and visual outcome, *J Cataract Refract Surg* 17:811-818, 1991.
41. Hassan TS, Soong HK, Sugar A et al: Implantation of Kelman-style, open-loop anterior chamber lenses during keratoplasty for aphakic and pseudophakic bullous keratopathy: a comparison with iris-sutured posterior chamber lenses, *Ophthalmology* 98:875-880, 1991.

Intraocular Lens–Related Opacifications: In Front Of, On, Within, Between, and Behind the Intraocular Lens

38

Rupal H. Trivedi, MD
Liliana Werner, MD, PhD
Suresh K. Pandey, MD
Qun Peng, MD
Stella Arthur, MD
Andrea M. Izak, MD
Tamer A. Macky, MD
David J. Apple, MD

It has been over 50 years since Harold Ridley's first implant, and today the cataract–intraocular lens (IOL) procedure has reached an extraordinarily high level of quality and performance.[1] This has no doubt been one of the most satisfying advances of medicine. Millions of individuals with visual disability or frank blindness from cataracts have benefited from this procedure. Ophthalmologists have reported that the modern cataract-IOL surgery is safe and complication free most of the time. This makes the watchword for any cataract surgeon to be "implantation," "implantation," "implantation."[2] In the mid-1980s, as IOLs were evolving rapidly, the watchword of the implant surgeon was "fixation," "fixation," "fixation."[3,4] Most techniques, lenses, and surgical adjuncts now allow us to achieve the basic requirement for successful IOL implantation, namely long-term stable IOL fixation in the capsular bag.

In this chapter, we would like to alert the reader to a new watchword, namely "opacification," "opacification," "opacification" (Figure 38-1).[5-11] Although opacification of the posterior capsule was always a concern after extracapsular cataract extraction (ECCE), in recent years efforts toward controlling and indeed eradicating posterior capsule opacification (PCO) have been explored in more depth. However, despite the finer and wondrous achievements of IOL implantation, a few items have "slipped through the cracks." In this text we detail several problematic issues regarding the opacification phenomena that should not be encountered at such a late stage in the evolution of IOL implantation. Many are related to unwanted and unacceptable opacifications of the IOL itself.[8-10]

Many of the complications discussed here are totally unexpected threats to vision and sometimes "blinding IOL opacifications" that should not be concerns within the current advanced stage in the evolution of the cataract-IOL procedure. Some of these are probably occurring because many surgical procedures today are often performed outside the realm of supervision of both nongovernmental and governmental authorities such as the Food and Drug Administration (FDA).

In this chapter we talk about the good, the bad, and the ugly. Examples of the "good" include the recent successes now being achieved in reducing the incidence of PCO. Examples of the "bad" include various proliferations of anterior capsule cells, problems caused by silicone oil adherence to IOLs, and problems with piggyback IOLs. The "ugly" include the sometimes striking and often visually disabling opacifications occurring on and within IOL optics, such as on some modern foldable IOLs, as well as polymethylmethacrylate (PMMA) optic degradation occurring with some models a decade or more after implantation. These are described in Table 38-1 according to the site of opacification.

Our research center was founded in 1983 by David J. Apple, MD, and Randall J. Olson, MD, in Salt Lake City, Utah. The research and specimens analysis during this early period were almost totally focused on cataract-IOL surgery; hence the center was named the Center for IOL Research. Following Apple's move to Charleston, S.C., in 1989 the scope of the work expanded, and we therefore changed the name to a more inclusive one, the Center for Research on Ocular Therapeutics and Biodevices.[12] As of December, 2000 we had accessioned more than 16,500

From the Center for Research on Ocular Therapeutics and Biodevices (Director: David J. Apple, MD), Storm Eye Institute, Medical University of South Carolina, Charleston, S.C.

The authors have no financial or proprietary interest in any product mentioned in this chapter.

This text was supported in part by an unrestricted grant from Research to Prevent Blindness, Inc., New York.

We acknowledge the help of our colleagues Mark P. Wimberly, BS, Josef M. Schmidbauer, MD, Luis G. Vargas, MD, Marcela Escobar-Gomez, MD, and Liwei Ma, MD, for their assistance. We give special thanks to the eye banks nationwide and to all the surgeons for submitting the explanted IOLs and supporting this effort.

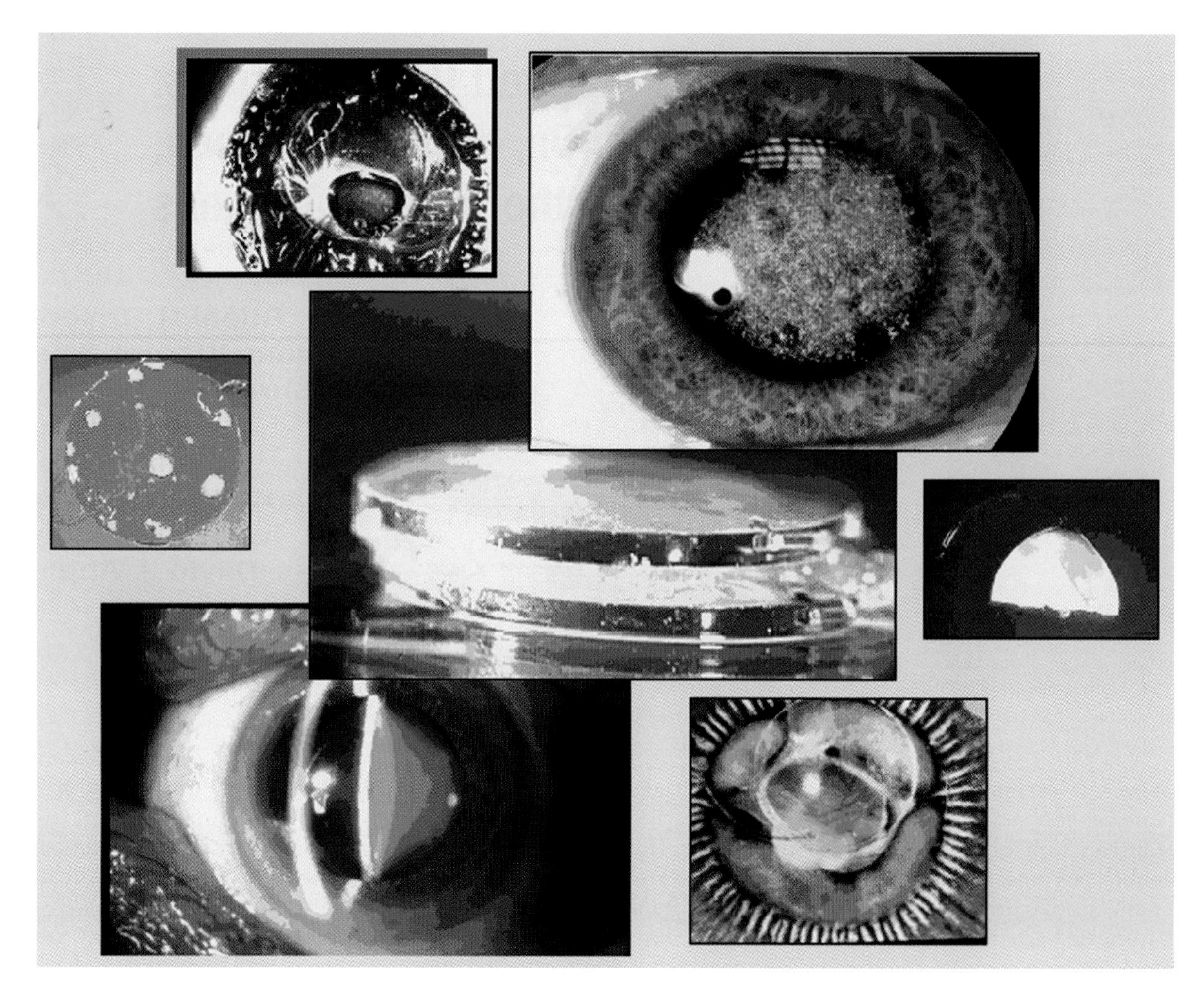

FIGURE 38-1 Photographs showing some of the IOL-related opacifications that are discussed in this chapter.

TABLE 38-1
IOL-Related Opacifications

Front (anterior)
- Anterior capsule opacification (ACO)
- Silicone oil adherence to IOLs

On (surface changes on the optical component of IOLs)
- Calcification on the surface of the Bausch & Lomb Hydroview IOL

Within (alteration inside the IOL optic)
- Degeneration of ultraviolet absorber material and calcium deposits within the optic of a hydrophilic IOL (manufactured by Medical Developmental Research)
- Glistening of the AcrySof IOL
- "Snowflake" or "crystalline" alteration of polymethylmethacrylate (PMMA) IOL optic: a syndrome caused by an unexpected late biodegradation of PMMA

Between (opacification between "piggyback" IOLs)
- Interlenticular opacification (IILO) of piggyback IOLs

Behind (posterior)
- Posterior capsule opacification (PCO)

IOL, Intraocular lens.

IOL-related specimens (Figure 38-2, *A*), including more than 7800 pseudophakic human globes. From January, 1988 through December, 2000, 6425 eyes with posterior chamber (PC) IOLs were analyzed, including 1109 eyes implanted with foldable IOLs (Figure 38-2, *B*).

Analysis of Pseudophakic Human Eyes Obtained Postmortem*

For future reference in this chapter, we first summarize how the specimens are accessioned and analyzed in our center. In general, the combination of both the anterior (surgeon's) view and the Miyake-Apple posterior photographic technique is used.[13,14]

*Based on the original work published by Miyake K, Miyake C: Intraoperative posterior chamber lens haptic fixation in the human cadaver eye, *Ophthalmic Surg* 16:230-236, 1985; Apple DJ, Lim E, Morgan R et al: Preparation and study of human eyes obtained postmortem with the Miyake posterior photographic technique, *Ophthalmology* 97:810-816, 1990.

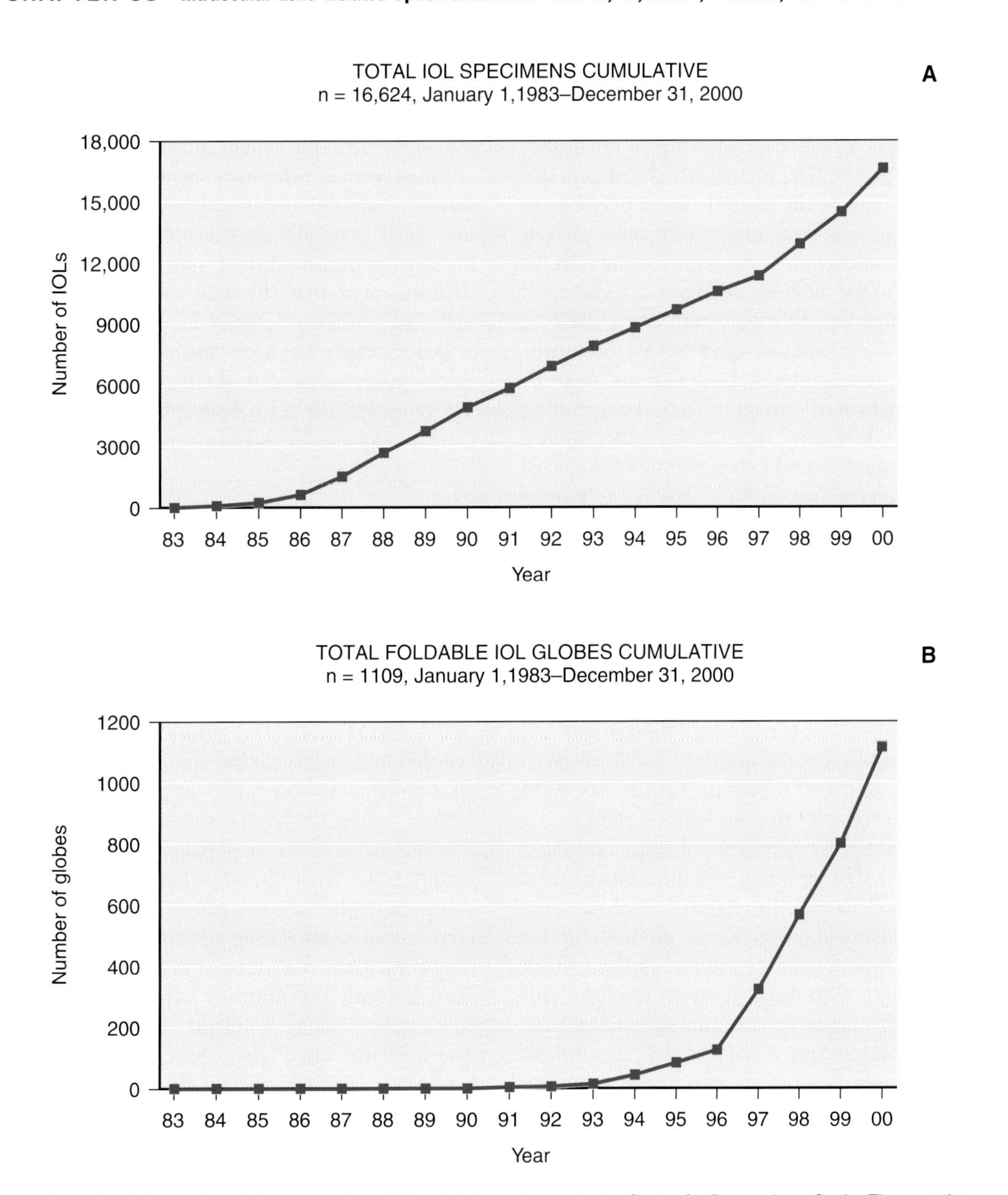

FIGURE 38-2 Cumulative accession of IOL-related specimens in the Center for Research on Ocular Therapeutics and Biodevices, January, 1983 through December, 2000. **A,** Total IOL specimens (n = 16,624). **B,** Foldable IOLs in globes obtained postmortem (n = 1109).

The former is the most direct way to measure rates and trends of anterior capsule opacification (ACO). The latter gives secure and easy determination of the presence of neodymium: yttrium-aluminum-garnet (Nd:YAG) posterior capsulotomies and PCO in autopsy eyes. We have analyzed six foldable IOL designs (one-piece silicone-plate large hole, one-piece silicone-plate small hole, three-piece silicone optic-Prolene haptics, three-piece silicone optic-PMMA haptics [Allergan SI 40], three-piece silicone optic-polyimide haptics, three-piece acrylic optic-PMMA haptics [Alcon AcrySof]) that appeared around 1989 and later and two types of rigid IOL designs (three-piece PMMA optic-Prolene haptics, one-piece PMMA optic-PMMA haptics) manufactured by several companies in use since the early 1980s. The accession rate of foldable IOLs began to increase in the early 1990s and has exponentially grown since about 1997. Lenses not implanted in the United States or not yet approved for domestic implantation could not be included in our analysis of ACO and PCO.

Each globe was received in 10% neutral buffered formalin and sectioned at the equator. Following gross examination from both front (surgeon's view) and from behind (Miyake-Apple posterior photographic technique), the globes were sectioned in the pupillo-optic nerve plane, with the cuts orientated parallel to the IOL haptics. This secures the entire IOL within the entire capsular bag. After dehydration and embedding in paraffin, the globes were sectioned, and the sections were stained with hematoxylin and eosin (H & E), periodic acid–Schiff (PAS), and Masson's trichrome stains for histopathologic evaluation. They were then examined under a light microscope (Olympus, Optical Co. Ltd., Japan), and photomicrographs were taken.

Analysis of Explanted IOLs*

The explanted IOLs were received in various media, including balanced salt solution (BSS) or 10% formaldehyde, or in a dry state. Depending on the type of the analysis to be performed, the IOLs were fixated in 10% neutral buffered formalin or not.

Pathologic evaluation of explanted rigid and foldable IOLs was performed according to the methods discussed elsewhere.[15,16] Gross analysis of the explanted IOLs was performed under a Leica/Wild MZ-8 Zoom Stereomicroscope (Vashaw Scientific, Inc., Norcross, Ga.), and gross photographs at various magnifications were taken using a 35-mm camera fitted to the operating microscope (Nikon N905 AF, Nikon Corporation, Tokyo, Japan). The lenses were also evaluated and photographed under an Olympus BX40F4 light microscope with an attached Olympus SC35 Type 12 camera (Olympus, Optical Co. Ltd., Japan). Depending on the type of analysis, the IOLs were then immersed in several histochemical agents, including H & E, PAS, alizarin red, Grocott's methenamine silver, Alcian blue, Congo red, Gram's stain, and so on.

Explanted hydrophilic acrylic foldable IOLs underwent histochemical analysis using special stains. For alizarin red staining (special stain for calcium [Ca]) the lenses were rinsed in distilled water, immersed in a 1% alizarin red solution for 2 minutes, rinsed again in distilled water, and reexamined under the light microscope. Ca salts stain red with this alizarin red stain.

Full-thickness sections through the optics of some explanted IOLs were also performed. The resultant cylindric blocks were dehydrated and embedded in paraffin. Sagittal sections were performed and stained using the von Kossa method for Ca (staining with nitrate solution for 60 minutes, exposure to a 100-watt lamp light, rinsing with distilled water, reaction with sodium [Na] thiosulfate solution for 2 minutes, rinsing with distilled water, and counterstaining in nuclear fast red solution for 5 minutes). Ca salts stain dark brown with this technique.

For scanning electron microscopy (SEM), IOLs were air-dried at room temperature for 7 days, sputter-coated with aluminum and/or gold/palladium, and examined under a JEOL JSM 5410LV scanning electron microscope. The specimens were further analyzed under a Hitachi 2500 Delta SEM equipped with a Kevex x-ray detector with light element capabilities for energy dispersive spectroscopy (EDS).

Anterior Capsule Opacification†

Introduction

When the anterior surface of the IOL optic biomaterial is in contact with the adjacent posterior aspect of the anterior capsule, the remaining anterior lens epithelial cells (A cells) may undergo fibrous metaplasia, leading to ACO or PCO.[17] When A cells are not surgically removed (in most cases it is neither necessary nor practical to attempt to remove these cells to achieve a satisfactory result), ACO may occur. Like PCO, ACO is also actually a misnomer because it is not the capsule that opacifies, but rather the cells lining the capsule. A more accurate term is *anterior subcapsular opacification*. However, the former term is firmly established in the literature and in clinical use. ACO generally occurs much earlier in comparison with PCO, sometimes within 1 month postoperatively. It has been demonstrated that the area of the anterior capsule opening seems to gradually decrease for up to 6 months postoperatively.

An excessive anterior capsule fibrosis or opacification may lead to major clinical problems and sequelae, such as difficulty in examining the retinal periphery, fibrous contraction of the capsule, capsulorhexis phimosis, and IOL decentration.

Pathogenesis

The cuboidal cells lining the anterior capsule (A cells) are the cells of origin of ACO. Results of Hara et al.[18] indicated that postoperative ACO is composed of fibroblast-like cells, derived from metaplastic lens epithelial cells, and collagen. Ishibashi et al.[19,20] studied the anterior capsule of cynomolgus monkeys obtained at different time points after ECCE with implantation of PC IOLs. The ACO was found to be composed of proliferated cellular and extracellular matrix. Because the proliferations were located between the anterior capsule and the anterior surface of the IOL optic, the authors stated that it should be referred to as anterior subcapsular opacification rather than simply ACO. Their ultrastructural analysis revealed that the cell components had two characteristics of epithelial cells: a basal lamina and desmosomes between adjacent cells. Also, some of the proliferated cells were directly connected to the lens epithelium beneath the anterior capsule. The extracellular matrix consisted of collagen fibrils, basal lamina–like material, and microfibrils. They also demonstrated two phases in the formation of ACO: an early phase consisting of proliferation of lens epithelial cells and a late phase involving degeneration or disappearance of lens epithelial cells and the presence of extracellular matrix.

Factors That May Contribute to ACO

Three major factors have been postulated to affect the degree of ACO: (1) the initial size of the continuous curvilinear capsulorhexis (CCC), (2) the IOL material and design, and (3) preexisting conditions, for example, the quality of the zonular support.

CAPSULORHEXIS SIZE

With a CCC smaller than the diameter of the IOL optic, the contact of the optic's biomaterial with the anterior capsule will induce fibrosis or opacification. The magnitude of the postoperative changes appears to be related to the initial CCC size,

*Based on the original work published by Apple DJ, Rabb M: *Ocular pathology: clinical applications and self-assessment,* St Louis, 1998, Mosby, pp 117-204; Apple DJ, Auffarth GU, Peng Q et al: *Foldable intraocular lenses: evolution, clinicopathologic correlation and complications,* Thorofare, NJ, 2000, Slack Inc.

†Based on the original work published by Werner L, Pandey SK, Escobar-Gomez M et al: Anterior capsule opacification: a histopathological study comparing different IOL styles, *Ophthalmology* 107:463-467, 2000; Werner L, Pandey SK, Apple DJ et al: Anterior capsule opacification: correlation of pathological findings with clinical sequelae, *Ophthalmology* 108:1675-1681, 2001.

although some authors did not find any correlation between these parameters.[21] Tsuboi et al.[22] have studied the influence of the CCC and IOL fixation on the blood-aqueous barrier. Their results indicate an unfavorable effect of in-the-bag fixation with a small CCC and thus a broad contact of the IOL optic with the anterior capsule. The important subset of ACO, capsular phimosis, relates to the CCC size. The sphincter effect of an intact capsulorhexis seems to be important in creating significant capsule shrinkage. Some authors believe that the size of the CCC is an important factor in the pathogenesis of this condition.[19,20] It is postulated that the more epithelium that is left, the greater the potential for capsule contraction. Although no correlation between the initial CCC size and the postoperative CCC constriction has been found by Gonvers, Sickenberg, and van Melle,[21] some authors have postulated that performing small, intact CCCs strongly increases the risk for capsule fibrosis and shrinkage. The relationship between the CCC size and PCO is discussed later in this chapter. Another phenomenon probably related to a small capsulorhexis size is the "capsular block syndrome," defined as a blockage of the contents within the capsular bag.

IOL MATERIAL AND DESIGN

Werner et al.[23,24] have performed extensive research regarding ACO. They compared at the microscopic level the influence of different IOL biomaterials and IOL designs on the development of anterior capsule fibrosis.[23] For this study, 460 globes accessioned from January 1995 to January 1999 were selected. After initial gross examination and preparation of the globes as mentioned previously, they were examined under a light microscope, and photomicrographs were taken at the CCC margin of each anterior capsule at a predetermined standard magnification of ×400. The anterior capsule fibrosis was scored under the light microscope according to the thickness of the fibrocellular tissue on the inner surface of the anterior capsule. Thickness measurements were done with a scale fitted to the eyepiece of the microscope. Table 38-2 shows the microscopic classification of ACO. The photomicrographs (Figure 38-3) demonstrate examples of all grades (0 to III) of ACO.

Table 38-3 presents the results concerning the histopathologic score of ACO obtained in each IOL group. The lenses are ranked according to the mean score, with the lowest score at the bottom (least amount of proliferation) and highest score at the top (most proliferation and thickness). Results of the histopathologic study confirm the observations of others that the rate of ACO is higher with silicone IOLs. Results of a macroscopic study performed by Werner et al.[24] (described later in text) also concur with histologic findings that the ACO score was highest with silicone IOLs. Among the four silicone IOL groups, plate-haptic silicone IOLs had higher scores than the three-piece designs. This difference was significant. Histopathologic findings concur with clinical findings in that the excessive CCC constriction observed with plate-haptic IOLs is probably due to the relatively large area of contact of the plate haptic silicone material with the anterior capsule, in sharp

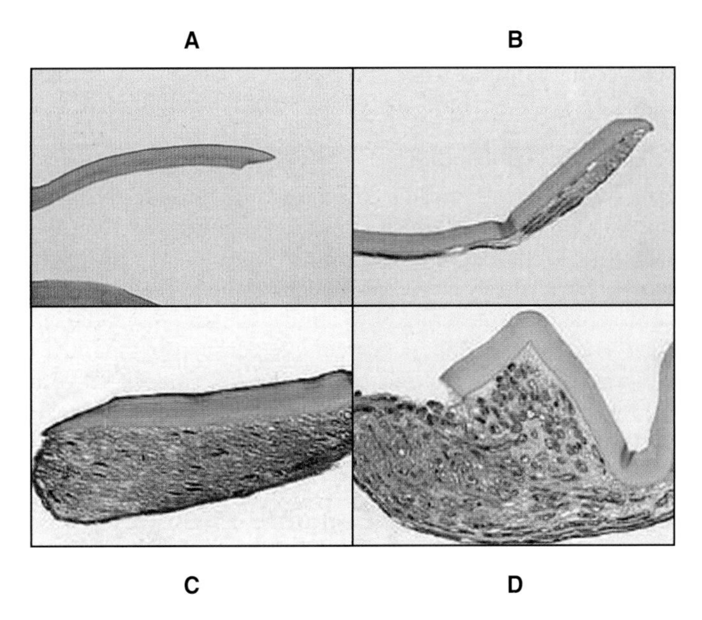

FIGURE 38-3 Photomicrographs taken at the CCC margin of pseudophakic human globes obtained postmortem (Masson's trichrome stain, original magnification ×400) showing anterior capsule fibrosis. **A,** Grade 0. **B,** Grade I. **C,** Grade II. **D,** Grade III.

TABLE 38-2

Microscopic Classification of ACO

Grade 0	No proliferating tissues or cells in the inner surface of the anterior capsule or only a single cell layer in the inner surface
Grade I	Proliferating tissues or cells with a thickness less than 60 μ or anterior capsule presenting at least two cell layers in the inner surface
Grade II	Proliferating tissues/or cells with a thickness from 60 to 120 μ
Grade III	Proliferating tissues/or cells with a thickness greater than 120 μ

ACO, Anterior capsule opacification.

TABLE 38-3

Histopathologic Scoring of ACO (from Grade 0 to III) in Human Globes Obtained Postmortem

IOL Style	Sample Size	Mean
One-piece silicone-plate, large hole	40	1.77 ± 0.86*
One-piece silicone-plate, small hole	67	1.28 ± 0.77
Three-piece silicone optic-PMMA haptics (Allergan SI40)	24	1.21 ± 0.72
Three-piece silicone optic-Prolene haptics	92	1.09 ± 0.65
Three-piece PMMA optic-PMMA/Prolene haptics	51	1.07 ± 0.84
One-piece PMMA optic-PMMA haptics	50	0.94 ± 0.68
Three-piece silicone optic-polyimide haptics	40	0.92 ± 0.76
Three-piece acrylic optic-PMMA haptics (Alcon AcrySof)	96	0.51 ± 0.52†

*Statistically significant when compared with all groups, except one-piece silicone-plate, small hole and three-piece silicone optic-PMMA haptics (Allergan SI40).
†Statistically significant when compared with all groups, except three-piece silicone optic-polyimide haptics.
ACO, Anterior capsule opacification; *IOL,* intraocular lens; *PMMA,* polymethylmethacrylate.

contrast to three-piece IOLs where the contact is limited to the surface of the optic. Thus the plate IOL has a large surface exposure that may stimulate cell proliferation and fibrosis.

PREEXISTING CONDITIONS

Cases of extreme capsule shrinkage are produced by an imbalance of forces in which a key factor appears to be zonular weakness. Weakened or absent zonular fibers may be unable to oppose the relatively increased strength of the centrally directed contractile forces generated by capsular fibrosis. In conditions such as pseudoexfoliation, the zonules can become markedly weakened. Capsular contraction has also been associated with other conditions such as diabetes, uveitis, myotonic muscular dystrophy, or retinitis pigmentosa.[25,26]

Sequelae of Anterior Capsular Shrinkage

Werner et al.[24] in their macroscopic study have evaluated the degree of ACO in human eyes obtained postmortem and compared the findings with sequelae of capsular shrinkage. Results of the study showed that the process of opacification of the anterior capsule may progress in four stages: (1) fibrosis or opacification of the capsulorhexis margin occurs at some places; (2) the entire anterior capsular edge in contact with the IOL optic's biomaterial becomes progressively opacified; (3) capsular folds form; and (4) advanced, excessive and/or asymmetric fibrosis and shrinkage may result in some complications, such as eccentric displacement of the CCC opening, IOL decentration, and capsulorhexis phimosis.

Only eyes with the IOL implanted in the capsular bag and with a capsulorhexis smaller than the IOL optic were included in this macroscopic study. Therefore, 300 eyes consecutively accessioned from January, 1996 to January, 2000 were selected. Following gross examination from a posterior view, the cornea and iris were excised to allow a better evaluation of the anterior capsule. From an anterior (surgeon's) view the ACO was scored under an operating microscope. Table 38-4 shows the classification used for the macroscopic study. Figure 38-4 shows examples of each grade of ACO.

The capsulorhexis diameter was measured in millimeters with calipers. The axis of PC-IOL decentration in the capsular bag was noted. The IOL decentration at this axis was then measured with calipers and expressed in millimeters. Table 38-5 presents the results concerning the score of ACO, capsulorhexis diameter, and IOL decentration obtained in each group. The groups are ranked according to the mean ACO score, with the highest score at the top and lowest score at the bottom.

Results regarding the CCC diameter have to be interpreted carefully. These suggest that the mean CCC opening was smallest with one-piece silicone plate lenses (a result of excessive capsular fibrosis and shrinkage) and largest with three-piece acrylic optic-PMMA haptic (AcrySof) lenses (which presented the least amount of ACO). Studies comparing the changes in capsulorhexis size after implantation of different IOLs have already demonstrated that CCC openings with plate-haptic silicone lenses have a marked tendency to constrict, whereas this tendency is least with AcrySof lenses.[27,28] Nevertheless, those studies take into account the initial size of the CCC. Information about the initial CCC size was not available in our series.[24]

TABLE 38-4
Macroscopic Classification of ACO

Grade 0	Clear (transparent) anterior capsule
Grade I	Opacification localized at the edge of the capsulorhexis
Grade II	Diffuse opacification, sometimes with areas of capsular folding
Grade III	Intense opacification, with areas of capsular folding
Grade IV	Constriction (phimosis) of the capsulorhexis opening (capsulorhexis diameter ≤3.5 mm)

ACO, Anterior capsule opacification.

Ten cases of capsulorhexis phimosis were observed in this study.[24] Seven cases were associated with three-piece silicone optic-Prolene haptic lenses (8.75%), and the three other cases were associated with one-piece silicone-plate lenses (8.57%). The mean decentration in these cases was 0.95 ± 0.9 mm for the first group and 0.4 ± 0.3 mm for the second. The difference in mean IOL decentration among the groups was found to be significant ($p = 0.01$). The hydrophobic acrylic lens (AcrySof) studied here presented the lowest mean decentration and ACO scores.

The intensity of these sequelae seems to be at least partially correlated with the IOL implanted. Nevertheless, because the data are not based on a clinical, follow-up study, we could not make definitive conclusions or establish a time line for the evolution of this process with different IOL materials or designs.

Clinical Significance

As mentioned earlier, the lowest mean decentration and ACO scores were found with AcrySof IOLs.[24] These findings may be of clinical significance in that, when using this IOL type, (1) anterior capsule polishing should not be necessary in most cases, (2) the incidence of decentration and capsulorhexis phimosis should be minimized, and (3) one might expect a better view of the peripheral retina through a clear anterior capsule during indirect ophthalmoscopy. Severe ACO may represent a significant clinical problem for the retinal surgeon because of difficulty in examining the retinal periphery. The large size of the capsulorhexis and implantation of hydrophobic acrylic IOL (AcrySof) are useful surgical pearls to overcome this problem.

Prevention

Several methods have been proposed to prevent CCC contraction and the resultant IOL decentration.[29] In routine cataract surgery, thorough polishing of the anterior capsule can be a useful procedure.[30] It is time consuming, somewhat impractical, and generally not necessary to achieve excellent results in most cases. However, anterior capsule polishing will make the onset of ACO less likely. Some authors recommend a careful anterior capsular polishing and removing of the anterior subcapsular epithelial cells. Nishi[31] proposed the use of a modified irrigating-aspirating tip with an abrasive surface. An effective hydrodissection helps to make lens substance removal easier, ensuring a more complete removal of masses of cortex and cells. Large CCC (>5.5 mm in diameter) was also found to be

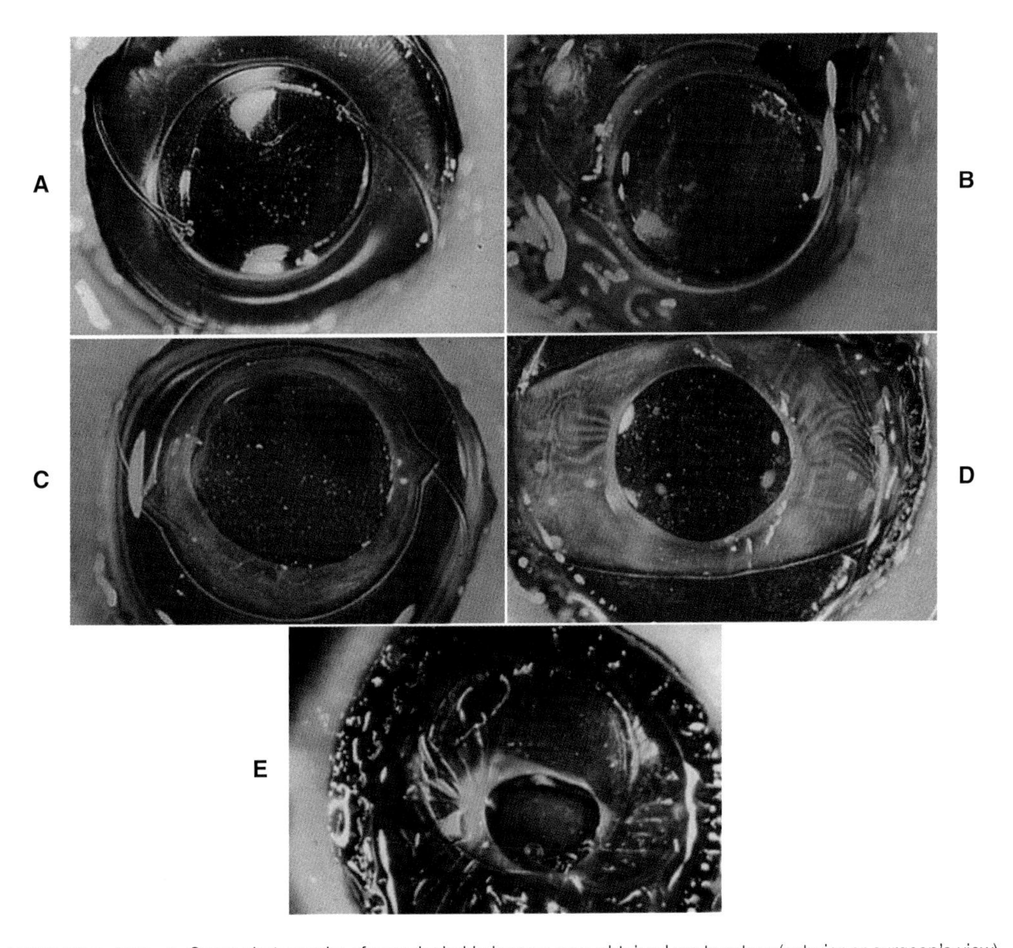

FIGURE 38-4 Gross photographs of pseudophakic human eyes obtained postmortem (anterior or surgeon's view) showing examples of grading system for anterior capsule opacification. **A,** Three-piece acrylic optic-PMMA haptic lens (Alcon AcrySof); ACO grade 0. **B,** Three-piece silicone optic-Prolene haptic lens; ACO grade I. **C,** Three-piece silicone optic-PMMA haptic lens (Allergan SI40); ACO grade II. **D,** One-piece silicone-plate, small hole lens; ACO grade III. **E,** Three-piece silicone optic-Prolene haptic lens; ACO grade IV (capsulorhexis phimosis).

TABLE 38-5

ACO Scoring (from Grade 0 to IV), Capsulorhexis Diameter, and IOL Decentration in Human Globes Obtained Postmortem

IOL Style	Sample Size	ACO Scoring	Capsulorhexis Diameter (mm)	Capsulorhexis Phimosis (n)	IOL Decentration (mm)
One-piece silicone-plate, large hole + One-piece silicone-plate, small hole	35	2.5 ± 0.9*	4.4 ± 0.6	3	0.2 ± 0.3
Three-piece silicone optic-Prolene haptics	80	1.9 ± 0.96	4.4 ± 0.65	7	0.4 ± 0.6
Three-piece silicone optic-PMMA haptics (Allergan SI40) + Three-piece silicone optic-polyimide haptics	30	1.7 ± 0.9	4.6 ± 0.7	0	0.2 ± 0.3
Three-piece PMMA optic-Prolene haptics	50	1.7 ± 0.9	4.55 ± 0.4	0	0.3 ± 0.4
One-piece PMMA optic-PMMA haptics	50	1.6 ± 0.7	4.6 ± 0.6	0	0.2 ± 0.3
Three-piece acrylic optic-PMMA haptics (Alcon AcrySof)	55	0.6 ± 0.7†	4.8 ± 0.7	0	0.08 ± 0.1

*Statistically significant when compared with all groups.
†Statistically significant when compared with all groups.
ACO, Anterior capsule opacification; *IOL,* intraocular lens; *PMMA,* polymethylmethacrylate.

correlated with less capsule contraction. However, it is not technically easy to perform large capsulorhexis, and it also hampers endocapsular phacoemulsification. Recently, the "initiative and definitive" concept of capsulorhexis has also been reported to have the advantage of the best of both worlds, endocapsular phacoemulsification and less ACO.[32]

Treatment

When capsular phimosis develops, radial anterior Nd:YAG capsulotomies can be performed to create four equally spaced radial cuts about 1 mm in length using an average power of 1.5 mJ.[33] It might be prudent to initiate linear cuts in all four quadrants, removing traction symmetrically, before completing the cuts. This technique may avoid extension of a radial tear from the first cut. Some authors recommend relaxing anterior capsulotomies immediately when capsule contraction is observed.[29] They postulate that active capsular fibrosis can be influenced with early YAG laser treatment, whereas later intervention may not help.[33] Although early Nd:YAG laser anterior capsulotomy presumably will prevent further lens decentration eventually associated with capsular phimosis and improve symptoms in most patients, it is not without risks. The IOL may dislocate posteriorly if a rupture in the posterior capsule is created.

Summary

ACO is actually a misnomer. The better term is anterior subcapsular opacification. The size of the CCC, as well as the IOL material and design, has a major influence on the development of ACO. According to recent studies, ACO was found to be lowest with hydrophobic acrylic lenses and highest with plate-haptic silicone IOLs.[5,23,24] The IOL design and material also influence the clinical presentation and sequelae of capsular shrinkage.

Silicone Oil Adherence to IOLs*

Introduction

The use of silicone oil in vitreoretinal microsurgery was reported in the literature.[34,35] However, intraocular use of silicone oil can lead to various complications. The very important issue that must be considered in vitrectomized, silicone oil–filled eyes undergoing cataract surgery with IOL implantation is the adhesion of silicone oil to the IOL surface, especially to silicone optic IOL designs.[36] Although the incidence of clinically significant silicone oil–IOL complication is reported to be relatively low, it is probably higher than what is generally assumed clinically because affected patients or potentially affected patients are usually seen later by a vitreoretinal surgeon rather than by the anterior segment surgeon. Also, this complication may be more common in countries outside of the United States because silicone oil is used more commonly.

Irreversible adherence of silicone oil to the IOL optic may lead to devastating sequelae, including visual disturbances and visual loss for the patient, as well as obstruction of the vitreoretinal surgeon's view into the eye. Therefore use of standard silicone optic IOL is not recommended in patients with either present or potential vitreoretinal disease that may require use of silicone oil as a tamponade.[36,37]

Silicone Oil Interaction with Different IOL Materials

The literature has reported that significant silicone oil coverage may occur on the surface of an IOL optic, especially one made from a hydrophobic material, as opposed to more hydrophilic materials.[36,37] Apple et al.[36,37] in two different studies have compared the degree of silicone oil adherence occurring with several IOLs fabricated from various biomaterials (Figure 38-5). These studies from our laboratory have demonstrated that the more hydrophobic materials with higher dispersive energy and relatively higher contact angles had more silicone oil adherence.[36,37] Hydrophilic biomaterial with relatively low contact angles and low dispersive surface energy demonstrated less silicone oil adherence. Furthermore, silicone oil coverage of PMMA IOLs was found to be significantly decreased once they were heparin-surface-modified (HSM).[38] This phenomenon might be explained by the fact that coating of PMMA IOLs with heparin converts their hydrophobic surface into a hydrophilic one. Some IOLs, for example, the hydrophobic-acrylic Alcon AcrySof and the Ciba Vision MemoryLens, show significantly less silicone oil coverage than standard silicone IOLs. The reason why these two IOL groups—one being relatively hydrophobic and the other relatively hydrophilic—have similar silicone oil adherence is not clear. Factors other than contact angle, such as surface energy, may play a role in this interaction. However, their values of percentage of silicone oil coverage are intermediate or higher than that of the crystalline lens, and they are also not immune to this complication. In another study from our laboratory,[6,39] we have reported that the interaction of silicone oil with a silicone IOL is dramatically decreased if the latter is surface modified with heparin (Figure 38-6).[6,39] Its hydrophilic chains that are bound to the surface of the IOL extend into the aqueous media and form a highly hydrated layer around the lens by trapping water molecules. This leads to reduction of silicone oil adherence to this kind of IOL as it has also been described with PMMA IOLs.

Mechanism of Action

The basis of silicone oil–IOL biomaterials interaction has been thoroughly explained by various authors. Apple et al.[36,37] and Cunanan et al.[40] explained the physicochemical basis of this phenomenon. Dick et al.[41] summarized the three main factors that influence silicone oil–IOL biomaterial interaction, in vitro and in vivo: (1) contact angle of the polymer—hydrophobic materials having higher contact angle than hydrophilic

*Based on the original work published by Apple DJ, Federman JL, Krolicki TJ et al: Irreversible silicone oil adhesion to silicone intraocular lenses: a clinicopathologic analysis, *Ophthalmology* 103:1555-1561, 1996; Apple DJ, Isaacs RT, Kent DG et al: Silicone oil adhesion to intraocular lenses: an experimental study comparing various biomaterials, *J Cataract Refract Surg* 23:536-544, 1997; Arthur SN, Peng Q, Apple DJ et al: Effect of heparin surface modification in reducing silicone oil adherence to various intraocular lenses, *J Cataract Refract Surg* 27:1662-1669, 2001.

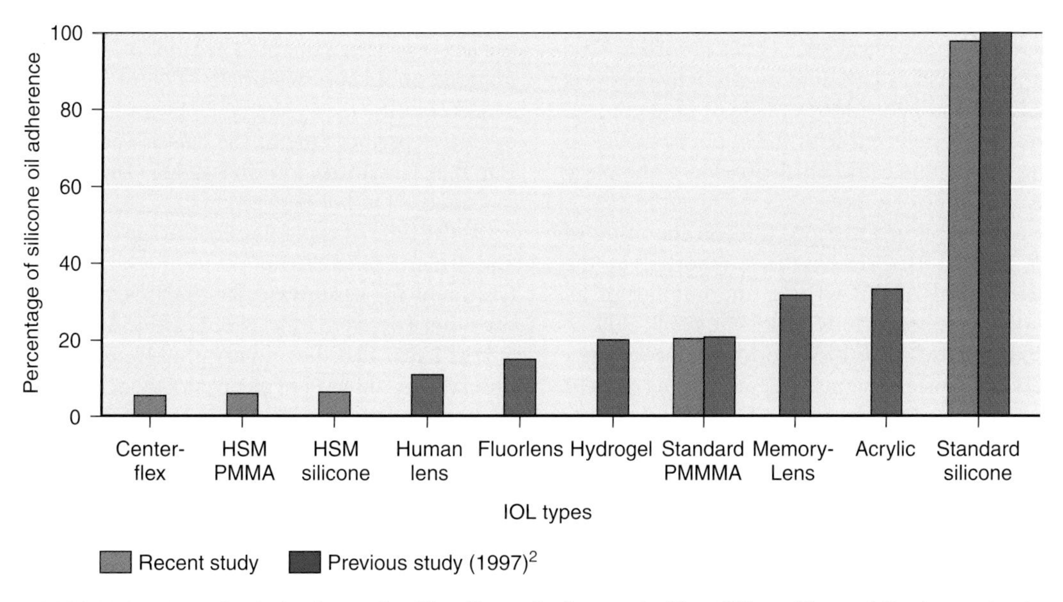

FIGURE 38-5 Graph showing results of the silicone oil adherence to different IOLs and the crystalline lens analyzed in two different studies performed in our center: the recent study *(red bars)* and the previous study *(blue bars)*.

materials; (2) free energy of the polymer—a sum of polar and dispersive components; and (3) surrounding biologic factors, such as body temperature, eye movements, and characteristics of the aqueous humor.

Treatment

In addition to appropriate IOL choice when addressing silicone oil–IOL interaction, investigators are finding new means to remove silicone oil from IOL surfaces in cases where the condition has become manifested. For example, Langefeld et al.[42] and Zeana et al.[43] demonstrated the effectiveness of perfluorhexyloctan ($C_{14}F_{13}H_{17}$ [F6H8]) in removing silicone oil from silicone IOL surfaces. Furthermore, Dick and Augustin[44] demonstrated that this solvent is more effective in removing silicone oil from an IOL with hydrophilic surfaces than from hydrophobic IOLs. This solvent appears to be tolerated by surrounding intraocular tissues. Hoerauf et al.[45] have reported on the effectiveness of using the solvent O44 for removal of silicone oil from the IOL surface. Kageyama and Yaguchi[46] have demonstrated a mechanical method of removing silicone oil from the IOL surfaces. Although effective, these procedures are invasive and require secondary surgical intervention.

Summary

Special care should be taken when selecting IOLs for patients who may be deemed to have a high propensity or potential for severe vitreoretinal disease that may require silicone oil treatment later. An awareness of clinically significant IOL–silicone oil interaction should be useful in lowering the incidence of such complications.

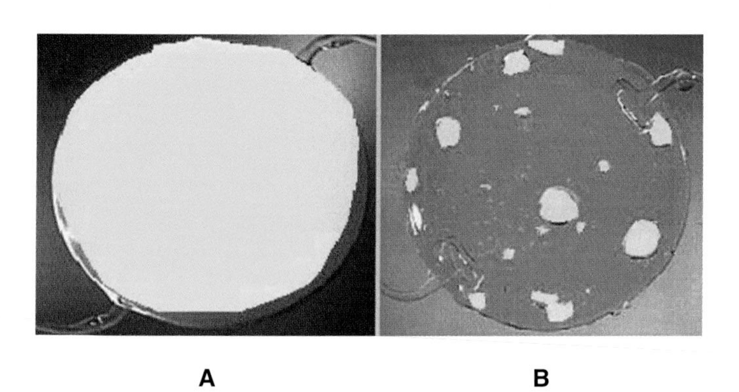

FIGURE 38-6 Gross photographs showing image analysis of silicone IOLs (Pharmacia Corporation, Peapack, NJ) after submersion in silicone oil. The yellow area indicates the silicone oil adherence to the IOL. **A,** Standard silicone IOL. **B,** HSM silicone IOL.

Calcification on the Surface of the Bausch & Lomb Hydroview IOL*

Introduction

The Bausch & Lomb Surgical (Rochester, NY) Hydroview IOL is a foldable hydrogel that has been implanted for several years in international markets; over 400,000 have been implanted worldwide. Although it was cleared for marketing in November, 1999 by the United States FDA, it has not yet been launched for general implantation in this country. The optic material of these

*Based on the original work published by Werner L, Apple DJ, Escobar-Gomez M et al: Postoperative deposition of calcium on the surfaces of a hydrogel intraocular lens, *Ophthalmology* 107:2179-2185, 2000; Pandey SK, Werner L, Apple DJ et al: Calcium precipitation on the surfaces of a foldable intraocular lens: a clinicopathological correlation, *Arch Ophthalmol* 120:391-393, 2002.

IOLs is composed of a cross-linked copolymer of 2-hydroxyethyl methacrylate (HEMA) and 6-hydroxyhexyl methacrylate, with a bonded benzotriazole-type ultraviolet (UV) absorber. The water content of this material is 18%, and the refractive index is 1.474. The haptics are modified C loops made of blue-colored PMMA, polymerically cross-linked with the optics by means of an interpenetrating polymer network, which provides a one-piece design with a true optic zone of 6 mm.

Relatively late postoperative Ca deposition on the optic of Hydroview lenses (model H60M) has been reported in the literature.[8,47-51] At the time of this writing, the number of all reported cases with complications is relatively small: 309 of approximately 400,000 lenses implanted worldwide. In 96 cases, the IOL changes were clinically significant, decreasing patient vision enough to result in lens explantation. The clinical reports have not been randomly distributed. Although this IOL model has been implanted in 3500 centers worldwide, reports have appeared in clusters. The majority has come from 31 ophthalmic practices in 11 countries. We have analyzed explanted opacified IOLs from several of these centers.[8,47-51]

Analyses of Explanted IOLs

R. I. Murray,[52] from Scotland, has reported two cases of late opacification of Hydroview lenses requiring explantation, but he did not perform pathologic analyses of the explanted lenses. We have recently reported analyses of the first six explanted Hydroview lenses that we received in our center.[47] In each case, the lens has been explanted because of deposition of crystalline material on its optical surfaces (Figure 38-7, *A*) associated with a decrease in visual acuity (VA) and glare in the late postoperative period. One of the lenses was explanted in Australia (Dr. B. B. Crayford), four in Sweden (Dr. A. Öhrström), and one in Canada (Dr. J. P. Gravel).

At the time of explantation, the age of the patients (2 women and 4 men) ranged from 70 to 85 years. Two patients were in treatment for cardiovascular diseases, two were diabetics, and the other two were otherwise healthy. All lenses were explanted at least 1 year after the primary procedure because of opacification observed at the level of the optics associated with a decrease in VA and significant glare. The surgeons described the findings as a "brown granularity" or "small red corpuscles" present on both external optical surfaces of the lenses. In some cases, the optic of the lenses was almost completely covered by those structures, giving them a "frosty" and very reflective appearance. Nd:YAG laser treatment was performed in all cases in an attempt to clean the optical surfaces, without success.

After initial primary gross and microscopic examination, the lenses were stained with alizarin red. Full-thickness sections were performed through the optic of two explanted Hydroview lenses and a control Hydroview lens. The resultant cylindric blocks were dehydrated and embedded in paraffin. Sagittal

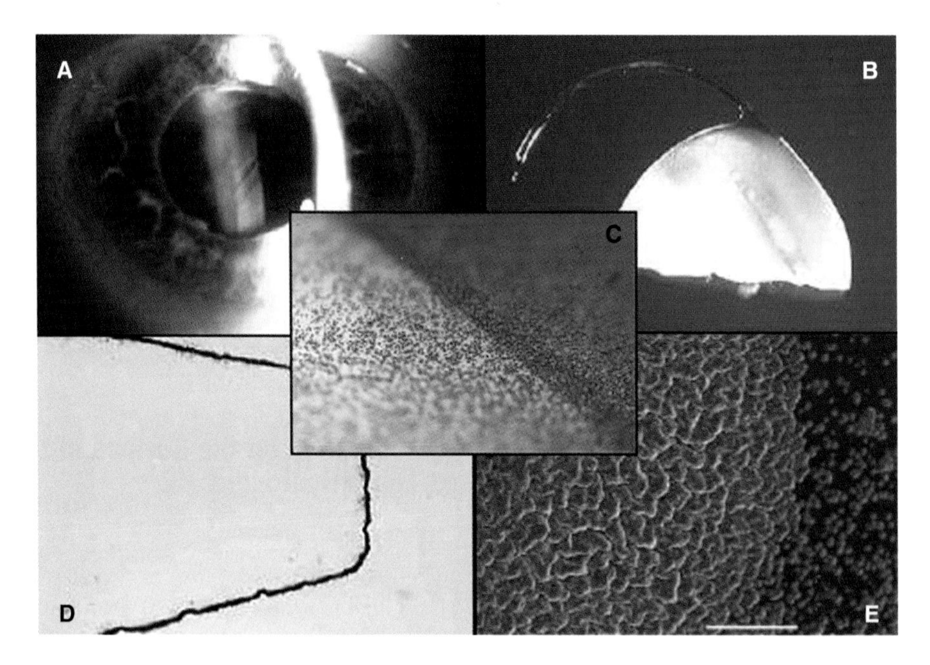

FIGURE 38-7 Calcification on the surface of Hydroview IOLs. **A,** Slit lamp photograph of an implanted Hydroview IOL showing the granularity present on the anterior surface of the lens. (Courtesy Dr. Arne Öhrström, Vasteras, Sweden.) **B,** Gross photograph showing an example of Hydroview IOL explanted because of optical opacification. **C,** Photomicrographs from the surface of an explanted Hydroview lens showing granular deposits. (Alizarin red; original magnification ×200.) **D,** Histologic sagittal section of the optic of one explanted Hydroview lens. The lens material itself was dissolved during the preparation for histologic examination, but the optic surface is delineated by a continuous layer of dark brown, irregular granules. (von Kossa's stain; original magnification ×200.) **E,** Scanning electron photomicrograph from the anterior optical surface of one explanted Hydroview lens. The deposits are composed of multiple globules of variable sizes, which are confluent in some areas.

sections were performed and stained using the von Kossa method for Ca.[53-55] One lens was analyzed under SEM as described previously. Incisional biopsies of conjunctiva and iris were also obtained from one of the patients during IOL removal and exchange to rule out the presence of dystrophic calcification in those tissues.[49]

Gross and microscopic evaluations of all of the explanted Hydroview lenses had almost identical findings. By gross evaluation the presence of the deposits on their optical surfaces was noted to cause different degrees of IOL haze or opacification, directly proportional to the amount of deposits on the IOL (see Figure 38-7, *B*). A layer of irregular granular deposits composed of multiple, fine, translucent spherical-ovoid granules covered the surfaces of the unstained IOLs. The deposits occurred on both anterior and posterior IOL optic surfaces, but not the haptics (see Figure 38-7, *B*). In some cases, both surfaces were almost completely covered by a confluent granular layer, whereas in other cases some intervening clear areas were observed. Multiple pits related to Nd:YAG laser treatment were observed on the posterior surface of the IOLs in all cases. Also, the deposits on the surfaces of the IOLs stained positive with alizarin red in all cases (see Figure 38-7, *C*). In some areas with scattered, small granules, only the deposits themselves stained red, whereas the IOL surface itself was not stained.

Sagittal histologic sections through the optic of two Hydroview lenses, stained using the von Kossa method, showed a continuous layer of dark brown, irregular granules on the anterior and posterior optical surfaces and the edges of the lenses (see Figure 38-7, *D*). Figure 38-7, *E*, shows the aspect of the deposits on the surface of one Hydroview lens under SEM. EDS performed on the deposits demonstrated the presence of peaks of Ca and phosphate. Histochemical evaluation of the conjunctival and iris biopsies from one of the patients, using alizarin red stain and von Kossa silver stain tests, did not reveal any evidence of Ca salts.

After completion of these analyses, we received eight other explanted Hydroview lenses in our center: three from Dr. J. P. Gravel (Canada), two from Dr. Sher (Canada), two from Dr. A Öhrström (Sweden), and one from Dr. A. Apel (Australia). The surgical, clinical, and pathologic features of these cases were similar to those described previously.

According to Dr. Crayford, infrared spectroscopic analyses performed on the surface of two other explanted lenses of the same model (not available to us) also revealed the presence of the same components (Basil B. Crayford, FRACO, personal communication, February 2000). Ca and phosphates were also found on the surfaces of three other Hydroview lenses explanted by Yu and Shek[56] using Raman spectra analysis and EDS.

Possible Factors Involved in the Pathogenesis

The mechanism of this complication is not fully understood, but it does not seem to be directly related to substances used during the surgery because it occurred in the late postoperative period. Also, the substances used during the surgery were not the same in all cases. The majority of the patients involved had an associated systemic disease; therefore the possibility of a patient-related factor, such as a metabolic imbalance, cannot be ruled out.

Ca deposition observed in the cases described here occurred in the late postoperative period. In the case of Hydroview IOLs, chemical removal of Ca phosphate revealed the presence of a few small pits and fissures with the SEM that were found to be artifactual, rather than permanent damage caused by the deposits on the IOLs surfaces (George Green, PhD, at Bausch & Lomb, personal communication, February, 2000). Yu and Shek[56] also confirmed that the deposits on their lenses were mainly localized on the external surfaces, but the polymer structure was not affected.

Lot history, component history, process changes, surgical setting and techniques, environmental factors, preexisting patient conditions, and packaging have been examined. According to Bausch & Lomb studies, part of the components of this packaging contains silicone, which may come off the packaging onto the optic of the lens. It then appears to be a catalyst for Ca precipitation. Fatty acids and silicone, perhaps in association with a metabolic disease in the affected patient, could result in the calcification. In a February, 2001 letter to surgeons who have implanted the Hydroview IOL, Bausch & Lomb described their investigation into the phenomenon. Surface chemistry studies identified the lens deposits as a layered mixture of octaCa phosphate, fatty acids, salts, and small amounts of silicone (Guttman C: Hydroview calcification resolved, *Ophthalmology Times* 26[4], 2001). An in vitro model was then constructed to find out how the material deposited onto the lens. This model, according to the manufacturer, revealed a migration of silicone from a gasket in the lens packaging onto the surface of the IOL. The manufacturer has correlated a change in packaging with the appearance of the opacification. In lenses placed into the current IOL packaging, trace amounts of low-molecular-weight silicone have been detected on some IOL surfaces. Although this substance was not present with the original packaging, the possible role of silicone in causing the complication remains unclear. The models also showed that in addition to silicone, fatty acids had to be present to attract Ca ions to the lens surface. A separate retrospective clinical case-control study was also conducted by the manufacturer at the sites where the highest incidences of calcification were reported. The manufacturer now believes that this problem is resolved. However, final verification will require a careful 1- to 2-year clinical study. Patients with these lenses must be carefully observed to determine the exact extent of this phenomenon.

Prevention and Treatment

It is important for the surgeons who implanted Hydroview lenses to recognize this condition. Excessive Nd:YAG laser treatment, in an attempt to clean the optical surfaces of the lenses, may jeopardize implantation of a new lens in the capsular bag after explantation of the Hydroview. Nd:YAG laser treatment was proven to be ineffective in cleaning the surfaces of the lenses. The cause of this condition seems to be multifactorial, and until the pathogenic mechanism is fully clarified, explantation and exchange of the IOL is the only available option. Methods for the prevention of this condition are also not completely defined to date. The manufacturer will make changes in the SureFold packaging, which will be produced with a gasket made from a nonsilicone material. Long-term clinical studies will determine the efficacy of this modification in the prevention of lens calcification.

Summary

The opacification of Hydroview lenses appears most commonly between 12 and 25 months postoperatively. Attempts to remove the opacity with an Nd:YAG laser have been unsuccessful. Analyses of opacified Hydroview lenses demonstrated that the deposit formation on their surfaces contains Ca.

Opacification Within the Optic of a Hydrophilic IOL*

Introduction

Foldable hydrogel (hydrophilic acrylic) IOLs are not yet available in the United States but have been marketed by several firms for several years in international markets. Late postoperative opacification within the optic substance of some IOLs manufactured from at least one source of a hydrophilic acrylic biomaterial has been reported recently[9,57,58] (Werner L, Apple DJ, Pandey SK: Late Postoperative opacification of 2 hydrophilic acrylic Intraocular lenses. Best paper of the session presented at the ASCRS Symposium on Cataract, IOL and Refractive Surgery, April/May 2001, San Diego, Calif.). The source of the polymer of this IOL, the SC60B-OUV design, was Vista Optics, United Kingdom; the manufacturer and distributor is Medical Developmental Research (MDR Inc., Clearwater, Fla.). As of May, 2000, MDR had announced 56 cases of late postoperative lens opacification of over 75,000 SC60B-OUV lenses implanted worldwide. In addition to the cases described here, the manufacturers were aware of at least 20 other cases that required explantation because of significant visual loss. The manufacturer withdrew all SC60B-OUV IOLs that have been fabricated from materials obtained from Vista Optics and sent in June of 2000 an informational letter to all lens users. All of these IOLs are now being manufactured from polymer material obtained from a new source, Benz Research, Sarasota, Fla. We analyzed the clinical, pathologic, histochemical, ultrastructural, and spectrographic features of these cases and tried to ascertain the nature of the intralenticular deposits in our center.[57-59]

Analysis of Explanted IOLs

All of the IOLs described here (n = 9) were explanted because of late postoperative opacification of the lens optic associated with decreased VA.[57] They were implanted and explanted by the same surgeon, Mahmut Kaskaloglu, MD, from the Ege University, Alsancak Izmir, Turkey. Each patient underwent uneventful phacoemulsification and implantation of the SC60B-OUV lens. Kaskaloglu has implanted 361 of these lenses between November 1997 and October 1999. He observed 18 cases of late postoperative opacification of the SC60B-OUV lens, 9 of which had associated visual symptoms sufficient to justify explantation and submit for pathologic analysis. Of the 18 cases of opacification, 5 patients were diabetics (2 explantations). Nevertheless, until now there is no information to establish a correlation between diabetics and postoperative opacification.

In general, the patients returned at around 24 months after the surgery complaining of a significant decrease in VA. The clinical characteristics of these lenses were different from the previously described "granularity" covering the optical surfaces of the Hydroview design. The clinical appearance was a clouding similar to a "nuclear cataract" (Figure 38-8, *A*). The lenses were explanted from 14 to 29 months postoperatively (24.42 ± 5.12). At the time of explantation, the ages of the patients ranged from 62 to 77 years (70.28 ± 5.76).

After initial gross and microscopic examination, we performed full-thickness sections through the optics of two of the explants (two sections each) and one of the controls. One of the resultant cylindric blocks from an explant in one of the cases and one from a control were directly stained with 1% alizarin red. A cylindric block from the explant in another case and another control were dehydrated and embedded in paraffin. Sagittal sections were performed and stained using the von Kossa method for Ca.[53-55] The other sagittal cut sections of the lens from both cases were prepared for SEM as described previously. One was sputter-coated with gold-palladium and the other with aluminum.

Gross and microscopic evaluations demonstrated that the optical surfaces and the haptics of some of the lenses were free of any deposits (see Figure 38-8, *B*). However, multiple small structures were initially noted to resemble "glistenings" within the central 5 mm of the IOL optical component. These were found to be the cause of each lens opacification. The edges of the optics and the haptics appeared clear. Alizarin red staining of the surfaces of all lenses was negative. Likewise, this stain was negative on the optical surfaces and haptics of the control IOLs.

Analysis of the cut sections (sagittal view) of the lens optics revealed multiple granules of variable sizes in a region beneath the external anterior and posterior surfaces of the IOLs. The granules were distributed in a line parallel to the anterior and posterior curvatures of the optics. In contrast to the findings of what morphologically resembled glistenings of the AcrySof IOL, light microscopic analyses revealed that the structures causing the opacification with these IOLs are not fluid-filled vacuoles but rather are granules of variable sizes. They stained positive with alizarin red (see Figure 38-8, *C*). Sagittal histologic sections stained with the von Kossa method also confirmed the presence of multiple dark brown-black granules mostly concentrated in a region immediately beneath the anterior and posterior optical surfaces (see Figure 38-8, *D*).

SEM analysis of a cut section (sagittal view) of the IOL optic (see Figure 38-8, *E*) confirmed that the region immediately subjacent to the IOLs' outer surfaces, as well as the central area of the optical cut section, were free of deposits. This also revealed the presence of the granules in the intermediate region beneath the anterior and posterior surfaces. EDS performed precisely on the deposits in the same section revealed the presence of Ca peaks. The central area of the optical cut section where no granules were present served as a control, showing only peaks of

*Based on the original work published by Werner L, Apple DJ, Kaskaloglu M et al: Dense opacification of the optical component of a hydrophilic acrylic intraocular lens: a clinicopathological analysis of 9 explanted lenses, *J Cataract Refract Surg* 27:1485-1492, 2001; Pandey SK, Werner L, Apple DJ et al: Hydrophilic acrylic intraocular lens optic and haptics opacification in a diabetic patient: Bilateral case report and clinicopathological correlation. *Ophthalmology* 109:2042-2051, 2002.

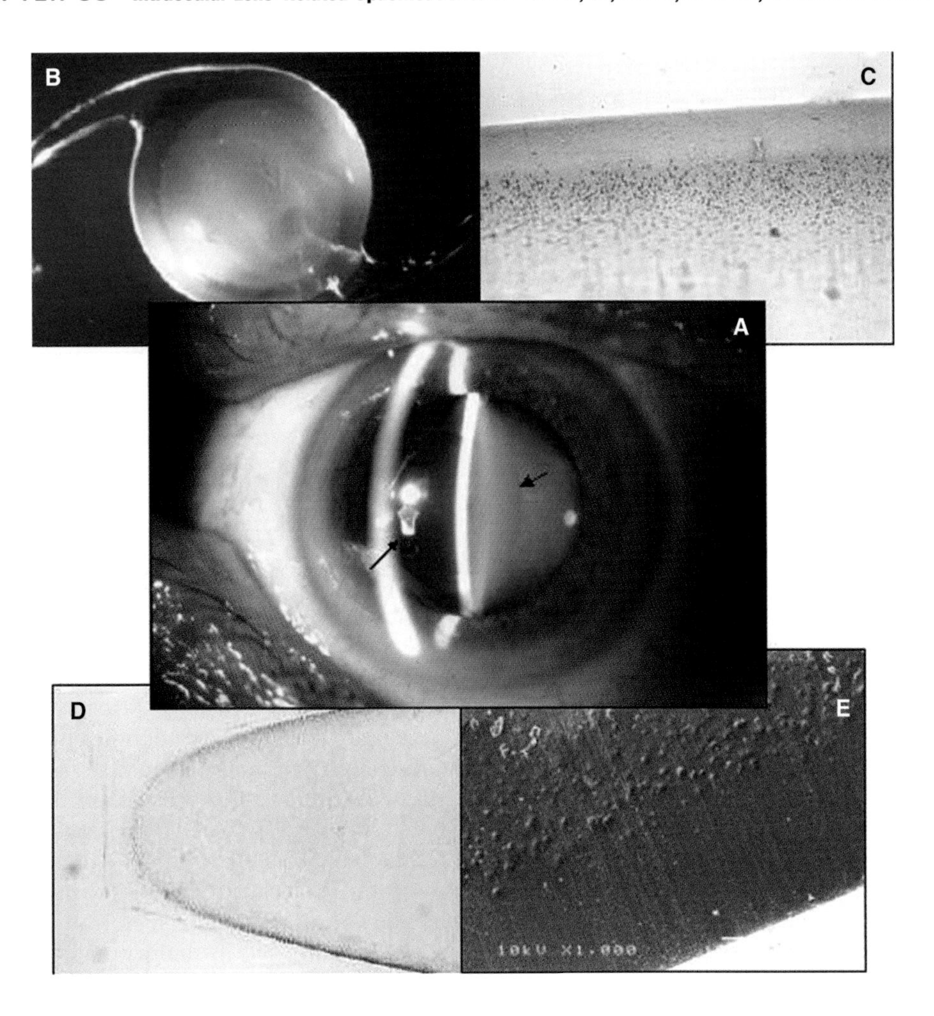

FIGURE 38-8 Opacification of SC60B-OUV IOLs. **A,** Clinical photograph of an implanted SC60B-OUV lens. The surgeon noted that the optic of the lens actually resembled a cataract. (Courtesy Dr. Mahmoud Soliman, Cairo, Egypt.) Arrows indicate the edge of capsulorhexis. **B,** Gross photograph of an explanted SC60B-OUV lens showing the central opacified optic area and an approximately 1-mm-wide clear band subtending the optic. The IOL haptics are also clear. **C,** Photomicrograph of a cut section of the lens optic (sagittal view) of an explanted SC60B-OUV lens showing the distribution of the deposits within its substance. The deposits stain positive with alizarin red. (Alizarin red; original magnification ×200.) **D,** Photomicrograph from a histologic sagittal section of the lens optic of an explanted SC60B-OUV lens showing the deposits that stained positive (dark brown-black) with the von Kossa method. (von Kossa stain; original magnification ×40.) **E,** Scanning electron photomicrograph from the cut section of the optic of an explanted SC60B-OUV lens. Note the presence of multiple granular deposits distributed in a line parallel to the external optical surfaces.

carbon and oxygen. EDS analysis of the deposits from the specimen obtained from one case, coated with aluminum, also demonstrated the presence of peaks of Ca and phosphate.

Three separate tests—the alizarin red stain, the von Kossa stain, and SEM analyses with EDS—strongly suggest that the granules are at least in part composed of Ca. Coating a specimen with aluminum instead of gold-palladium enhanced identification of the substances by EDS. EDS analysis of the former demonstrated the presence of Ca and phosphates peaks. This suggests that the deposits within the IOL optics are composed of hydroxyapatite. Hydroxyapatite is the thermodynamically stable phase of Ca phosphate in biologic systems. EDS demonstrated the presence of Ca peaks only at the level of the deposits, not in the center of the optic and not in the region immediately subjacent to the surface.

Frohn et al.[60] have studied explants of this IOL model and have noted that the opacification within the optics may be related to the presence of unbound UV absorbers (monomers). According to these researchers, spectroscopic findings indicated premature aging of the UV blocking agent incorporated in the lens biomaterial. Indeed, the material of these IOLs, composed of a cross-linked copolymer of poly 2-HEMA and methyl methacrylate (MMA), does contain an incorporated UV absorber that functions to protect the retina from UV radiation in the 300- to 400-nm range. This range of protection is normally provided by the crystalline lens. Their findings and the calcification process demonstrated by us may be correlated, although our data do not allow us to make definitive conclusions.

At the time of this writing, we are in the process of analyzing 24 more IOLs of the same model that we recently have received in our center from different countries. In rare cases, the opacification was observed as early as 3 months postoperatively. Also, in some cases the opacification extended toward the haptics, which were completely opacified in one case. As noted before, a large percentage of the patients appeared to be diabetic.

Summary

Analysis of explanted SC60B-OUV lenses because of opacification has demonstrated the cause to be the presence of granular deposits within the optics. The mechanism is not fully understood. The opacification does not seem to be directly related to substances used during the surgery because it always occurred in the late postoperative period. The possibility of a patient-related factor, such as a metabolic imbalance, cannot be ruled in or out. We have noted material positive for Ca in the deposits,[57] and Frohn et al.[60] have noted unbound UV-absorber monomers. Further biochemical studies are necessary to reveal the complete biochemical profile of these alterations. It is now important to carefully follow clinical outcomes of this lens to ensure that this phenomenon will disappear following this change in polymer source.

Glistening of the AcrySof IOL

Introduction

Glistening related to the AcrySof IOL (Figure 38-9) is well described in the literature as an acute onset of intralenticular, small, refractile, fluid-filled vacuoles present inside the optic of the Alcon AcrySof.[61,62] Glistenings have been reported to occur as soon as 1 week after surgery. The occurrence of some degree of glistening formation has been reported in all eyes implanted with an AcrySof lens for at least 6 months postoperatively. Some authors could not find a statistically significant relationship between the time and severity of glistenings. However, 93% of the IOLs that had more than trace glistenings had been in the eye for more than 1 year postoperatively.[62] Mitooka and associates reported a prevalence of nearly 60% glistening formation 4 to 22 months postoperatively in 144 patients with AcrySof IOLs (K. Mitooka, MD, et al: Poster presented at the Symposium on Cataract, IOL and Refractive Surgery, Seattle, Wash., April 1999).

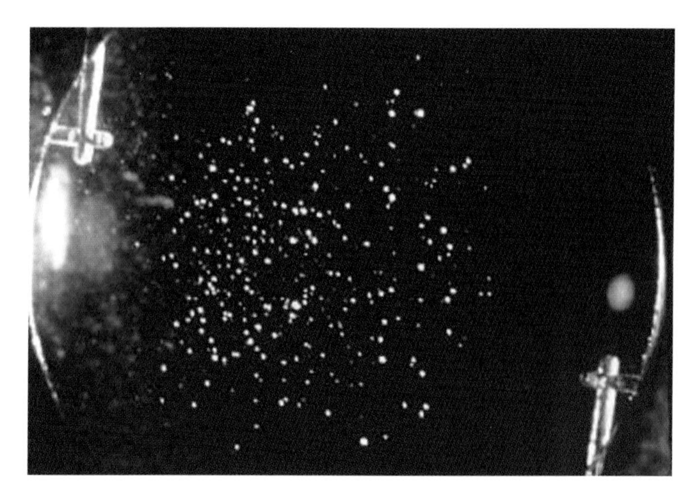

FIGURE 38-9 Gross photograph showing the glistenings within an AcrySof IOL.

Pathogenesis

In vitro studies have suggested that the occurrence of glistenings (microvacuoles) in AcrySof IOLs may be related to variations in the temperature (Δt). The formation of vacuoles within the submersed acrylic polymer is observed when there is a transient increase in temperature above the glass transition temperature, which is approximately 18.5° C for AcrySof (Apple DJ: Clinicopathological correlation of vacuoles in an acrylic IOL. Best paper of the session, presented at the ASCRS Symposium on Cataract, IOL and Refractive Surgery, April 1998, San Diego, Calif.). Glistenings may subsequently form from anterior chamber fluid. The vacuoles have the characteristics of fluid rather than air bubbles.

Another in vitro study has demonstrated that when maintained at a constant temperature, Wagon Wheel (WW) packaged IOLs showed no glistening formation, and the AcryPak (AP) packaged IOLs showed significant glistening formation.[62] Glistenings were noted with WW packaged IOLs only under fluctuating temperature conditions. It has been reported that the IOL packaging, the AP packaging, and the sterilization technique used with that system may have made the IOL susceptible to the microvacuole formation. In vitro studies have also demonstrated that the temperature at which the IOLs were stored and shipped in the dry state had no influence on the glistenings and was thus unrelated to this phenomenon. In another in vitro study, glistenings initially progressed in size and density, gradually stabilizing in size with increasing density throughout the study period.[63]

The voluntary withdrawal of the AP packaged IOLs seems to have cured the glistening problem for this lens. However, in a recent retrospective study, Christiansen et al.[64] have reported the appearance of glistenings in many patients with the AcrySof IOL even after the change to the WW packaged IOLs.

Impact on Visual Function

Clinical studies on the AcrySof IOL have demonstrated that contrast sensitivity has been decreased in some patients, but clinically significant decrease on VA in association with glistenings has been rare. However, a recent study has demonstrated a statistically significant difference in VA between eyes with mild and severe glistening,[62] but for glare and contrast sensitivity, no significant difference was found.

Summary

Glistening or vacuoles are described in the literature as acute onset of intralenticular, small, refractile, fluid-filled vacuoles inside the optic of the Alcon AcrySof IOL.[61-65] It has been reported to occur as early as 1 week postoperatively. Although initially reported to occur with only the AP packaging system, recently literature has reported its occurrence with WW packaging also.

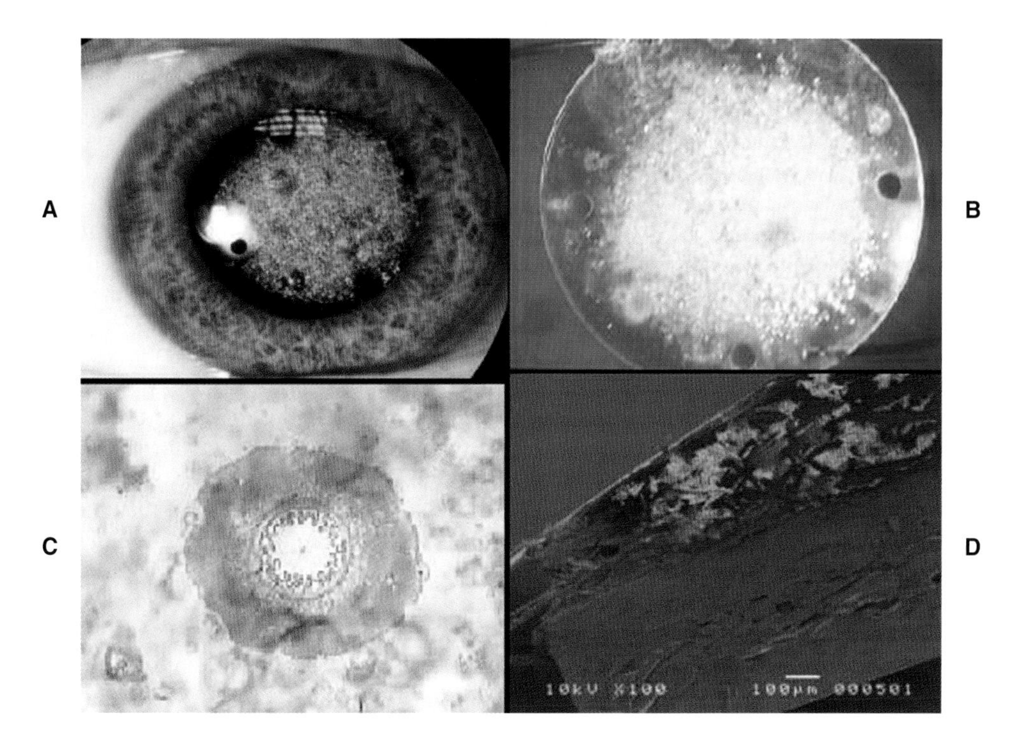

FIGURE 38-10 Snowflake" or crystalline opacification of PMMA IOLs. **A,** Clinical picture of an eye implanted with a PMMA IOL. Note the dense lesions covering the central part of the IOL optic. The peripheral optic protected by the iris is clear of the lesions. **B,** Gross photograph of a rigid three-piece PMMA lens affected with snowflake degradation, demonstrating that most of the involvement is within the central core of the lens optic, with sparing of the outer periphery of the optic. **C,** High-power three-dimensional light photomicrograph of a rigid three-piece PMMA lens affected with snowflake degradation showing an individual snowflake lesion. There is an empty central space containing few particles of PMMA convoluted material (fragmented PMMA) surrounded by a dense outer pseudocapsule. **D,** Scanning electron microscopic analysis of the cut edge of one affected lens shows that lesions are present within the one third of the anterior stroma of the optic; the posterior part remains free of lesions.

"Snowflake" or Crystalline Opacification of PMMA IOL Optic Biomaterial*

Introduction

PMMA was used as an optic biomaterial in Sir Harold Ridley's original IOL (manufactured by Rayner Intraocular Lenses Ltd, London, United Kingdom) and first implanted in 1949.[66] Although surgeons in the industrialized world and in selected areas in the developing world have largely transitioned to foldable IOL biomaterials, PMMA does remain in widespread use in many regions. Over the past 50 years, PMMA has been rightly considered a safe, tried and true material for IOL manufacturing with good and high-quality control. Biomaterial studies on PMMA IOL optics were rarely required. Until now, any untoward complications such as PMMA-optic material alteration or breakdown have not been seen with this material and its fabrication. However, we recently have reported gradual but progressive late postoperative alteration or destruction of PMMA optic biomaterial causing significant decrease in VA, sometimes to a severity that requires IOL explantation.

Dr. Jean Champbell sent the first explant with this phenomenon to us in 1991. Subsequently and at an increased rate over the past 4 years, 25 cases including 9 explanted IOLs were submitted to our laboratory.[10,67]

Analysis of Explanted IOLs

All of the explanted IOLs in this study were three-piece PC IOLs with rigid PMMA optical components and blue polypropylene or extruded PMMA haptics. These had been implanted in the early 1980s to early 1990s in most cases, and the clinical symptoms appeared late postoperatively, about 8 to 15 years after the implantation. The clinical, gross, light, and electron microscopic profiles of all the cases showed almost identical findings, differing only in the degree of intensity of the "snowflake" lesions that in turn reflected the severity and probably the duration of the opacification. In the early stages of many of the cases, the lesions were first noted clinically by a routine slit lamp examination, in the absence of visual disturbances. Most examiners described the white-brown opacities within the IOL optics as "crystalline deposits" (Figure 38-10, A). They appeared to progress gradually in most cases. Clinically, the slowly progressive opacities of the IOL optics usually start as scattered white-brown spots within

*Based on the original work presented by Apple DJ, Peng Q, Arthur SN et al: Snowflake degeneration of polymethyl methacrylate posterior chamber intraocular lens optic material: a newly described clinical condition caused by an unexpected late opacification of polymethyl methacrylate, *Ophthalmology* 109:1666-1675, 2002.

the substance of the IOL optic. These usually do not have an impact on the patients' VA. They gradually increase in intensity and number, eventually reaching a point where the VA loss necessitates removal or exchange of the IOL. In addition to visual loss, the symptoms included decrease in contrast sensitivity and various visual disturbances and aberrations, including glare.

The snowflake lesions were most commonly observed in the central and midperipheral portion of the IOL optics (see Figure 38-10, *B*). The peripheral 0.5- to 1-mm rim of the lens optic appeared to be free of opacification. Views of the cut edges of the bisected optic specimens prepared for SEM confirmed that the snowflake lesions were all within the substance of the IOL. Many were focal and discrete, with intervening clear areas, but some appeared coalescent. In at least some cases there was an uninvolved space between the front IOL surface and the actual lesions, which involved the anterior one third of the optic's substance. The opacifications showed no birefringence in polarized light. All histochemical and EDS analyses were negative, indicating no infiltration of exogenous material. Although various miscellaneous changes, such as surface protein depositions, were noted on some cases, SEM revealed that no other surface changes correlated with the opacification could be identified. Confocal microscopy of one IOL confirmed the spherical (circular) nature of the lesions as observed under light microscopy and SEM (see Figure 38-10, *C* and *D*). Under higher magnification, the individual opacities revealed a distinct pattern consisting of a pseudocapsule surrounding the core of the lesion, which appeared to be "empty" except for the fragments of convoluted material. The examinations performed to identify the nature of the deposits, including EDS, did not document any exogenous chemicals apart from the lens optic's PMMA itself. High-power three-dimensional light microscopy and SEM of bisected IOL optics were the most informative examinations with regard to illustrating the structural nature of the opacifications.

Mechanism of Action

The manufacturing variations in some lenses fabricated in the 1980s to early 1990s, especially those made with molding processes (injection, compression, cast), may be responsible for the snowflake lesions. PMMA is a polymer of MMA. It is manufactured by additional polymerization using the MMA monomer, the process being started by an initiator substance.[68-70] A frequently used initiator is azo-*bis*-isobutyryl nitrile (ABIN). It can be postulated that PMMA disruption might be related to a specific manufacturing problem, such as leaving the residual initiator substance (ABIN) embedded in the substance of the PMMA optic. This can occur during a molding process. The two double-bonded units of the ABIN initiator may be broken by gradual UV stimulation, with a release of nitrogen gas (N_2). Either heat or UV light exposure can cause such gas formation. Indeed the normal polymerization process for PMMA synthesis in part consists of a heat-induced N_2 formation. During this normal process the N_2 escapes from the mixture. However, with a poor manufacturing process, for example, using excessive initiator more than the fractional amount required, unwanted initiator might be entrapped in the PMMA substance. Therefore the double bonds of the initiator might leave to a continuous UV radiation, thereby releasing gaseous N_2 within the PMMA substance. This would explain the formation of loculated cavitations in the lesions, in which the outer pseudocapsule consists of PMMA material compressed outwardly from the cavity, the central spaces containing the N_2 gas, and the convoluted material within the spaces consisting of disrupted PMMA. Because there is no route for aqueous ingress into the optic (e.g., pores), a permeation of aqueous into the parenchyma forming the cavities is unlikely. The molding procedure, in which each mold is made one at a time, would more likely be prone to manufacturing problems within the individual molds.

Two pathologic observations of the snowflake phenomenon suggest that the lesions may be sensitive to long-term solar (UV) exposure. First, opacities are often situated in the center of the optic, extending to the midperipheral portion but often leaving the distal peripheral rim free of the opacities. Furthermore, the opacities are present most commonly and intensely on the anterior one third of the IOL's thickness, the stratum that might be expected to have more interaction with UV radiation.

Although UV radiation might be a contributing factor, the exact pathogenesis as of now only can be hypothesized. Potential causes of the development of a snowflake lesion include poor filtrations of the precured monomeric components (MMA, UV blocker, thermal initiator); nonhomogeneous dispersement of the UV chromophore and/or thermal initiator into the polymer chain; excessive thermal energy during the curing process, leaving voids in the polymer matrix; and insufficient post-annealing of the cured PMMA polymer.

These hypothetical mechanisms have the potential to form microheterogeneity within the PMMA polymer that, over time and potentially with exposure to UV radiation, could result in a lesion within the polymer. Additional experimentation is necessary to determine if any of these proposed mechanisms for the formation of a snowflake lesion are realized.

Summary

As a footnote to the description of this condition, these late-occurring lesions may be viewed as representing a "time bomb" effect, indeed so designated by some authorities in the 1990s. This syndrome, referred to as snowflake opacification, occurs unexpectedly long after the implantation and in some ways provides a partial vindication of those who spoke with concern about this possibility. Therefore today's ophthalmologists must be aware of, diagnose, and know when to explant and exchange these lenses. Recognizing the nature of this syndrome is important to spare patients and their doctors unwarranted worries about the cause of visual problems or loss and also to obviate unwarranted diagnostic testing. Awareness of this delayed complication may also be warranted in developing countries, where PMMA IOLs are still used in the majority of cases. Virtually all IOLs manufactured today seem to be satisfactory. However, many such early designs from American manufacturers, as described in this report, have been delivered to the developing world over the years, sometimes implanted without regard to expiration dates on the packaging. It would be very unfortunate to see this complication showing up in underprivileged areas where patients have little resources for managing this type of visual loss or blindness.

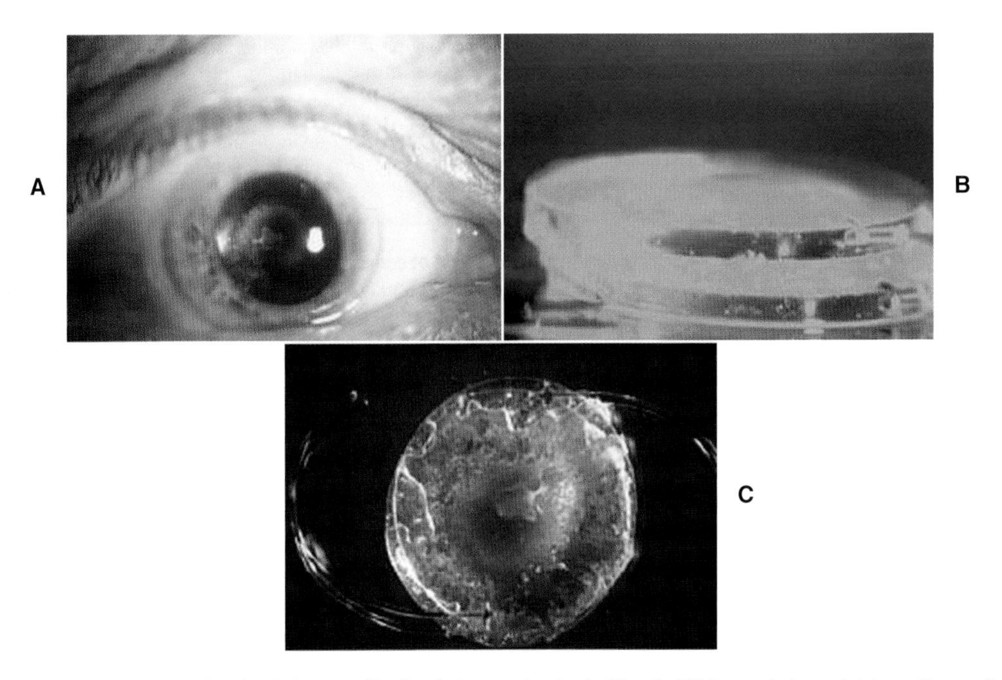

FIGURE 38-11 Interlenticular opacification between piggyback IOLs. **A,** Slit lamp photograph taken after pupil dilation, showing the opacification between the lenses, 27 months postoperatively. **B,** Gross photograph from a pair of explanted piggyback lenses (sagittal view) showing the membranelike formation sandwiched between the lenses. **C,** Frontal view of the same pair of lenses. Note the white opacification between the two implants. There are some clear areas, including the central zone, where a depression on the anterior surface of the anterior lens can be observed.

Interlenticular Opacification of "Piggyback" IOLS*

Introduction

One of the most important complications related to the implantation of multiple PC IOLs (piggyback IOL or polypseudophakia) is interlenticular opacification (ILO), also named interpseudophakos Elschnig pearls or "red rock syndrome" (Stasiuk R: "Red rock syndrome: interlenticular opacification with piggyback IOL implantation. Presented at the ESCRS Symposium on Cataract, IOL and Refractive Surgery, September 1999, Vienna, Austria).[71-75] Together with surgeons performing piggyback implantation, we have been devoting constant efforts to determine the pathogenesis and management of this complication.[7,74-76] Recently we have proposed clinical and pathologic lessons for prevention and management of this entity (Pandey SK, Snyder ME, Werner L et al: Interlenticular opacification (ILO): clinical and pathological lessons for prevention and management. Prize winning video; Pandey SK, Werner L, Apple DJ et al: Interlenticular opacification after piggyback intraocular lens implantation. Best cataract poster, presented at the ASCRS Symposium on Cataract, IOL and Refractive Surgery, April-May 2001, San Diego, Calif.). The technique of piggyback IOLs is used relatively often now, and it will increase in use during the next decades. Therefore an awareness of this new condition, as well as of the surgical methods to prevent its development, is warranted.

*Based on the original work published by Gayton JL, Apple DJ, Peng Q et al: Interlenticular opacification: a clinicopathological correlation of a new complication of piggyback posterior chamber intraocular lenses, *J Cataract Refract Surg* 26:330-336, 2000; Werner L, Shugar JK, Apple DJ et al: Opacification of piggyback IOLs associated with an amorphous material attached to interlenticular surfaces, *J Cataract Refract Surg* 26:1612-1619, 2000; Werner L, Apple DJ, Pandey SK et al: Analysis of elements of interlenticular opacification, *Am J Ophthalmol* 133:320-326, 2002.

Analysis of Explanted IOLs

With the first two specimens we received in our laboratory, surgeons had exhaustively tried to clean the interface between the lenses before explantation.[74,75] However, we have recently received four new pairs of acrylic piggyback lenses explanted because of ILO. Three of these new cases shared the common aspect that exhaustive attempts to clean the interface between the lenses were not performed by the surgeons before explantation, probably because ILO is now a well-known entity. This fact allowed us to analyze new explanted piggyback lenses with all the original components of ILO in situ, which helped us better understand the pathogenesis of this complication.[76]

After macroscopic and microscopic analysis, lenses from some cases had their surfaces directly stained with H & E and were reexamined under the light microscope. The posterior lens of one case was processed for histopathologic examination (dehydration in ethanol, embedding in paraffin, section) and the resultant tissue sections were stained with H & E, PAS, and Masson's trichrome. The anterior lens of another specimen was prepared for SEM.

In our first clinicopathologic report (Dr. Gayton's cases), the opaque, membranelike material localized between the piggyback lenses (Figure 38-11) was histopathologically demonstrated to be composed of retained/regenerative cortex and proliferating lens epithelial cells, including bladder (Wedl) cells. This profile

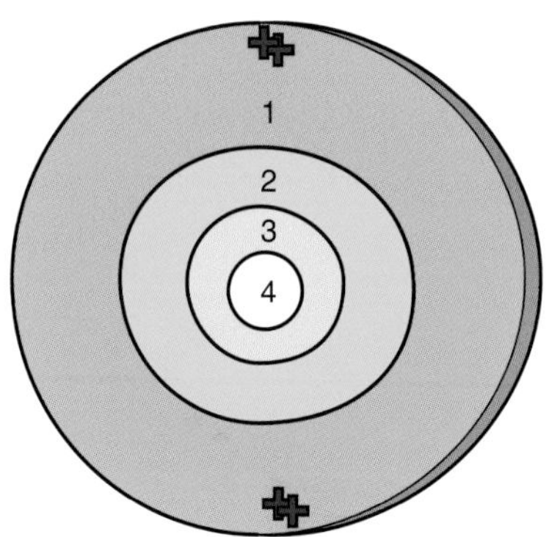

(1) Zone with thick, retained/regenerative cortical material and pearls in the peripheral interlenticular space.

(2) Zone of breakdown/degeneration of retained/regenerative cortical material and pearls, forming clusters of small round structures.

(3) Zone of compression of round structures, forming an amorphous layer.

(4) Central zone of IOL contact, presenting few or no deposits.

FIGURE 38-12 Schematic drawing representing a frontal view of a pair of AcrySof piggyback lenses. The interlenticular space was divided in four zones, according to its thickness and the aspect of the material attached to the IOLs' opposing surfaces. (Schematic drawing by Liliana Werner, MD, PhD, Charleston, SC.)

is virtually identical to the pathologic process seen in posterior subcapsular cataracts and in the typical "pearl" form of PCO.[74]

In our second report (Dr. Shugar's case), the surgeon could not aspirate the paracentral material attached mostly to the anterior surface of the posterior IOL, which was amorphous, compact, and completely acellular. He could only aspirate the pearls and retained/regenerative cortex in the peripheral interface. The cases described in the two aforementioned reports were considered as different forms of ILO at that time.[75]

However, further analysis of the lenses explanted without previous attempts to clean their opposing surfaces and thus with the ILO components in situ helped us to understand its pathogenesis.[76] It shows that the classification of ILO in different forms may be artificial. The material opacifying the interlenticular space was composed mostly of retained/regenerative cortical material in all cases. From the peripheral interface toward the central interface, the aspect of the opacifying material changed as the interlenticular space was progressively narrower. Figure 38-12 is a schematic drawing showing a frontal view of a pair of AcrySof piggyback lenses separated in the periphery and almost fused together in the center summarizes it. The material attached to the peripheral interface (zone 1), where the interlenticular space is wider was very thick. At the midperipheral interface (zone 2), the thick cortical material was broken into multiple small, round structures. At the paracentral zone (zone 3) the round structures were progressively compressed until only a flat, compact layer of an amorphous material could be observed. SEM photographs clearly demonstrated this fact. At the central interface (zone 4) where the lenses were in close opposition, almost no material could be found.[76]

Histologic sections obtained from the posterior lens in one case and stained with H & E, PAS, and Masson's trichrome demonstrated the breakdown of residual/regenerative cortical material into multiple, small globules. Compression of the globules in the paracentral area because of the narrower interlenticular space was demonstrated by SEM analysis of the posterior surface of the anterior lens in another case. EDS analysis performed on the deposits demonstrated the presence of peaks of sodium.

Pathogenesis

To date, all cases of ILO we analyzed in our laboratory seemed to be related to two PC IOLs being implanted in the capsular bag through a small capsulorhexis, with its margins overlapping the optic edge of the anterior IOL for 360 degrees. There may also be a specific interaction with the AcrySof material itself as it has been found to present adhesive properties in vitro. When two AcrySof lenses are implanted in the capsular bag, there is a bioadhesion of the anterior surface of the front lens to the anterior capsule edge and of the posterior surface of the back lens to the posterior capsule. In this scenario, the two IOLs are sequestered together with aqueous and lens epithelial cells in a hermetically closed microenvironment. The migration of the cells from the equatorial bow is then directed toward the interlenticular space (Figure 38-13). Changes in pH and oxygen content may promote liquefactive degeneration of the retained/regenerative cortical material, with the formation of clusters of small, round structures. Cortical liquefactive degeneration with the formation of "globules," similar to the round structures

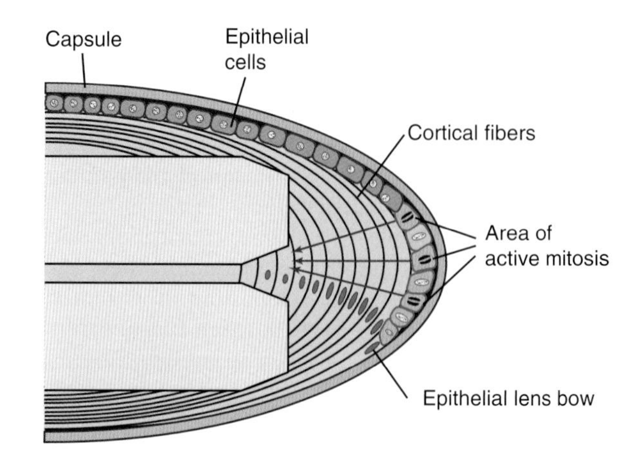

FIGURE 38-13 Schematic illustration showing two intraocular lenses placed in the capsular bag. Note the potential ingrowth of lens epithelial cells from the equatorial lens bow in the interlenticular space. (Schematic drawing by Nithi Visessook, MD, Charleston, SC.)

observed in our last few ILO cases, is an important histopathologic indication of cataractous changes.

Findl et al.[77,78] studied the morphologic appearance and size of contact zones of piggyback IOLs. Changes in the morphology and the size of the contact zone of the piggyback IOLs of different materials and optic designs were analyzed prospectively. The contact zone between the anterior and posterior IOLs was photodocumented from day 1 to 1 year after surgery using specular microscopy. A contact zone was present with all IOL materials studied. The area of contact, however, differed significantly. With PMMA IOLs, the contact zone was small and surrounded by Newton rings, indicating the tiny gap between the IOLs. With IOLs of soft material, such as silicone and hydrogel, it was larger than with PMMA IOLs and had a slightly irregular shape. With foldable acrylic IOLs, it was regular, round, and slightly larger than with the other soft materials. The contact area enlarged primarily during the first 3 months after surgery. After 1 year, two eyes with acrylic piggyback IOLs had a membrane formation around the contact zone, and two eyes developed Elschnig pearls between the IOLs. Contact area enlargement appears to be induced by capsular shrinkage.

Surgical Prevention

Based on the common features of ILO cases, some surgical methods were proposed for its prevention (Figure 38-14). The first option would be to implant both IOLs in the capsular bag but with a relatively large-diameter capsulorhexis. In this scenario, there is a possibility that the cut edge of the rhexis may fuse with the posterior capsule. This should help sequester the

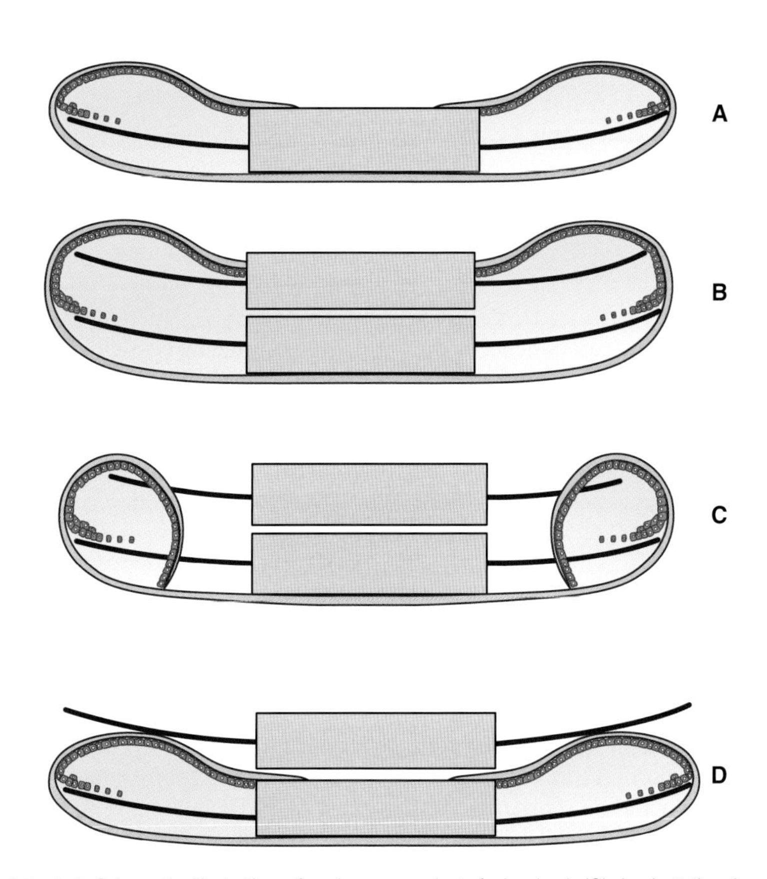

FIGURE 38-14 Schematic illustration of various scenarios of piggyback IOL implantation (suggested by the authors and other surgeons in consultation, including Johnny L. Gayton, MD, Paul Ernest, MD, and Ron Stasiuk, MD). IOL optic = gray; IOL haptic = blue; lens capsule and retained/proliferative equatorial cells = red. With the Alcon AcrySof IOL the anterior lens epithelial cells usually atrophy, and the capsule adheres to the anterior capsule. (Schematic drawing by Beau B. Evans, BM, Charleston, SC.) **A,** Control: Implantation of a single IOL with a relatively small CCC. The cut edge of the CCC is in contact with the anterior surface of the IOL optic. **B,** Piggyback IOLs: Both IOLs implanted are in the capsular bag with a relatively small-diameter CCC. The edge of the CCC rests in the front of the IOL optic. This sequesters both lenses totally within the capsular bag compartment. With this scenario, retained/proliferative equatorial lens epithelial cells have direct access to the interlenticular space (ILS). **C,** Piggyback IOLs: Both IOLs implanted are in the capsular bag but with a relatively larger-diameter CCC. In this scenario, the cut edge of the CCC possibly may fuse with the posterior capsule as shown here. This fusion process should help sequester the retained/proliferative equatorial lens epithelial cells within the equatorial fornix and prohibit growth toward the ILS. This should thus lessen the likelihood of migration of cells into this space. **D,** Piggyback IOLs: The posterior (rear) IOL is implanted in the capsular bag with the cut edge of the relatively small-diameter CCC resting on its anterior optical surface. The anterior (front) IOL is placed in the ciliary sulcus, anterior to the CCC. Retained/proliferative lens epithelial cells are confined to the compartment of the capsular bag around the rear IOL, but the ILS in front of the CCC is sequestered with this scenario.

retained/proliferated equatorial lens epithelial cells within the equatorial fornix. The other possibility is to implant the anterior IOL in the sulcus and the posterior IOL in the bag with a small rhexis. The rhexis margin will adhere to the anterior surface of the posterior IOL, and the cells within the equatorial fornix will also be sequestered. Careful follow-up of the cases implanted using these techniques will indicate their effectiveness in the prevention of ILO. We have recently evaluated the efficacy of the second surgical option. Dr. M. Edward Wilson from Charleston, SC, implanted piggyback AcrySof lenses in infantile eyes to manage the changing refractive status of these patients. This procedure, called "temporary polypseudophakia," may help in the prevention and treatment of amblyopia by avoiding residual hyperopia. The posterior lens is implanted in the capsular bag through a capsulorhexis that is smaller than the IOL optic, and the anterior lens is implanted in the ciliary sulcus. Within 12 to 24 months after the primary surgical procedure, the lens implanted in the ciliary sulcus is explanted and exchanged. To date, 15 infantile eyes have had this procedure performed successfully without significant clinical complications, and 7 AcrySof lenses have already been explanted. After almost 2 years of follow-up, no significant ILO was observed in any of these cases.[79]

Summary

Analyses of new ILO cases in which all the components of the opacifying material were in situ allowed us to confirm that the pathogenesis of this complication is similar to that of PCO. The aspect of this material varies according to the space available in the interlenticular interface. Surgeons should be aware that careful cortical cleanup is mandatory in piggyback IOL implantation.

Posterior Capsule Opacification*

Introduction

PCO has been well known since ECCE was introduced in cataract surgery. Indeed Ridley noted it in his very first IOL implantation. PCO was the most common complication of cataract surgery.[66,80] It occurred at an incidence of between 30% to 50% through the 1980s and early 1990s, when the surgical importance of cortical and cell cleanup was less understood than it is now.[81] In a 1998 meta-analysis, PCO rates of 11.8% after 1 year, 20.7% after 3 years, and 28.4% after 5 years have been reported.[82] However, the incidence of PCO is rapidly decreasing. Dr. David Spalton (London, United Kingdom) has rightly mentioned that "PCO was a disease of 2000." Our current data show that with modern surgical techniques, IOL designs, and materials, the Nd:YAG laser treatment rate for PCO is decreasing downward to a rate of single digits.[83-90] The validity of this observation can be at least partially verified and documented by tying the information and conclusions gained from clinical studies with the PCO/Nd:YAG laser data.

Pathogenesis

Although all of the lens epithelial cells are a continuous single cell line, in terms of function and pathologic processes, it is useful to divide these into two different functional groups: the A cells and the E cells. The primary type of response of the A cells to any stimulus is to proliferate and form fibrous tissue by undergoing fibrous metaplasia, sometimes called "pseudofibrous metaplasia" by Font and Brownstein.[17] The E cells comprise the germinal cells, which are the primary cells in the origin of PCO. They normally migrate centrally from the lens equator and contribute to the formation of the nucleus, epinucleus, and cortex throughout life. E cells are the primary source of the pearl form of PCO. In contrast to the A cells, which, when disturbed, tend to remain in place and not migrate, the E cells of the equatorial lens bow tend to migrate posteriorly along the posterior capsule. Therefore the term *PCO* is a misnomer. It is not the capsule that opacifies. The opaque membrane ensues as retained cells proliferate and migrate onto the posterior capsule. The resulting opacity usually takes one or two morphologic forms or a mixture of the two. The first is clusters of swollen, opacified epithelial "pearls" or clusters of proliferated and posterior migrated E cells (bladder or Wedl cells). It is probable that both the A and the E cells have the capability to contribute to the pearl form of PCO, as well as the second form, the fibrous form. A cells probably are more implicated in the pathogenesis of the fibrotic form of PCO because the primary type of response of these cells is fibrous metaplasia. Although the preferred type of growth of the E cells is in the direction of bullouslike bladder (Wedl) cells, they may also contribute to the formation of the fibrous form of PCO by undergoing a fibrous metaplasia. The E cells within the Soemmerring's ring are the source of PCO in most cases. Therefore it is important to note that Soemmerring's ring is a direct precursor to PCO. If surgeons were able to prevent Soemmerring's ring formation by any means, then a decrease in PCO rates would follow.

Analysis of Nd:YAG Posterior Capsulotomy Rates in Rigid and Foldable IOL Designs

Table 38-6 shows the ranking of the Nd:YAG laser posterior capsulotomy rates for eight lens designs as of December, 2000, with the lens showing the lowest percentage at the top and the highest rate at the bottom (Figure 38-15). Note that the four lenses with the lowest rates ranging between 3.3% and 20.7% are modern designs mostly implanted after 1992, in contrast to the four lenses with the higher rates ranging between 23.3% and 33.7%. These were all older designs, already in the database before 1992. The difference in the Nd:YAG laser rates between the acrylic IOLs and the other IOL types was found to be

*Based on the original work published by Apple DJ, Solomon KD, Tetz MR et al: Posterior capsule opacification, *Surv Ophthalmol* 37:73-116, 1992; Apple DJ, Peng Q, Visessook N et al: Surgical prevention of posterior capsule opacification. Part 1: How are we progressing in eliminating this complication of cataract surgery? *J Cataract Refract Surg* 26:180-187, 2000; Part 2: Enhancement of cortical clean up by increased emphasis and focus on the hydrodissection procedure, *J Cataract Refract Surg* 26:188-197, 2000; Part 3: The intraocular lens barrier effect as a second line of defense, *J Cataract Refract Surg* 26:198-213, 2000; Apple DJ, Peng Q, Visessook N et al: Eradication of posterior capsule opacification: documentation of a marked decrease in neodymium:yttrium-aluminium-garnet laser posterior capsulotomy rates noted in an analysis of 5416 pseudophakic human eyes obtained postmortem, *Ophthalmology* 108:505-518, 2001.

TABLE 38-6
Nd: YAG Rate (%) January 1, 1988 to December 31, 2000

IOL	Total	Nd: YAG	YAG %	IOL	Total	Nd: YAG	YAG %
Three-piece acrylic-PMMA (AcrySof)	361	12	3.3	All lenses since January 1988	6425	1892	29.4%
Three-piece silicone-PMMA	110	16	14.5	Foldable lenses	1109	170	15.3%
One-piece silicone plate, large hole	85	13	15.3	Rigid lenses	5316	1722	32.3%
Three-piece silicone-polyimide	82	17	20.7				
Three-piece silicone-prolene	347	81	23.3				
One-piece silicone, plate, small hole	124	31	25.0				
One-piece all-PMMA (rigid)	2128	647	30.4				
Three-piece PMMA (rigid)	3188	1075	33.7				

IOL, Intraocular lens; *Nd: YAG,* neodymium:yttrium = aluminum = garnet; *PMMA,* polymethylmethacrylate.

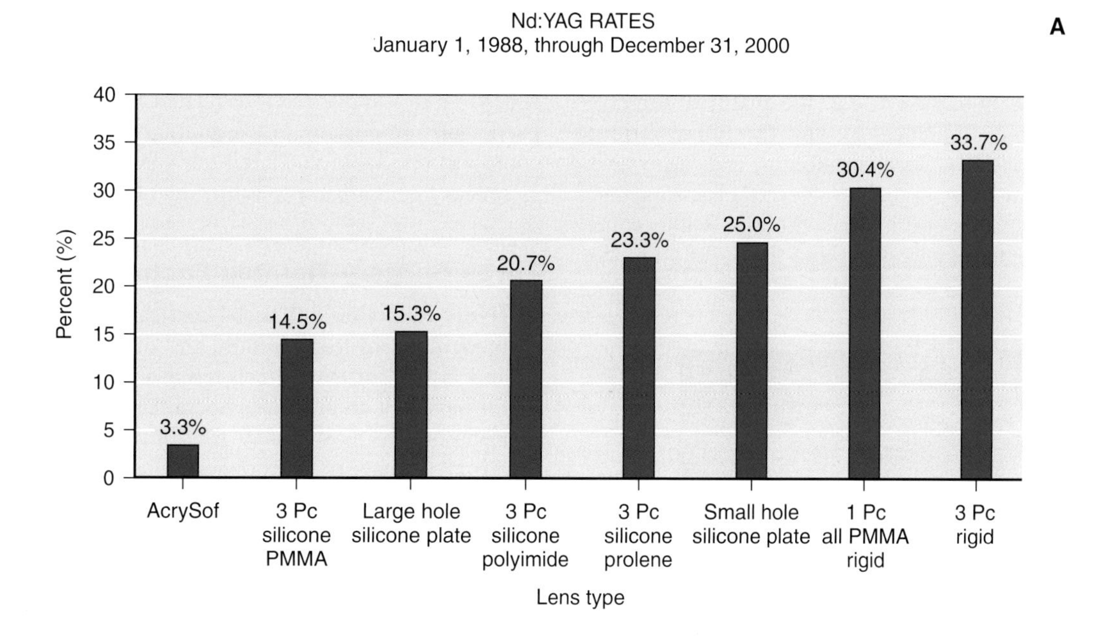

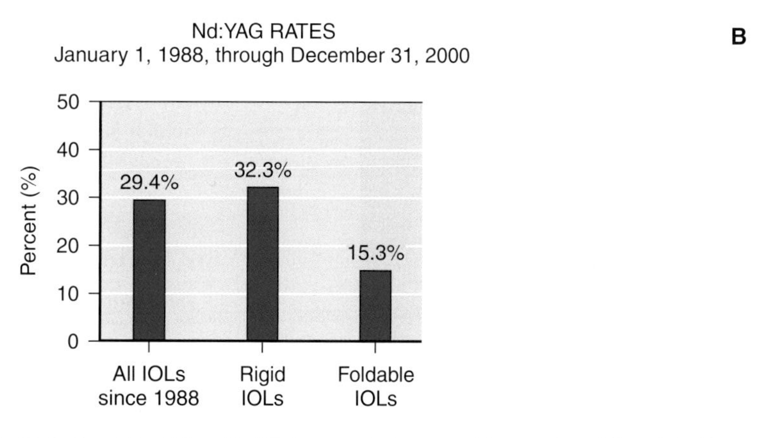

FIGURE 38-15 A, Bar graph showing relative Nd:YAG laser posterior capsulotomy rates of the eight IOLs described in this chapter. Note the low rate (3.3%) of the acrylic-PMMA (Alcon AcrySof) lens. The four lenses with the lowest rates were all relatively new, compared with the four lenses with the highest rates. This suggests that the differences in Nd:YAG laser rates between the two groups at least in part relate to variations in surgical technique, with obvious information on small-incision surgery helping create the efficient results of the newer lenses. **B,** Nd:YAG posterior capsulotomy rate of all lenses in this study was 29.4%. The rate of the rigid lenses was 32.3%. Note, in sharp contrast, that the rate for the foldable lenses taken together was only 15.3%. This efficacious result is based on the combination of high-quality modern "capsular" surgery associated with high-quality modern foldable IOLs.

statistically significant (p <0.05, for all comparisons, Chi square test). The Nd:YAG laser rate of all six foldable IOLs collectively, 15.3% (170/1109), was significantly lower than the rate of the rigid IOLs (Figure 38-16) (32.3%; 1722/5316; p <0.05, Chi square test). If the AcrySof IOL is removed from the group, the rate noted amongst the other foldable IOLs studied increases to 158/748 (21.1%).

To evaluate the influence of lens quality versus the influence of the surgical technique on the PCO/Nd:YAG laser posterior capsulotomy rates, it is useful to follow a trend line over a long-term period. Under optimal conditions, but not possible in this analysis, the information should be viewed considering the age and the duration of each implant. However, the dates of implantation or the time between implantation and death were difficult to determine because of ethical considerations. These variables are going to factor out over time as larger numbers are obtained and the "trend time line" is extended.

Tracking the trend time lines for each lens design will be necessary to help rule out other factors in addition to the duration of each implant in the eye (e.g., the quality of surgery) to properly assess the differences among the IOLs. Various surgeons' criteria for Nd:YAG laser capsulotomy (e.g., aggressive, conservative) also play a role in the rate. Nevertheless surgeons' criteria, surgical technique, and implant duration will become equalized as the number of accessions and the duration of the study increase.

A

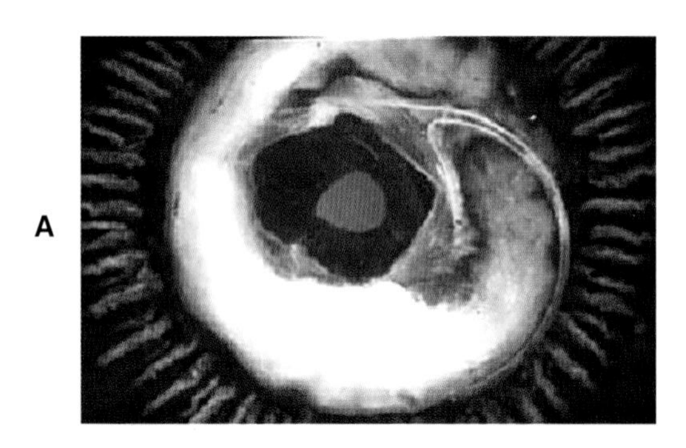

B

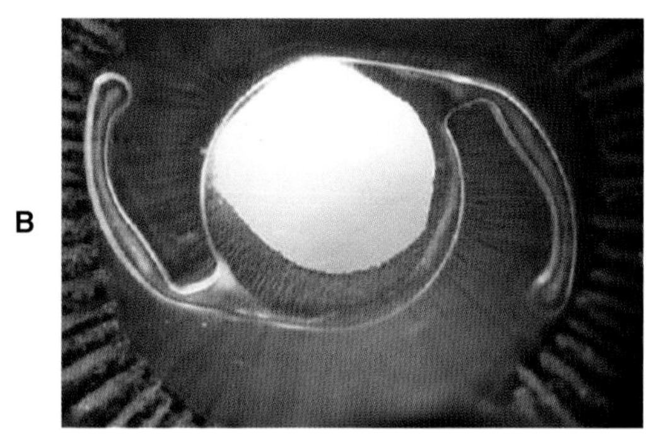

FIGURE 38-16 Posterior capsule opacification. **A,** Miyake-Apple view of a rigid one-piece PMMA IOL in situ, following Nd:YAG capsulotomy. Note the polygonal rim of the capsulotomy and the dense aspect of the PCO. **B,** Miyake-Apple view of a foldable one-piece Alcon AcrySof lens showing excellent centration and clarity of the media with perfect symmetric in-the-bag fixation. There is slight contact of the iris at the upper left edge of the IOL optic, but otherwise this represents an excellent result. This is the first pseudophakic human eye obtained postmortem implanted with this design that we received in our center, as it has only recently been introduced in the market.

Two Principles of PCO Prevention

The principles of PCO prevention can be subdivided into two categories:

1. **Primary line of defense:** The first line of defense is to minimize the number of retained/regenerated cells and cortex in the capsular bag.
2. **Secondary line of defense:** If some cells do remain, the barrier effect works as a second line of defense and helps to prevent PCO by blocking the growth of the cells from the equatorial region toward the center of the visual axis.

After conducting several experimental studies on the pathogenesis and treatment of PCO and after compiling information derived from other laboratories and clinical studies from several centers worldwide, we have ascertained various factors that help bring about the very positive conclusion that surgeons now have the sufficient tools and appropriate IOLs to help reduce the incidence of PCO.[11,83-90]

Although all steps of the cataract operation are important in reducing any complication, we have identified three surgery-related factors and three IOL-related factors that stand out as particularly important in preventing or at least delaying this complication (Table 38-7). It is our goal to show that all of these factors as a unit are key to achieving PCO reduction.

Three Surgery-Related Factors to Reduce PCO

1. **Hydrodissection-enhanced cortical cleanup:** With careful, meticulous hydrodissection, the operation is much easier and faster, cortex and cell removal is more thorough, and formation of an unwanted Soemmerring's ring is minimized. Recently, we have shown this important additional long-term advantage of hydrodissection, namely, a means of more efficient removal of cortex and cells, that in turn is essential in reducing PCO.[88]
2. **In-the-bag (capsular) fixation:** The hallmark of modern cataract surgery is the achievement of consistent and secure in-the-bag (capsular) fixation. The most obvious advantage of in-the-bag fixation is the sequestration of the IOL from adjacent uveal tissues. This is also extremely important in reducing the amount of PCO. The primary function of in-the-bag fixation is enhancing the IOL-optic barrier effect, which is functional and maximal when the lens optic is fully

TABLE 38-7
Six Factors to Reduce PCO

Three Surgery-Related Factors "Capsular" Surgery	Three IOL-Related Factors "Ideal" IOL
1. Hydrodissection-enhanced cortical cleanup	1. Biocompatible IOL to reduce stimulation of cellular proliferation
2. In-the-bag fixation	2. Maximal IOL optic–posterior capsule contact, angulated haptic, "adhesive" biomaterial to create a "shrink wrap"
3. Small CCC with edge on IOL surface	3. IOL optic geometry, square truncated edge

CCC, Continuous curvilinear capsulorhexis; *IOL,* intraocular lens; *PCO,* posterior capsule opacification.

in-the-bag with direct contact with the posterior capsule. In case one or both haptics are not placed in the bag, a potential space is created, allowing an avenue for cells to grow posteriorly toward the visual axis.

3. **Capsulorhexis edge on IOL surface:** A less obvious but significant addition to precise in-the-bag fixation is creating a CCC diameter slightly smaller than that of the IOL optic. For example, if the IOL optic were 6 mm, the capsulorhexis diameter would ideally be slightly smaller, perhaps 5 to 5.5 mm. This places the cut anterior capsule edge on the anterior surface of the optic, providing a tight fit (analogous to a "shrink wrap"), therefore helping to sequester the optic in the capsular bag from the surrounding aqueous humor. This mechanism may protect the milieu within the capsule from at least some potentially deleterious factors within the aqueous, especially some macromolecules, and some inflammatory mediators. The concept of capsular sequestration based on the CCC size and shape is subtle, but more surgeons appear to be applying this principle and seeing its advantages.

Three IOL-Related Factors to Reduce PCO

1. **Biocompatibility:** Lens material biocompatibility is an often-misunderstood term. It may be defined by many criteria, such as the ability to inhibit stimulation of epithelial cellular proliferation: the less the cell proliferation, the less the chance for secondary cataract formation. The Alcon AcrySof IOL scored well with these criteria, with respect to Soemmerring's ring formation, PCO, and ACO. In addition, the amount of cell proliferation is greatly influenced by surgical factors, such as copious cortical cleanup. Furthermore, the time factor plays a role, such as the duration of the implant in the eye. Additional long-term studies are required to assess the overall role of biocompatibility in the pathogenesis of PCO.
2. **Maximal IOL optic–posterior capsule contact:** Other contributing factors in reducing PCO are posterior angulation of the IOL haptic and posterior convexity of the optic. These are due to the creation of a shrink wrap, or a tight fit of the posterior capsule against the back of the IOL optic. The relative stickiness of the IOL optic biomaterial probably helps to produce an adhesion between the capsule and IOL optic. Preliminary evidence shows that the Alcon AcrySof IOL biomaterial provides such enhanced adhesion, or "bioadhesion,"[91,92] although further study is required.
3. **IOL optic geometry, square truncated edge:** The IOL optic barrier effect plays an important role as a second line of defense against PCO, especially in cases where retained cortex and cells remain following ECCE ("no space, no cells"). A lens with one or both haptics "out-of-the-bag" has much less of a chance to produce a barrier effect. Indeed, the IOL optic's barrier function has been one of the main reasons that PC IOLs implanted after ECCE throughout the decades did not produce an unacceptably high incidence of florid PCO. Actually, the barrier effect has enabled the success of IOL implantation after ECCE during the past decades.

A subtle difference between classic optics with a round tapered edge and optics with a square truncated edge became evident recently. The effect of a square-edge optic design as a barrier was first reported by Nishi in the rabbit model (Nishi O: Presented at the Fifteenth Congress of the European Society of Cataract and Refractive Surgeons, Prague, Czech Republic, September, 1997). In a clinicopathologic study, our laboratory was the first to confirm this phenomenon in human eyes (Apple DJ: Optic geometry in relation to posterior capsule opacification. Presented at the Chicago Ophthalmology Society, Chicago, Ill., November, 1997). We reported our results of a large histopathologic analysis covering the IOL barrier effect, with special reference to the efficacy of the truncated edge.[89] A truncated, square-edged optic rim appears to cause a complete blockade of cells at the optic edge, preventing epithelial ingrowth over the posterior capsule. The enhanced barrier effect provided by this optic geometry probably functions as an "icing on the cake." It seems to provide another reserve factor, in addition to the five aforementioned factors, contributing in diminishing the overall incidence of visually significant PCO.

Our studies up to date have shown that the Alcon AcrySof IOL best achieves the goals of these three IOL-related factors. Recently Nishi et al.[93] have reported that the AcrySof lens lost its preventive effect on PCO when the optic was rounded. According to the same authors, the effect of the AcrySof lens in preventing PCO is mainly a result of its rectangular, sharp-edged optic design. The acrylic material may play a complementary role by helping to create a sharp capsular bend. Capsular bend formation would be the key to the PCO preventive effect of the IOL. Other IOL designers are rapidly moving to provide comparable features, especially a conversion to sharp edges. A major disadvantage of the truncated edge is the possible formation of clinical visual aberration such as glare, halos, and crescents. Subtle changes in manufacturing are now helping to alleviate these complications.

Summary

A major reduction of Nd:YAG laser capsulotomy rates toward single digits is now possible because of application of these surgical factors and modern lenses, at least in the industrialized world. This will be of great benefit to patients in achieving improved long-term results and avoidance of Nd:YAG laser capsulotomy complications. Eradication of the Nd:YAG laser procedure will help control what has been the second most expensive cost to the U.S. Medicare System.

To date, we cannot precisely determine the relative proportion or contribution of IOL design versus surgical techniques to the decrease of Nd:YAG laser rates observed here. However, this could be possible with continuing analysis including annual updates and increasing numbers of pseudophakic autopsy eyes. The tools, surgical procedures, skills, and appropriate IOLs are now available to eradicate PCO. Continued motivation to apply the six factors noted in this chapter, the efficacy of which have been further suggested in a recent study, will help diminish this final major complication of cataract-IOL surgery exactly 50 years after Ridley's first encounter with this complication.

Implanting an IOL into an adult eye is an extremely successful procedure. However, decreased incidence of postoperative complications of cataract-IOL surgery led us to become complacent and less vigilant regarding assessment and careful testing of new ocular prostheses and surgical procedures. Despite the positive evolution of cataract-IOL surgery, but concurrent with this era of probably decreased vigilance, we are now unfortunately iden tifying some serious problems. Therefore ophthalmic surgeons have responded to this challenge, and continued research is ongoing that will further improve the outcome of the cataract-IOL operation and help surgeons to provide better care for patients.

REFERENCES

1. Apple DJ, Ridley H: A golden anniversary celebration and a golden age, *Arch Ophthalmol* 117:827-828, 1999 (editorial).
2. Apple DJ, Kincaid MC, Mamalis N et al: *Intraocular lenses: evolution, designs, complications, and pathology,* Baltimore, Md, 1989, Williams & Wilkins.
3. Apple DJ, Mamalis N, Loftfield K et al: Complications of intraocular lenses: a historical and histopathological review, *Surv Ophthalmol* 29:1-54, 1984.
4. Apple DJ, Reidy JJ, Mamalis N et al: A comparison of ciliary sulcus and capsular bag fixation of posterior chamber intraocular lenses, *J Am Intraocul Implant Soc* 11:44-63, 1985.
5. Mackey TA, Pandey SK, Werner L et al: Anterior capsule opacification. *Int Ophthalmol Clin* 41:17-31, 2001.
6. Arthur SN, Peng Q, Escobar-Gomez M et al: Silicone oil adherence to silicone intraocular lenses. *Int Ophthalmol Clin* 41:33-45, 2001.
7. Trivedi RH, Izak AM, Werner L et al: Interlenticular opacification of piggy-bank intraocular lenses. *Int Ophthalmol Clin* 41:47-62, 2001.
8. Izak AM, Werner L, Pandey SK et al: Calcification on the surface of the Bausch & Lomb Hydroview intraocular lens. *Int Ophthalmol Clin* 41:63-77.
9. Macky TA, Trivedi RH, Werner L et al: Degeneration of ultraviolet absorber material and calcium deposits within the optic of a hydrophilic intraocular lens. *Int. Ophthalmol Clin* 41:79-90, 2001.
10. Peng Q, Apple DJ, Arthur SN et al: Snowflake opacification of poly(methyl methacrylate) intraocular lens optic biomaterial: a newly described syndrome. *Int Ophthalmol Clin* 41:91-107, 2001.
11. Schmidbauer JM, Vargas LG, Peng Q et al: Posterior capsule opacification, *Int Ophthalmol Clin* 41:109-131, 2001.
12. Apple DJ: Center for Intraocular Lens Research transfers to Medical University of South Carolina, *J Cataract Refract Surg* 14:481-482, 1988.
13. Miyake K, Miyake C: Intraoperative posterior chamber lens haptic fixation in the human cadaver eye, *Ophthalmic Surg* 16:230-236, 1985.
14. Apple DJ, Lim E, Morgan R et al: Preparation and study of human eyes obtained postmortem with the Miyake posterior photographic technique, *Ophthalmology* 97:810-816, 1990.
15. Apple DJ, Rabb MF: *Ocular pathology: clinical applications and self-assessment,* St Louis, 1998, Mosby.
16. Apple DJ, Auffarth GU, Peng Q et al: *Foldable intraocular lenses: evolution, clinicopathologic correlation and complications,* Thorofare, NJ, 2000, Slack.
17. Font RL, Brownstein S: A light and electron microscopic study of anterior subcapsular cataracts, *Am J Ophthalmol* 78:972-984, 1974.
18. Hara T, Azuma N, Chiba K et al: Anterior capsular opacification after endocapsular cataract surgery, *Ophthalmic Surg* 23:94-98, 1992.
19. Ishibashi T, Araki H, Sugai S et al: Anterior capsule opacification in monkey eyes with posterior chamber intraocular lenses, *Arch Ophthalmol* 111: 1685-1690, 1993.
20. Ishibashi T, Araki H, Sugai S et al: Histopathologic study of anterior capsule opacification in pseudophakic eyes, *Nippon Ganka Gakkai Zasshi* 97: 460-466, 1993.
21. Gonvers M, Sickenberg M, van Melle G: Change in capsulorhexis size after implantation of three types of intraocular lenses, *J Cataract Refract Surg* 23:231-238, 1997.
22. Tsuboi S, Tsujioka M, Kusube T et al: Effect of continuous circular capsulorhexis and intraocular lens fixation on the blood-aqueous barrier, *Arch Ophthalmol* 110:1124-1127, 1992.
23. Werner L, Pandey SK, Escobar-Gomez M et al: Anterior capsule opacification: a histopathological study comparing different IOL styles, *Ophthalmology* 107:463-467, 2000.
24. Werner L, Pandey SK, Apple DJ et al: Anterior capsule opacification: correlation of pathological findings with clinical sequelae, *Ophthalmology* 108:1675-1681, 2001.
25. Davison JA: Capsule contraction syndrome, *J Cataract Refract Surg* 19: 582-589, 1993.
26. Hayashi H, Hayashi K, Nakao F et al: Anterior capsule contraction and intraocular lens dislocation in eyes with pseudoexfoliation syndrome, *Br J Ophthalmol* 82:1429-1432, 1998.
27. Hayashi K, Hayashi H, Nakao F et al: Reduction in the area of the anterior capsule opening after polymethylmethacrylate, silicone, and soft acrylic intraocular lens implantation, *Am J Ophthalmol* 123:441-447, 1997.
28. Dahlhauser KF, Wroblewski KJ, Mader TH: Anterior capsule contraction with foldable silicone intraocular lenses, *J Cataract Refract Surg* 24:1216-1219, 1998.
29. Shammas HJ: Relaxing the fibrosed capsulorhexis rim to correct induced hyperopia after phacoemulsification, *J Cataract Refract Surg* 21:228-229, 1995.
30. Mathey CF, Kohnen TB, Ensikat HJ et al: Polishing methods for the lens capsule: histology and scanning electron microscopy, *J Cataract Refract Surg* 20:64-69, 1994.
31. Nishi O: Removal of lens epithelial cells by ultrasound in endocapsular cataract surgery, *Ophthalmic Surg* 18:577-580, 1987.
32. Vasavada AR, Shastri L: Initial and definitive capsulorhexes: an extended application, *J Cataract Refract Surg* 26:634, 2000.
33. Chambless WS: Neodymium:YAG laser anterior capsulotomy and a possible new application, *J Am Intraocul Implant Soc* 11:33-34, 1985.
34. Cox MS, Trese MT, Murphy PL: Silicone oil for advanced proliferative vitreoretinopathy, *Ophthalmology* 93:648-650, 1986.
35. Lean JS, Leaver PK, Cooling RJ et al: Management of complex retinal detachments by vitrectomy and fluid/silicone exchange, *Trans Ophthalmol Soc U K* 102:203-205, 1982.
36. Apple DJ, Federman JL, Krolicki TJ et al: Irreversible silicone oil adhesion to silicone intraocular lenses: a clinicopathologic analysis, *Ophthalmology* 103:1555-1561, 1996.
37. Apple DJ, Isaacs RT, Kent DG et al: Silicone oil adhesion to intraocular lenses: an experimental study comparing various biomaterials, *J Cataract Refract Surg* 23:536-544, 1997.
38. Batterbury M, Wong D, Williams R et al: The adherence of silicone oil to standard and heparin-coated PMMA intraocular lenses, *Eye* 8:547-549, 1994.
39. Arthur SN, Peng Q, Apple DJ et al: Effect of heparin surface modification in reducing silicone oil adherence to various intraocular lenses, *J Cataract Refract Surg* 27:1662-1669, 2001.
40. Cunanan CM, Ghazizadeh M, Buchen SY et al: Contact-angle analysis of intraocular lenses, *J Cataract Refract Surg* 24:341-351, 1998.
41. Dick B, Greiner K, Magdowski G et al: Long-term stability of heparin-coated PMMA intraocular lenses: results of an in-vitro study, *Ophthalmologe* 94:920-924, 1997.
42. Langefeld S, Kirchhof B, Meinert H et al: A new way of removing silicone oil from the surface of silicone intraocular lenses, *Graefes Arch Clin Exp Ophthalmol* 237:201-206, 1999.
43. Zeana D, Schrage N, Kirchhof B et al: Silicone oil removal from a silicone intraocular lens with perfluorohexyloctane, *J Cataract Refract Surg* 26: 301-302, 2000.
44. Dick H, Augustin AJ: Solvent for removing silicone oil from intraocular lenses: experimental study comparing various biomaterials, *J Cataract Refract Surg* 26:1667-1672, 2000.
45. Hoerauf H, Menz DH, Dresp J et al: [O44-a solvent for silicone oil adhesions on intraocular lenses], *Klinische Monatsblatter fur Augenheilkunde* 214:71-76, 1999.
46. Kageyama T, Yaguchi S: Removing silicone oil droplets from the posterior surface of silicone intraocular lenses, *J Cataract Refract Surg* 26:957-959, 2000.
47. Werner L, Apple DJ, Escobar-Gomez M et al: Postoperative deposition of calcium on the surfaces of a hydrogel intraocular lens, *Ophthalmology* 107:2179-2185, 2000.
48. Apple DJ, Werner L, Escobar-Gomez M et al: Deposits on the optical surfaces of Hydroview intraocular lenses, *J Cataract Refract Surg* 26:796-797, 2000 (letter).
49. Pandey SK, Werner L, Apple DJ et al: Calcium precipitation on the surfaces of a foldable intraocular lens: a clinicopathological correlation, *Arch Ophthalmol* 120:391-393, 2001.
50. Apple DJ, Werner L, Pandey SK: Newly recognized complications of posterior chamber intraocular lenses, *Arch Ophthalmol* 119:581-582, 2001 (editorial).
51. Werner L, Apple DJ, Izak AM: Discoloration/opacification of modern foldable intraocular lens designs. In Buratto L, Werner L, Zanini M, Apple DJ, eds: Phacoemulsification: principles and techniques. Thorofare, NJ, 2002, Slack Inc., pp 659–670.
52. Murray RI: Two cases of late opacification of the Hydroview hydrogel intraocular lens, *J Cataract Refract Surg* 26:1272-1273, 2000 (letter).
53. McGee Russell SM: Histochemical methods for calcium, *J Histochem Cytochem* 6:22-42, 1958.
54. Carr LB, Rambo ON, Feichtmeir TV: A method of demonstrating calcium

in tissue sections using chloranilic acid, *J Histochem Cytochem* 9:415-417, 1961.

55. Pizzolato P: Histochemical recognition of calcium oxalate, *J Histochem Cytochem* 12:333-336, 1964.
56. Yu AFK, Shek TWH: Hydroxyapatite formation on implanted hydrogel intraocular lenses, *Arch Ophthalmol* 107:2179-2185, 2001.
57. Werner L, Apple DJ, Kaskaloglu M et al: Dense opacification of the optical component of a hydrophilic intraocular lens: a clinicopathological analysis of 9 explants, *J Cataract Refract Surg* 27:1485-1492, 2001.
58. Pandey SK, Werner L, Apple DJ, et al: Hydrophilic acrylic intraocular lens optic and haptics opacification in a diabetic patient: Bilateral case report and clinicopathological correlation. *Ophthalmology* 109:2042-2051, 2002.
59. Apple DJ, Werner L, Pandey SK: The opalescence of hydrogel intraocular lens, *Eye* 15:817-819, 2001 (letter).
60. Frohn A, Dick HB, Augustin AJ et al: Eintrubungen bei Acryllisen Typ SC60B-OUV der Firma MDR, *Ophthalmo-Chirurge* 2:173-175, 2000.
61. Dhaliwal DK, Mamalis N, Olson RJ et al: Visual significance of glistenings seen in the AcrySof intraocular lens, *J Cataract Refract Surg* 22:452-457, 1996.
62. Omar O, Pirayesh A, Mamalis N et al: In vitro analysis of AcrySof intraocular lens glistenings in AcryPak and Wagon Wheel packaging, *J Cataract Refract Surg* 24:107-113, 1998.
63. Dogru M, Tetsumoto K, Tagami Y et al: Optical and atomic force microscopy of an explanted AcrySof intraocular lens with glistenings, *J Cataract Refract Surg* 26:571-575, 2000.
64. Christiansen G, Durcan FJ, Olson RJ et al: Glistenings in the AcrySof intraocular lens: pilot study, *J Cataract Refract Surg* 27:728-733, 2001.
65. Dick HB, Olson RJ, Augustin AJ et al: Visual acuity vacuoles in the Acrysof intraocular lens as factor of the presence of serum in aqueous humor, *Ophthalmic Res* 33:61-67, 2001.
66. Ridley NHL: Artificial intraocular lenses after cataract extraction, St. *Thomas Hospital Reports* 7:12-14, 1951.
67. Apple DJ, Peng Q, Arthur SN et al: Snowflake degeneration of polymethyl methacrylate posterior chamber intraocular lens optic material: a newly described clinical condition caused by an unexpected late opacification of polymethyl methacrylate, *Ophthalmology* 109:1666-1675, 2002.
68. Park JB: *Biomaterials: an introduction,* New York, 1979, Plenum Press.
69. Sugaya H, Sakai Y: Polymethylmethacrylate: from polymer to dialyzer, *Contrib Nephrol* 125:1-8, 1999.
70. Christ FR, Buchen SY, Deacon J et al: Biomaterials used for intraocular lenses. In Wise DL, et al, editors: *Encyclopedic handbook of biomaterials and bioengineering,* New York, 1995, Marcel Dekker.
71. Gayton JL, Sanders VN: Implanting two posterior chamber intraocular lenses in a case of microphthalmos, *J Cataract Refract Surg* 19:776-777, 1993.
72. Stasiuk R: Interface Elschnig pearl formation with piggyback implantation, *J Cataract Refract Surg* 26:158-159, 2000 (letter).
73. Shugar JK, Keeler S: Inter-pseudophakos intraocular lens surface opacification as a late complication of piggyback acrylic posterior chamber intraocular lens implantation, *J Cataract Refract Surg* 26:448-455, 2000.
74. Gayton JL, Apple DJ, Peng Q et al: Interlenticular opacification: a clinicopathological correlation of a new complication of piggyback posterior chamber intraocular lenses, *J Cataract Refract Surg* 26:330-336, 2000.
75. Werner L, Shugar JK, Apple DJ et al: Opacification of piggyback IOLs associated with an amorphous material attached to interlenticular surfaces, *J Cataract Refract Surg* 26:1612-1619, 2000.
76. Werner L, Apple DJ, Pandey SK et al: Analysis of elements of interlenticular opacification, *Am J Ophthalmol* 133:320-326, 2002.
77. Findl O, Menapace R, Rainer G et al: Contact zone of piggyback acrylic intraocular lenses, *J Cataract Refract Surg* 25:860-862, 1999.
78. Findl O, Menapace R, Georgopoulos M et al: Morphological appearance and size of contact zones of piggyback intraocular lenses, *J Cataract Refract Surg* 27:219-223, 2001.
79. Wilson ME, Peterseim MW, Englert JA et al: Pseudophakia and poly-pseudophakia in the first year of life, *J AAPOS* 5:238-245, 2001.
80. Apple DJ, Sims JC: Harold Ridley and the invention of the intraocular lens, *Surv Ophthalmol* 40:279-292, 1995.
81. Apple DJ, Solomon KD, Tetz MR et al: Posterior capsule opacification, *Surv Ophthalmol* 37:73-116, 1992.
82. Schaumberg DA, Dana MR, Christen WG et al: A systematic overview of the incidence of posterior capsular opacification, *Ophthalmology* 105:1213-1221, 1998.
83. Apple DJ, Peng Q, Visessook N et al: Eradication of posterior capsule opacification: documentation of a marked decrease in neodymium:yttrium-aluminium-garnet laser posterior capsulotomy rates noted in an analysis of 5416 pseudophakic human eyes obtained postmortem, *Ophthalmology* 108:505-518, 2001.
84. Werner L, Apple DJ, Pandey SK: Postoperative proliferation of anterior and equatorial lens epithelial cells. In Buratto L, Osher RH, Masket S, editors: *Cataract surgery in complicated cases,* Thorofare, NJ, 2000, Slack, pp 399-417.
85. Ram J, Apple DJ, Peng Q et al: Update on fixation of rigid and foldable posterior chamber intraocular lenses. Part II. Choosing the correct haptic fixation and intraocular lens design to help eradicate posterior capsule opacification, *Ophthalmology* 106:891-900, 1999.
86. Ram J, Pandey SK, Apple DJ et al: Effect of in-the-bag intraocular lens fixation on the prevention of posterior capsule opacification, *J Cataract Refract Surg* 27:1039-1046, 2001.
87. Apple DJ, Peng Q, Visessook N et al: Surgical prevention of posterior capsule opacification. Part I. How are we progressing in eliminating this complication of cataract surgery? *J Cataract Refract Surg* 26:180-187, 2000.
88. Peng Q, Apple DJ, Visessook N et al: Surgical prevention of posterior capsule opacification. Part II. Enhancement of cortical clean up by increased emphasis and focus on the hydrodissection procedure, *J Cataract Refract Surg* 26:188-197, 2000.
89. Peng Q, Visessook N, Apple DJ et al: Surgical prevention of posterior capsule opacification. Part III. The intraocular lens barrier effect as a second line of defense, *J Cataract Refract Surg* 26:198-213, 2000.
90. Apple DJ: Influence of intraocular lens material and design on postoperative intracapsular cellular reactivity, *Trans Am Ophthalmol Soc* 98:257-283, 2000.
91. Linnola RJ, Werner L, Pandey SK et al: Adhesion of fibronectin, vitronectin, laminin and collagen type IV to intraocular lens materials in pseudophakic human autopsy eyes. Part I. Histological sections, *J Cataract Refract Surg* 26:1792-1806, 2000.
92. Linnola RJ, Werner L, Pandey SK et al: Adhesion of fibronectin, vitronectin, laminin and collagen type IV to intraocular lens materials in pseudophakic human autopsy eyes. Part II. Explanted IOLs, *J Cataract Refract Surg* 26:1807-1818, 2000.
93. Nishi O, Nishi K, Akura J et al: Effect of round-edged acrylic intraocular lenses on preventing posterior capsule opacification, *J Cataract Refract Surg* 27:608-613, 2001.

Intraoperative Complications of Phacoemulsification Surgery

39

Robert H. Osher, MD
Robert J. Cionni, MD
Scott E. Burk, MD, PhD

The successful management of intraoperative complications requires a combination of recognition, knowledge, skill, and judgment. The surgeon must respond almost automatically because the intense stress of the moment may impair clear, rapid thinking. Therefore the best approach to the management of intraoperative complications is thorough preparation for all possibilities. This chapter focuses on a constellation of intraoperative complications. Because the majority of these complications will be encountered by every cataract surgeon, a well-prepared and knowledgeable response will usually result in a successful visual outcome.

Patient Movement

The primary drawback of local anesthesia is the patient's ability to move during surgery. Although most movement occurs from talking, coughing, or simply fidgeting, an occasional patient will abruptly sit up and try to leave the operating room while the surgeon is still working.

Prevention

As always, the best solution to a problem is its prevention. Taping the forehead to the operating table helps decrease small movements by patients with head tremors and for those who lack the concentration to lie still. This is best accomplished before surgery begins, so it is better to evaluate the patient's mobility before beginning the operation. If a significant head tremor or movement disorder is noted at the preoperative examination, it may be wise to consider general anesthesia.

Allowing the patient to become overly sedated or to fall asleep is also dangerous. The patient may suddenly awaken in a disoriented state and violently thrust the head, resulting in severe intraocular damage. A periodic reminder may aid the somnolent patient in staying awake. Coughing can also cause sudden head movement, as well as significant positive pressure. We ask the patient to warn us if he or she feels a cough coming. A box of cough drops located at the microscope has been helpful on numerous occasions.

To minimize restlessness, it is best to be certain that the patient is comfortable before surgery begins. This includes ample ventilation beneath the drapes, placement of supporting pillows, and a proper configuration of the table or stretcher.

Management

The anesthesiologist can be invaluable in decreasing excessive patient movement by administering appropriate medications when indicated during the procedure. Although the surgeon should always be kind and courteous, it may occasionally become necessary for the surgeon to be stern with the patient to prevent damage to the eye. The self-sealing nature of modern phacoemulsification incisions is particularly advantageous when patient movement becomes excessive. With a self-sealing incision the surgeon always has the luxury of briefly halting surgery. Although it is almost always possible to resume surgery after the patient's anxiety or discomfort has been alleviated, the nature of modern self-sealing incisions can permit the surgeon to suspend surgery and correct a serious problem before returning to the operating room at a later time or even on another day.

Retrobulbar Hemorrhage

Severe retrobulbar hemorrhage may necessitate cancellation of intraocular surgery.[1,2] High orbital or intraocular pressure significantly increases the likelihood of complications, including iris prolapse, posterior capsule rupture, and vitreous loss. Anticoagulant therapy increases the risk of a serious retrobulbar hemorrhage, and we routinely ask our patients to check with their internist regarding the safety of discontinuing anticoagulant use before surgery. In many cases, topical anesthesia may be preferred to avoid the possibility of retrobulbar hemorrhage.

In many instances of limited retrobulbar hemorrhage, we have found that phacoemulsification with posterior chamber intraocular lens (IOL) implantation can be performed safely, provided that several criteria are met. First, active bleeding must be appropriately managed with immediate, direct orbital pressure to expedite clotting and limit the volume of blood behind the globe. Once this is accomplished, the surgeon should evaluate the extent of the hemorrhage. Surgery can proceed if the globe is soft and easily retropulsed, the lids are loose and mobile, and proptosis is not excessive. If one or more of these parameters are not met, either digital massage or placement of a mercury bag against the orbit for 5 to 10 minutes may adequately reduce the pressure so that these parameters are fulfilled. It may also be necessary to perform a lateral canthotomy to reduce lid tightness. If the surgeon remains uncertain about the safety of proceeding after 30 minutes, it is best to reschedule the surgery rather than forge ahead and face severe positive pressure.

In rare cases, the accumulation of orbital blood may elevate the intraocular pressure enough to threaten vision. The intraocular pressure can be measured quickly using the Schiotz tonometer or tonopen. However it is more important to know the retinal perfusion status than the exact intraocular pressure. For this reason we keep a special lens (Osher panfundus lens, manufactured by Ocular Instruments) readily available, that can be used to quickly view the fundus through the operating microscope. If the central retinal artery is pulsating, its diastolic pressure has been exceeded and vision may be threatened. The combination of progressive proptosis, a tight orbit, central retinal artery pulsation, progressive corneal epithelial edema, and high intraocular pressure requires the surgeon to act quickly and dissect into the periocular space with a scissors to release an expanding hematoma. If this fails to decompress the globe, the lower and upper lids should be disinserted by an emergency lateral canthotomy and cantholysis.

In a series of 60 cases of retrobulbar hemorrhage related to the anesthetic injection, only 3 cases required cancellation because they failed to satisfy the previously mentioned criteria for proceeding with surgery.[3] With few exceptions, the eyes undergoing surgery did not develop intraocular complications, and the postoperative visual results were similar to a control group of patients in whom retrobulbar hemorrhage had not developed.

Although small-incision surgery allows one to deal more easily with the complications associated with a retrobulbar hemorrhage, it does not eliminate them completely. The surgeon who proceeds with surgery in the face of a limited retrobulbar hemorrhage should be comfortable managing an eye with significant positive pressure.

Complications of Topical Anesthesia

Although this topic is covered elsewhere in this book, several important points deserve repeating. The experienced surgeon realizes that excellent anesthesia requires appropriate preoperative counseling so that the patient's natural fear of eye surgery is minimized. Confirming adequate topical anesthesia before beginning the operation and then reassuring the patient in a gentle, caring voice are worth the time and effort. We instruct the patient to inform us if he or she feels anything uncomfortable, emphasizing that any discomfort can be promptly "numbed" by a few extra eye drops.

While some surgeons find supplement intracameral anesthesia to be helpful, the most important factor when using topical anesthesia is appropriate patient selection. In addition, to prevent unexpected movements, the eye should be "stabilized" by a second instrument through the stab incision during delicate intraocular maneuvers. Finally, repeated phrases of reassurance contribute to the safety and comfort of the patient.

Incision

Developments in incision design and construction offer the surgeon choices among scleral tunnel, near-clear, or clear corneal incisions with steep axis or temporal placement and frown, straight, smile, or even radial incision configurations.[4-6] Although each has its own advantages and disadvantages, which are covered elsewhere in this book, they all share in common the goal of obtaining a well-sealed wound that is either astigmatically neutral or in some cases designed to counteract preexisting astigmatism. A poorly constructed incision will make a routine case difficult. Likewise, a carefully planned and precise incision may convert an extremely difficult case into an enjoyable and successful procedure. The following generalities about the incision are discussed to help prevent avoidable complications.

Placement

The first consideration is axis placement. The foremost determinant of axis placement is ease of access to the globe so that a prominent superior orbital rim will not interfere. This often necessitates a superotemporal or temporal approach. The other factors involved in axis placement are astigmatism and, occasionally, anatomic landmarks such as vessels, peripheral anterior synechiae, corneal opacity, or a preexisting filter.

The distance the incision is placed from the cornea must also be determined, and several factors must be considered. Given the same incision size, the closer the incision is to the central cornea, the greater the tendency for cylindric alteration at that axis.[7,8] In addition, wound placement affects the tunnel length. Clear corneal incisions require a shorter tunnel to avoid working too close to the central cornea, whereas scleral tunnel incisions must have a greater length to avoid premature entry. Thus tunnel length is a variable that also deserves consideration. A wound with too short a length may be more difficult to close or fail to be watertight without sutures because there is less flap surface for appositional closure. An example of this is a short clear corneal incision, which might be watertight with increased intraocular pressure but leaks with pressure on the posterior lip of the incision.[9] By contrast, a well-constructed incision more posterior may provide a better seal. However, a tunnel that is too long can hinder motion of the phacoemulsification tip, causing excessive globe movement during phacoemulsification and undesirable corneal distortion. When creating a scleral wound, the surgeon must be careful to avoid excessive bleeding and premature entry. The posterior scleral incision also results in a more difficult, "uphill" approach, which may simulate scleral depression during the procedure, leading to significant positive pressure.

Young patients with low scleral rigidity are more likely to experience molding or scleral shrinkage around the shaft of the

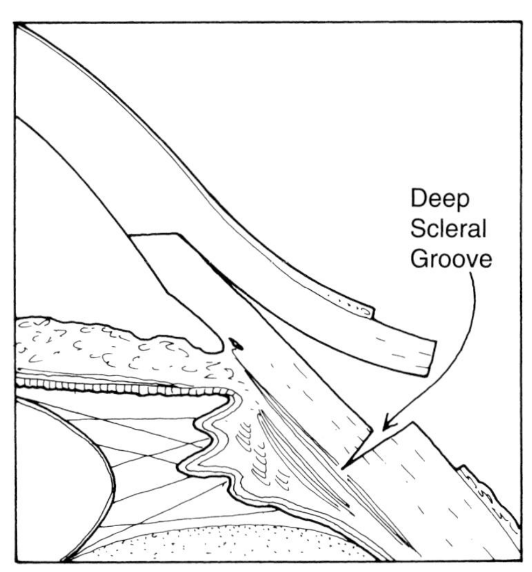

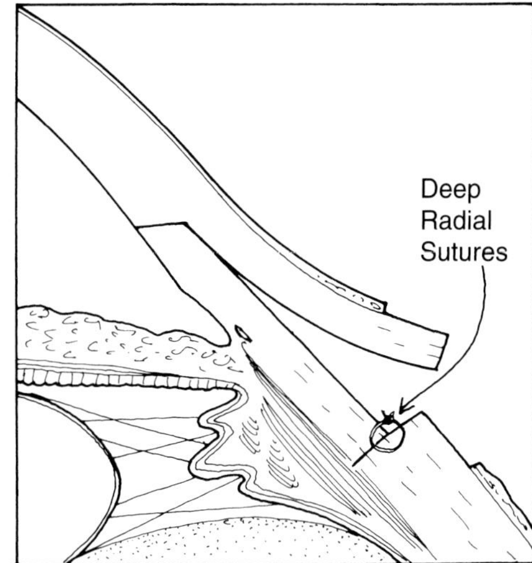

FIGURE 39-1 Placement of deep sutures when the scleral groove is too deep.

phacoemulsification needle. Therefore a less tight incision may occasionally be desirable and is more likely to allow watertight closures. This is especially true if the surgeon is also attempting to reduce plus cylinder in the axis of the incision.

Depth

When a scleral tunnel approach is too deep, an incision may result in entry into the suprachoroidal space or premature entry into the chamber angle. The former may be associated with bleeding and hypotony, whereas the latter is associated with iris prolapse. If the suprachoroidal space is entered, placement of deep sutures may prevent prolonged hypotony following surgery (Figure 39-1). A guarded knife for performing the incision is helpful, and it is unnecessary to exceed the depth of one half the scleral thickness.

Anterior Chamber Entrance

The size of the entrance into the anterior chamber must allow easy entry of the phacoemulsification needle and therefore must be tapered to its dimensions. Too large an entrance may result in a leaky incision with constant chamber shallowing throughout the operation, requiring a temporary suture (Figure 39-2). An undersized wound will not permit sufficient sliding of the phacoemulsification needle shaft, causing eye rotation during phacoemulsification and possibly constricting irrigation flow around the needle, which increases the chances of thermal injury with resulting wound gape. In addition, too small an incision is more likely to result in trauma to the Descemet's membrane. A certain amount of "snugness" is desirable, but the wound should be extended if it is excessively tight.

The location of the entrance into the anterior chamber is also important. A more anterior entrance affords a more watertight wound yet causes more corneal striae during phacoemulsification, making visualization difficult and adding to the endothelial cell loss. Moreover, an anterior entry makes manipulation of the proximal pole of the nucleus and subincisional cortex more difficult. Too posterior an entrance invites iris prolapse. In addition, as mentioned previously, because there is less tissue apposition, a watertight wound is less likely.

Wound Leak

If the incision is not watertight at the conclusion of the operation, the surgeon may select among several choices. First, a 30-gauge cannula may be used to inject balanced salt solution (BSS) into the lateral borders of the incision. This maneuver causes hydration of the stroma and enough swelling to stop a mild wound leak. Second, it is easy to pass a 10-0 nylon suture that can be either tied and cut or looped for temporary closure with subsequent removal in the office.

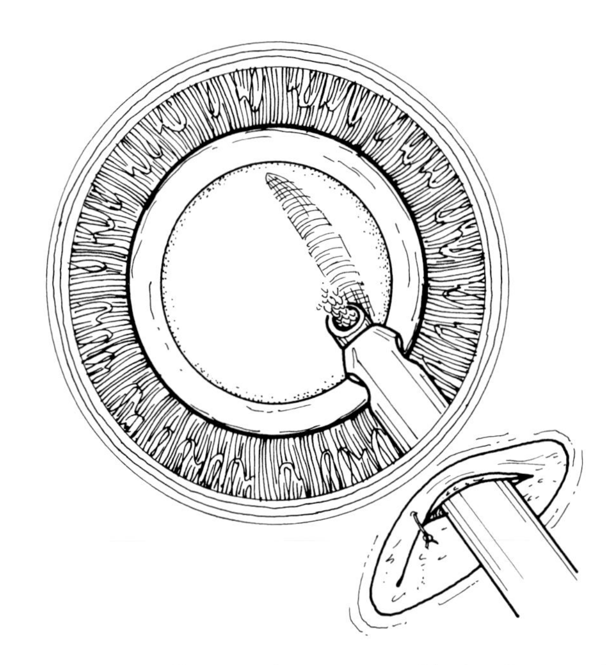

FIGURE 39-2 Placement of a temporary radial suture for an oversized phacoemulsification incision.

Finally, if the wound leak is secondary to gaping from thermal injury, special suturing techniques described by Osher may be required. A radial 10-0 nylon suture is passed from the corneal tissue through the floor and tied, not crossing the incision to incorporate the distal wound margin. Alternatively, a horizontal 10-0-nylon suture can be passed, bringing the posterior roof to the anterior floor. Each of these techniques helps to compensate for tissue shrinkage and minimize induced cylinder.[10,11]

Tear of the Descemet's Membrane

A tear of the Descemet's membrane at the anterior chamber entry site can be caused by improper insertion of an instrument through the incision. To avoid this occurrence, the leading tip should be directed posteriorly whenever inserting an instrument. The ability to do so can be compromised in eyes with shallow chambers in which a posteriorly directed passage would engage the iris. The use of a viscoelastic agent to deepen the chamber before entry with a keratome or a phacoemulsification tip will aid the surgeon in preventing this complication. As mentioned earlier, an adequate incision size will also minimize the likelihood of a Descemet's membrane tear.

The most important step in managing a tear in the Descemet's membrane is recognizing its presence. If unnoticed, continued instrument manipulation may increase the extent of the detachment. Inadvertent injection of a viscoelastic agent into the separation can also extend the detachment. Once recognized, the Descemet's membrane can usually be reattached by one or two simple maneuvers. Placing pressure on the posterior lip of the wound at the site of the tear will generate an egress of fluid, which will reposition a small Descemet's membrane flap in most instances. Alternatively, a small air bubble or viscoelastic agent can be used to tamponade a Descemet's membrane flap into position where an optional suture may help.

A larger tear may require more extensive suturing. The needle should pass through clear cornea central to the "hinge" of the tear and then be directed peripherally to splint the Descemet's membrane into position. We have not needed to use gas or tissue glue although others have reported success with these modalities.

Iris Prolapse

Prolapse of the iris may lead to postoperative pupil irregularity, iris transillumination defects, peripheral anterior synechiae, or uveal incarceration into the wound. Intraoperatively, acute prostaglandin release may cause constriction of the pupil, whereas rupture of vessels from the minor iris circle may result in intraocular bleeding further complicating the operative procedure.

PREVENTION

A well-constructed incision that extends "uphill" in the clear cornea will help to prevent iris prolapse, whereas a posterior entry will ensure its occurrence (Figure 39-3). Efforts to both minimize iris trauma and reduce positive pressure will decrease the likelihood of iris prolapse. In addition, because acutely elevating the intraocular pressure may also cause iris prolapse, care should be taken to avoid excessive injection of fluid or viscoelastic agents into the eye.

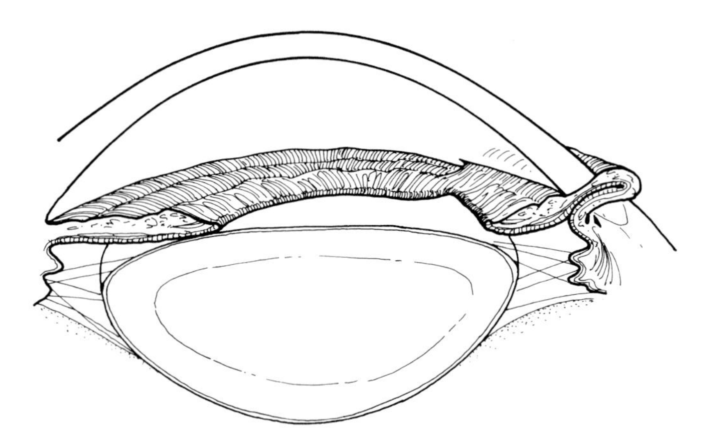

FIGURE 39-3 Iris prolapse through a posteriorly placed entrance into the anterior chamber.

MANAGEMENT

The surgeon should try to identify the cause of the prolapse to manage the underlying problem properly. Excessive intraocular pressure can be reduced by eliminating sources of external pressure, such as proper speculum positioning and release of a bridle suture if used. The intraocular pressure can be further lowered by aspirating fluid or viscoelastic material from the anterior chamber, preferably via the second incision site. The iris can be gently repositioned in most cases by the cannula on the viscoelastic syringe, leaving some viscoelastic agent on the iris surface. If these attempts fail, the surgeon should not hesitate to perform a small peripheral iridectomy at the site of prolapse to neutralize the pressure gradient between the anterior and posterior chambers. Repeated iris manipulation should be avoided because the iris becomes increasingly more frayed and flaccid. At the end of the case a drop of an intracameral miotic agent, judicious use of a viscoelastic, a peripheral iridotomy, and deeply placed sutures can help reduce the possibility of iris incarceration in the wound.

Intraocular Hemorrhage

Hemorrhage from the wound may compromise visibility and obscure the surgical events within the eye. Blood may also accumulate behind an IOL or dissect through the zonules into the vitreous cavity. Although intraocular hemorrhage will invariably absorb, it may acutely reduce vision, stimulate inflammation, accelerate capsular opacification, and prevent pupillary movement by clot formation, leading to posterior synechiae. For these reasons, we encourage the discontinuation of anticoagulant therapy before surgery, with the approval of the patient's internist. If anticoagulant therapy cannot be discontinued, a clear corneal approach with topical anesthesia is preferred.

We have found that intraocular hemorrhage occurs more commonly when the incision is placed more temporal, more posterior, and deeper than usual. In these locations, larger blood vessels are encountered, and bleeding is often more brisk.

Because of its space-occupying properties, viscoelastic material will often limit the amount of intraocular bleeding and may serve to tamponade the bleeding site. In addition, elevating the intraocular pressure by overfilling the chamber with adrenalized BSS can often stop bleeding, and point cautery to a feeder vessel, away from the wound itself, can be helpful. After the source of the bleeding has been addressed and the bleeding has stopped, the surgeon should evacuate any intraocular blood before clot formation occurs.

The evacuation of blood from the anterior chamber can be done by simply depressing the posterior lip of the wound with a cannula. However, to prevent additional bleeding it is probably best to aspirate the blood while infusing BSS in a "closed" system, thereby maintaining the intraocular pressure. This can be done through the main incision with a miniature irrigation-aspiration tip or through two side port incisions using separate irrigation and aspiration. The likelihood of postoperative hyphema can be reduced in sutureless procedures by firming the globe with BSS at the end of the procedure to attain a high normal intraocular pressure. This maneuver will seal the anterior lip of the wound more tightly, preventing entrance of blood into the anterior chamber.

Anterior Capsulectomy

Most surgeons have adopted capsulorhexis as their preferred anterior capsulectomy technique. This type of capsulectomy is much stronger and resistant to peripheral extension during nucleus manipulation, cortical removal, and IOL implantation.[12-14] Not only has the incidence of anterior capsular tears been reduced, but we have also found that the incidence of posterior capsule tears has also been reduced (0.2%) since incorporating capsulorhexis into our surgical technique.[15] Moreover, if a tear in the posterior capsule should occur, there is a greater likelihood of being able to place a posterior chamber IOL into the capsular bag or into the ciliary sulcus over an intact rim of anterior capsule.

Osher has developed the concept of the "safety rhexis" to have a "second chance" if the capsulorhexis is faulty. A 22-gauge needle slash results in an anterior capsular tear with two arms. The lower arm is redirected opposite the orientation of the upper arm, which prevents it from running with the primary tear. The upper arm of the tear is then directed clockwise around the anterior capsule, finishing the capsulorhexis outside of the original starting point.[16] If a problem occurs with the upper arm, the surgeon may resume the capsulorhexis by tearing the second edge counterclockwise until it connects with the first arm. There are several different variations of this theme, but the important concept is that the capsulorhexis that misbehaves can be corrected (Figure 39-4).

Peripheral Extension

The surgeon just learning capsulorhexis will encounter peripheral extension more often than one who is more experienced with this technique. Certain conditions predispose to this event. Anterior bowing of the lens-iris diaphragm will encourage peripheral extension. This condition is more common in patients with shallow anterior chambers and in those with positive pressure. This is caused by the curvature of the anterior lens capsule that can be conceptualized as a "hill." If the capsular tear runs over the "edge of the hill," it will continue to pursue a "downhill" course, resisting attempted redirection uphill (Figure 39-5).

In young patients, the leading edge of the anterior capsular tear also has a tendency to run peripherally. This may be due to the elastic forces of the zonulocapsular apparatus, the intralenticular pressure, and anterior chamber shallowing associated with lower scleral rigidity. The widely dilated pupil of a young patient may also lend itself to a larger capsulectomy, and if the zonular insertions are encountered, the tear will have a strong tendency to follow the radial course of the zonule, rather than the desired circumferential course.

A conscious effort is made to perform a slightly smaller capsulectomy in the young patient, but not so small as to compromise nuclear manipulation or subincisional cortical aspiration. Moreover, it is imperative to retroplace the lens-iris diaphragm with a generous amount of viscoelastic material in the young patient and in those with either shallow anterior chambers or positive pressure. If the viscoelastic material is extruded, refilling the chamber may be required; alternatively, selecting a more retentive viscoelastic agent, such as Healon5, may be effective. It may be helpful to attach a bent needle or cystotome to the viscoelastic syringe, thereby eliminating the tendency for the viscoelastic agent to escape as one enters and exits the anterior chamber. Once the chamber deepens, the capsulorhexis will be easier to guide in the desired direction (Figure 39-6).

Occasionally, even in experienced hands the anterior capsular tear will extend too far peripherally to redirect. Persistent heroic attempts to force the tear centrally may cause it to further extend around the equator into the posterior capsule. The experienced surgeon will know when the location of the tear is too peripheral by the "feel" of resistance to his or her efforts to redirect the tear. The surgeon should return to the starting point and proceed with a second continuous tear using the "safety" capsulorhexis strategy or switch to a can-opener technique until the capsulectomy is completed (Figure 39-7).

If the anterior capsule tear has extended peripherally or if the capsulorhexis is finished inside the starting point, creating a "notch" in the anterior capsule ring, phacoemulsification should be performed with extreme care to avoid stress to the capsular bag. The second instrument is used to manipulate the nucleus away from the area of peripheral extension without generating forces that may extend the tear further. A low aspiration and vacuum system allows phacoemulsification to occur slowly, without sudden chamber shallowing or excessive fluid movement through compromised zonules. Aspiration of cortex is also performed gently and lastly in the area of the peripheral extension. The IOL selected should have soft haptics and should be inserted with minimal force exerted on the capsule, and the haptics should be maneuvered away from the area of the weakened capsular bag.

In cases in which a notch in the capsulorhexis exists, a better approached involves notch management. A fine intraocular scissors can be used to make an angulated cut lateral to the notch. Intraocular forceps are used to grasp the resulting flap

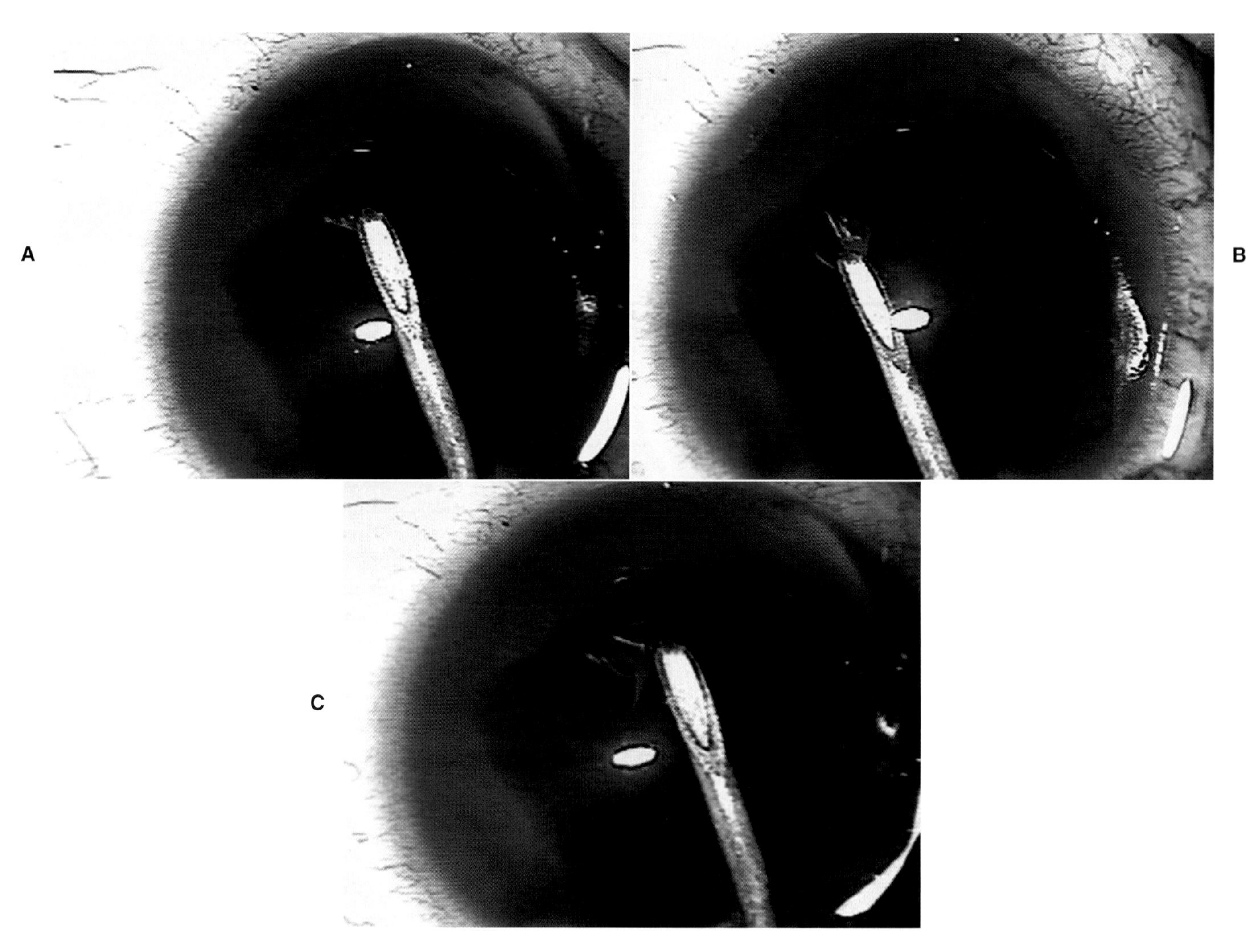

FIGURE 39-4 Operating microscope view of an eye with aniridia. Trypan blue has been applied to the anterior capsule. **A,** Capsulorhexis is initiated with a bent 22-gauge needle. **B,** The 22-gauge needle is used to reverse the direction of the lower arm of the capsular tear. **C,** The remainder of the capsulorhexis proceeds normally; however, should the surgeon encounter a problem with the capsulorhexis, it can be restarted easily in the opposite direction.

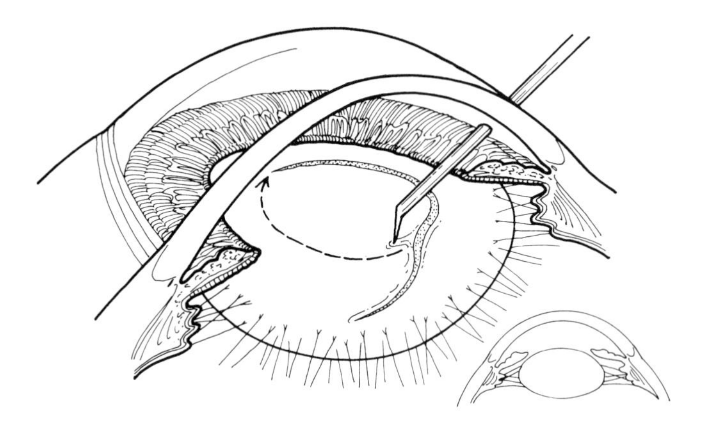

FIGURE 39-5 Shallowing of the anterior chamber causes the capsule tear to run peripherally "downhill," instead of following the intended course *(broken line).*

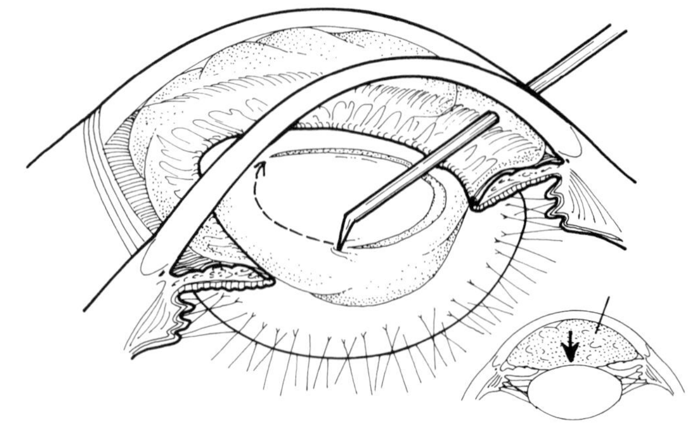

FIGURE 39-6 Deepening the anterior chamber with viscoelastic allows the capsule to tear along the desired course *(broken line).*

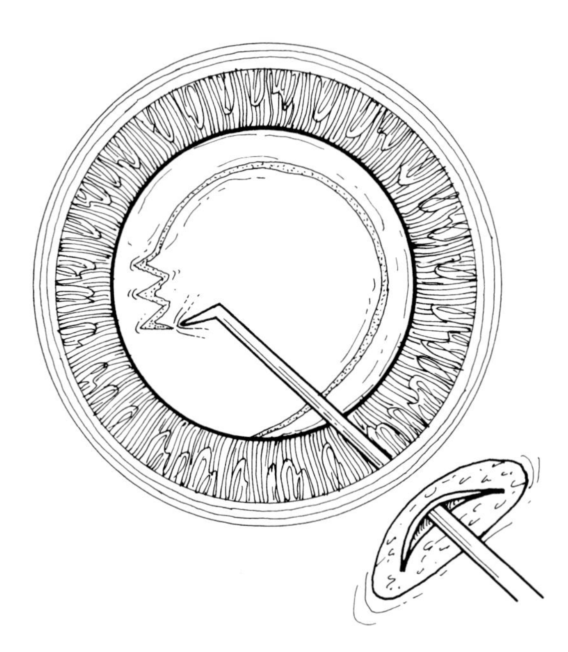

FIGURE 39-7 Conversion of a capsulorhexis that ran peripherally into a can-opener capsulotomy.

and enlarge the capsulorhexis to create a smooth, continuous tear peripheral to the notch. (See Figure 39-8, which depicts a similar maneuver for enlarging the capsular opening.) If the notch is proximal, either a reverse cutting scissors (Duckwort and Kent) is necessary or the capsule is button-holed with a blade. A scissors is introduced into the hole, and a snip is made, creating a reverse-angled flap as the button hole is connected to the edge of the capsulorhexis. The flap is grasped, and the capsulorhexis is enlarged, thereby excising the notch and replacing it with a continuous edge.

Small Capsulectomy

Although too large a capsulorhexis may lead to peripheral extension, a capsulectomy that is too small makes manipulation of the nucleus and cortex more difficult. A small anterior capsular opening will particularly frustrate surgeons who favor a nucleus tipping or prolapsing technique. However, the well-prepared surgeon may select a number of maneuvers that will facilitate phacoemulsification, even when the capsulectomy is small. Two popular maneuvers involve either grooving then dividing the nucleus within the capsular bag or simply chopping the nucleus into sections.

A small capsulectomy also makes cortical aspiration beneath the incision more difficult. In some cases it may be necessary to maneuver the irrigation-aspiration tip so that it is nearly vertical while rotating the eye to reach the subincisional cortex. Therefore we believe that it is easier and safer to start cortex removal in the subincisional area while the capsular bag is held open by the remainder of the cortex.

Despite starting cortex removal in the subincisional area, this maneuver can still be challenging, thus the prepared surgeon should have an alternate method available, such as an angled or steerable irrigation-aspiration tip, bimanual aspiration, or aspiration with a curved cannula introduced through either the main incision or a side port incision.

A small capsulectomy may also lead to "capsular block syndrome" described by Masket.[17] In this syndrome, viscoelastic material trapped in the capsular bag by adhesion of the anterior capsule to the anterior surface of the IOL breaks down and causes an increasing osmotic gradient with excessive expansion of the capsular bag. A laser capsulotomy, preferably in the anterior capsule beyond the edge of the implant, relieves the osmotic imbalance, thereby resolving this complication.

An excessively small capsulorhexis may also result in the capsulophimosis syndrome, with opacification and contraction of the anterior capsular opening. In severe cases capsulophimosis syndrome can result in zonular stripping and a decentered IOL requiring surgical intervention.

When necessary to enlarge a capsulectomy, a Vannas scissors can be used to create a tear orienting the cut in the desired direction and then enlarging the capsulorhexis with the capsule forceps (Figure 39-8). This is safest when performed under the protection of a viscoelastic agent and after the IOL has been implanted. The proximal edge of the anterior capsule is the most difficult to enlarge and requires a reverse cutting scissors. Alternatively, a small tear can be created with a sharp blade immediately adjacent to the capsular margin. The edge can then be grasped with a forceps, completing the enlargement.

The White Cataract

Historically, the white cataract has been a notorious cause of a torn capsulorhexis. Not only is the visualization of the rhexis edge a factor, but also there is an elevated endocapsular pressure due to cortical liquefaction, which tends to cause an extension of the tear. Horiguchi and co-workers introduced the concept of anterior capsular staining, which has become invaluable in visualizing the rhexis edge.[18-25] Osher developed the following three-step method to avoid using an air bubble in the anterior chamber as advocated by other groups.

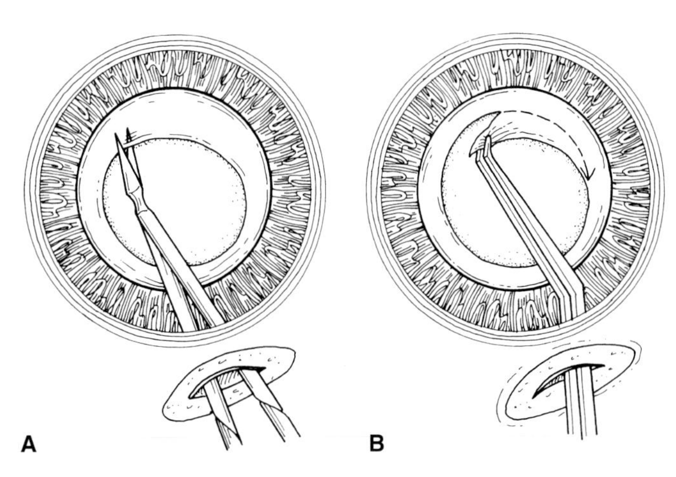

FIGURE 39-8 Enlargement of the capsulorhexis. **A,** Capsular edge is incised with intraocular scissors to create a small flap. **B,** Flap is grasped with forceps, and the new tear is directed to rejoin the capsulorhexis *(broken line)*. This technique may be used to enlarge the capsular opening or to excise a capsular notch and provide a new continuous capsular edge.

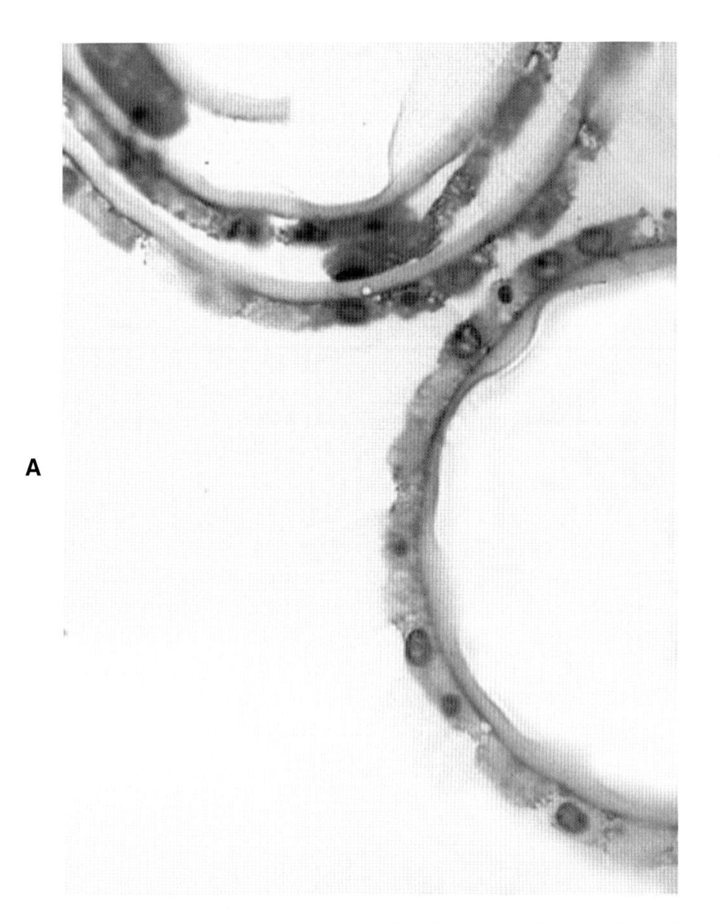

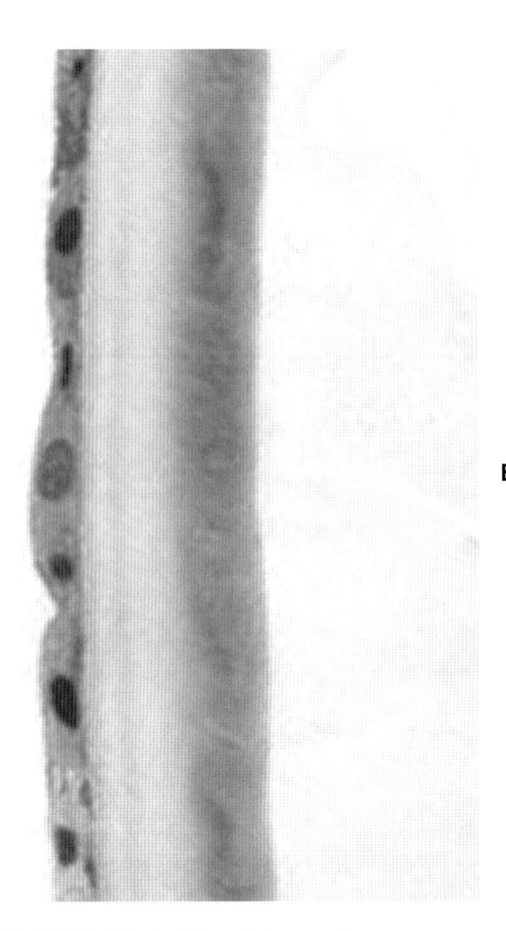

FIGURE 39-9 A, Anterior capsule from a patient with congenital aniridia (200×). Note the thin anterior capsule and curling nature, as compared to **B,** the anterior capsule from a patient without aniridia (200×).

Healon5 is initially injected into the anterior chamber. Next a gentle stream of BSS is instilled along the anterior capsule, which lifts the Healon5 toward the corneal dome and creates a wafer-thin layer of space. Finally, indocyanine green (ICG) or trypan blue dye is injected directly onto the anterior capsule, "painting" the intended rhexis size. This technique protects the corneal endothelium, avoids accumulation of dye within the viscoelastic material, and provides superior staining of the anterior capsule, thereby enhancing the visualization of the capsulorhexis edge.

Congenital Aniridia

The surgeon should be aware of the extreme fragility of the anterior capsule in some patients with aniridia. Osher initially identified the fragile behavior of these anterior capsules intraoperatively, and histopathologic analysis has demonstrated that the clinically fragile anterior capsules are remarkably thin (Figure 39-9).[26]

Phacoemulsification

A variety of complications can occur during phacoemulsification, some of which are discussed in the following paragraphs.

Insertion of the Handpiece

Careless insertion of the phacoemulsification tip can damage Descemet's membrane, chafe the iris stroma, and even cause an iridodialysis. These complications are more likely to occur in eyes with shallow chambers in which there is little room between the iris and the cornea. If the incision is made properly and the instruments are carefully angled toward the pupil, these complications can be avoided. An effective technique in decreasing iris chafing is to introduce the phacoemulsification tip bevel down and then rotate the bevel upward during the insertion.

The technique must be modified if there is iris prolapse plugging the incision before or during the phacoemulsification entry. The prolapsed iris is repositioned as described earlier. A viscoelastic agent is then instilled onto the adjacent iris. If an attempt is made to insert the phacoemulsification tip with irrigation on, prolapse will inevitably recur. Instead, the irrigation should be off until the phacoemulsification tip has completely entered the anterior chamber, at which point it is safe to resume infusion.

Excessive Globe Movement

An incision that is too tight or improper manipulation of the phacoemulsification handpiece can lead to excessive globe movement. In addition, a longer tunnel makes excessive globe movement more likely, whereas a shorter tunnel or a clear corneal incision lessens its occurrence. If the surgeon's movements are adjusted so that the wound site acts as a fulcrum for the handpiece, excessive movement of the globe should not occur. If the problem persists, the incision should be enlarged slightly.

Shallow Anterior Chamber

The presence of a shallow anterior chamber makes phacoemulsification extremely difficult. Descemet's membrane detachments and difficulty reaching the subincisional cortex are more likely to occur as the surgeon tends to direct the wound more anteriorly to avoid the iris. As described earlier, whenever the lens-iris diaphragm is relatively forward, peripheral extensions are more likely to occur during the capsulorhexis. In addition, iris prolapse and damage to both the iris and corneal endothelium may occur during insertion of the phacoemulsification needle. Spontaneous prolapse of the nucleus can be minimized by carefully sizing the capsulorhexis and avoiding excessive hydrodissection in these cases. The use of a higher-viscosity viscoelastic agent will often help to maintain a deeper anterior chamber. Fortunately, the anterior chamber will usually deepen significantly on completion of the emulsification.

Chamber Collapse

When sudden chamber collapse occurs, there is a risk of iris or posterior capsule damage. In addition, repeated episodes with corneal folding may damage corneal endothelial cells and lead to increased postoperative corneal edema. There are several different causes of chamber collapse.

FOOT SWITCH INATTENTIVENESS

The anterior chamber will routinely become shallow if the surgeon is so preoccupied with intraocular maneuvering that he or she forgets to control the foot switch. Continuous low irrigation, even in foot position zero, helps to maintain the anterior chamber depth, although not all phacoemulsification units are capable of this setting.

INSUFFICIENT INFLOW

As a general rule, the irrigation stream should be just enough to maintain the depth of the anterior chamber because excessive irrigation can be traumatic to the corneal endothelium. If the infusion is insufficient, however, shallowing of the chamber will occur. When prompt elevation of the bottle height fails to increase the infusion, an air block, a venting problem, faulty tubing, or even an error in preparation is probably responsible. A wound of insufficient size might compress the collapsible sleeve that accompanies some systems. Kinking of this sleeve may also compromise infusion, resulting in chamber shallowing.

EXCESSIVE OUTFLOW

In contrast to a tight incision, too large an incision allows fluid to escape. A more subtle problem is a tendency for the surgeon to elevate the instrument, which causes the wound to gape and the chamber to empty. This error tends to occur in patients with deep orbits because it is quite easy to inadvertently distort and lift open the wound, especially if the surgeon is operating over a high brow. If too large an incision is made, placement of a single radial suture will often tighten the wound enough to inhibit egress of fluid. Alternatively, a new incision site may be selected.

EXTERNAL GLOBE COMPRESSION

Compression against the sclera from any source may cause the anterior chamber to shallow. Possible causes include retrobulbar hemorrhage, excessive retrobulbar anesthesia, tight lids, pressure from the lid speculum, and traction from a rectus fixation suture. If the shaft of an instrument is inadvertently pressed against the sclera while the surgeon is working, problems maintaining the chamber will occur. A longer scleral tunnel approach often will result in globe compression when the surgeon attempts to reach the proximal nuclear edge and the subincisional cortex.

FLUID PARAMETERS

Chamber collapse is more likely to occur when the technique selected uses a high aspiration rate and a high vacuum level. In addition, these parameters require a higher bottle height, which may raise the intraocular pressure. When the aspiration port is occluded, vacuum levels rise to the maximal level until the ultrasound abruptly clears the occlusion. Fluid immediately rushes into the port, driven not only by the high aspiration rate but also by the high intraocular pressure and the elastic forces of the stretched scleral walls. This results in a chamber-collapsing tendency and a more volatile anterior chamber. We have advocated a technique using a lower aspiration rate, vacuum, and bottle heights, which results in a more stable chamber.[27,28]

Positive Pressure

The presence of positive pressure makes phacoemulsification a more difficult procedure with a higher incidence of complications. The chamber will tend to become shallow, leaving less room and less margin for error during the phacoemulsification. Iris prolapse and progressive miosis are more likely. The nucleus may spontaneously prolapse forward, and it may be difficult to reposition, forcing the surgeon to perform emulsification in the anterior chamber. The posterior capsule assumes a convex configuration, which makes it more prone to tears. Moreover, the capsular bag closes, making cortical aspiration and IOL placement more challenging. If positive pressure is encountered, the surgeon must take all steps necessary to identify the cause and, if possible, to correct it.[29]

CAUSES OF POSITIVE PRESSURE

External compression of the globe is a common cause of positive pressure that is often preventable or easily resolved. An excessive volume of retrobulbar or peribulbar anesthesia in a small orbit can cause globe compression. A poorly designed lid speculum, or one that is improperly placed, can result in positive pressure. However, one that is designed to lift the lids off the globe may not only avoid positive pressure in routine cases but also prevent it in patients with tight lids.

Tight lids associated with narrow palpebral fissures act to tether the globe, leading to positive pressure. The surgeon should always do everything he or she can to reduce the pressure that the lids exert on the globe. Several clues indicate excessive lid pressure. When the eyelids are opened for insertion of the speculum, the surgeon may observe narrowed fissures with little visible sclera, or a blunted lateral canthal angle may be restricting the width of the fissure. Taught lids will also tend to snap closed when opened. Another sign of potential lid pressure is indentation of the conjunctiva by either the lid margin or the speculum. If a bridle suture is being placed, resistance of globe rotation may also be an indication of tight lids. Obviously, blepharospasm can cause tight lids, which should be respected by the surgeon because patients with blepharospasm have been known to expel the lid speculum.

After the speculum has been inserted and adequate anesthesia has been obtained, it may be necessary to perform a lateral canthotomy. A hemostat is used to clamp a few millimeters of the lateral canthal angle for 1 or 2 minutes. After releasing the hemostat, a horizontal incision is made with scissors through the canthus, and little if any bleeding results.

Excessive traction from a fixation suture may increase the intraocular pressure by either excessive downward rotation of the globe or actually lifting the globe from the orbit. Therefore, if a traction suture is used, the minimal force required to maintain the globe in its primary position is desirable.

Several specific circumstances that originate within the eye cause positive pressure. If the posterior capsule has been ruptured or a zonular dialysis has occurred, persistent irrigation may cause expansion of fluid pockets within the vitreous gel, resulting in anterior displacement of the capsule and iris. High infusion is to be avoided when a zonular dialysis or posterior capsule rent is present. Air may also shallow the anterior chamber by getting behind the iris and producing air-induced pupillary block. Scleral collapse can result in chamber shallowing, especially in eyes of young patients, in eyes that have undergone previous vitrectomy, or in eyes that have been "oversoftened." Finally, choroidal hemorrhage or effusion can cause positive pressure and will often shallow or flatten the anterior chamber.

Another cause of positive pressure is body habitus. When lying flat, obese patients have a tendency toward increased intraocular pressure. By elevating the head and chest of the patient to a level comfortable for both the patient and surgeon, the positive pressure can be significantly diminished.

Any condition leading to a Valsalva maneuver may obstruct venous return, elevating orbital and intraocular pressure. Straining with a full bladder, coughing, discomfort, or anxiety must be managed properly. After appropriate communication, the surgeon should address the specific problem by allowing the patient to urinate, offering the patient a cough drop, or repositioning the patient until he or she is comfortable.

Performing phacoemulsification when positive pressure is present can be difficult, yet several maneuvers may decrease the risks of complications. Capsulorhexis and proper phacoemulsification insertion techniques in the face of shallow chamber have already been described. Excessive hydrodissection should be avoided to prevent spontaneous prolapse of the nucleus. The aspiration level should be reduced, and it may be necessary to elevate the bottle. Short rather than long bursts of ultrasound may be advantageous. It may also be necessary to use a dull second instrument to either hold the nucleus posteriorly or to restrain the posterior capsule while performing the emulsification in the safe zone immediately above it. Adjusting the handpiece angle within the incision may decrease its tendency toward scleral depression, gaping, or twisting of the wound. The surgeon should suppress the reflex request for intravenous hypertonic solutions because shrinkage of the vitreous may actually worsen scleral collapse, leading to an even shallower chamber. The use of a more highly retentive viscoelastic agent such as Healon5 should aid in maintaining a deeper chamber. Excessive chamber collapse may even require the instillation of the viscoelastic agent and removal of the cortex by a "dry" manual technique.

Rarely, IOL implantation will be jeopardized by persistent chamber collapse despite the use of viscoelastic material. Under these circumstances, the surgeon should be familiar with emergency maneuvers. First, if the implant can be introduced into the anterior chamber under viscoelastic protection without risking injury to the cornea, then the IOL can be rotated into the capsular bag by working through the side port incision(s). Such a closed system generally allows maintenance of the anterior chamber space by instilling a highly retentive viscoelastic material. However, if the chamber collapse is so great that the lens implant cannot be introduced into the eye safely, the surgeon can deepen the chamber by aspirating fluid vitreous using a 25-gauge needle via an external approach at the pars plana. Because vitreous aspiration increases the risk of hemorrhage, as well as retinal tear or detachment, this maneuver should be used only when clearly necessary. Of course, if the chamber shallowing is progressive and the surgeon suspects a suprachoroidal hemorrhage, rapid closure of the eye followed by ophthalmoscopy is essential. The management of this severe complication is discussed later in this chapter.

Thermal Burn

Regardless of whether a piezoelectric crystal or a magnetostrictive design is operative, the phacoemulsification transducer converts energy into acoustic waves, moving the hollow titanium tip back and forth at excursions of approximately 100 μm at a specified frequency. Both shock and fluid waves are generated when transient micron-sized bubbles implode within a few acoustic cycles, resulting in the mechanical emulsification of the cataract.[30] A portion of the energy is lost as heat, which is conducted into the eye via the titanium tip, where it is cooled and removed from the eye by the irrigation-aspiration exchange.

If for any reason this exchange is hampered, the potential for thermal damage can rapidly occur within 1 to 3 seconds. Inadequate inflow of fluid may be due to kinking of tubing or insufficient irrigation. Outflow may be compromised by faulty preparation of tubing, pump failure, or viscoelastic obstruction. In any case the critical warning sign of inadequate fluid exchange is the production and stagnation of lens milk around the tip. Immediate cessation of the emulsification is indicated while the surgeon and the operating room personnel make every effort to identify the source of the problem.

Several quick maneuvers will serve as prophylaxis against thermal burn. The surgeon should check the phacoemulsification function and confirm that irrigation and aspiration are

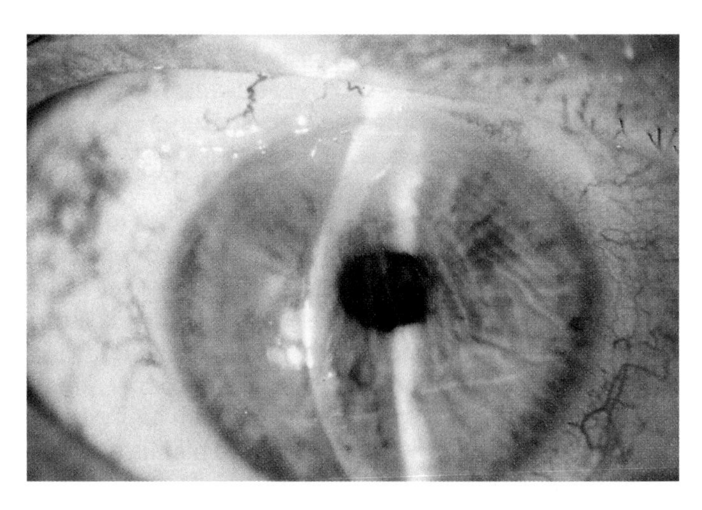

FIGURE 39-10 Slit lamp photograph of a thermal burn from phacoemulsification. Note the marked edema and opacification of the superior stroma. Striae extend from the burn in a radial pattern because of heat-induced contraction of the collagen. (Courtesy Roger F. Steinert, MD.)

occurring within the test chamber before entering the eye. If the anterior chamber has been filled with a viscoelastic agent, aspirating a small amount just around the tip adjacent to the anterior cortex will ensure adequate exchange unobstructed by even the most retentive viscoelastic agent. The incision size and length of the tunnel must be adequate to avoid kinking and torquing of the tubing. Although cooling the BSS and using pulsed ultrasound have been advocated by some surgeons, others prefer an ultrasound needle designed to maintain fluid either through an inner metal sleeve (MacKool), through metallic grooves (Barret), or using an aspiration bypass hole (Alcon). A more significant advance will be the introduction of a temperature-sensitive transducer in the future.

Should a thermal burn occur, the surgeon must select a suturing technique to minimize the risk of faulty closure, wound leak, and excessive cylinder. A radial suture (gape stitch) passed through the anterior lip and then through the floor but avoiding the distal lip or a horizontal suture (Osher stitch) bringing together the posterior roof and the anterior floor will serve this purpose.[10,11] A typical thermal burn is illustrated in Figure 39-10.

Iris Trauma and Pupillary Constriction

Damage to the iris during phacoemulsification can be caused by either iris prolapse or direct injury from the tip of the ultrasonic handpiece. Iris prolapse or injury may cause loss of pigment, flaccidity, bleeding, pupillary irregularity, or even cystoid macular edema.

Direct trauma to the iris from the phacoemulsification tip can be prevented in most, if not all, cases. Insertion techniques to decrease iris chafing have already been presented. By using low aspiration rates during phacoemulsification, events occur more slowly, and the iris is much less likely to "jump" suddenly into the phacoemulsification port. Using lower vacuum levels and ultrasound power levels will minimize damage if the iris is encountered inadvertently. Once the iris has been injured, it may be necessary to use a second instrument as a retractor to prevent additional damage, which becomes more difficult to avoid when the iris tissue is fraying and flaccid.

Often overlooked is the damage to the iris caused by contact with the exposed metal of the titanium tip that extends beyond the silicone sleeve. For this reason, it is best to minimize the metal exposure when performing phacoemulsification in an eye with a small pupil.

Any trauma to the iris may release prostaglandins and stimulate the iris sphincter to contract. Contact with an instrument, the nucleus, or an implant, as well as multiple chamber collapses, will result in pupillary constriction. Preoperative topical nonsteroidal antiinflammatory agents, in combination with intraoperative epinephrine added to the BSS infusion, may help to maintain pupillary dilation.[31]

Several small pupil phacoemulsification techniques are very effective,[32] yet the surgeon must be experienced in using these techniques. Radial iridotomy, multiple sphincterotomies, Frye sphincter stretching, and the use of iris retracting hooks are all techniques for managing the small or constricting pupil.[33-42] Recently, Healon5 has been introduced, and its capability to achieve viscomydriasis has given us another pupil-expanding option.

Posterior Capsule Tears

The torn posterior capsule is probably the most frequent significant complication encountered by the surgeon learning phacoemulsification, and it continues to occur, albeit rarely, in even the expert's hands. An open posterior capsule may increase the risk of cystoid macular edema and retinal detachment.[43] In most instances, posterior capsule rupture can be prevented. However, if a tear does occur, proper management will usually allow a successful procedure with safe placement of a posterior chamber IOL.[44]

Prevention

Fortunately, the incidence of a torn posterior capsule decreases with the increasing experience of the surgeon. The most severe posterior capsule tears occur during attempted emulsification of the nucleus. A continuous circular capsulorhexis can greatly diminish this complication because the stability of the anterior capsule edge prevents peripheral extension into the posterior capsule. The use of low-vacuum, low-aspiration phacoemulsification will also reduce the likelihood of a torn posterior capsule because the tendency toward sudden chamber shallowing or collapse is minimized. Low-power phacoemulsification also adds to the safety because there is less chance of piercing through the nucleus and rupturing the posterior capsule. Emulsification techniques that fracture or chop the nucleus may also reduce the risk of posterior capsule rupture.

As the emulsification progresses, a second instrument may be placed behind the remaining nucleus to hold the posterior capsule back and physically prevent it from contacting the phacoemulsification tip when the anterior chamber is shallowing. We use a dull, fingered instrument which functions as a nucleus manipulator or chopper (Duckworth and Kent) for this purpose and find it to be both safe and effective.

A recent development is the introduction of the silicone I/A tip by Alcon. This soft, smooth material provides superior capsular protection compared to traditional metallic tip designs.

Different types of cataracts may require specific modifications in surgical techniques because they may be associated with a higher risk of posterior capsule tearing or other complications. The brunescent cataract acts like a bowling ball, with its nucleus indistinguishable from the cortex. If too mobile, its large size and firm consistency can easily lead to a zonular dialysis. The surgeon may avoid performing hydrodissection initially, taking advantage of the firm grip that the cortex has on the nucleus. After the central nucleus is debulked and a very deep groove is made, late hydrodissection either under the anterior capsule or through a nuclear crack loosens the remaining peripheral shell from the capsule, which can be emulsified as it is rotated and chopped. Posterior lamellae can be lifted with a second instrument away from the posterior capsule, where the emulsification can be completed safely.

The young patient with a very soft cataract is also at greater risk for a torn posterior capsule because the second instrument, or phacoemulsification tip, will readily penetrate this cataract. Moreover, low scleral rigidity results in a tendency for anterior chamber shallowing, so a lower aspiration rate, reduced vacuum, and less phacoemulsification power are safer.

The posterior polar cataract and the cataract associated with posterior lenticonus or lentiglobus may be associated with a weakened or defective posterior capsule. Hydrodissection may be all that is needed to rupture a thinned posterior capsule in these patients or extend an already defective capsular opening. Here, low chamber pressure; gentle and limited multimeridianal hydrodissection loosening equatorial cortex; and reduced aspiration rate, vacuum, ultrasound power, and infusion may be the safest approach to these patients. It is best to assume that the posterior capsule is already open. Minimal nuclear manipulation in a closed system and the skillful use of viscoelastic material for dry cortical removal and tamponade of the tear, as well as converting a tear to a posterior capsulorhexis, are helpful principles in managing the posterior polar cataract.[45-50]

A morgagnian cataract is associated with a dramatic escape of liquefied cortex from the capsular bag when the initial puncture is made into the proximal anterior lens capsule. Careful aspiration of the liquefied cortex will prevent it from obstructing the surgeon's view for the rest of the procedure. As the intumescence is relieved and the liquid cortex removed, the capsular bag will become shallow, bringing the anterior and posterior capsule leaflets closer to each other and placing the posterior capsule at risk for being torn during the anterior capsulectomy. Therefore a viscoelastic agent should be injected through the initial puncture site to refill the capsular bag before proceeding with this challenging capsulorhexis. The use of a capsular dye such as trypan blue or ICG is recommended for improved capsular visualization in any white cataract[18,19,22-25] (Figure 39-11).

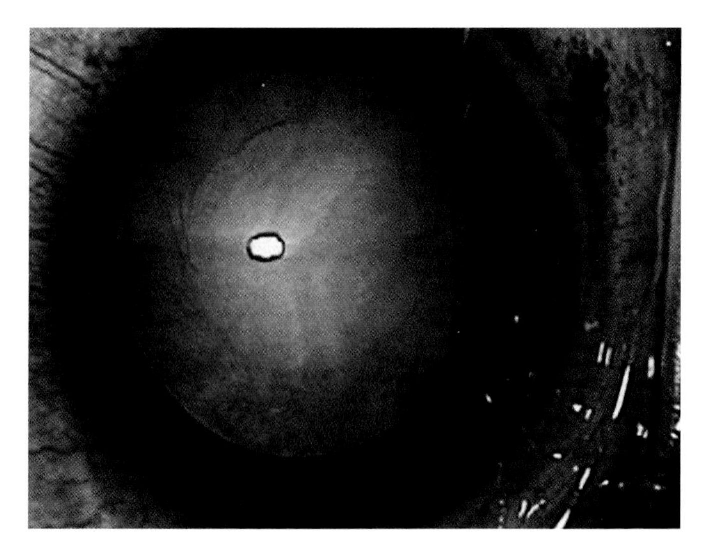

FIGURE 39-11 Operating microscope view of an ICG-assisted continuous capsulorhexis in an eye with an opalescent cataract. Note that the zonules, which are very anteriorly placed zonules, stain slightly darker green.

Management

Knowledgeable and skillful management of a posterior capsule tear is essential to the successful outcome of the procedure. At whatever stage the tear is discovered, establishment of a semi-closed pressurized system is necessary. Allowing the anterior chamber to collapse will promote forward movement of the vitreous, with possible extension of the tear.

If a tear is discovered during phacoemulsification, residual nuclear material may be removed by either emulsification or converting to an extracapsular technique. If most of the nucleus has already been emulsified, the surgeon may use the second instrument to move the remaining nucleus away from the tear to complete the emulsification. Infusion should be lowered to prevent increasing the pressure in the anterior segment and driving the nucleus back into the vitreous cavity. Viscoelastic material or the second instrument may be placed behind the nuclear fragment over a smaller rent to prevent loss of lens material. Short bursts of low-energy ultrasound with low aspiration, effective vacuum, and reduced irrigation will decrease the risk of nuclear loss, chamber shallowing, and vitreous prolapse. Once the nucleus has been emulsified, the phacoemulsification handpiece should not be removed without simultaneously injecting viscoelastic material through the second stab site to prevent vitreous prolapse and extension of the tear. This is a critical maneuver and may be the deciding factor in whether or not a vitrectomy must be performed, as well as whether or not an IOL can be implanted into the capsular bag.

Cortical removal can be safely accomplished without extending the tear by following several surgical principles. Low-flow irrigation will not excessively expand or displace vitreous and will minimize the likelihood of vitreous prolapse through the tear. The cortex remote from the tear should be removed initially so that the majority of cortex will have been removed before manipulating cortex near the rent. Cortex should be stripped toward the rent because any force generated away from it will cause its extension. The removal of as much cortex as possible is desirable, yet heroic efforts to remove all cortex should be avoided because such attempts might extend the tear and further compromise the integrity of the capsular bag. The same warning applies to vacuuming the central posterior capsule when the tear is peripheral because the yttrium-aluminum-garnet laser can be safely used following surgery. Withdrawal of the irrigation-aspiration handpiece should be accompanied by further reduction of irrigation and simultaneous injection of air or viscoelastic into the eye to maintain the anterior chamber depth. An alternative and perhaps safer method of cortical removal is manual aspiration using both a bent cannula and a J-shaped cannula under the protection of viscoelastic material. This manual technique of "dry" aspiration of cortex is more time consuming but decreases the risk of extending the tear and vitreous loss.

If vitreous is encountered at any point in the procedure, a low-flow bimanual vitrectomy may be performed while avoiding traction on the vitreous. This is best accomplished by using a cannula for infusion at the second stab site in combination with a separate automated vitrector, which is passed through the capsular tear to perform the anterior vitrectomy. The infusion is not placed into the vitreous cavity because removing just the prolapsed anterior vitreous is preferable to a massive vitrectomy. An alternative technique is a "dry" (no infusion) vitrectomy that uses a viscoelastic agent to maintain the anterior segment while the vitrectomy is performed through the opening in the torn capsule.[51] Recently, there has been a trend toward performing vitrectomy by passing the vitreous cutter through a pars plana incision, and this technique, although it carries the increased risk of vitreous hemorrhage, may be more effective at clearing vitreous from the anterior segment.

A new technique for staining the vitreous has been introduced by Burk and colleagues. Kenalog (triamcinolone acetonide) is diluted and then injected into the anterior chamber, which results in a dramatic visibility of the vitreous to aid in a more effective vitrectomy (Figure 39-12).[52]

Three Special Maneuvers

If the tear is identified when both the nucleus and vitreous are present in the anterior segment, the Posterior Assisted Levitation (PAL) technique may be helpful if the surgeon fears loss of the nucleus. Developed by Charles Kelman, an emergency stab incision is placed through the pars plana, and a spatula is introduced. The nucleus is lifted into the anterior chamber from behind, where it can be emulsified or expressed.[53]

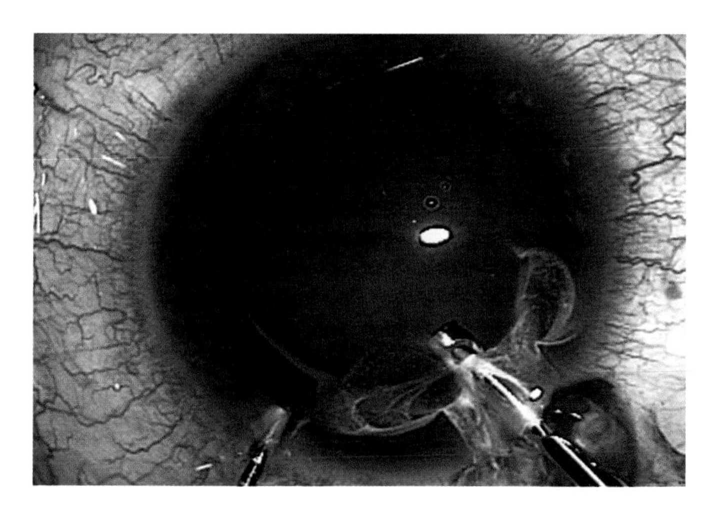

FIGURE 39-12 Vitreous gel made clearly visible by the injection of Kenalog particles seen streaming into the vitrectomy port.

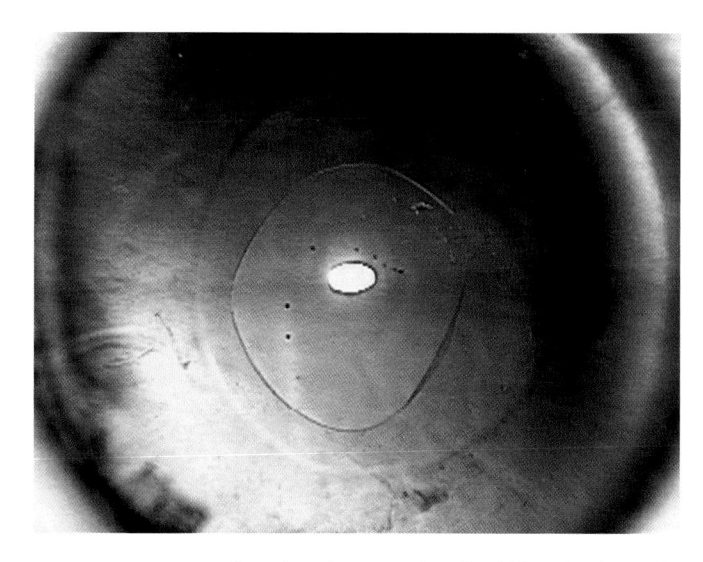

FIGURE 39-13 Operating microscope view of an ICG-assisted posterior capsulorhexis in a cadaver eye. Note the light green staining of the capsular bag and the intact anterior capsular rim in the foreground.

Another option developed by Mark Michaelson is to introduce a Sheets glide between the nucleus and the tear. This allows the surgeon to either emulsify or express the nucleus with less fear of losing the nucleus. A retentive viscoelastic agent placed behind the nucleus for increased safety may be useful in cases of small posterior capsular tears and may be used in combination with the previous maneuvers, but it should seldom be used alone with large posterior capsular tears because the nucleus may still sublux backward if either the vitreous cavity creates an inviting vacuum or if the pressure in the anterior chamber is elevated.

Finally, the surgeon must be capable of converting a limited linear tear into a posterior capsulorhexis. In this maneuver the vitreous face is retroplaced with viscoelastic, and a fine Utrata forceps is used to grasp the edge of the tear and redirect it until a continuous edge is achieved. Although it is not always possible, the strength of the capsular bag is best guaranteed if this maneuver is successfully accomplished (Figure 39-13).

Intraocular Lens Placement

The key to successful placement of an IOL in the presence of a posterior capsule tear is clear visualization of the capsulozonular anatomy. Only by determining the exact anatomy of the tear can the integrity of the capsular support be understood. After viscoelastic material is instilled, the iris is gently retracted with a collar-button instrument (Figure 39-14).* The most desirable location and orientation of the lens, its design, and the optimal insertion technique should become evident to the surgeon. It is better for a surgeon either to suture fixate a PC IOL or not to

*Osher Iris Retractor, Duckworth and Kent.

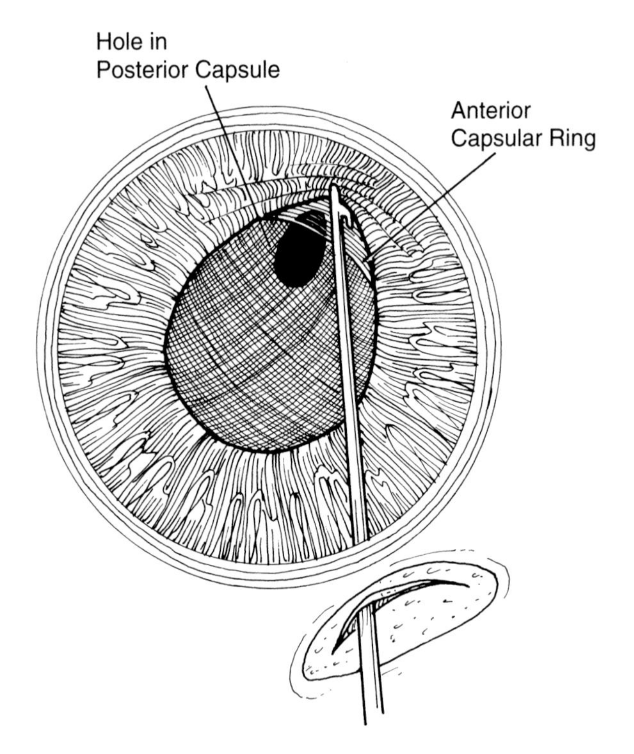

FIGURE 39-14 Retraction of the iris to visualize the extent of a posterior capsular tear.

implant a posterior chamber lens if he or she is unsure of the anatomy than to rely on chance alone for proper fixation and enduring centration.

Several guidelines have emerged for implanting posterior chamber IOLs in these challenging eyes. When the opening in the posterior capsule is small with well-defined borders, the bag can be inflated with viscoelastic material, and a capsule forceps can be used to convert the tear to a continuous posterior capsulorhexis.[54] The tear is then less likely to extend if the bag is stretched by placement of the IOL. Placement of the IOL using a dialing technique may exert more force in the capsular bag, causing extension of the tear. Therefore a superior haptic compression maneuver or a slowly unfolding lens in the capsular bag may be safer. If the tear is large, with peripheral extension and poorly defined borders, viscoelastic agent is placed over the anterior capsule rim to collapse the bag and allow implantation into the ciliary sulcus, however the IOL power for the ciliary sulcus should be decreased by 0.5 diopters from the capsular bag calculation. Another option is to place the haptics in the ciliary sulcus and capture the optic in the capsulorhexis opening. Perhaps the single-piece AcrySof SA60AT IOL from Alcon is the safest IOL to implant into the capsular bag when the posterior capsule is open. This IOL has a very small mass when injected, and its haptics open slowly and gently, especially when the capsular bag is filled with Healon5. Therefore the lens can be rotated without placing excessive force on the equatorial capsule. Even when the lens has unfolded, the haptic is uniquely soft. Moreover, there is a rapid postoperative bioadhesive effect caused by fibronectin, which seals the IOL to the capsule. However, this IOL is not intended for sulcus placement.

Whether the lens is placed within the bag or into the ciliary sulcus, it should be positioned with the haptics oriented for best support, which is usually 90 degrees away from the axis of the tear. Once the lens is centered, its fixation should be evaluated by slightly decentering the lens toward each haptic and releasing it to observe for spontaneous recentering. If it does not recenter itself, the haptic should be rotated to a different axis. If the lens still shows signs of poor fixation and will not center itself, it can be repositioned from the capsular bag into the ciliary sulcus, sutured into the ciliary sulcus, or removed and exchanged for an anterior chamber IOL provided there are no relative contraindications, such as poorly controlled glaucoma, significant peripheral anterior synechiae, or iris loss. If an anterior chamber lens is used, each haptic should always be flexed, lifted, and allowed to reseat itself in the angle to prevent inadvertent iris entrapment.

Once the lens is well centered and its stability has been confirmed, acetylcholine may be instilled onto the pupillary sphincter because miosis will both retard late vitreous prolapse and make any residual vitreous easier to visualize. Either air or a viscoelastic agent will help to establish a formed, pressurized chamber for precise wound closure and control the vitreous position. Air does have the advantages of allowing any vitreous to fall back and delineating any transcameral vitreous strands by their interruption of a smooth round bubble in the anterior chamber. Sweeping the pupil with a microhook is always recommended to ensure that there is no prolapsed vitreous remaining. If the posterior capsule was torn but a vitrectomy was not performed, a peripheral iridectomy should be considered depending on the circumstances as a prophylactic measure against vitreous-induced pupillary block.

At the conclusion of the procedure, protective viscoelastic material can be removed manually or with an irrigation-aspiration tip. However, if the chamber collapses, one risks further vitreous prolapse. Therefore the irrigation-aspiration tip should not simply be withdrawn from the incision. Air should be injected through the stab incision simultaneously with tip withdrawal to prevent momentary chamber collapse and late vitreous prolapse. The air can then be removed in small aliquots and exchanged for a buffered saline solution so that the anterior chamber depth is maintained.

Zonular Dialysis

A zonular dialysis may be present before surgery either as a result of preexisting trauma or in association with specific disorders (i.e., Marfan syndrome, Weill-Marchesani syndrome). Phacodonesis, iridodonesis, vitreous in the anterior chamber, visibility of the lens equator. A slit view of the nucleus that appears off center or a "gap" between the iris border and the lens may provide important clues to this diagnosis. Pseudoexfoliation is another condition that has a propensity for weakened zonules. Surgical management of these challenging cases is beyond the scope of this chapter and is reviewed elsewhere.[55-66]

An intraoperative zonular dialysis may result from a traumatic capsulectomy, excessive maneuvering of the nucleus, or aspiration of either the anterior or the posterior capsule with

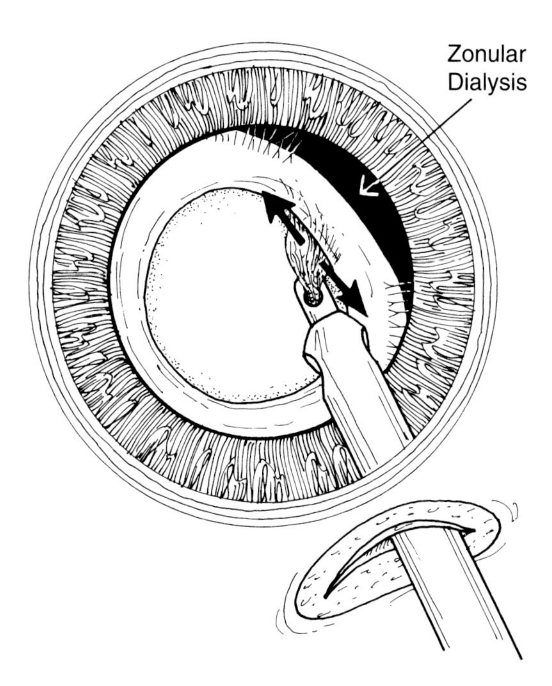

FIGURE 39-15 Cortical stripping in the presence of a zonular dialysis should always be done using gentle tangential movements *(black arrows)*. Radial forces should be avoided to prevent enlarging the zonular dialysis.

the irrigation-aspiration tip. Prompt recognition and the avoidance of further trauma are the best response. A highly retentive viscoelastic agent placed over the area of dialysis will act to restrain the vitreous, reducing the possibility of prolapse. Similar principles apply to the torn posterior capsule in that all forces generated within the eye should be directed toward rather than away from the zonular dialysis to avoid "unzippering" of the adjacent intact zonules.

Capsulorhexis, nuclear removal, and cortical removal may be very difficult when a loose capsular bag cannot exert countertraction. Stabilizing a loose capsular bag with Prolene iris retractors and even a capsular tension ring may be necessary and has proven very helpful in removing the nucleus and cortex in some patients. Cortical stripping may require frequent foot pedal reflux if the capsule is drawn into the aspiration port. The last cortex to be removed should be that in proximity to the zonular dialysis. It should not be stripped radially but rather parallel to the dialysis (Figure 39-15). If cortex adheres tightly to the capsule, viscodissection may facilitate separation. Heroic perseverance in the removal of every last bit of cortex should be avoided to preserve capsulozonular support for the IOL.

If vitreous presents through the dialysis, either a low-infusion bimanual or dry anterior vitrectomy should be performed. Alternatively, the vitreous cutter can be introduced through the pars plana. Once the anterior segment is free of vitreous, an IOL can be implanted into the capsular bag as long as the anterior capsule ring is intact and zonular dialysis is not in excess of about 4 hours. There is some debate regarding the optimal orientation of the IOL. We have placed it both parallel and perpendicular to the zonular dialysis (Figure 39-16). Perpendicular haptic orientation (see Figure 39-16, *B*) may help resist postoperative capsular contracture that causes the IOL to decenter. A larger, holeless optic is recommended because a slight decentration

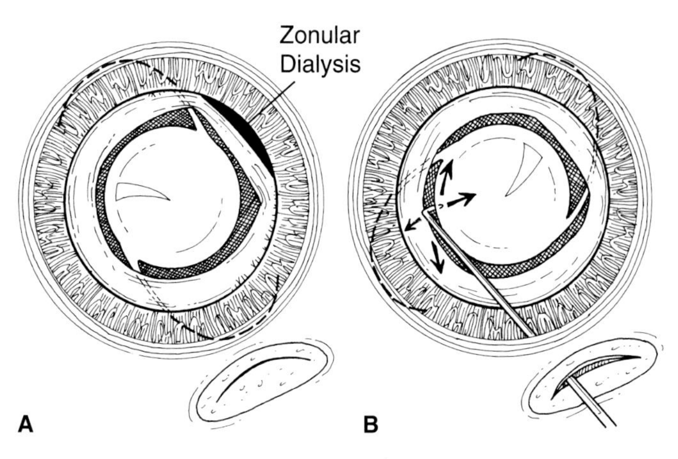

FIGURE 39-16 Orientation of the IOL parallel to **(A)** or perpendicular to **(B)** the zonular dialysis. The "bounce" test is performed with an IOL hook to determine stability *(arrows)*.

may occur as postoperative forces generated by the remaining intact zonules come into play.

If the zonular dialysis is severe, the surgeon who wishes to implant an IOL has several choices. An older technique involves the instillation of alpha-chymotrypsin, allowing delivery of the entire capsular bag and its contents, followed by either a sutured posterior chamber lens or an anterior chamber lens. Conversely, if the surgeon has been successful at removing nuclear and cortical material, the remaining capsule may be left alone because it probably does have some stabilizing effect. Suturing of one or both haptics through the ciliary sulcus may be sufficient if there is some residual capsulozonular support. However, these options are not our preference.

We strongly believe that the patient with a severe zonular dialysis should have the benefit of a capsular tension ring, and there are numerous publications supporting this conclusion since 1993.[56-66] Cionni[66] designed a modification with an eyelet on a hook that allows permanent suture fixation through the ciliary sulcus while the attached capsular tension ring is within the bag. Only by reexpanding the loose bag, refixating it to the sclera, and implanting an IOL in the capsular bag is the patient with severe zonular dialysis optimally managed (Figures 39-17 and 39-18).

Dropped Nucleus

Posterior dislocation of a partially emulsified nucleus into the vitreous cavity is a complication dreaded by every phacoemulsification surgeon. Its most common cause is excessive infusion, which raises the anterior chamber pressure, literally pushing the nucleus through an opening in the posterior capsule.

If the nucleus suddenly falls back into the vitreous but remains in view, the PAL technique may be performed or a viscoelastic agent may be injected quickly behind the nucleus, which may buy time for retrieval with a lens loop. If the lens disappears altogether, the cortex should be removed and a gentle bimanual vitrectomy performed through either the limbus or pars plana. If the nucleus does not present during vitrectomy, the surgeon may attempt to float it forward by

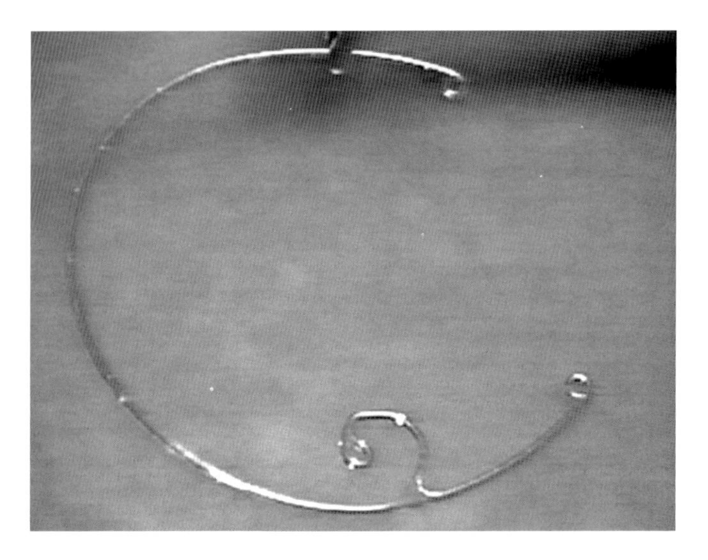

FIGURE 39-17 Cionni modified endocapsular tension ring. The ring expands the capsular bag and has an eyelet for permanent fixation to the sclera.

directing a gentle stream of irrigation fluid through a 22-gauge cannula posteriorly into the vitreous cavity. If the nucleus becomes visible, it can be recovered by sliding a loop beneath. Delivery of the nucleus from the eye must be preceded by liberally enlarging the size of the incision and possibly the capsulorhexis opening.

When the nucleus fails to present, the surgeon should remove as much cortex as possible, and the patient should be referred to a vitreoretinal specialist. Heroic attempts to retrieve the nucleus should be avoided because excessive intravitreal maneuvers by an anterior segment surgeon have the propensity to do more harm than good and openly invites litigation. Intravitreal emulsification or flotation of the dropped nucleus with perfluorocarbon is well within the expertise of the vitreoretinal surgeon. Whether the original surgeon elects to implant an IOL before closing the eye or leaves this task to the vitreoretinal specialist must be considered on an individual basis. Traditionally, if the nucleus was very brunescent, the IOL was not implanted initially because the nucleus had to be brought forward if intravitreal fragmentation was not possible. However, newer vitrectomy machines are capable of emulsifying even the most mature lenses. Accompanying the vitreoretinal surgeon to the operating room to assist with IOL implantation should be considered by the cataract surgeon because he or she is more experienced in anterior segment surgery.

Intraoperative Pupillary Block

During the phacoemulsification or I/A step, an unusual deepening of the chamber and posterior displacement of the iris border can occur as a sign of intraoperative pupillary block. Rarely, this can also occur during the removal of a viscoelastic agent after the IOL is in the capsular bag. A second instrument placed into the pupil under the iris results in the reversal of these findings as the capsular block is broken.

Acute Corneal Clouding

There is always the remote possibility that the surgeon can inject either the wrong concentration of a drug or even the wrong solution into the eye. We have seen the cornea become opaque when an inappropriate mixture of Miochol was instilled, and we are aware of a case where distilled water was substituted for BSS.

Prompt recognition followed by immediate intracameral irrigation with BSS is indicated. The vital communication

A

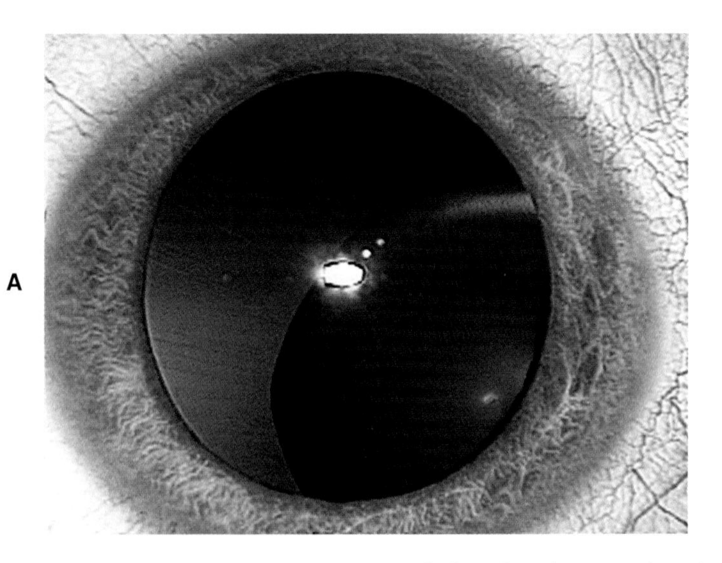

B

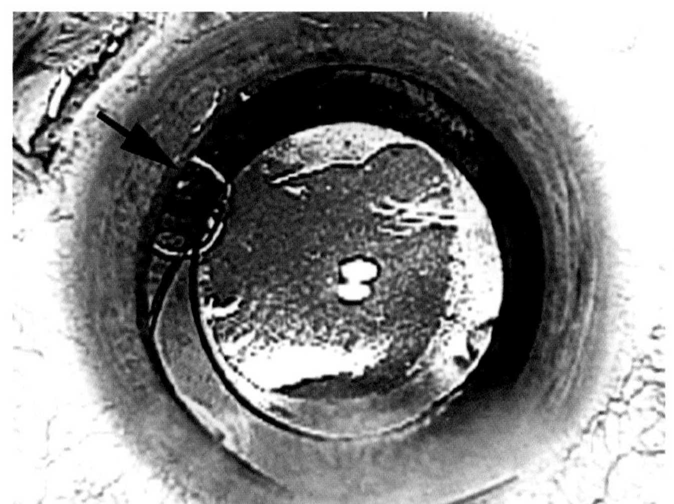

FIGURE 39-18 A, Operating microscope view of severe zonular laxity in a patient with Marfan syndrome. **B,** Operating microscope view following phacoemulsification and intraocular lens implantation. Note the fixation loop with eyelet of the Cionni modified endocapsular tension ring *(black arrow)*.

between members of the well-trained operation team will minimize the risk of the potentially disastrous complication.

Expulsive Hemorrhage

The catastrophic complication of expulsive hemorrhage is more likely to occur in older patients with brunescent lenses, preexisting uveitis, glaucoma, high myopia, or systemic hypertension or in those receiving anticoagulation therapy.[67,68] Early recognition is the key to successful management. Chamber shallowing with positive pressure may be the first sign of a choroidal hemorrhage. The surgeon may notice a loss of the red reflex, and the patient may complain of pain despite adequate anesthesia. If the surgeon suspects this diagnosis, ophthalmoscopy should be performed to determine whether a choroidal hemorrhage is developing. Although the indirect ophthalmoscope should be readily available, a lens has been developed by Ocular Instruments (Osher Panfundus lens) that can be kept sterile on the surgeon's tray and allows a quick view of the fundus through the operating microscope.

The globe that becomes firm abruptly demands immediate closure of the eye. If the surgeon is unable to close the wound because of extensive pressure, he or she should tamponade the incision with a finger while mannitol is being given.[69] Once the incision has been closed, uveal tissue that has prolapsed can be repositioned, and the anterior chamber can be deepened with air, BSS, or a viscoelastic material. If the anterior chamber fails to deepen or if closure of the incision is unsuccessful, the surgeon should urgently attempt to drain the choroidal hemorrhage via a posterior sclerotomy 3.5 to 4 mm posterior to the limbus.

The importance of cortical removal or IOL implantation pales in relation to the crisis at hand because the singular goal is to save the eye. A secondary procedure can always be performed at a later date. Fortunately, this complication is extraordinarily rare in phacoemulsification surgery because the small wound is protective against this disastrous event. Moreover, the use of a self-sealing incision provides an obvious advantage in this situation. In several of our cases, this watertight incision has permitted the completion of cortical removal by a manual technique using a 27-gauge cannula through a stab incision. Following the resolution of the choroidal hemorrhage, these patients underwent successful secondary IOL implantation several weeks later.

Conclusions

Phacoemulsification is an elegant and safe procedure that is rewarding to both the patient and the surgeon. Complications will be encountered by every cataract surgeon, and their management will depend on experience, skill, and sound judgment. We have presented a spectrum of intraoperative complications and offered our perspective in preventing and managing these situations.

As phacoemulsification techniques change, so also will the types and frequency of complications. We encourage surgeons to modify these basic principles and apply them to new techniques that will be introduced in the future.

REFERENCES

1. Feibel RM: Current concepts in retrobulbar anesthesia, *Surv Ophthalmol* 30:102-110, 1985.
2. Ellis P: Retrobulbar injection, *Surv Ophthalmol* 18:425-430, 1974.
3. Cionni R, Osher R: Retrobulbar hemorrhage, *Ophthalmology* 98:1153-1155, 1991.
4. Koch D: Standard analysis of cataract incision construction, *J Cataract Refract Surg* 17:661-667, 1999.
5. Ernest P, Kiesslue L, Lowery K: Relative strength of cataract incisions in cadaver eyes, *J Cataract Refract Surg* 17:668-671, 1991.
6. Singer J: Frown incisions for minimizing individual astigmatism after small incision cataract surgery with rigid optic intraocular lens implantation, *J Cataract Refract Surg* 17:677-688, 1991.
7. Jaffe N, Claymann H: The pathophysiology of corneal astigmatism after cataract extraction, *Trans Am Acad Ophthalmol Otolaryngol* 79:615-630, 1975.
8. Masket S: Nonkeratometric control of post-operative astigmatism, *Am Intraocular Implant Soc J* 11:134-147, 1985.
9. Ernest P: Cadaver eye study of the relative stability of clear corneal incisions and scleral corneal incisions used in small incision cataract surgery. Presented at the American Society of Cataract and Refractive Surgery Meeting, Seattle, Wash, May 1993.
10. Osher R: New suturing techniques, *Audiovisual J Cataract Implant Surg* 6(3), 1990.
11. Osher R: Thermal burns, *Audiovisual J Cataract Implant Surg* 9, 1993.
12. Thim K, Grag S, Corydon L: Stretching capacity of capsulorhexis and nucleus delivery, *J Cataract Refract Surg* 17:27-31, 1991.
13. Wasserman D, Apple D, Castaneda V et al: Anterior capsular tears and loop fixation of posterior chamber intraocular lenses, *Ophthalmology* 98:425-432, 1991.
14. Assia E, Apple D, Tsai J et al: The elastic properties of the lens capsule in capsulorhexis, *Am J Ophthalmol* 3:628-632, 1991.
15. Osher R, Cionni R: The torn posterior capsule: its intraoperative behavior, surgical management and long term consequences, *J Cataract Refract Surg* 16:459-494, 1990.
16. Osher RH, Falzoni W, Osher JM: Our phacoemulsification technique. In L Buratto, L Werner, M Zanini et al (eds), *Phacoemulsification principles and techniques*, ed 2, Thorofare, NJ, 2003, SLACK, Inc.
17. Masket S: Postoperative complications of capsulorhexis, *J Cataract Refract Surg* 19:721-724, 1993.
18. Horiguchi M, Miyake K, Ohta I, Ito Y: Staining of the lens capsule for circular continuous capsulorrhexis in eyes with white cataract, *Arch Ophthalmol* 116:535-537, 1998.
19. Pandey SK, Werner L, Escobar-Gomez M et al: Dye-enhanced cataract surgery. Part I. Anterior capsule staining for capsulorhexis in advanced/white cataract, *J Cataract Refract Surg* 26:1052-1059, 2000.
20. Werner L, Pandey SK, Escobar-Gomez M et al: Dye-enhanced cataract surgery. Part II. Learning critical steps of phacoemulsification, *J Cataract Refract Surg* 26:1060-1065, 2000.
21. Pandey SK, Werner L, Escobar-Gomez M, et al: Dye-enhanced cataract surgery. Part III. Posterior capsule staining to learn posterior continuous curvilinear capsulorhexis, *J Cataract Refract Surg* 26:1066-1071, 2000.
22. Newsom TH, Oetting TA: Indocyanine green staining in traumatic cataract, *J Cataract Refract Surg* 26:1691-1693, 2000.
23. Pandey SK, Werner L, Apple DJ: Staining the anterior capsule, *J Cataract Refract Surg* 27:647-648, 2001.
24. Sturmer J: Cataract surgery and the "Blue Miracle," *Klin Monatsbl Augenheilkd* 219:191-195, 2002.
25. de Waard PW, Budo CJ, Melles GR: Trypan blue capsular staining to "find" the leading edge of a "lost" capsulorhexis, *Am J Ophthalmol* 134:271-272, 2002.
26. Schneider S, Osher RH, Burk SE et al: Thinning of the anterior capsule: a new finding associated with congenital aniridia. *J Cataract Refract Surg* 2003 (in press).
27. Wilbrandt H, Wilbrandt T: Evaluation of intraocular pressure fluctuations with differing phacoemulsification approaches, *J Cataract Refract Surg* 19:223-231, 1993.
28. Osher R: Slow motion phacoemulsification approach, *J Cataract Refract Surg* 19:667, 1993.
29. Cionni R: Review of positive pressure, *Audiovisual J Cataract Implant Surg* 8(4), 1992.
30. Davis P: Phaco transducers: basic principles and corneal thermal injury, *Eur J Implant Ref Surg* 5:109, 1993.
31. Keates R, McGowan K: Clinical trial of flurbiprofen to maintain pupillary dilation during cataract surgery, *Ann Ophthalmol* 16:919-921, 1984.

32. Osher R, Gimbel H, Galand A et al: Small pupil phacoemulsification, *Audiovisual J Cataract Implant Surg* 7, 1991.
33. Mackool RJ: Small pupil enlargement during cataract extraction: a new method, *J Cataract Refract Surg* 18:523-526, 1992.
34. Nichamin LD: Enlarging the pupil for cataract extraction using flexible nylon iris retractors, *J Cataract Refract Surg* 19:793-796, 1993.
35. Shepherd DM: The pupil stretch technique for miotic pupils in cataract surgery, *Ophthalmic Surg* 24:851-852, 1993.
36. Koch PS: Techniques and instruments for cataract surgery, *Curr Opin Ophthalmol* 5:33-39, 1994.
37. Fry L: Pupil stretching, *Video J Cataract Refractive Surg* 9, 1995.
38. Masket S: Avoiding complications associated with iris retractor use in small pupil cataract extraction, *J Cataract Refract Surg* 22:168-171, 1996.
39. Dinsmore SC: Modified stretch technique for small pupil phacoemulsification with topical anesthesia, *J Cataract Refract Surg* 22:27-30, 1996.
40. Novak J: Flexible iris hooks for phacoemulsification, *J Cataract Refract Surg* 23:828-831, 1997.
41. Barboni P, Zanini M, Rossi A, Savini G: Monomanual pupil stretcher, *Ophthalmic Surg Lasers* 29:772-773, 1998.
42. Oetting TA, Omphroy LC: Modified technique using flexible iris retractors in clear corneal cataract surgery, *J Cataract Refract Surg* 28:596-598, 2002.
43. Jaffe H: *Cataract surgery and its complications,* ed 3, St Louis, 1981, Mosby, pp 368, 576-579.
44. Gimble H: Divide and conquer nucleofractis phacoemulsification: development and variations, *J Cataract Refract Surg* 17:281-291, 1991.
45. Osher RH, Yu BC, Koch DD: Posterior polar cataracts: a predisposition to intraoperative posterior capsular rupture, *J Cataract Refract Surg* 16:157-162, 1990.
46. Cheng KP, Hiles DA, Biglan AW, Pettapiece MC: Management of posterior lenticonus, *J Pediatr Ophthalmol Strabismus* 28:143-149, 1991.
47. Vasavada A, Singh R: Phacoemulsification in eyes with posterior polar cataract, *J Cataract Refract Surg* 25:238-245, 1999.
48. Allen D, Wood C: Minimizing risk to the capsule during surgery for posterior polar cataract, *J Cataract Refract Surg* 28:742-744, 2002.
49. Fine IH, Packer M, Hoffman RS: Management of posterior polar cataract, *J Cataract Refract Surg* 29:16-19, 2003.
50. Hayashi K, Hayashi H, Nakao F, Hayashi F: Outcomes of surgery for posterior polar cataract, *J Cataract Refract Surg* 29:45-49, 2003.
51. Osher R: Dry vitrectomy, *Audiovisual J Cataract Refract Surg* 8, 1992.
52. Burk SE, Da Mata AP, Schneider S et al: Visualizing vitreous using Kenalog suspension, *J Cataract Refract Surg* 2003 (in press).
53. Kelman C: PALTechnique, *Video J Cataract Refractive Surg* 12, 1996.
54. Castaneda V, Tegler U, Tsai J et al: Posterior continuous curvilinear capsulorhexis, *Ophthalmology* 99:45, 1992.
55. Osher R: Surgical approach to the traumatic cataract, *Audiovisual J Cataract Implant Surg* 3, 1987.
56. Osher R, Cionni R, Gimbel H et al: Cataract surgery in patients with pseudoexfoliation: cataract surgery in patients with pseudoexfoliation syndrome, *Eur J Implant Refract Surg* 5:46-50, 1993.
57. Cionni RJ, Osher RH: Endocapsular ring approach to the subluxed cataractous lens, *J Cataract Refract Surg* 21:245-249, 1995.
58. Fine IH, Hoffman RS: Phacoemulsification in the presence of pseudoexfoliation: challenges and options, *J Cataract Refract Surg* 23:160-165, 1997.
59. Gimbel HV, Sun R, Heston JP: Management of zonular dialysis in phacoemulsification and IOL implantation using the capsular tension ring, *Ophthalmic Surg Lasers* 28:273-281, 1997.
60. Cionni RJ, Osher RH: Management of profound zonular dialysis or weakness with a new endocapsular ring designed for scleral fixation, *J Cataract Refract Surg* 24:1299-1306, 1998.
61. Menapace R, Findl O, Georgopoulos M et al: The capsular tension ring: designs, applications, and techniques, *J Cataract Refract Surg* 26:898-912, 2000.
62. Menkhaus S, Motschmann M, Kuchenbecker J, Behrens-Baumann W: Pseudoexfoliation (PEX) syndrome and intraoperative complications in cataract surgery, *Klin Monatsbl Augenheilkd* 216:388-392, 2000.
63. Ahmed II, Crandall AS: Ab externo scleral fixation of the Cionni modified capsular tension ring, *J Cataract Refract Surg* 27:977-981, 2001.
64. Bayraktar S, Altan T, Kucuksumer Y, Yilmaz OF: Capsular tension ring implantation after capsulorhexis in phacoemulsification of cataracts associated with pseudoexfoliation syndrome: intraoperative complications and early postoperative findings, *J Cataract Refract Surg* 27:1620-1628, 2001.
65. Gimbel HV, Sun R: Clinical applications of capsular tension rings in cataract surgery, *Ophthalmic Surg Lasers* 33:44-53, 2002.
66. Cionni RJ, Osher RH, Snyder ME: Five years experience with the Cionni modified capsular tension ring, *Video J Cataract Refractive Surg* 18, 2002.
67. Riderman J, Harbin T, Campbell D: Post-operative suprachoroidal hemorrhage following filtrating procedures, *Arch Ophthalmol* 194:201-205, 1986.
68. Speaker M, Guerleio P, Riet J et al: A case control study of risk factors for intraoperative suprachoroidal expulsive hemorrhage, *Ophthalmology* 98:202-210, 1991.
69. Osher M: Emergency treatment of vitreous bulge and wound gaping complicating cataract surgery, *Am J Ophthalmol* 44:409-411, 1957.

40 Surgical Repositioning and Explantation of Intraocular Lens

Robert H. Osher, MD
Robert J. Cionni, MD
Robert E. Foster, MD
Mark S. Blumenkrantz, MD
Andrea P. Da Mata, MD

Although most eyes that undergo cataract extraction and intraocular lens (IOL) implantation are rapidly rehabilitated from an anatomic and visual standpoint, a small percentage develops complications that require repositioning, replacement, or removal of the pseudophakos. Occasionally, the cause is faulty lens design, which results in chronic inflammation. In other cases, a lens of an inappropriate size leads to unacceptable lens mobility and an uncomfortable, inflamed eye. Incorrect dioptric power may result in anisometropia, asthenopia, or other refractive symptoms. Iris tuck and uveal irritation may follow improper intraoperative positioning of an anterior chamber lens. A posterior chamber lens may decenter because of a number of reasons, including asymmetric haptic placement, inadequate capsular or zonular support, pseudoexfoliation, progressive posterior synechiogenesis with pupillary capture, endocapsular fibrosis, late zonular dehiscence, enlargement of the neodymium:yttrium-aluminum-garnet laser posterior capsulotomy incision, or postoperative trauma to the eye.[1,2]

Complications of malpositioned and dislocated anterior chamber IOLs (AC IOLs) include uveitis, glaucoma, hyphema, cystoid macular edema (CME), and corneal decompensation. In contrast, complications of dislocated posterior chamber IOLs (PC IOLs) tend to be less severe and are primarily optical in character. These include the development of anisokonia, blurred vision, diplopia induced by prismatic image displacement, and glare, which may occur as a result of diffractive effects on the lens edge or positioning holes.

Although surgical intervention is definitive, it is not the only approach available in the management of difficult IOL cases. Conservative observation and pharmacologic therapy should always be considered.[2,3] Many eyes with IOLs that are dislocated into the vitreous cavity during the earlier days of implant surgery have maintained excellent vision with no surgical intervention. The course of action must reflect the type and location of the lens, the age of the patient, the symptoms, the visual acuity, the corneal endothelial health, the presence and severity of intraocular inflammation, and the status of the fellow eye. When surgical intervention is under consideration, a decision must be made with regard to the timing of surgery, the approach (anterior versus posterior), the composition of the surgical team (cataract surgeon, vitreoretinal surgeon, or both) and the disposition of the pseudophakos (repositioning, replacement, or removal.)

Conservative therapy such as observation may be appropriate for an eye with an anterior chamber lens that is associated with a peaked or oval pupil as long as signs and symptoms of intraocular inflammation are absent. Pharmacologic management consisting of topical steroids may be indicated in the case of mild cell and flare that is unassociated with symptoms or with reduced vision. A trial with a nonsteroidal antiinflammatory agent in combination with a steroid is justified as a first step in symptomatic pseudophakic CME. Edge-related reflections, diplopia, or glare may in some cases be managed successfully by topical pilocarpine. Topical sodium chloride might be preferable to surgery in treating peripheral corneal edema associated with incipient corneal decompensation in an elderly patient who has a low endothelial cell count.[4] The malpositioned iris-supported lens associated with refractive or inflammatory symptoms is less commonly managed by conservative measures because of our recognition that this design is inferior when compared with both open-loop anterior chamber and most other styles of posterior chamber lenses. However, the posterior dislocation of a single haptic of the Copeland lens or the loop of a Binkhorst or Medallion lens may be associated with posterior synechiae or a fixed pupil that acts to prevent dislocation of the optic. Sequential pharmacologic manipulation of the pupil can result in successful repositioning of the lens in selected instances.[4-6]

Decentered and dislocated PC IOLs have become more prevalent because these lenses account for more than 95% of all lenses implanted in the United States today. The most common presenting complaint is unwanted optical images caused by either a centering hole or the edge of the optic within the pupil. If the symptoms are infrequent and limited to the evening when the pupil is more dilated, the surgeon may elect to manage these patients conservatively by using a topical miotic. More severe or disabling symptoms can be managed by repositioning, explanting, or exchanging the IOL. When complete dislocation of a posterior chamber lens has occurred outside the visual axis, several options exist, including (1) observation and correction of monocular aphakia by external means (2) IOL repositioning, and (3) IOL exchange.[6-8] Effective suturing techniques both for secondary placement of posterior chamber lenses and for repositioning of dislocated lenses have further increased the available options.[9-14]

In this chapter we discuss methods and results of treatment for IOL problems that require surgical intervention.

Patient Education

The patient should be thoroughly advised of the management alternatives in cases of IOL dislocation, which include spectacle or contact lens aphakic correction, repositioning, exchange, or removal in the event that a relative contraindication to IOL implantation is encountered intraoperatively. The patient should also be apprised of the short- and long-term complications of this technique, including IOL redislocation; residual refractive error; or symptoms related to the presence of a decentered edge, vitreous hemorrhage, retinal tear, retinal detachment, CME, and endophthalmitis. Some patients, when fully informed of all potential risks and benefits, may elect to receive more conservative forms of management. Conservative management is appropriate in the absence of any absolute indications for removal, such as infection or mechanical retinal damage.

General Methods

Preoperative Evaluation

All patients being considered for surgical correction of IOL problems require thorough preoperative evaluation, which includes the determination of a bilateral best-corrected visual acuity, slit lamp biomicroscopy, gonioscopy, and dilated fundus ophthalmoscopy. Keratometry, ultrasonography, specular microscopy with endothelial cell count, and, in some instances, potential acuity meter testing should be performed. A review of the original operative report and knowledge of the lens power and postoperative refraction may be useful. On reviewing this information, a preliminary decision can be made to reposition, remove, and/or exchange the IOL. The procedure chosen to correct a malpositioned posterior chamber lens cannot always be finalized at the time of the preoperative examination and should be reassessed during surgery when the pupil is maximally dilated to allow direct visualization of the anatomic relationships. If the pupil fails to dilate, a stab incision at the corneoscleral junction permits entry of a microhook to retract the iris. Adequate visualization is essential for understanding the pathophysiology of the malpositioned posterior chamber lens and for correcting the underlying problem.

Another benefit of surgical intervention is the achievement of a more desirable refractive error. Reviewing the original keratometry and ultrasound measurements along with the postoperative refractive data may help the surgeon reconstruct the original pseudophakic status. Knowledge of the IOL style, its A-constant, and the location in which it was originally placed allows refinements in the selection of a new IOL. In addition, moderate or high astigmatism can be reduced by incision placement, astigmatic keratotomy, or limbal relaxing incisions.

Postoperative Follow-Up

The best-corrected visual acuity is measured at each visit, and the outcome of other surgical goals, which include the resolution of residual refractive error, iritis, glaucoma, corneal edema, visual distortion, and/or CME, is evaluated. Additional specialized studies may include comparative endothelial cell counts and fluorescein angiography when indicated.

Surgical Techniques

Anterior Chamber Intraocular Lens

Repositioning of an anterior chamber lens should be performed when a haptic incarcerates iris tissue or when iris is prolapsed into the wound or into the peripheral iridectomy. If it is diagnosed early, iris incarceration and haptic malposition can be corrected by flexing, lifting, and repositioning the offending haptic. Intolerable aberrant optical images might occasionally be corrected by adroit repositioning of the iris and AC IOL; however, some may only be alleviated by explantation.

Although repositioning might suffice in selected cases, lens explantation is necessary when excessive mobility or "propellering" is observed, indicating that the lens is too small, or when severe tenderness, iris ovalization, and indentation of the ciliary body suggest that the lens is too large and rigid. Explantation of an AC IOL is also necessary when the lens is associated with chronic uveitis-glaucoma-hyphema (UGH) syndrome that is resistant to medical therapy.[6,7]

The closed filamentous anterior chamber lenses, most notably the Azar (91Z), the Leiske, and the Stableflex, have filamentous haptics that may become enveloped by peripheral anterior synechiae. When synechiae are present, the explantation technique involves severing the haptics from the optic to remove the lens in pieces, thereby avoiding bleeding, iridodialysis, and severe damage to the angle. The optic should be manipulated carefully because the severed haptics are sharp and potentially hazardous. With viscoelastic material filling the anterior chamber, a spatula placed under the optic serves as a ramp to prevent snagging of the posterior wound lip during removal.

Once the optic has been explanted, the remaining filamentous haptics are threaded back through the synechial tunnels until they are free in the anterior chamber, where they can be easily removed (Figures 40-1 and 40-2). See also Chapter 42, Corneal Edema.

If a posterior capsular remnant is present and offers adequate peripheral support, the AC IOL may be exchanged for a PC IOL. Suturing a posterior chamber lens to either the iris or through the ciliary sulcus offers additional techniques for lens exchange, especially in a patient with glaucoma or with an abnormal anterior segment (e.g., extensive synechiae, angle recession).[9-14]

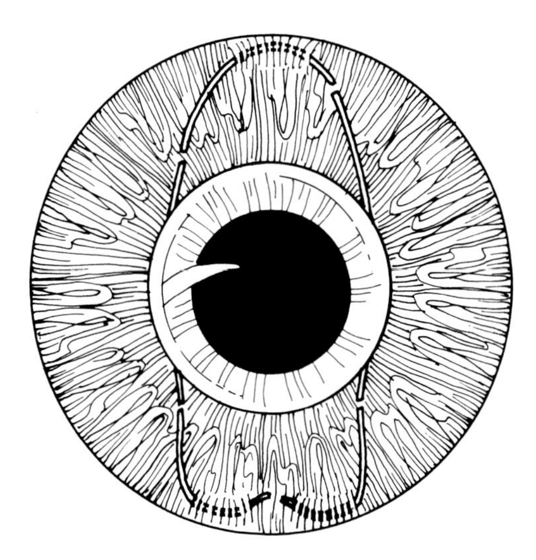

FIGURE 40-1 Anterior chamber lens with filamentous haptics encased by peripheral anterior synechiae. Scissors are used to sever the haptic from the optic.

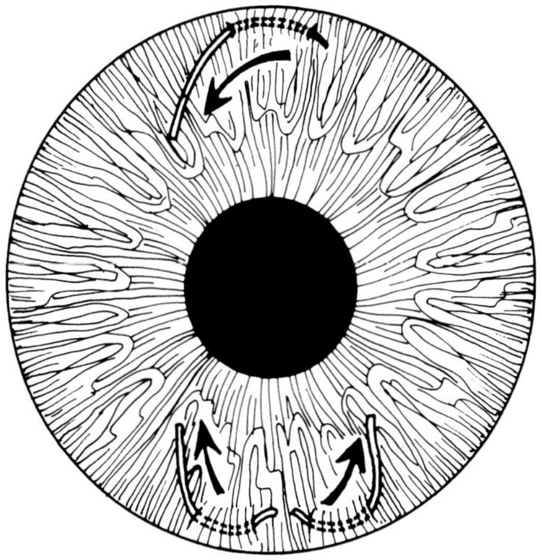

FIGURE 40-2 After removal of the optic, the severed haptics are back-threaded into the anterior chamber and removed.

Iris-Supported Lenses

As a general rule, dislocated and malpositioned iris-supported lenses should be either explanted or exchanged for anterior or posterior chamber lenses. Surgical repositioning of these lenses can be considered in situations where a more extensive explantation-exchange procedure may be risky, such as in an elderly patient with a dangerously low endothelial cell count. In such an instance, the main surgical principle in these eyes (which have invariably undergone previous intracapsular surgery) is to perform minimal manipulation under air within a closed system. Viscoelastic material should be avoided if possible because it is difficult to remove without disturbing the vitreous. Using fluid may also be relatively undesirable because hydration of the vitreous body can lead to either anterior chamber shallowing or vitreous prolapse. Two microhooks introduced through strategically placed limbal stab incisions are effective for haptic manipulation. These incisions are made just anterior to the corneoscleral junction to avoid bleeding into the eye. One hook is used to retract and depress the iris, while the other elevates and decenters the optic in the opposite direction. The haptics are repositioned, and the pupil is pharmacologically constricted to ensure IOL fixation.

When an iris-fixated IOL is associated with chronic irritation or progressive endothelial cell loss, explantation is the procedure of choice. Separation of posterior synechiae, often in conjunction with an anterior vitrectomy, aids explantation. Retrieval of lenses dislocated into the anterior vitreous can be accomplished using a two-stab anterior approach by ensnaring the visible haptic with a C-shaped hook and ushering the lens back through the pupil and into the anterior chamber. A second hook is then placed under the lens, which reduces the possibility of "losing" the lens. Once the lens is forward, the pupil is constricted with an intracameral miotic trapping the lens in the anterior chamber. At this point, it is safe to open the eye and to remove the lens using a second instrument as a ramp and relieving all vitreous adhesions with a mechanical cutter. More posteriorly dislocated iris IOLs can be removed by vitrectomy techniques identical to those described for dislocated posterior chamber lenses in a subsequent section. Following removal of a dislocated iris-supported lens, either anterior chamber lens implantation or posterior chamber lens implantation with scleral or iris suture support can be performed at the surgeon's discretion (Figure 40-3).

Posterior Chamber Intraocular Lenses

When asymmetric haptic fixation is the underlying cause of IOL decentration and the capsule is intact, rotation of the lens with a one- or preferably a two-hook technique results in each of the haptics assuming a new position within the ciliary sulcus. However, sulcus fixation is not recommended for single-piece acrylic style IOLs. If the capsular bag is intact with a previous capsulorhexis, a viscoelastic can be injected through a 30-gauge cannula placed strategically at the optic-haptic junction. It is often surprising to observe the separation of the fused anterior and posterior capsules as the capsular bag opens despite years of closure. Cortical material can be aspirated, the posterior capsule can be vacuumed, and the IOL can be rotated and recentered inside the bag. If either a can-opener capsulotomy has been

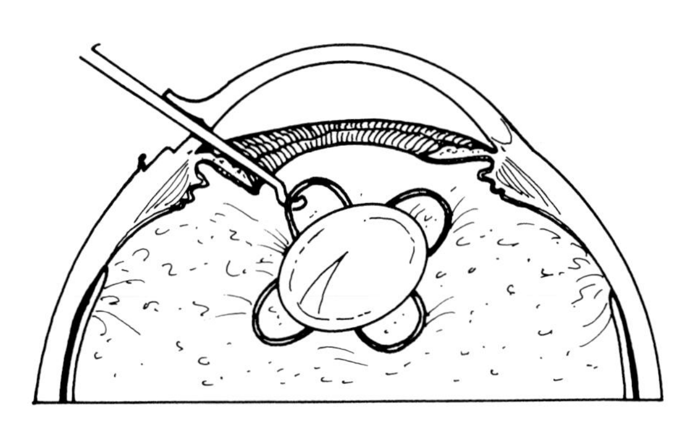

FIGURE 40-3 Removal of the dislocated iris-fixated lens from the anterior vitreous cavity by a limbal approach using a C-hook.

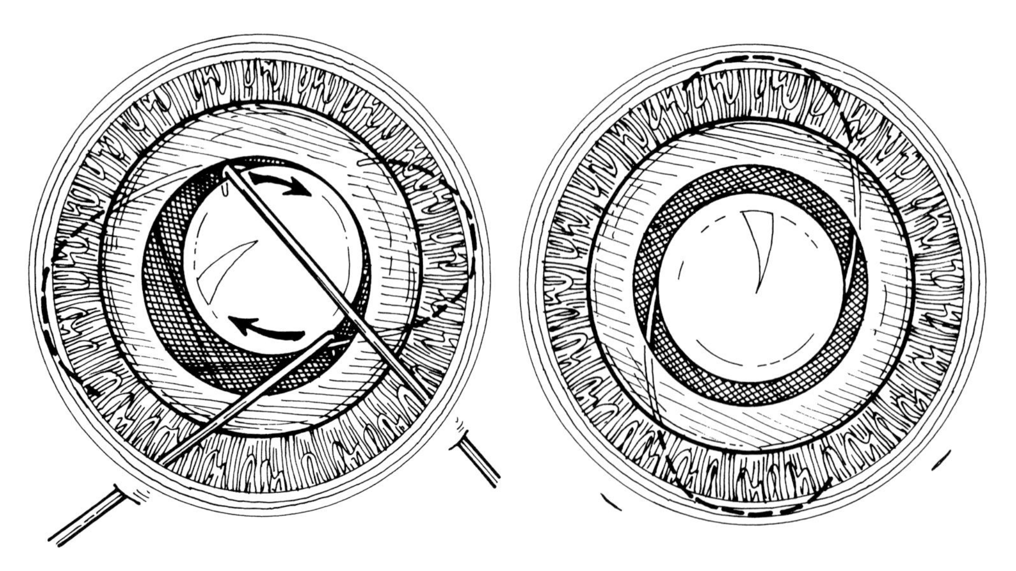

FIGURE 40-4 Two-hook rotation of a malpositioned PC IOL in the ciliary sulcus.

performed or the posterior capsule has been opened, it is safer to rotate the IOL until centered within the ciliary sulcus. Once the lens is centered, the Osher "bounce test" is performed by gently and deliberately decentering the optic toward each haptic to ensure spontaneous recentration. Failure to recenter indicates either a serious problem with the capsular support or permanent deformation of the lens haptic and may indicate the need for suture fixation, explantation, or exchange depending on the nature of the problem (Figures 40-4 and 40-5).

If a lens with know filamentous haptics fails to easily rotate, it is likely that the haptic is either snagged within the zonules or protruding through a tear in the zonules or the capsular bag. Reverse rotation followed by decentration toward the ensnared haptic and then rerotation can sometimes free it. The lens can then be rotated 90 degrees and "bounce tested" for centration and fixation. Continued resistance to rotation indicates that haptic amputation is necessary and the piecemeal removal of the lens may be required. When the severed haptic is stuck within the bag, an attempt should be made to inject viscoelastic material under an edge, which often opens the bag, allowing retrieval. If a lens has haptics with an eyelet or bulbous tip, gentle perseverance under the protection of a viscoelastic agent may enable successful removal, although amputation of the haptic, leaving it behind, is preferable to causing irrevocable damage to the capsular bag. Rarely, the entire lens within the capsule may require explantation.

Exchange implantation is performed in cases of a subluxed posterior chamber lens when adequate residual peripheral capsulozonular support is present. This can best be determined after all posterior synechiae between iris and capsule are separated intraoperatively to reconstruct a full-sized posterior chamber. Direct inspection of the peripheral retroiridal anatomy indicates the best axis for implantation and where best fixation may be achieved. Provided there is sufficient residual capsular support, three-piece Acrylic foldable or a single-piece all-polymethylmethacrylate (PMMA) IOL with a large optic

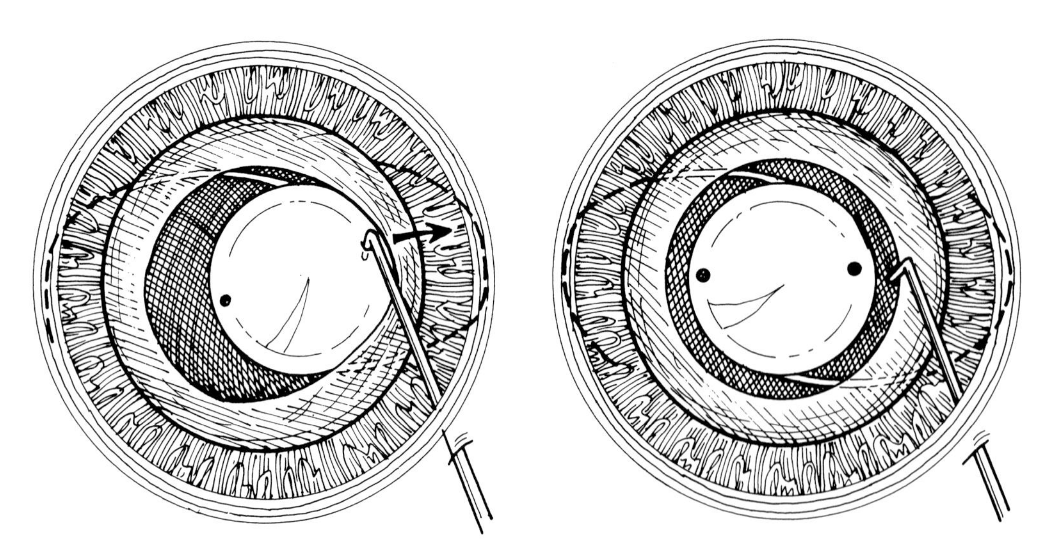

FIGURE 40-5 The "bounce" test used to ensure that a repositioned PC IOL spontaneously recenters.

(6 to 6.5 mm) without positioning holes and with a large diameter (12.5 to 13.5 mm) is preferable to either an anterior chamber lens or a sutured posterior chamber lens. Today it would be rare to explant a lens without also performing an exchange.

If the procedure is to be carried out solely by a limbal approach, careful management of the vitreous is very important. If vitreous fills the anterior chamber, a bimanual vitrectomy with low-flow irrigation through a second stab incision can be performed.[15] If minimal vitreous prolapse is present, a dry vitrectomy can be performed by filling the chamber with a viscoelastic, through which the vitrectomy handpiece is inserted. This vitrectomy technique produces a more limited vitrectomy, with less tendency toward collapse of the globe.

At the conclusion of the procedure, protective viscoelastic material can be removed manually or with a miniature irrigation-aspiration tip. Careful maintenance of the anterior chamber is necessary to prevent additional vitreous prolapse. Therefore the miniature irrigation-aspiration tip should not simply be withdrawn from the incision. It is a better technique to insert a 30-gauge cannula on a 3-ml air syringe through the second stab incision, injecting air as the irrigation-aspiration tip is removed. The air bubble in the anterior chamber maintains a deep chamber and can be safely exchanged for balanced salt solution in small aliquots.

Foldable lenses can be explanted by different techniques than the traditional hard lenses because the optic can be refolded or cut and removed through a small incision. Transection with either a scissors or a snare can be achieved under viscoelastic protection before removing each half. Jack Dodick popularized the Hinge technique, in which the optic is partially transected leaving the distal fifth intact. When one half of the optic is grasped and ushered into the incision, the other half hinges open and follows.[16]

Paul Ernst[17] developed a clever method for intraocular folding of the IOL. First, the superior haptic is prolapsed out of the incision under viscoelastic protection. Next, a spatula is passed under the optic from a stab incision placed across from the primary incision, and a lens insertion forceps is introduced over the optic. Upward force of the spatula combined with the downward force of the forceps results in refolding of the optic, which can then be explanted.

A final innovative technique was developed by Shuichiro Eguchi. After prolapsing the proximal haptic into the anterior chamber, a radial scissors cut is made. The lens is then rotated, and a second radial cut is made 90 degrees away. A quarter of the lens is explanted, and the remainder of the lens is rotated out through the wound.

Dislocation of Posterior Chamber Lens into the Vitreous

Before repositioning is attempted, the precise lens type and dioptric power should be ascertained to arrange for alternate lens implantation in the event that repositioning cannot be successfully achieved. Considerations in the decision to reposition or replace a lens include the structural stability of the lens, the size, and the haptic design. As an example, foldable silicone lenses are less amenable to repositioning than all-PMMA lenses because of their greater inherent structural instability. Lenses with smaller optical zones and interhaptic distances are more likely to produce optical edge effects and to be less stable when suspended by scleral sutures than other styles. Similarly, very thin or shortened haptics, particularly older-style J loops, are less amenable to primary suture fixation than other styles. A variety of techniques have been described for repositioning lenses that are displaced into the vitreous.[18-31] These include iris fixation,[18-20] scleral suture or residual capsular fixation,[20-22,25-30] and temporary liquid perfluorocarbon flotation with permanent scleral suture fixation.[24]

SCLEROTOMY PLACEMENT

Sclerotomies for suture fixation of PC IOLs are made in the ciliary sulcus, typically 1 mm posterior to the limbus. Separate sclerotomies 3 mm posterior to the surgical limbus are used for the purpose of vitrectomy and other intraoperative maneuvers to avoid damage to the fixation sutures, iris root, and ciliary body.

SUTURE FIXATION

A 9-0 or 10-0 monofilament nonabsorbable suture should be used for long-term fixation. Polypropylene (Prolene) is preferable to nylon because of a lower frequency of a late breakage.

In cases of limited subluxation or when the peripheral aspect of the haptic cannot be visualized, it is easiest to pass one arm of a double-armed suture above the haptic and the other below, each exiting the eye at the level of the ciliary sulcus, approximately 1 mm apart. When the sutures are tightened, the loop will have ensnared the haptic, which can then be pulled to the sulcus.

When the lens is completely dislocated into the posterior segment, it may be easier and less traumatic to pass a Prolene loop suture over one haptic and to bring this to the ciliary sulcus region (Figures 40-6 and 40-7). The second haptic can then be grasped with a second loop passed through a sclerotomy that is 180 degrees away and used to center the lens. In addition to grasping the suture with an intraocular forceps, the suture can also be passed through a hollow-bore 25-gauge needle as described by William E. Smiddy.[32]

In some instances, it may be difficult to grasp the second dangling haptic with a suture loop because of visualization problems related to pupil size, illumination, and the close proximity of the haptic to the peripheral retina. In such instances, the use of pupillary stretching techniques, an illuminated pick to centrally displace the haptic, and wide-angle viewing systems, such as the AVI system, may facilitate this maneuver. Occasionally, passing the suture loop over the haptic is problematic, and the surgeon should be certain that all vitreous gel adherent to the haptic has been cut and, if necessary, should fixate the haptic with an illuminated pick or forceps. Other authors have recommended temporary externalization of the haptic through the sclerotomy for suture knot fixation or other related techniques.[23]

Perfluorocarbon liquids have been successfully used by surgeons experienced in vitreoretinal techniques to elevate posteriorly dislocated lenses (Figure 40-8). Once the lens is immediately posterior to the iris plane, placement of loop sutures around the haptics or, alternatively, placement of single-armed

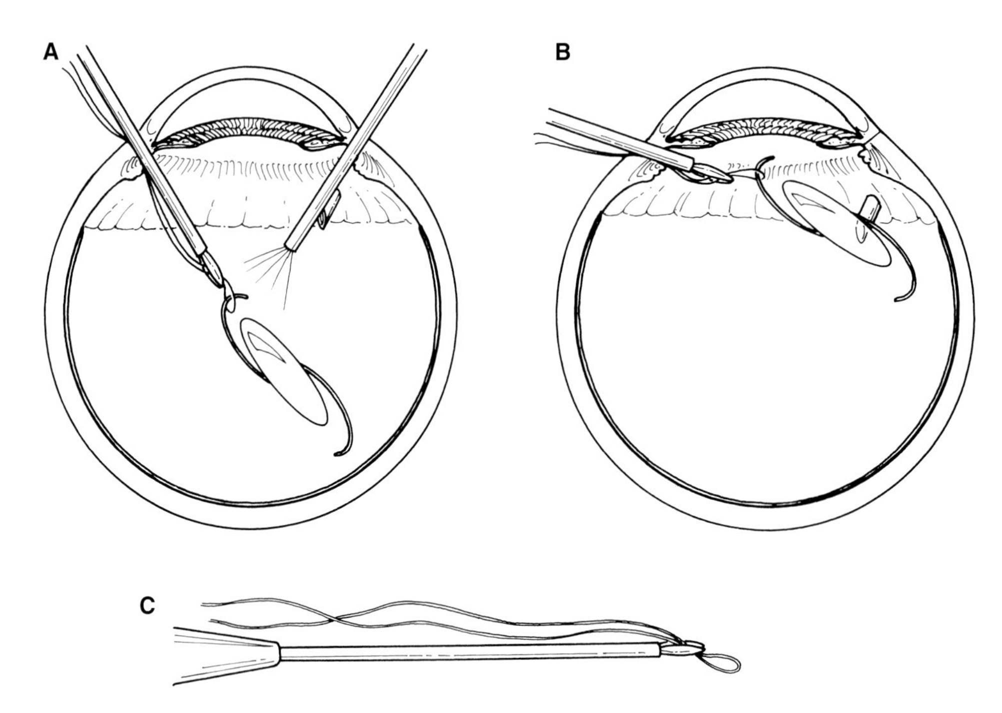

FIGURE 40-6 **A,** Placement of polypropylene suture around haptic of dislocated PC IOL in vitreous cavity. **B,** Suture loop is withdrawn, bringing haptic into position in the ciliary sulcus. **C,** Correct size of a suture loop held by the intraocular forceps.

Prolene sutures through positioning holes (if they are present) can be performed. After the fixation sutures are placed, the surgeon removes the residual perfluorocarbon liquid. The surgeon must take care not to let the IOL slide off the dome of the perfluorocarbon liquid bubble because it can be difficult to retrieve and may damage the peripheral retina. Of note, perfluorocarbon liquid should only be used in conjunction with complete posterior vitrectomy because inadvertent retention and secondary glaucoma can result if the substance is not completely removed.[33]

Following fixation, care must be taken to prevent exposure of the Prolene suture. This is often done by working under a

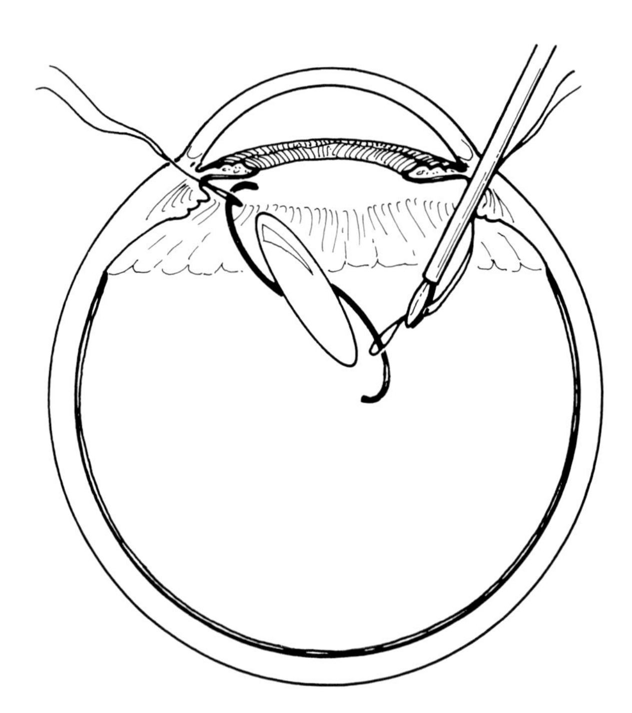

FIGURE 40-7 Repositioning of haptic in ciliary sulcus by tension on the second polypropylene suture.

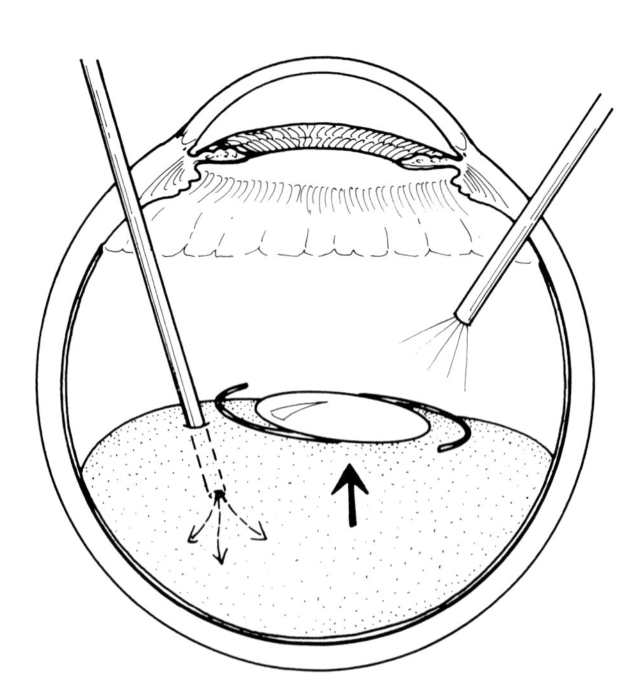

FIGURE 40-8 Perfluorocarbon liquid flotation of dislocated PC IOL into anterior vitreous cavity.

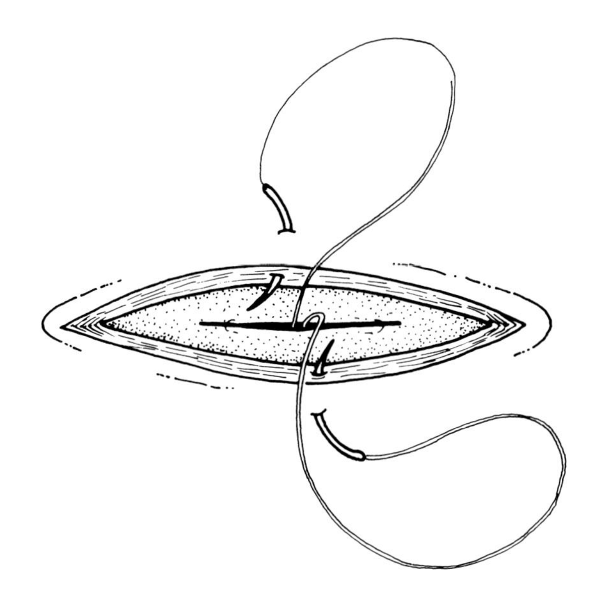

FIGURE 40-9 Closure of sclerotomy by oversewing and suture inversion beneath scleral flap.

preplaced partial-thickness scleral flap. The edges of the Prolene suture can also be inverted with the sclerotomy wound and oversewn with absorbable suture, with care being taken to not sever the Prolene fixation suture (Figure 40-9).

Alternatively, the Prolene suture can be placed within a half-thickness scleral groove and tied to itself after inverted passage of the suture through the lips of the groove in a mattress fashion (Figure 40-10).

Intraocular Lens Exchange

In many instances, repositioning a dislocated PC IOL may not be possible or desirable. This may be related either to structural abnormalities of the implant or to coexisting ocular conditions that necessitate removal and/or exchange. The dislocated lens may have preexisting structural damage to the haptic, as a result of haptic distortion or breakage precluding adequate refixation. In some instances, haptics may break as a result of intraocular manipulation or may be extruded through a sclerotomy as a result of excessive suture tension. In other instances, a haptic may appear unstable or decentered with transscleral suspension and require replacement with an alternate-style lens.

Techniques for secondary IOL implantation are discussed in Chapter 37.

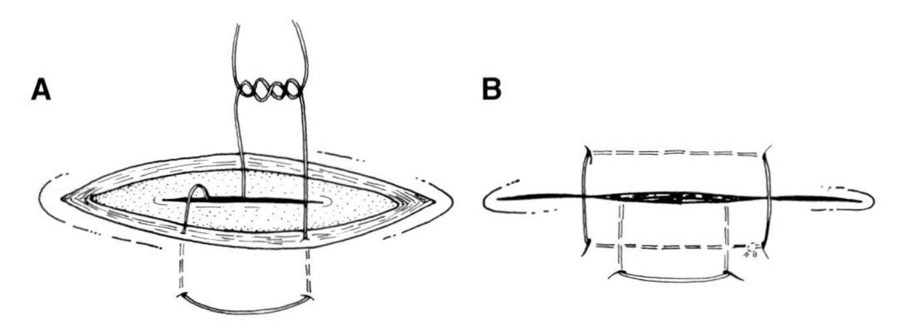

FIGURE 40-10 **A** and **B,** Two alternate methods for closure of suture site within partial-thickness scleral groove.

TABLE 40-1
Intraocular Lens (IOL) Type

Lens Type	Number
Anterior chamber lens	24
Iris-supported lens	11
Posterior chamber (PC) lens	33*

*One lens was a sutured PC IOL.

Anterior (Limbal) Approach: Surgical Results

Sixty-eight eyes of 67 patients who were referred to the Cincinnati Eye Institute between 1983 and 1990 underwent IOL repositioning, removal, or exchange by an anterior approach without pars plana vitrectomy. The average age of the patients was 69 years and ranged from 39 to 87 years. The types of lenses that required intervention are shown in Table 40-1. Today the ratios would be quite different because the majority of lens exchanges involve posterior chamber IOLs, reflecting their dominance.

ANTERIOR CHAMBER INTRAOCULAR LENSES

The underlying causes that necessitated surgical intervention are listed in Table 40-2. Seven of the nine undersized lenses were in contact with the cornea, causing corneal edema. Six of eight eyes with chronic uveitis also had glaucoma (modified UGH syndrome). Chronic CME was present in five eyes, four of which showed evidence of vitreous traction and adherence to the implant. Iris tuck secondary to an oversized IOL was identified in five eyes. The chief complaint of one patient with an undersized lens was some visual distortion secondary to lens decentration. Incorrect lens power was not a problem identified in this group.

The procedures that were performed are shown in Table 40-3. Most lenses were exchanged, although seven eyes with malpositioned anterior chamber lenses were left aphakic because of the presence of glaucoma with extensive peripheral synechiae. (Today, a sutured posterior chamber lens would be preferable to aphakia, but these cases underwent surgery before 1989 when we began suturing posterior chamber lenses to achieve ciliary sulcus fixation.) The average interval between the primary operation and surgical intervention was 4.2 years

TABLE 40-2
Anterior Chamber Lenses (24 Eyes)

Indications for Surgery*	Patients (n)
Undersized	9
Corneal touch	7
Chronic uveitis	8
Uveitis-glaucoma-hyphema (UGH) syndrome	6
Cystoid macular edema (CME)	5
Iris tuck/oversize	5
Optical	1
Wrong power	0

*Some patients had multiple diagnoses.

TABLE 40-3
Anterior Chamber Lenses (24 Eyes)

Surgical Procedure	Number
Reposition	2
Explantation	22
Exchange (AC IOL)	7
Exchange (PC IOL)	3
Exchange (PC IOL sutured)	5

TABLE 40-4
Anterior Chamber Lenses (24 Eyes)

Reason for Intervention	Rate of Success
Fixation	8/9*
Corneal edema	7/7
Uveitis	8/8
Elevated intraocular pressure	3/4†
Cystoid macular edema	5/5
Tuck	5/5
Optical	1/1

*Decentration recurred at 5 weeks in one patient, and the lens was then removed.
†Off medicines.

TABLE 40-5
Anterior Chamber Lenses: Visual Result (24 Eyes)

Patients (n)	Change in Lines of Vision
1	−4*
10	0
5	+1
2	+2
2	+3
2	+4
1	+5
1	+6

*Retrocorneal membrane.

TABLE 40-6
Iris-Supported Lenses (11 Eyes)

Indications for Surgery	Patients (n)
Posterior dislocation	8
Anterior dislocation	2
Corneal edema	2
Uveitis	2

and ranged from 2 months to 13 years. Postoperatively, the patients were observed for an average of 19.1 months, with follow-up ranging from 2 to 65 months. The surgical results are listed in Table 40-4. One repositioned lens decentered and was subsequently removed without reimplantation. All eyes with corneal edema, uveitis, optical aberration, CME, or iris tuck improved after surgery. One patient with lens-induced glaucoma had a trabeculectomy performed at the time of surgery and has subsequently remained off of medications. One patient with advanced UGH syndrome developed epithelial downgrowth and uncontrolled intraocular pressure that required several filtering procedures and necessitated cyclocryotherapy 7 months following surgery.

The visual results are shown in Table 40-5. Eight of the 24 eyes improved two lines or more on Snellen acuity testing. The visual acuity in 15 eyes improved by only one line of Snellen visual acuity or remained unchanged. One patient with epithelial downgrowth lost four lines at 6 months. One patient developed CME 5 weeks after surgery, which resolved after weeks of topical and periocular steroid treatment. The patient ultimately attained a visual acuity of 20/30. No other complications were present in this group.

IRIS-SUPPORTED INTRAOCULAR LENSES

Eleven iris-supported lenses required surgical intervention for the complications shown in Table 40-6. Most of these eyes presented with anterior or posterior dislocation of one or more haptics, and two developed corneal edema from haptic contact with the corneal endothelium.

The surgical procedures performed are shown in Table 40-7. Of the 11 lenses, 8 were simply repositioned through a stab incision because these patients were elderly with low endothelial cell counts. The average interval between surgeries was 4.1 years, with a range of 2 days to 7 years. The average length of follow-up was 9.3 months, with a range between 1 and 27 months.

One lens, a Binkhorst style that was repositioned, again dislocated anteriorly 5 months after surgery. The lens was removed and exchanged for an AC IOL. Another patient with an unstable iris-supported lens underwent exchange for a sulcus-fixated posterior chamber lens, which subsequently dislocated through an unrecognized zonular dialysis. The lens was explanted and was replaced with an anterior chamber lens, but one haptic was later found protruding through the peripheral iridectomy. Once again, the lens was exchanged, this time for a larger-diameter anterior chamber lens. Although the lens has remained stable, the patient has experienced recurrent episodes of CME that has been very responsive to topical steroids. Another patient with corneal edema, a cell count of 400 mm, and an anterior displaced Copeland lens showed some reduction in the amount of edema but did not experience complete clearing. The surgical results are summarized in Table 40-8.

TABLE 40-7
Iris-Supported Lenses (11 Eyes)

Surgical Procedure	Patients (n)
Repositioned	8
Explantation	3
Exchange (AC IOL)	2
Exchange (PC IOL)	1

TABLE 40-8
Iris-Supported Lenses (11 Eyes)

Reason for Intervention	Success Rate
Position	10/10*
Uveitis	2/2
Corneal edema	2/2†

*Dislocation recurred twice.
†One incomplete resolution of corneal edema.

TABLE 40-9
Iris-Supported Lenses: Visual Results (11 Eyes)

Patients (n)	Change in Lines of Vision
5	0
3	+1
2	+2
1	+6

No loss of acuity occurred in the group, and three eyes demonstrated an improvement of two or more lines of acuity by Snellen testing (Table 40-9). Except for one case of recurrent CME that was responsive to steroids, no long-term complications were associated with these procedures.

POSTERIOR CHAMBER INTRAOCULAR LENSES (ANTERIOR APPROACH)

Surgical intervention was required in 33 eyes with posterior chamber lenses. The most common reasons to operate were optical symptoms—typically, edge glare, monocular diplopia, and unwanted optical images from a decentered or subluxed lens (Table 40-10). Three of these cases were associated with ocular trauma.

The procedures performed are shown in Table 40-11. Although the majority of lenses were exchanged for another posterior chamber lens, two lenses were simply repositioned, both after a relatively short interval from the initial surgery (2 to 4 months). The other 31 lenses were removed after a longer interval, averaging 1.8 years with a range between 1 month and 7 years.

The most striking surgical finding was how often the Prolene haptics were severely deformed, making explantation rather than repositioning necessary. Three of the lenses exchanged were replaced with an AC IOL because inadequate capsulozonular support for a posterior chamber lens was present, and much of the study was performed before development of scleral suturing techniques in 1989. Two other cases were left aphakic for the same reason and neither patient was a candidate for an anterior chamber lens.

The surgical results for this group are summarized in Table 40-12. The average length of follow-up was 8.3 months, with time ranging from 2 to 46 months. All predetermined surgical goals were attained except in the group with coexisting glaucoma. Trabeculectomy performed at the time of the lens exchange lowered the intraocular pressure in one eye. Spontaneous lowering of the intraocular pressure occurred in a second eye, and medical control using a topical beta-blocker was successful in a third eye. In the fourth eye with glaucoma, a second trabeculectomy was required to control the intraocular pressure 1 year after lens exchange.

The visual results are illustrated in Table 40-13. An improvement in Snellen acuity of two lines or greater was documented in 11 eyes, whereas the acuity remained unchanged in 20 eyes. No patient lost vision, and no serious intraoperative or postoperative complications occurred in this group.

TABLE 40-10
Posterior Chamber Lenses (33 Eyes)

Indications for Surgery	Patients (n)
Optical	23
Chronic uveitis	5
Extrusion	2
Glaucoma	4
Wrong power	2

TABLE 40-11
Posterior Chamber Lenses (33 Eyes)

Surgical Procedure	Patients (n)
Repositioned	2
Explantation	31
Exchange (AC IOL)	3
Exchange (PC IOL)	25
Exchange for sutured PC IOL	1

TABLE 40-12
Posterior Chamber Lenses: Surgical Results

Reason for Intervention	Success Rate
Optical	23/23
Uveitis	5/5
Glaucoma	3/4
Malposition	1/1
Wrong power	2/2

TABLE 40-13
Posterior Chamber Lenses: Visual Results (33 Eyes)

Patients (n)	Change in Lines of Vision
20	0
2	+1
9	+2
1	+4
1	+7

TABLE 40-14

Results of Vitrectomy and Repositioning for Posteriorly Dislocated IOLs

Authors	Patients (n)	Method	VA ≥20/40	Comments
Sternberg and Michels (1986)	5	Iris/haptic fixation	5/5	
Smiddy and Flynn (1991)	4	Sclera/haptic fixation	3/4	
Maguire et al (1991)	6	Sclera/haptic fixation	4/6	Prior retinal damage in 2/6 eyes
Chan (1992)	12	Sclera/haptic fixation	11/12	CME in 3/12 eyes
Lewis and Sanchez (1993)	8	Sclera/positioning hole fixation; temporary perfluorocarbon	6/8	
Mello et al (2000)	110 (72 in posterior segment)	Sclera or capsule/haptic fixation	63/110	Postoperative RD in 7/110 eyes CME 19/110 eyes
Thach et al (2000)	78	Sclera/haptic fixation after temporary externalization of haptic		Postoperative RD in 5/78 eyes CME in 20/78 eyes
Sarrafizadeh et al (2001)	59	Repositioned with (16) or without (13) sutures with scleral or capsule/haptic fixation Exchanged for sutured PC IOL (13) or AC IOL (17)	12/29 repositioned 19/30 exchanged	Nonrandomized case series comparing repositioning versus exchange of dislocated PC IOL; similar complication rates

CME, Cystoid macular edema; *RD,* retinal detachment; VA, visual acuity.

POSTERIOR CHAMBER LENSES (PARS PLANA RESULTS)

When posterior chamber lenses are completely dislocated into the vitreous cavity, resulting in optical symptoms of aphakia rather than edge effects or diplopia, a pars plana approach is typically employed for retrieval. The surgeon then has the option either to place the primary lens into the ciliary sulcus with suture support if no structural damage has occurred to the lens and no sizing abnormality is present or, conversely, to remove and replace the lens by an anterior approach, as previously outlined.

The results of several published surgical series of primary positioning by a pars plana route are summarized in Table 40-14. Of 282 eyes with dislocated IOLs, treated by either exchange or repositioning with either scleral or iris fixation to supplement sulcus repositioning, 165 (58%) achieved 20/40 or better final vision. Fifty seven of 282 (20%) developed CME, which was usually transient and responsive to medical therapy, and 19 (6.7%) developed a retinal detachment postoperatively. Postoperative retinal detachments developed between 10 days and 2 years after surgery, although most occurred in the first 2 months following IOL repositioning or exchange. Other reported complications of ciliary sulcus repositioning by a pars plana route with scleral fixation sutures include lens tilt, redislocation, suture erosion, retinal phototoxicity, persistent intraocular pressure elevation, corneal opacification, iris capture, epiretinal membrane formation, suture exposure, persistent uveitis, wound leak, and vitreous hemorrhage.

Conclusions

Surgical treatment of malpositioned and dislocated IOLs remains an important and challenging clinical problem. Several previous publications have summarized the reasons for IOL removal. Kraff et al.[34] reported their results of explantation surgery in 1986, at which time anterior chamber lenses were most often removed as a result of corneal decompensation and chronic inflammation. Apple et al.[35] showed that many anterior chamber lenses were explanted because of poor manufacturing, characterized by rough optic and haptic edges, which resulted in chronic iris chafing. Posterior chamber lenses, which represented only 20% of those explanted in the survey by Kraff et al., were removed because of dislocation, decentration, or incorrect power. Similar data were reported by Solomon et al.[36] in a series of 2500 explant cases evaluated at the Center for Intraocular Lens Research between 1982 and 1988. Anterior chamber lenses accounted for 59% and were usually explanted because of pseudophakic bullous keratopathy or inflammatory complications. Iris-fixated lenses represented 21%, whereas posterior chamber lenses accounted for 20%. The latter were most frequently explanted because of decentration, malposition, or inflammation. Mamalis et al[37] reviewed 102 explanted lenses between 1982 and 1989. Anterior chamber lenses, which represented 66.7% of the series, were removed because of pseudophakic bullous keratopathy, UGH syndrome, and CME. Iris-supported lenses made up 17.6%, with pseudophakic bullous keratopathy representing the most frequent reason for removal. PC IOLs represented 15.7% of the explanted lenses, and the underlying cause was most often lens dislocation or decentration. Although approximately 70% of these patients underwent IOL exchange, the overall visual outcome showed that 39% experienced improvement, 46% were unchanged, and 15% showed a worsening of vision following surgery. The most common cause for further visual deterioration was corneal decompensation followed by glaucoma and CME. It was noteworthy that 90% of patients who underwent exchange with a PC IOL had a successful clinical outcome.

In a series of 1400 implant cases published in 1980, Kline and Yang[38] found a 1.7% incidence of lens removal. Corneal edema, CME, uveitis, and iris erosion were the most common causes for explantation. Smiddy and Flynn[21] reviewed 32 cases of posterior dislocation of posterior chamber lenses. Management consisted of conservative observation without surgery in 2 eyes, repositioning in 19 eyes, exchange in 8 eyes, and explantation without exchange in 3 eyes. The visual acuity of 20/40 or better was achieved in 69% of eyes in their study. Doren, Stern, and Driebe[39] reviewed 101 consecutive explantations performed between 1983 and 1987. The majority of lenses removed were anterior chamber styles (53.9%) and iris-fixated lenses (33.7%). Pseudophakic bullous keratopathy was the main reason for explantation (69%) followed by UGH syndrome (9%) and IOL instability (7%). The best visual outcome was attained in eyes with an unstable IOL, half of which attained visual acuity of 20/40 or better. The poorest visual outcome was seen in eyes with UGH syndrome. Although 83% of the eyes in the latter group failed to attain acuity better than 20/200, even these patients benefited by the resolution of pain and better control of the intraocular pressure.

Sinskey, Amin, and Stoppel[40] conducted a retrospective review of 79 patients who underwent IOL exchange. Sixty-one percent were posterior chamber lenses, and 39% were anterior chamber lenses; these were replaced by posterior chamber (76%) and anterior chamber (24%) lenses. Indications for lens exchange included eccentric or displaced IOL (42%), endothelial decompensation (28%), incorrect IOL power (13%), and UGH syndrome (10%). The postoperative visual acuity was better than or equal to 20/30 in 72%, whereas 8% had a loss of one or more lines of visual acuity. Complications encountered following lens exchange included retinal detachment in 4 eyes, glaucoma in 14 eyes, corneal decompensation in 3 eyes, and anisometropia in 1 eye.

A series of 31 consecutive subluxed posterior chamber lenses referred to the Wilmer Institute between 1983 and 1991 was evaluated.[41] Presumed anatomic causes of IOL subluxation were identified in 90%, including capsular or zonular rupture (18 eyes), vitreous loss (11 eyes), asymmetric haptic fixation (5 eyes), haptic deformation (2 eyes), cortical remnants with progressive posterior synechiae (1 eye), problems related to a previously sutured PC IOL (3 eyes), and the IOL resting on the anterior hyaloid face in 2 eyes with no remaining posterior capsule. The primary direction of the IOL subluxation was classified as sunset syndrome (16 eyes), lateral decentration (8 eyes), sunrise syndrome (5 eyes), and IOL tilt (2 eyes). Thirty patients had an optic edge, and 12 had a positioning hole in the pupillary space. One patient had severe sunset syndrome with only a visible haptic in the pupil. The reported symptoms included decreased visual acuity (19 patients), glare (13 patients), monocular diplopia (13 patients), streaks of light (6 patients), halos (4 patients), unstable vision (4 patients), photosensitivity (3 patients), and ghost images (2 patients). One of three surgical procedures was used to correct the implant subluxation: modified McCannel sutures (19 eyes), IOL exchange (8 eyes), or IOL rotation (4 eyes).

The results showed that a Snellen visual acuity of 20/40 or better was achieved in 94%. Compared with the preoperative acuity, 2 patients lost one line, 15 patients remained at the same level or gained one line, and 14 patients improved two or more lines. CME was diagnosed angiographically in 5 patients and clinically in 2 patients, improved in 4 patients, and persisted in 3 patients. No new cases of CME were identified, and surgical complications were limited to peaking of the pupil (three eyes) and increased capsular opacification (two eyes). Complete symptomatic improvement was achieved in 87%.

Lyle and Jin[42] analyzed a large series of eyes undergoing IOL exchange with and without penetrating keratoplasty. In the 56 eyes that underwent IOL exchange without penetrating keratoplasty, the type of lens explanted was an AC IOL in 41%, an iris-supported IOL in 14%, and a PC IOL in 45%. The most frequent indications were dislocation of the lens in 20 eyes (36%), incorrect power in 14 eyes (25%), and CME in 11 eyes (20%). The geometric mean visual acuity improved from 20/61 preoperatively to 20/43 postoperatively. A visual acuity of 20/40 or better was attained in 69%, and 46% of eyes gained two or more lines. The main reason for a visual acuity of less than 20/200 was CME (four eyes). The authors noted a better prognosis if either the original lens was a PC IOL or if the original lens was exchanged for a PC IOL. The most frequent complications following explantation included hyphema (23%), CME (18%), posterior capsule opacification (13%), and glaucoma (9%). Isolated cases of choroidal detachment, endophthalmitis, retinal detachment, and lens dislocation also occurred.

Our experience has been similar and is summarized in the preceding section and tables. The types of lenses that were included in our studies were 33 posterior chamber lenses (49%), 24 anterior chamber lenses (35%), and 11 iris plane lenses (16%). Several AC IOLs were used for exchanges early in our study; however, this reflects that we initiated this study in the mid-1980s. Today our strong preference is for posterior chamber lenses when a lens exchange is required. In addition, the percentage of PC IOLs explanted in our study appears higher than in previous studies,[21,35-39] This may be due to the longer follow-up of a large number of posterior chamber lenses, the reduction of anterior chamber lenses being implanted, and the discontinuation of iris plane lenses.

Thirty-two eyes (47%) showed improved Snellen acuity, whereas only one eye (2%) with severe UGH syndrome developed worse vision related to epithelial downgrowth and corneal edema following surgery. Although 35 patients (51%) experienced no change in visual acuity, many had 20/20 acuity before surgery and therefore were not expected to improve.

The surgical goals were successfully achieved in 94% of the cases. The goals included correction of malposition or unstable fixation; elimination of optical aberrations; and resolution of corneal edema, uveitis, elevated intraocular pressure, or CME. Although chronic CME can cause permanent damage to the retinal architecture, visual acuity actually improved in 30 of the 47 eyes (64%) with concomitant CME. The resolution of preexisting corneal edema was also found to occur if an offending haptic or unstable lens was removed before irrevocable endothelial cell damage. In a large series of 102 eyes undergoing anterior chamber and iris plane IOL exchange for early corneal decompensation, resolution of edema occurred in 34%.[43] Postoperative endothelial cell counts stabilized in several patients who previously had a progressive decline in the endothelial cell count before IOL exchange.

Explantation of an IOL is always challenging, yet armed with knowledgeable preparation and meticulous operative technique, the results may be satisfying to both the patient and the surgeon.

REFERENCES

1. Brown, DC, Swead JW: Intraocular lens implant exchanges, *J Am Intraocul Implant Soc* 11:376-379, 1985.
2. Flynn HW Jr: Management and repositioning of posteriorly dislocated intraocular lenses. In Stark WJ, Terry AC, Maumenee AE, editors: *Anterior segment surgery: oils, lasers, and refractive keratoplasty,* Baltimore, 1987, William & Wilkins, pp 321-329.
3. Blumenkranz M, Maguire A: Modern management considerations in dislocation of crystalline and intraocular lenses. In Stirpe M, editor: *Advances in vitroretinal surgery,* Rome, 1992, Fondazione GB Bietti/Ophthalmic Communications Society, 1992, pp 39-46.
4. Insler M, Benefield D, Ross V: Topical hyperosmolar solution in the reduction of corneal edema, *LAO J* 13:149, 1987.
5. Osher RH: Surgical management of the malpositioned posterior chamber lens, *Audiovisual J Cataract Implant Surg* VII, 1991.
6. Ellington FR: The uveitis-glaucoma-hyphema syndrome associated with the Mark VIII anterior chamber lens implant, *Am Intracellular Implant Soc J* 4:50, 1978.
7. Keates RH, Ehrlich DR: "Lenses of change": complications of anterior chamber implants, *Ophthalmology* 85:408, 1978.
8. Percival SPK, Das SK: UGH syndrome after posterior chamber lens implantation, *J Am Intraocul Implant Soc* 9:200, 1983.
9. Koch DD: Scleral fixation of posterior chamber implants, *Audiovisual J Cataract Implant Surg* VI, 1990.
10. Price FW: Iris fixation of posterior chamber implants, *Audiovisual J Cataract Implant Surg* VI, 1990.
11. Moretsky SL: Suture fixation technique for subluxated posterior chamber IOL through stab wound incision, *J Am Intraocular Implant Soc* 10:455-480, 1984.
12. Girard LJ, Nino N, Wesson M et al: Scleral fixation of subluxed posterior chamber intraocular lens, *J Cataract Refract Surg* 14:326-337, 1986.
13. Anand R, Bowman RW: Simplified technique for suturing dislocated posterior chamber intraocular lens to the ciliary sulcus, *Arch Ophthalmol* 108:1205-1206, 1990 (letter).
14. Lubniewski AJ, Holland EJ, Van Meter WS et al: Histologic study of eyes with transsclerally sutured posterior chamber intraocular lens, *Am J Ophthalmol* 110:237-243, 1990.
15. Snyder ME, Foster RE: Anterior vitrectomy, *Comp Ophthalmol Update* 2:149-158, 2001.
16. Batlan SJ, Dodick JM: Explantation of foldable silicone intraocular lens, *Am J Ophthalmol* 122:270-272, 1996.
17. Ernst P: Intraocular refolding. *Video J Cataract Refractive Surg* XII(4), 1996.
18. Sternberg P, Michels RG: Treatment of dislocated posterior chamber intraocular lenses, *Arch Ophthalmol* 104:1391-1393, 1986.
19. Flynn HW, Buus D, Culbertson WW: Management of subluxated and dislocated intraocular lenses using pars plana vitrectomy instrumentation, *Cataract Refract Surg* 16:51-56, 1990.
20. Smiddy WE, Flynn HW: Needle assisted scleral fixation technique for relocating posteriorly dislocated IOLs, *Arch Ophthalmol* 111:161-162, 1993.
21. Smiddy W, Flynn H: Management of dislocated posterior chamber intraocular lenses, *Ophthalmology* 98:889-894, 1991.
22. Maguire AM, Blumenkranz MS, Ward TG et al: Scleral loop fixation for posteriorly dislocated intraocular lenses, *Arch Ophthalmol* 109:1754-1758, 1991.
23. Chan CK: An improved technique for management of dislocated posterior chamber implants, *Ophthalmology* 99:51-57, 1992.
24. Lewis H, Sanchez G: The use of liquid perfluorocarbon in the repositioning of posteriorly dislocated intraocular lenses, *Ophthalmology* 100:1055-1059, 1993.
25. Smiddy WE, Ibanez GV, Alfonso E et al: Surgical management of dislocated intraocular lenses, *J Cataract Refract Surg* 21:64-69, 1995.
26. Mello MO, Scott IU, Smiddy WE et al: Surgical management and outcomes of dislocated intraocular lenses, *Ophthalmology* 107:62-67, 2000.
27. Thach AB, Dugel PU, Sipperley JO et al: Outcome of sulcus fixation of dislocated posterior chamber intraocular lenses using temporary externalization of the haptics, *Ophthalmology* 107:480-484, 2000.
28. Sarrafizadeh R, Ruby AJ, Hassan TS et al: A comparison of visual results and complications in eyes with posterior chamber intraocular lens dislocation treated with pars plana vitrectomy and lens repositioning or lens exchange, *Ophthalmology* 108:82-89, 2001.
29. Wong KL, Grabow HB: Simplified technique to remove posteriorly dislocated lens implants, *Arch Ophthalmol* 119:273-274, 2001.
30. Kokame GT, Atebara NH, Bennett MD: Modified technique of haptic externalization for scleral fixation of dislocated posterior chamber lens implants, *Am J Ophthalmol* 131:129-31, 2001.
31. Johnson MW, Schneiderman TE: Surgical management of posteriorly dislocated silicone plate intraocular lenses, *Curr Opin Ophthalmol* 9:11-15, 1998.
32. Smiddy WE: Management of posterior chamber intraocular lens dislocation, *Comp Ophthalmol Update* 2:1-16, 2001.
33. Foster RE, Smiddy WS Alfonso EC et al: Secondary glaucoma associated with retained perfluorophenanthrene, Am J Ophthalmol 118:253-255, 1994.
34. Kraff M, Sanders DR, Lieberman HL et al: Secondary intraocular lens implantation, *Ophthalmology* 90:324-326, 1983.
35. Apple DJ, Brems RN, Park RD et al: Anterior chamber lenses. Part I. Complications and pathology and a review of designs, *J Cataract Refract Surg* 13:157-173, 1987.
36. Solomon K, Apple D, Mamalis N et al: Complications of intraocular lenses with special reference to an analysis of 2500 explanted intraocular lenses (IOLs), *Eur J Implant Ref Surg* 3:195-200, 1991.
37. Mamalis N, Crandall A, Pulsipher M et al: Intraocular lens explantation and exchange: a review of lens styles, clinical indications, clinical results, and visual outcome, *J Cataract Refract Surg* 17:810-818, 1991.
38. Kline OR, Yang HK: A review of 1400 intraocular lens implant cases, *Contact Lens* 7:262-278, 1981.
39. Doren G, Stern G, Driebe W: Indications for and results of intraocular lens exchanges, *J Cataract Refract Surg* 18:79-85, 1992.
40. Sinskey RM, Amin P, Stoppel JO: Indications for and results of a large series of intraocular lens exchanges, *J Cataract Refract Surg* 19:68-71, 1993.
41. Panton RW, Sulewski ME, Parker JS et al: Surgical management of subluxed posterior-chamber intraocular lens, *Arch Ophthalmol* 111:919-926, 1993.
42. Lyle W, Jin JC: An analysis of intraocular lens exchange, *Ophthalmic Surg* 23:453-458, 1992.
43. Coli AF, Price FW Jr, Whitson WE: Intraocular lens exchange for anterior chamber intraocular lens-induced corneal endothelial damage, *Ophthalmology* 100:384-393, 1993.

Wound Dehiscence Following Cataract Surgery

41

Douglas D. Koch, MD
Li Wang, MD
Kenneth D. Novak, MD

Wound dehiscence is incisional weakness that compromises the structural integrity or optical quality of the eye. It is one of the rare causes of blindness following cataract surgery. Although the actual incidence of wound dehiscence is likely to vary moderately depending on multiple factors, the shift to small-incision surgery and the evolution in techniques of wound design have reduced the incidence markedly, with recent reports indicating a range of 0.02% to 1.5%.[1-6] For example, Quraishy and Casswell[4] reported an incidence of traumatic wound dehiscence of 0.4% (21/5600) following extracapsular cataract extraction (ECCE) from 1986 to 1993. From the same hospital, only one case of traumatic wound dehiscence (0.02%) was identified in 4200 phacoemulsification procedures from 1996 to 1998.[5]

Wound construction is the critical determinant of wound integrity, and the two key elements of the wound are its size and architecture.[6-10] The traditional limbal or scleral incision was designed for ready access to the anterior chamber and simple closure with radially oriented sutures. Two or three planes were incorporated into the incision, but the intrascleral (or intralimbal) portion was short, and the site of entry into the anterior chamber was located near the iris root. Key elements of the scleral tunnel incision include a long (>2 mm) intrascleral component and an anterior entry into the chamber.[7,11] The latter creates an internal corneal valve that is closed by intraocular pressure.

Stimulated in part by advances in foldable lens design, small-incision surgery (3.5 mm or less) has largely supplanted the traditional 6- to 7-mm incision. Initially, these incisions were simply small scleral tunnels, but the scleral tunnel has in turn largely been supplanted by clear corneal incisions. Advantages of the clear corneal incision include avoidance of the conjunctiva and sclera, allowing virtually bloodless surgery; easier access to the eye; safer surgery; and reduced operating time.

The principles of clear corneal wound construction remain the same: create adequate tunnel length with an internal corneal valve to create a self-sealing wound. Several corneal incision constructions have been used: paracentesis incision, two-plane or grooved incision, hinged incision, and three-plane incision. Ernest et al.[12] showed that clear corneal incisions demonstrated resistance to leakage comparable to similarly constructed scleral tunnel incisions.[10] In an animal model, Ernest et al.[12] evaluated the role of the site of external opening of the incision on incision healing and stability. They found that starting incisions in the vascular region (limbus) resulted in a fibroblastic response that enhanced incision stability and allowed rapid incision healing within 7 days postoperatively, compared with the 60 days' healing time required for incisions started in the avascular region (cornea). Their findings are compelling, but clinical studies have not yet been performed of the effect of the incision site on factors such as wound integrity and induced astigmatism.

To understand the pathogenesis of wound dehiscence, it is important to review the mechanisms of wound healing and the factors that can predispose to wound compromise.

The Wound Healing Process

A scleral, limbal, or corneal incision creates a tissue gape that initiates a process of repair by tissue addition. For scleral and limbal incision, active wound healing begins within 48 hours of surgery; the initial phase is the ingrowth of episcleral vascular tissue.[13,14] Over the next several weeks, this tissue fills the entire incision, creating a fibrovascular plug. Over the ensuing 2 or more years, remodeling occurs, resulting in reorientation of the wound healing collagen so that it becomes parallel to existing scleral collagen. Concurrently, vascularization and cellularity diminish.

At 1 week postoperatively, wound strength is approximately 10% of that found in normal nonincised tissue.[15-17] By 8 weeks postoperatively, this value is roughly 40%, and by 2 years postoperatively, the wound has regained approximately 75% to 80% of its original strength. Therefore, although the wound is most vulnerable to dehiscence early in the postoperative period, depending on its size and construction, the cataract incision retains a permanent susceptibility to traumatic dehiscence.[18-20]

Corneal incisions heal by ingrowth of keratocytes,[12] which initially are oriented parallel to the incision and therefore perpendicular to lamellae of the corneal stroma. These keratocytes then undergo fibroblastic transformation and, over months, reorient themselves to become parallel to the corneal lamellae. Compared with scleral and limbal wound healing, the wound healing process of the corneal incision is much slower and ultimately produces a weaker incision, as attested by the relative fragility of corneal graft wounds.

The clinical impact of this slower healing of corneal wounds is not fully understood. For standard 3- to 3.5-mm corneal tunnel incisions, the small incision size and wound construction appear to largely or even fully compensate for the deficiencies in the corneal wound healing process. However, it is probable that the slower healing of corneal incisions may predispose to problems with dehiscence in poorly constructed small incisions and in incisions longer than 4 mm. It is possible (but unproven to date) that there is greater against-the-wound astigmatic shift with corneal incisions compared with limbal or scleral wounds of the same size.

Factors Predisposing to Wound Dehiscence

The surgical incision and its closure are only as reliable as the corneoscleral tissue substrate (Figure 41-1). Particularly for larger incisions, wound healing may be delayed or incomplete in the setting of profound systemic illness[3] and malnutrition (particularly vitamin C deficiency).

An unusual example of the role of systemic factors in wound healing occurs with Werner's syndrome, which is an autosomal recessive condition of premature aging associated with cataract formation by the age of 20 to 40 years. Jonas et al.[21] reported that wound dehiscence occurred in 10 out of 18 cataract wounds at 2.5 to 21 weeks postoperatively. The cause is a presumed deficiency in fibroblast growth potential.

Peripheral ulcerative keratitis and scleritis associated with underlying collagen vascular disease can produce marked scleral and/or corneal thinning, rendering wound closure extremely difficult. These entities also may flare after surgery, leading to melting of the tunnel incision.

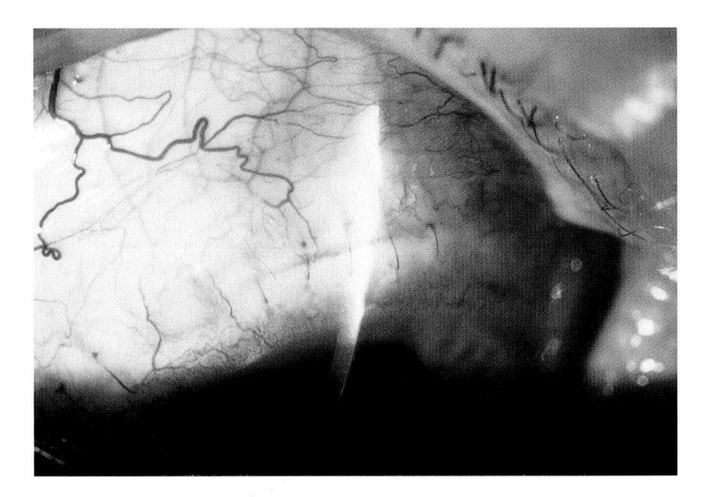

FIGURE 41-1 Scleral "melting" and 6 diopters (D) of against-the-wound astigmatism developed in a 68-year-old woman 3 weeks following uncomplicated planned extracapsular cataract extraction. The wound was resutured, but within 4 weeks there was spontaneous loosening of all sutures and recurrence of 4 D of against-the-wound astigmatism. Note wound gape, scleral edema, and loose sutures. Because of poor scleral integrity, no further wound revision was attempted.

At multiple junctures during cataract surgery, the corneal or scleral tunnel incision may be subject to compromise that can predispose to later dehiscence. Excessive episcleral cautery may devitalize the flap, delaying tissue ingrowth essential to wound healing and in extreme cases precipitating flap necrosis. Tearing or buttonholing of the roof of the tunnel can make closure difficult, and a groove or dissection into the ciliary body, if sufficiently anterior, can create a deep channel into the anterior chamber. False passages in the tunnel itself with multiple levels of anterior chamber entry may also arise and escape detection and closure. Even the ideal 50% thickness flap may be damaged intraoperatively by excessive handling or by heating from the phacoemulsification tip, causing a corneoscleral burn.

At the close of surgery, a seton may be left in the tunnel, creating a wound fistula.[22] This may occur with capsular or cortical remnants, vitreous, or prolapsed iris. Incorrect suture placement and tying may distort wound architecture and predispose to leakage.

The seal of the internal corneal valve is intraocular pressure dependent, and an apparently watertight wound can leak as a result of postoperative hypotony. The latter, in turn, can be caused by insufficient chamber inflation at the conclusion of surgery, sluggish ciliary body function (itself often caused by hypotony), or accidental wound lip compression (e.g., eye rubbing) that leads to aqueous egress.

Perioperative systemic steroid exposure may predispose to dehiscence of large incisions. Fechner and Wichmann[23] reported a 10% incidence of wound dehiscence in 100 phakic myopic eyes treated with high-dose systemic steroids directly before and after implantation of iris-fixated lenses. The intended suppression of postoperative inflammation apparently interfered with the initial stages of wound healing. Not surprisingly, there is also some evidence that topical corticosteroids may also delay wound healing. Barba et al.[24] reported that corneas treated with topical corticosteroids had less wound healing at 7 days after surgery than untreated corneas or corneas treated with nonsteroidal antiinflammatory drugs. However, the relevance of these findings to small-incision surgery is unclear, and we are unaware of cases of actual wound dehiscence precipitated by topical corticosteroid use.

Manifestations of Wound Dehiscence

Wound healing can present in a variety of ways, and each has different prognostic significance and therapeutic implications.

Wound Leak

The most obvious presentation of wound dehiscence is a frank wound leak. A wound leak that occurs in the first several days postoperatively is usually due to inadequate suture closure for the particular wound configuration. Although perhaps not a true wound "dehiscence," it nevertheless falls within the purview of this discussion. Wound leaks that develop later—after the wound has been documented to be closed at one or more postoperative visits—are due primarily to trauma or, less commonly, spontaneous loosening or breakage of a suture or tissue melting or necrosis.

The clinical signs of wound leak include poor vision, ocular hypotony, broad corneal folds, shallow anterior chamber, hyphema, choroidal effusions, choroidal folds, and optic nerve edema. The intraocular pressure typically ranges from 0 to 6 or 7 mm Hg but occasionally can be higher. The definitive diagnosis is made by instilling concentrated fluorescein, using either fluorescein strips or 2% fluorescein solution. Although both methods are equally effective, use of the solution avoids the sometimes cumbersome act of "painting" the incision with the fluorescein strip. One sign that we find particularly helpful is evaluation of the internal corneal valve: in the presence of a wound leak, the valve can be seen to be gaping with posterior displacement of the posterior portion of the wound. Gimbel, Sun, and DeBroff[25] recommended the use of gonioscopy to recognize internal wound gape during and after surgery. Ultrasound biomicroscopy has been reported helpful in detecting a subtle wound leak as a cause of chronic hypotony in a patient 1 year after cataract surgery by phacoemulsification.[26]

Management depends on several factors, including etiology, timing, severity, and the structural appearance of the incision. Wound leaks that are noted in the first or second day postoperatively often seal on their own as a result of the postoperative inflammatory process. Adjunctive medical management can include the following:

1. *Decreasing or stopping corticosteroid therapy*. This is a logical, if unproven, maneuver to eliminate pharmacologic inhibition of wound healing.
2. *Prophylactic administration of topical antibiotics*. Our preference is one with a broad spectrum of coverage, such as a fluoroquinolone.
3. *Cycloplegia, preferably with a long-acting agent such as atropine or scopolamine*. This may improve ciliary body function by minimizing hypotony-induced ciliary body detachment.
4. *Full-time patching*. This is usually reserved for persistent (>5 days) or severe (<2 mm Hg intraocular pressure and/or shallow anterior chamber) cases.
5. *Use of a 48- or 72-hour collagen shield or disposable soft contact lens*. The indications for this are similar to those for patching, and selection is sometimes based on the patient's preferences. In evaluating lens fit, it is important to ensure that the lens covers the incision.
6. *Topical administration of aqueous inhibitors (e.g., beta-blockers)*. Theoretically, this will diminish the flow of aqueous through the incision, hastening wound closure.

Resuturing of an early postoperative wound leak may be indicated in several circumstances: (1) if the anterior chamber is flat; (2) if intraocular pressure remains low for several days, particularly in the presence of a shallow anterior chamber; (3) if iris prolapse occurs, or (4) if there is extensive external wound gape, particularly if excessive flattening along the meridian of the incision has developed.

Wound leaks that occur after the first several days can sometimes be managed medically, particularly if wound apposition is generally good and the integrity of the eye is unaffected. Unfortunately, in our experience this is not often the case, and these cases generally fit into the category of wound rupture requiring surgical repair (discussed later in the chapter).

Inadvertent Filtering Bleb

A wound leak under sealed conjunctiva results in formation of a filtering bleb. The management is again highly dependent on the timing and severity. Filtering blebs noted in the first few days postoperatively typically resolve. This process can be hastened using the medical measures discussed earlier for management of a wound leak.

Filtering blebs that develop after the first several postoperative days usually reflect the breakdown of an initially well-apposed wound, which can occur from trauma, suture breakage or loosening, or scleral melting. Spontaneous resolution of blebs with this cause is less likely because there is insufficient inflammation to promote closure of the incisional gaping.

Regardless of the time of onset and the cause, blebs that persist beyond several days can undergo epithelialization of the fistulous tract. This channel is resistant to medical treatment and many forms of surgical intervention.

Treatment of persistent filtering blebs depends on the level of the intraocular pressure, the overall integrity of the wound, and patient comfort. Surgical repair is indicated in eyes with poorly tolerated hypotony. Large, thin-walled blebs that "weep" aqueous may predispose to the development of endophthalmitis, and surgical closure should be considered. Filtering blebs accompanied by poor wound apposition typically induce against-the-wound astigmatism, and, if this is excessive for the patient's needs, it is a relative indication for surgical repair. Dellen can form adjacent to large blebs, and these can be resistant to standard therapy with topical lubricants.[27] Some patients are uncomfortable because of lid contact with the filtering bleb or may have cosmetic concerns when the bleb is large and cystic; in these situations, bleb repair may be indicated (Figure 41-2).

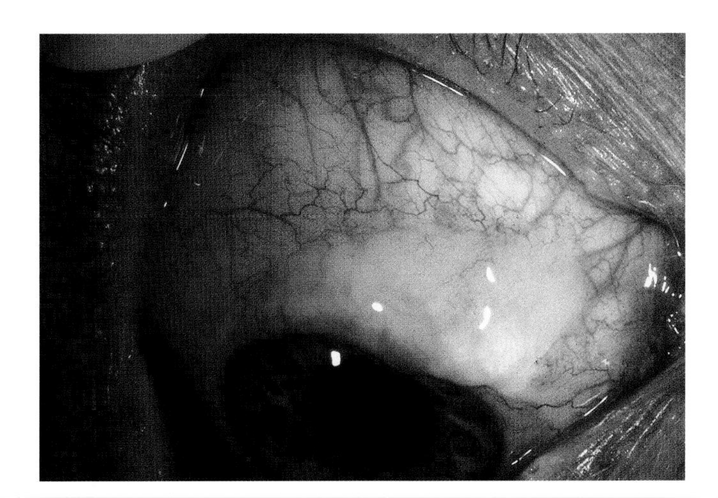

FIGURE 41-2 Persistent inadvertent filtering bleb 2 years following cataract surgery. Intraocular pressure was 11 mm Hg in this eye and 19 mm Hg in the fellow eye. Patient complained of progressive, severe eye irritation and tearing. Surgical repair consisted of excision of cystic conjunctiva, scraping of fistulous track, closure of the track with interrupted 9-0 nylon sutures, and coverage of the track with a half-thickness scleral flap. The bleb recurred, but at less than 50% of original size, and the intraocular pressure was 14 mm Hg.

Closure of a long-standing filtering bleb is complicated by epithelialization of the fistula.[28] Relatively noninvasive methods to close or shrink chronic blebs include cryotherapy, chemical cauterization with trichloroacetic acid, argon laser treatment following application of methylene blue or rose bengal dye (Steinert RF, personal communication, 1994), neodymium:yttrium-aluminum-garnet (Nd:YAG) laser,[29] and diathermy.[30,31]

Surgical closure of the fistula requires either its excision or sufficient compression and inflammation to foster cicatricial closure. We recommend excision of all conjunctiva that was involved in the filtering bleb to eliminate these channels. The wound must be carefully explored and the fistula identified. The fistulous tract can be scraped or excised, and, if necessary, the remaining hole covered or filled with a scleral graft or a folded half-thickness scleral flap.[32,33] The wound is then meticulously resutured. If the sutures appear to induce excessive astigmatism, this can be minimized by placing a scleral relaxing incision just posterior to the sutures. This incision is placed at a depth of around 300 μm and should extend the length of the sutured region. Finally, the conjunctiva and Tenon's capsule are advanced and meticulously sutured. Postoperative anti-inflammatory treatment is kept to a minimum. Even with these steps, complete closure of a bleb is not always successful. However, a large bleb can sometimes be dramatically reduced in size and low pressure ameliorated, thereby achieving partial surgical success.

Patients with persistent filtering blebs should be warned of the risk of development of bleb-induced endophthalmitis. The incidence and severity of postcataract endophthalmitis are increased in patients with filtering blebs,[34-36] and early detection is desirable.

Wound Rupture

One of the most severe sight-threatening presentations of wound dehiscence is frank wound rupture,[19,20,37,38] which is the traumatic reopening of a wound that had previously been sealed, usually accompanied by extrusion of intraocular contents. Susceptibility to traumatic wound rupture is presumably highly dependent on the size and architecture of the incision, exacerbated by any of the patient's predisposing factors. Indeed, wound failure can occur without apparent precipitating trauma in patients with abnormal sclera or poor healing. Conversely, in patients with small self-sealing incisions, a traumatic rupture of the globe without compromise of the incision is even possible.

Most traumatically induced wound ruptures have extensive structural disruption of the incision with poor wound edge apposition and iris prolapse (Figure 41-3). The amount of damage to the wound is almost always much more widespread than is evident preoperatively. The initial steps of surgical repair consist of dissecting free the conjunctival flap, exploring the incision, reopening of the wound beyond the margin of dehiscence, and freshening of the wound edges by scraping them with a sharp blade.

Iris prolapse occurs in the majority of eyes that sustain late postoperative wound rupture. This may in part be due to the infrequent use of peripheral iridectomy, which predisposes to a large disparity in pressure between the posterior and anterior chambers at the moment of traumatic wound opening. Iris that is frankly necrotic should be excised and cultured. A viable iris can usually be repositioned after it is meticulously scraped to remove any adherent epithelial cells. There is some controversy over the management of iris that has been prolapsed over 24 hours because of concern about the introduction of epithelium or microorganisms; excision may be preferred in these instances.[39,40] Epithelial downgrowth has been reported after repositioning an iris that was prolapsed for 7 days. It is often easiest to reposition an iris through a separate stab incision. The surgeon should be cautious to avoid exerting excessive traction on the iris root, which could create an iridodialysis, hemorrhage, or both.

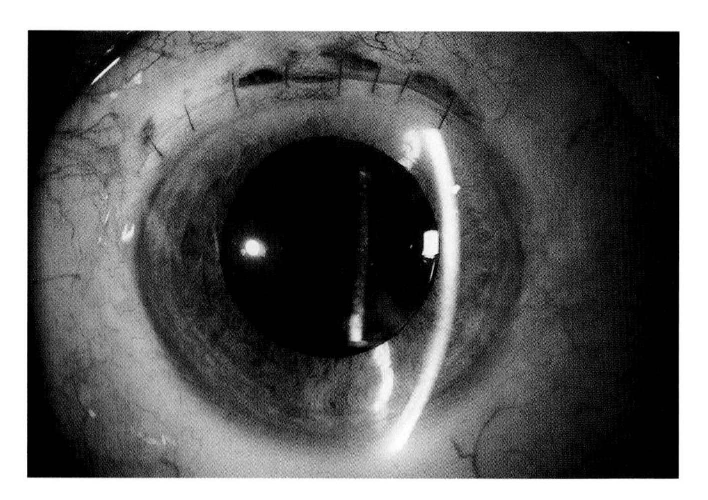

FIGURE 41-3 Presumed traumatic wound dehiscence that was detected 3 weeks following uncomplicated extracapsular cataract extraction. The patient indicated that he had rubbed the eye. Note iris prolapse; no wound leak occurred.

Vitrectomy is performed as needed, and the intraocular lens is repositioned or exchanged as necessary. The wound is then meticulously resutured; our preference is interrupted 10-0 or 9-0 nylon sutures. Topical and broad-spectrum intravenous antibiotics are usually recommended for 2 to 5 days following wound repair, possibly followed by several days of oral antibiotic administration.

Epithelial Downgrowth and Fibrous Ingrowth

One of the most insidious manifestations of wound dehiscence is epithelial downgrowth.[41,42] This is a rare complication of cataract surgery and has multiple presentations, including corneal decompensation, severe glaucoma with or without obvious angle closure, chronic anterior uveitis, and the presence of a retrocorneal membrane with a demarcated leading edge[42] (Figure 41-4). The presence of epithelial downgrowth can sometimes be confirmed by irradiating the affected iris with an argon laser. Using laser settings of 300 to 700 mW and 500-μm spot size, a white blanching is seen at the site of laser treatment, as opposed to a standard burn or brown color change of the normal iris surface. Epithelial downgrowth can sometimes be diagnosed with specular endothelial microscopy; a demarcation line can be seen separating endothelial cells (which are often abnormal in size

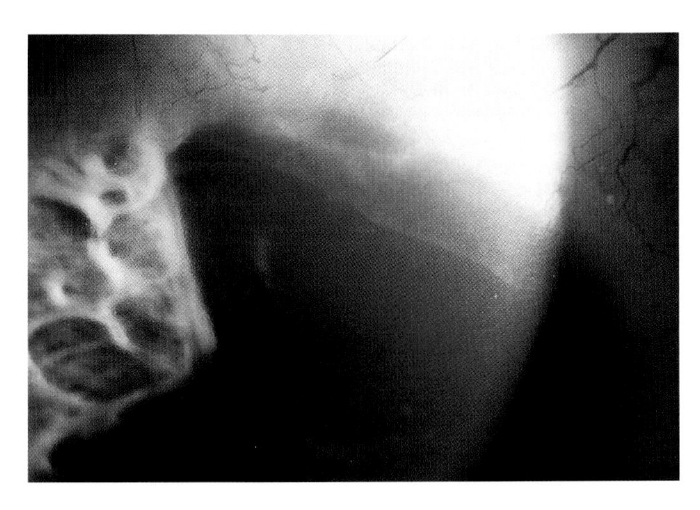

FIGURE 41-4 Epithelial downgrowth with membrane on corneal endothelial surface 21 months following traumatic wound rupture; note prominent leading edge. Diagnosis was confirmed by frozen section obtained at the time of iridocyclectomy.

and configuration) from dark, poorly defined cells representing the epithelium.[43,44] Definitive diagnosis depends on histopathologic confirmation of the presence of epithelial tissue in the eye.

Another manifestation of epithelial downgrowth is the presence of an intraocular cyst (Figure 41-5).[45] This usually involves the iris and is often adherent to the posterior surface of the cornea. The cyst is slowly expansile and readily transilluminates. An epithelial implantation cyst can readily be transformed into true epithelial downgrowth if the cyst is inadvertently lysed.[46]

The time of onset of epithelial downgrowth is highly variable, but it typically presents within months of the surgery. It appears to be more common in patients who have undergone multiple procedures or in patients who have experienced postoperative complications with wound closure.

Definitive treatment of epithelial downgrowth consists of complete destruction or excision of all intraocular epithelial tissue. Surgical techniques include some combination of cryotherapy of the involved cornea with the anterior chamber filled with air; iridocyclectomy with excision of the internal corneal flap in the affected region; and pars plana vitrectomy with removal of all involved iris, ciliary body, and lens with endolaser of any other suspected involved areas.[22] Unfortunately, the prognosis is poor.[47]

Fibrous ingrowth is the abnormal invasion of the anterior chamber by connective tissue from the incision.[48-50] This condition is uncommonly diagnosed clinically, and it occurs in eyes with deficient wound closure, possibly in the presence of abnormal endothelium. By slit lamp biomicroscopy, it appears as a thick, opaque membrane on the posterior surface of the cornea. Vascularization is sometimes evident. It tends to be slower growing and more clearly demarcated than epithelial downgrowth. It is typically detected histopathologically in tissue from eyes that have undergone incisional repair or in enucleated specimens.

Against-the-Wound Astigmatism

One of the most subtle but perhaps most common manifestations of wound dehiscence is excessive flattening along the meridian of the incision.[51] This condition can begin at any time in the first 2 years postoperatively and can progress for years thereafter. A precise definition of this condition is difficult to formulate, in part because the determination of excessive flattening along the meridian of the incision depends on incision size. Shifts of unusual magnitude would include flattening of greater than or equal to 1.5 diopters for a 5-mm or smaller incisions, greater than or equal to 2 diopters for 6- to 7-mm incisions, and greater than or equal to 3 diopters for extracapsular incisions. This process is usually detected first by keratometry, refraction, or computerized videokeratography (Figure 41-6). With computer videokeratography, characteristic asymmetric flattening can often be seen in the semimeridian adjacent to the incision.

A

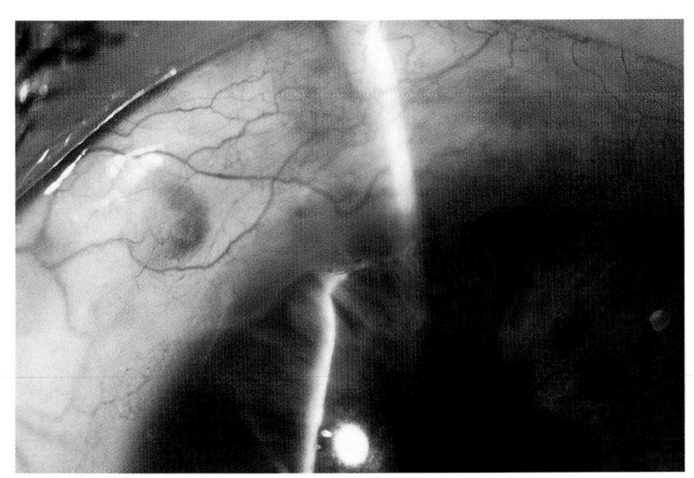

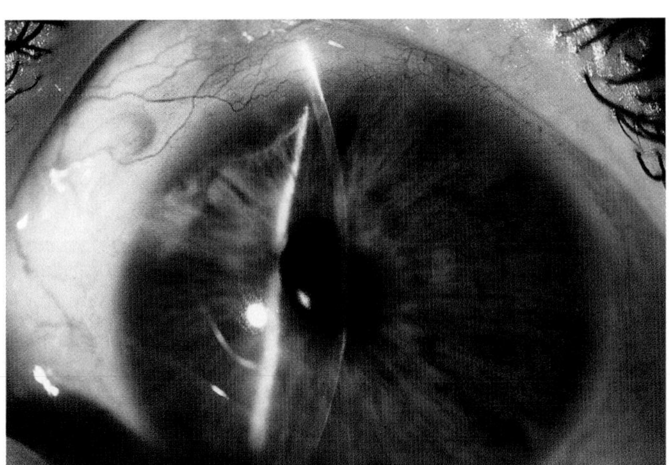

B

FIGURE 41-5 **A,** Iris epithelial cyst that was noted 18 months following intraocular lens exchange and scleral flap recession. **B,** High-magnification detail of the cyst. Patient has done well with 20/40 vision 18 months following iridocyclectomy and suture fixation of a posterior chamber lens.

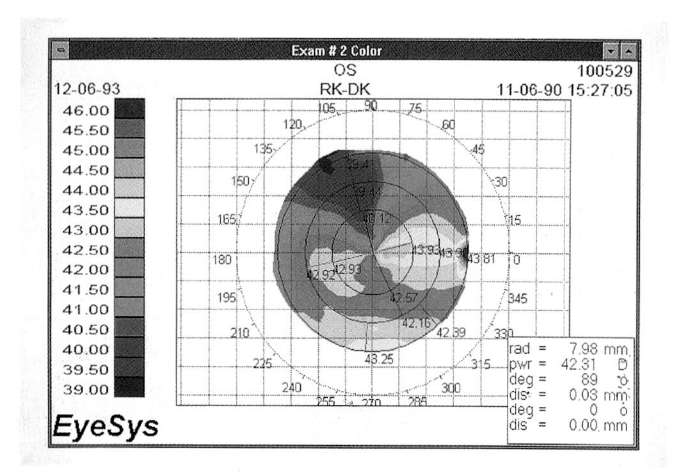

FIGURE 41-6 Computerized videokeratographic map showing against-the-wound astigmatism (2.75 D by keratometry) 4 years following secondary intraocular lens implantation through a superior 7-mm incision. Note asymmetric flattening greater in the semimeridian adjacent to the incision.

Excessive against-the-wound astigmatism is fostered by the tissue addition that occurs as part of the natural wound healing process, but additional elements are required. Wound construction is important. Predisposition to excessive flattening along the meridian of the incision increases with longer wounds and shorter tunnels. This problem certainly is more common in superior incisions and indeed is rarely seen with temporal incisions. Intrinsic patient factors, perhaps labeled "poor healing" for want of a better term, often seem to play a major role (see Figure 41-1).

Treatment in most instances is directed at reducing the induced astigmatism. Although the cause is incisional weakness or dehiscence, surgical repair of the incision is fraught with difficulties and is generally reserved for selected cases detected in the first 2 to 4 weeks postoperatively. Wound resuturing can induce excessive with-the-wound astigmatism, requires reentry of the eye, and provides no certainty that the process will not recur. For most patients, our preference is first to attempt conservative management with glasses or, in rare instances, contact lenses. Astigmatic keratotomy or peripheral corneal relaxing incisions are offered to patients who poorly tolerate the strong refractive correction required or who keenly desire improved uncorrected vision.

Conclusions

Wound dehiscence is a relatively uncommon but potentially devastating complication of cataract surgery. It has multiple manifestations requiring a wide spectrum of therapeutic responses. Advances in wound construction techniques and small-incision surgery have greatly reduced the prevalence and magnitude of this surgical complication.

REFERENCES

1. Swan KC, Campbell L: Unintentional filtration following cataract surgery, *Arch Ophthalmol* 71:77-83, 1964.
2. Lambrou FH, Kozarsky A: Wound dehiscence following cataract surgery, *Ophthalmic Surg* 18:738-740, 1987.
3. Arango JL, Margo CE: Wound complications following cataract surgery: a case-control study, *Arch Ophthalmol* 116:1021-1024, 1998.
4. Quraishy MM, Casswell AG: May I bend down after my cataract operation, doctor? *Eye* 10:92-94, 1996.
5. Ball JL, McLeod BK: Traumatic wound dehiscence following cataract surgery: a thing of the past? *Eye* 15:42-44, 2001.
6. Anders N, Pham DT, Wollensak J: Etiology of insufficient wound sealing in cataract operation with the no-stitch technique, *Ophthalmologe* 92:270-273, 1995.
7. Ernest PH, Lavery KT, Kiessling LA: Relative strength of scleral corneal and clear corneal incisions constructed in cadaver eyes, *J Cataract Refract Surg* 20:626-629, 1994.
8. Heier JS, Walton WT, Enzenauer RW et al: Wound strength comparison of a 5.1-millimeter no-stitch with a 7.0-millimeter sutured incision in human cadaver globes, *Ophthalmic Surg* 25:685-687, 1994.
9. Ernest PH, Fenzl R, Lavery KT et al: Relative stability of clear corneal incisions in a cadaver eye model, *J Cataract Refract Surg* 21:39-42, 1995.
10. Mackool RJ, Russell RS: Strength of clear corneal incisions in cadaver eyes, *J Cataract Refract Surg* 22:721-725, 1996.
11. Koch PS: Structural analysis of cataract incision construction, *J Cataract Refract Surg* 17(suppl):661-667, 1991.
12. Ernest P, Tipperman R, Eagle R et al: Is there a difference in incision healing based on location? *J Cataract Refract Surg* 24:482-486, 1998.
13. Flaxel JT, Swan KC: Limbal wound healing after cataract extraction, *Arch Ophthalmol* 81:653-659, 1969.
14. Flaxel JT: Histology of cataract extractions, *Arch Ophthalmol* 83:436-444, 1970.
15. Gliedman ML, Karlson KE: Wound healing and wound strength of sutured limbal wounds, *Am J Ophthalmol* 39:859-865, 1955.
16. Masuda K: Tensile strength of corneoscleral wounds repaired with absorbable sutures, *Ophthalmic Surg* 12:110-114, 1981.
17. Koch DD, Smith SH, Whiteside SB: Limbal and scleral wound healing. In: *Healing processes in the cornea*, The Woodlands, 1989, Portfolio Publishing, pp 165-181.
18. Hurvitz LM: Late clear corneal wound failure after trivial trauma, *J Cataract Refract Surg* 25:283-284, 1999.
19. Pham DT, Anders N, Wollensak J: Wound rupture 1 year after cataract operation with 7 mm scleral tunnel incision (no-stitch technique), *Klin Monatsbl Augenheilkd* 208:124-126, 1996.
20. Routsis P, Garston B: Late traumatic wound dehiscence after phacoemulsification, *J Cataract Refract Surg* 26:1092-1093, 2000.
21. Jonas JB, Ruprecht KW, Schmitz-Valckenberg P et al: Ophthalmic surgical complications in Werner's syndrome: report on 18 eyes of nine patients, *Ophthalmic Surg* 18:760-764, 1987.
22. Schaeffer AR, Nalbandian RM, Brigham DW et al: Epithelial downgrowth following wound dehiscence after extracapsular cataract extraction and posterior chamber lens implantation: surgical management, *J Cataract Refract Surg* 15:437-441, 1989.
23. Fechner PU, Wichmann W: Retarded corneoscleral wound healing associated with high preoperative doses of systemic steroids in glaucoma surgery, *Refract Corneal Surg* 7:174-176, 1991.
24. Barba KR, Samy A, Lai C, Perlman JI et al: Effect of topical anti-inflammatory drugs on corneal and limbal wound healing, *J Cataract Refract Surg* 26: 893-897, 2000.
25. Gimbel HV, Sun R, DeBroff BM: Recognition and management of internal wound gape, *J Cataract Refract Surg* 21:121-124, 1995.
26. Machemer HF, Roters S: Ultrasound biomicroscopy of chronic hypotony after cataract extraction, *J Cataract Refract Surg* 27:327-329, 2001.
27. Soong HK, Quigley HA: Dellen associated with filtering blebs, *Arch Ophthalmol* 101:385-387, 1983.
28. Soong HK, Meyer RF, Wolter JR: Fistula excision and peripheral grafts in the treatment of persistent limbal wound leaks, *Ophthalmology* 95:31-36, 1988.
29. Geyer O: Management of large, leaking, and inadvertent filtering blebs with the neodymium:YAG laser, *Ophthalmology* 105:983-987, 1998.
30. Cleasby GW, Fung WE, Webster RG: Cryosurgical closure of filtering blebs, *Arch Ophthalmol* 87:319-323, 1972.
31. Yannuzzi LA, Theodore FH: Cryotherapy of post-cataract blebs, *Am J Ophthalmol* 76:217-222, 1973.
32. Clinch TE, Kaufman H: Repair of inadvertent conjunctival filtering blebs with a scleral flap, *Arch Ophthalmol* 110:1652-1653, 1992.
33. Rao SK, Padmanaban P: An unusual complication of a postcataract filtering bleb, *Ophthalmic Surg Lasers* 28:601-602, 1997.

34. Mandelbaum S, Forster RK: Endophthalmitis associated with filtering blebs, *Int Ophthalmol Clin* 27:107-111, 1987.
35. Dickens A, Greven CM: Posttraumatic endophthalmitis caused by lactobacillus, *Arch Ophthalmol* 111:1169, 1993.
36. Phillips WB II, Wong TP, Bergren RL et al: Late onset endophthalmitis associated with filtering blebs, *Ophthalmic Surg* 25:88-91, 1994.
37. Kass MA, LaHav M, Albert DM: Traumatic rupture of healed cataract wounds, *Am J Ophthalmol* 81:722-724, 1976.
38. Johns KJ, Sheils P, Parrish CM et al: Traumatic wound dehiscence in pseudophakia, *Am J Ophthalmol* 108:535-539, 1989.
39. Orlin SE, Farber MG, Brucker AJ et al: The unexpected guest: problem of iris reposition, *Surv Ophthalmol* 35:59-66, 1990.
40. Menapace R: Delayed iris prolapse with unsutured 5.1 mm clear corneal incisions, *J Cataract Refract Surg* 21:353-357, 1995.
41. Maumenee AE: Treatment of epithelial downgrowth and intraocular fistula following cataract extraction, *Trans Am Ophthmol Soc* 62:153-162, 1964.
42. Kuchle M, Green WR: Epithelial ingrowth: a study of 207 histopathologically proven cases, *Ger J Ophthalmol* 5:211-223, 1996.
43. Smith RE, Parrett C: Specular microscopy of epithelial downgrowth, *Arch Ophthalmol* 96:1222-1224, 1978.
44. Liang RA, Sandstrom MM, Leibowitz HM, Berrospi AR: Epithelialization of the anterior chamber: clinical investigation with the specular microscope, *Arch Ophthalmol* 97:1870-1874, 1979.
45. Knauf HP, Rowsey JJ, Margo CE: Cystic epithelial downgrowth following clear-corneal cataract extraction, *Arch Ophthalmol* 115:668-669, 1997.
46. Orlin SE, Raber IM, Laibson PR et al: Epithelial downgrowth following the removal of iris inclusion cysts, *Ophthalmic Surg* 22:330-335, 1991.
47. Stark WJ, Michels RG, Maumenee AE et al: Surgical management of epithelial ingrowth, *Am J Ophthalmol* 85:772-780, 1978.
48. Bloomfield SE, Jakobiec FA, Iwamoto T: Fibrous ingrowth with retrocorneal membrane, *Ophthalmology* 88:459-465, 1981.
49. McDonnell PJ, de la Cruz Z, Green WR: Vitreous incarceration complicating cataract surgery: a light and electron microscopic study, *Ophthalmology* 93:247-253, 1986.
50. Kremer I, Zandbank J, Barash D et al: Extensive fibrous downgrowth after traumatic corneoscleral wound dehiscence, *Ann Ophthalmol* 23:465-468, 1991.
51. Gelender H: Management of corneal astigmatism after cataract surgery, *Refract Corneal Surg* 7:99-102, 1991.

Corneal Edema After Cataract Surgery

42

Roger F. Steinert, MD

Corneal endothelial decompensation after cataract extraction is a well-known although rare complication of all types of cataract surgery. The overall incidence is less than 1%. This chapter reviews the differential diagnosis and treatment of corneal edema after cataract surgery. Chapter 21 addresses combined penetrating keratoplasty and cataract surgery in patients with preoperatively compromised corneas.

Pathophysiology

The final common pathway of corneal stromal edema after cataract surgery is inadequate endothelial pump function to keep the corneal stroma and epithelium in their relatively dehydrated and clear state.[1] Elevated intraocular pressure can overwhelm the corneal endothelial pump. Reduction in intraocular pressure will reverse the edema in such cases. In a marginally compensated endothelium, lowering of intraocular pressure with antiglaucomatous medications from a high-normal to a low-normal reading can make a critical difference in corneal clarity.

The corneal endothelium acts to dehydrate the cornea both actively through an adenosine triphosphate–driven bicarbonate ion pump[2-4] and passively through the integrity of the cellular membrane barrier.[5,6] The adult human corneal endothelium has little ability to replicate to replace damaged cells.[7-10] Endothelial cells do migrate, enlarge, and undergo fibroblastic metaplasia in an effort to cover denuded areas of Descemet's membrane to reestablish the intercellular junctions.[10-12] An adaptive increase in the number of pump sites per cell may occur in diseased corneas.[1] Therefore some cases of corneal edema will improve over several weeks to months. Inflammation may also transiently reduce endothelial pump function.[13] Elimination of the inflammation may be accompanied by restoration of corneal clarity.

Differential Diagnosis of Postoperative Corneal Edema

Table 42-1 lists the principal causes of postoperative corneal edema after cataract surgery.

Surgical trauma is often the culprit in unexpected postoperative corneal endothelial decompensation. Direct local injury to the endothelium with an instrument or a portion of the intraocular lens (IOL) implant will result in a discrete patch of edema. Over time, the migration of adjacent endothelial cells can restore corneal clarity if the area of injury is not overly large. Diffuse edema may result from difficulty in delivering the nucleus in extracapsular cataract extraction or prolonged ultrasound in phacoemulsification, particularly if all or part of the nucleus is fragmented in the anterior chamber. A high volume of balanced salt solution infusion alone is generally well tolerated by the corneal endothelium, but prolonged infusion studies have demonstrated a difference between regular balanced salt solution and enhanced balanced salt solution formulas in endothelial injury.[14-18]

Toxicity from a variety of chemical contaminants may result in diffuse endothelial decompensation. It is frequently but not always accompanied by other evidence of intraocular toxicity, most notably a fixed and dilated pupil and elevated intraocular pressure.[19,20] This syndrome is often called *toxic anterior segment syndrome* (TASS). In more extreme cases, toxicity will result in an excessive inflammatory reaction, ciliary body shutdown and hypotony, or acute retinal inflammation or retinal necrosis, or both.

When toxicity is suspected, all intraocular solutions and medications are suspect and should be reviewed. More commonly, toxicity results from agents not intended for use inside the eye or agents used in excessive concentration. Examples include detergents used in cleaning reusable instruments, incorrect concentrations of additives, addition of preserved instead of nonpreserved additives to infusions, or confusing an intended intraocular medication for some other substance that is toxic. Antibiotics are particularly suspect. Errors in dilution medications may occur. External antibiotics may also inadvertently enter the anterior chamber, particularly through an unsutured wound. A subconjunctival bolus superiorly overlying a superior corneal scleral tunnel may be expressed into the anterior chamber through lid pressure, for example. Aminoglycoside antibiotics, in particular, have profound retinal toxicity at all but extremely low concentrations.

Detachment of the Descemet's membrane is usually recognized intraoperatively. If not, slit lamp examination postoperatively is diagnostic.[12,21-24] A glassy membrane similar to the lens capsule will be seen separated from the posterior stroma. If extensive, the exact configuration of the detached membrane can be

TABLE 42-1

Principal Causes of Corneal Edema After Cataract Surgery

Cause
Surgical trauma
Instruments
IOL
Irrigating solutions
Ultrasonic vibrations
Nuclear fragments
Prior surgery
Primary corneal endothelial disease
Fuchs' dystrophy
Low enthothelial cell density without guttae
Chemical injury
Preservations in solutions
Residual toxic chemicals on instruments (e.g., detergents, dried solutions)
Improper concentrations of solutions (e.g., antibiotics)
Osmotic damage
Direct toxicity
Mistakenly used toxic chemicals, expired agents, or incorrect solutions (e.g., normal saline instead of balanced salt solution)
IOL syndromes
Direct endothelial touch
Long-term toxicity (? inflammatory)
Contact with other ocular tissues
Flat chamber
Iris bombé
Suprachoroidal effusion-hemorrhage
Detachment of Descemet's membrane
Trauma from retained foreign material
Nuclear chips
Particulate matter
Postoperative glaucoma
Inflammation
Membranous ingrowth or downgrowth
Epithelial downgrowth
Fibrous ingrowth
Endothelial proliferation
Vitreous touch-adherence
Absence of IOL and capsule
Brown-McLean syndrome

IOL, Intraocular lens

difficult to interpret. Localized detachments are often in close proximity to their proper anatomic location. If the Descemet's membrane can be brought back into proper anatomic apposition with the posterior stroma, and the endothelium itself has not been irreversibly damaged, the endothelial pump function will itself reattach the Descemet's membrane because of the relative vacuum created by the endothelial pump. This is best accomplished surgically by introduction of an air bubble through a paracentesis wound inferiorly. This can be performed intraoperatively or postoperatively in the operating room or at the slit lamp microscope in favorable cases. Only when the Descemet's membrane is held away from the stroma by traction is a suture needed. A full-thickness through-and-through 10-0 nylon suture can forcefully reappose an area of intractable detachment (Figure 42-1). Instrumentation of the membrane itself should be avoided if possible because of the local injury to the endothelium that will occur. Use of viscoelastic agents should be avoided in an effort to reappose the Descemet's membrane. If the viscoelastic agent enters between the posterior corneal stroma and the Descemet's membrane, it will prevent reattachment of the membrane and may remain as a barrier indefinitely. Finally, although reattachment of the Descemet's membrane and restoration of corneal clarity is urgent, it is not a true emergency. The endothelium is bathed in aqueous, even in the detached form. The endothelium will remain viable while an orderly reintervention is planned. Abnormal endothelial proliferation will occur with prolonged detachment or improper adhesion.[12,25,26]

Unsuspected Low Preoperative Endothelial Cell Density

A small portion of the population has a low endothelial cell density not heralded by the presence of corneal guttae.[27,28] To detect these patients preoperatively, some cataract surgeons perform routine preoperative specular microscopy with endothelial cell counts. Other surgeons argue against this routine testing in view of its expense and the fact that a low cell count should not alter the surgical technique; in all cases, the surgeon presumably employs the best available technique to minimize endothelial cell injury. Careful inspection with a broad oblique beam at high magnification under the slit lamp biomicroscope can, in fact, disclose the endothelial cell pattern. With practice, the surgeon can make a good estimate of the endothelial cell density and pattern. Formal specular microscopy with endothelial cell photography can then be reserved for cases of probable abnormality rather than used as a screening tool.

An occasional patient will experience unexpected corneal edema after apparently atraumatic surgery. In the absence of preoperative specular microscopy, the status of the endothelium in the fellow eye should be examined. A case of naturally low cell density will almost always be bilateral. Examination of the fellow eye will therefore help in the differential diagnosis of unexpected postoperative corneal edema.

Intraocular lens syndromes are a leading cause of corneal decompensation many years after the surgery. A loose anterior chamber IOL or a large or loose pupillary-supported iris plane IOL will directly traumatize the corneal endothelium, cause a progressive attrition of endothelial cells, and ultimately lead to clinically evident corneal edema. The edema will characteristically begin in a localized zone over the area of trauma but will progress as the remaining endothelial cells migrate into the area of damage.

Corneal edema beginning many years after IOL implantation may be due to excessive loss of endothelium at the time of surgery, followed by ongoing normal or accelerated attrition of the remaining endothelium. So-called closed-loop anterior chamber IOLs (Azar 91Z from IOLAB, Leiske Surgidev Style 10, Stableflex from Optical Radiation Corporation, Hesburg

A

B

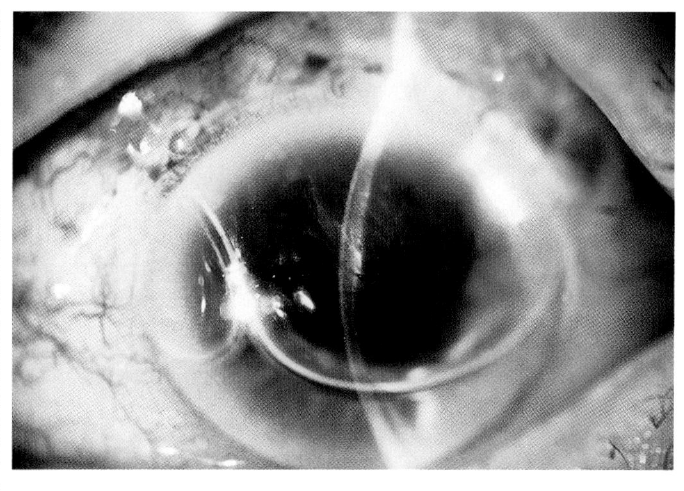

C

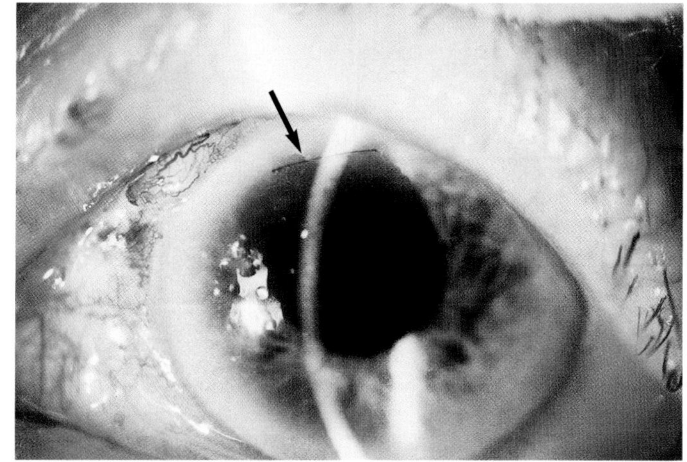

FIGURE 42-1 A, Detached Descemet's membrane is seen as a glassy membrane in the anterior chamber behind an area of corneal edema. The detachment may be extensive with curling of the Descemet's membrane on itself well away from the area of edema, or it may be a shallow detachment only seen with a thin slit beam. Often a small amount of blood is trapped at the edge of the inferior detachment *(arrows).* **B,** Most Descemet's membrane detachments can be reapposed by placing a large air bubble in the anterior chamber through an inferior paracentesis. **C,** Particularly where extensive detachment or traction on the membrane exists that cannot be fully relieved, a through-and-through 10-0 nylon suture is needed to forcefully reappose the Descemet's membrane and prevent aqueous access into the space between the posterior corneal stroma and the separated membrane *(arrow).* After several weeks, the suture may be removed in most cases.

from IntraOptics) have a much higher rate of late corneal decompensation than any other anterior chamber lenses, especially the Kelman three-foot (Omnifit) and four-foot (Multiflex) styles.[29-31] Many surgeons suspect that all anterior chamber lenses have a higher rate of long-term complications than do posterior chamber lenses, whereas other surgeons believe that this perception arises because anterior chamber lenses are typically employed in complicated cases in which posterior capsule support has been compromised. Adequate data to prove or disprove these viewpoints may never be available.

Late-onset corneal edema associated with anterior chamber lenses is often preceded by or accompanied by cystoid macular edema, a phenomenon that has been termed the *cornea-retina syndrome.* A generally accepted explanation for this syndrome is that the anterior chamber IOL causes chronic subclinical inflammation. Prostaglandins are the inflammatory mediators most often suspected as capable of causing both cystoid macular edema and corneal endothelial cell loss.

The anterior chamber IOLs in these cases of cornea-retina syndrome are typically not loose. In fact, gonioscopy reveals peripheral iris synechiae around the closed-loop haptics (Figure 42-2). Special techniques are required to explant these

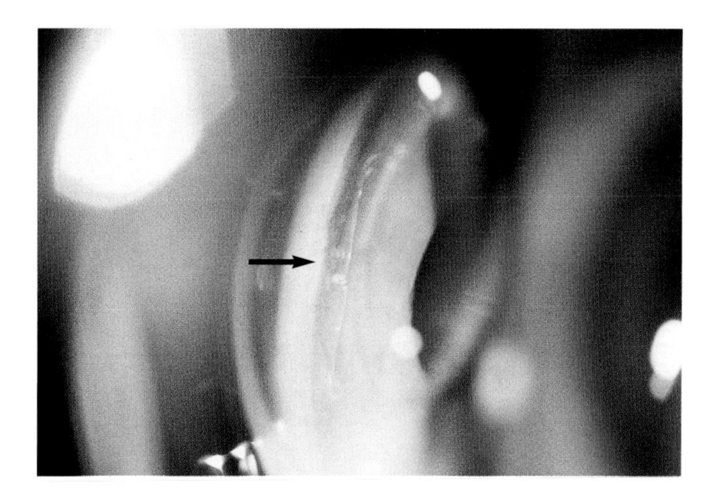

FIGURE 42-2 Gonioscopic examination of a Stableflex anterior chamber lens shows typical peripheral anterior synechia formation around the distal haptic loop *(arrow).*

closed-loop anterior chamber IOLs, as detailed in Figures 42-3 and 42-4 (see also Chapter 40). Simple traction on incarcerated haptic will cause iridodialysis and severe bleeding.

A loose IOL causing corneal edema can be differentiated from the cornea-retina syndrome in two ways. Clinical examination with gonioscopy usually is diagnostic. Specular microscopy also is often diagnostic when the corneal edema is localized to a peripheral area. If the localized edema is due to trauma from a loose IOL, the endothelial cell density increases with increasing distance from the area of edema. In contrast, in the cornea-retina syndrome, the corneal endothelial density will be very low and borderline to maintain compensation throughout the remaining clear cornea.

If the cornea decompensates centrally and penetrating keratoplasty is performed, most surgeons will exchange a closed-loop anterior chamber IOL for either an open-loop anterior chamber IOL or a suture-fixated posterior chamber IOL.[32-38] The best type of replacement IOL remains undetermined in regard to both short-term complications and long-term graft survival and recovery of vision.

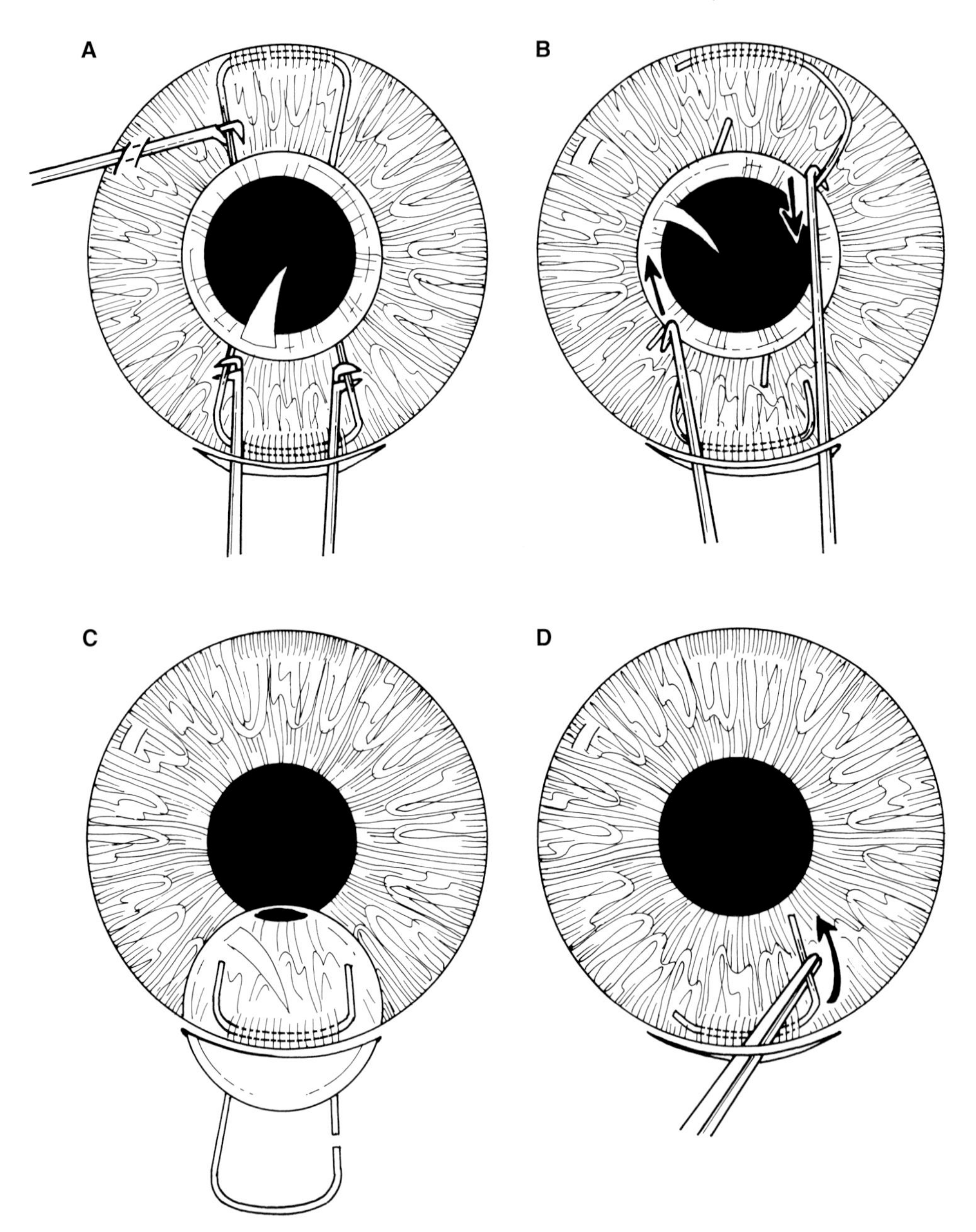

FIGURE 42-3 Technique for explantation of a Surgidev Style 10 (Leiske) anterior chamber IOL. **A,** Through an inferotemporal paracentesis, a haptic cutting instrument (Rapazzo haptic cutter, Storz Instruments) is introduced to cut one arm of the inferior haptic. Through the superior wound, with the anterior chamber maintained by viscoelastic solution, both arms of the superior haptic are cut. **B,** Using two IOL manipulating hooks, the IOL is then rotated gently. The inferior haptic uncurls and is drawn through the inferior peripheral anterior synechia without tearing the synechia, which would result in bleeding and an iridodialysis. **C,** The rotated IOL is then delivered through the superior wound, taking care not to snag the iris or the wound on the transected haptic. **D,** The remaining superior haptic is then grasped with a forceps and rotated out of the superior peripheral anterior synechia.

Management of a patient with late-onset cystoid macular edema or localized corneal edema in the presence of an anterior chamber IOL is problematic. In most cases of late-onset cystoid macular edema and essentially all cases of localized corneal edema, the endothelium will be severely depleted even when the cornea remains clinically clear. Nevertheless, the longer cystoid macular edema persists, the more likely that it will cause irreversible macular damage even if acute leakage resolves. My approach to new late-onset cystoid macular edema is an intense course of topical steroids and nonsteroidal antiinflammatory agents (e.g. dexamethasone, 0.1%, or prednisolone acetate, 1%, combined with ketorolac, 0.5% [Acular], or diclofenac, 0.1% [Voltaren], both four times daily). If the cystoid macular edema does not improve over 1 month, or resolves but then recurs, I believe that exchange of the closed-loop anterior chamber IOL is strongly indicated. Improvement may occur with a replacement Kelman-style anterior chamber IOL, but I favor scleral suture fixation of a posterior chamber IOL for the best long-term

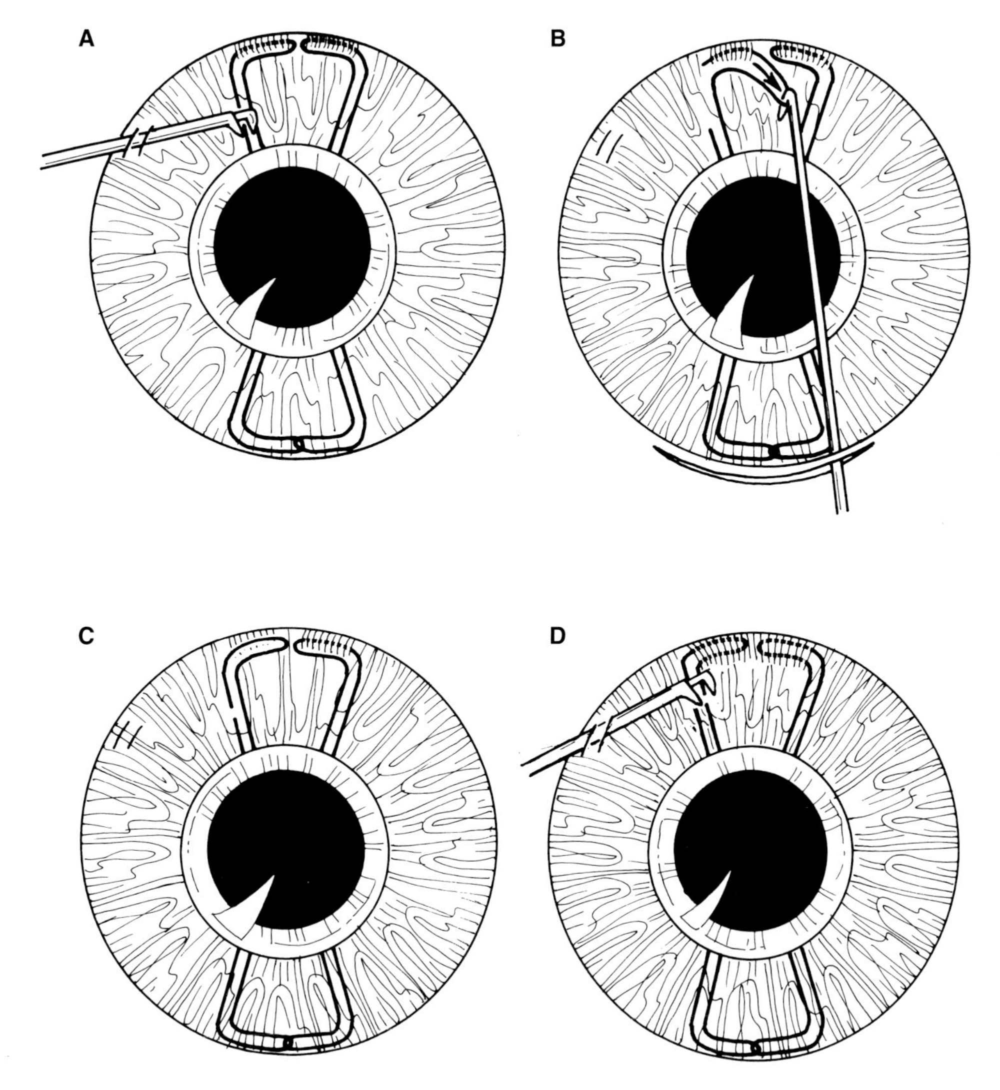

FIGURE 42-4 Technique for explantation of a Stableflex-style anterior chamber IOL. **A,** Through an inferotemporal paracentesis, a haptic cutter transects the lateral arm of the haptic. **B,** Sinskey-style hook engages the "toe" of the haptic by direct visualization if possible or by carefully passing it within the two haptic struts. With gentle traction on the "toe," the haptic unfolds and is drawn through the inferior peripheral anterior synechia, avoiding bleeding or iridodialysis. **C,** Freed from the peripheral anterior synechia, the haptic is now loose within the anterior chamber. The same maneuver is now performed on the remaining haptics that are entrapped in peripheral anterior synechia. This should be determined by preoperative gonioscopic inspection and confirmed directly at surgery. Not all four haptics are necessarily engaged in peripheral anterior synechia. Sometimes the "toes" cross, as illustrated in the superior haptics (6 o'clock position in the figure). The IOL hook must engage only the desired haptic and avoid engaging the wrong haptic or both haptics simultaneously. After freeing all of the haptics, the IOL is delivered through the wound. **D,** In occasional cases of extreme inflammatory reaction, the peripheral anterior synechia entirely covers the "toe" of the haptic or both arms of the haptic. In this case, it is best to simply transect the two arms of the haptic as distal as possible and leave the remaining haptic in the angle. The acute angle of the "toe" does not allow a haptic to "uncurl" out of the synechia with traction on the "heel" or upper "leg" of the haptic.

TABLE 42-2
Treatment of Corneal Edema

Eliminate cause
Treat inflammation
Lower intraocular pressure
Remove tissue-IOL contact
Reattach Descemet's membrane
Enhance surface dehydration
Evaporate
Hypertonic agents
Treat pain
Lubricants
Soft contact lenses
Cautery of the Bowman's layer
Conjunctival flap
Restore anatomy
Penetrating keratoplasty

IOL, Intraocular lens

results. The surgeon must perform atraumatic surgery if the fragile cornea is to remain compensated. Explantation must use the techniques outlined in Figures 42-3 and 42-4. Secondary IOL implantation is reviewed in Chapter 37. Cystoid macular edema is covered in detail in Chapter 47, and management of intraocular inflammation is discussed in Chapter 50.

Table 42-2 outlines the decision-making steps for managing complications of closed-loop anterior chamber IOLs.

Peripheral Corneal Edema

Perhaps the rarest and most benign form of corneal edema is the syndrome described by Brown and McLean.[39,40] In the classic syndrome, an aphakic patient experiences peripheral corneal stromal and epithelial edema that spares the superior cornea. Pigment deposits are present on the underlying endothelium. A central zone of 5 to 7 mm remains clear and compact indefinitely despite the peripheral edema. The peripheral iris may show transillumination, but the trabecular meshwork is not necessarily hyperpigmented. If the patient is bilaterally aphakic, the syndrome is usually present in both eyes. There is no clinical inflammation, and the cause is unknown. Although the classic presentation is following intracapsular cataract extraction, it may occur after extracapsular cataract extraction.[41] Moreover, although the syndrome is said to occur only 6 years or more postoperatively, I have seen the syndrome appear 3 months after sulcus suturing of a posterior chamber lens in a 40-year-old patient with prior extracapsular extraction of a traumatic cataract (Figure 42-5).

Treatment of Postoperative Corneal Edema

Hypertonic Solutions

Hypertonic solutions, typically 5% sodium chloride ophthalmic preparations, can improve the visual function of a patient with mild, predominantly microcystic epithelial edema. This will be particularly beneficial to the patient on awakening in the morning, when edema is maximal because of lack of evaporation during the night when the eyelids are closed. Use of a 5% sodium chloride ointment at bedtime will also help reduce the accumulation of edema while the eyelids are closed during sleep. However, the use of hypertonic solutions is only palliative. It does not improve or restore endothelial pump function or the integrity of the cell barrier.

Antiinflammatory Therapy

Reduction of intraocular inflammation may be of benefit in some cases of postoperative edema. Inflammation can cause transient dysfunction of the endothelial pump. Moreover, inflammation may cause some degree of endothelial cell death. By extrapolation, pharmacologic treatment of inflammation

A

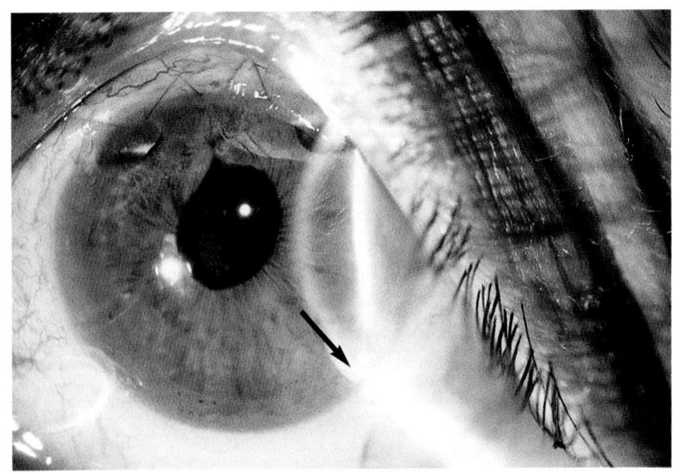

B

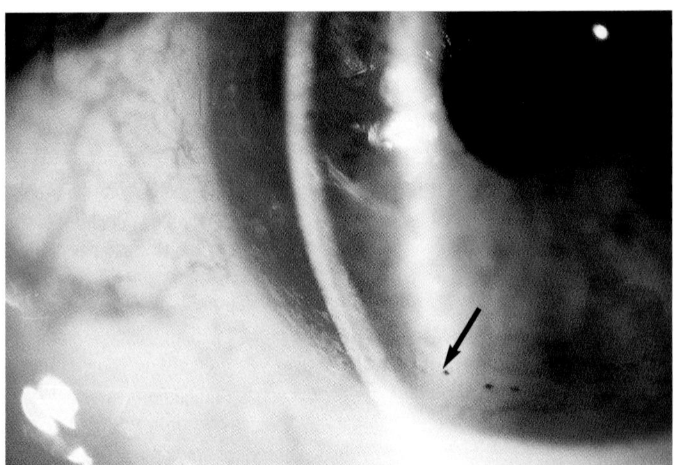

FIGURE 42-5 A, Slit lamp photomicrograph of a patient with Brown-McLean syndrome of peripheral corneal edema *(arrow)*. **B,** High magnification reveals classic pigment deposits on the endothelium underlying the area of edema *(arrow)*.

with topical steroids and perhaps nonsteroidal antiinflammatory drugs may help maximize the surviving endothelium, improving the chance that corneal clarity will ultimately return postoperatively. This supposition has not been rigorously proved, but most clinicians will treat patients with strong topical steroids such as prednisolone acetate, 1%, or dexamethasone, 0.1%, as often as every 1 to 2 hours in cases of acute postoperative corneal edema. Steroid therapy may be of no benefit in noninflammation-related corneal edema, however. Topical dexamethasone did not differ from placebo in the rate of occurrence of corneal edema in a controlled study of patients with Fuchs' dystrophy.[42]

Penetrating Keratoplasty

Restoration of vision in an eye with irreversible corneal edema requires penetrating keratoplasty. A final decision about proceeding with penetrating keratoplasty should usually be deferred 2 to 3 months postoperatively in case of acute decompensation after cataract surgery. In some cases of marginal corneal endothelial function, clarity is regained within this time frame. If there is active ongoing inflammation, the decision to proceed with penetrating keratoplasty should be deferred while intense antiinflammatory therapy continues, to enhance the probability of transplant survival and restoration of the patient's own corneal clarity. In occasional cases of severe striae with both stromal and epithelial edema, the situation may be so clearly irreversible that it is in the patient's best interest to proceed with penetrating keratoplasty earlier than 3 months after the original cataract extraction.

The treatment options for corneal edema are listed in Table 42-2.

REFERENCES

1. Waring GO, Bourne WM, Edelhauser HF et al: The corneal endothelium: normal and pathologic structure and function, *Ophthalmology* 1982; 89:531.
2. Maurice DM, Riley MV: The cornea. In Graymore CN, editor: *Biochemistry of the eye,* New York, 1970, Academic Press.
3. Kaye GI, Tice LW: Studies on the cornea. V. Electron microscopic localization of adenosine trisphosphatase activity in the rabbit cornea in relation to transport, *Invest Ophthalmol* 5:22, 1966.
4. Barfort P, Maurice D: Electrical potential and fluid transport across the corneal endothelium, *Exp Eye Res* 19:11, 1974.
5. Maurice DM: Cornea and sclera. In Davson H, editor: *The eye,* ed 3, New York, 1984, Academic Press.
6. Kreutziger GO: Lateral membrane morphology and gap junction structure in rabbit corneal endothelium, *Exp Eye Res* 23:285, 1976.
7. Flaxel JT, Swan KC: Limbal wound healing after cataract extraction: a histological study, *Arch Ophthalmol* 81:653-659, 1969.
8. Kloucek F: The corneal endothelium, *Acta Univ Carol [Med] (Praha)* 123:321-373, 1967.
9. Van Horn DL, Edelhauser HF, Aaberg TM et al: In vivo effects of air and sulfur hexafluoride gas on rabbit corneal endothelium, *Invest Ophthalmol* 11:1038-1036, 1972.
10. Capella JA: Regeneration of endothelium in diseased and injured corneas, *Am J Ophthalmol* 74:810-817, 1972.
11. Iwamoto T, DeVoe AG: Electron microscopic studies on Fuchs' combined dystrophy. I. Posterior portion of the cornea, *Invest Ophthalmol* 10:9-28, 1971.
12. Waring GO, Laibson PR, Rodriques M: Clinical and pathologic alterations of Descemet's membrane: with emphasis on endothelial metaplasia, *Surv Ophthalmol* 18:325-368, 1973-1974.
13. Dohlman CH, Hyndiuk RA: Subclinical and manifest corneal edema after cataract extraction. In *Transactions of the New Orleans Academy of Ophthalmology, Symposium on the Cornea,* St Louis, 1972, Mosby, p 214.
14. Edelhauser HF, Van Horn DL, Hyndiuk RA et al: Intraocular irrigating solutions: their effect on corneal endothelium, *Arch Ophthalmol* 93:658-657, 1975.
15. Dikstein S, Maurice DM: The metabolic bases to the fluid pump in the cornea, *J Physiol* 221:29-41, 1972.
16. Dikstein S: Efficiency and survival of the corneal endothelial pump, *Exp Eye Res* 15:639-644, 1973.
17. Anderson EI, Fischbarg J, Spector A: Fluid transport, ATP level, and ATPase activities in isolated rabbit endothelium, *Biochem Biophys Acta* 307:557-562, 1973.
18. Anderson EI, Fischbarg J, Spector A: Disulfide stimulation of fluid transport and effect on ATP level in rabbit endothelium, *Exp Eye Res* 19:1-10, 1974.
19. Breebaart AC, Nuyts RMMA, Pels E et al: Toxic endothelial cell destruction of the cornea after routine extracapsular cataract surgery, *Arch Ophthalmol* 108:1121-1125, 1990.
20. Nuyts RMMA, Edelhauser HF, Pels EII et al: Toxic effects of detergents on the corneal endothelium, *Arch Ophthalmol* 108:1158-1162, 1990.
21. Samuels B: Detachment of Descemet's membrane, *Trans Am Ophthalmol Soc* 26:427-437, 1928.
22. Scheie HG: Stripping of Descemet's membrane in cataract extraction, *Trans Am Ophthalmol Soc* 62:140-152, 1964.
23. Sparks GM: Descemetopexy: surgical reattachment of stripped Descemet's membrane, *Arch Ophthalmol* 78:31-34, 1967.
24. Zeiter HJ, Zeiter JT: Descemet's membrane separation during five hundred forty-four intraocular lens implantations, *J Am Intraocul Implant Soc* 9: 36-39, 1983.
25. Donaldson DD, Smith TR: Descemet's membrane tubes, *Trans Am Ophthalmol Soc* 64:89-109, 1966.
26. Kroll AJ: Proliferation of Descemet's membrane, *Arch Ophthalmol* 82: 339-343, 1969.
27. Kayes J, Holmberg A: The fine structure of the cornea in Fuchs' endothelial dystrophy, *Invest Ophthalmol* 3:47-67, 1964.
28. Stocker FW: *The endothelium of the cornea and its clinical implications,* ed 2, Springfield, Ill, 1971, Charles C. Thomas.
29. Solomon KD, Apple DJ, Mamalis N et al: Complications of intraocular lenses with special reference to an analysis of 2500 explanted intraocular lenses (IOLs), *Eur J Implant Refract Surg* 3:195, 1991.
30. Lim ES, Apple DJ, Tsai JC et al: An analysis of flexible anterior chamber lenses with special reference to the normalized rate of lens explantation, *Ophthalmology* 98:243, 1991.
31. Price FW Jr: Factors contributing to corneal decompensation with the Stableflex lens, *J Cataract Refract Surg* 14:53-57, 1988.
32. Kozarsky M, Stopak S, Waring GO et al: Results of penetrating keratoplasty for pseudophakic corneal edema with retention of intraocular lens, *Ophthalmology* 91:1141, 1984.
33. Speaker MG, Lugo M, Laibson PR et al: Penetrating keratoplasty for pseudophakic bullous keratopathy, *Ophthalmology* 95:1260, 1988.
34. Kornmehl EW, Steinert RF, Odrich MG et al: Penetrating keratoplasty for pseudophakic bullous keratopathy edema associated with closed-loop anterior chamber intraocular lenses, *Ophthalmology* 97:407-414, 1990.
35. Schein OD, Kenyon KR, Steinert RF et al: A randomized trial of intraocular lens fixation techniques with penetrating keratoplasty, *Ophthalmology* 100:1437-1443, 1993.
36. Price FW Jr, Whitson WE: Visual results of suture-fixated posterior chamber lenses during penetrating keratoplasty, *Ophthalmology* 96:1234-1240, 1989.
37. Soong HK, Meyer RF, Sugar A: Posterior chamber IOL implantation during keratoplasty for aphakic or pseudophakic corneal edema, *Cornea* 6:306-312, 1987.
38. Soong HK, Musch DC, Kowal V et al: Implantation of posterior chamber intraocular lenses in the absence of lens capsule during penetrating keratoplasty, *Arch Ophthalmol* 107:660-665, 1989.
39. Brown SI, McLean JM: Peripheral corneal edema after cataract extraction: a new clinical entity, *Trans Am Acad Ophthalmol Otolaryngol* 73:465-470, 1969.
40. Brown SI: Peripheral corneal edema after cataract extraction, *Am J Ophthalmol* 70:326-329, 1970.
41. Flaxel JT, Swan KC: Limbal wound healing after cataract extraction: a histological study, *Am J Ophthalmol* 81:653-659, 1969.
42. Wilson SE, Bourne WM, Brubaker RF: Effect of dexamethasone on corneal endothelial Fuchs' dystrophy, *Invest Ophthalmol Vis Sci* 29:357, 1988.

Glaucoma After Cataract Surgery

43

Paul H. Kalina, MD
Bradford J. Shingleton, MD

Advances in instrumentation and cataract surgical techniques have resulted in shorter operating time, smaller incisions, and earlier visual rehabilitation. However, glaucoma following cataract surgery is still a common problem. Elevation in intraocular pressure (IOP) may occur early or late in the postoperative course and can be either open or closed angle. Many causes exist for IOP elevation after cataract surgery, and it is inappropriate to categorize them all under the terms *aphakic* or *pseudophakic* glaucoma.

As cataract surgery has evolved, so have the types of postoperative glaucoma. With the decline in intracapsular cataract surgery and rigid anterior chamber lenses, enzyme glaucoma and the uveitis-glaucoma-hyphema (UGH) syndrome are rarely seen. Extracapsular cataract surgery and posterior chamber lens implants brought a rise in pigmentary glaucoma as a result of pigment release from the ciliary sulcus and posterior iris. The widespread use of viscoelastic agents with cataract surgery plays a significant role in early postoperative IOP elevation. More recently, phacoemulsification and clear corneal incisions have lessened glaucoma from wound compression caused by tight suture closure. Clear corneal phacoemulsification also allows cataract surgery to be done in normal and glaucomatous eyes with less risk of postoperative IOP worsening. The use of topical anesthesia now allows glaucoma patients to continue using their antiglaucoma medications without interruption. At the same time, new types of postoperative anterior segment complications, such as capsular block, are being seen.

Surgeons must also realize that glaucoma after cataract surgery does not always result directly from the surgery itself but may occur after postoperative interventions, such as neodymium: yttrium-aluminum-garnet (Nd:YAG) posterior capsulotomy.

This chapter reviews the wide-ranging differential diagnosis of glaucoma after cataract surgery (Table 43-1) and presents the therapeutic options for the ophthalmologist.

Open-Angle Glaucomas

Primary Open-Angle Glaucoma

Primary open-angle glaucoma may first become apparent following cataract surgery secondary to anatomic alterations, the natural evolution of the disease, or both. In the early era of cataract surgery, incomplete wound closure with aqueous leakage and low pressure (hypotony) were common. Today, the incidence of inadvertent aqueous leakage is low because of finer suture material and more advanced closure techniques. Particularly in planned extracapsular surgery, tight closure techniques,[1,2] suture compression,[3] and edema[4] may mechanically distort the filtration angle and further compromise aqueous outflow, leading to elevated IOP. Scleral tunnel and clear cornea phacoemulsification techniques reduce but do not eliminate this problem.[2] Even if preoperative IOP control is satisfactory, the risk of an acute pressure rise following uncomplicated intracapsular or extracapsular cataract surgery is greater in eyes with preexisting glaucoma than in healthy eyes.[5,6]

Besides alterations in angle configuration, early open-angle postoperative IOP increase after cataract surgery may be the result of retained viscoelastic, postoperative inflammation, bleeding, or pigment dispersion.[7]

The long-term effect of cataract surgery on glaucoma control varies depending on the method of cataract extraction. Following intracapsular and extracapsular surgery, several studies have reported IOP reduction for weeks to months.[8,9] Other groups have found no long-term pressure reduction.[5,6,10] With clear corneal phacoemulsification, several authors have shown an associated reduction in IOP in normal and glaucoma suspect eyes.[11-16] Patients with glaucoma were shown to have a reduction in IOP plus a lowering in the number of medications necessary to control postoperative IOP.[11] However, clear corneal phacoemulsification should not be performed with the intent of achieving better IOP control, but with the thought that IOP will likely remain stable or be slightly reduced at 1 year.

Cataract surgery in eyes with preexisting filtration blebs may result in IOP elevation and decrease in bleb size.[6,17]

The presence of a properly positioned posterior chamber intraocular lens (IOL) implant does not affect IOP. Although closed-loop, anterior chamber IOLs occasionally produce significant IOP elevation, the current semiflexible, one-piece, open-loop style lenses are associated with fewer problems.[18]

An early postoperative rise in IOP may be minimized with topical beta-blockers,[19] topical apraclonidine,[20] systemic carbonic anhydrase inhibitors,[21] topical prostaglandin analogues,[22] and intracameral carbachol.[21] In addition, judicious use and removal of viscoelastic substances are recommended (see Viscoelastic

TABLE 43-1
Glaucoma After Cataract Surgery

Open-angle Glaucomas	
• Primary open-angle glaucoma	• Dislocated nuclear fragments
• Blood-induced glaucomas	• Corticosteroids
Hyphema	• Viscoelastics
Ghost cell glaucoma	• Nd:YAG laser capsulotomy
• Uveitis	• Vitreous in anterior chamber
• UGH syndrome	• Cyclodialysis cleft closure
• Lens particle	• Alpha-chymotrypsin
Closed-Angle Glaucomas	
• Preexisting angle-closure glaucoma	
• Pupillary block	
• Malignant glaucoma	
• Neovascular glaucoma	
• Epithelial/fibrovascular ingrowth	

UGH, Uveitis-glaucoma-hyphema.

Agents). Nonsteroidal antiinflammatory drugs are ineffective in preventing or decreasing the magnitude of the pressure elevation.[23]

Persistent postoperative IOP elevation resulting from primary open-angle glaucoma mandates standard treatment protocols. Earlier and more aggressive management is indicated in patients with significant preexisting glaucomatous optic nerve damage.

Blood-Induced Glaucomas

HYPHEMA

Blood in the anterior chamber during the early postoperative period typically originates from the scleral cataract incision, an iridectomy, or pupillary sphincter tears.

Patients with postoperative hyphemas may be asymptomatic or have decreased vision. Circulating or layered red blood cells, or both, are seen in the anterior chamber with an open angle. An endocapsular location is an unusual type of postoperative hemorrhage.[24] Pupillary block is uncommon but may develop if bleeding extends into the posterior chamber, occludes an iridectomy, or both. If the anterior hyaloid face is not intact, blood may be seen in the vitreous cavity.

Open-angle glaucoma occurs from trabecular meshwork obstruction by red blood cells, platelets, fibrin, and hemosiderin-filled macrophages. Secondary angle-closure glaucoma results from peripheral anterior synechiae that may develop in the setting of persistent large hyphemas and inflammation.

Any amount of intraocular bleeding may elevate IOP, but larger hyphemas usually cause higher IOPs.[25] Postoperative hyphemas and glaucoma resulting from them are generally self-limited and resolve without complications. Management depends on the degree of IOP elevation, the status of the optic nerve, and the presence or absence of sickle cell anemia. A healthy optic nerve can withstand a moderate IOP rise without damage and does not require antiglaucoma therapy. Medical treatment is favored if the IOP is acutely elevated to greater than 40 mm Hg or persistently elevated to greater than 30 mm Hg for 2 weeks.[25] In the presence of preexisting glaucomatous optic nerve damage or sickle cell disease, earlier and more aggressive management is required.[25] Aqueous suppressants, especially topical beta-blockers and topical or oral carbonic anhydrase inhibitors (avoided in sickle cell patients) are the preferred medical approach. Hyperosmotic agents may be helpful (e.g., oral isosorbide, 2 ml/kg, or intravenous mannitol, 20% solution, 2 ml/kg over 30 minutes). It is best to avoid using miotics and prostaglandin analogues, which may exacerbate intraocular inflammation, as well as adrenergic agents, which cause vasoconstriction. Additional therapeutic measures include frequent administration of topical corticosteroids (every 1 to 2 hours) to decrease inflammation; elevating the head of the bed to minimize posterior blood layering; and, if medically possible, avoiding aspirin, aspirin-containing products, sodium warfarin (Coumadin), and nonsteroidal antiinflammatory agents. Cycloplegics, systemic steroids, and aminocaproic acid are not commonly used for postsurgical hyphemas.

Despite medical therapy, surgical intervention may be required in the situations of uncontrolled IOP, corneal blood staining, or a clot of prolonged duration.[25] Traditional IOP criteria for surgical intervention to avoid optic nerve damage in hyphemas are an IOP greater than 50 mm Hg for 5 days or greater than 35 mm Hg for 7 days. Preexisting optic nerve damage or sickle cell disease warrants earlier interventions,[24,26] an IOP lower than 25 mm Hg is desirable in these circumstances. Any sign of corneal blood staining warrants surgical intervention.[25] Patients with compromised endothelial cell function may require earlier intervention. Large clots that persist longer than 10 days or total hyphemas lasting more than 5 days are often evacuated to avoid peripheral anterior synechiae and corneal blood staining.

Surgical techniques for hyphema evacuation include anterior chamber washout with or without coaxial irrigation-aspiration, automated cutting-aspiration of clot material, or clot expression (Figure 43-1). Simple removal of circulating red blood cells and debris often suffices for IOP control, but visual rehabilitation is hastened by clot removal. If vitreous is admixed with blood in the anterior chamber, automated cutting-aspiration equipment is required for surgical removal.

LATE HYPHEMAS (SWAN SYNDROME)

Anterior segment hemorrhage months to years after cataract surgery may arise from neovascularization at the surgical incision site,[27-32] vascular iris tufts in contact with anterior chamber IOL haptics in the ciliary sulcus, or blood vessels in contact with posterior chamber IOL haptics in the ciliary sulcus (see also Uveitis-Glaucoma-Hyphema Syndrome and Neovascular Glaucoma). Patients typically have painless, transient blurring of vision. Visual acuity and IOP depend on the amount of bleeding and trabecular meshwork function. Diagnosis of anterior chamber bleeding sites is made by gonioscopic identification of neovascularization at the previous wound site or in areas of peripheral anterior synechia formation. It is uncommon to see bleeding directly from these vessels, but red blood cell "dusting" on the corneal endothelium may be present.

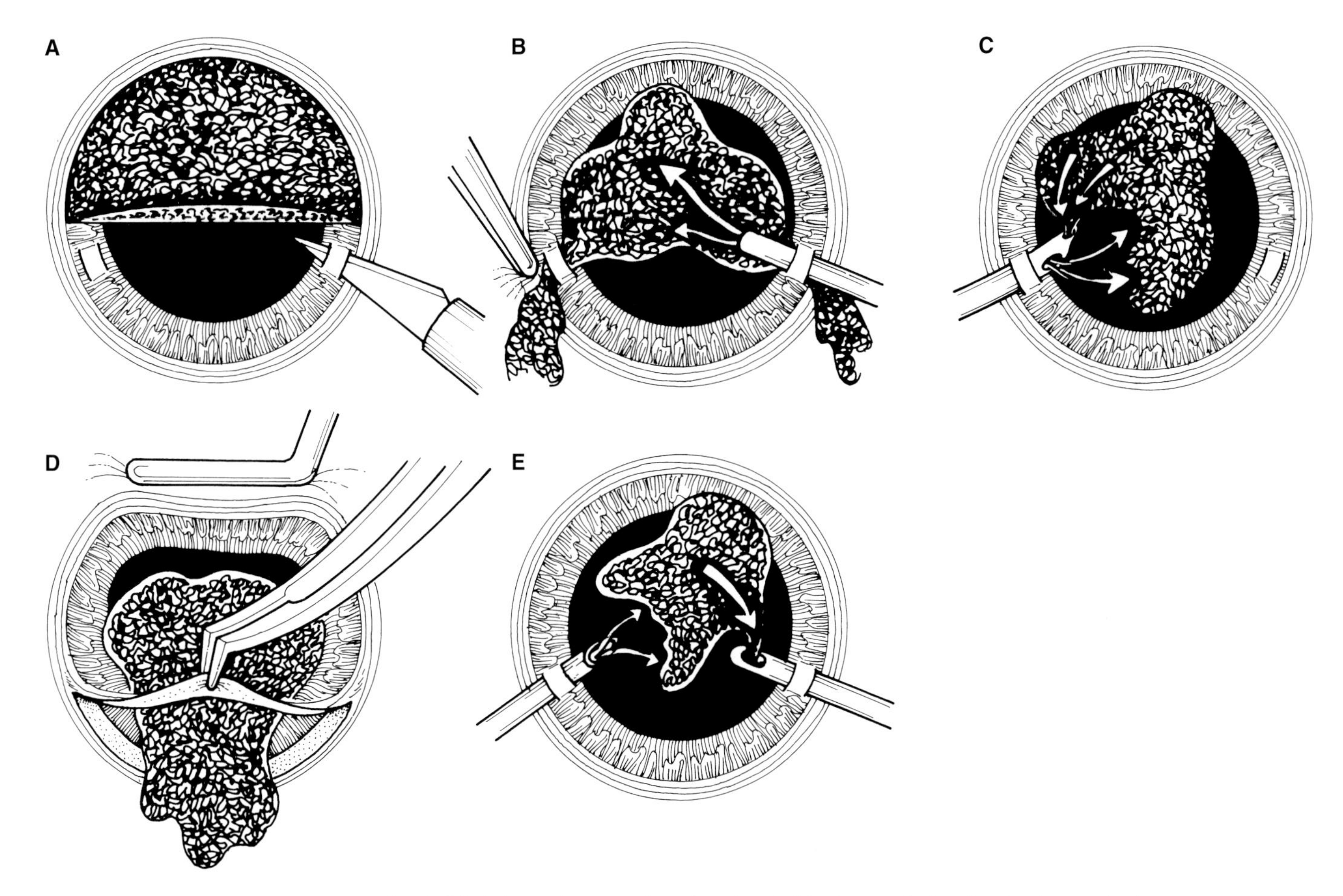

FIGURE 43-1 Surgical techniques for evacuation of postsurgical hyphemas. **A,** Anterior chamber washout. **B,** Irrigation and aspiration of blood. **C,** Coaxial automated cutting and aspiration of clot. **D,** Clot expression. **E,** Bimanual irrigation and automated cutting.

Treatment is often limited to topical medications as needed to control inflammation and IOP. Many eyes have only a single, isolated incident. Recurrent hemorrhages are best managed by laser goniophotocoagulation to the offending vessel when visible, although success with limbal cryopexy has also been reported.[28,33] Long-term acuity deficits or intractable glaucoma are uncommon.[28]

Recurrent bleeding that is related to the haptic placement of an anterior chamber lens typically requires an IOL exchange. Posterior chamber lenses without haptic notches or bulbs can often be rotated 90 degrees to position the haptics away from vessels. Haptic cutting and IOL exchange may also be required.

GHOST CELL GLAUCOMA

Erythrocytes begin degenerating within a few days after a vitreous hemorrhage.[34] After 1 to 3 weeks, they are tan and khaki colored, less pliable, spherical, devoid of intracellular hemoglobin, and freely mobile.[34] These cells are called "ghost cells." After cataract surgery, an intact anterior hyaloid face largely prevents movement of cells into the anterior chamber, but any disruption allows easy access (Figure 43-2). Secondary open-angle glaucoma is produced from obstruction of the trabecular meshwork by the ghost cells. IOP may be normal or may rise rapidly to high levels if large numbers of cells are present.[34] Elevated pressure can persist for several months. A fine dusting of ghost cells may be seen on the corneal endothelium, and a layering of cells in the anterior chamber has the appearance of a tan hypopyon (Figure 43-3). The angle is normal or shows a slight khaki discoloration to the trabecular meshwork.

Standard medications are often ineffective in lowering IOP until the number of ghost cells in the anterior chamber has decreased. If the IOP remains persistently elevated despite maximally tolerated medical therapy, an anterior chamber washout should be considered. Recurrent IOP elevation is common even with repeated anterior chamber washouts, and a vitrectomy to remove the reservoir of posterior segment ghost cells may be required.[35]

Uveitis

Glaucoma rarely results from the mild postoperative inflammation that is routinely seen after cataract surgery. More commonly, glaucoma occurs in eyes with preexisting uveitis or in eyes with a more severe inflammatory response. Uveitic glaucoma can be open angle, closed angle, or a combination of both. Open-angle glaucoma results from inflammation-related alterations in the trabecular meshwork. Changes include swelling of the trabecular matrix, endothelial cell dysfunction, or

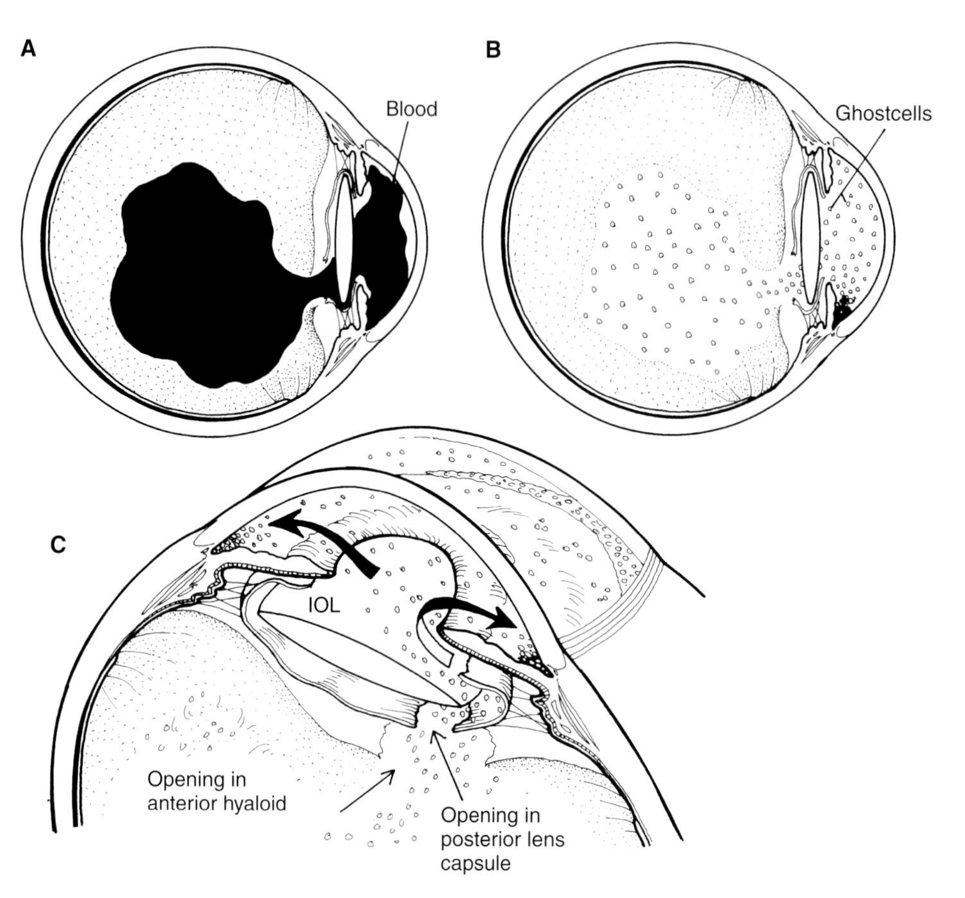

FIGURE 43-2 Mechanism of ghost cell glaucoma. **A,** Clotted blood in the anterior and posterior chamber. **B,** Erythrocytes degrade to ghost cells. **C,** Rigid khaki-colored ghost cells enter the anterior chamber from the reservoir in vitreous humor through disrupted posterior capsule and anterior hyaloid face. Obstruction of the trabecular meshwork leads to glaucoma.

accumulation of inflammatory cells and debris.[36] Corticosteroid treatment and endogenous prostaglandins may also contribute.[37] Angle-closure glaucoma can occur from peripheral anterior synechiae, posterior synechiae, or rubeosis iridis.

Cataract surgery in patients with heterochromic iridocyclitis may be associated with secondary open-angle glaucoma.[38] In these eyes, gonioscopy typically discloses an open angle with fine, iris blood vessels that differ from the coarse, arborizing vessels associated with neovascular angle closure.[39] On entering the anterior chamber, bleeding may occur from these vessels. A secondary open-angle glaucoma has also been reported in conjunction with episcleritis in a patient with a transscleral-fixated posterior chamber implant.[40]

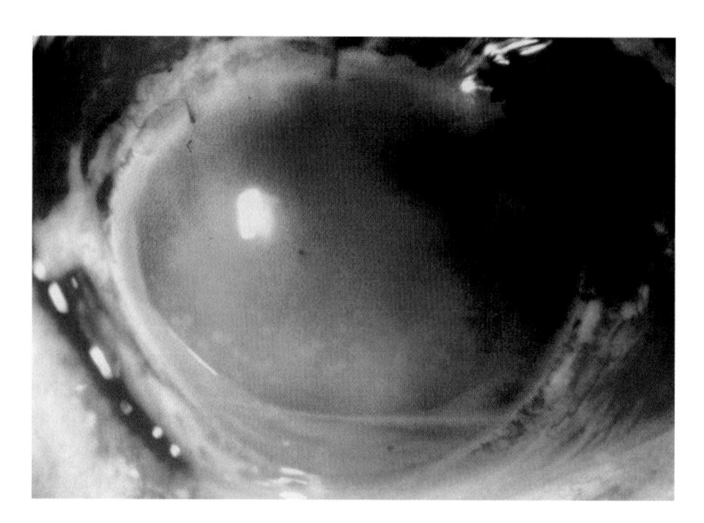

FIGURE 43-3 Tan "hypopyon" characteristic of ghost cell glaucoma.

Clinical symptoms of uveitis include pain, photophobia, and decreased vision. Findings on examination may include miosis, perilimbal injection, keratic precipitates, cells and flare in the anterior chamber, and, occasionally, fibrin.

Postoperative uveitic glaucoma is managed medically by controlling inflammation with frequent corticosteroid use. Cycloplegic and sympathomimetic agents are given to prevent or break posterior synechiae. For severe intraocular inflammation, periocular or systemic antiinflammatory medication may be needed. Elevated IOP is treated with topical beta-blockers, topical or systemic carbonic anhydrase inhibitors, and hyperosmotic agents. Miotic agents and prostaglandin analogues are avoided. Iridectomies should be created to relieve pupillary block when indicated. Laser trabeculoplasty is largely ineffective. If medical therapy fails, filtration surgery with adjunctive antifibrotic treatment or seton placement is indicated.

Rarely, noninflammatory pigment cells circulating in the anterior chamber after posterior chamber IOL implant surgery may be associated with glaucoma.[41] This typically arises with sulcus-fixated IOLs and resultant haptic erosion of pigment from the ciliary body or posterior iris. Iris transillumination may be seen in the area of iris-haptic contact. On gonioscopy, the trabecular meshwork demonstrates dense pigmentation similar to pigment dispersion syndrome. Standard antiglaucoma therapy is instituted, but rarely IOL rotation, removal, or exchange is required.

Uveitis-Glaucoma-Hyphema Syndrome

Uveitis combined with glaucoma and hyphema results from an IOL implant rubbing against the iris. It was a more frequent problem with early versions of iris-fixated and anterior chamber IOLs[18,42-47] but is also reported with posterior chamber implants.[41,48-50] Causes include imperfections in implant construction, improperly sized lenses, or imperfectly positioned lenses. Initially, patients are treated conservatively with ocular antiinflammatory and antiglaucoma medications. Patients with persistent glaucoma, recurrent hemorrhage, or endothelial decompensation require removal of the implant. If the trabecular meshwork has not been irreversibly damaged, the glaucoma will subside.[42,44,47]

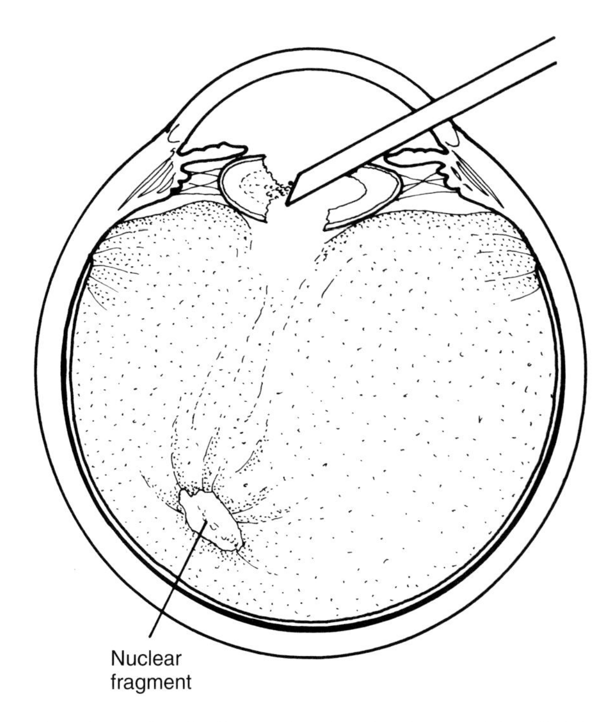

FIGURE 43-4 Dislocated nucleus fragment in vitreous humor.

Lens Particle Glaucoma

Residual cortical material after cataract extraction can cause significant IOP elevation by either open- or closed-angle mechanism.[51] This glaucoma typically occurs early in the postoperative period, although it can occur years later if a Soemmerring's ring cataract suddenly opens. Nd:YAG laser rupture of an epithelial pearl may be the precipitating factor. The patient presents with a red, painful eye. Keratic precipitates, anterior chamber inflammation, and retained lens material are seen.

Lens material causes severe obstruction of trabecular outflow channels,[52] but unlike phacolytic glaucoma, heavy molecular weight proteins are lacking. Obstruction to outflow may also result from macrophages filled with lens material, inflammatory cells, or persistent inflammation. Treatment with topical corticosteroids and antiglaucoma medications, excluding miotic and prostaglandin agents, is usually sufficient until IOP normalizes. Severe inflammation or persistent pressure elevation, or both, may require surgical removal of the residual lens material.

Dislocated Nuclear Fragments

With the rise in popularity of phacoemulsification as the preferred method for cataract surgery, the incidence of inadvertent posterior capsule tear and loss of nuclear fragments into the vitreous cavity has increased (Figure 43-4).[53-58] Lens dislocation into the vitreous most often occurs during lens emulsification or cortical cleanup.[54,58-61] It tends to be inversely correlated with the experience of the surgeon performing the phacoemulsification. Other risk factors include inadequate zonular support (pseudoexfoliation, trauma, previous vitrectomy), very hard nuclei, deep-set eyes, poorly dilated pupils, or patient movement during surgery.[54,58,59,62-64]

Lens fragments in the vitreous are a serious problem. Lens particles left in the eye during cataract surgery seem to induce an inflammatory reaction that is somewhat proportional to the size of the displaced fragment.[55] Patients may develop significant visual loss, chronic uveitis, secondary glaucoma, corneal edema, and retinal detachment.[55,65-69] One study reported a 52% incidence of glaucoma in eyes with retained lens fragments.[55]

Small pieces of lens cortex or a small chip of nucleus without significant corneal edema or glaucoma may only require medical management with topical corticosteroids.[70] However, larger lens fragments are best managed by consultation with a vitreoretinal surgeon. Removal of large lens fragments by an anterior segment approach is not recommended. Aggressive attempts at lens fragment removal with lens loops, forceps, anterior vitrectomy, or phacoemulsification handpiece should not be done. These maneuvers typically result in vitreoretinal traction and carry a higher risk of retinal tears, retinal detachment, and potential corneal edema or decompensation. The best approach by the cataract surgeon is to perform a thorough cleanup of the vitreous and cortex using appropriate automated vitrectomy cutting instrumentation. An IOL, either anterior or posterior depending on the available capsular support, may be placed. The presence of an IOL does not interfere with the vitrectomy or removal of lens fragments.[55,67,68] The cataract incision should then be tightly closed with sutures. The patient should be referred in a timely fashion to a vitreoretinal surgeon for a three-port pars plana vitectomy-fragmentectomy.[55,69]

Studies on the timing of vitrectomy for removal of retained lens fragments allow some general conclusions to be drawn. Vitrectomy need not be performed the same day. A reasonable time frame for vitrectomy is within 1 to 2 weeks. Visual acuity is generally improved with vitrectomy within this time frame.[55,58,65-73] A tendency toward a less likely chance of elevated eye pressure may occur in eyes undergoing early vitrectomy.[63,69,71,73] However, a delay in vitrectomy allows time for corneal edema to clear, elevated eye pressure to be treated, and the patient to be prepared for further surgery.[74,75] Although retinal detachment is the major source of poor visual outcome, excellent visual results are typically achieved. Elevated eye pressure is managed with standard antiglaucoma medications. Several studies have shown that removal of lens fragments has a beneficial effect on the secondary glaucoma.[67-69,73,76]

See Chapter 39, Intraoperative Complications of Phacoemulsification Surgery, for further discussion of displaced lens fragments after cataract surgery.

Corticosteroids

Postoperative administration of topical, periocular, or systemic corticosteroids may produce secondary open-angle glaucoma.[77-85] Topical corticosteroids, a mainstay of postoperative cataract care, are most commonly implicated. Although a less frequent cause of IOP elevation, administration of periocular repository corticosteroids can result in a significant IOP rise that is often delayed.[77,82-85] These depot preparations are used in the treatment of cystoid macular edema or uveitis to increase intraocular drug concentrations and reduce the need for frequent instillation of drops.[77,82-85]

Corticosteroid-induced glaucoma is related to the drug preparation, potency, frequency of administration, and duration of application. With depot preparations, drug release is primarily regulated by the biochemical composition of the corticosteroid. Highly water-soluble compounds diffuse rapidly and are short acting, whereas water-insoluble preparations persist longer.

Individuals with primary open-angle glaucoma,[86] their first-degree relatives,[87] diabetics,[88] and patients with high myopia[89] seem to be at higher risk for steroid-related IOP elevation. In patients without these predisposing factors, the clinician cannot predict which patients will have a pressure rise. Patients of any age may be affected. IOP elevation can occur in the presence of a functioning filter or seton device.[90,91]

Corticosteroids raise IOP by reducing aqueous outflow[92] through effects on glycosaminoglycan metabolism.[93] The release of enzymes that depolymerize glycosaminoglycans is inhibited, and glycosaminoglycans accumulate within the trabecular meshwork.

Diagnosis requires a high index of suspicion and careful questioning. The predominant clinical finding is IOP elevation. The onset of IOP elevation is variable and can be significantly delayed. It may rise within the first week after the start of corticosteroid treatment or not until months or years later. Patients are usually asymptomatic. Eyes generally are not inflamed despite an increased IOP. Depending on the degree and duration of IOP elevation, optic nerve head cupping and visual field loss may or may not be present.

The first step in the management of corticosteroid glaucoma is to stop topical steroid therapy. Clinically significant IOP elevation is treated with the standard antiglaucoma medications. Careful follow-up and monitoring are required. In most cases, IOP returns to normal within days to weeks, although persistent elevation can occur. If corticosteroid medications must be continued, decreasing the strength and frequency or changing the type of corticosteroid and mode of administration may be useful.[94] If periocular corticosteroids have been given, excision of residual steroid material should be considered if IOP cannot be controlled medically.[81,82,84,85] Biochemical analysis of excised depots has shown that significant amounts of periocular corticosteroids can remain for long periods. Laser trabeculoplasty is generally not helpful. If IOP is medically uncontrolled or progressive optic nerve damage occurs, patients require filtering surgery.

Viscoelastic Agents

Viscoelastic agents were introduced into ophthalmic surgery in 1972[95] and have greatly expanded the options available to ophthalmic surgeons by protecting tissue surfaces from mechanical damage, maintaining anterior chamber depth, and assisting in hemostasis. Since then, many materials with varying physical and biochemical properties have become commercially available. Some of these agents include Healon (1% sodium hyaluronate), Healon GV (1.4% sodium hyaluronate), Healon 5 (2.3% sodium hyaluronate), Viscoat (3% sodium hyaluronate/4% chondroitin sulfate), and OcuCoat (2% hydroxypropylmethylcellulose). Orcolon, a polyacrylamide polymer, was removed from the market because of severe uveitis and secondary glaucoma[96] resulting from contamination with microspheres that obstructed outflow.

The most common complication from use of viscoelastic in cataract surgery is a significant and potentially dangerous IOP elevation in the early postoperative period.[97-101] The IOP rise peaks between 4 and 7 hours postoperatively and returns to normal within 24 to 72 hours.[102-105] Ocular pain and blurred vision are common presenting symptoms. Corneal edema and stagnation of circulating cells in the anterior chamber may be seen on the slit lamp examination. The angle is open.

Viscoelastic substances leave the eye through the trabecular meshwork as relatively unchanged large molecules. Even in the presence of intraocular inflammation, little degradation of the viscoelastic substance occurs.[106] Studies demonstrate that these molecules elevate IOP by impairing aqueous humor outflow.[106] Eyes with Eyes with insufficient trabecular meshwork function before surgery are more likely to have a significant elevation of IOP.[107]

IOP changes after viscoelastic use in cataract surgery have been studied by numerous clinicians. Lane et al.[108] compared early postoperative IOP after use of Healon, Viscoat, and OcuCoat. All three agents produced significant IOP elevation at 4 hours postoperatively. Holzer et al.[105] found a moderate increase in IOP postoperatively for Healon 5, Viscoat, OcuCoat, and Healon GV. The highest mean IOP was at 4 hours, with the highest to lowest IOP by agent being Healon 5, Viscoat, OcuCoat, and Healon GV. At 24 hours postoperatively, all groups had a mean IOP less than 20 mm Hg.

To reduce the incidence of postoperative IOP elevation, ophthalmic surgeons evacuate the viscoelastic agent at the completion of the procedure. However, removal of the viscoelastic only lessens, not eliminates, the incidence of IOP elevation.[99,100,102] Rates of removal vary from agent to agent. Highly viscous agents, such as Healon, Healon GV, and Healon 5, can cause significant IOP increases but require significantly less time to remove from the eye. Conflicting reports exist on the effectiveness of prophylactic treatment with topical beta-adrenergic agents and systemic carbonic anhydrase inhibitors.[109,110]

In the early postoperative period after cataract surgery, IOP should be monitored closely. A clinically significant IOP rise should be treated with either simple release of aqueous via the paracentesis site[111] or antiglaucoma medications. If IOP elevation persists, surgical evacuation of the viscoelastic agent or filtration/seton surgery may be necessary to prevent visual loss.

See Chapter 5 for a detailed discussion of viscoelastic agents.

Capsular Block Syndrome (or Capsular Bag Distension Syndrome)

Capsular block syndrome occurs in patients who have had cataract removal with implantation of a posterior chamber IOL in the capsular bag after an anterior continuous curvilinear capsulorhexis.[112-116] Most cases occur immediately postoperatively, but capsular block has been observed as long as 5 years after surgery.[115]

Clinical features of this syndrome include an unexpected myopic overrefraction, anterior displacement of the optic and iris diaphragm, shallowing of the anterior chamber, increased space between the optic and posterior capsule, adherence of the anterior capsule to the IOL, and occasionally a persistent uveitis. Early postoperatively, the IOP may be normal or elevated. If untreated, eyes with capsular block syndrome develop glaucoma, posterior synechiae, and/or posterior capsule opacification with debris within the capsular bag.

To develop this problem, the anterior capsulorhexis must be smaller than the IOL optic and a viscoelastic used. The condition results from a blockage of the contents within the capsular bag. Lens particulates and viscoelastic material are prevented from passing between the IOL optic and the anterior capsule. It is not exactly clear what mechanism draws fluid into the capsular bag and results in its distension.

Postoperatively, capsular block is relieved by performing an anterior capsulotomy peripheral to the edge of the IOL, if observable, or a posterior capsulotomy if the pupil cannot be dilated past the edge of the IOL.[116] Although uncommon, persistent IOP elevation is treated with standard antiglaucoma medications.

Neodymium:Yttrium-Aluminum-Garnet (Nd:YAG) Laser Capsulotomy

Short-term increases in IOP after an Nd:YAG capsulotomy are well documented[117-120] and can result in significant and vision-threatening IOP elevation in both aphakic and pseudophakic patients.[121,122] IOP elevation commonly occurs in the first 2 hours after the procedure but may occur later. The rise is typically transient but may persist.[123] The new onset of glaucoma or the worsening of preexisting glaucoma can occur.[124] Patients with preexisting glaucoma appear to be more susceptible to a rise in IOP[125] and should be monitored with extra caution and over the long term after the procedure.[126]

Intermediate and long-term changes in IOP following Nd:YAG capsulotomy also occur.[126-129] Long-term IOP problems after Nd:YAG capsulotomy appear to be correlated with the IOP measurement 1 hour following the procedure. Therefore any patient who has a short-term rise in IOP should be checked regularly thereafter for the possibility of developing long-term IOP problems.[126]

The IOP elevation is caused by reduced facility of outflow from plugging of the trabecular meshwork with capsular particles, inflammatory cells, and protein, as well as from prostaglandin-mediated effects.[130] The number of laser pulses and total energy delivered do not appear to be contributing factors.[124]

Patients undergoing Nd:YAG capsulotomy require close medical observation to detect and treat postoperative pressure elevation. Although varying results have been reported, prophylactic use of timolol,[131] pilocarpine, topical dorzolamide,[132] acetazolamide,[133,134] and topical apraclonidine[135] has been shown to be highly effective in preventing acute pressure spikes following laser treatment. Persistent IOP elevation is managed with standard antiglaucoma medications.

See Chapter 44 for an extensive discussion of Nd:YAG laser capsulotomy.

Vitreous in the Anterior Chamber

Secondary open-angle glaucoma from vitreous in the anterior chamber is uncommon. It may occur (1) after intracapsular surgery with iatrogenic or spontaneous breakage of the anterior hyaloid face, (2) after extracapsular surgery with iatrogenic capsular rupture and incomplete vitrectomy, or (3) after posterior capsulotomy.[136,137]

Vitreous within the anterior chambers of enucleated eyes results in trabecular meshwork obstruction and secondarily a decrease in aqueous outflow[136] (Figure 43-5). In human eyes, uncertainty exists as to whether vitreous alone, inflammation, or a combination of factors actually causes glaucoma.

IOP elevation is seen a few weeks or months after surgery. Anterior segment inflammation is often minimal. Pressure elevation is treated with standard antiglaucoma therapy. Hyperosmotic and mydriatic agents may help by retracting vitreous from the angle. The effect of miotic agents is variable. Anterior vitrectomy may be successful for medically uncontrolled

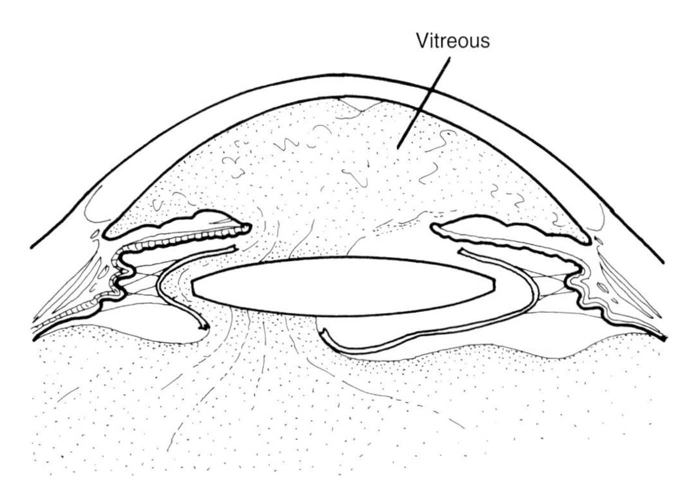

FIGURE 43-5 Vitreous humor filling the anterior chamber through the posterior capsule opening, leading to obstruction of trabecular meshwork.

glaucoma.[136] However, even total removal of vitreous from the anterior chamber and angle does not ensure resolution of the glaucoma.

Cyclodialysis Cleft Closure

A cyclodialysis cleft is a separation between the scleral spur and ciliary body that produces a direct communication between the anterior chamber and the suprachoroidal space. Cleft formation may occur as an inadvertent complication from cataract surgery. It is fortunately an uncommon problem.

Clefts vary in size, and small ones are especially difficult to see with gonioscopy. The size of the cleft is not related to the degree of hypotony.[138]

Postoperative ocular hypotony is the initial typical clinical presentation. Other clinical features include reduced visual acuity, anterior chamber shallowing, choroidal effusions, optic nerve edema, and macular edema.

Treatment is directed at partial or complete closure of the cyclodialysis cleft. Conservative medical management involves atropine 1% drops twice daily. Cycloplegia helps to promote contact between the sclera and choroid. Miotics and topical steroids are avoided. If medical therapy fails, cyclodialysis clefts can be closed with argon laser, cryotherapy, or placement of sutures.[138,139]

IOP may acutely rise to high levels from either spontaneous or therapeutic closure of the cleft.[140,141] The pressure rise is usually rapid and severe but generally transient. Management of IOP elevation includes topical beta-adrenergic blockers, topical alpha-2 agonists, topical or systemic carbonic anhydrase inhibitors, and hyperosmotic agents.

Alpha-Chymotrypsin (Enzyme) Glaucoma

Although rarely seen today, alpha-chymotrypsin glaucoma was very common following enzyme zonulolysis in intracapsular cataract extraction.[142] In 1964, Kirsch[143] first reported glaucoma from the use of alpha-chymotrypsin in human cataract extraction.

This condition results from acute obstruction of the trabecular meshwork outflow channels by zonular fragments. Scanning electron microscopy of animal eyes demonstrates particulate material blocking the trabecular meshwork near Schlemm's canal and within the uveal meshwork; saline-perfused control eyes show no material.[144] Particles vary in size and shape. Transmission electron microscopy identifies them as zonular fragments and not alpha-chymotrypsin or its by-products. Zonular fragments have also been documented in human eyes.[145] Tonography studies document an impaired facility to outflow. Pilocarpine lowers pressure and improves outflow except during peak pressure rise.[142]

The onset of the IOP rise occurs during the first several days after cataract surgery and may last days to weeks.[47] Clinical findings include mild to severe elevation in IOP, corneal edema, normal anterior chamber depth, and an open angle. IOP elevation is dose dependent. Patients with preexisting glaucoma have a slightly greater or no greater incidence of this glaucoma. Tonography shows no long-term alteration in trabecular meshwork outflow between 2 and 6 months postoperatively in patients who had previously demonstrated a postoperative pressure increase.[146]

The pressure rise may be prevented or minimized by using a 1:10,000 enzyme dilution instead of 1:5000, limiting the volume used, and irrigating the anterior chamber. Prophylactic use of timolol and acetazolamide may also be of benefit.[33,147] Any postoperative pressure rise should be managed conservatively with antiglaucoma medications until spontaneous resolution occurs, which is usually within 1 week.

Closed-Angle Glaucomas

Preexisting Angle Closure

A previous history of angle-closure glaucoma increases the risk of glaucoma following cataract surgery, especially if significant angle closure is present preoperatively. However, the degree of preoperative synechial closure is not proportional to the potential severity of postoperative glaucoma. Intense postoperative inflammation and/or prolonged flattening of the anterior chamber can result in permanent peripheral anterior synechiae. A shallow or flat anterior chamber following cataract extraction is commonly associated with a wound leak, choroidal detachment, or both. Medical therapy is initiated, but early surgical intervention may be required to prevent, reduce, or avoid synechial closure, as well as other complications.

Pupillary Block

Pupillary block represents blockage of aqueous humor flow from the posterior chamber to the anterior chamber. It develops when the pupillary space and iridectomies are occluded with vitreous,[148-152] gas,[153] blood,[25] inflammatory materials,[37] capsule,[154] lens cortical material, IOL,[155] or silicone oil.[156] This entity is the most common cause of angle-closure glaucoma following cataract surgery with or without IOL implantation and may complicate both intracapsular[157] and extracapsular cataract extraction.[155,158-160] Anterior chamber, iris plane, and posterior chamber IOL implants have been reported with pupillary block. In addition, pupillary block may occur in the presence of peripheral and sector iridectomies.[155,158-161]

Aphakic pupillary block glaucoma presents days to weeks following surgery with a shallow or flat anterior chamber, elevated IOP, and occlusion of the pupillary space, iridectomies, or both. Pseudophakic block with an anterior chamber implant presents the same way except that (1) the central anterior chamber is deep (the optic holds the iris under it posteriorly), and the peripheral chamber is shallow or flat with an iris bombé configuration (Figure 43-6); or (2) the chamber is uniformly shallow. Although dependent on the stage of glaucoma development, gonioscopy usually shows the filtration angle to be closed.

Medical and laser therapies are used to break pupillary block, deepen the anterior chamber, and prevent chronic angle-closure glaucoma. Iris dilation with cycloplegic-mydriatic agents often eliminates pupillary block. Pupillary block from air can be treated with patient positioning and mydriasis. Elevated IOP is treated with topical beta-adrenergic blockers, topical or systemic carbonic anhydrase inhibitors, and hyperosmotic agents, as needed. Prostaglandin analogues are typically not recommended

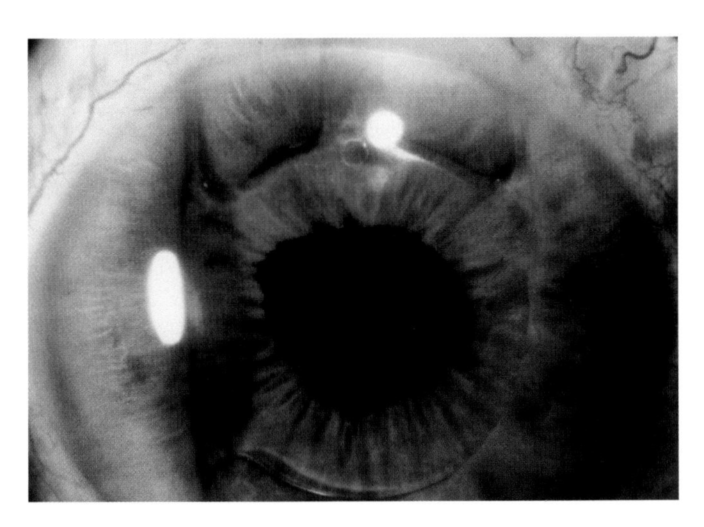

FIGURE 43-6 Iris bombé with pupillary block.

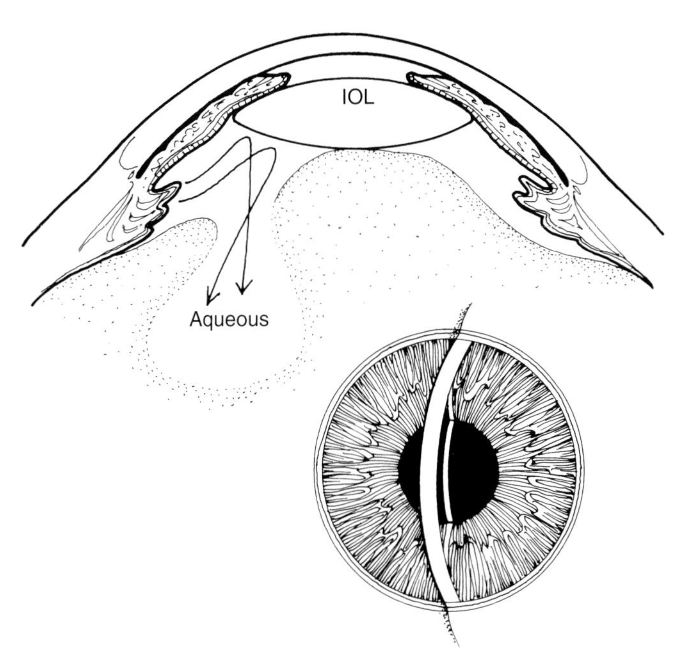

FIGURE 43-7 Malignant glaucoma with posterior aqueous diversion and shallowing of anterior chamber.

for angle closure glaucoma. A laser iridectomy is recommended in conjunction with medical therapy to prevent recurrence. The laser iridectomy is often easier to create before pupillary dilation. Gonioscopy should be performed soon after elimination of pupillary block to assess for residual angle closure. If peripheral anterior synechiae persist, argon laser gonioplasty may be helpful to reduce synechiae and should be performed promptly to maximize success.[162] Surgical goniosynechialysis,[163] filtration surgery, or seton placement may be required for cases of extensive synechiae and high IOP (Table 43-2). The role of routine surgical iridectomy with posterior chamber implants is controversial. Because the risk of pupillary block is low, the general tendency with phacoemulsification and self-sealing incisions (corneal or scleral) is to not perform an iridectomy.[159,164,165]

Reverse pupillary block or "sticky pupil" syndrome may be noted intraoperatively. This blockage of communication between the anterior chamber and the posterior chamber is due to a seal of viscoelastic agent between the iris and the IOL. Chamber deepening results in an exaggerated concave configuration. Blockage is relieved by removal of the viscoelastic agent.

Malignant Glaucoma (Posterior Aqueous Diversion)

The term *malignant glaucoma* conveys the message of a serious form of glaucoma that responds poorly to conventional glaucoma therapy and may result in serious vision loss. The terms *ciliary block glaucoma* and *posterior aqueous diversion* are also used to describe this condition. Both of these terms better describe the pathophysiology, which is blockage of anterior movement of aqueous humor near the junction of the ciliary processes, lens equator, and anterior vitreous face. Aqueous humor is then diverted posteriorly into and behind the vitreous cavity with resultant forward movement of the vitreous and shallowing of the anterior chamber (Figure 43-7). Impermeability of the anterior hyaloid membrane and vitreous body to the anterior flow of aqueous humor has been found as perfusion pressure is elevated.[166] Impermeability may be increased by hyaloid to ciliary body apposition. The sequence of events in malignant glaucoma is thought to be initiated by increased pressure behind a posteriorly detached vitreous, compaction of the vitreous, and further decreased fluid movement through it.

Malignant glaucoma may occur following cataract surgery with or without associated trabeculectomy.[167,168] Phakic eyes with a history of angle-closure glaucoma and a degree of closed angle at the time of surgery are at highest risk.[169] Onset may occur intraoperatively or months after surgery.

Clinical characteristics and response to medical therapy, surgery, or both, distinguish malignant glaucoma from choroidal detachment, pupillary block, and suprachoroidal hemorrhage (Table 43-3; see Figure 43-7). In malignant glaucoma, both the central and peripheral anterior chambers are shallow or flat. IOP may be normal or elevated. Choroidal detachment is not seen. Unlike pupillary block glaucoma, clinical findings persist despite having a patent iridectomy. If patency of the iridectomy is questioned, an additional iridectomy should be made to definitively rule out pupillary block. Serous and hemorrhagic choroidal detachments have a characteristic fundus appearance, and a choroidal tap confirms the presence of fluid or blood in the suprachoroidal space.

Medical therapy for malignant glaucoma includes mydriatic-cycloplegic agents (1% atropine, 0.25% scopolamine, 10%

TABLE 43-2
Treatment Sequence for Pupillary Block

- Laser indectomy
- Pupillary dilation
- Reduce IOP medically
- Argon laser gonioplasty—residual synechiae
- Surgical goniosynechialysis—synechiae with ↑ IOP
- Filtration/seton surgery

TABLE 43-3
Distinguishing Characteristics of Shallow or Flat Anterior Chamber

	Malignant Glaucoma	Serous Choroidal Detachment	Pupillary Block	Suprachoroidal Hemorrhage	Wound Leak
Onset	Intraoperatively or any time thereafter	Within first postoperative week	Early or late postoperatively	Intraoperatively or within the first week	Within the first postoperative week
Anterior chamber	Shallow or flat	Shallow or flat	Shallow or flat	Shallow or flat	Shallow or flat
Intraocular pressure	Normal or elevated	Low	Normal or elevated	Normal or elevated	Low
Fundus	No choroidal detachment	Smooth, light brown choroidal elevations	Normal	Dark brown or red choroidal elevation	Choroidal detachment may or may not be present
Patient iridectomy present	Yes	Yes	No	Yes	Yes
Relief by indectomy	No	No	Yes	No	No
Relief by suprachoroidal fluid drainage and anterior chamber reformation	No	Yes	No	Yes	No

phenylephrine[170]), topical or systemic carbonic anhydrase inhibitors, hyperosmotic agents, and topical beta-blockers.[171] Mydriatic-cycloplegic agents presumably act by tightening the lens-iris diaphragm and pulling the lens back against the vitreous, thus stopping the cycle of posterior fluid migration. Miotic or prostaglandin therapy is ineffective and may precipitate or aggravate malignant glaucoma. Medical therapy is continued until the IOP is satisfactorily reduced and the anterior chamber deepens. If treatment is successful, all medications except cycloplegic agents are gradually discontinued. Indefinite continuation of cycloplegia is essential to prevent relapse. If medical treatment is unsuccessful after a few days, further therapy with laser or surgery is indicated. In cases of aphakia or pseudophakia, the Nd:YAG laser may be used to disrupt the anterior hyaloid face.[162,168,172] Surgical intervention involves pars plana aspiration of liquid vitreous and restoration of the anterior chamber depth with or without goniosynechialysis.[173,174] (See also Chapter 45.)

Neovascular Glaucoma

Neovascular glaucoma is a secondary angle-closure glaucoma that results from the growth of new blood vessels on the anterior surface of the iris and across the anterior chamber angle. These vessels grow rapidly and may lead to complete synechial closure of the angle. Iris neovascularization results from retinal hypoxia, typically seen in diabetes mellitus, central retinal vein occlusion, and carotid occlusive disease.[175] Hypoxia leads to the production of a soluble angiogenic factor that causes the proliferation of new blood vessels.[176] The presence of an intact posterior capsule or anterior hyaloid appears to prevent anterior movement of this factor.[177-179] Disruption of the capsule is associated with an increased incidence of rubeosis. The preoperative presence of proliferative diabetic retinopathy also carries a significantly greater risk of the development of neovascular glaucoma following cataract surgery.[177,180]

Several stages exist in the development of rubeosis and neovascular glaucoma. Neovascularization typically begins at the pupillary margin and progresses toward the root of the iris. Interestingly, new vessels may first form around peripheral iridectomies.[181] Patients may have few early symptoms. With advanced disease, the eye becomes very painful with poor vision, conjunctival injection, corneal edema, and very high IOPs. Gonioscopy in early cases shows a normal and open angle, but as the condition progresses, abnormal vessels and areas of synechial closure are seen across the angle. Blood vessels that cross the scleral spur and arborize onto the trabecular meshwork are definitely abnormal.[175] Rubeotic glaucoma can progress to total angle closure within days. Distinguishing between an open and closed angle is important because an open angle signifies an opportunity for achieving vessel regression with panretinal photocoagulation. Panretinal photocoagulation should be performed in rubeotic eyes with retinal ischemic disorders.[181]

Elevated IOP is treated with topical and systemic aqueous suppressants. Because of the presence of inflammation, miotic and prostaglandin agents are avoided. Cycloplegics and topical corticosteroids are used to reduce inflammation. In the early stages of disease, panretinal photocoagulation is performed with the hope of causing vessel regression and preservation of an open angle. It may be possible to avoid glaucoma surgery. Laser goniophotocoagulation appears to be of little value. If pressure is significantly elevated despite medical treatment and vision is endangered, urgent filtering surgery with antimetabolite supplementation is required. If this surgery is unsuccessful, seton devices or cyclodestructive procedures have shown some success. The rate of phthisis following cyclodestructive procedures may approximate 10%. Eyes with neovascular glaucoma and no vision are not candidates for surgical therapy. Comfort is best achieved with chronic use of cycloplegic agents and topical steroids.

Epithelial and Fibrovascular Ingrowth

Epithelial and fibrovascular ingrowth result from either epithelial or connective tissue growth into the anterior chamber and across the trabecular meshwork. Both conditions were

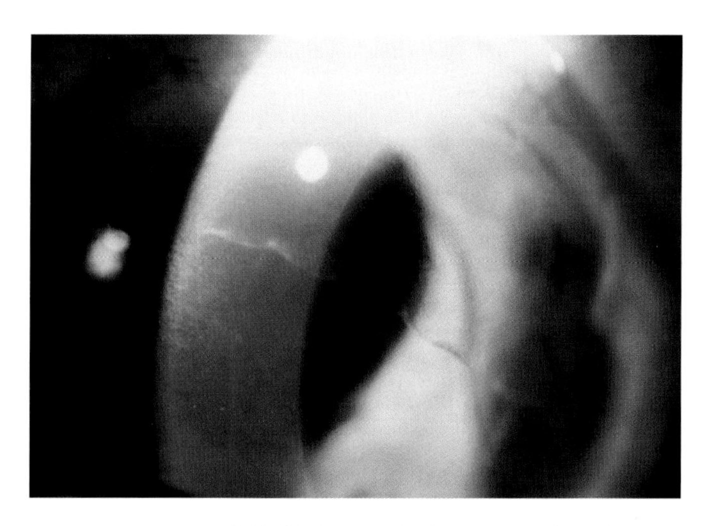

FIGURE 43-8 Epithelial downgrowth with retrocorneal membrane.

more common with intracapsular cataract extraction and early surgical techniques. The incidence has significantly decreased over the past decade.[182,183] Associated risk factors include complicated or difficult surgery and poor wound construction or closure with leakage.

The diagnosis of epithelial downgrowth is often delayed. Symptoms may be vague and include tearing, dull pain, redness, photophobia, and blurred vision.[184] Examination may show wound gape, a filtering bleb, and a fistulous tract with positive Seidel testing. Retroillumination of the cornea shows a translucent membrane that is demarcated by a gray line. The leading edge of this line often has a thickened and scalloped appearance (Figure 43-8). Unlike corneal graft rejection, keratic precipitates are not associated with this line. Corneal edema and deep corneal vascularization may be present. Anterior segment cells and flare are seen. Iris involvement is often extensive and can be delineated with the argon laser. Gonioscopy also helps to assess the extent of epithelialization. Membranes may also grow over the pupil, vitreous face, or IOL implants.

The clinical picture for fibrous ingrowth differs slightly, with membranes appearing gray or white and demonstrating more irregular leading edges. Vascularization is more commonly present.

Histopathologic studies and electron microscopy show that nonkeratinized, stratified squamous epithelium grows over the posterior cornea, angle, iris, ciliary body, vitreous, and retina.[185] Epithelium is also usually seen along the surgical wound, which may or may not have incarcerated tissue. A chronic inflammatory cell infiltrate is frequently present within the tissues.

Glaucoma almost invariably occurs with downgrowth[183] and may result from synechial closure of the angle, pupillary block, and inflammation-related changes. Hypotony may also occur secondary to a fistula and wound leak.

No medical therapy exists to stop progression from either epithelial or fibrovascular ingrowth.[186] Surgery is the mainstay of treatment. Before surgery is performed, the extent of ingrowth on the iris is delineated with the argon laser. White burns indicate the presence of epithelium. Surgical therapy requires removal of the involved iris, vitreous, and implant. Cryotherapy is applied to the cornea, angle, and ciliary body to devitalize remaining epithelium. Salvage of the globe is the prime consideration. Filtration with antifibrotic agents or seton devices may be needed for pressure control.

See Chapter 46 for a detailed discussion of epithelial and fibrous ingrowth.

Treatment of Glaucoma After Cataract Surgery: General Principles

As noted previously, all efforts are made to determine the cause of the IOP elevation that develops after cataract surgery. Therapy is directed toward elimination or treatment of the specific cause (Table 43-4). In general, mainstays of therapy include topical and systemic aqueous suppressants. Miotic and prostaglandin agents may be helpful in open-angle glaucomas when there is no inflammation or chamber shallowing. However, disruption of the blood-aqueous barrier[181] and cystoid macular edema in the early postoperative period have been reported after cataract surgery in patients receiving topical latanoprost.[187-196] Adrenergic agents are generally avoided because of the possibility, albeit small, of cystoid macular edema that may develop after cataract surgery. Apraclonidine and brimonidine are helpful adjuncts for acute therapy of high IOP spikes and are beneficial for short-term IOP treatment from days to weeks. Oral and intravenous osmotic agents are occasionally needed for profound IOP elevations. Eye surgeons should always be alert to the possibility of corticosteroid- or cycloplegic-induced glaucoma that may require cessation of steroid and cycloplegic therapy.

Conventional laser treatment for glaucoma after cataract surgery generally involves laser iridectomy for pupillary block and laser trabeculoplasty for open-angle glaucoma. Argon laser trabeculoplasty may not be as effective in the pseudophakic patient as it is in the phakic patient, but it is still a helpful treatment modality for many patients. Laser therapy is also indicated for malignant glaucoma and neovascular glaucoma, as noted earlier.

Surgery for glaucoma is occasionally required in aphakic and pseudophakic patients. Decisions concerning surgical technique and location of surgery depend largely on the status of the conjunctiva, vitreous, and IOL. Most surgeons prefer to operate in areas of conjunctiva that have not been disrupted by previous surgery. At the same time, it is generally preferable to perform surgery superiorly rather than inferiorly to avoid exposing filtration blebs to a greater risk of infection. Filtration surgical techniques may be either partial thickness or full

TABLE 43-4

Glaucoma After Cataract Surgery: Treatment Sequence

- Identify and treat specific cause
- Add standard glaucoma medications
- Laser therapy
- Filtration surgery with antimetabolite
- Seton (tube/shunt)
- Cycloablation

thickness. Vitreous must be removed if it is present in the area of the sclerectomy. The position of the IOL may direct the surgeon's choice of operative location.

If surgery is required for IOP control, a filtration procedure with intraoperative antifibrotics may be preferred. A limbal-based conjunctival flap is preferred to reduce leaks, but a fornix-based conjunctival flap may be used if necessary. Tight scleral flap closure is favored to minimize the risk of suprachoroidal hemorrhage. Selective laser suture lysis or releasable sutures are used postoperatively to facilitate aqueous egress. Supplemental use of 5-fluorouracil is also added postoperatively if necessary.

If standard filtration surgery with mitomycin-C fails, a tube-shunt seton device is often the next option. Deep sclerectomy procedures (viscocanalostomy and others) may be effective, particularly in eyes with minimal limbal scarring from previous procedures. Aphakic and pseudophakic eyes undergoing laser and surgical procedures more commonly require supplemental glaucoma medications for IOP control postoperatively than do phakic eyes. Because of the risk of visual loss and phthisis, cyclodestructive procedures are reserved for patients in which filtration or tube-shunt procedures fail. Transscleral cyclophotocoagulation is our preferred ciliary body destructive procedure of choice.

REFERENCES

1. Rich WJ: Further studies on early postoperative ocular hypertension following cataract extraction, *Trans Ophthalmol Soc U K* 89:639-645, 1969.
2. Rothkoff L, Beidner B, Glumenthal M: The effect of corneal section on early increased intraocular pressure after cataract extraction, *Am J Ophthalmol* 85:337-338, 1978.
3. Kirsch RE, Levine O, Singer JA: Further studies on the ridge at the internal edge of the cataract incision, *Trans Am Acad Ophthalmol Otolaryngol* 83:224-231, 1977.
4. Lee PF, Trotter RR: Tonographic and gonioscopic studies before and after cataract extraction, *Arch Ophthalmol* 58:407-416, 1957.
5. McGuigan LJB, Gottsch J, Stark WJ et al: Extracapsular cataract extraction and posterior chamber lens implantation in eyes with preexisting glaucoma, *Arch Ophthalmol* 104:1301-1308, 1986.
6. Savage JA, Thomas JV, Belcher CD et al: Extracapsular cataract extraction and posterior chamber intraocular lens implantation in glaucomatous eyes, *Ophthalmology* 92:1506-1516, 1985.
7. Fang EN, Kass MA: Increased intraocular pressure after cataract surgery, *Semin Ophthalmol* 9:235-242, 1994.
8. Bigger JF, Becker B: Cataracts and primary open angle glaucoma: the effect of uncomplicated cataract extraction on glaucoma control, *Trans Am Acad Ophthalmol Otolaryngol* 75:260-272, 1971.
9. Linn JG: Cataract extraction in management of glaucoma, *Trans Am Acad Ophthalmol Otolaryngol* 75:273-280, 1971.
10. Kaufman IH: Intraocular pressure after lens extraction, *Am J Ophthalmol* 59:722-723, 1965.
11. Shingleton BJ, Gamell LS, O'Donoghue MW et al: Long-term changes in intraocular pressure after clear corneal phacoemulsification: normal patients versus glaucoma suspect and glaucoma patients, *J Cataract Refract Surg* 25:885-876, 1999.
12. Tong JT, Miller KM: Intraocular pressure change after sutureless phacoemulsification and foldable posterior chamber lens implantation, *J Cataract Refract Surg* 24: 256-262, 1998.
13. Kim DD, Doyle JW, Smith MF: Intraocular pressure reduction following phacoemulsification cataract extraction with posterior chamber lens implantation in glaucoma patients, *Ophthalmic Surg Lasers* 30:37-40, 1999.
14. Schwenn O, Dick B, Krummenauer F et al: Intraocular pressure after small incision cataract surgery: temporal sclerocorneal versus clear corneal incision, *J Cataract Refract Surg* 27:421-425, 2001.
15. Tennen DG, Masket S: Short- and long-term effect of clear corneal incisions on intraocular pressure, *Ophthalmology* 102:863-867, 1995.
16. Pohjalainen T, Vesti E, Uusitalo RJ et al: Intraocular pressure after phacoemulsification and intraocular lens implantation in nonglaucomatous eyes with and without exfoliation, *J Cataract Refract Surg* 27:26-431, 2001.
17. Lamping KA, Bellows AH, Hutchinson BT et al: Long-term evaluation of initial filtration surgery, *Ophthalmology* 93:91-101, 1986.
18. Berger RO: Fox shield treatment of the UGH syndrome, *J Cataract Refract Surg* 12:419-421, 1986.
19. Haimann MH, Phelps CD: Prophylactic timolol for prevention of high intraocular pressure after cataract extraction: a randomized, prospective, double-blind trial, *Ophthalmology* 88:233-238, 1981.
20. Prata JA Jr, Rehder JR, Mello PA: Apraclonidine and early postoperative intraocular hypertension after cataract extraction, *Acta Ophthalmol* 70:434-439, 1992.
21. Fry LL: Comparison of the postoperative intraocular pressure with Betagan, Betoptic, Timoptic, Iopidine, Diamox, Pilopine Gel, and Miostat, *J Cataract Refract Surg* 18:14-19, 1992.
22. Scherer WJ, Mielke DL, Tidwell PF et al: Efficacy of latanoprost on intraocular pressure following cataract extraction, *J Cataract Refract Surg* 1999; 25:304.
23. Strelow SA, Sherwood MB, Broncato LJ et al: The effect of diclofenac sodium ophthalmic solution on intraocular pressure following cataract extraction, *Ophthalmic Surg* 23:170-175, 1992.
24. Hagen JC III, Gaasterland DE: Endocapsular hematoma: description and treatment of a unique form of postoperative hemorrhage, *Arch Ophthalmol* 109:514-518, 1991.
25. Shingleton BJ, Hersh PJ: Traumatic hyphema. In Shingleton BJ, Hersh PJ, Kenyon KR, editors: *Eye trauma,* St Louis, 1991, Mosby.
26. Deutsch TA, Weinreb RN, Goldberg MF: Indications for surgical management of hyphema in patients with sickle cell trait, *Arch Ophthalmol* 102:566-569, 1984.
27. Benson WE, Karp LA, Nichols CW et al: Late hyphema due to vascularization of the cataract wound, *Ann Ophthalmol* 10:1109-1111, 1978.
28. Jarstad JS, Hardwig PW: Intraocular hemorrhage from wound neovascularization years after anterior segment surgery (Swan syndrome), *Can J Ophthalmol* 22:271-275, 1987.
29. Speakman JS: Recurrent hyphema after surgery, *Can J Ophthalmol* 10:299-304, 1975.
30. Swan KC: Hyphema due to wound vascularization after cataract extraction, *Arch Ophthalmol* 89:87-90, 1973.
31. Swan KC: Late hyphema due to wound vascularization, *Trans Am Acad Ophthalmol Otolaryngol* 81:138-144, 1976.
32. Watzke RC: Intraocular hemorrhage from wound vascularization following cataract surgery, *Trans Am Ophthalmol Soc* 72:242-248, 1974.
33. Barraquer J, Rutlan J: Enzymatic zonulysis and postoperative ocular hypertension, *Am J Ophthalmol* 63:159, 1967.
34. Campbell DG, Simmons RJ, Grant WM: Ghost cells as a cause of glaucoma, *Am J Ophthalmol* 81:441-450, 1976.
35. Summers CG, Lindstrom RI: Ghost cell glaucoma following lens implantation, *J Am Intraocul Implant Soc* 9:428-433, 1983.
36. Kass MA, Podos SM, Moses RA et al: Prostaglandin E1 and aqueous humor dynamics, *Invest Ophthalmol Vis Sci* 2:1022-1027, 1992.
37. Kass MA, Johnson T: Corticosteroid-induced glaucoma. In Ritch R, Shields MB, Krupin T, editors: *The glaucomas,* St Louis, 1989, Mosby, pp 1161-1168.
38. Hart CT, Wrad DM: Intra-ocular pressure in Fuchs' heterochromic uveitis, *Br J Ophthalmol* 51:739-743, 1967.
39. Lerman S, Levy C: Heterochromic iritis and secondary neovascular glaucoma, *Am J Ophthalmol* 57:479-481, 1964.
40. Leo RJ, Palmer DJ: Episcleritis and secondary glaucoma after transscleral fixation of a posterior chamber intraocular lens, *Arch Ophthalmol* 109:617, 1991.
41. Masket S: Pseudophakic posterior iris chafing syndrome, *J Cataract Refract Surg* 12:252-256, 1986.
42. Alpar JJ: Glaucoma after intraocular lens implantation: survey and recommendations, *Glaucoma* 7:241-245, 1985.
43. Choyce DP: Complications of the anterior chamber implants of the early 1950s and the UGH syndrome or Ellingson syndrome of the late 1970s, *J Am Intraocul Implant Soc* 4:22-29, 1978.
44. Ellingson FT: The uveitis-glaucoma-hyphema syndrome associated with the Mark VIII anterior chamber lens implant, *J Am Intraocul Implant Soc* 4:50-53, 1978.
45. Moses L: Complications of rigid anterior chamber implants, *Ophthalmology* 91:819-825, 1984.
46. Nicholson DH: Occult iris erosion: a treatable cause of recurrent hyphema in iris-supported intraocular lenses, *Ophthalmology* 89:113-120, 1982.

47. Obstbaum SA: Management of glaucoma in the implanted patient, *J Am Intraocul Implant Soc* 7:252-259, 1981.
48. Apple DJ, Mamalis N, Loftfield K et al: Complications of intraocular lenses: a historical and histopathological review, *Surv Ophthalmol* 29:1-54, 1984.
49. Pazandak B, Johnson S, Kratz R: Recurrent intraocular hemorrhage associated with posterior chamber lens implantation, *J Am Intraocul Implant Soc* 9:327-329, 1983.
50. Percival SPB, Das SK: UGH syndrome after posterior chamber lens implantation, *J Am Intraocul Implant Soc* 9:200-201, 1983.
51. Epstein DL: Diagnosis and management of lens-induced glaucoma, *Ophthalmology* 89:227-230, 1982.
52. Epstein DL, Jedziniak JA, Grant WM: Obstruction of aqueous outflow by lens particles and by heavy-molecular-weight soluble lens proteins, *Invest Ophthalmol Vis Sci* 17:272-277, 1978.
53. Emery JM, Wilhelmus KA, Rosenberg S: Complications of phacoemulsification, *Ophthalmology* 85:141-150, 1978.
54. Monshizadeh R, Samiy N, Haimovici R: Management of retained intravitreal lens fragments after cataract surgery, *Surv Ophthalmol* 43:397-404, 1999.
55. Gilliland GD, Hutton WL, Fuller DG: Retained intravitreal lens fragments after cataract surgery, *Ophthalmology* 99:1263-1269, 1992.
56. Irvine WD, Flynn HW, Murray TG: Retained lens fragments after phacoemulsification manifesting as marked intraocular inflammation with hypopyon, *Am J Ophthalmol* 114:610-614, 1992.
57. Pande M, Dabbs TR: Incidence of lens matter dislocation during phacoemulsification, *J Cataract Refract Surg* 22:737-742, 1996.
58. Tommila P, Immonen I: Dislocated nuclear fragments after cataract surgery, *Eye* 9:437-441, 1995.
59. Allinson RW, Metrikin DC, Fante RG: Incidence of vitreous loss among third-year residents performing phacoemulsification, *Ophthalmology* 99:726-730, 1992.
60. Gonvers M: New approach to managing vitreous loss and dislocated lens fragments during phacoemulsification, *J Cataract Refract Surg* 20:346-349, 1994.
61. Leaming DV: Practice styles and preferences of ASCRS members: 1994 survey, *J Cataract Refract Surg* 21:378-385, 1995.
62. Guzek JP, Holm M, Cotter JB et al: Risk factors for intraoperative complications in 1000 extracapsular cataract cases, *Ophthalmology* 94:461-466, 1987.
63. Margherio RR, Margherio AR, Pendergast SD et al: Vitrectomy for retained lens fragments after phacoemulsification, *Ophthalmology* 104:1426-1432, 1997.
64. Streeten BW: Pathology of the lens. In Albert DM, Jakobiec FA, editors: *Principles and practices of ophthalmology: clinical practice,* Philadelphia, 1994, WB Saunders, pp 2180-2239.
65. Hutton WL, Snyder WB, Vaiser A: Management of surgically dislocated intravitreal lens fragments by pars plana vitrectomy, *Ophthalmology* 85:176-189, 1978.
66. Fastenberg DM, Schwartz PL, Shakin JL et al: Management of dislocated nuclear fragments after phacoemulsification, *Am J Ophthalmol* 112: 535-539, 1991.
67. Lambrou FH Jr, Steward MW: Management of dislocated lens fragments after cataract surgery, *Ophthalmology* 1260-1262, 1992.
68. Kim JE, Flynn HW Jr, Smiddy WE et al: Retained lens fragments after phacoemulsification, *Ophthalmology* 101:1827-1832, 1994.
69. Blodi BA, Flynn HW Jr, Blodi CF et al: Retained nuclei after cataract surgery, *Ophthalmology* 99:41-44, 1992.
70. Wong D, Briggs MC, Hickey-Dwyer MU et al: Removal of lens fragments from the vitreous cavity, *Eye* 11:37-42, 1997.
71. Yeo LMW, Charteris DG, Bunce C et al: Retained intravitreal lens fragments after phacoemulsification: a clinicopathological correlation, *Br J Ophthalmol* 83:1135-1138, 1999.
72. Watts P, Hunter J, Bunce C: Vitrectomy and lensectomy in the management of posterior dislocation of lens fragments, *J Cataract Refract Surg* 26: 832-837, 2000.
73. Vilar NF, Flynn HW Jr, Smiddy WE et al: Removal of retained lens fragments after phacoemulsification reverses secondary glaucoma and restores visual acuity, *Ophthalmology* 104:787-792, 1997.
74. Stilma JS, van der Sluijs FA, van Meurs JC et al: Occurrence of retained lens fragments after phacoemulsification in the Netherlands, *J Cataract Refract Surg* 23:1177-1182, 1997.
75. Topping TM: Discussion of paper by Gilliland GD, Hutton WL, Fuller DG, *Ophthalmology* 99:1268-1269, 1992.
76. Borne MJ, Tasman W, Regillo C et al: Outcomes of vitrectomy for retained lens fragments, *Ophthalmology* 103:971-976, 1996.
77. Brubaker RF, Halpin JA: Open-angle glaucoma associated with topical administration of flurandrenolide to the eye, *Mayo Clin Proc* 50:322-326, 1975.
78. Eisenlohr JE: Glaucoma following the prolonged use of topical steroid medication to the eyelids, *J Am Acad Dermatol* 8:878-881, 1983.
79. Covell LL: Glaucoma induced by systemic steroid therapy, *Am J Ophthalmol* 45:108-109, 1958.
80. McDonnell PJ, Kerr Muir MG: Glaucoma associated with systemic corticosteroid therapy, *Lancet* 2:386-387, 1985.
81. Herschler J: Intractable intraocular hypertension induced by repository triamcinolone acetonide, *Am J Ophthalmol* 74:501-504, 1972.
82. Herschler J: Increased intraocular pressure induced by repository corticosteroids, *Am J Ophthalmol* 82:90-93, 1976.
83. Kalina R: Increased intraocular pressure following subconjunctival corticosteroid administration, *Arch Ophthalmol* 81:788-790, 1969.
84. Mills DW, Siebert LF, Climenhaga DB: Depot triamcinolone-induced glaucoma, *Can J Ophthalmol* 21:150-152, 1986.
85. Kalina PH, Erie JC, Rosenbaum L: Biochemical quantification of triamcinolone in subconjunctival depots, *Arch Ophthalmol* 113:867-869, 1995.
86. Armaly MF: Effect of corticosteroids on intraocular pressure and fluid dynamics. II. The effect of dexamethasone in the glaucomatous eye, *Arch Ophthalmol* 70:492-499, 1963.
87. Becker B, Hahn KA: Topical corticosteroids and heredity in primary open-angle glaucoma, *Am J Ophthalmol* 57:543-551, 1964.
88. Becker B: Diabetes mellitus and primary open angle glaucoma: the XXVII Edward Jackson memorial lecture, *Am J Ophthalmol* 71:1-16, 1971.
89. Podos SM, Becker B, Morton WR: High myopia and primary open-angle glaucoma, *Am J Ophthalmol* 62:1039-1043, 1966.
90. Mermoud A, Salmon JF: Corticosteroid-induced ocular hypertension in draining Molteno single-plate implants, *J Glaucoma* 2:32-36, 1993.
91. Wilensky JT, Snyder D, Gieser D: Steroid-induced ocular hypertension in patients with filtering blebs, *Ophthalmology* 87:240-244, 1980.
92. Armaly MF: Effects of corticosteroids on intraocular pressure and fluid dynamics. I. The effect of dexamethasone in the normal eye, *Arch Ophthalmol* 70:482-491, 1963.
93. Spaeth GL, Rodrigues MM, Weinreb S: Steroid-induced glaucoma. A. Persistent elevation of intraocular pressure. B. Histopathologic aspects, *Trans Am Ophthalmol Soc* 75:353-381, 1977.
94. Mindel JS, Goldberg J, Tavitian HO: Similarity of the intraocular pressure response to different corticosteroid esters when compliance is controlled, *Ophthalmology* 86:99-107, 1979.
95. Balazs EA, Freeman MI, Kloti R et al: Hyaluronic acid and replacement of vitreous and aqueous humor, *Mod Prob Ophthalmol* 10:3-21, 1972.
96. Seigel MJ, Spiro HJ, Miller JA et al: Secondary glaucoma and uveitis associated with Orcolon, *Arch Ophthalmol* 109:1496-1497, 1991.
97. Binkhorst CD: Inflammation and intraocular pressure after the use of Healon in intraocular lens surgery, *J Am Intraocul Implant Soc* 6:340-341, 1980.
98. Genstler DE, Keates RH: Amvisc in extracapsular cataract extraction, *J Am Intraocul Implant Soc* 9:317-320, 1983.
99. Glasser DB, Matsuda M, Edelhauser HF: A comparison of the efficacy and toxicity of and intraocular pressure response to viscous solutions in the anterior chamber, *Arch Ophthalmol* 104:1819-1824, 1986.
100. Obstbaum SA: Glaucoma and intraocular lens implantation, *J Cataract Refract Surg* 12:257-261, 1986.
101. Olivius E, Thorburn W: Intraocular pressure after surgery with Healon, *J Am Intraocul Implant Soc J* 11:480-482, 1985.
102. Cherfan GM, Rich WJ, Wright G: Raised intraocular pressure and other problems with sodium hyaluronate and cataract surgery, *Trans Ophthalmol Soc U K* 103:277-279, 1983.
103. Henry JC, Olander K: Comparison of the effect of four viscoelastic agents on early postoperative intraocular pressure, *J Cataract Refract Surg* 22:960-966, 1996.
104. Kohnen T, von Her M, Schutte E et al: Evaluation of intraocular pressure with Healon and Healon GV in sutureless cataract surgery with foldable lens implantation, *J Cataract Refract Surg* 22:227-237, 1996.
105. Holzer MP, Tetz MR, Auffarth GU et al: Effect of Healon 5 and 4 other viscoelastic substances on intraocular pressure and endothelium after cataract surgery, *J Cataract Refract Surg* 27:213-218, 2001.
106. Berson FG, Patterson MM, Epstein DL: Obstruction of aqueous outflow by sodium hyaluronate in enucleated human eyes, *Am J Ophthalmol* 68:1037-1050, 1983.
107. Handa J, Henry JC, Krupin T et al: Extracapsular cataract extraction with posterior chamber lens implantation in patients with glaucoma, *Arch Ophthalmol* 105:765-769, 1987.

108. Lane SS, Naylor DW, Kullerstrand LJ et al: Prospective comparison of the effects of Occucoat, Viscoat, and Healon on intraocular pressure and endothelial cell loss, *J Cataract Refract Surg* 17:21-26, 1991.
109. Anmarkrud N, Bergaust B, Bulie T: The effect of Healon and timolol on early postoperative intraocular pressure after extracapsular cataract extraction with implantation of a posterior chamber lens, *Acta Ophthalmol* 70:96-100, 1992.
110. Paper LG, Balasz EA: The use of sodium hyaluronate (Healon) in human anterior segment surgery, *Ophthalmology* 87:699-705, 1980.
111. Calhoun FR Jr: The clinical recognition and treatment of epithelialization of the anterior chamber following cataract extraction, *Trans Am Ophthalmol Soc* 47:498-553, 1949.
112. Davison JA: Capsular bag distension after endophacoemulsification and posterior chamber intraocular lens implantation, *J Cataract Ref Surg* 16:99-108, 1990.
113. Holtz SJ: Postoperative capsular bag distension, *J Cataract Ref Surg* 18:310-317, 1992.
114. Miyake K, Ota I, Ichihashi S et al: New classification of capsular block syndrome, *J Cataract Ref Surg* 24:1230-1234, 1998.
115. Nishi O, Nishi K, Takahasi E: Capsular bag distension syndrome noted 5 years after intraocular lens implantation, *Am J Ophthalmol* 125:545-547, 1998.
116. Theng JTS, Jap A, Chee SP: Capsular block syndrome: a case series, *J Cataract Ref Surg* 26:462-467, 2000.
117. Stark WJ, Worthen D, Holladay JT et al: Neodymium:YAG lasers: an FDA report, *Ophthalmology* 92:209-212, 1985.
118. Channell MM, Beckman H: Intraocular pressure changes after neodymium-YAG laser posterior capsulotomy, *Arch Ophthalmol* 102:1024-1026, 1984.
119. Flohr MJ, Robin AJ, Kelley JS: Early complications following Q-switched neodymium:YAG laser posterior capsulotomy, *Ophthalmology* 92:60-363, 1985.
120. Slomovic AR, Parrish RK: Acute elevations of intraocular pressure following Nd:YAG laser posterior capsulotomy, *Ophthalmology* 92: 973-976, 1985.
121. Vine AK: Ocular hypertension following Nd:YAG laser capsulotomy: a potentially blinding complication, *Ophthalmic Surg* 15:283-284, 1984.
122. Richter CU, Arzeno G, Pappas H et al: Intraocular pressure elevation following Nd:YAG laser posterior capsulotomy, *Ophthalmology* 92:636, 1985.
123. Demer JL, Koch DD, Smith JA et al: Persistent elevation in intraocular pressure after Nd:YAG laser treatment, *Ophthalmic Surg* 17:465-466, 1986.
124. Steinert RF, Puliafito CA, Kumar SR et al: Cystoid macular edema, retinal detachment, and glaucoma after Nd:YAG laser posterior capsulotomy, *Am J Ophthalmol* 112:373-380, 1991.
125. Keates RH, Steinert RF, Puliafito CA et al: Long-term follow-up of Nd:YAG laser posterior capsulotomy, *J Am Intraocul Implant Soc* 10: 164-168, 1984.
126. Ge J, Wand M, Chiang R et al: Long-term effect of Nd:YAG laser posterior capsulotomy on intraocular pressure, *Arch Ophthalmol* 118:1334-1337, 2000.
127. Leys M, Pameijer JH, deJong P: Intermediate-term changes in intraocular pressure after neodymium-YAG laser posterior capsulotomy, *Am J Ophthlamol* 100:332-333, 1985.
128. Fourman S, Apisson J: Late-onset elevation of intraocular pressure after neodymium-YAG laser posterior capsulotomy, *Arch Ophthalmol* 109:511-513, 1991.
129. Jahn C, Emke M: Long-term elevation of intraocular pressure after Nd:YAG laser posterior capsulotomy, *Ophthalmologica* 210:85-89, 1996.
130. Altamirano D, Mermoud A, Pittet N et al: Aqueous humor analysis after Nd:YAG laser capsulotomy with the laser flare-cell meter, *J Cataract Refract Surg* 18:544-558, 1992.
131. Rakofsky S, Koch D, Faulkner et al: Levobunolol 0.5% and timolol 0.5% to prevent intraocular pressure elevation after neodymium:YAG laser posterior capsulotomy, *J Cataract Refract Surg* 23:1975-1080, 1997.
132. Hartenbaum D, Wilson H, Maloney S, et al, and the Dorzolamide Laser Study Group: a randomized study of Dorzolamide in the prevention of elevated intraocular pressure after anterior segment laser surgery, *J Glaucoma* 8:273-275, 1999.
133. Parker WT, Clorfeine GS, Stocklin RD: Marked intraocular pressure rise following Nd:YAG laser capsulotomy, *Ophthalmic Surg* 15:103-104, 1984.
134. Richter CU, Arzeno G, Pappas HR et al: Prevention of intraocular pressure elevation following neodymium-YAG laser posterior capsulotomy, *Arch Ophthalmol* 103:912, 1985.
135. Pollack IP, Brown RH, Crandall AS et al: Prevention of the rise in intraocular pressure following neodymium-YAG posterior capsulotomy using topical 1% apraclonidine, *Arch Ophthalmol* 106:754-757, 1988.
136. Grant WM: Open-angle glaucoma with vitreous filling the anterior chamber following cataract extraction, *Trans Am Ophthalmol Soc* 61: 196-218, 1963.
137. Samples JR, Van Buskirk EM: Open-angle glaucoma associated with vitreous humor filling the anterior chamber, *Am J Ophthalmol* 102:759-761, 1986.
138. Epstein DL: Cyclodialysis. In Epstein DL, Allingham RR, Schuman JS, editors: *Chandler and grant's glaucoma*, ed 4, Baltimore, 1997, Williams & Wilkins, pp 573-379.
139. Dreyer EB, Aquino NM: Cyclodialysis cleft in anterior chamber area. In F. Hampton Roy, editor: *Master techniques in ophthalmic surgery*, Baltimore, 1995, Williams & Wilkins, pp 3-8.
140. Harbin TS Jr: Treatment of cyclodialysis clefts with argon laser photocoagulation, *Ophthalmology* 89:1082-1083, 1982.
141. Ormerod LD, Baerveldt G, Green RL: Cyclodialysis clefts: natural history, assessment and management. In Weinstein GW, editor: *Open angle glaucoma*, New York, 1986, Churchill Livingstone, pp 201-205.
142. Kirsch RE: Further studies on glaucoma following cataract extraction associated with the use of alpha-chymotrypsin, *Trans Am Acad Ophthalmol Otolaryngol* 69:1011-1023, 1965.
143. Kirsch RE: Glaucoma following cataract extraction associated with use of alpha chymotrypsin, *Arch Ophthalmol* 72:612-620, 1964.
144. Anderson DR: Experimental alpha chymotrypsin glaucoma studied by scanning electron microscopy, *Am J Ophthalmol* 71:470-476, 1971.
145. Worthen DM: Scanning electron microscopy after alpha chymotrypsin perfusion in man, *Am J Ophthalmol* 73:637-642, 1972.
146. Jocson VL: Tonography and gonioscopy: before and after cataract extraction with alpha chymotrypsin, *Am J Ophthalmol* 60:318-322, 1965.
147. Packer AJ, Fraioli AJ, Epstein DL: The effect of timolol and acetazolamide on transient intraocular pressure elevation following cataract extraction with alpha-chymotrypsin, *Ophthalmology* 88:239-243, 1981.
148. Allen JC: Surgical treatment pupillary block, *Ann Ophthalmol* 9:661-664, 1977.
149. Anderson DR, Forster RK, Lewis ML: Laser iridotomy for aphakic pupillary block, *Arch Ophthalmol* 93:343-346, 1975.
150. Chandler PA: Glaucoma from pupillary block in aphakia, *Arch Ophthalmol* 67:14-17, 1962.
151. Hitchings RA: Aphakic glaucoma: prophylaxis and management, *Trans Ophthalmol Soc U K* 98:118-123, 1978.
152. Reese AB: Herniation of the anterior hyaloid membrane following uncomplicated intracapsular cataract extraction, *Trans Am Ophthalmol Soc* 46:73-96, 1948.
153. Chang S, Lincoff HA, Coleman DJ et al: Perfluorocarbon gases in vitreous surgery, *Ophthalmology* 92:651-656, 1985.
154. Tomey KF, Traverso CE: Neodymium-YAG posterior capsulotomy for the treatment of aphakic and pseudophakic pupillary block, *Am J Ophthalmol* 104:502-507, 1987.
155. Samples JR, Bellows AR, Rosenquist RC et al: Pupillary block with posterior chamber intraocular lenses, *Arch Ophthalmol* 105:335-337, 1987.
156. Burk LL, Shields MB, Proia AD et al: Intraocular pressure following intravitreal silicone oil injection, *Invest Ophthalmol Vis Sci* 26(suppl):159, 1985.
157. Sheie HG, Ewing MQ: Aphakic glaucoma, *Trans Ophthalmol Soc U K* 98:111-117, 1978.
158. Bellows AR, Johnstone MA: Surgical management of chronic glaucoma in aphakia, *Ophthalmology* 90:807-813, 1983.
159. Cohen JS, Osher RH, Weber P et al: Complications of extracapsular cataract surgery: the indications and risks of peripheral iridectomy, *Ophthalmology* 91:826-829, 1984.
160. Van Buskirk EM: Pupillary block after intraocular lens implantation, *Am J Ophthalmol* 95:55-59, 1983.
161. Forman JS, Ritch R, Dunn MW et al: Pupillary block following posterior chamber lens implantation, *Ophthalmic Laser Ther* 2:85-97, 1987.
162. Halkias A, Magauran DM, Joyce M: Ciliary block (malignant) glaucoma after cataract extraction with lens implant treated with YAG laser capsulotomy and anterior hyaloidotomy, *Br J Ophthalmol* 76:569-570, 1992.
163. Weiss HS, Shingleton BJ, Bellows AR et al: Argon laser gonioplasty in the treatment of angle closure glaucoma, *Am J Ophthalmol* 114:14-18, 1992.
164. Schulze RR, Copeland JR: Posterior chamber intraocular lens implantation without peripheral iridectomy: a preliminary report, *Ophthalmic Surg* 13:567, 1982.
165. Simel PF: Posterior chamber implants without iridectomy, *J Am Intraocul Implant Soc* 8:141-143, 1982.

166. Epstein DL, Hashimoto JM, Anderson PJ et al: Experimental perfusions through the anterior and vitreous chambers with possible relationships to malignant glaucoma, *Am J Ophthalmol* 88:1078-1086, 1979.
167. Duy TP, Wollensak J: Ciliary block (malignant) glaucoma following posterior chamber lens implantation, *Ophthalmic Surg* 18:741-744, 1987.
168. Tomey KF, Senft SH, Antonios SR et al: Aqueous misdirection and flat chamber after posterior chamber implants with and without trabeculectomy, *Arch Ophthalmol* 105:770-773, 1987.
169. Simmons RJ, Thomas JV, Yaqub MK: Malignant glaucoma. In Ritch R, Shields MB, Krupin T, editors: *The glaucomas*, St Louis, 1989, Mosby, pp 1251-1263.
170. Chandler PA, Grant WM: Mydriatic-cycloplegic treatment in malignant glaucoma, *Arch Ophthalmol* 68:353-359, 1962.
171. Dickens CJ, Shaffer RN: The medical treatment of ciliary block glaucoma after extracapsular cataract extraction, *Am J Ophthalmol* 103:237, 1987.
172. Epstein DL, Steinert RF, Puliafito CA: Neodymium-YAG laser therapy to the anterior hyaloid in aphakic malignant (cilio-vitreal block) glaucoma, *Am J Ophthalmol* 98:137-143, 1984.
173. Chandler PA, Simmons RJ, Grant WM: Malignant glaucoma: medical and surgical treatment, *Am J Ophthalmol* 66:496-502, 1968.
174. Lynch MG, Brown RH, Michels RG et al: Surgical vitrectomy for pseudophakic malignant glaucoma, *Am J Ophthalmol* 102:149-153, 1986.
175. Wand M: Neovascular glaucoma. In Ritch R, Shield MB, Krupin T, editors: *The glaucomas,* St Louis, 1989, Mosby, pp 1063-1110.
176. Gu QX, Fry GL, Lata GF et al: Ocular neovascularization, *Arch Ophthalmol* 103:111-117, 1985.
177. Poliner LS, Christianson DJ, Escoffery RF et al: Neovascular glaucoma after intracapsular and extracapsular cataract extraction in diabetic patients, *Am J Ophthalmol* 100:637-643, 1985.
178. Wand M: Hyaloid membrane vs. posterior capsule as a protective barrier, *Arch Ophthalmol* 103:1112, 1985.
179. Weinreb RN, Wasserstrom JP, Parker W: Neovascular glaucoma following neodymium-YAG laser posterior capsulotomy, *Arch Ophthalmol* 104:730-731, 1986.
180. Aiello LM, Wand M, Liang G: Neovascular glaucoma and vitreous hemorrhage following cataract surgery in patients with diabetes mellitus, *Ophthalmology* 90:814-819, 1983.
181. Wand M, Dueker DK, Aiello LM et al: Effects of panretinal photocoagulation on rubeosis iridis, angle neovascularization, and neovascular glaucoma, *Am J Ophthalmol* 86:332-339, 1978.
182. Bernardino VB, Kim JC, Smith TR: Epithelialization of the anterior chamber after cataract extraction, *Arch Ophthalmol* 82:742-750, 1969.
183. Weiner MJ, Trentacoste J, Pon DM et al: Epithelial downgrowth: a 30-year clinicopathological review, *Br J Ophthalmol* 73:6-11, 1989.
184. Smith MF, Doyle JW: Glaucoma secondary to epithelial and fibrous downgrowth, *Semin Ophthalmol* 9:248-253, 1994.
185. Zavala EY, Binder PS: The pathologic findings of epithelial ingrowth, *Arch Ophthalmol* 98:2007-2014, 1980.
186. Stark WJ, Michels RG, Maumenee AE et al: Surgical management of epithelial downgrowth, *Am J Ophthalmol* 85:772-780, 1978.
187. Miyake K, Ota I, Maekubo K et al: Latanoprost accelerates disruption of the blood-aqueous barrier and the incidence of angiographic cystoid macular edema in early postoperative pseudophakias, *Arch Ophthalmol* 117:34-40, 1999.
188. Lima MC, Paranhos A Jr, Salim S et al: Visually significant cystoid macular edema in pseudophakic and aphakic patients with glaucoma receiving latanoprost, *J Glaucoma* 9:317-321, 2000.
189. Rowe JA, Hattenhauer MG, Herman DC: Adverse side effects associated with latanoprost, *Am J Ophthalmol* 124:683-685, 1997.
190. Heier JS, Steinert RF, Frederick AR: Cystoid macular edema associated with latanoprost use, *Arch Ophthalmol* 116:680-682, 1998.
191. Avakian A, Renier SA, Butler PJ: Adverse effects of latanoprost on patients with medically resistant glaucoma, *Arch Ophthalmol* 116:679-680, 1998.
192. Ayyala RS, Cruz DA, Margo CE et al: Cystoid macular edema associated with latanoprost in aphakic and pseudophakic eyes, *Am J Ophthalmol* 126:602-604, 1998.
193. Callanan D, Fellman RL, Savage JA: Latanoprost-associated cystoid macular edema, *Am J Ophthalmol* 126:134-135, 1998.
194. Thorne JE, Maguire AM, Lanciano R: CME and anterior uveitis with latanoprost use, *Ophthalmology* 105:1981-1983, 1998.
195. Warwar RE, Bullock JD, Ballal D: Cystoid macular edema and anterior uveitis associated with latanoprost use: experience and incidence in a retrospective review of 94 patients, *Ophthalmology* 105:263-268, 1998.
196. Moroi SE, Gottfredsdottir MS, Schteingart MT et al: Cystoid macular edema associated with latanoprost therapy in a case of patients with glaucoma and ocular hypertension, *Ophthalmology* 106:1024-1029, 1999.

Neodymium:Yttrium-Aluminum-Garnet Laser Posterior Capsulotomy

44

Roger F. Steinert, MD
Claudia U. Richter, MD

The neodymium:yttrium-aluminum-garnet (Nd:YAG) laser is a solid-state laser with a wavelength of 1064 mm that can disrupt ocular tissues by achieving optical breakdown with a short, high-power pulse. Optical breakdown results in ionization, or plasma formation, in the ocular tissue. This plasma formation then causes acoustic and shock waves that disrupt tissue.[1,2]

The development of the Nd:YAG laser as an ophthalmic instrument and its application in discussion of the posterior capsule coincided with the conversion from intracapsular to extracapsular surgical techniques in cataract surgery. Before the introduction of the Nd:YAG laser, only surgical cutting or polishing of the posterior capsule could manage opacification of the posterior capsule following extracapsular cataract extraction. Nd:YAG laser posterior capsulotomy introduced a technique for closed-eye, effective, and relatively safe opening of the opacified posterior capsule, and laser capsulotomy rapidly became the standard of care.[3]

Capsular Opacification

Postoperative opacification of initially clear posterior capsules occurs frequently in patients after extracapsular extraction of senile cataracts, although the time to opacification is highly variable. In adults, the time from surgery to visually significant opacification varies from months to years,[4,5] and the rate of opacification declines with increasing age.[6,7] In younger age groups, almost 100% opacification occurs within 2 years after surgery.

The incidence of posterior capsule opacification varies with different studies. Sinskey and Cain[8] reported that 43% of their patients required discussion, with an average follow-up of 26 months and a range from 3 months to 4 years. Emery, Wilhelmus, and Rosenberg[6] found opacification in 28% of their patients with 2 to 3 years of follow-up. Late opacification of the posterior capsule after 3 to 5 years has been reported to be approximately 50%.[9,10] Several studies have reported that the incidence of posterior capsule opacification is lower if a posterior chamber intraocular lens (IOL) is inserted with a convex posterior configuration in close apposition to the posterior capsule.[11-14] Phacoemulsification is associated with lower rates of posterior capsule opacification than extracapsular cataract extraction.[15]

A study of posterior capsule opacification in 5416 postmortem pseudophakic eyes by Apple et al.[16,17] and Peng et al.[18,19] identified six factors associated with reduced posterior capsule opacification:

1. Hydrodissection-associated cortical cleanup
2. In-the-bag IOL fixation
3. Continuous circular capsulorhexis diameter slightly smaller than the IOL optic
4. IOL material associated with reduced cellular proliferation. Hydrogel IOLs are associated with the highest rate of posterior capsule opacification; polymethylmethacrylate (PMMA) is intermediate; and silicone and acrylic optic material, the lowest.[20,21]
5. Maximal IOL optic to posterior capsule opacification
6. IOL optic geometry with a square, truncated edge[22,23]

Diabetes mellitus may reduce the rate of posterior capsule opacification compared with nondiabetic patients.[24]

Experimental and pathologic studies indicated that posterior capsule opacification occurs as a result of the formation of opaque secondary membranes by active lens epithelial proliferation, transformation of lens epithelial cells into fibroblasts with contractile elements, and collagen deposition.[25-30] The anterior lens epithelial cells proliferate onto the posterior capsule at the site of apposition of the anterior capsule flaps to the posterior capsule.[31] The contraction caused by the myoblastic features of the lens epithelial cells produces wrinkling of the posterior capsule.

Collagen deposition results in white fibrotic opacities. Mitotic inhibitors instilled into the anterior chamber after extracapsular cataract extraction have been shown to reduce capsular opacification dramatically, but pharmacologic inhibition of capsular opacification has yet to be successfully introduced into clinical practice.[32,33]

The finding that posterior capsule opacification results from lens epithelial cells proliferating onto the posterior capsule at the site of apposition of the anterior capsule flaps explains the inability of polishing the capsule at surgery to delay the onset or

Figures and portions of the text were previously published in Steinert RF, Puliafito CA: *The Nd:YAG laser in ophthalmology: principles and clinical applications of photodisruption,* Philadelphia, 1985, WB Saunders.

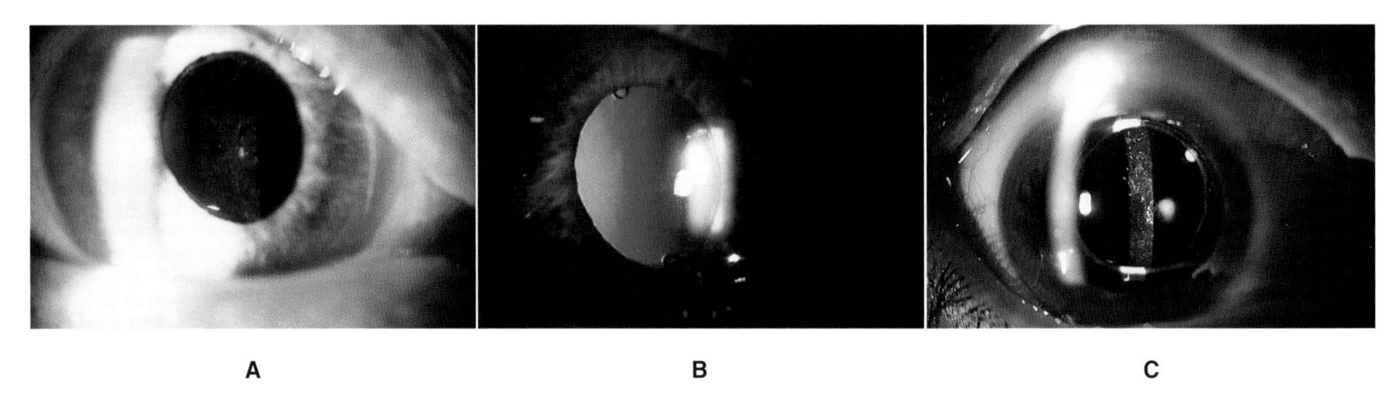

FIGURE 44-1 A and **B,** Fine fibrosis of the posterior capsule seen at the second postoperative examination represents cortical lamellae left at the time of surgery. The fibrosis is evident with oblique slit lamp illumination **(A)** but is optically insignificant when viewed with a red reflex **(B)**. **C,** Fine fibrosis may also develop months or years after cataract surgery on an initially clear capsule. This eye is shown 2.5 years after phacoemulsification cataract extraction with implantation of a one-piece polymethylmethacrylate IOL within the capsular bag. (From Steinert RF, Puliafito CA: *The Nd:YAG laser in ophthalmology: principles and clinical applications of photodisruption,* Philadelphia, 1985, WB Saunders, p 74.)

reduce the frequency of late capsular opacification,[4,6-8] because polishing the posterior capsule cannot remove the epithelial cells from the anterior capsule flaps. A peripheral ring in the capsular bag may reduce opacification, however.[34]

Additional clinical evidence that (1) a convex posterior chamber IOL can inhibit posterior capsule opacification and (2) close apposition of peripheral anterior and posterior capsule flaps leads to posterior capsule opacification was provided in an early study by Tan and Chee.[35] They reported an unusual form of early central posterior capsule fibrosis that occurred when a posteriorly vaulted biconvex optic IOL was positioned with the optic anterior to a capsulorhexis opening smaller than the optic diameter. This positioning, usually with haptic fixation in the ciliary sulcus, allowed the anterior capsule flaps to be apposed to the posterior capsule and the IOL not to be in close apposition to the central posterior capsule. Migration of lens epithelial cells onto the posterior capsule then resulted in early central opacification.

Clinically, optical degradation of initially clear posterior capsules takes several forms. *Fibrosis* connotes a gray-white band or plaquelike opacity that may be recognized in the early postoperative period or may occur later. Fibrosis that is present in the first days to weeks postoperatively probably most often represents cortical lamellae left at the time of surgery (Figure 44-1). Fibrosis that develops months to years postoperatively is caused by migration of anterior lens epithelium, fibroblastic metaplasia, and collagen production.[31] Figure 44-2 shows a dense fibrinous plaque. Heavy fibrosis occurs frequently at the edge of a posterior chamber IOL placed in the bag with apposition of anterior and posterior capsules (Figure 44-3).

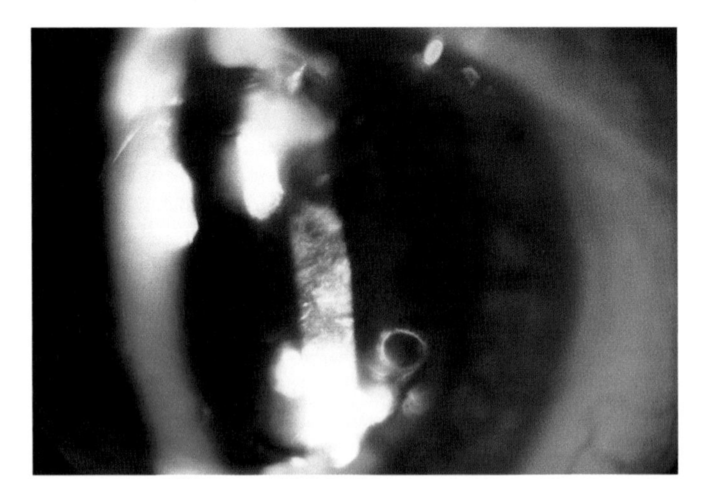

FIGURE 44-2 Heavy diffuse fibrosis of a posterior capsule behind a posterior chamber IOL. (From Steinert RF, Puliafito CA: *The Nd:YAG laser in ophthalmology: principles and clinical applications of photodisruption,* Philadelphia, 1985, WB Saunders, p 74.)

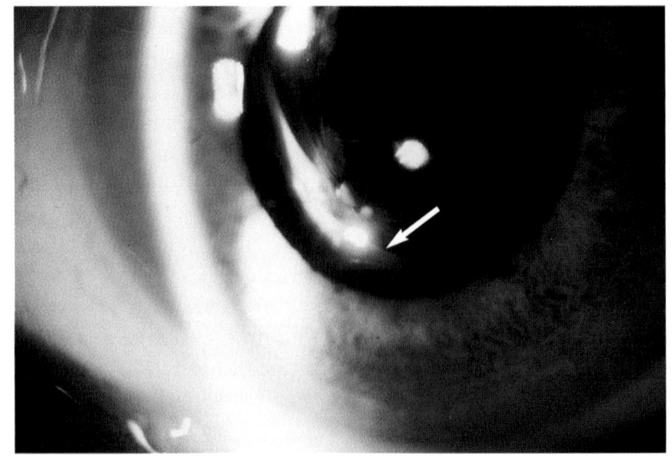

FIGURE 44-3 Dense fibrosis at the edge of a posterior chamber IOL optic placed in the bag *(arrow)* in which an anterior capsular flap is apposed to the posterior capsule. (From Steinert RD, Puliafito CA: *The Nd:YAG laser in ophthalmology: principles and clinical applications of photodisruption,* Philadelphia, 1985, WB Saunders, p 75.)

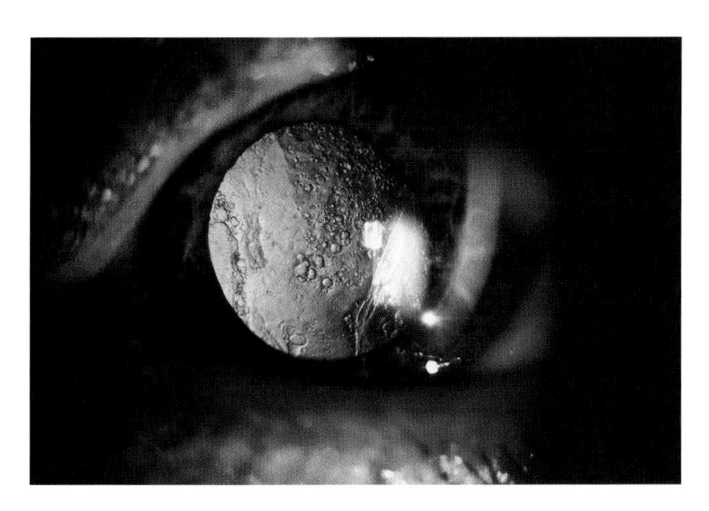

FIGURE 44-4 Red reflex view shows formation of multiple small epithelial pearls after anterior epithelial cells migrate centrally from peripheral areas of apposition of anterior capsular flaps to the posterior capsule. (From Steinert RF, Puliafito CA: *The Nd:YAG laser in ophthalmology: principles and clinical applications of photodisruption,* Philadelphia, 1985, WB Saunders, p 75.)

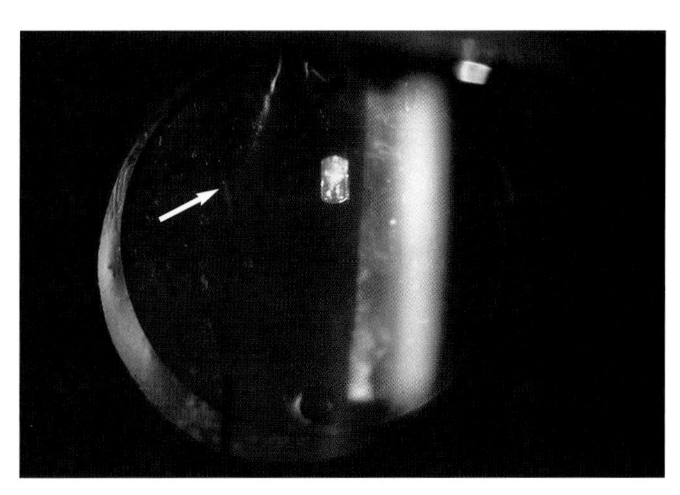

FIGURE 44-5 Broad wrinkles of the clear posterior capsule *(arrow)* are seen on red reflex, with numerous small epithelial pearls. (From Steinert RF, Puliafito CA: *The Nd:YAG laser in ophthalmology: principles and clinical applications of photodisruption,* Philadelphia, 1985, WB Saunders, p 76.)

Formation of small *Elschnig pearls* and *bladder cells* (Figure 44-4), the second major form of opacity, occurs months to years after surgery. This type of opacity occurs from proliferating lens epithelial cells, which can form layers several cells thick.[31]

Capsular wrinkling can have two manifestations. Broad undulations of clear capsule are particularly common in the early postoperative period before the capsule becomes tense. Posterior chamber lens haptics may induce these broad wrinkles along the axis of the haptic orientation. Conversely, a posterior chamber lens may tend to flatten broad wrinkles if the optic body presses on the capsule. Fibrotic contraction can also induce wrinkles (Figure 44-5). Broad, undulating wrinkles of clear capsule rarely are visually disturbing to the patient; an occasional patient may perceive linear distortion or shadows that correspond to the wrinkles and that are relieved by capsulotomy. In contrast, fine wrinkles or folds in the capsule, caused by myoblastic differentiation, can result in marked optical disturbance (Figure 44-6). These fine wrinkles are caused by myofibroblastic differentiation on the migrating lens epithelial cells, which acquire contractile properties, resulting in the wrinkles.[31]

If the iris forms synechiae to the capsule, reactive pigment epithelial hyperplasia and migration onto the capsule may occur. Most often these adhesions occur if large amounts of cortex are

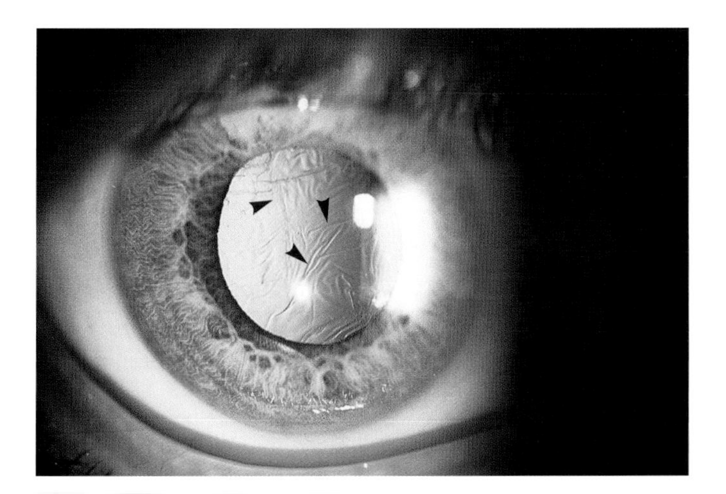

FIGURE 44-6 Fine wrinkles in the posterior capsule are evident on red reflex *(arrowheads).* These wrinkles alone can be visually disturbing and can reduce acuity by several lines or cause Maddox rod light streaks. (From Steinert RF, Puliafito CA: *The Nd:YAG laser in ophthalmology: principles and clinical applications of photodisruption,* Philadelphia, 1985, WB Saunders, p 76.)

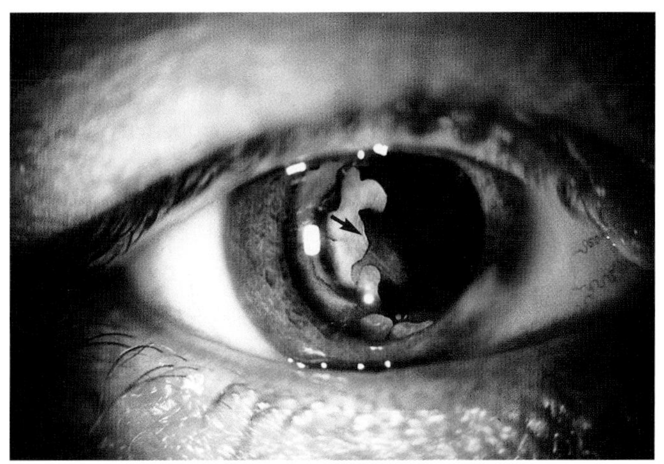

FIGURE 44-7 Pigment from proliferating uveal melanocytes has covered a large portion of this dense pupillary membrane, which formed after a traumatic cataract 40 years previously. The border of the pigment has a sharp scalloped configuration *(arrow).* (From Steinert RF, Puliafito CA: *The Nd:YAG laser in ophthalmology: principles and clinical applications of photodisruption,* Philadelphia, 1985, WB Saunders, p 77.)

left at the time of surgery, which is particularly common with traumatic cataracts. Figure 44-7 shows dense melanin deposition on a pupillary membrane after an old traumatic cataract. Localized pigmented precipitates on the capsule and IOL can occur spontaneously or after hemorrhage or inflammation.

Posterior Capsulotomy

Indications

Nd:YAG laser capsulotomy is indicated for treatment of opacification of the posterior capsule resulting in decreased visual acuity or visual function, or both, for the patient. Careful assessment is necessary to be certain that the posterior capsule opacification is the cause of decreased visual acuity. Some patients may particularly complain of difficulty with glare despite what appears to be minimal capsular opacification. Glare testing can be helpful in validating these symptoms.[36]

Contraindications

Attempted Nd:YAG laser capsulotomy is contraindicated if corneal scars, irregularity, or edema preclude adequate visualization of the target aiming beam or degrade the Nd:YAG laser beam optics, preventing reliable and predictable optical breakdown. The procedure is also contraindicated if the patient proves unable or unwilling to fixate adequately, with the threat of inadvertent damage to adjacent intraocular structures.

The presence of a glass IOL, few of which remain, is a relative contraindication because of the possibility of causing a complete fracture in the glass optic.[37] The merits of surgical discission in this instance should be carefully weighed.

Known or suspected active cystoid macular edema (CME) is a relative contraindication, given evidence regarding a beneficial effect of the barrier function of an intact posterior capsule and rare cases of clinical CME that occur after Nd:YAG laser capsulotomy.[38] Conservative practice suggests avoidance of capsulotomy in an eye with active inflammation until the visual impairment becomes functionally unacceptable to the patient.

Nd:YAG laser posterior capsulotomy rarely may be complicated by a retinal tear or detachment. Despite a lack of clinical data establishing a correlation between the number or energy level of laser pulses and retinal detachment, prudence dictates that in eyes already at high risk for retinal detachment, the least amount of energy and the lowest possible number of shots should be used to accomplish the capsulotomy, and only a small opening should be made (Table 44-1). The alternative of repolishing the capsule may be considered.

Technique

PREOPERATIVE ASSESSMENT

All patients require a complete ophthalmic history and examination before treatment, including notation of medical history and systemic medications, vision, intraocular pressure in both eyes, slit lamp examination, and fundus examination. Judging the contribution of a capsular opacity to a patient's overall visual deficit may be difficult. Table 44-2 lists useful techniques. Some capsular opacities are impressive in oblique slit lamp illumination but are insignificant when viewed against the red reflex. In general, these opacities cause little visual difficulty. The single most reliable technique for assessing capsular opacity is direct ophthalmoscopy because the surgeon's view of retinal details generally correlates with the patient's view of the world. Retinoscopy and the red reflex seen at the slit lamp examination or with a direct or indirect ophthalmoscope also reveal significant optical disturbances. The fundus view with the Hruby lens or 90-diopter lens may also allow accurate assessment of capsular clouding, whereas the indirect ophthalmoscope can penetrate significant capsular opacity.

The laser interferometer and the potential acuity meter should penetrate mild to moderate capsular opacity and be able to predict macular function. However, both instruments may give false-positive ("good") acuity prediction in the presence of CME,[39] which is the most common cause of postcataract visual impairment besides capsular opacity itself. False-negative acuity predictions may also occur because of diffuse posterior capsule opacification, poor pupillary dilation, poor patient posture at the slit lamp examination, communication problems, alphabet illiteracy, nystagmus, tremor, senility, poor patient cooperation, and fatigue.[40,41]

Unless the capsule is extremely dense, adequate visualization may be present for fluorescein angiography or angioscopy. In

TABLE 44-1
Contraindications to Laser Capsulotomy

ABSOLUTE CONTRAINDICATIONS
Corneal scars, irregularities, or edema that:
Interferes with target visualization
Makes optical breakdown unpredictable
Inadequate stability of the eye
RELATIVE CONTRAINDICATIONS
Glass intraocular lens
Known or suspected cystoid macular edema
Active intraocular inflammation
High risk for retinal detachment

TABLE 44-2
Assessment of Significance of Capsular Opacity

Direct ophthalmoscopic visualization of fundus structures
Retinoscopy
Red reflex evaluation by:
Slit lamp examination
Direct ophthalmoscopic examination
Indirect ophthalmoscopic examination
Hruby lens view of fundus
Laser interferometer evaluation
Potential acuity meter evaluation
Fluorescein angiography

A B

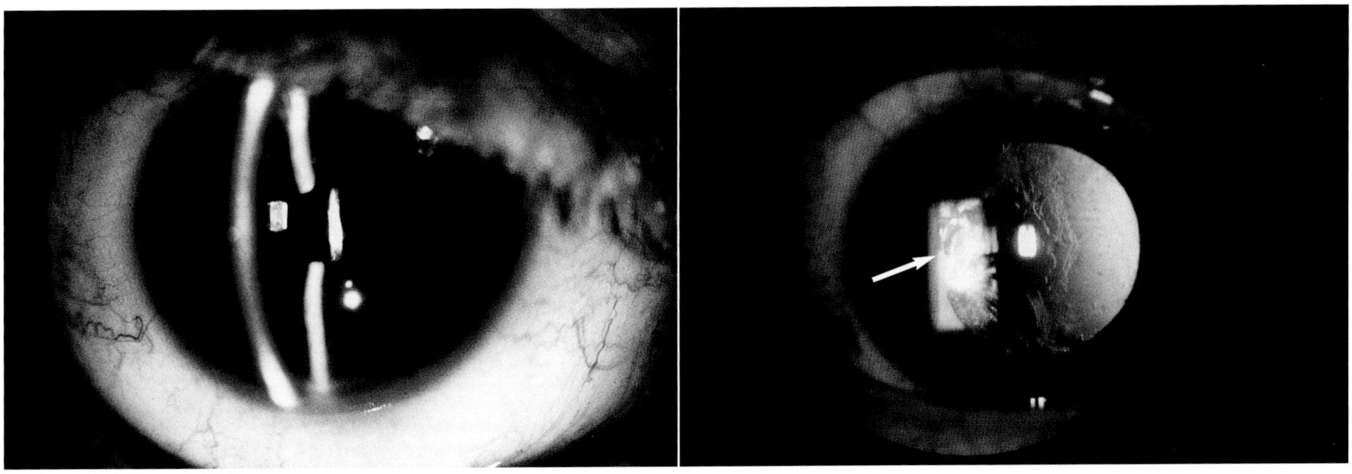

FIGURE 44-8 A, Typical capsular opacity before dilation. **B,** Capsulotomy appears eccentric because of uneven pupillary dilation caused by posterior synechia to the capsule *(arrow).* The capsular opening is properly centered for the undilated pupil. (From Steinert RF, Puliafito CA: *The Nd:YAG laser in ophthalmology: principles and clinical applications of photodisruption,* Philadelphia, 1985, WB Saunders, p 81.)

patients in whom the capsular opacity seems inadequate to explain the quality of vision, CME should be anticipated and documented so that unnecessary and possibly deleterious capsulotomy can be avoided.

PREPARATION OF THE PATIENT

The purpose and nature of the procedure should be explained to the patient and *informed consent* obtained beforehand. At the time of treatment, the patient usually is reassured by the familiar presence of the slit lamp delivery system. The surgeon should remind the patient that the procedure is painless. The patient may hear small clicks or pops, but the patient must simply maintain steady fixation. The procedure is completed in a matter of minutes.

Brimonidine, apraclonidine, or a *beta-blocking agent* should be administered in the eye immediately on completion of the Nd:YAG laser posterior capsulotomy to minimize a post-operative intraocular pressure spike. If the administration of these agents is contraindicated, a topical or systemic carbonic anhydrase inhibitor, prostaglandin analogue, or, in a case of an extremely vulnerable optic nerve, oral hyperosmotic agent may be used to prevent or treat any intraocular pressure elevation following laser therapy.

Dilation of the pupil facilitates visualization of the capsule over a broad expanse. Except in cases of an iris-clip lens, dilation is helpful for a surgeon inexperienced with laser capsulotomy. In the absence of a miotic pupil, however, dilation may be omitted when an experienced surgeon is performing the procedure.

If the pupil is to be dilated, the landmarks of the pupillary zone of the capsule should be sketched beforehand. Pupils are often eccentric or may dilate eccentrically, as shown in Figure 44-8. Inattention to the pupillary zone may result in an eccentric capsulotomy and may necessitate a second session at the laser to induce the surgeon to perform an overly large capsulotomy to prevent this possibility. If the laser is available, the patient can be brought to the laser before dilation, and a single "marker" shot can be placed in the capsule near the middle of the pupillary axis. When the pupil is subsequently dilated, the marker shot accurately reminds the surgeon of the patient's true visual axis.

For routine dilation, we recommend only a single drop of 2.5% phenylephrine. If this is inadequate, a drop of 0.5% or 1% tropicamide may be added. Weak dilation is intended to prevent iris capture of a posterior chamber IOL (Figure 44-9), which may be difficult to properly reposition.

No anesthesia is generally required for capsulotomy unless a contact lens is used. In that case, a drop of topical anesthetic is applied to the cornea immediately before the beginning

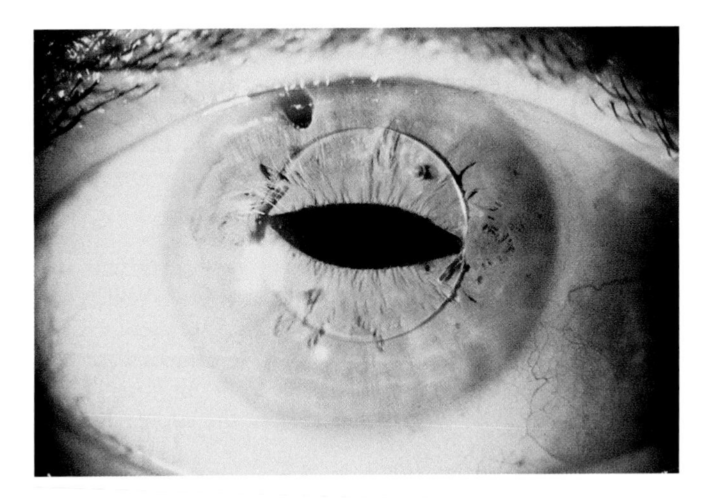

FIGURE 44-9 Iris capture of a ciliary sulcus–fixated planar haptic posterior chamber IOL. This phenomenon can occur after wide dilation for posterior capsulotomy. If dilation is necessary at all, weak mydriatics and cycloplegics should be employed. (From Steinert RF, Puliafito CA: *The Nd:YAG laser in ophthalmology: principles and clinical applications of photodisruption,* Philadelphia, 1985, WB Saunders, p 81.)

TABLE 44-3

Preparation of the Patient

BEFORE THE TREATMENT SESSION
Complete ophthalmic history and examination
Discussion of proposed procedure, including risks, benefits, and alternatives; signing of informed consent form
Apraclonidine or beta-adrenergic blocking agent
Pupillary dilation (optional)
Determination of visual axis and normal pupillary size: sketch and preliminary laser marker shot
Weak mydriatic and cycloplegic agents: 2.5% phenylephrine or 0.5% or 1% tropicamide
AT THE LASER
Review of the procedure, the expected pop or click, and the importance of fixation
Application of topical anesthetic if contact lens is to be used
Adjustment of stool, table, chin rest, and footrest for optimal patient comfort
Application of head strap to maintain forehead position
Darkening of the room (optional)
Provision of fixation target for fellow eye (illumination of target if room is darkened)

of the procedure. In rare circumstances, such as nystagmus, a retrobulbar injection to establish akinesia may be helpful. If a topical anesthetic is applied in advance of the procedure for examination or instillation of painful mydriatic and cycloplegic agents, the patient should be instructed to keep the eyes closed during the interval while waiting for the laser treatment to maintain the surface integrity and optical quality of the corneal epithelium.

The patient must be seated comfortably with properly adjusted stool, table, and chin rest heights and a footrest when appropriate. A strap that passes from the headrest behind the patient's head is useful to counteract the tendency of many patients to move back during the course of the treatment. The surgeon's visualization of the target is usually improved in a darkened room. If a patient is expected to fixate with the other eye, however, an illuminated fixation target should be provided. Table 44-3 summarizes the steps in patient preparation.

PROCEDURE

A contact lens such as the Peyman or central Abraham lens may be used to stabilize the eye, improve the laser beam optics, and facilitate accurate focusing. The Abraham Nd:YAG laser increases the convergence angle to 24 degrees from 16 degrees, decreases the area of laser at the posterior capsule to 14 μm from 21 μm, and increases the beam diameter at both the cornea and the retina. The Abraham Nd:YAG laser lens must be used with care because it is a modified posterior pole lens; if the Nd:YAG laser is not sent through the lens button, but rather the peripheral "carrier" portion of the lens, the Nd:YAG laser may be focused on the retina and cause damage.[42]

The minimal amount of energy necessary to obtain breakdown and rupture the capsule is desired. With most lasers, a typical capsule can be opened by using 1 to 2 mJ/pulse.

TABLE 44-4

Posterior Capsulotomy Technique

Use minimum energy: 1 mJ if possible
Identify and cut across tension lines
Perform a cruciate opening:
Begin at the 12 o'clock position in the periphery
Progress toward the 6 o'clock position
Cut across at the 3 and 9 o'clock positions
Clean up any residual tags
Avoid freely floating fragments

The capsule is examined for wrinkles that indicate tension lines. Shots placed across tension lines result in the largest opening per pulse because the tension causes the initial opening to widen.

Figure 44-10 shows an actual capsulotomy, photographed sequentially and drawn from the photographs, showing the opening as it develops and the location of the next laser shot. Table 44-4 outlines the basic technique. The usual strategy is to create a cruciate opening, beginning superiorly near the 12 o'clock position and progressing downward toward the 6 o'clock position. Unless a wide opening has already developed, shots are then placed at the edge of the capsule opening, progressing laterally toward the 3 and 9 o'clock positions. If any capsular flaps remain in the pupillary space, the laser is fired specifically at the flaps to cut them and cause them to retract and fall back to the periphery.

The goal is to achieve flaps based in the periphery inferiorly. Free-floating fragments should be avoided because they may remain and cause visual interference. Cutting in a circle ("can-opener" style) tends to create large fragments that may not sink from the visual axis or that may settle against the endothelium or angle structures. A large "vitreous floater" of residual capsule may bother the patient.

Beginning the cruciate opening in the superior periphery has several advantages. The initial shots are in the periphery so that if the patient becomes startled and an adjacent IOL is marked, the mark appears in the periphery. Both the patient and surgeon can have settled down before the more critical central area is treated. Furthermore, as the flaps develop, gravity aids in pulling them toward the inferior periphery. In contrast, it can be much more difficult to cause a flap that is hanging down from above to retract.

An IOL may be marked in the course of the capsulotomy. This is particularly true for posterior chamber lenses for which there is little or no separation of the capsule from the IOL. The issue of laser damage to the IOL is discussed under Complications. Figure 44-11 shows a capsulotomy without damage to an overlying posterior chamber IOL.

Visually significant pits and cracks can be minimized and avoided through careful techniques, as outlined in Table 44-5. The minimal amount of energy must be employed. With a typical capsule and careful focusing, 1 to 2 mJ is usually adequate. The capsule should be carefully examined for an area of separation from the IOL in which to begin the capsulotomy. Once the capsulotomy has begun, further areas of separation usually develop.

A

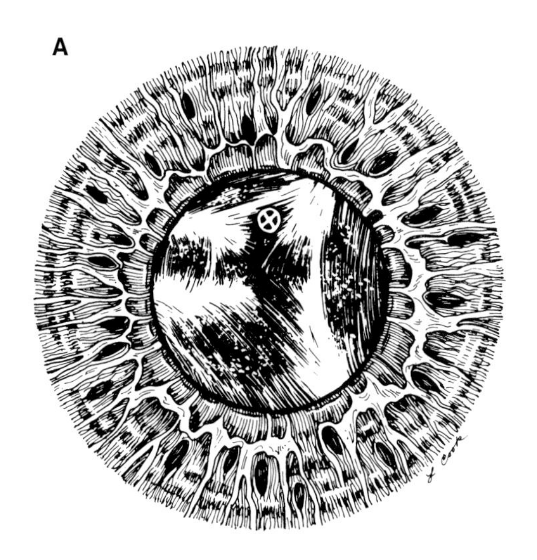

B

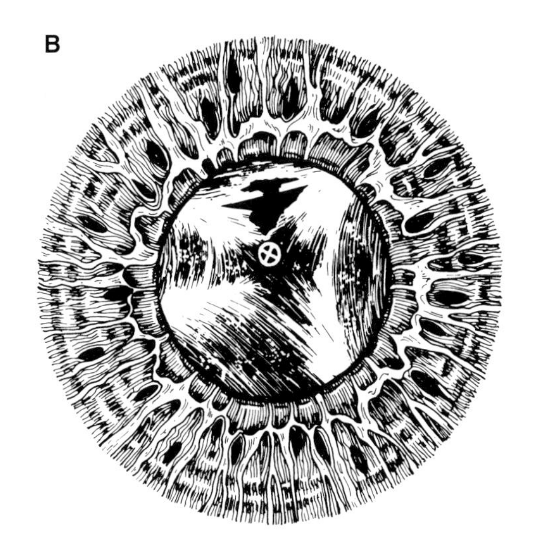

C

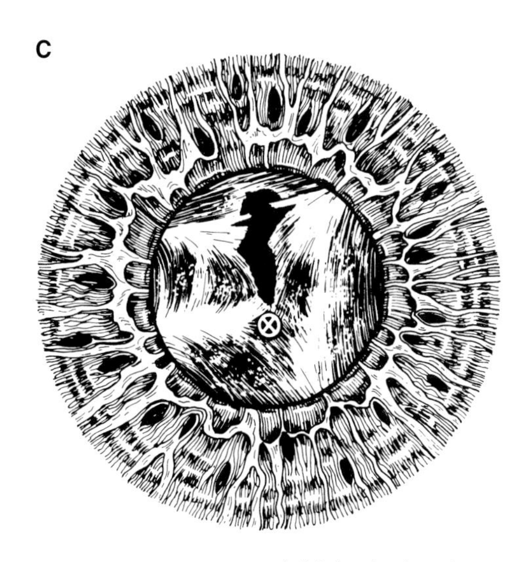

D

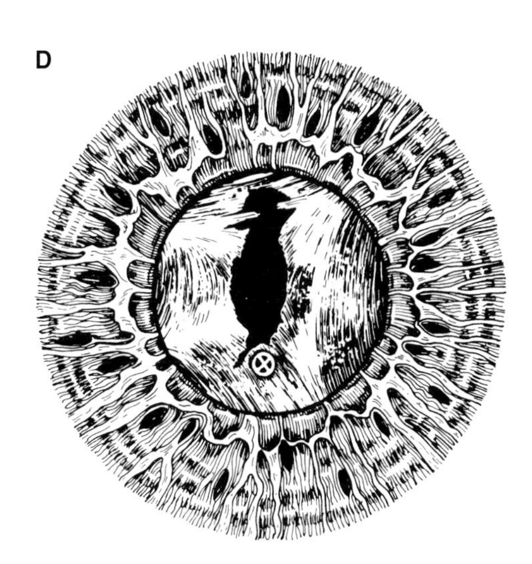

FIGURE 44-10 Artist drawing based on sequential capsulotomy photographs. The capsulotomy is developed in a cruciate pattern. **A,** The first shot is made superiorly in the location of some fine tension lines. **B,** The second shot is aimed inside the inferior edge of the initial opening. **C,** The next shot again is made at the 6 o'clock position of the capsulotomy border. **D,** The fourth shot is made across inferior tension lines to allow the capsulotomy to widen.

(Continued)

Following the usual strategy of beginning the capsulotomy in the 12 o'clock periphery gives an indication of the tendency for IOL marking in a noncritical area. If there is a tendency for unavoidable repeated marks, the usual cruciate pattern should be modified. Instead of progressing from the 12 o'clock to the 6 o'clock position across the visual axis, the cut should be made nasally and temporally, staying in the periphery of the optical zone. The capsule can then be opened in a "Christmas-tree" fashion, based inferiorly, without any shots in the central visual axis.

One other technique is very helpful in avoiding IOL marks. The laser can be intentionally focused posterior to the capsule, causing optical breakdown in the anterior vitreous. The shock wave then radiates forward and ruptures the capsule. Optical breakdown just at the capsule and IOL surface, with resultant IOL marking, is avoided. Because the breakdown threshold is higher in the anterior vitreous than at an optical interface like the capsule, higher energy is required to use this technique, usually a minimum of 2 mJ. Therefore care must be taken to focus consistently at an area posterior to the capsule so that the breakdown is not allowed to come up to the back of the IOL, which would result in a larger mark. Because this technique traumatizes the vitreous, we prefer to reserve the deep focus technique for cases in which IOL marks are occurring with focus directly on the capsule.

In aphakic eyes, the reverse of a deep focus approach, namely, deliberate focus anterior to the capsule, has been advocated by

E

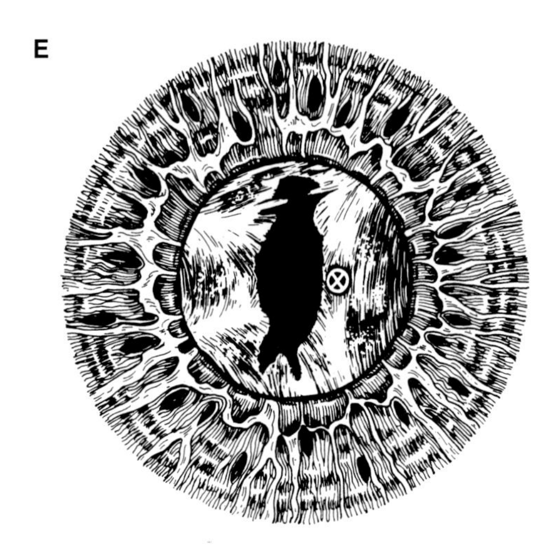

F

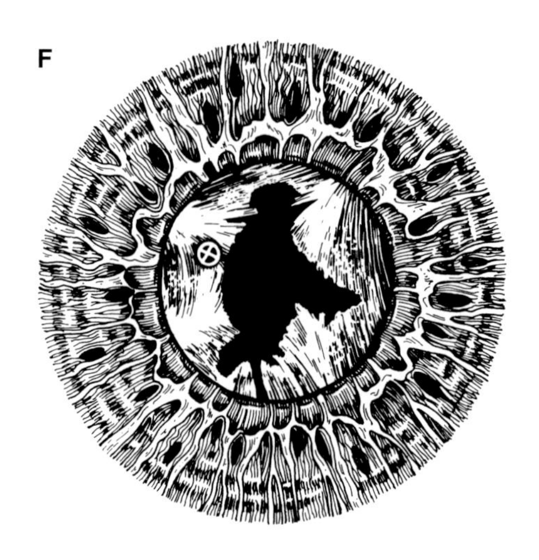

G

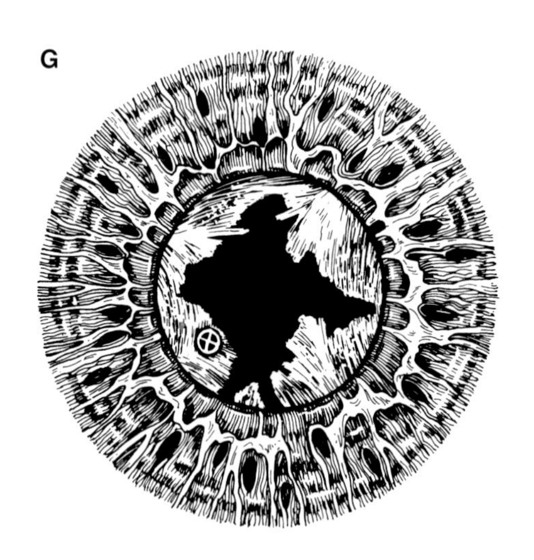

H

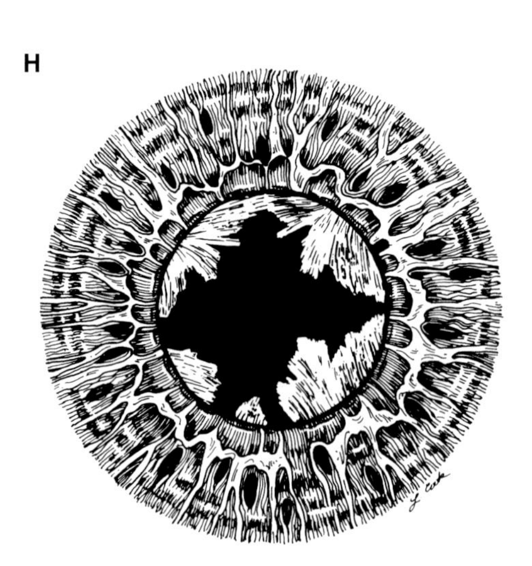

FIGURE 44-10, cont'd, Artist drawing based on sequential capsulotomy photographs. The capsulotomy is developed in a cruciate pattern. **E,** The opening is nearly 3 mm wide. It is widened by a shot at the 3 o'clock capsulotomy margin. **F,** The opening now needs to be directed to the left, with a shot at the 9 o'clock position. **G,** The cruciate opening has been accomplished, but a triangular flap extends into the pupillary space from the 7:30 region in the left inferior pupil. A shot is applied to the flap both to cut it and to push it toward the periphery. **H,** The capsulotomy is complete, and the pupil will be clear of capsule after the dilation wears off. (From Steinert RF, Puliafito CA: *The Nd:YAG laser in ophthalmology: principles and clinical applications of photodisruption,* Philadelphia, 1985, WB Saunders, pp 84-85.)

some as a mechanism for opening the capsule while leaving the anterior hyaloid intact.

CAPSULOTOMY SIZE

In the absence of a specific reason for a small opening, such as concern for a patient at high risk of retinal detachment, the capsulotomy should be as large as the pupil in isotopic conditions, such as driving at night, when glare from the exposed capsulotomy edge is most likely. A small opening in a dense membrane results in excellent optics, analogous to those of a small pupil (Figure 44-12). When the capsule is only hazy and transmits images to the retina, however, a small opening is an improvement but is still suboptimal. The hazy membrane continues to transmit a poor quality image that mixes at the retina with the image transmitted through the clear opening. The patient may experience symptoms of blur, glare, or decreased contrast sensitivity.

Figure 44-13 shows an example of a posterior capsulotomy performed without dilation. As the patient looks up, down, left, and right, the laser can be applied to capsular edges behind the sphincter so that the capsulotomy can be perfectly centered. The slit lamp illumination should be with a narrow beam, angled obliquely, to minimize miosis and indicate average pupillary size with ambient dim lighting.

Capsulotomies may also spontaneously enlarge postoperatively. Capone et al.[43] demonstrated that capsulotomies may increase

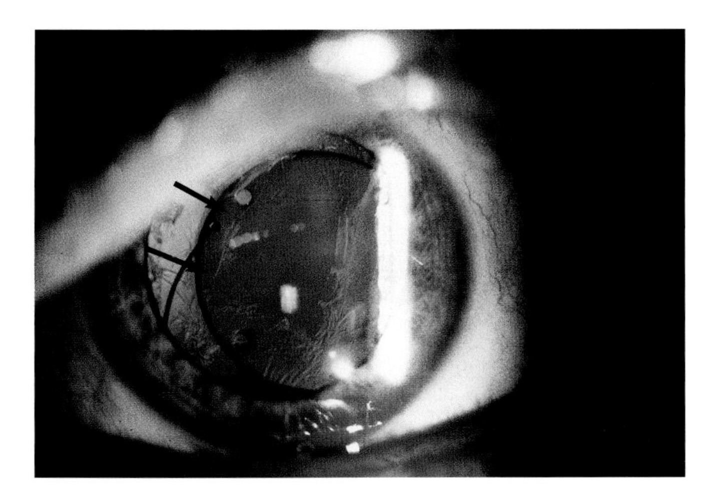

FIGURE 44-11 Posterior capsulotomy performed on a capsule in direct apposition to a lathe-cut posterior chamber IOL. Figure 44-6 is the pretreatment photograph of the same eye. Note the eccentric location of the optic caused by the displacement of the inferior haptic in the bag and the superior haptic in the ciliary sulcus. The capsulotomy is properly located in the visual axis, but care is taken not to extend the opening beyond the edge of the optic to avoid vitreous herniation around the optic *(arrow)*. (From Steiner RF, Puliafito CA: *The Nd:YAG laser in ophthalmology: principles and clinical applications of photodisruption,* Philadelphia, 1985, WB Saunders, p 86.)

in mean area by 32% within 6 weeks and that the capsular enlargement tended toward sphericity with capsular tag retention. Tension created by contractile properties of myofibroblastic lens epithelial cells or by IOL haptics, or both, may cause this alteration in capsulotomy contour.

A capsule with residual haze not only impairs vision under standard conditions but also produces glare. A clinical study of glare after extracapsular cataract extraction substantiated the deleterious effect of capsular opacification.[36] Steinert and Puliafito[44] demonstrated that glare and haze continue to be a problem for 1- and 2-mm capsular openings, decrease with a 3-mm opening, and fully resolve only with a 4-mm capsular opening.

TABLE 44-5
Minimizing Intraocular Lens Laser Marks

Use minimum energy
Use a contact lens to:
Stabilize the eye
Improve laser beam optics
Facilitate accurate focusing
Identify and areas of intraocular lens–capsule separation and begin treatment there
If lens making is occurring, make an opening in the shape of a Christmas tree from the 12 o'clock to the 4:30 position and from the 12 o'clock to the 7:30 position without placing any shots in the central optical zone
Use deep focus techniques:
Optical breakdown occurs in the anterior vitreous
The shock wave radiates forward and ruptures the capsule
Higher energy (2 mJ or more) must be used

POSTOPERATIVE CARE

After Nd:YAG laser posterior capsulotomy in all patients, brimonidine, apraclonidine, or a beta-blocker should be administered topically to minimize any intraocular pressure increase. For high-risk patients, intraocular pressure may be measured again 1 hour following laser treatment. If the patient has significant preexisting glaucomatous disc damage or the intraocular pressure is increased 5 mm Hg or more at 1 hour, the intraocular pressure should also be remeasured at 4 hours.

An increased intraocular pressure may be treated with further brimonidine, apraclonidine, topical beta-adrenergic antagonists, prostaglandin analogue, topical pilocarpine, topical or systemic carbonic anhydrase inhibitor, or hyperosmotic agents. The patient's medical history, allergies, and current ocular therapy

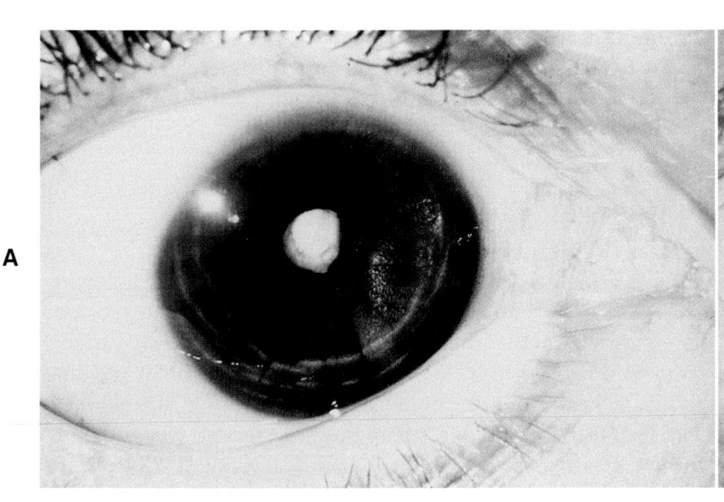

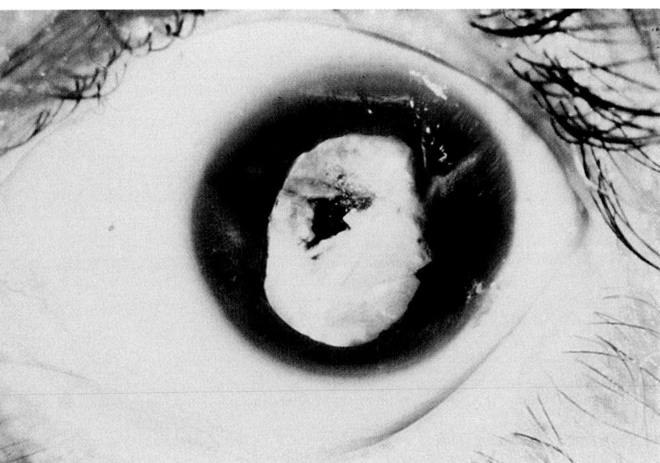

FIGURE 44-12 A, Dense retropupillary membrane after complicated extracapsular cataract extraction. **B,** An adequate membrane opening is well centered on the pupillary axis. (From Steinert RF, Puliafito CA: *The Nd:YAG laser in ophthalmology: principles and clinical applications of photodisruption,* Philadelphia, 1985, WB Saunders, p 92.)

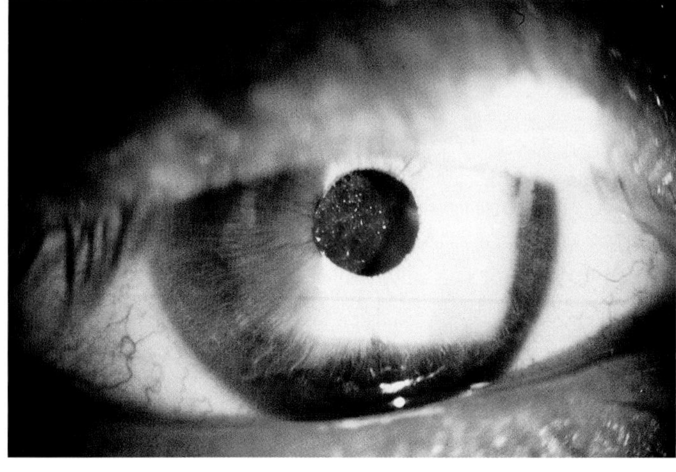

A

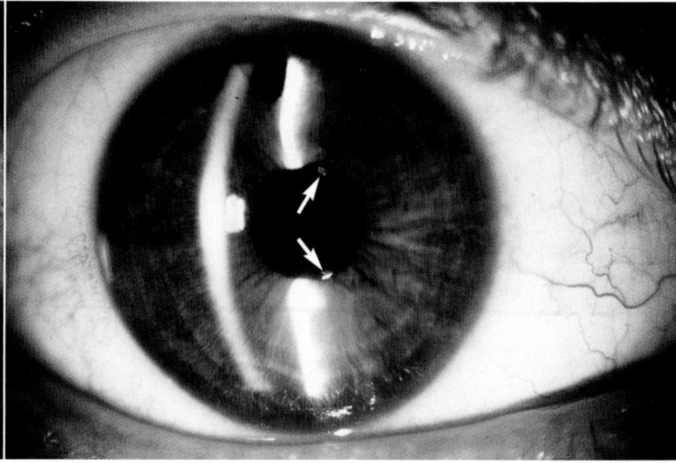

B

FIGURE 44-13 Posterior capsulotomy performed without pupillary dilation. **A,** Hazy capsule before treatment. **B,** After laser application, the pupillary zone is clear. Two tags of capsule at the edge of the pupil can be seen *(arrows)*. These could be easily exposed to the laser by having the patient look up and down. (From Steinert RF, Puliafito CA: *The Nd:YAG laser in ophthalmology: principles and clinical applications of photodisruption,* Philadelphia, 1985, WB Saunders, p 82.)

should be reviewed before determining the appropriate acute antiglaucoma therapy. If the intraocular pressure has increased following the posterior capsulotomy, antiglaucoma therapy should be continued for at least 1 week to prevent a delayed pressure elevation. Intraocular pressure should be measured again about 1 week after laser surgery and sooner if indicated by a pressure increase or preexisting glaucomatous optic nerve damage or visual field loss.

Treatment following laser therapy (Table 44-6) with topical steroids and cycloplegic agents varies widely according to the individual surgeon's experience. Many patients may be managed easily with no therapy following laser treatment. Because a few patients experience iritis, some surgeons favor topical steroids four times daily for one or more postoperative weeks. The topical steroids may usually be discontinued at that point, although some patients may require a tapered dosage.

TABLE 44-6
Care Following Capsulotomy

MEDICATION
Antiglaucoma medications
Apraclonidine immediately following capsulotomy
Optional additional antiglaucoma therapy (beta-adrenergic antagonist, pilocarpine, carbonic anhydrase inhibitor, hyperosmotic agents) as needed for intraocular pressure control
Cycloplegics (optional)
1% cyclopentolate at time of treatment
Steroids (optional)
1% prednisolone or 0.1% dexamethasone four times a day. tapered as needed
MINIMAL SUGGESTED FOLLOW-UP PROTOCOL
1 to 4 hr
Pressure rise to 5 mm Hg: treatment should be given
1 day
1 wk
1 mo
3 mo
6 mo

Results

Nd:YAG laser posterior capsulotomy results in improved visual acuity in 83% to 96% of eyes.[38,45-52] Failure of vision to improve following Nd:YAG laser posterior capsulotomy is often due to preexisting ocular disease, including age-related macular degeneration, CME, other macular disease, retinal detachment, corneal edema, glaucoma, ischemic optic neuropathy, and amblyopia.

Complications

Complications of Nd:YAG laser posterior capsulotomy causing decreased vision are uncommon but include elevated extraocular pressure, CME, retinal detachment, IOL damage, endophthalmitis, iritis, vitritis, macular holes, and corneal edema.

Intraocular Pressure Elevation

Elevated intraocular pressure is recognized as the most common, although usually transient, complication following Nd:YAG laser capsulotomy. The frequency of intraocular pressure elevations greater than 10 mmHg has been variably observed in 15% to 67% of eyes.[53-59] The intraocular pressure typically begins to rise immediately after the laser capsulotomy, peaks at 3 to 4 hours, decreases but may remain elevated at 24 hours, and usually returns to baseline at 1 week.[54] Rarely, the intraocular pressure may remain persistently elevated, causing visual field loss[60,61] or requiring glaucoma surgery, or both. The acute intraocular pressure increase may also be high enough to cause loss of light perception vision.[62] The elevated intraocular pressure following Nd:YAG laser posterior capsulotomy has been associated with preexisting glaucoma,[54,55] capsulotomy size, lack of a posterior chamber IOL,[53,54,57-59] sulcus fixation of a posterior chamber IOL,[63] laser energy required for the capsulotomy,[54-56] myopia,[58] and preexisting vitreoretinal disease.[58] Although not well studied, most surgeons believe that reliable in-the-bag fixation of posterior chamber IOLs has vastly reduced the incidence of clinically significant elevation of intraocular pressure after Nd:YAG laser capsulotomy.

Increased intraocular pressure following Nd:YAG laser capsulotomy is associated with a reduced facility for aqueous humor outflow.[54,64] This reduced facility has been attributed to capsular debris,[65] acute inflammatory cells, liquid vitreous,[58,66] and shock wave damage to the trabecular meshwork.[38] Laboratory studies have demonstrated pigment granules, erythrocytes, fibrin, lymphocytes, and macrophages within the trabecular meshwork after laser capsulotomy,[64] supporting the proposal that acute inflammatory cells and capsular debris are the cause of the increased intraocular pressure. Eyes with preexisting glaucoma may have an increased frequency and magnitude of intraocular pressure elevation following laser treatment because the glaucomatous eyes already have a reduced outflow facility, and further obstruction of the trabecular meshwork results in a marked intraocular pressure increase.

Liquid vitreous as the cause of outflow obstruction has been supported by the clinical association between increased intraocular pressure following laser treatment and myopia,[58] preexisting vitreoretinal disease,[58] lack of a posterior chamber IOL,[53,54,57-59] and sulcus-fixated posterior chamber IOLs.[63] A capsule-fixated posterior chamber IOL and a smaller capsulotomy may provide a barrier effect, preventing liquid vitreous from reaching the anterior chamber and trabecular meshwork. Experimentally, liquid vitreous injected into the anterior chamber in owl monkey eyes was found to increase intraocular pressure.[66]

Nd:YAG laser–induced shock waves causing increased intraocular pressure resulting in damage to the trabecular meshwork is supported clinically by the association between increased intraocular pressure and higher total laser energy used to create the capsulotomy.[54,56] However, photodisruption pulses in the aqueous of the midanterior chamber have not been associated with increased intraocular pressure,[66] nor has there been microscopic evidence of damage to the trabecular cords.[64]

Because increased intraocular pressure is a common complication following laser therapy and can result in permanent loss of vision, prevention of the intraocular pressure increase is appropriate. Apraclonidine,[67,68] brimonidine,[69] timolol,[59,70,71] levobunolol,[71,72] and pilocarpine[57] have been shown to decrease the frequency and magnitude of intraocular pressure increases following laser treatment, although apraclonidine is the most effective. Apraclonidine, timolol, levobunolol, or other beta-adrenergic antagonists are all administered 1 hour before the Nd:YAG laser posterior capsulotomy and again following the procedure. Because of its miotic effect, pilocarpine should only be administered postoperatively. Patients at high risk for intraocular pressure elevation or those with vulnerable optic nerves should be carefully monitored following the laser capsulotomy because prophylactic therapy may not prevent late intraocular pressure increases.[59]

The intraocular pressure following Nd:YAG laser capsulotomy may also be elevated by vitreous obstruction of a sclerostomy,[73] the development of neovascular glaucoma,[74] or pupillary block glaucoma.[75,76]

Ge et al.[77] found evidence that the long-term intraocular pressure may remain elevated above precapsulotomy baseline in patients with existing glaucoma or for whom a high intraocular pressure developed acutely after capsulotomy.

Cystoid Macular Edema

CME has been reported to develop in 0.55% to 2.5% of eyes following Nd:YAG laser posterior capsulotomy.[38,49-51,78-80] CME may occur between 3 weeks and 11 months after the capsulotomy.[80] One prospective study examined fluorescein angiography before and 4 to 8 weeks after Nd:YAG laser posterior capsulotomy in 136 patients and found no CME.[58] This study provides evidence that the incidence of new CME is low following laser capsulotomy, although some patients may acquire CME at a later date than the follow-up fluorescein angiograms performed n this study. Stark et al.[50] concluded that the risk of CME could be lowered by a longer interval between extracapsular cataract extraction and laser capsulotomy, although other studies have not confirmed this.[80] Treatment of CME following Nd:YAG laser posterior capsulotomy is identical to its treatment following cataract extraction and is discussed in Chapter 47.[81]

RETINAL DETACHMENT

Retinal detachment may complicate Nd:YAG laser posterior capsulotomy in 0.08% to 3.6% of eyes.* A retrospective analysis of Medicare claims found that the cumulative probability of retinal detachment over 36 months following cataract surgery was 1.6% to 1.9% in patients who had laser capsulotomy versus 0.8% to 1% in patients undergoing cataract surgery alone.[84] However, this retrospective study could not distinguish if the same or fellow eye had cataract surgery, capsulotomy, and retinal detachment, nor could it determine the sequence. A retinal detachment may occur early after the laser capsulotomy or more than a year later.[80] Asymptomatic retinal breaks were found at a rate of 2.1% within 1 month of posterior capsulotomy in one study.[85] Myopia,[86-89] a history of retinal detachment in the other eye,[88,90] younger age,[86,88] and male sex[88] are risk factors following Nd:YAG laser posterior capsulotomy.

Intraocular Lens Damage

Pitting of IOLs occurs in 15% to 33% of eyes during Nd:YAG laser posterior capsulotomy.[38,50] The pitting usually is not visually significant, although rarely the damage may cause sufficient glare and image degradation that the damaged IOL must be explanted.[91]

The type and extent of lens damage depend on the material used in the IOL. Glass IOLs may be fractured by the Nd:YAG laser.[37,92] PMMA IOLs sustain cracks and central defects with radiating fractures.[93] Molded PMMA IOLs are more easily damaged than higher-molecular-weight lathe-cut lenses.[94]

*References 38 ,47, 49-51, 78-80, 82, 83.

Damage to silicone lenses is characterized by blistered lesions and localized pits surrounded by multiple tiny pits.[93,95]

The damage threshold is lowest for silicone, intermediate for PMMA, and highest for acrylic materials.[96,97] The frequency of the damage depends on the IOL style. IOLs designed with a ridge separating the posterior capsule from the IOL sustain less damage than lenses with a convex posterior surface and close apposition between the posterior chamber IOL and the posterior capsule.[96]

Endophthalmitis

Several cases of *Propionibacterium acnes* endophthalmitis have been reported following Nd:YAG laser posterior capsulotomy.[98-100] The patients were reported to have decreased vision caused by posterior capsular opacification and an otherwise quiet eye. Following the laser capsulotomy, the eyes developed significant uveitis and loss of vision. Presumably, the capsulotomy created an opportunity for the organisms sequestered within the capsule to reach the vitreous and develop into endophthalmitis.

Other Complications

Iritis persisting for 6 months after laser capsulotomy has been reported in less than 1% of eyes.[12,84] Macular holes have rarely been reported to develop after capsulotomy.[78,101] Specular microscopic studies have reported corneal endothelial cell loss of 2.3% to 7% following Nd:YAG laser posterior capsulotomy.[49,102,103]

REFERENCES

1. Aron-Rosa D, Aron JJ, Griesemann M et al: Use of the neodymium-YAG laser to open the posterior capsule after lens implant surgery: a preliminary report, *J Am Intraocul Implant Soc* 6:352, 1980.
2. Aron-Rosa D, Griesemann JC Aron JJ: Use of a pulsed neodymium-YAG laser (picosecond) to open the posterior lens capsule in traumatic cataract: a preliminary report, *Ophthalmic Surg* 12:496, 1981.
3. Fankhauser F, Lortscher J, Van der Zypen E: Clinical studies on high and low power laser radiation upon some structures of the anterior and posterior segments of the eye, *Int Ophthalmol* 5:15, 1982.
4. Wilhelmus KR, Emery JM: Posterior capsule opacification following phacoemulsification. In Emery JM, Jacobson AC, editors: *Current concepts in cataract surgery: selected proceedings of the Sixth Biennial Cataract Surgical Congress,* St Louis, 1980, Mosby, pp 304-380.
5. Baratz KH, Cook BE, Hodge DO: Probability of Nd:YAG laser capsulotomy after cataract surgery in Olmsted County, Minnesota, *Am J Ophthalmol* 131:161-166, 2001.
6. Emery JM, Wilhelmus KR, Rosenberg S: Complications of phacoemulsification, *Ophthalmology* 85:141, 1978.
7. Coonan P, Fung WE, Webster RG et al: The incidence of retinal detachment following extracapsular cataract extraction: a ten-year study, *Ophthalmology* 4:206, 1985.
8. Sinskey RM, Cain W: The posterior capsule and phacoemulsification, *J Am Intraocul Implant Soc* 4:206, 1978.
9. Kraff MC, Sanders DR, Lieberman HL: Total cataract extraction through a 3 mm incision: a report of 650 cases, *Ophthalmic Surg* 10:46, 1979.
10. Wilhelmus KR, Emery JM: Posterior capsule opacification following phacoemulsification, *Ophthalmic Surg* 11:264-267, 1980.
11. Sterling S, Wood TO: Effect of intraocular lens convexity on posterior capsule opacification, *J Cataract Refract Surg* 12:651, 1986.
12. Downing JE: Long term discission rate after placing posterior chamber lenses with the convex surface posterior, *J Cataract Refract Surg* 12:651, 1986.
13. Frezzotti R, Caporossi A: Pathogenesis of posterior capsule opacification. Part I. Epidemiological and clinico-statistical data, *J Cataract Refract Surg* 16:347, 1990.
14. Born CP, Ryan DK: Effect of intraocular lens optic design on posterior capsular opacification, *J Cataract Refract Surg* 16:188, 1990.
15. Davidson MG, Morgan DH, McGahan MC: Effect of surgical technique on in vitro posterior capsule opacification, *J Cataract Refract Surg* 26:1550-1554, 2000.
16. Apple DA, Peng Q, Visessook N et al: Eradication of posterior capsule opacification: documentation of a marked decrease in Nd:YAG laser posterior capsulotomy rates noted in an analysis of 5416 pseudophakic human eyes obtained postmortem, *Ophthalmology* 108: 505-518, 2001.
17. Apple DA, Peng Q, Visessook N et al: Surgical prevention of posterior capsule opacification. Part 1. Progress in eliminating this complication of cataract surgery, *J Cataract Refract Surg* 26:180-187, 2000.
18. Peng Q, Apple DA, Visessook N et al: Surgical prevention of posterior capsule opacification. Part 2. Enhancement of cortical cleanup by focusing on hydrodissection, *J Cataract Refract Surg* 26:188-197, 2000.
19. Peng Q, Visessook N, Apple DA et al: Surgical prevention of posterior capsule opacification. Part 3. Intraocular lens optic barrier effect as a second line of defense, *J Cataract Refract Surg* 26:198-213, 2000.
20. Hollick EJ, Spalton DJ, Ursell PG et al: Posterior capsule opacification with hydrogel, polymethylmethacrylate, and silicone intraocular lenses: two-year results of a randomized prospective trial, *Am J Ophthalmol* 129:577-584, 2000.
21. Wang M-C, Woung L-C: Digital retroilluminated photography to analyze posterior capsule opacification in eyes with intraocular lenses, *J Cataract Refract Surg* 26:56-61, 2000.
22. Hollick EJ, Spalton DJ, Ursell PG et al: The effect of polymethylmethacrylate, silicone, and polyacrylic intraocular lenses on posterior capsule opacification 3 years after cataract surgery, *Ophthalmology* 106:49-55, 1999.
23. Nishi O, Nishi K, Wickstrom K: Preventing lens epithelial cell migration using intraocular lenses with sharp rectangular edges, *J Cataract Refract Surg* 26:1543-1549, 2000.
24. Zaczek A, Zetterstrom C: Posterior capsule opacification after phacoemulsification in patients with diabetes mellitus, *J Cataract Refract Surg* 25:233-237, 1999.
25. Roy FH: After-cataract: clinical and pathological evaluation, *Ann Ophthalmol* 3:1364, 1971.
26. Hiles DA, Johnson BL: The role of the crystalline lens epithelium in post-pseudophakos membrane formation, *J Am Intraocul Implant Soc* 6:141, 1980.
27. McDonnell PJ, Green WR, Maumenee AE et al: Pathology of intraocular lenses in 33 eyes examined postmortem, *Ophthalmology* 90:386, 1983.
28. McDonnell PJ, Stark WJ, Green WR: Posterior capsule opacification: a specular microscopic study, *Ophthalmology* 91:853, 1984.
29. Cobo ML, Ohsawa E, Chandler D et al: Pathogenesis of capsular opacification after extracapsular cataract extraction: an animal model, *Ophthalmology* 91:851, 1984.
30. Nishi O: Posterior capsule opacification. Part 1. Experimental investigations, *J Cataract Refract Surg* 25:106-117, 1999.
31. McDonnell PJ, Zarbin MA, Green WR: Posterior capsule opacification in pseudophakic eyes, *Ophthalmology* 90:1548, 1983.
32. Chan RY, Emery JM, Kretzer F: Mitotic inhibitors in preventing posterior lens capsule opacification. In Emery JM, Jacobson AC, editors: *Current concepts in cataract surgery: selected proceedings of the Seventh Biennial Cataract Surgical Congress,* New York, 1982, Appleton-Century-Crofts, pp. 217-224.
33. Clark DS, Emery JM, Munsell MF: Inhibition of posterior capsule opacification with an immunotoxin specific for lens epithelial cells: 24 month clinical results, *J Cataract Refract Surg* 24:1614-1620, 1998.
34. Nishi O, Nishi K, Menapace R: Capsule-bending ring for the prevention of capsule opacification: a preliminary report, *Ophthalmic Surg Lasers* 29:749-753, 1998.
35. Tan DTH, Chee SP: Early central posterior capsular fibrosis in sulcus-fixated biconvex intraocular lenses, *J Cataract Refract Surg* 19:471, 1993.
36. Nadler DJ, Jaffee NS, Clayman HM et al: Glare disability in eyes with intraocular lenses, *Am J Ophthalmol* 97:43, 1984.
37. Riggins J, Pedrotti LS, Keates RH: Evaluation of the neodymium:YAG laser for treatment of ocular opacities, *Ophthalmic Surg* 14:675, 1983.
38. Keates RH, Steinert RF, Puliafito CA et al: Long-term follow-up of Nd-YAG laser posterior capsulotomy, *J Am Intraocul Implant Soc* 10:164, 1984.
39. Faulkner W: Laser interferometric prediction of postoperative visual acuity in patients with cataracts, *Am J Ophthalmol* 95:626, 1983.
40. Klein TB, Slomovic AR, Parrish RK II et al: Visual acuity prediction before neodymium-YAG laser posterior capsulotomy, *Ophthalmology* 93:808, 1986.

41. Smiddy WE, Radulovic D, Yeo JH et al: Potential acuity meter for predicting visual acuity after neodymium:YAG posterior capsulotomy, *Ophthalmology* 93:397, 1986.
42. Dickerson DE, Gilmore JE, Gross J: The Abraham lens with the neodymium-YAG laser, *J Am Intraocul Implant Soc* 9:438, 1983.
43. Capone A, Rehkopf PG, Warnicki JW et al: Temporal changes in posterior capsulotomy dimensions following neodymium:YAG laser discission, *J Cataract Refract Surg* 16:451, 1990.
44. Steinert RF, Puliafito CA: Posterior capsulotomy and pupillary membranectomy. In Steinert RF, Puliafito CA, editors: *The Nd-YAG laser in ophthalmology: principles and clinical applications of photodisruption,* Philadelphia, 1985, WB Saunders, pp 72-95.
45. Aron-Rosa DS, Aron J-J, Cohn HC: Use of a pulsed picosecond Nd:YAG laser in 6,664 cases, *J Am Intraocul Implant Soc* 10:35, 1984.
46. Aron-Rosa DS: Posterior capsulotomy and picosecond pulsed YAG laser influence on eye pressure, *Cataract* 1:13, 1983.
47. Aron-Rosa DS: Pulsed picosecond pulsed and nanosecond YAG lasers: principles and uses, *Cataract* 1:9, 1984.
48. Terry AC, Apple DJ, Price FW, et al: Neodymium-YAG laser for posterior capsulotomy, *Am J Ophthalmol* 96: 716, 1983.
49. Johnson SH, Kratz RP, Olson PF: Clinical experience with the Nd:YAG laser, *J Am Intraocul Implant Soc* 10:452, 1984.
50. Stark WJ, Worthen D, Holladay JT et al: Neodymium:YAG lasers: an FDA report, *Ophthalmology* 92:209, 1985.
51. Bath PE, Fankhauser F: Long-term results of Nd:YAG laser posterior capsulotomy with the Swiss laser, *J Cataract Refract Surg* 12:150, 1986.
52. Wasserman EL, Axt JC, Sheets JH: Neodymium-YAG laser posterior capsulotomy, *J Am Intraocul Implant Soc J* 11:245, 1985.
53. Slomovic AR, Parrish RK II: Acute elevations of intraocular pressure following Nd:YAG laser posterior capsulotomy, *Ophthalmology* 92:973, 1985.
54. Richter CU, Arzeno G, Pappas H et al: Intraocular pressure elevation following Nd:YAG laser posterior capsulotomy, *Ophthalmology* 92:636, 1985.
55. Flohr MJ, Robin AL, Kelley JS: Early complications following Q-switched neodymium:YAG laser posterior capsulotomy, *Ophthalmology* 92:360, 1985.
56. Chanell MM, Beckman H: Intraocular pressure changes after neodymium:YAG laser posterior capsulotomy, *Arch Ophthalmol* 102:1024, 1984.
57. Brown SVL, Thomas JV, Belcher CD et al: Effect of pilocarpine in treatment of intraocular pressure following neodymium:YAG laser posterior capsulotomy, *Ophthalmology* 392:354, 1985.
58. Schubert HD: Vitreoretinal changes associated with rise in intraocular pressure after Nd:YAG laser capsulotomy, *Ophthalmic Surg* 18:19, 1987.
59. Migliori ME, Beckman H, Channell MM: Intraocular pressure changes after following neodymium:YAG laser capsulotomy in eyes pretreated with timolol, *Arch Ophthalmol* 105:473, 1987.
60. Demer JL, Koch DD, Smith JA et al: Persistent elevation in intraocular pressure after Nd:YAG laser treatment, *Ophthalmic Surg* 17:465, 1986.
61. Kurata F, Krupin T, Sinclair S et al: Progressive glaucomatous visual field loss after neodymium:YAG laser capsulotomy, *Am J Ophthalmol* 98:632, 1984.
62. Vine AK: Ocular hypertension following Nd-YAG laser capsulotomy: a potentially blinding complication, *Ophthalmic Surg* 15:283, 1984.
63. Gimbel HV, Van Westenbrugge JA, Sanders DR et al: Effects of sulcus vs. capsular fixation on YAG-induced pressure rises following posterior capsulotomy, *Arch Ophthalmol* 108:1126, 1990.
64. Lynch MG, Quigley HA, Green WR et al: The effect of neodymium:YAG laser capsulotomy on aqueous humor dynamics in the monkey eye, *Ophthalmology* 93:1270, 1986.
65. Altamirano D, Mermoud A, Pittet T et al: Aqueous humor analysis after Nd:YAG laser capsulotomy with the laser flare-cell meter, *J Cataract Refract Surg* 18:554, 1992.
66. Schubert HD, Morris WJ, Trokel SL et al: The role of the vitreous in the intraocular pressure rise after neodymium-YAG laser capsulotomy, *Arch Ophthalmol* 103:1538, 1985.
67. Pollack IP, Brown RH, Crandall AS et al: Prevention of the rise in intraocular pressure following neodymium-YAG laser posterior capsulotomy using topical 1% apraclonidine, *Arch Ophthalmol* 106:754, 1988.
68. Rosenberg LF, Krupin T, Ruderman J et al: Apraclonidine and anterior segment surgery: comparison of 0.5% vs 1.0% apraclonidine for prevention of postoperative intraocular pressure rise, *Ophthalmology* 102:1312-1318, 1995.
69. Gartaganis SP, Mela EK, Katsimpris JM et al: Use of topical brimonidine to prevent intraocular pressure elevations following Nd:YAG laser posterior capsulotomy, *Ophthalmic Surg Lasers* 30:647-652, 1999.
70. Richter CU, Arzeno G, Pappas HR et al: Prevention of intraocular pressure elevation following neodymium-YAG laser posterior capsulotomy, *Arch Ophthalmol* 103:912, 1985.
71. Rakofsky S, Koch DD, Faulkner JD et al: Levobunolol 0.5% and timolol 0.5% to prevent intraocular pressure elevation after neodymium:YAG laser posterior capsulotomy, *J Cataract Refract Surg* 23:1075-1080, 1997.
72. Silverstone DE, Novack GD, Kelley EP et al: Prophylactic treatment of intraocular pressure elevations after neodymium-YAG laser posterior capsulotomies and extracapsular cataract extractions with levobunolol, *Ophthalmology* 95:713, 1988.
73. Schrader CE, Belcher CD III, Thomas JV et al: Acute glaucoma following Nd-YAG laser membranotomy, *Ophthalmic Surg* 14:1015, 1983.
74. Weinreb RN, Wasserstrom JP, Parker W: Neovascular glaucoma following neodymium-YAG laser posterior capsulotomy, *Arch Ophthalmol* 104:730, 1986.
75. Gstalder RJ: Pupillary block with anterior chamber lens following Nd:YAG laser capsulotomy, *Ophthalmic Surg* 17:249, 1986.
76. Ruderman JM, Mitchell PG, Kraff M: Pupillary block following Nd-YAG laser capsulotomy, *Ophthalmic Surg* 14:1418, 1983.
77. Ge J, Wand M, Chiang R, Paranhos A et al: Long-term effect of Nd:YAG laser posterior capsulotomy on intraocular pressure, *Arch Ophthalmol* 118:1334-1337, 2000.
78. Winslow RL, Taylor BC: Retinal complications following YAG capsulotomy. *Ophthalmology* 92:785, 1985.
79. Chambless WS: Neodymium:YAG laser posterior capsulotomy results and complications, *J Am Intraocul Implant Soc* J 11:31, 1985.
80. Steinert RF, Puliafito CA, Kumar SR et al: Cystoid macular edema, retinal detachment, and glaucoma after Nd:YAG laser posterior capsulotomy, *Am J Ophthalmol* 112:373, 1991.
81. Lewis H, Singer TR, Hanscom TA et al: A prospective study of cystoid macular edema after neodymium:YAG laser posterior capsulotomy, *Ophthalmology* 94:478, 1987.
82. Liesegang TJ, Bourne WM, Ikstrup DM: Secondary surgical and neodymium:YAG laser discissions, *Am J Ophthalmol* 100:510, 1985.
83. Rickman-Barger L, Florine CW, Larson RS et al: Retinal detachment after neodymium:YAG laser posterior capsulotomy, *Am J Ophthalmol* 107:531, 1989.
84. Javitt JC, Tielsch JM, Canner JK et al: National outcomes of cataract extraction: increased risk of retinal complications associated with Nd:YAG laser posterior capsulotomy, *Ophthalmology* 99:1487, 1992.
85. Ranta P, Tommila T, Immonen I, Summanen P et al: Retinal breaks before and after neodymium:YAG laser posterior capsulotomy, *J Cataract Refract Surg* 26:1190-1197, 2000.
86. Koch DD, Liu JF, Gill EP et al: Axial myopia increases the risk of retinal complications after neodymium:YAG laser posterior capsulotomy, *Arch Ophthalmol* 107:986, 1989.
87. Dardenne MU, Gerten GJ, Kokkas K et al: Retrospective study of retinal detachment following neodymium:YAG laser posterior capsulotomy, *J Cataract Refract Surg* 15:676, 1989.
88. Davison JA: Retinal tears and detachments after extracapsular cataract surgery, *J Cataract Refract Surg* 14:624, 1988.
89. Jacobi FK, Hessemer V: Pseudophakic retinal detachment in high axial myopia, *J Cataract Refract Surg* 23:1096-1102, 1997.
90. Shah GR, Gills JP, Durham DG et al: Three thousand YAG lasers in posterior capsulotomies: an analysis of complications and comparing to polishing and surgical discission. *Ophthalmic Surg* 17:473, 1986.
91. Bath PE, Hoffer KJ, Aron-Rosa D et al: Glare disability secondary to YAG laser intraocular lens damage, *J Cataract Refract Surg* 13:309, 1987.
92. Fritch CD: Neodymium:YAG laser damage to glass intraocular lens, *J Am Intraocul Implant Soc* 10:225, 1984.
93. Joo C-K, Kim J-H: Effect of neodymium:YAG laser photodisruption on intraocular lenses in vitro, *Am J Cataract Refract Surg* 18:562, 1992.
94. Downing JE, Alberhasky JT: Biconvex intraocular lenses and Nd:YAG capsulotomy: experimental comparison of surface damage with different poly(methylmethacralate) formulations, *J Cataract Refract Surg* 16:732, 1990.
95. Keates RH, Sall KN, Kreter JK: Effect of the Nd:YAG laser on polymethylmethacrylate, HEMA copolymer, and silicone intraocular materials, *J Cataract Refract Surg* 13:401, 1987.
96. Fallor MK, Hoft RK: Intraocular lens damage associated with posterior capsulotomy: a comparison of intraocular lens designs and four different Nd:YAG laser instruments, *J Am Intraocul Implant Soc J* 11:564, 1985.
97. Newland TJ, McDermott ML, Eliott D et al: Experimental neodymium:YAG laser damage to acrylic, poly(methylmethacrylate), and silicone intraocular lenses, *J Cataract Refract Surg* 25:72-76, 1999.

98. Tetz MR, Apple DJ, Price FW et al: A newly described complication of neodymium:YAG laser capsulotomy: exacerbation of an intraocular infection, *Arch Ophthalmol* 105:1324, 1987.
99. Piest KL, Kincaid MC, Tetz MR et al: Localized endophthalmitis: a newly described cause of the so-called toxic lens syndrome, *J Cataract Refract Surg* 13:498, 1987.
100. Carlson AN, Koch DD: Endophthalmitis following Nd:YAG laser posterior capsulotomy, *Ophthalmic Surg* 19:168, 1988.
101. Blacharski, PA, Newsome DA: Bilateral macular holes after Nd:YAG laser posterior capsulotomy, *Am J Ophthalmol* 105:417, 1988.
102. Slomovic AR, Parrish RK II, Forster RK et al: Neodymium-YAG laser posterior capsulotomy: central corneal endothelial cell density, *Arch Ophthalmol* 104:536, 1986.
103. Schrems W, Belcher CD III, Tomlinson CP: Changes in the human central corneal endothelium after neodymium:YAG laser surgery, *Ophthalmic Laser Ther* 1:143, 1986.

Neodymium:Yttrium-Aluminum-Garnet Laser in the Management of Postoperative Complications of Cataract Surgery

45

Roger F. Steinert, MD

Photodisruption with the neodymium:yttrium-aluminum-garnet (Nd:YAG) laser can effectively treat a number of disorders arising after cataract surgery and intraocular lens (IOL) implantation. The pressure wave generated by optical breakdown of an Nd:YAG laser pulse allows the surgeon to cut and manipulate intraocular structures in a variety of postoperative disorders.

Pupillary Block Glaucoma

Acute angle closure glaucoma in aphakia and pseudophakia may take several forms, as outlined in Table 45-1.[1,2] Corneal edema and haze, anterior chamber reaction, and iris congestion may make argon laser iridectomy impossible. Even if a patent iridectomy is formed, an argon laser iridectomy may not relieve the glaucoma because of the role of the vitreous. In many cases, the Nd:YAG laser can better treat these conditions and is the treatment of first choice.[3] The success of the Nd:YAG laser "anterior hyaloidotomy" in curing ciliovitreal block glaucoma, in which surgical and argon iridectomies have failed, demonstrates the pathophysiologic role of the anterior hyaloid face in many cases of pupillary block glaucoma.

Figure 45-1 illustrates a case of pupillary block in a patient who had an iridectomy and antibiotic therapy for endophthalmitis after complex extracapsular cataract extraction with an anterior chamber IOL (AC IOL). The surgical iridectomy became occluded postoperatively, but an argon laser iridotomy succeeded in relieving the resultant iris bombé. Within weeks, the argon laser iridotomy closed, and the iris bombé recurred with an intraocular pressure of 50 mm Hg. The Nd:YAG laser at 4 mJ readily created several new iridotomies with permanent relief of the iris bombé and pressure elevation. The pupillary membrane also was cleared by the Nd:YAG laser.

The most common setting for pseudophakic block is after placement of an AC IOL, typically after complicated extracapsular cataract extraction or phacoemulsification. The risk of pupillary block is heightened when the surgeon fails to place a large surgical iridectomy. Even after a large anterior vitrectomy, further vitreous may prolapse and occlude the pupil against the optic of the AC IOL. A large surgical iridectomy may also be occluded by prolapsing vitreous, of course, as well as by capsular and cortical remnants.

The role of the hyaloid face in aphakic malignant glaucoma is clearly illustrated by the case shown in Figure 45-2. Three months after complicated cataract extraction and subsequent IOL removal in a patient who also had a large superior loss of iris, the chamber nevertheless became shallow, and the pressure rose to 34 mm Hg over several days, with the onset of deep pain. A thin, intact hyaloid face or inflammatory membrane was present. The patient was treated with the Nd:YAG laser, which was focused and fired at 3 mJ on the hyaloid face through the mild corneal edema despite less than 1 mm of residual anterior chamber depth. The anterior chamber deepened immediately.

Technique for Aphakic and Pseudophakic Iridectomy and Anterior Hyaloid Vitreolysis

Preparation of the Patient

In many cases, the patient will have been treated maximally with miotic agents. If not, application of a miotic agent such as pilocarpine 2% is advisable to place the iris on maximal stretch.

Procedure

Four to 8 mJ is usually adequate to perforate the iris in one pulse. Corneal edema or an anterior chamber reaction may necessitate higher energy to obtain the same optical breakdown cutting power. In most cases, at least three iridotomies should be made to ensure full relief of aqueous entrapment, which may be localized into sectors around an AC IOL, and to increase the chance of maintaining at least one long-term patent iridotomy. Iridotomies tend to shrink as bombé is relieved, and the iris falls back. Inflammation also may close iridotomies postoperatively.

If the chamber is markedly shallow or flat, the haptic of an AC IOL, when present, usually provides a small area of clearance from the cornea. The first laser shots can be made immediately adjacent to such a haptic insertion to avoid corneal injury.

After the iridotomy has been completed or when a patent basal surgical iridectomy is already present, the Nd:YAG laser should be fired into the anterior vitreous through the iridectomy

Portions of the text and figures have previously been published in Steinert RF, Puliafito CA: *The Nd:YAG laser in ophthalmology: principles and clinical applications of photodisruption,* Philadelphia, 1985, WB Saunders.

TABLE 45-1
Classification of Acute Aphakic and Pseudophakic Glaucoma

PUPILLARY BLOCK (IRIDOVITREAL BLOCK)
Absent, imperforate, or secluded peripheral Iridectomies Inflammatory adhesion of intact hyaloid face to iris
Anterior chamber hemorrhage and exudate
APHAKIC MALIGNANT GLAUCOMA (CILIOVITREAL BLOCK)
Posterior diversion of aqueous

or the pupil. This procedure ruptures the hyaloid face and relieves any malignant glaucoma component caused by the intact hyaloid face.

Postoperative Care

Intense topical steroid therapy such as prednisolone acetate 1%, or dexamethasone 0.1%, is used at least four times daily and more often as inflammation requires. Inflammation and a tendency for synechia formation also require cycloplegia and mydriasis. Intraocular pressure must be monitored and treated appropriately

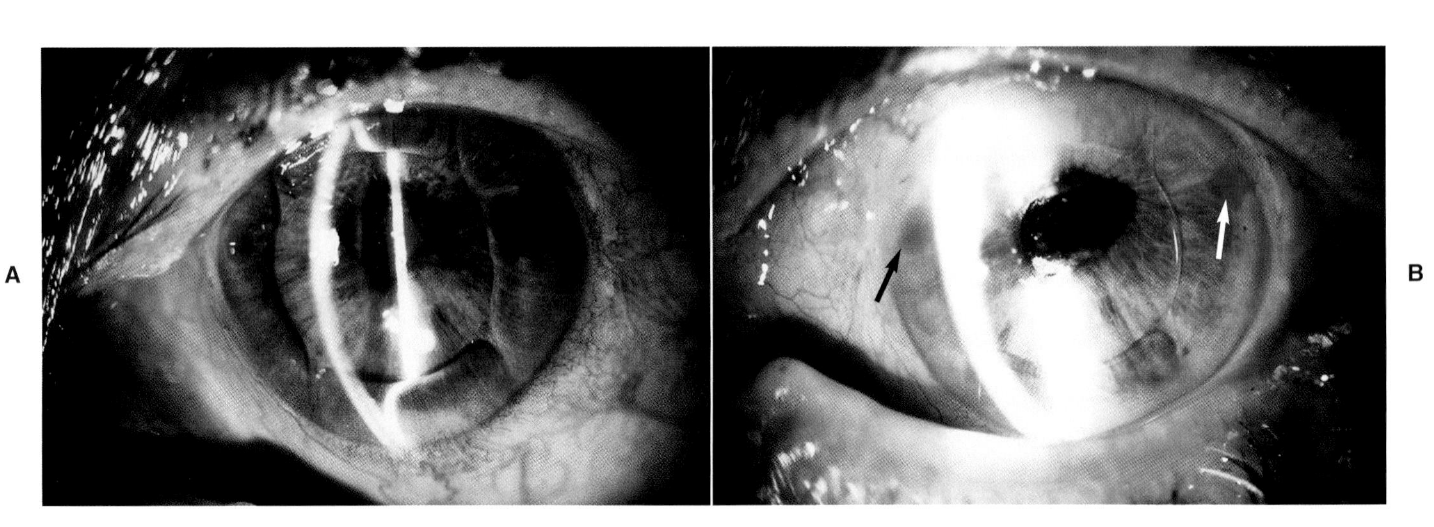

FIGURE 45-1 A, Recurrent pseudophakic pupillary block with iris bombé after endophthalmitis and closure of argon laser iridectomy. **B,** Nd:YAG laser at 4 mJ readily created several iridectomies *(arrows)* with permanent relief of the iris bombé. A pupillary membranectomy was also performed. (From Steinert RF, Puliafito CA: *The Nd:YAG laser in ophthalmology: principles and clinical application of photodisruption,* Philadelphia, 1985, WB Saunders, p 106.)

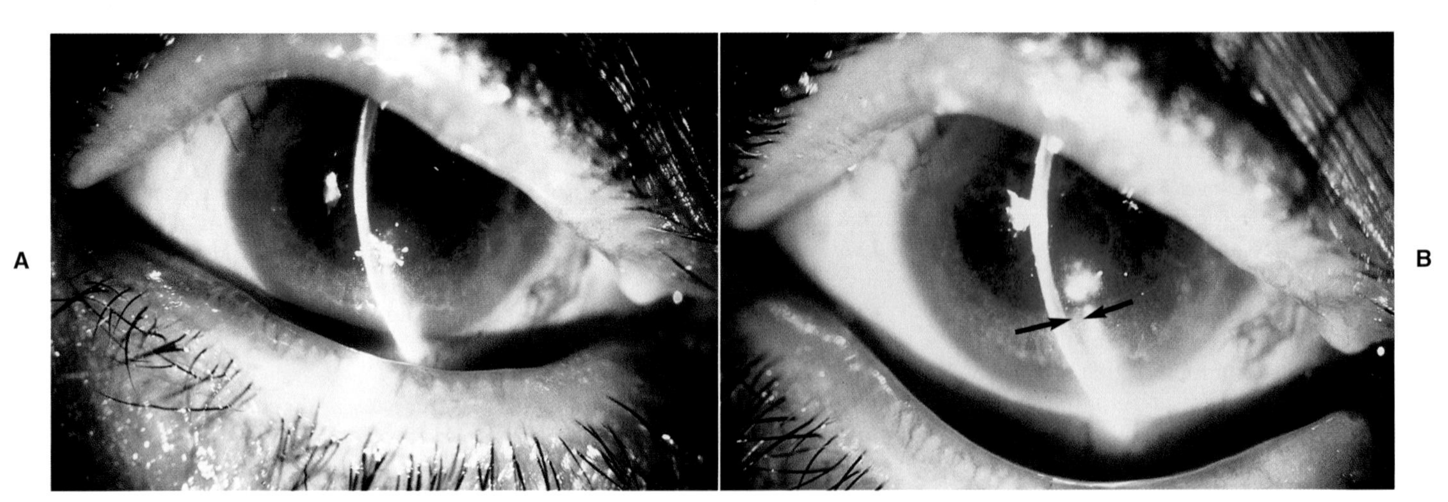

FIGURE 45-2 A, Aphakic malignant glaucoma with apposition of inferior iris to edematous cornea. **B,** Depth is restored to the anterior chamber immediately after Nd:YAG laser pulses have opened the anterior hyaloid face. *Arrows* show separation of iris and cornea, in comparison with part **A.** (From Steinert RF, Puliafito CA: *The Nd:YAG laser in ophthalmology: principles and clinical applications of photodisruption,* Philadelphia, 1985, WB Saunders, p XII.)

Anterior Vitreolysis and Cystoid Macular Edema

Vitreous strands and bands to the wound may cause eccentric pupils and can be associated with cystoid macular edema (CME) (Irvine-Gass CME).[4,5] Iliff[6] first reported visual improvement after surgical section of such vitreous bands to the wound. He coined the term *vitreous-tug syndrome*, although no evidence was given that tugging on the vitreous body was, in fact, present or responsible for the visual loss.

Katzen, Fleischman, and Trokel[7] first reported the use of the Nd:YAG laser to lyse strands of vitreous to cataract wounds in their series. Vision improved by variable amounts in all 14 patients treated. However, the presence of CME was judged clinically, and the results of fluorescein angiography before and after laser treatment were not reported for 13 of the eyes.

Because of the unpredictable natural history of aphakic CME, with erratic response to antiinflammatory agents and frequent spontaneous improvement,[8,9] small and controlled series cannot unequivocally prove the efficacy of a given technique. However, my clinical experience has confirmed a high rate of visual improvement after anterior segment vitreolysis, particularly in favorable cases.[10] In that series of 29 patients, 22 of the patients had fluorescein angiographic confirmation of the presence of CME before laser treatment. The interval between cataract extraction and treatment averaged 10 months, with a range of 1 to 42 months; average follow-up after laser vitreolysis was also 10 months, with a range of 3 to 27 months.

The change in best-corrected Snellen acuity is shown in Figure 45-3. No patient had loss of vision after laser vitreolysis.

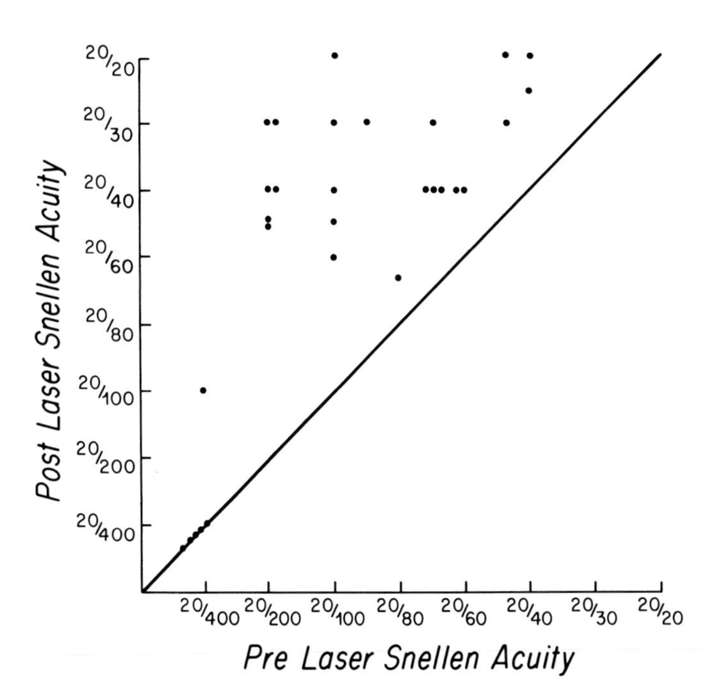

FIGURE 45-3 Scattergram of visual acuity level before and after Nd:YAG laser vitreolysis. Points above the diagonal line represent improvement. (From Steinert RF, Wasson PJ: Neodymium:YAG laser anterior vitreolysis for Irvine-Gass cystoid macular edema, *J Cataract Refract Surg* 15:304-307, 1989.)

The visual acuity in 16 of the 29 patients (55%) improved by two or more lines, with stable acuity following treatments. Five (17%) patients' vision improved by at least two lines, but they experienced ongoing fluctuation of acuity. Vision in 8 patients (28%) showed less than two lines of improvement. Of these 8 patients, 2 had progressive maculopathy in addition to the CME (1 had an epiretinal membrane and one had progressive diabetic maculopathy), 2 had severe glaucoma with loss of central vision in addition to the CME, and 2 had persistent CME. Two other patients were lost to follow-up without documentation of the basis for persistent unimproved acuity. Of note, patients who did not respond to vitreolysis had the poorest pretreatment visual acuity measurements.

Postlaser fluorescein angiography was performed on nine eyes. Three eyes showed complete resolution of the CME, two showed improvement but persistent leakage, one showed an unimproved appearance of the fluorescein angiographic leakage but still experienced improved acuity, and three had persistent CME and less than two lines of visual improvement.

Techniques for Anterior Vitreolysis

Preoperative Assessment

The evaluation and medical treatment of CME are reviewed in detail in Chapter 47. A comprehensive examination including fluorescein angiography should be performed to establish a definitive diagnosis of CME.

Small vitreous strands may be missed on casual examination. The strand is usually best seen on slit lamp examination with a narrow slit beam in a darkened room. Careful gonioscopy may be necessary to visualize the strand, particularly if the vitreous enters the anterior chamber through the area of a peripheral iridectomy. The most favorable cases for Nd:YAG laser vitreolysis are those with relatively discrete strands under tension. Broad bands are most difficult to fully transect. Amorphous vitreous herniation is extremely difficult to cut with a laser approach. In general, the larger the amount of vitreous involvement, the more consideration should be given to pars plana vitrectomy for definitive removal of all pathologic vitreous.

Pupillary distortion may be subtle. Figure 45-4, *A*, shows mild peaking of a pupil, indicating a vitreous strand coming around the pupil. After vitreolysis, less peaking is present, although some permanent change has occurred in the sphincter, preventing complete rounding of the pupil, as seen in Figure 45-4, *B*. Permanent changes in the iris stroma are frequent in cases of long duration. Figure 45-5 shows the decreased but persistent oval shape of the pupil after lysis of a vitreous strand. The iris stroma is partially depigmented locally, perhaps indicating chafing of the iris by the vitreous strand. The vitreous band may distort the pupil in several ways, depending on the angle, direction, and number of vitreous strands under tension. Figure 45-6 shows a "hammock" effect by two separate strands.

Preparation of the Patient

The procedure should be explained beforehand and informed consent obtained. The patient should be told that the procedure often requires more than one session.

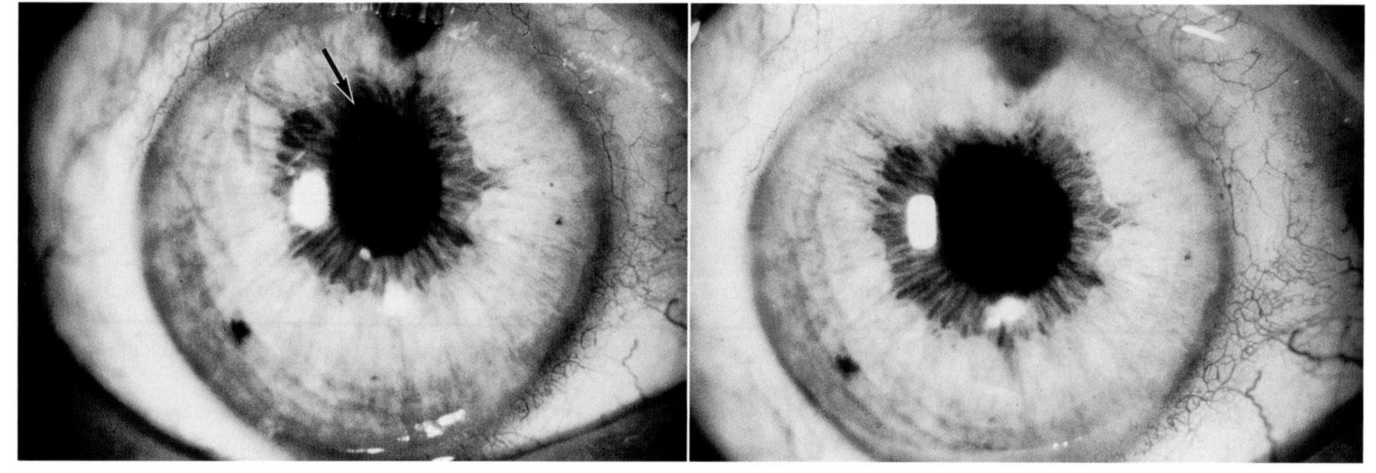

FIGURE 45-4 **A,** Fine vitreous strand caused mild peaking of the pupil *(arrow)*. Gonioscopy showed a fine vitreous strand to the wound. **B,** After laser vitreolysis, less peaking is present, but chronic change in the sphincter prevents a completely normal pupillary contour. (From Steinert RF, Puliafito CA: *The Nd:YAG laser in ophthalmology: principles and clinical applications of photodisruption,* Philadelphia, 1985, WB Saunders, p 120.)

When the vitreous strand or band passes through the pupil, treatment is often facilitated by administration of pilocarpine 2% every 10 minutes for three or four drops preoperatively. Inducing stretch of the vitreous through miosis facilitates identification of the strand. Moreover, release of tension when the laser transects the strand is shown more definitively.

Procedure

Figure 45-7 illustrates the three most common configurations of vitreous to the wound: (1) a small discrete strand, (2) a broad band, and (3) a band with either adhesions to the iris or iris entrapment behind the band.

The laser can be directed at a vitreous strand in four general areas (*inset*, Figure 45-7, *A*). The most reliable landmark during vitreolysis is the cataract wound because the vitreous band or strand has to terminate at that location. The cataract wound is visualized with a gonioscopy lens (pathway 1 on figure), and the laser can be fired at the wound area with a reasonable chance of successful vitreolysis. Because of the contact lens and mirror optics, the energy settings are usually in the 6- to 12-mJ range to obtain adequate cutting power. The disadvantages of this technique include the requirement of a gonioscopy lens, which involves some extra manipulation and positioning requirements, and the subsequent commitment to use a contact lens for the completion of the treatment session, even if a different approach is needed later in the session, because of the application of gonioscopy fluid to the cornea.

If the cornea is clear near the limbus and a vitreous strand can be visualized with some clearance from the iris stroma,

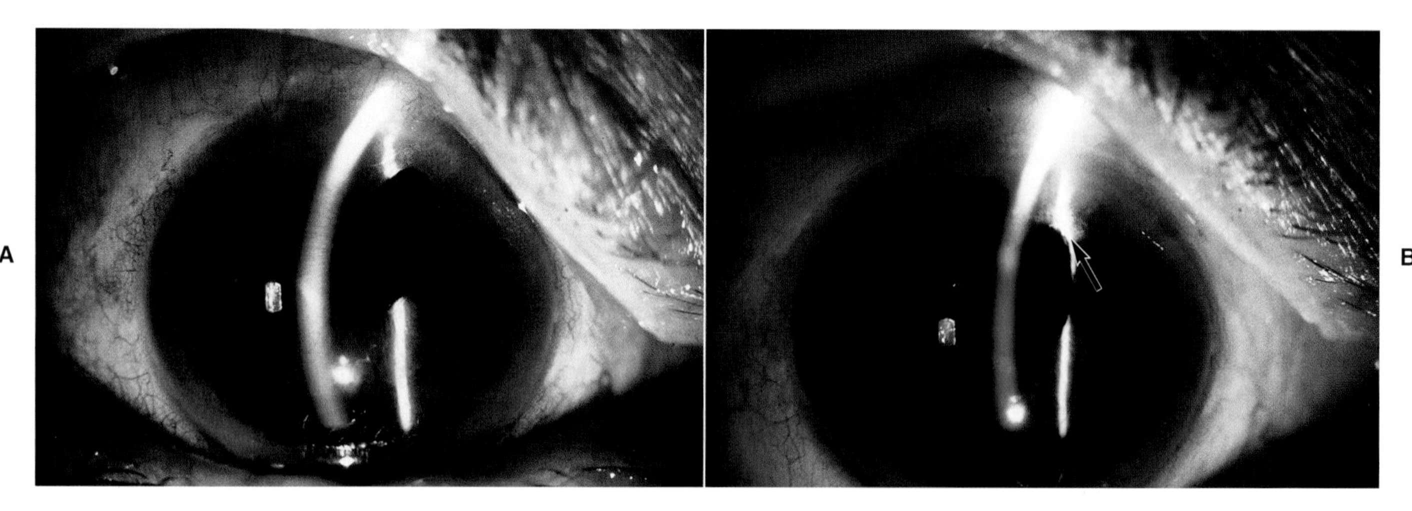

FIGURE 45-5 **A,** Eccentric pupil caused by a vitreous strand. **B,** After vitreolysis, depigmentation of the underlying iris stroma, present before the laser treatment, is more readily seen *(arrow)*, and the pupil remains partially distorted. (From Steinert RF, Puliafito CA: *The Nd:YAG laser in ophthalmology: principles and clinical applications of photodisruption,* Philadelphia, 1985, WB Saunders, p 120.)

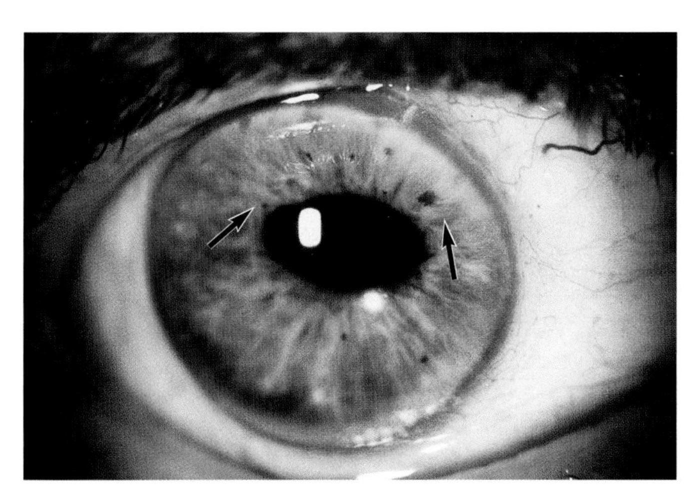

FIGURE 45-6 Pupillary distortion caused by two separate strands of vitreous to the wound *(arrows)*. The pupil became round after treatment. Despite CME of 57 months' duration, vision improved from counting-fingers level to 20/50. (From Steinert RF, Puliafito CA: *The Nd:YAG laser in ophthalmology: principles and clinical applications of photodisruption,* Philadelphia, 1985, WB Saunders, p 116.)

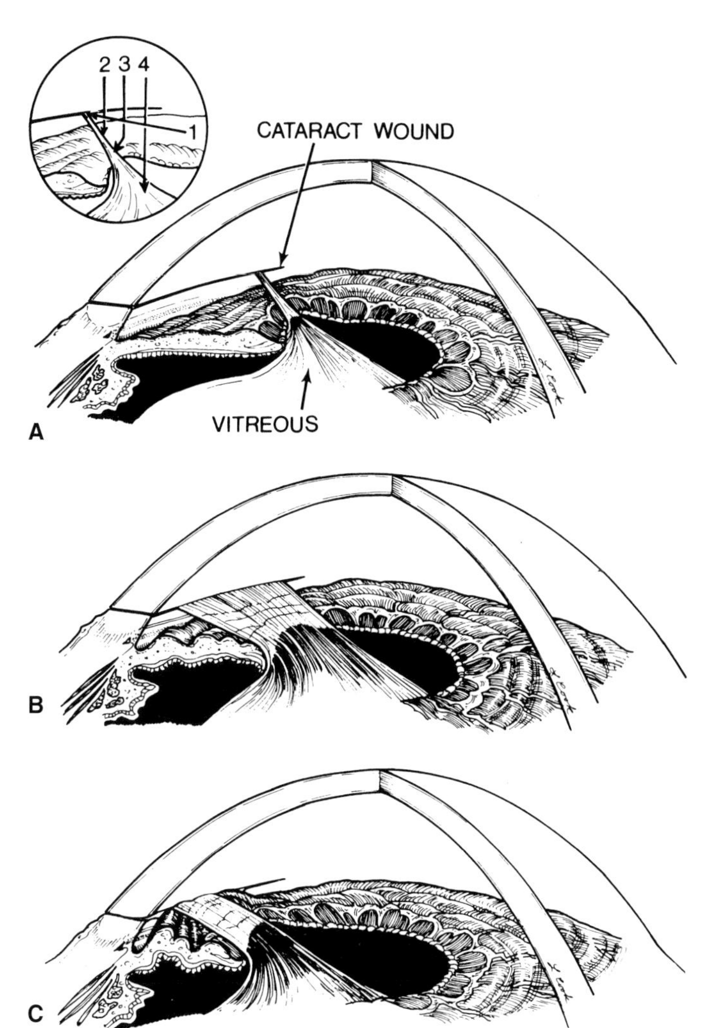

FIGURE 45-7 **A,** A narrow vitreous strand to a cataract wound. The inset shows possible laser pathways for vitreolysis: (1) a gonioscopic approach, directed at the cataract wound—the location at which the vitreous strand is often the most discrete; (2) a direct approach near the limbus; (3) a direct approach in the region of the collarette; and (4) a direct approach at the pupil. This last approach is rarely successful. **B,** A broad vitreous band at the wound. **C,** Iris pulled upward in a tentlike configuration and entrapped by the vitreous incarceration in the wound. (From Steinert RF, Puliafito CA: *The Nd:YAG laser in ophthalmology: principles and clinical applications of photodisruption,* Philadelphia, 1985, WB Saunders, p 122.)

direct cutting without a contact lens or with a peripheral button Abraham lens may be successful along pathway 2 (see Figure 45-7). Usually 4 to 8 mJ is required. In the course of dozens to hundreds of shots along this pathway, considerable pigment may be liberated from the underlying iris stroma, which will ultimately obscure the surgeon's view. Misfocused shots can cause local damage to the underlying or overlying stroma.

Occasionally the use of pathway 3 (see Figure 45-7), directed at the vitreous passing over the iris collarette, can be helpful. This is particularly true when the vitreous has formed adhesions to the collarette, pulling it forward in a tentlike formation. Close proximity of vitreous and iris makes damage to the underlying iris stroma likely, but this may be clinically tolerable.

The use of pathway 4 (see Figure 45-7), directed at the vitreous as it passes around the pupil, is tempting but rarely successful. Vitreous traction components are poorly defined as they come around the pupil. The shock wave is ineffective at rupturing vitreous strands except directly at the laser focal point. Firing the laser immediately adjacent to the pupillary border inevitably causes low-grade capillary hemorrhage, as well as the release of pigment, obscuring further visualization of the area.

Successful treatment releases the tension and converts a discrete strand or band to an amorphous gelatinous appearance. Observation of the change and any iris deformation is the best indicator of a successful release of tension. Hundreds of shots over several treatment sessions may be necessary to cut a large band.

Postoperative Care

Strong topical steroids such as prednisolone acetate 1% or dexamethasone 0.01% are given four times daily until visual improvement occurs, typically in 2 to 3 months. Topical non-steroidal antiinflammatory drugs may well be of further benefit alone or in conjunction with topical steroids. Typically, ketorolac or diclofenac drops are administered four times daily.

Intraocular pressure elevation following vitreolysis has not been well documented. A drop of a beta-blocker or brimonidine at the time of treatment probably provides adequate prophylaxis if desired.

In recalcitrant cases, the addition of a systemic nonsteroidal antiinflammatory drug can be considered.

"Prophylactic" Vitreolysis

With the availability of laser vitreolysis, the surgeon may treat vitreous strands to the wound in the absence of CME in an effort to prevent its later development. Only a large, long-term randomized treatment trial can scientifically determine the usefulness of this approach, and such a study is unlikely.

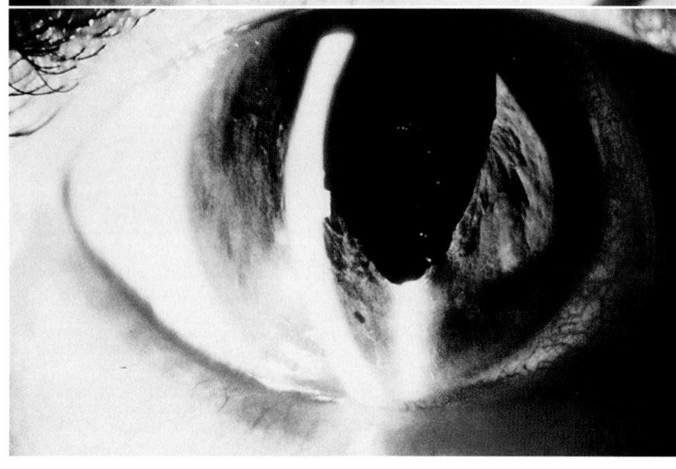

FIGURE 45-8 A, Updrawn pupil after intracapsular cataract extraction. **B,** Immediately after sphincterotomy, a candle wax–like trickle of blood was seen clotted at the inferior margin of the sphincterotomy *(arrow)*. A light reflection from the lid margin gave an appearance similar to hypopyon *(arrowhead)*, but no gross hemorrhage or inflammation occurred. **C,** One week later, the clot had cleared, and the central cornea was in the optical axis. (From Steinert RF, Puliafito CA: *The Nd:YAG laser in ophthalmology: principles and clinical applications of photodisruption,* Philadelphia, 1985, WB Saunders, p 108.)

Certainly, some patients with vitreous strands to the wound never acquire CME.

In patients with vitreous to the wound and good visual acuity, a baseline fluorescein angiogram is recommended to document the macular status. If CME is detected, laser vitreolysis is probably indicated even in the presence of good acuity. If visual loss later develops in conjunction with the new onset of CME, the baseline angiogram will be a useful reference to further support therapeutic intervention.

Coreoplasty

The Nd:YAG laser can cut through iris stroma or the pupillary sphincter to open an occluded visual axis. Indications for coreoplasty including pupillary enlargement for restoration of vision or improvement of the fundus view for examination and treatment. Synechialysis can also affect a pupillary configuration, as discussed in the next section.

Figure 45-8 illustrates a case in which the pupil became updrawn after intracapsular cataract extraction many years earlier. The upper lid covered the pupil. Unless the lid was elevated, vision was limited to counting fingers. The Nd:YAG laser cut through the sphincter with only a localized, self-limited hemorrhage. Vision improved to 20/70 and was limited only by preexisting maculopathy.

In Figure 45-9, postoperative inflammation has caused nearly complete seclusion of the pupil over a posterior chamber IOL (PC IOL). Dense associated fibrosis was present with thickening of the iris stroma. Six mJ pulses directed through a central button Abraham lens successfully enlarged the pupil with a resultant improvement in acuity from 20/80 to 20/30.

Technique

PREPARATION OF THE PATIENT

In addition to a comprehensive eye examination and informed consent, information regarding the presence of bleeding abnormalities must be specifically elicited in the history because clotting abnormalities increase the risk of a large hyphema.

Preparatory thermal iris photocoagulation with an argon laser has not been necessary or helpful in most cases. Very heavy and extensive iris coagulation is necessary to prevent bleeding when the pulsed Nd:YAG laser is subsequently used. The pressure wave after optical breakdown radiates over several millimeters with enough shearing force to cause a capillary oozing. Thus it is difficult to eliminate bleeding without widespread intense preparatory coagulation. An exception to this principle is a visible blood vessel whose patch cannot be avoided; it would be folly to cut such a vessel with the Nd:YAG laser without prior photocoagulation. Patients in whom preparatory laser coagulation

FIGURE 45-9 A, Nearly total seclusion of the pupil secondary to postoperative inflammation after extracapsular cataract extraction with posterior chamber IOL implantation. **B,** Coreoplasty with the Nd:YAG laser resulted in little improvement superiorly, inferiorly, and nasally (to the right). However, in the temporal zone, to the left, the sphincter was successfully transected, and a clear visual axis was restored.

has been performed generally state that the photocoagulation is more painful than the photodisruption.

Procedure

Six to 10 mJ is the usual setting. Numerous shots are required to cut across 3 to 5 mm of sphincter and stroma.

The sphincter is the most difficult region to cut and, with the minor arterial circle, the most prone to hemorrhage. If the surgeon starts at the pupil and cuts across the sphincter first, gross hemorrhage and free red blood cells and fibrin in the anterior chamber may prevent completion of the treatment in one session. To avoid significant hemorrhage until nearly the end of the session, the treatment should begin in the peripheral iris stroma and progress toward the sphincter and pupil. Figure 45-10 illustrates a sequential sphincterotomy.

If bleeding begins without clotting and does not cease rapidly, pressure should be applied to the globe through a contact lens, if one is being used, by a finger through the eyelids, or with a cotton-tipped swab applied to the globe. Pressure adequate to stop the bleeding is maintained for several minutes until effective iris intravascular coagulation has time to occur.

Because the damage zone from optical breakdown ("plasma growth") occurs backward along the beam path toward the Nd:YAG laser source, it is possible to perform sphincterotomy and coreoplasty over a PC IOL without damaging the underlying lens. However, it is *not* advisable to perform this procedure in a phakic patient. The pressure wave generated can rupture the anterior capsule of the natural crystalline lens, inducing immediate cataract formation.

Postoperative Care

A strong topical steroid (typically prednisolone acetate 1% or dexamethasone 0.1%) is given four times daily initially, with the dosage tapered as inflammation subsides. Cycloplegia is usually unnecessary. Intraocular pressure elevation is monitored and treated appropriately.

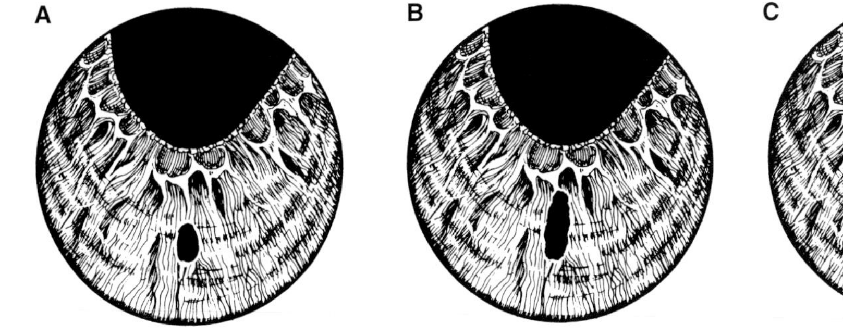

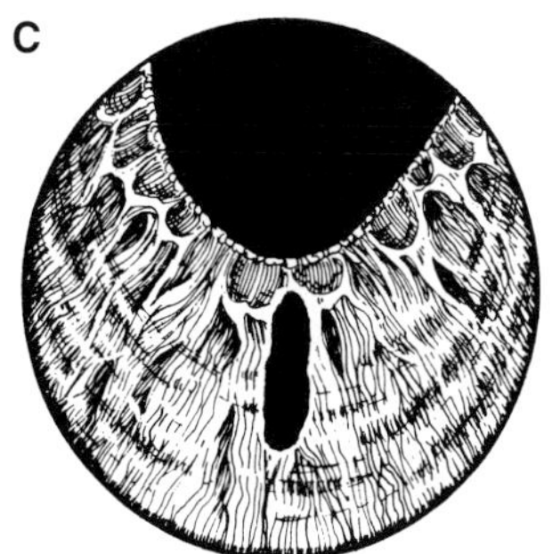

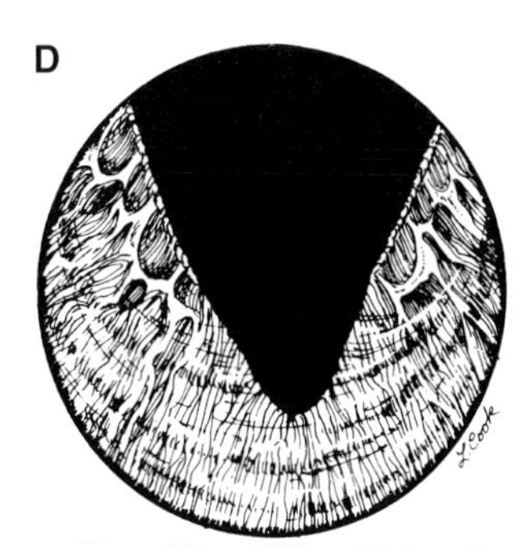

FIGURE 45-10 Technique for Nd:YAG laser sphincterotomy. **A,** Treatment is begun in the peripheral iris stroma. **B** and **C,** Progressive cutting is made toward the iris sphincter. **D,** Sphincter is cut last so that bleeding is minimized for as long as possible to increase the chance of completing the treatment in one session. (From Steinert RF, Puliafito CA: *The Nd:YAG laser in ophthalmology: principles and clinical applications of photodisruption,* Philadelphia, 1985, WB Saunders, p 110.)

Synechialysis

Localized synechiae with associated pigment may be broken by photocoagulation with the argon laser. Generally, however, the Nd:YAG laser is more successful than the argon laser in synechialysis because pigmentation of the target is not required and forceful rupture of adhesions can be achieved.

The most common synechiae are to the anterior or posterior capsule, or both. Often a tag of anterior capsule, such as is typically present after a can-opener anterior capsulotomy, adheres to the underside of the iris. As progressive fibrosis and adhesion between the anterior and posterior capsule occur, the iris adhesion is brought posteriorly. This process can exert sufficient force to bring the iris sphincter around the edge of a PC IOL, leading to iris capture of the IOL optic. In Figure 45-11, *A*, the iridocapsular adhesion has exposed the superior edge of the PC IOL. This is more evident after dilation. Two-millijoule shots applied to the area of adhesion both freeze the adhesion and rupture the posterior capsule in that area. Following treatment (Figure 45-11, *C*), the iris sphincter is back in proper position anterior to the PC IOL.

Another cause of iridocapsular adhesion is a retained fragment of anterior capsule that becomes incarcerated in the cataract wound. The appearance will simulate a vitreous strand to the wound as shown in Figure 45-12, *A*. Careful examination will disclose a typically grayish membrane resulting from fibrosis of the epithelial cells on the anterior capsule, distinctly different from the appearance of a vitreous strand. After dilation, the capsular origin can be seen (Figure 45-12, *B*). The capsular fragment is disrupted with the laser at approximately 2 to 3 mJ if the laser is used and approximately 6 mJ if the laser is used gonioscopically. Extra energy is needed because of the thickened fibrotic nature of the capsule.

If the capsular fragment is not disrupted within several months postoperatively, however, additional adhesions may form because of the proliferation of the cells present on the anterior capsule fragment. In one case, shown in Figure 45-12, *C*, the pupillary position has improved with photodisruption of the capsule strand incarcerated in the wound, but the pupil remains partially eccentric. The edge of the PC IOL is exposed and a source of functionally significant glare for the patient. This was addressed with further Nd:YAG laser pulses to the epithelial pearl adhesion underlying the iris superiorly. This succeeded in further freeing the sphincter and resulting in a nearly round pupil (see Figure 45-12, *D*).

Removal of the Intraocular Lens Precipitates

Inflammatory precipitates on the IOL surface are not usual. They may consist of both pigmented and nonpigmented, relatively

A

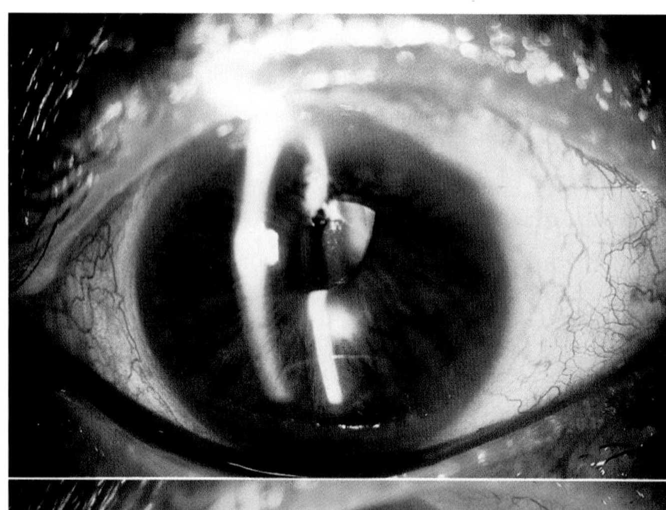

B

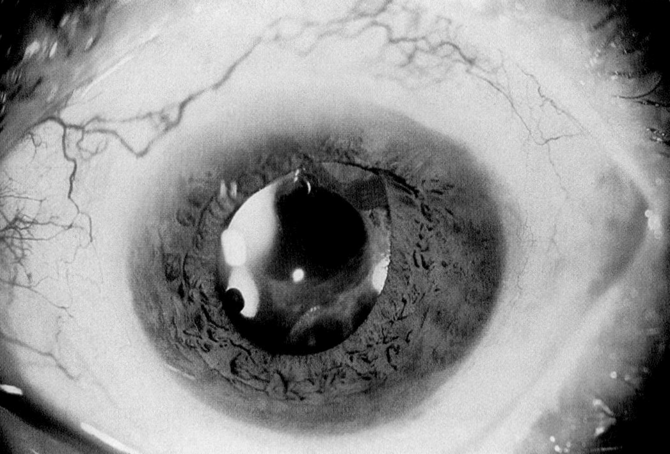

C

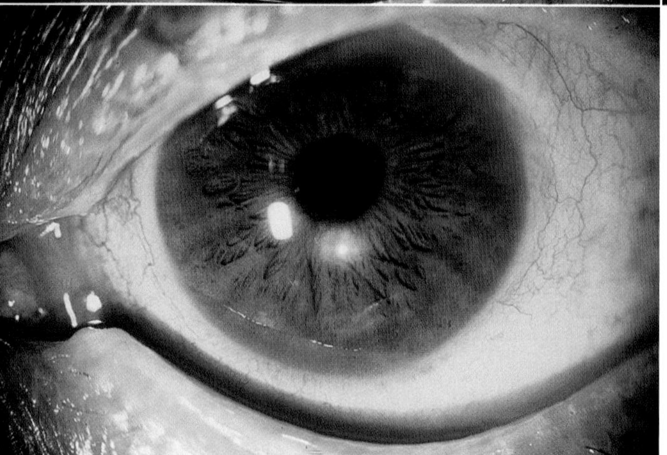

FIGURE 45-11 A, Iris capture of a PC IOL secondary to iridocapsular adhesions in an undilated patient. **B,** Adhesion of the iris to the anterior capsular edge is seen clearly after dilation. **C,** IOL capture is released, and the pupil becomes round after Nd:YAG laser capsulotomy releases the iridocapsular adhesions.

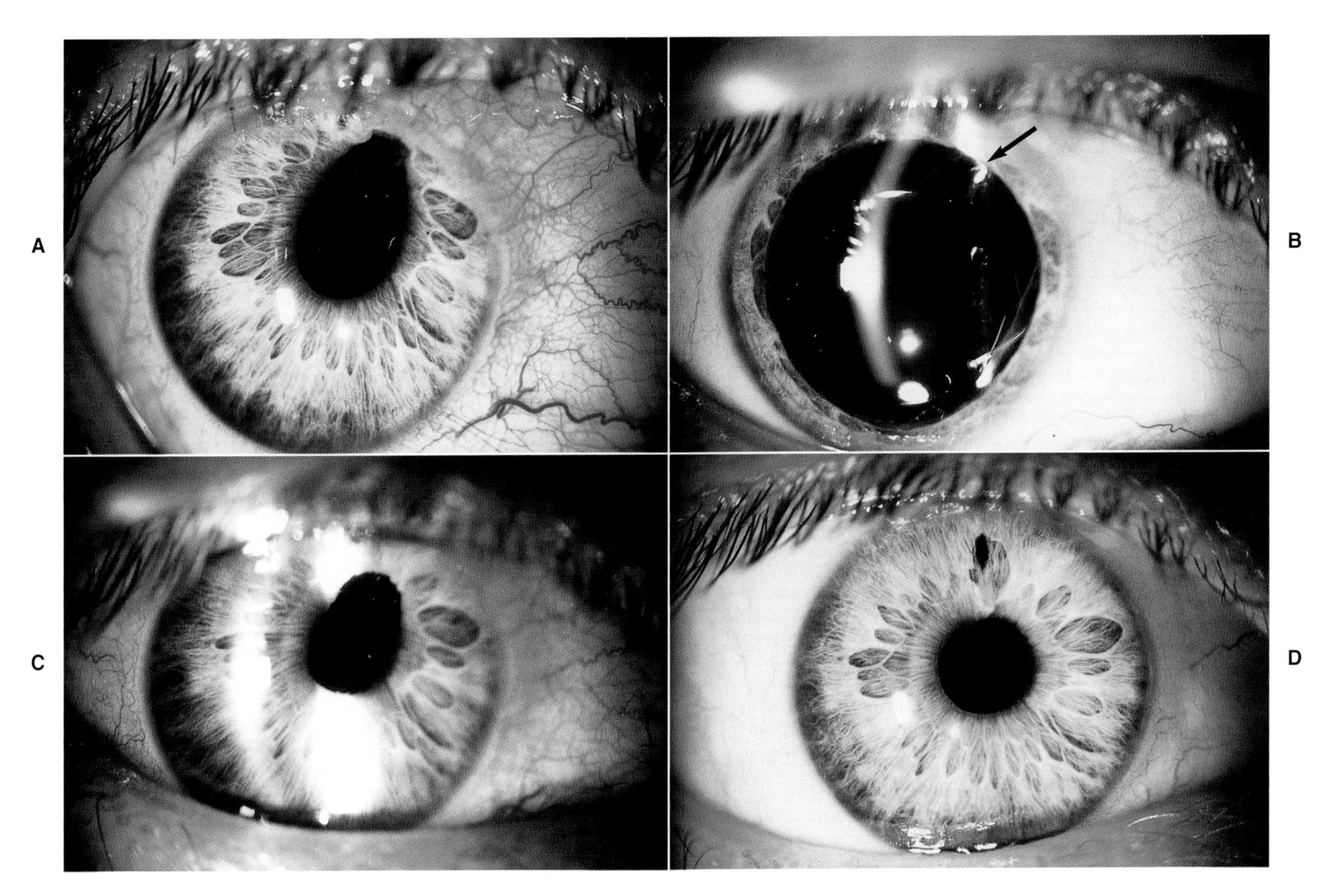

FIGURE 45-12 **A,** Iridocapsular adhesion simulating pupillary distortion seen with vitreous incarceration in the wound. **B,** After dilation, the iridocapsular adhesion is better seen *(arrow)*. **C,** After lysis of the anterior capsular fragment, improvement in the pupillary position is seen compared with the preoperative photo **(A),** but the iris distortion continues to expose the edge of the IOL optic, giving glare symptoms. **D,** After gonioscopic application of Nd:YAG laser pulses to the iridocapsular adhesions posterior to the iris, the pupil becomes central, and the glare symptoms are resolved.

round precipitates similar in appearance to keratic precipitates or the inflammation may cause the deposition of a more fibrinous gray sheet.

In some cases, these precipitates will respond to appropriate antiinflammatory therapy. In some cases, however, visually significant precipitates remain after the inflammation is quiet.

As shown in Figure 45-13, *A,* a mixture of localized dense inflammatory precipitates and a sheetlike precipitate remain after a severe postoperative inflammation. Marked clearing of the IOL optics is evident in Figure 45-13, *B,* following Nd:YAG laser therapy.

To remove IOL precipitates, the Nd:YAG laser is set at an energy level adequate to create optical breakdown in the aqueous. This is typically about 2 to 3 mJ. The Nd:YAG laser aiming beams are first focused on the anterior IOL surface. The laser is then slightly defocused by withdrawing the laser slightly toward the beam origin and away from the beam target. The abrupt pressure wave generated by the subsequent optical breakdown in front of the IOL precipitate liberates inflammatory debris into the aqueous humor, leaving a cleaned IOL.

Anterior Capsule

The lens anterior capsule becomes hazy postoperatively because of the epithelial cells present on the inner surface of the anterior capsule. Retained anterior capsule in the pupillary zone will invariably become opaque. Fortunately, retained capsule does not become strongly adherent to the underlying IOL.

In Figure 45-14, *A,* a large remnant of anterior capsule remained after implantation of a PC IOL and significantly opacified. The pupillary zone was cleared with Nd:YAG laser photodisruptive pulses of 2 to 3 mJ. These pulses were applied beginning in the upper left corner and were then carried in the direction of the lower right corner (Figure 45-14, *B*). The capsular membrane was not fully liberated but rather was left adherent at the lower right to curl up on itself. Damage to the underlying PC IOL is avoided by focusing on the anterior capsule and then withdrawing the laser focus slightly anterior to the target. The propagation of the laser plasma is toward the laser source. Accordingly, the damage to the underlying IOL can be avoided

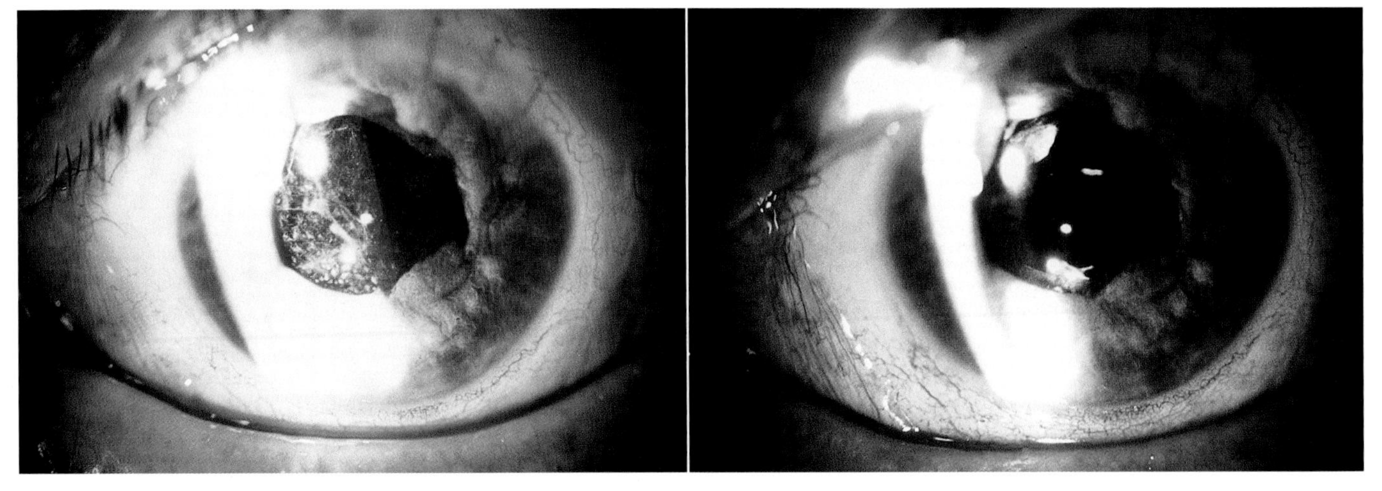

FIGURE 45-13 A, After complicated extracapsular cataract extraction with PC IOL implantation and prolonged postoperative inflammation, fibrinous and cellular debris persist on the anterior IOL optic. **B,** Nd:YAG laser photodisruptive pulses have cleared most of the debris from the IOL surface.

as long as the photodisruptive optical breakdown is not focused within the IOL itself.

Contracture of a continuous curvilinear capsulorhexis may cause progressive blockage of an initially clear pupillary zone. This may be due to eccentric contracture of an anterior capsule, as shown in Figure 45-15, *A*, or a more symmetric contracture, as shown in Figure 45-16, *A*. This "capsule contraction syndrome"[11] or "capsular phimosis syndrome" is seen more commonly when the diameter of the original cataract surgical capsulorhexis is 4 mm or smaller. It is attributed to contracture of the structurally strong round anterior capsule opening by the lens epithelial cells that have undergone myofibroblastic differentiation. In addition to causing pupillary obstruction, the capsular contracture stretches the peripheral zonules, with the risk of frank rupture of the zonules and potential weakening of the IOL support. Capsular contracture is best avoided by keeping the diameter of continuous curvilinear capsulorhexis to 5 mm or greater.

As soon as the capsular contracture syndrome is recognized postoperatively, Nd:YAG laser photodisruption of the capsular margin should be undertaken. This will prevent further contraction of the capsule because the disrupted anterior capsule no longer has mechanical integrity. In addition, the pupillary zone is clear of the opaque capsule.

The technique typically consists of 2- to 3-mJ pulses at the edge of the capsulorhexis, transecting the round capsulorhexis edge into at least four quadrants. The capsule will then contract and eventually resume a relatively round appearance with a much larger opening (see Figure 45-16, *B*).

Damage to the underlying PC IOL is avoided by deliberate anterior defocusing of the laser beam as described earlier for

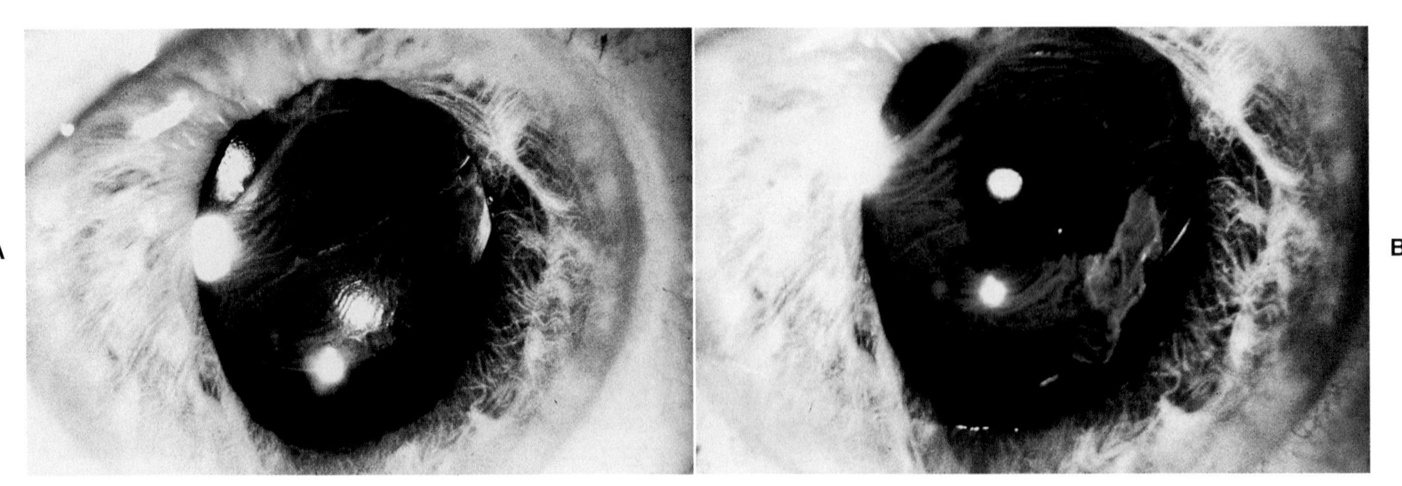

FIGURE 45-14 A, Anterior capsule was inadvertently retained after PC IOL implantation. Opacification of the anterior capsule occurred rapidly. **B,** A window has been cut in the anterior capsule with the Nd:YAG laser, with a small amount of the anterior capsule remaining attached in the lower right to avoid a free-floating capsular remnant in the anterior chamber. No damage has occurred to the anterior IOL surface.

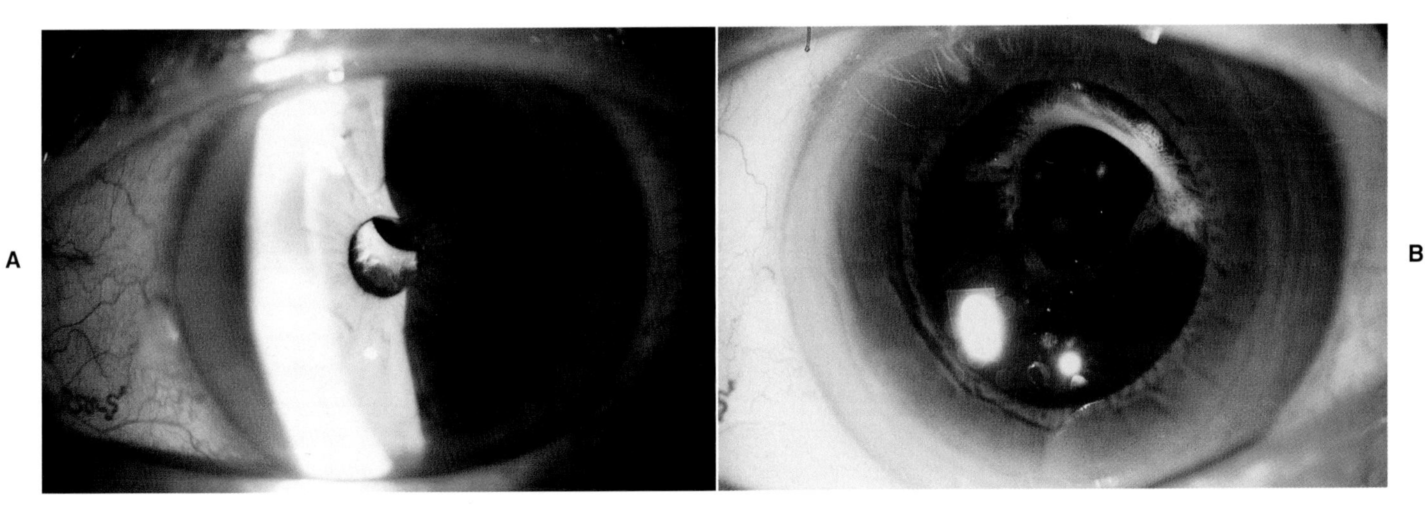

FIGURE 45-15 A, Contracture of the anterior capsule inferiorly has nearly occluded the optical zone. **B**, Nd:YAG laser cutting of the inferior capsule adhesion restores an adequate visual axis.

removal of the IOL precipitates and opening of retained anterior capsule.

Retained Cortical Material

Occasionally, cortex is retained postoperatively. It may be unrecognized initially or may be deliberately left because of a defect in the posterior capsule or a difficult-to-reach location, particularly under the incision. Cortex will become hydrated in the hours after surgery, swelling and loosening its position. Occasionally, on the day after surgery the visual axis has been occluded by such hydrated retained cortical material (Figure 45-17, *A*).

Retained cortex may slowly resorb, but this process is particularly slow when the cortex is trapped between the posterior capsule and the PC IOL anteriorly. With essentially no aqueous turnover, the gradual clearing of this material can take a number of months. Moreover, rather than clearing fully, the retained material may slowly become a dense fibrotic sheet that is difficult to open with laser techniques and may require more invasive surgery.

In such a case, the hydrated opaque cortical material can be liquefied with photodisruptive laser pulses. A minimal amount of laser energy is used, just adequate to cause optical breakdown within the cortical material. A typical amount of energy would be 2 mJ. The pressure wave from Nd:YAG pulses within the cortex will emulsify the hydrated cortex, creating an appearance of a more uniform lens "milk." Within 24 hours, this more liquefied material will usually clear, restoring a good visual zone (see Figure 45-17, *B*).

The rapid liberation of lens protein through photodisruption may cause secondary inflammation and pressure elevation. Prophylactic antiglaucoma medical therapy is indicated, as is

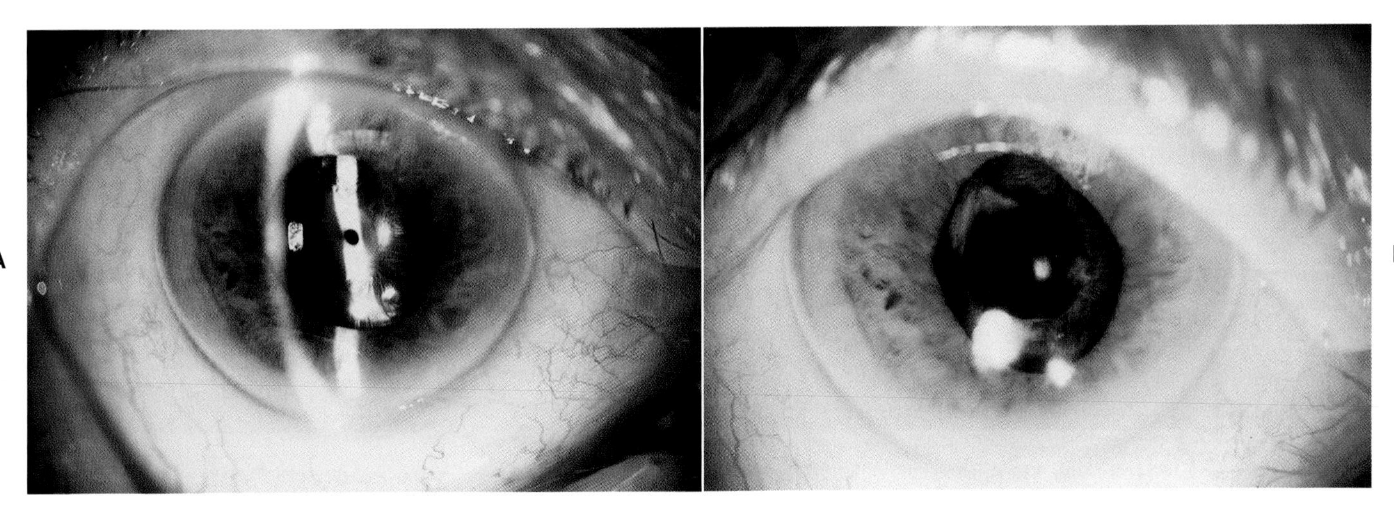

FIGURE 45-16 A, Symmetric contracture of the anterior capsulorhexis leaves an inadequate visual axis. **B,** Photodisruption of the anterior capsulotomy edge restores an adequate visual axis.

A

B

FIGURE 45-17 **A,** Retained cortex is hydrated but trapped behind the posterior chamber IOL optic. **B,** Nd:YAG laser pulses have disrupted the retained cortex in the pupillary zone.

close monitoring of the patient. The surgeon should be prepared to surgically irrigate the retained cortical material if a clinically intolerable level of inflammation or pressure elevation occurs.

Intraocular Lens Repositioning

In rare circumstances, Nd:YAG laser photodisruption can be used to manipulate the position of an IOL. The pressure wave from optical breakdown can shift an IOL optic if the optic is sufficiently mobile.

One special case is illustrated in Figure 45-18, *A*. A previously well-centered ciliary sulcus–fixated PC IOL became captured in the pupil after pupillary dilation. The pupil could not be redilated beyond the border of the IOL optic. Mechanical manipulation of the IOL optic by placing the patient in the supine position or with pressure of a cotton-tipped applicator over the ciliary sulcus failed to cause the IOL optic to shift posteriorly.

A 6-mJ pulse from an Nd:YAG laser was then applied to the peripheral edge of the IOL. The laser was focused just anterior to the anterior IOL surface. This anterior pressure wave caused the IOL optic to shift posteriorly, just behind the pupillary sphincter. The sphincter was then constricted with pilocarpine, successfully maintaining the PC IOL in the posterior chamber (see Figure 45-18, *B*).

Conclusions

Nd:YAG laser photodisruption allows a surgeon to effectively reach inside the eye with a pair of microscissors delivered on a beam of light. In rare circumstances, photodisruptive laser energy

A

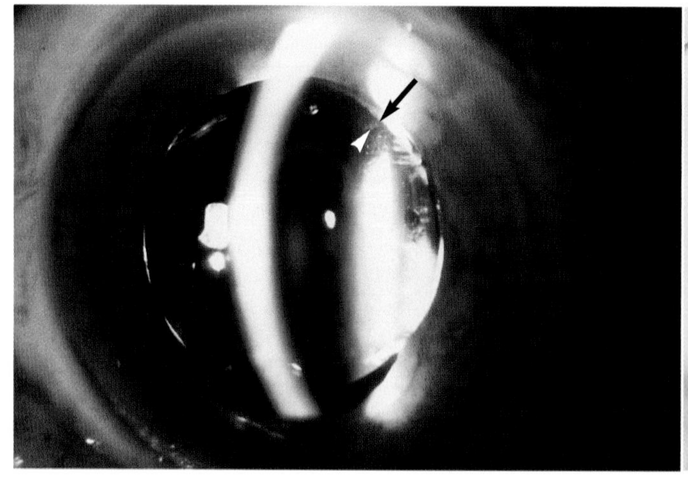

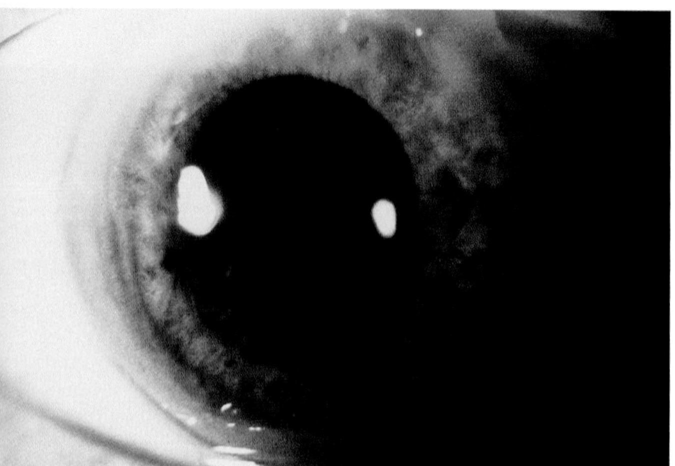

B

FIGURE 45-18 **A,** Iris capture of the optic of a PC IOL *(arrow)*. A single 6-mJ pulse focused at an area just anterior to the lens surface, approximately 1 mm centrally from the optic edge *(arrowhead)*, retropulsed the optic behind the iris. **B,** IOL is now in proper position behind the iris. (From Steinert RF, Puliafito CA: *The Nd:YAG Laser in Ophthalmology: Principles and Clinical Applications of Photodisruption,* Philadelphia, 1985, WB Saunders, p 130.)

can be constructively used to push and cut. Photodisruption therefore gives the surgeon additional options in the correction of a wide range of complications following cataract surgery.

REFERENCES

1. Shaffer RN: The role of vitreous detachment in aphakic and malignant glaucoma, *Trans Am Ophthalmol Otolaryngol* 28:217-231, 1954.
2. Shaffer RN: A suggested anatomic classification to define the pupillary block glaucomas, *Invest Ophthalmol* 12:540-542, 1973.
3. Epstein DL, Steinert RF, Puliafito CA: Neodymium-YAG laser therapy to the anterior hyaloid in aphakic malignant (ciliovitreal block) glaucoma, *Am J Ophthalmol* 98:137-143, 1984.
4. Irvine SR: A newly defined vitreous syndrome following cataract surgery, *Am J Ophthalmol* 36:599-619, 1953.
5. Gass JDM, Norton EWD: Cystoid macular edema and papilledema following cataract extraction, *Arch Ophthalmol* 76:646-661, 1966.
6. Iliff CE: Treatment of vitreous tug syndrome, *Am J Ophthalmol* 162:856-859, 1966.
7. Katzen LE, Fleischman JA, Trokel S: YAG laser treatment of cystoid macular edema, Am J Ophthalmol 95:589-592, 1983.
8. Gass JDM, Norton EWD: Follow-up study of cystoid macular edema following cataract extraction, *Trans Am Acad Ophthalmol Otolaryngol* 73:665-682, 1969.
9. Jacobson DR, Dellaporta A: Natural history of cystoid macular edema after cataract extraction, *Am J Ophthalmol* 77: 445-447, 1974.
10. Steinert RF, Wasson PJ: Neodymium:YAG laser anterior vitreolysis for Irvine-Gass cystoid macular edema, J Cataract Refract Surg 15:304-307, 1989.
11. Davison JA: Capsule contraction syndrome, *J Cataract Refract Surg* 19: 582-589, 1993.

Epithelial and Fibrous Invasion of the Eye

46

Alex P. Hunyor, MB, BS
C. Davis Belcher III, MD

Epithelial and fibrous invasions into the anterior chamber have long been recognized as complications of cataract surgery, other anterior segment surgery, and trauma. These conditions, particularly the former, continue to pose a significant diagnostic and management problem for ophthalmic surgeons, despite their decreasing incidence resulting from advances in surgical technique.

Epithelial Invasion

Historical Perspective

In 1830 Mackenzie[1] described the occurrence of a posttraumatic iris inclusion cyst. Rothmund[2] in 1872 reported a study of 37 cases of epithelial cysts of the anterior chamber, with two occurring after cataract extraction and the remainder following trauma. He proposed that these cysts resulted from implantation of epithelium at the time of trauma or surgery. Collins and Cross[3] in 1892 demonstrated histopathologically the presence of epithelium in the anterior chamber in two cases of epithelial implantation cyst after cataract extraction. The work of Guaita[4] and Meller[5] emphasized poor wound healing in allowing entry of epithelial cells. Perera[6] in 1937 reviewed numerous reports, differentiating cystic epithelial lesions from sheetlike epithelial ingrowth, noting the importance of incarceration of iris or lens capsule and of hypotony in favoring epithelial invasion. He proposed a classification of epithelial invasion into (1) "pearl" tumors of the iris, (2) epithelial (inclusion) cysts of the iris, and (3) epithelialization (also referred to as epithelial ingrowth or downgrowth) of the anterior chamber. This classification remains useful in differentiating these three entities with related etiologies but clearly different clinical course, treatment and outcome.

Pearl Tumors

Pearl tumors (pearl cysts) are rare, opaque, cystic or solid "pearly" lesions that usually occur after trauma but have been described after intraocular surgery.[7] They result from traumatic implantation of skin or hair follicles into the anterior chamber and usually form a small, circumscribed lesion that is not connected with the entry site and confined to the iris (Figure 46-1). These lesions grow slowly and rarely exceed 2 to 3 mm in diameter. Histologically, they are encapsulated structures of cuboidal or stratified epithelial cells with a central mass of keratinized cells, cholesterol crystals, and necrotic debris; hair follicles and foreign bodies have also been found. In the uncommon instances that these cysts significantly enlarge or cause iridocyclitis, en bloc excision usually yields good results.

Epithelial Inclusion Cysts

Of the two major forms of epithelial invasion resulting from implantation of surface epithelium into the anterior chamber, epithelial inclusion (or implantation) cysts tend to follow a more benign, although quite variable, clinical course.

INCIDENCE

There are no figures for the incidence of epithelial cyst as a separate entity. The overall incidence of cystic and sheetlike epithelial invasion after accidental and surgical penetration of the anterior segment has been estimated in early studies[8,9] at 0.06% to 0.11%, and cysts are considered the more common form.

PREDISPOSING FACTORS AND PATHOGENESIS

Epithelial inclusion cysts have been reported after cataract extraction, penetrating keratoplasty, and other forms of surgery and trauma to the anterior segment, as summarized by Farmer and Kalina.[10] In cases following cataract surgery, there is usually evidence of poor wound closure, often with incarcerated iris, lens matter, or vitreous. Rarely, cysts are discontinuous with the wound from their onset and are presumably due to implantation of surface epithelium by intraocular instruments, as discussed by Ferry.[11] Experimental evidence[12,13] points to contact with the iris and exposure to plasmoid aqueous (containing proliferative factors) as determinants of the development and size of epithelial cysts.

The factors regulating development of implanted or ingrowing epithelial cells into cysts, as opposed to sheetlike ingrowths, are unclear. The number of cells, initial morphology of the ingrowth (a bilayer or loop as opposed to a single layer), degree of attachment to iris and angle structures, vascular supply, and duration of exposure to plasmoid aqueous (a longer exposure favoring progressive sheetlike ingrowth) may all play a role.

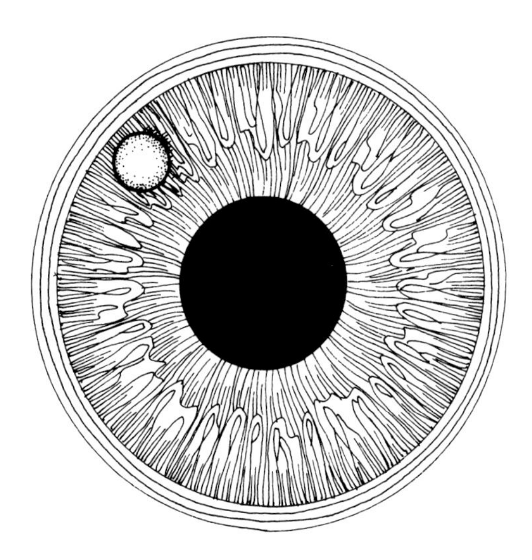

FIGURE 46-1 "Pearl" tumor of the iris.

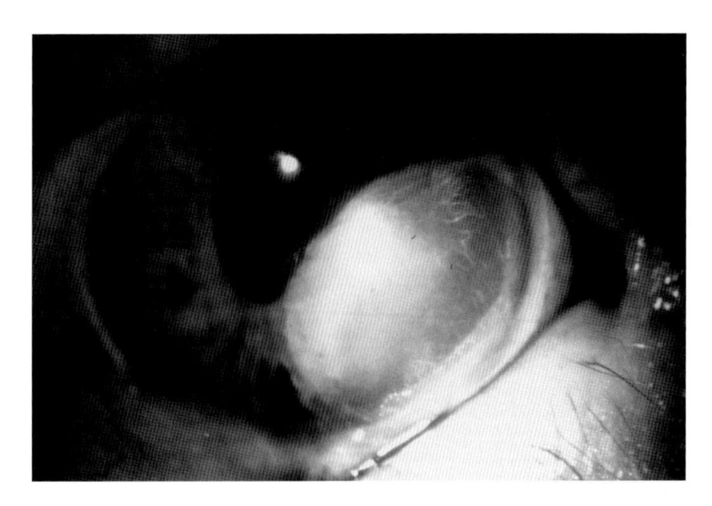

FIGURE 46-2 Epithelial inclusion cyst of the anterior chamber.

As discussed later on, in some cases epithelial cysts may be converted into sheetlike downgrowth if treated with surgery or laser.

PRESENTATION, CLINICAL FEATURES, AND DIAGNOSIS

Cysts may remain quiescent for many years before enlarging and/or causing symptoms. Patients may seek treatment because of recognition or noticeable enlargement of an otherwise asymptomatic lesion, visual symptoms caused by extension into the visual axis, or symptoms of intraocular inflammation and secondary glaucoma that may accompany periods of cyst growth.

Epithelial inclusion cysts are typically translucent or gray in appearance and usually are associated with the anterior surface of the peripheral iris. There may be displacement of an iris pillar or distortion of the pupil (Figure 46-2). Cysts may grow through an iridotomy or peripheral iridectomy into the posterior chamber and appear to arise from the iris itself. For a review of the differential diagnosis of cystic lesions of the iris, see Shields, Sanborn, and Augsburger.[14] Signs of anterior uveitis, sometimes with secondary glaucoma, may be present. Sympathetic ophthalmia associated with secondary glaucoma from cystic epithelial invasion of the anterior chamber has been reported,[15] as has mucogenic open-angle glaucoma resulting from a goblet cell cyst of the anterior chamber.[16] Subluxation of an anterior chamber intraocular lens (IOL) by a large epithelial cyst has also been noted.[17] Massive enlargement of cysts may cause corneal decompensation by extensive contact with the corneal endothelium.

The diagnosis of epithelial inclusion cyst is suggested by the history or signs of surgery or trauma; contact with the surgical or traumatic wound; characteristics of cystic lesions such as transillumination, occasionally mobility, and tremulousness; scant pigmentation; lack of vascularity; superficial relationship to the iris; and signs of associated uveitis.

HISTOPATHOLOGIC FEATURES

Cysts are typically thin-walled structures lined with squamous or cuboidal epithelium, sometimes including goblet cells (Figure 46-3). Electron microscopic studies[18] demonstrate epithelial cells with a thin basal lamina, desmosomal junctions, cytoplasmic filaments, scant mitochondria, terminal bars, and apical microvilli, characteristic of ocular surface epithelium, most likely conjunctival. They contain straw-colored, turbid, or mucinous fluid. There may be pigmentation, particularly of the posterior portion of the cyst. Often there is evidence of contact between the cyst and the traumatic or surgical wound, which may be lost later in its development.

MANAGEMENT

Although some authors have advocated early surgical intervention for epithelial cysts, they follow a highly variable clinical course (from spontaneous regression[19] to rapid growth), and there is a well-established risk of conversion to sheetlike epithelial downgrowth after surgery and laser treatment. There is general agreement that the most appropriate management includes periodic observation at 3- to 4-month intervals with serial anterior segment photography and prompt intervention in cases in which vision is impaired by encroachment on the visual axis, uveitis, glaucoma, or corneal edema.

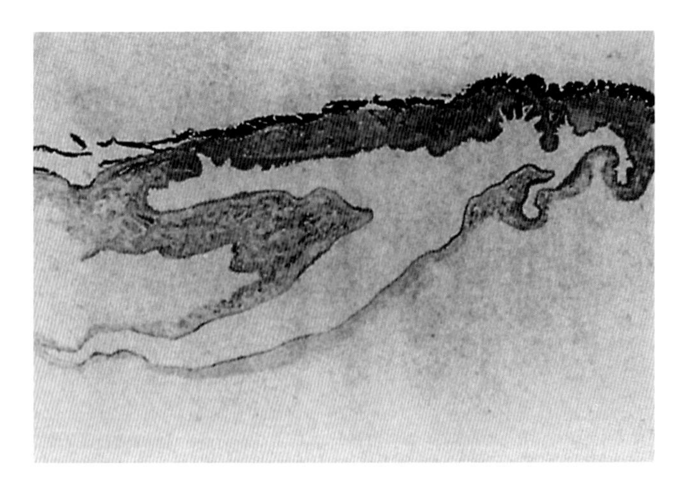

FIGURE 46-3 Light microscopy of an epithelial inclusion cyst, showing a clear lumen lined by nonkeratinized squamous epithelium. (Hematoxylin and eosin stain; ×40.) (From Orlin SE, Raber IM, Laibson PR et al: Epithelial downgrowth following the removal of iris inclusion cysts, *Ophthalmic Surg* 22:330-335, 1991.)

Various treatment modalities have been employed, including needle aspiration, injection with radioactive and sclerosing substances, diathermy, cryotherapy, electrolysis, radiotherapy, photocoagulation, numerous surgical approaches, and combinations of the preceding methods. In the absence of any large series, comparison of the efficacy of these techniques is difficult. The management of epithelial cysts of the anterior chamber remains a difficult balance between the need for elimination of the cyst with low risk of recurrence and minimization of complications of the treatment itself. As yet, no single treatment modality has provided this combination.

Radiotherapy, despite the initial enthusiasm of Perera[6] and others, has been abandoned because of variable results and lack of safety. Diathermy coagulation[20,21] has largely been supplanted by laser photocoagulation.

Ferry and Naghdi[22] successfully treated a large cyst by insertion of a cryostylet into the cyst (via a needle puncture), freezing it to –10° to 0° F for 15 seconds, and exteriorization and excision of the cyst and adherent iris tissue. Cyst aspirations with injection of astatine,[23] iodine,[24] and other sclerosing agents have also been reported, with varying degrees of success and safety. Cyst aspiration with laser photocoagulation and/or cryotherapy, and surgical techniques, are the mainstay of current therapy and will be discussed in more detail.

CURRENT TECHNIQUES

For small unpigmented cysts, aspiration followed by cryotherapy to the collapsed cyst is our preferred treatment. For unpigmented cysts too large for cryotherapy and for all pigmented cysts, aspiration followed by argon laser photocoagulation is favored. Large unpigmented cysts, if fully aspirated and collapsed against the iris with the technique to be described, are usually successfully photocoagulated using the heat sink effect of the underlying iris pigment.

Aspiration and photocoagulation. Meyer-Schwickerath,[25] Okun and Mandell,[26] and others have described treatment of epithelial cysts with xenon arc photocoagulation. Multiple treatments were required, and cysts were collapsed and fibrosed, preventing further growth. In 1975 L'Esperance and James[27] first described successful treatment of epithelial cysts by argon laser photocoagulation. The authors' preferred method of treatment for pigmented epithelial inclusion cysts and larger unpigmented cysts is argon laser photocoagulation, with a technique similar to that described by Thomas, Lederer, and Simmons,[28] as outlined next.

In a minor operating room under topical anesthesia (or peribulbar anesthesia in less cooperative patients), the affected eye is prepared as for cataract surgery with skin sterilization and draping, and a lid speculum is inserted. A first paracentesis through clear cornea is performed well away from the cyst with an angled 15-degree disposable blade (Figure 46-4). The second paracentesis is made into the cyst at its base, via its attachment to the anterior chamber angle where present (Figure 46-5), avoiding cyst puncture within the anterior chamber, which can potentially increase the risk of conversion to sheetlike ingrowth.

A 27-gauge intraocular cannula attached to a syringe is inserted into the cyst cavity via the second paracentesis, and the cyst contents are aspirated to collapse the cyst (Figure 46-6). Cytologic examination of the aspirated fluid (for epithelial cells) may be performed. The anterior chamber is re-formed with air, which promotes the collapse of the cyst against its posterior wall (Figure 46-7). Blunt dissection of the anterior cyst wall from the posterior cornea, with a spatula inserted via the first paracentesis, may also be required (Figure 46-8). Physiologic saline solution is then exchanged for the air in the anterior chamber. Routine postoperative topical antibiotics are instilled in the eye.

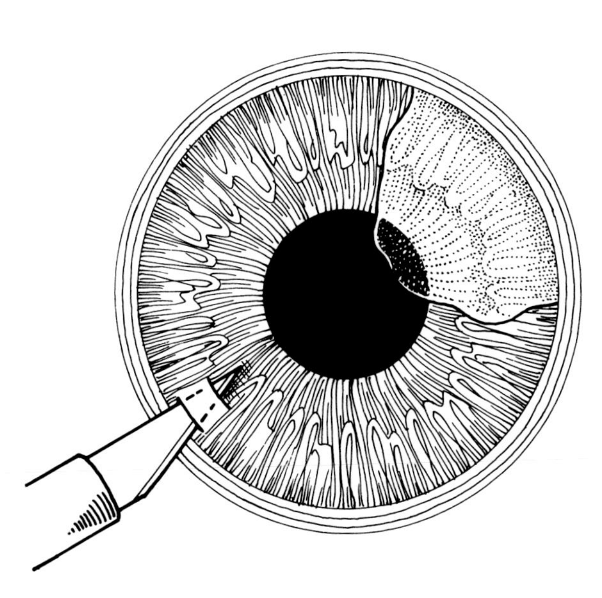

FIGURE 46-4 Initial anterior chamber paracentesis is performed well away from the cyst.

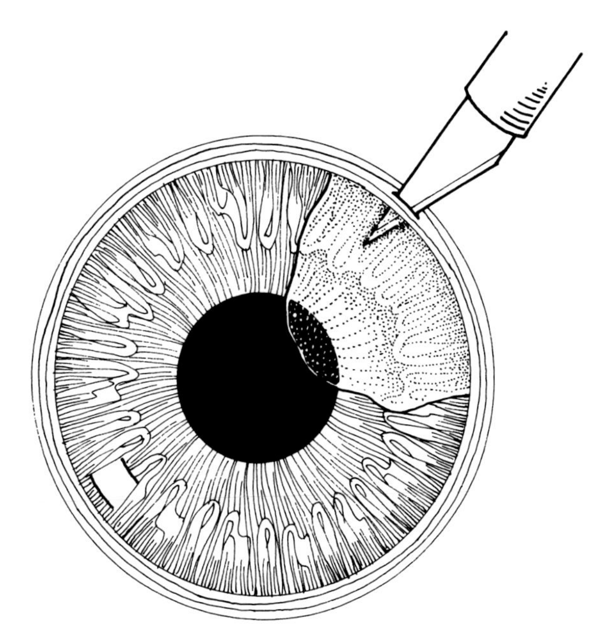

FIGURE 46-5 Second paracentesis enters the base of the cyst, avoiding cyst puncture that communicates with the anterior chamber.

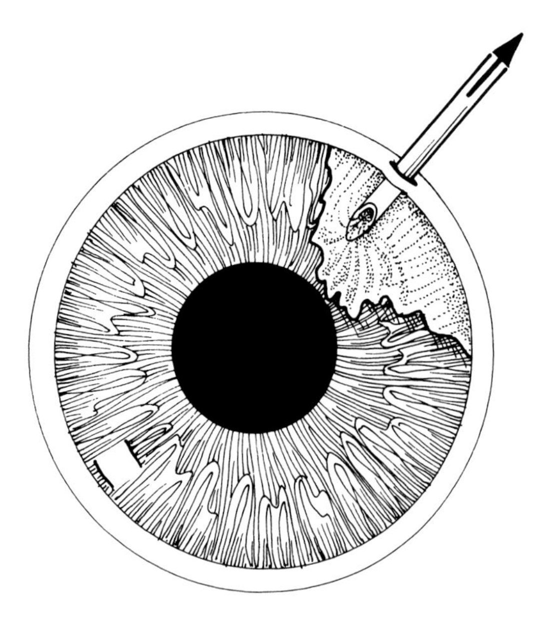

FIGURE 46-6 Cyst contents are aspirated with a 27-gauge intraocular cannula.

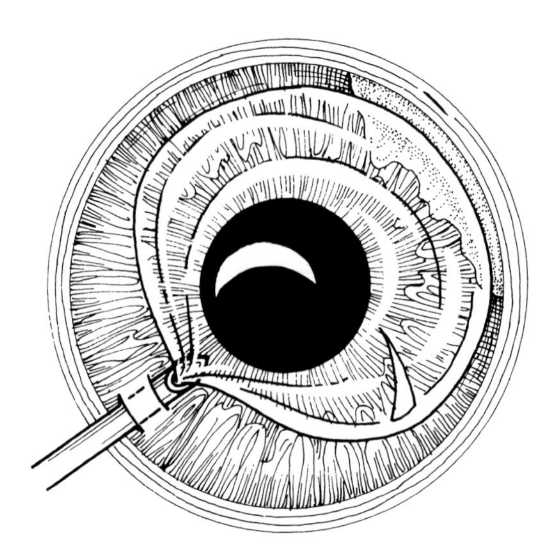

FIGURE 46-7 Anterior chamber is re-formed with air, promoting cyst collapse against the iris.

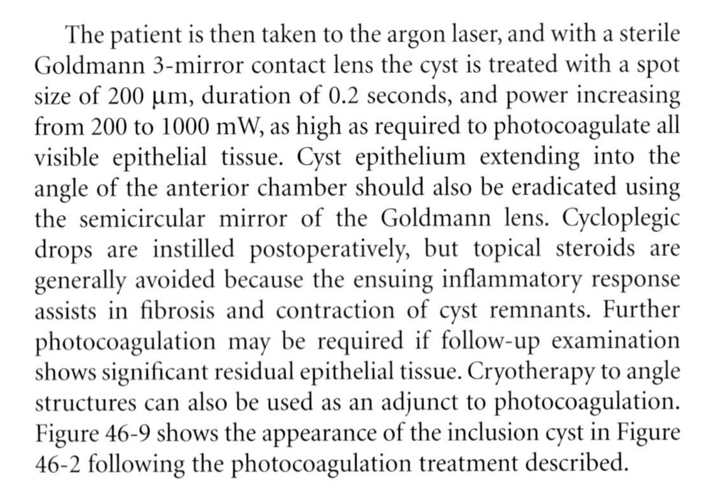

The patient is then taken to the argon laser, and with a sterile Goldmann 3-mirror contact lens the cyst is treated with a spot size of 200 μm, duration of 0.2 seconds, and power increasing from 200 to 1000 mW, as high as required to photocoagulate all visible epithelial tissue. Cyst epithelium extending into the angle of the anterior chamber should also be eradicated using the semicircular mirror of the Goldmann lens. Cycloplegic drops are instilled postoperatively, but topical steroids are generally avoided because the ensuing inflammatory response assists in fibrosis and contraction of cyst remnants. Further photocoagulation may be required if follow-up examination shows significant residual epithelial tissue. Cryotherapy to angle structures can also be used as an adjunct to photocoagulation. Figure 46-9 shows the appearance of the inclusion cyst in Figure 46-2 following the photocoagulation treatment described.

L'Esperance and James[27] reported shrinkage and disappearance of four cysts over a 6-week period following argon laser photocoagulation (without prior aspiration). Scholz and Kelly[29] and Sugar, Jampol, and Goldberg[30] reported successful eradication of epithelial cysts with the same technique. The authors prefer the technique outlined earlier, with aspiration before photocoagulation, because it facilitates more complete photocoagulation and theoretically reduces the likelihood of leaving a free epithelial edge, which may progress to sheetlike epithelial ingrowth. Honrubia, Brito, and Grijalbo[31] reported elimination of several epithelial cysts, with no recurrence or significant complications, using this technique.

The complications of photocoagulation include iritis, which may be marked; a transient rise in intraocular pressure resulting from outflow obstruction by protein and cellular debris, which

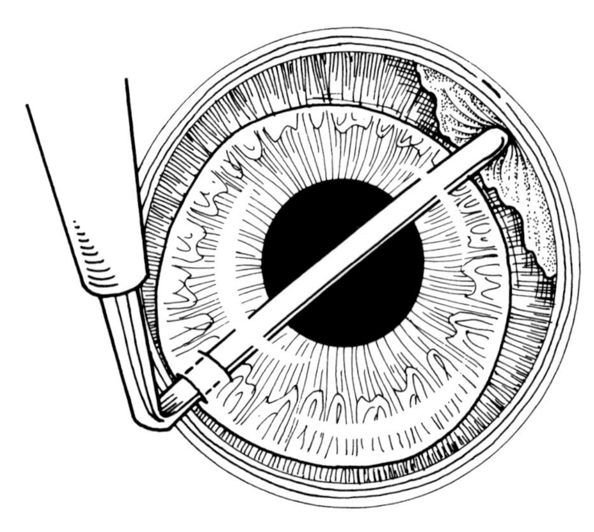

FIGURE 46-8 Blunt dissection of the cyst wall from the posterior cornea may be performed via the first paracentesis.

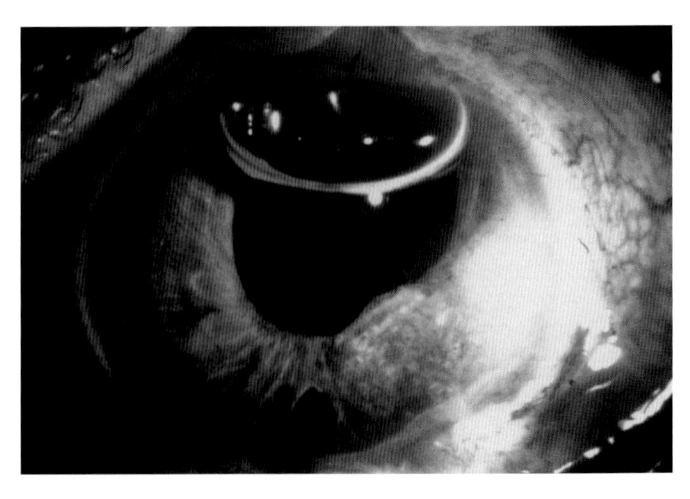

FIGURE 46-9 Appearance of the cyst from Figure 46-2 following aspiration and photocoagulation.

usually responds to medical treatment and resolves within 2 weeks; corneal opacity from photocoagulation of cyst material adjacent or adherent to the posterior cornea (largely avoidable by posterior displacement of the cyst and angling of the laser beam); hemorrhage from iris vessels (rarely, hemorrhage into a cyst may facilitate argon laser absorption); cataract induction in the phakic eye; and conversion to sheetlike epithelial ingrowth.[32] Treatment of epithelial implantation cysts with the Nd:YAG laser is not recommended because without accompanying cryotherapy or photocoagulation to ensure fibrosis of cyst remnants, the risk of sheetlike ingrowth with such a procedure seems high. Recurrence of such cysts after Nd:YAG treatment is also likely.[33]

Surgery. Surgery for epithelial inclusion cysts has ranged from excision by iridectomy[10] following cryotherapy[22] or aspiration, including debridement or alcohol swabbing of the involved cornea,[34] to block excision with cryotherapy (with or without vitrectomy)[35] and more radical excision including lamellar corneal excision[36] or corneal and corneoscleral grafting.[37,38] A summary of surgical techniques is given in Table 46-1. Some authors still advocate en bloc excision as the treatment of choice for epithelial inclusion cysts. Surgical approaches, particularly more extensive procedures, carry considerable risks of complications, such as conversion to sheetlike ingrowth, glaucoma, corneal edema, vitreous loss and hemorrhage, and cystoid macular edema. Such procedures may often be avoided by thorough treatment with aspiration followed by cryotherapy with or without photocoagulation, depending on cyst size.

Regardless of technique, the aim of treatment should be complete eradication of the epithelial cells, as incomplete treatment carries a significant risk of conversion to sheetlike epithelial ingrowth. Early detection of treatment failures with more conservative techniques should allow consideration of more aggressive surgery, such as block excision, before ingrowth is too advanced. Long-term follow-up is required in all cases, as recurrences or conversion to sheetlike epithelial ingrowth may be detected years after initial apparently successful treatment.

PROGNOSIS

The long-term outlook for eyes with epithelial inclusion cysts is far better than for sheetlike ingrowth; however, the visual results from published cases of surgical treatment of such cysts are generally poor. There is clearly considerable bias toward a poorer prognosis group in such reports, as the large number of epithelial cysts that require no intervention have not been included. Those eyes that develop complications of treatment (particularly sheetlike epithelial ingrowth and cystoid macular edema) and those with preexisting poor visual acuity make up the majority of those with poor visual outcome. Corneal decompensation from causes other than sheetlike ingrowth is usually successfully treated with penetrating keratoplasty. Ideally a large prospective study of such cysts, both treated and untreated, would give a more accurate assessment of the optimal treatment modality and overall prognosis.

Epithelial Ingrowth

Since the 1800s, the grim visual prognosis of eyes with epithelial ingrowth, which almost invariably progressed to intractable glaucoma and blindness, was recognized. This condition is also referred to as epithelial downgrowth, epithelialization of the anterior chamber, and diffuse or sheetlike epithelial ingrowth (to distinguish it from the cystic form described earlier). It may be difficult to diagnose, and despite the use of multiple therapies including aggressive surgical approaches, its treatment remains challenging, and good visual outcomes are few.

INCIDENCE

The quoted clinical incidence of epithelial ingrowth has long been accepted as an underestimate, owing to lack of recognition

TABLE 46-1

Chronology of Surgical Techniques for Epithelial Inclusion Cyst*†

Year	Author(s)	Technique/Comments
1955	Maumenee, Shannon[34]	Eleven cases; subtotal/total cyst removal, large iridectomies, denudation of involved posterior cornea; no recurrence, complications, downgrowth
1955	Rizzuti[39]	Aspiration-excision by iridectomy-iridodialysis; postoperative VA, 20/30
1962	Sugar, Willenz[36]	Excision of cyst, involved iris, posterior corneoscleral lamella; VA 20/25
1974	Harbin, Maumenee[40]	Reported 6 cases of conversion to epithelial downgrowth after cyst excision; urged conservative management (cyst aspiration with cryotherapy to angle and photocoagulation to cyst remnants on iris)
1981	Bruner et al[35]	Closed-eye approach in aphakic patients: cyst aspiration/cryotherapy. Open-sky cyst excision/transscleral cryotherapy in phakic patients. Seven cases: 4 uncomplicated, 2 persistent CME, 1 sheetlike ingrowth, 1 persistent corneal edema; VA better than 20/60 in 43%
1981	Eiferman, Rodrigues[18]	Iridocyclectomy/penetrating keratoplasty; wound dehiscence and graft failure from unrelated cause (no recurrence)
1981	Farmer, Kalina[10]	Excision by iridectomy-iridodialysis; postoperative VA 20/20
1992, 1996	Naumann, Rummelt[37,38]	Forty-five cases; block excision by sector iridectomy with excision of cornea, sclera and ciliary body and tectonic corneoscleral grafting; 28% vitreous hemorrhage; 22% corneal decompensation; VA 20/60 or better in 43%; no recurrences; no conversion to sheetlike ingrowth

*This table is a summary only. The reader should consult the appropriate sources as referenced.
†Single case reports unless otherwise indicated.
CME, Cystoid macular edema; *PPV,* pars plana vitrectomy; *VA,* visual acuity (postoperative).

and the difficulty of making the diagnosis on clinical, rather than pathologic, grounds. As mentioned earlier, the overall incidence of cystic and sheetlike epithelial invasion of the anterior segment after trauma and surgery in earlier studies[8,9] was 0.06% to 0.11% (up to 1.1% in one study[41]), and in a clinicopathologic review by Weiner et al.,[42] the incidence after cataract surgery was 0.12% overall from 1953 to 1983, dropping to 0.076% in the period 1973 to 1983.

More important than the incidence of this condition is its occurrence in eyes enucleated after cataract surgery—an average of 16% and 17%, respectively, in the large series compiled by Maumenee[43] and Jaffe et al.[44] A review of eyes enucleated more recently (1962-1976) by Merenmies and Tarkkanen[45] demonstrated epithelial ingrowth in 10.6% of eyes enucleated following cataract surgery; they noted that all cases of ingrowth occurred before 1969.

The decreasing incidence of epithelial ingrowth has been attributed to the use of the operating microscope; improvements in surgical technique (modern extracapsular and phacoemulsification surgery, with smaller incisions); and the use of finer, higher quality suture material. There are now several reports of epithelial ingrowth following sutureless small incision cataract surgery, both with scleral tunnel and clear corneal incisions.[46-49] Despite the impression of a decreasing incidence of epithelial ingrowth, it is of significant concern that the proportion of cases that are clinically unrecognized appears to be increasing, which suggests a lower awareness by clinicians of this potentially devastating condition.[50]

PREDISPOSING FACTORS AND PATHOGENESIS

Epithelial ingrowth has most commonly been reported following intracapsular and extracapsular cataract surgery (with or without IOL implantation), trauma, and penetrating keratoplasty. In a series by Weiner et al.,[42] 15% of cases followed trauma, and 85% followed surgery (86% cataract surgery, 12% penetrating keratoplasty, 2% other). In a series of 207 histopathologically proven cases of epithelial ingrowth, Kuchle and Green found cataract surgery was the cause in 59.4% of cases.[50] Ingrowth has also been described after surgery for epithelial inclusion cyst (as discussed earlier), Nd:YAG laser treatment of inclusion cyst,[32] pterygium excision,[42] glaucoma filtration procedure,[9] transcorneal (McCannel) suture,[50] discission of posterior capsule,[51] and aspiration of aqueous.[52]

Predisposing factors. Factors predisposing to the development of epithelial ingrowth include technically difficult or complicated surgery (particularly with capsular rupture and vitreous loss); incomplete or delayed wound healing; hypotony; wound fistula; inadvertent filtering bleb; chronic inflammation; and incarceration of iris, vitreous, or lens remnants in the wound. Paufique and Hervouët[53] found that young, highly myopic or diabetic patients were at higher risk of developing ingrowth—the known poor wound healing of diabetics and the relative thinness of ocular tissues in young and highly myopic patients may account for these findings.

There is experimental evidence[54,55] that anticoagulants inhibit the formation of the usual fibrinous barrier to epithelial migration, and 5 of Weiner's 124 cases were in anticoagulated patients; however, the significance of these findings is unclear. No other medications have been proposed to influence ingrowth.

Previous assertions that epithelial ingrowth was less likely with a limbus-based than a fornix-based flap, not supported in larger series,[42,56] are largely inconsequential in view of modern wound closure techniques. Similarly, corneoscleral sutures per se have been dismissed as a potential cause,[57] and catgut and silk sutures in cataract incisions (previously implicated in epithelial ingrowth) are essentially obsolete. In a considerable number of cases of epithelial ingrowth, surgery and the postoperative period appeared uneventful and no predisposing factors were identified.

Pathogenesis. Most attempts to further understand the pathogenesis of epithelial ingrowth, by the use of animal experimental models, have met with little success. For a review of experimental work in this area, which is beyond the scope of this chapter, see Burris, Nordquist, and Rowsey[58] and Regan.[13] Burris, Nordquist, and Rowsey[58-60] developed a cat model of epithelial ingrowth that correlates well both clinically and histologically with the features of the human condition. Despite its potential for evaluation of treatment modalities for epithelial ingrowth, we could find no reports of its use after 1986.[61]

It has generally been accepted that epithelial ingrowth largely results from suboptimal surgical technique, allowing a free edge of surface epithelium to proliferate into the anterior chamber. It is equally clear that implantation of epithelial cells alone will not produce ingrowth. The following factors are recognized as being significant in the pathogenesis of epithelial ingrowth; however, none are invariably present in cases of ingrowth, and, conversely, they may be present in the absence of ingrowth.

Poor wound healing, with or without a clinically evident fistula, may result from poor incision or suturing technique or incarceration of iris, vitreous, or lens remnants. Persistence of plasmoid or secondary aqueous, which contains proliferative factors not found in normal aqueous (which may not sustain the invading epithelium, let alone allow proliferation), appears important in establishing and maintaining ingrowth—its persistence may be due to hypotony or chronic inflammation. Approximation of iris tissue to the wound (even without incarceration) is frequently seen and provides a rich vascular bed for the epithelium. Damage to the underlying corneal endothelium may in part be a prerequisite for migration of the epithelial membrane (by loss of the usual cell contact inhibition) and to a larger extent may represent a cytotoxic effect of the extension of pseudopodia by the epithelial cells, causing disruption of the endothelial plasma membrane.[51,59]

Many features of the pathogenesis of epithelial ingrowth remain unclear, particularly how in some eyes there can be relentless progression of the epithelial membrane in the absence of a fistula, hypotony, or signs of inflammation.

PRESENTATION, CLINICAL FEATURES, AND DIAGNOSIS

Patients often present within weeks to months after surgery or trauma, but there are reports of presentations as early as 4 days[5] and as late as 38 years[50] following surgery. Weiner et al.[42] found the most common symptoms (in decreasing order of frequency) to be decreasing visual acuity, red eye, painful eye, tearing, photophobia, and foreign body sensation. Patients may have been labeled as having "uveitis" that failed to respond to topical corticosteroids.

The clinical signs at first presentation of epithelial ingrowth may individually be nonspecific (particularly in the absence of

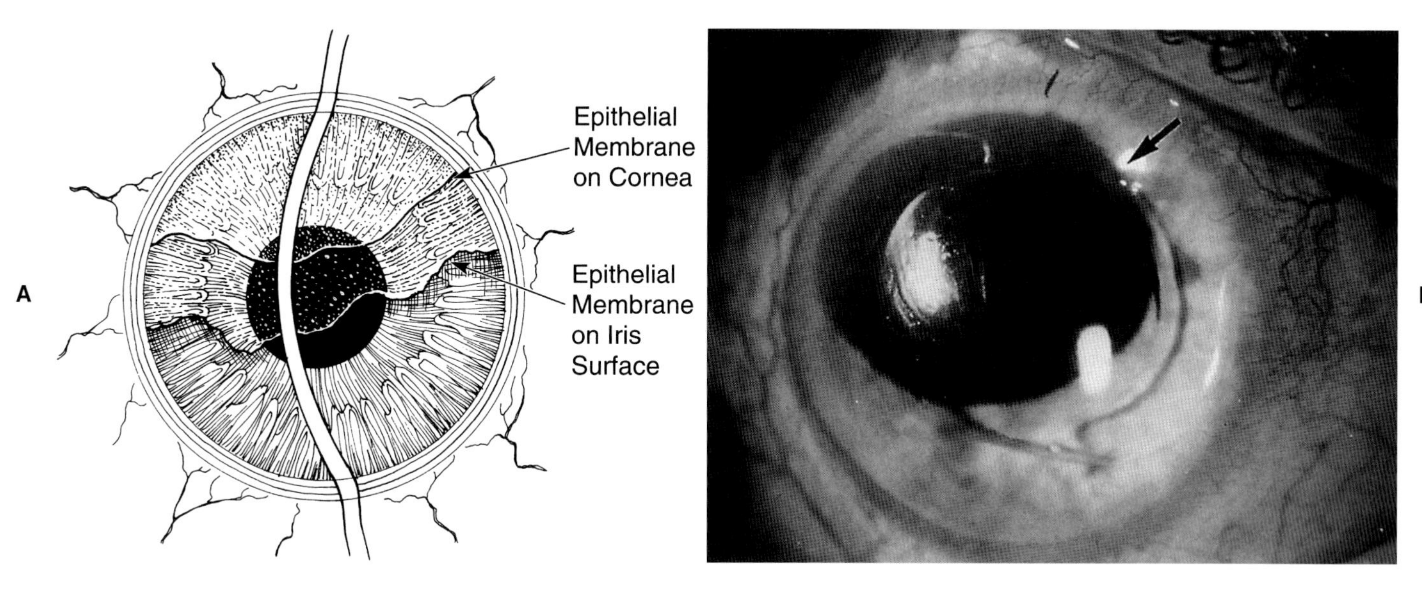

FIGURE 46-10 A, Ingrowing epithelial membrane on the posterior corneal surface. **B,** Ingrowing epithelial membrane. *Arrow* indicates the leading edge of the epithelium.

an obvious retrocorneal membrane), and a high index of suspicion is required to make an early diagnosis. A gaping wound, inadvertent filtering bleb, or an obvious wound fistula should arouse such suspicions.

The epithelial sheet (shown in Figure 46-10, *A*) is most often seen as a retrocorneal membrane with a "gray line" at the leading edge (Figure 46-10, *B*), sometimes with focal "pearl-like" regions resulting from clustering of epithelial cells. These features are best appreciated with retroillumination (Figure 46-11). The involved cornea is frequently clear, although there may be epithelial edema or prominent corneal vascularization. There is clinical evidence of stromal vascularization in approximately half of cases (which Calhoun[62] equated with more rapid progression of ingrowth) and histopathologic evidence in almost all (see further on). Burris, Nordquist, and Rowsey[58] identified pre-Descemet's vascularization as "a harbinger of occult epithelial downgrowth" in their cat model. Descemet's folds may be evident in hypotonous eyes, particularly those with corneal edema. Less common corneal findings include bullous keratopathy, band keratopathy, and a variable level of reduction in corneal sensation.

There may be signs of iridocyclitis, and the membrane may be visible on the surface of the iris. Often iris involvement is manifest as loss of the usual iris contour and mobility or pupillary distortion. Advancement of epithelial ingrowth is usually more rapid over the richly vascular iris than the posterior cornea, and thus progression or otherwise of the retrocorneal membrane is not a reliable indicator. Gonioscopy (Figure 46-12) often reveals peripheral anterior synechiae, a degree of epithelialization of the angle, or incarcerated iris, lens remnants, or vitreous. An epithelialized communication with a fistula or bleb may also be evident.

Intraocular pressure is abnormal in the majority of affected eyes, partly depending on the extent of disease on presentation. Hypotony is documented in up to one third of cases and is highly suggestive of a wound fistula. A significant number of patients with a clinically demonstrable fistula have normal intraocular pressures. Glaucoma is present in approximately half of cases and is almost invariably present in advanced epithelial ingrowth.

The epithelial membrane may extend over the pupil, vitreous face, ciliary body, and retina and may cause retinal detachment.

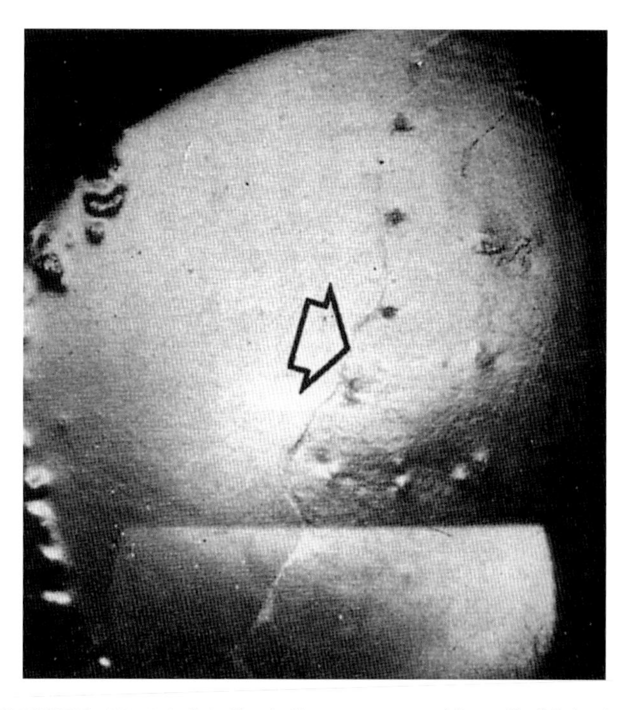

FIGURE 46-11 Retroillumination appearance of the epithelial sheet on the posterior corneal surface, with thickened and irregular leading edge *(arrow)*. (From Stark WJ, Michels RG, Maumenee AE et al: Surgical management of epithelial ingrowth, *Am J Ophthalmol* 85:772-780, 1978. Published with permission from the *American Journal of Ophthalmology*. Copyright by the Ophthalmic Publishing Company.)

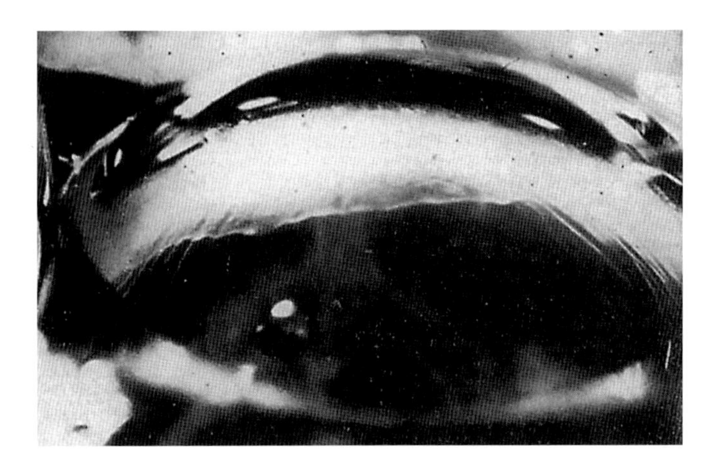

FIGURE 46-12 Gonioscopic view of the superior angle of the left eye, showing the ingrowing membrane throughout the entire view. A large strand of vitreous extends into the cataract incision at 12 o'clock. (From Zavala EY, Binder PS: The pathologic findings of epithelial ingrowth, *Arch Ophthalmol* 98:2007-2014, 1980. Copyright 1980, American Medical Association.)

Epithelial ingrowth has been reported, primarily involving the anterior and posterior lens capsule[63] and proliferating over the surface of an IOL.[64-66] Cystoid macular edema may be present, particularly in eyes with long-standing inflammation. The use of topical steroid medications may temporarily ameliorate some of the symptoms and signs associated with epithelial ingrowth, sometimes delaying the diagnosis.

Diagnostic adjuncts. The diagnosis of epithelial ingrowth requires a combination of awareness of the condition, history and thorough examination for the clinical signs outlined earlier, and the use of additional diagnostic procedures.

Noninvasive procedures

Seidel's test. To perform Seidel's test, 2% fluorescein drops are instilled into the eye, and gentle pressure is applied to the globe. Using the slit lamp with the cobalt blue filter, aqueous flowing from a fistula appears as a lighter stream of fluid in the pool of green fluorescein. Up to one third of eyes have a fistula demonstrable in this fashion on presentation, although presumably all have a fistula at some stage in the development of ingrowth.

Specular and confocal microscopy. At the level of the endothelium, a sharply defined border may be seen between areas of normal endothelium and the epithelial membrane[51,67] (Figure 46-13), and there is usually evidence of endothelial cell loss, reflected in the large size of the remaining endothelial cells, which also appear morphologically abnormal.[68] Confocal microscopy has also been used to identify epithelial ingrowth on the corneal endothelium.[69]

Argon laser photocoagulation. Application of a 500-μm spot size, 100- to 300-mW intensity burn for 0.1 second will produce a characteristic white fluffy appearance if invading epithelium is present on the iris, and a slight focal burn on normal iris (Figure 46-14).

Invasive procedures

Iris biopsy. First advocated by Verhoeff,[70] full-thickness biopsy of iris adjacent to the wound, which is invariably involved in ingrowth if present, may be performed to confirm the diagnosis.

Curettage of the posterior corneal surface. Calhoun[71] described curettage of the posterior corneal surface in a region of suspected downgrowth. He used a 1-mm serrated curette to procure a specimen for microscopy, which can easily differentiate between regular, evenly spaced endothelial cells and epithelial cells that are closely packed, spindled, and less regular and have denser cytoplasm. This technique is used infrequently.

Anterior chamber paracentesis. This technique[72] along with cytologic examination of aqueous for epithelial cells has been used but has a relatively poor yield, and it is unhelpful if negative.

Differential diagnosis. As outlined by Maumenee,[43] the differential diagnosis of epithelial ingrowth includes:

1. Reduplication of Descemet's membrane, which appears as a glassy membrane on the posterior cornea, anterior iris, and angle. This usually occurs in eyes with chronic iridocyclitis and is the condition most likely to resemble epithelialization, but photocoagulation does not produce the appearance described earlier.
2. Fibrous ingrowth, which may have a similar retrocorneal membrane but tends to be slower growing and display more prominent vascularity.
3. Vitreocorneal adhesions, which may appear grayish and may cause corneal edema; however, their slit lamp appearance is characteristic, and they and do not progress in the same fashion as ingrowth.
4. Anterior shelved clear corneal or scleral tunnel incision.
5. Detachment of Descemet's membrane.
6. Peripheral corneal edema.

HISTOPATHOLOGIC FEATURES

Microscopic examination of tissue involved in epithelial ingrowth typically reveals 1 to 12 layers of irregularly arranged, stratified squamous ocular surface epithelium.[50] Goblet cells are sometimes seen, and even in their absence, the electron microscopic characteristics of the epithelium suggest conjunctiva rather than cornea as the source in many cases.[51,59,60,73]

The epithelium is usually present as a membrane of one to three cell layers over the posterior cornea, almost invariably with evidence of stromal vascularization, particularly along the tract of the wound or incision.[74] Weiner et al.[42] found concomitant stromal (fibrous) ingrowth in 55% of postsurgical cases of epithelial ingrowth. The "gray line" that may be seen clinically corresponds to heaped up epithelial cells at the margin of the epithelial sheet. At the leading edge there is a sloping appearance, as observed in epithelial wound healing[75] (Figure 46-15). The irregular arrangement of epithelial cells at the margin gives rise to the scalloped edge seen on slit lamp examination.

In the majority of cases, there is extension of the membrane as a "more luxuriant" growth averaging three to five cell layers[42] on the anterior surface of the iris and angle (or false angle created by peripheral anterior synechiae). The membrane may extend over the posterior iris, anterior vitreous face, ciliary body, and retina. Fibrous contraction resulting from concomitant rubeosis may cause ectropion uveae. Ocular surface epithelium usually extends well into the surgical or traumatic wound, and fine sectioning of enucleated specimens often reveals continuity of the epithelial lining of the anterior chamber with the surface epithelium. There is often incarceration of iris, lens remnants, or vitreous in the wound.

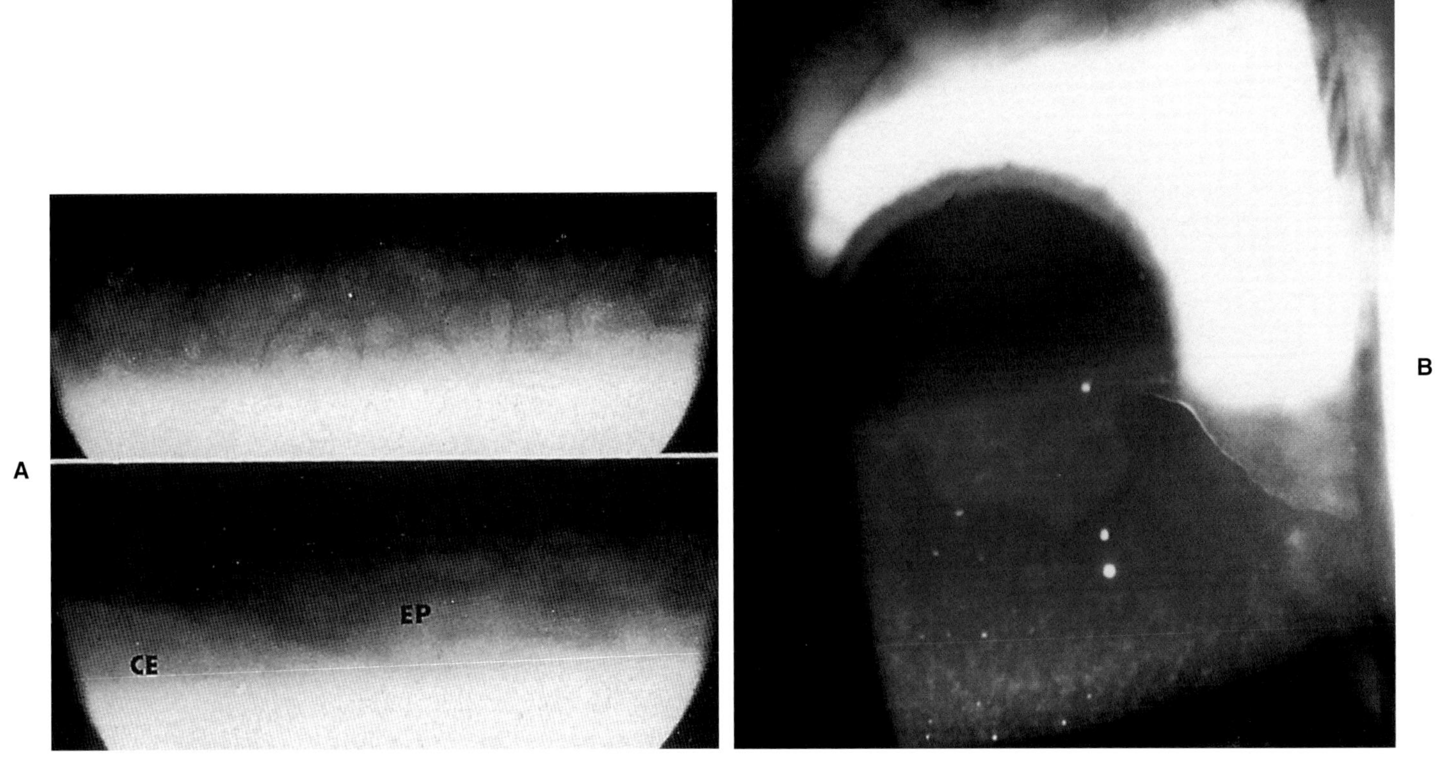

FIGURE 46-13 A, Specular microscopy of epithelial ingrowth (×400). *Top,* Specular micrograph of inferior central (clear) part of corneal endothelium. Cells are grossly enlarged and distorted, and nuclei are prominent. Cell count is 600 per square millimeter. *Bottom,* Specular micrograph of leading edge of epithelial ingrowth. The membrane edge is sharp, and individual epithelial cells cannot be delineated in the area of epithelial ingrowth *(EP)*. With careful focusing, individual enlarged, distorted corneal endothelial *(CE)* cells can be visualized. (From Zavala EY, Binder PS: The pathologic findings of epithelial ingrowth, *Arch Ophthalmol* 98:2007-2014, 1980. Copyright 1980, American Medical Association.) **B,** Leading edge of epithelium ingrowth clearly seen advancing over corneal endothelium. (Courtesy Ann M. Bajart, MD.)

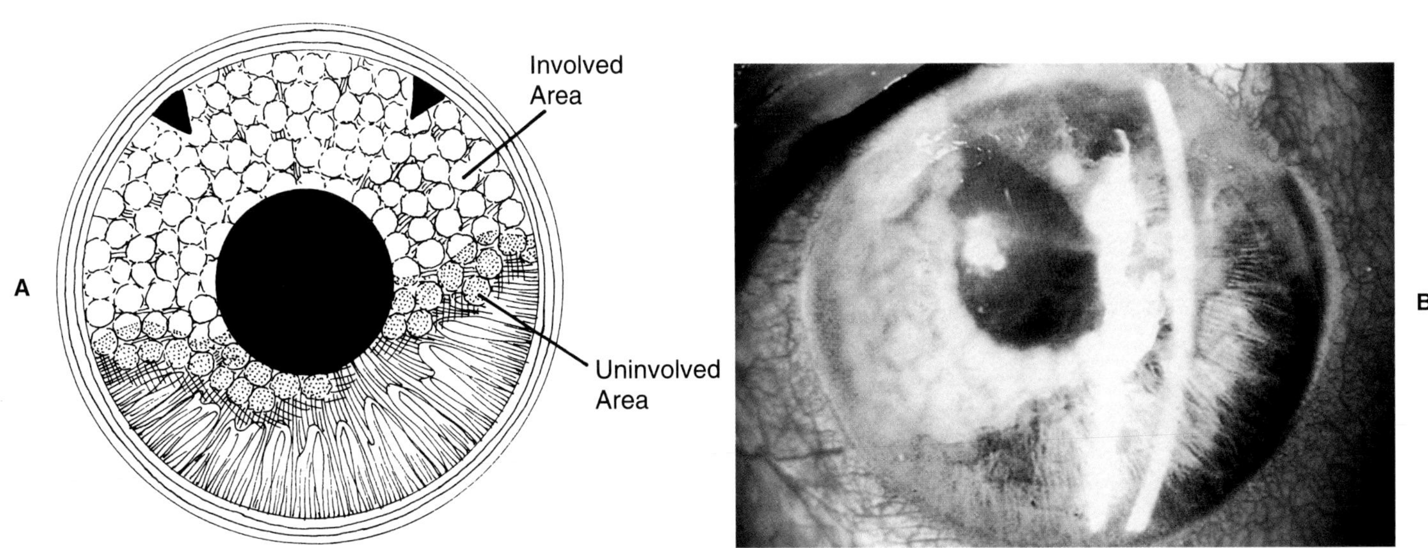

FIGURE 46-14 A, Argon laser photocoagulation produces characteristic fluffing of iris involved with epithelial ingrowth and a slight focal burn on normal iris. **B,** Argon laser photocoagulation of iris involved in epithelial ingrowth.

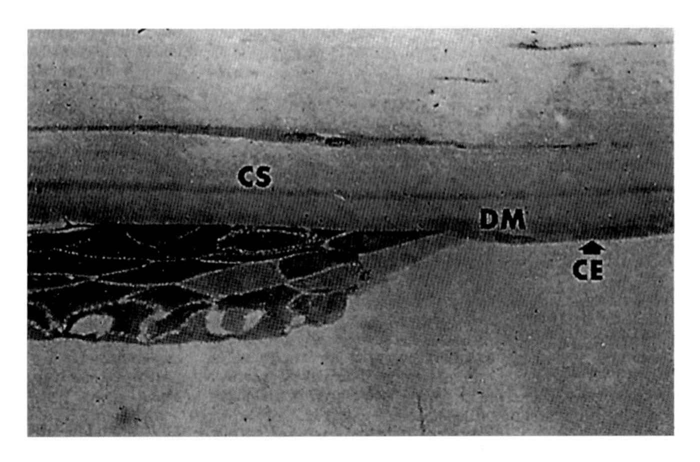

FIGURE 46-15 Light microscopy of ingrowing epithelium on the posterior corneal surface (corneal endothelium *[CE]*), with a tapered leading edge. The most superficial ingrowing cells are edematous and vacuolated. Descemet's membrane *(DM)* and the corneal stroma *(CS)* appear unaffected. (Basic fuchsin stain, ×400.) (From Zavala EY, Binder PS: The pathologic findings of epithelial ingrowth, *Arch Ophthalmol* 98:2007-2014, 1980. Copyright 1980, American Medical Association.)

The mechanisms of glaucoma in epithelial ingrowth, as discussed by Smith et al.,[76] include secondary angle closure by contraction of the epithelial and fibrous tissue lining the false angle; obstruction of outflow by epithelium lining the entire angle; pupillary block from occlusion by the epithelial sheet; obstruction of the trabecular meshwork by macrophages and desquamating epithelial cells; chronic uveal inflammation, leading to trabeculitis and decreased outflow; and the rare mucogenic glaucoma resulting from goblet cell secretion.[77] An infiltrate of chronic inflammatory cells is commonly seen in the ciliary body, iris, and episclera. Cystoid macular edema may also be present in eyes with long-term inflammation.

MANAGEMENT

Although surgical eradication of epithelial ingrowth is the only widely accepted therapeutic modality capable of curing this condition, the results are modest even in the most experienced of hands. A chronologic summary of surgical techniques used in the management of epithelial ingrowth is given in Table 46-2.

Radiotherapy was first used in 1924[78] but was abandoned by the late 1960s because of questionable efficacy, unclear guidelines regarding dosage, and its high potential for damage to ocular structures. Reports of success with radiotherapy were also criticized for the lack of a tissue diagnosis in many cases. Early experience with surgery was so discouraging that it was considered to accelerate the progression of the disease,[79] which (treated or untreated) resulted in blindness and often in enucleation.

There was renewed interest in surgical treatment of epithelial ingrowth in the 1950s[80-82] (see Table 46-2), and Maumenee[43] in 1964 was the first to publish a large series (26 cases) of surgically treated ingrowths. His technique involved identification and excision of any fistula; wide excision of all involved iris tissue;

TABLE 46-2
Chronology of Surgical Techniques for Epithelial Ingrowth*

Year	Author(s)	Technique/Comments
1957	Maumenee[82]	Single case; alcohol/curettage of epithelium from posterior cornea; iridectomy/anterior vitrectomy; VA 20/20 at 2½ years, no recurrence
1958	Sullivan[81]	Four cases; corneoscleral excision/grafting; membrane excised from iris, ciliary body, vitreous; 1 enucleation; VA, 2 count fingers, one 20/100
1964	Maumenee[43]	Conjunctival flap; identify/excise any fistula; excision of all involved iris; involved posterior cornea curetted, débrided, swabbed with 70% alcohol; 26 cases; 3 enucleations, 3 RD, 13 CO, 6 VA 20/50 or better (23%)
1970	Maumenee et al[56]	Preceding technique with excision/cryotherapy of involved ciliary body, anterior vitrectomy, either cryotherapy/curettng or alcohol to involved cornea; 40 cases; 5 enucleations, 20 CE, 17 glaucoma, 5 hypotony (3 phthisis), 1 RD, 11 successes (27.5%)
1973	Brown[83]	Three cases (advanced ingrowth); modification of Maumenees technique, with deep lamellar scleral/angle excision; cryotherapy to involved cornea; 1 subsequent PK; no recurrences; all 3 had postoperative (controlled) glaucoma; all achieved ambulatory vision (best 20/80)
1977	Friedman[84]	Three cases; en bloc excision of cornea, sclera, iris, ciliary body, vitreous; repair with corneoscleral graft; VAs 20/50, 20/60, 20/100; no recurrence
1978	Stark et al[85]	Ten cases; argon laser to define iris involvement; surgical technique as described in text; 4 PKs; VA improved in 8/10; 4 successes† (40%)
1979	Brown[64]	Fourteen cases of advanced ingrowth; 9 cases, technique as preceding (1973); 4 PKs; 3 recurrences, 1 success†; 5 cases, cornea debrided (not cryotherapy); 2 PKs; 1 recurrence, 1 success†; 6 required cyclocryotherapy for glaucoma (not caused by recurrence)
1992	Naumann, Rummelt[37]	Four cases; excision cornea, sclera, iris, ciliary body; anterior vitrectomy; tectonic corneoscleral grafting; complications: VH, CE, glaucoma; VA, 2 patients 20/100, 2 patients LP
2002	Lai, Haller[88]	Fluid-gas exchange with intraocular 5-FU; 2 treatments; VA 20/200 with no recurrence at 8 months
2002	Shaikh et al[89]	Intraocular 5-FU mixed with sodium hyaluronate–viscodissection of retrocorneal epithelial membrane; no recurrence at 14 months

*This table is a summary only. Please consult the appropriate sources as referenced.
†Defined as VA 20/50 or better, normal intraocular pressure on topical or no medication, no recurrence. *CE*, Corneal edema; *CO*, corneal opacification; *5-FU*, 5-fluorouracil; *LP*, light perception; *PK*, penetrating keratoplasty; *RD*, retinal detachment; *SO*, sympathetic ophthalmia; *VA*, visual acuity (postoperative); *VH*, vitreous hemorrhage.

and treatment of the involved area of posterior cornea with curettage, debridement, or swabbing with 70% alcohol. Subsequent modifications to this technique by Maumenee and coworkers have resulted in the currently accepted surgical approach, as outlined here.

In his 1970 series of 40 cases, Maumenee established stringent criteria for success in treating epithelial ingrowth[56]: postoperative visual acuity 20/50 or better, no recurrence of ingrowth, and intraocular pressure controlled on topical or no medication. Limited anterior vitrectomy was added to excision of involved iris and ciliary body, with cryotherapy to the involved posterior corneal surface becoming preferred to other methods of epithelial eradication. Success was achieved in 27.5% of cases, enucleation was required in 12.5%, and complications included corneal edema, hypotony, glaucoma, vitreous opacity, and retinal detachment.

Alterations to Maumenee's technique (see Table 46-2) have included deep lamellar excision of sclera and angle structures,[83] cryotherapy to suspected areas of angle/ciliary body involvement,[64] corneoscleral excision and grafting,[39,81,84] and the modifications of Stark et al.[85] (see further on). The more surgically destructive approaches, in an attempt to more thoroughly eradicate invading epithelium, have not achieved any higher success rates; however, they have included small numbers of patients or, in the case of Brown's series, involved more advanced cases of ingrowth (involving at least 50% of the cornea, iris, or both).

CURRENT TECHNIQUES

The most widely accepted surgical approach is the modification of Maumenee's technique by Stark et al.[85] Preoperative argon laser photocoagulation is used to delineate the extent of iris involvement. This is best performed within 24 hours of surgery, as this degree of photocoagulation usually results in significant anterior chamber inflammation.

Rectus muscle traction sutures are placed transconjunctivally after conjunctival peritomy. A limbal or fornix-based conjunctival flap is dissected to expose the superior corneoscleral limbus. A careful search for aqueous leakage from a fistula (which may not have been evident with Seidel's test at the slit lamp examination) is performed, using 2% fluorescein and external pressure on the globe. If a fistula is found, it is excised and closed with sutures; or a scleral flap, hinged anteriorly, is prepared for later closure of larger fistulae. The leading edge of the epithelial sheet on the posterior surface of the cornea may be marked with a blade.

In cases where a pars plana vitrectomy approach is used, sclerotomies are performed 3 to 4 mm posterior to the limbus, and the vitrectomy instrument is used to excise involved iris and vitreous. Bleeding is controlled with bipolar diathermy or by transiently increasing intraocular pressure. Excised tissue is studied cytologically to confirm the diagnosis of epithelial ingrowth. As complete a vitrectomy as possible should be performed, to allow space for fluid-air exchange to enhance the effects of cryotherapy, and minimise the risk of vitreous prolapse or incarceration.

If a large fistula is present, its site is sealed by suturing the previously prepared scleral flap to the peripheral cornea. Indirect ophthalmoscopy with scleral indentation is performed, and any retinal tears are treated with cryotherapy, laser, and/or

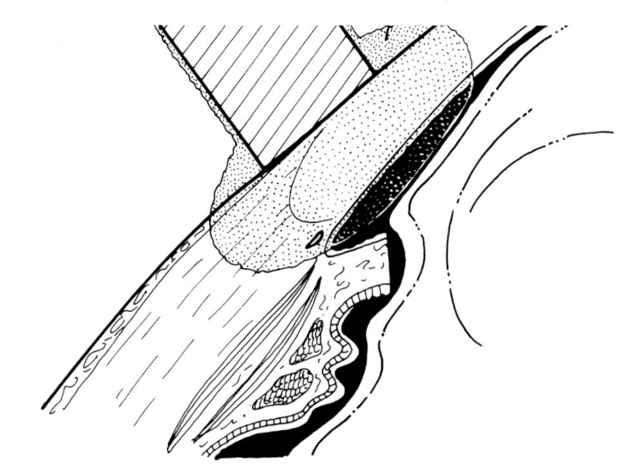

FIGURE 46-16 Transcorneal and transscleral cryotherapy is used to eliminate residual ingrowing epithelium.

scleral buckling as required. After fluid-air exchange, transcorneal and transscleral cryotherapy is then performed to eliminate residual epithelium on the posterior cornea, angle, and ciliary body (Figure 46-16). Stark et al.[85] recommend that a single freeze is adequate if air insulation is used. Unless required for tamponade of retinal breaks, the air bubble is replaced with physiologic saline solution. Frequent topical corticosteroid drops are used postoperatively. The treated epithelium on the cornea usually sloughs after a few days.

Stark et al.[85] achieved impressive results in their report of 10 consecutive patients treated with this technique (average 23 months' follow-up), with improvement in visual acuity in 8 of 10 cases and four eyes with 20/40 or better vision. Four eyes required penetrating keratoplasty: one eye had residual epithelial cells on examination of the corneal button, and all grafts remained clear during the follow-up period. Brown,[64] who used a similar technique with more extensive excision of angle structures, also reported favorable results from keratoplasty in eyes treated for ingrowth. As emphasized by previous authors, patients with epithelial ingrowth must be observed for some years after treatment before recurrence can be ruled out.

Most contemporary cases of epithelial ingrowth that we have seen as a complication of cataract surgery have involved aphakic eyes with secondary anterior chamber IOLs. The IOL is usually removed as part of the surgical management of this condition, although there are no data to suggest the optimal surgical management in these circumstances. Experience with posterior chamber IOLs is limited.

In eyes with extensive involvement from epithelial ingrowth not amenable to curative surgery, particularly in very elderly patients, it is reasonable to aim for control of intraocular pressure, preservation of some functional vision, and avoidance of enucleation. Fish et al.[86] reported nine cases in which Molteno implants were used for intractable secondary glaucoma caused by epithelial ingrowth, achieving control of intraocular pressure in seven, comfort in six, and maintenance of formed vision (at least 1/200) in five patients. The use of a Krupin-Denver valve for control of glaucoma in this condition has also been described.[87] Closure of a fistula is contraindicated if curative surgery is not possible because intraocular pressure will almost certainly become uncontrollable.

The most promising recent advance in the treatment of diffuse epithelial ingrowth is the use of intraocular 5-fluorouracil (5-FU).[88,89] Loane and Weinreb[90] reported the use of subconjunctival 5-FU, but this had only a temporary effect in halting the progress of the epithelial membrane, and the eye was ultimately enucleated. Lai and Haller[88] treated an aphakic patient with fluid-gas exchange and 500 μg of 5-FU injected into the anterior chamber, followed by face-down positioning to concentrate the 5-FU in the retrocorneal space. After a second injection of 5-FU, the epithelial membrane was no longer visible. There was no recurrence at 8 months' follow-up. Shaikh et al.[89] used 1 mg of 5-FU mixed with sodium hyaluronate, to viscodissect an epithelial ingrowth membrane from the posterior corneal surface. Repeat penetrating keratoplasty was required for graft failure, but no recurrence was observed at 14 months' follow-up.

The use of 5-FU (and possibly other antimetabolites) may offer a less invasive approach, or act as a useful adjunct to surgical intervention, for management of these challenging cases. Even if corneal endothelial toxicity and corneal decompensation occurs, penetrating keratoplasty has a reasonable chance of success if the ingrowth has been eliminated. Further experience and long-term follow-up are required to establish the role of this treatment modality.

PROGNOSIS

Even if clinically recognized and surgically treated, epithelial ingrowth carries a poor prognosis. Patients with fistulae were recognized by Maumenee[43] as having a worse outcome. Even in patients with ultimately poor visual acuity, surgery improves outcome in terms of comfort and avoidance of enucleation, compared with medical management (topical antibiotics and steroids) or no treatment. In the series by Weiner et al.,[42] 52% of patients with epithelial ingrowth after surgery eventually required enucleation; only 19% of patients treated with iridectomy and surgical excision had enucleations, compared with all patients treated medically and 95% of those not treated.

Fibrous Ingrowth

In contrast to epithelial ingrowth, there has been relatively little attention given to fibrous ingrowth in the ophthalmic literature. It is often an incidental pathologic finding and infrequently behaves in the aggressive, almost malignant fashion of epithelial ingrowth. Alternative expressions for fibrous ingrowth include fibrous overgrowth, fibrous metaplasia, fibrocytic ingrowth, fibroblastic ingrowth, stromal ingrowth, and stromal overgrowth. Some authors also use the term *retrocorneal membrane* interchangeably with *fibrous ingrowth,* particularly in cases following penetrating keratoplasty.

HISTORICAL PERSPECTIVE

Early in twentieth century, fibrous ingrowth was included in discussions of the complications of cataract surgery, with Henderson[91] emphasizing the role of incarceration of iris, lens capsule, or lens debris in allowing entry of connective tissue to the anterior chamber, paralleling epithelial invasion, and Collins[92] asserting that fibrous ingrowth was invariably a result of infection. In 1947, Levkoieva[93] highlighted the incidence of fibrous ingrowth in eyes enucleated after penetrating injury. He and others have debated the likely source of the ingrowing fibrous tissue (see Predisposing Factors and Pathogenesis)

INCIDENCE

Fibrous ingrowth is usually diagnosed on pathologic grounds, and estimates of its clinical incidence have not been reported. Its incidence in enucleated eyes after cataract surgery is as high as 36% in some series[94] and has generally been found to be more common than epithelial ingrowth. Despite this, fibrous ingrowth is a less frequent cause of enucleation than is epithelial ingrowth. Weiner et al.[42] found concomitant fibrous ingrowth in 55% of cases of epithelial ingrowth following cataract surgery.

PREDISPOSING FACTORS AND PATHOGENESIS

Similar factors predispose to fibrous ingrowth as those discussed earlier under epithelial ingrowth, namely technically difficult or complicated surgery (particularly with capsular rupture and vitreous loss); incomplete or delayed wound healing; hypotony; uveitis; and incarceration of iris, vitreous, or lens remnants in the wound. Swan[95] emphasizes recurrent hemorrhage as a predisposing factor to fibrous ingrowth and states that more posterior incisions, which may damage the deep scleral plexus, are more likely to cause hemorrhage. The importance of incarceration of material in the cataract wound was emphasized by findings of McDonnell, de la Cruz, and Green[96]: 84% of cases with vitreous incarceration after cataract surgery studied histopathologically showed evidence of fibrous ingrowth. Swan[95] noted that ingrowth along incarcerated tissue is unlikely if the outer wound edges are in good apposition.

The exact source of fibroblasts in fibrous ingrowth remains a contentious issue. Swan[95] confirmed the observations of Henderson[91] that subepithelial connective tissue is most likely the major source of fibroblasts that invade the anterior chamber in fibrous ingrowth (rather than being overgrowth of corneal, scleral, or limbal stroma, as is often stated). He also observed that the usual physiologic degree of fibroblastic ingrowth, as part of wound healing, may extend further than usual if the endothelium (which usually bridges the inner wound margin) has been damaged. This is supported by the studies of Brown and Kitano[97] in rabbits. The degree of perforation of Descemet's membrane (which may determine the likelihood of invasion of fibrous tissue) has been highlighted by some authors[98,99] as an important pathogenetic factor.

Blood-derived mononuclear cells[95] and metaplastic endothelial cells have also been proposed as sources of fibroblasts. Retrocorneal/posterior corneal membranes resulting from fibrous metaplasia of endothelial cells, such as those following penetrating keratoplasty and clear corneal cataract incisions, differ in histologic appearance to those of fibrous ingrowth from limbal incisions and should be considered separately. One report[100] describes a "double membrane" composed of a anterior, vascularized fibrous ingrowth, apparently arising from subepithelial connective tissue, and a posterior, relatively amorphous and acellular layer, which appeared to arise from fibroblastic transformation of endothelial cells. Production of extracellular matrix by endothelial cells in response to disease and injury is well established and has been discussed in detail by Waring et al.[101-103] Their classification of abnormal collagenous tissue in the region of the posterior cornea into three types of "posterior collagenous layer of the cornea" is a useful and more accurate method of describing this fibrous tissue, regardless of its cell(s) of origin.

PRESENTATION, CLINICAL FEATURES, AND DIAGNOSIS

Fibrous ingrowth has been observed following penetrating anterior segment trauma, cataract surgery, glaucoma filtering surgery, and penetrating keratoplasty. It has some features in common with epithelial ingrowth, but as a rule runs a self-limiting course, and the ingrowing membrane has a different appearance (Figure 46-17).

The clinical course of fibrous ingrowth is highly variable and depends on extent of the factors promoting ingrowth. Frequently it runs an insidious course with little discomfort, and if the condition is diagnosed clinically, the membrane is often noted as an incidental finding. Less commonly, patients present with decreased visual acuity caused by the fibrous membrane or symptoms related to uveitis, glaucoma, or (rarely) retinal detachment.

Typically, the membrane of fibrous ingrowth is gray or white and has a less well-defined border than that of epithelial ingrowth. It is well described by Swan[104] as an interlacing meshwork of fine fibers, with the appearance of woven cloth, and fine tonguelike strands of fibrous tissue extending from the leading edge. Any extension over the angle, iris, and vitreous is usually identifiable as a thick fibrous membrane. It may also appear as a fine gray sheet over the vitreous face, resembling the membrane associated with postoperative iridocyclitis or hyphema. In cases associated with recurrent hyphema, the membrane may be straw colored as a result of blood pigment deposition. The membrane on the posterior cornea may also be translucent, with a relatively well-defined margin and a similar appearance to the membrane of epithelial ingrowth, especially in regions of stripping of Descemet's membrane, or vitreous touch.

There is usually corneal edema overlying the affected area of cornea, and bullous keratopathy is also common. An updrawn pupil resulting from contraction of fibrous tissue may be evident. Glaucoma is a frequent finding and may be due to overgrowth of the anterior chamber angle or peripheral anterior synechiae associated with chronic inflammation. The degree of inflammation tends to parallel the behavior of the fibrous proliferation, from self-limited fibrous ingrowth with minimal inflammation to extensive proliferation of fibrous tissue, which may be accompanied by marked uveitis. As noted by Duke-Elder,[105] there may be an absence of marked inflammatory changes if the uveal structures are enveloped in fibrous tissue. Subsequent contraction of this tissue may result in retinal detachment, hypotony, and phthisis bulbi. Conversely, fibrous ingrowth is a common finding in phthisical eyes enucleated after cataract surgery.[99]

The diagnosis of fibrous ingrowth should be made on the basis of the preceding clinical features and awareness of the factors predisposing to the development of fibrous ingrowth in the setting of previous anterior segment surgery or trauma. There are no specific recommended diagnostic adjuncts, although if there is sufficient suspicion of epithelial ingrowth on clinical grounds, the further tests recommended on p. 566 may be useful. The differential diagnosis of fibrous ingrowth corresponds to that of epithelial ingrowth, as detailed earlier (see p. 566). Clearly, if surgery is performed for one of the complications mentioned previously, a histopathologic diagnosis should be made on examination of the excised tissue.

HISTOPATHOLOGIC FEATURES

Externally there may be evidence of poor apposition of wound edges. Similar inadequate apposition internally is reflected in a larger gap between the cut edges of Descemet's membrane, filled with advancing fibrous tissue. The source of this fibrous tissue (subepithelial connective tissue, corneal/limbal stroma, or metaplastic endothelium) is usually not apparent. The corneal stroma may show deep vascularization and a chronic inflammatory cell

A

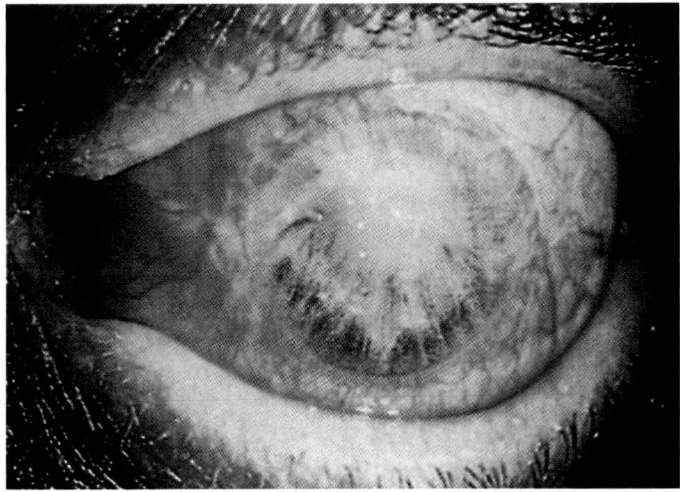

B

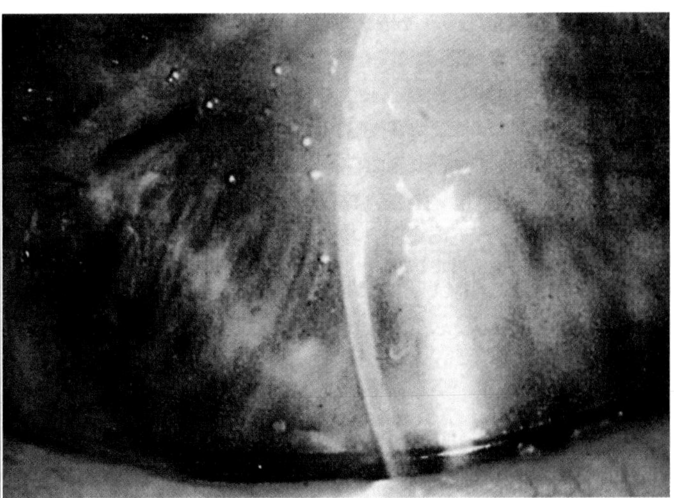

FIGURE 46-17 **A,** Marked corneal opacity resulting from fibrous ingrowth. **B,** Magnified view demonstrating the irregular serrated margin of the fibrous membrane. (From Bloomfield SE, Jakobiec FA, Iwamoto T: Fibrous ingrowth with retrocorneal membrane, *Ophthalmology* 88:459-465, 1981.)

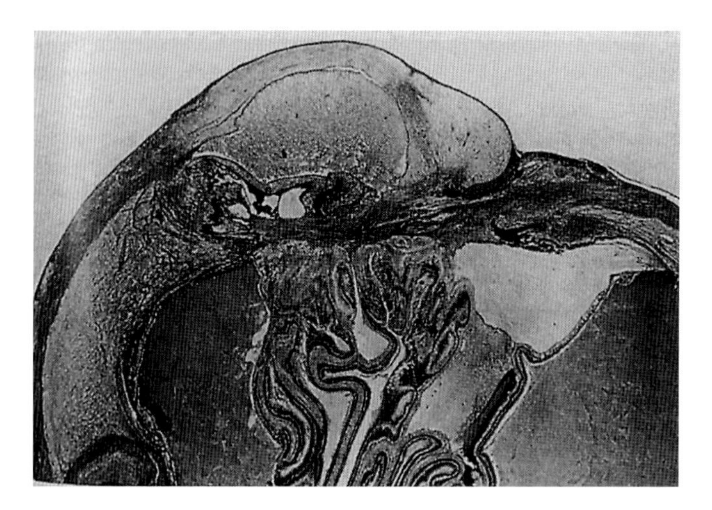

FIGURE 46-18 Light microscopy of massive fibrous ingrowth through a cataract incision forming a dense secondary membrane and causing retinal detachment. (Hematoxylin and eosin stain; ×10.) (From Allen JC: Epithelial and stromal ingrowth, *Am J Ophthalmol* 65:179-182, 1968. Published with permission from the *American Journal of Ophthalmology*. Copyright by the Ophthalmic Publishing Company.)

infiltrate. There may be evidence of suture-related inflammation, and poorly placed or improperly tensioned sutures, resulting in poor wound coaptation, may be seen.

There is usually damage to the endothelium and stripping of Descemet's membrane adjacent to the wound. The anterior chamber angle may be closed by peripheral anterior synechiae or a fibrocellular sheet; the trabecular meshwork in eyes with long-standing fibrous ingrowth appears atrophic or sclerotic. There may be incarceration of iris, lens capsule, lens cortical remnants, or vitreous, as discussed earlier. A pupillary membrane may be present, and contraction of fibrous tissue may lead to pupillary distortion, or, in cases of extensive ingrowth, retinal detachment (Figure 46-18). Wound fistulae appear less common in cases of fibrous ingrowth (without concomitant epithelial ingrowth) than in epithelial ingrowth alone.

MANAGEMENT

As for epithelial ingrowth, modern surgical technique has led to a reduction in risk factors for the development of fibrous ingrowth. Prevention of these conditions is far more effective than attempts at cure. Treatment of the underlying ingrowth itself is not nearly so important in fibrous as in epithelial ingrowth; as many eyes remain stable or progress little over the years, treatment is usually confined to managing specific sequelae of ingrowth. This may include treatment for corneal edema or uveitis (although it is generally accepted that topical steroids will not halt progression of membrane itself); retrocorneal membrane excision with or without penetrating keratoplasty; surgical or Nd:YAG cutting of pupillary membranes; release of vitreous and retinal traction, which may require vitrectomy and scleral buckling; and management of secondary glaucoma. Viscoelastic displacement of a retrocorneal membrane due to fibrous ingrowth has also been recently described.[106] Although Friedman and Henkind[107] proposed radiotherapy in progressive fibrous ingrowth, there are no clinical reports of its use.

PROGNOSIS

In the absence of any large clinical series of cases of fibrous ingrowth, the prognosis of this condition is based largely on anecdotal experience. The overall outlook is considerably better than that of epithelial ingrowth because many cases of fibrous ingrowth are self-limited. Eyes with more extensive or progressive forms of fibrous ingrowth have a poor prognosis, similar to that of epithelial ingrowth, and surgery may be of benefit in treatment of specific complications, although results are modest at best.

REFERENCES

1. Mackenzie W: *A practical treatise on the diseases of the eye,* London, 1830, Longman, Rees, Orme, Brown and Green.
2. Rothmund A: Ueber Cysten der Regenbogenhaut, *Klin Monatsbl Augenheilkd* 10:189-223, 1872.
3. Collins ET, Cross FR: Two cases of epithelial implantation cyst in the anterior chamber after extraction of cataract, *Trans Ophthalmol Soc UK* 12:175, 1892.
4. Guaita M: Proliferation de l'endothélium cornéen sur l'iris et le champ pupillaire aprés l'extraction de la cataracte, *Arch d'Ophth* 13:507, 1893.
5. Meller J: Ueber Epitheleinsenkung und Cystenbildung im Auge, *Arch F Ophth* 52:436, 1901.
6. Perera CA: Epithelium in the anterior chamber of the eye after operation and injury, *Trans Am Acad Ophthalmol Otolaryngol* 42:142-164, 1937.
7. Sitchevska O, Payne BF: Pearl cysts of the iris, *Am J Ophthalmol* 34: 833-839, 1951.
8. Terry TL, Chisholm JF, Schonberg AL: Studies on the surface-epithelium invasion of the anterior segment of the eye, *Am J Ophthalmol* 22:1083-1110, 1939.
9. Theobald GD, Haas JS: Epithelial invasion of the anterior chamber follow ing cataract extraction, *Trans Am Acad Ophthalmol Otolaryngol* 52:470-485, 1948.
10. Farmer SG, Kalina RE: Epithelial implantation cyst of the iris, *Ophthalmology* 88:1286-1289, 1981.
11. Ferry AP: The possible role of epithelial-bearing surgical instruments in pathogenesis of epithelialization of the anterior chamber, *Ann Ophthalmol* 3:1089-1093, 1971.
12. Cogan DG: Experimental implants of conjunctiva into the anterior chamber, *Am J Ophthalmol* 39:165-172, 1955.
13. Regan EF: Epithelial invasion of the anterior chamber, *Arch Ophthalmol* 60:907, 1958.
14. Shields JA, Sanborn GE, Augsburger JJ: The differential diagnosis of malignant melanoma of the iris: a clinical study of 200 patients, *Ophthalmology* 90:716, 1983.
15. Schwartzenberg T, Cahnita M: Sympathetic ophthalmitis associated with cystic epithelial invasion of the anterior chamber: a clinical case, *J Fr Ophtalmol* 5:831-837, 1982.
16. Layden WE, Torczynsk E, Font RL: Mucogenic glaucoma and goblet cell cyst of the anterior chamber, *Arch Ophthalmol* 96:2259-2263, 1978.
17. Ruiz-Moreno T, Cortes-Valdes E, Zazurca-Muinos J: Luxation of an anterior chamber lens caused by secondary serous epithelial cyst, *J Fr Ophtalmol* 12:313-315, 1989.
18. Eiferman RA, Rodrigues MM: Squamous epithelial implantation cyst of the iris, *Ophthalmology* 88:1281, 1981.
19. Winthrop SR, Smith RE: Spontaneous regression of an anterior chamber cyst: a case report, *Ann Ophthalmol* 13:431-432, 1981.
20. Vail D: Treatment of cysts of the iris with diathermy coagulation, *Trans Am Ophthalmol Soc* 51:371-383, 1953.
21. Hogan MJ, Goodner EK: Surgical treatment of epithelial cysts of the anterior chamber, *Arch Ophthalmol* 64:286-291, 1960.
22. Ferry AP, Naghdi MR: Cryosurgical removal of epithelial cyst of iris and anterior chamber, *Arch Ophthalmol* 77:86-87, 1967.
23. Shaffer RN: Alpha Irradiation: effect of astatine on the anterior segment and on an epithelial cyst, *Trans Am Ophthalmol Soc* 50:607, 1952.
24. Fralick FB: Management of complications after cataract extraction, *Trans Pac Coast Otoophthalmol Soc* 32:42-53, 1951.
25. Meyer-Schwickerath G: *Light coagulation,* St Louis, 1960, Mosby.
26. Okun E, Mandell A: Photocoagulation treatment of epithelial implantation

cysts following cataract surgery, *Trans Am Ophthalmol Soc* 72:170-183, 1974.
27. L'Esperance FA, James WA: Argon laser photocoagulation of iris abnormalities, *Trans Am Acad Ophthalmol Otolaryngol* 79:321-339, 1975.
28. Thomas JV, Lederer CM, Simmons RJ: Photocoagulation for epithelial ingrowth and cysts of the anterior chamber. In Belcher CD, Thomas JV, Simmons RJ, eds: *Photocoagulation in glaucoma and anterior segment disease,* Baltimore, 1984, Williams & Wilkins, pp 196-205.
29. Scholz RT, Kelly JS: Argon laser photocoagulation treatment of iris cysts following penetrating keratoplasty, *Arch Ophthalmol* 100:926-927, 1982.
30. Sugar J, Jampol LM, Goldberg MF: Argon laser destruction of anterior chamber implantation cysts, *Ophthalmology* 91:1040-1044, 1984.
31. Honrubia FM, Brito C, Grijalbo MP: Photocoagulation of iris cyst, *Trans Ophthalmol Soc UK* 102:184-186, 1982.
32. Orlin SE, Raber IM, Laibson PR et al: Epithelial downgrowth following the removal of iris inclusion cysts, *Ophthalmic Surg* 22:330-335, 1991.
33. Cahane M, Rosner M, Avni I et al: Nd-YAG laser treatment of anterior chamber implantation cysts, *Metab Syst Pediatr Ophthalmol* 11:47-49, 1988.
34. Maumenee AE, Shannon CR: Epithelial invasion of the anterior chamber, *Trans Pac Coast Otoophthalmol Soc* 36:107-135, 1955.
35. Bruner WE, Michels RG, Stark WJ et al: Management of epithelial cysts of the anterior chamber, *Ophthalmic Surg* 12:279-285, 1981.
36. Sugar HS, Willenz AL: Posterior lamellar resection of the cornea for epithelial implantation cyst in the anterior chamber, *Am J Ophthalmol* 54:800-803, 1962.
37. Naumann GOH, Rummelt V: Block excision of cystic and diffuse epithelial ingrowth of the anterior chamber, *Arch Ophthalmol* 110:223-227, 1992.
38. Rummelt V, Naumann GO: Block excision with tectonic corneoscleroplasty for cystic and/or diffuse epithelial invasion of the anterior eye segment: report of 51 consecutive patients (1980-1996), *Klin Monatsbl Augenheilkd* 211:312-323, 1997.
39. Rizzuti AB: Traumatic implantation cysts of the iris with special emphasis on surgical aspects, *Am J Ophthalmol* 39:13-20, 1955.
40. Harbin TS, Maumenee AE: Epithelial downgrowth after surgery for epithelial cyst, *Am J Ophthalmol* 78:1-4, 1974.
41. Christensen L: Epithelialization of the anterior chamber. In *Transactions of the New Orleans Academy of Ophthalmology: symposium on cataracts,* St Louis, 1965, Mosby.
42. Weiner MJ, Trentacoste J, Pon DM et al: Epithelial downgrowth: a 30-year clinicopathological review, *Br J Ophthalmol* 73:6-11, 1989.
43. Maumenee AE: Treatment of epithelial downgrowth and intraocular fistula following cataract extraction, *Trans Am Ophthalmol Soc* 62:153-166, 1964.
44. Jaffe NS, Jaffe MS, Jaffe GF: Epithelial invasion of the anterior chamber. In *Cataract surgery and its complications,* ed 5, St Louis, 1989, Mosby, pp 582-613.
45. Merenmies L, Tarkkanen A: Causes of enucleation following cataract extraction, *Acta Ophthalmol* 55:47-352, 1977.
46. Holliday JN, Buller CR, Bourne WM: Specular microscopy and fluorophotometry in the diagnosis of epithelial downgrowth after a sutureless cataract operation, *Am J Ophthalmol* 116:238-240, 1993.
47. Knauf HP, Rowsey J, Margo C: Cystic epithelial downgrowth following clear-corneal cataract extraction, *Arch Ophthalmol* 115:668-669, 1997.
48. Lee BL, Gaton DD, Weinreb RN: Epithelial downgrowth following phacoemulsification through a clear cornea, *Arch Ophthalmol* 117:283, 1999.
49. Vargas LG, Vroman DT, Solomon KD, Holzer MP, Escobar-Gomez M, Schmidbauer JM, Apple DJ, Epithelial downgrowth after clear cornea phacoemulsification: report of 2 cases and review of the literature, *Ophthalmology* 109:2331-2335, 2002.
50. Kuchle M, Green WR: Epithelial ingrowth: a study of 207 histopathologically proven cases, *German J Ophthalmol* 5:211-223, 1996.
51. Abbott RL, Spencer WH: Epithelialization of the anterior chamber after transcorneal (McCannel) suture, *Arch Ophthalmol* 96:482-484, 1978.
52. Zavala EY, Binder PS: The pathologic findings of epithelial ingrowth, *Arch Ophthalmol* 98:2007-2014, 1980.
53. Paufique L, Hervouët F: L'invasion épithéliale de la chambre antérieure après opération de cataracte, *Ann Oculist* 197:105-129, 1964.
54. Binder R, Binder H: Experimentelle Untersuchungen über den Einfluss von Anticoagulatien auf die Heilung von Hornhautschnittwunden, *Graefes Arch Ophthalmol* 155:337-344, 1954.
55. Bick MN: Heparinization of the eye, *Am J Ophthalmol* 32:663-670, 1949.
56. Maumenee AE, Paton D, Morse PH et al: Review of 40 histologically proven cases of epithelial downgrowth following cataract extraction and suggested surgical management, *Am J Ophthalmol* 69:598-603, 1970.
57. Allen JC, Duehr PA: Sutures and epithelial downgrowth, *Am J Ophthalmol* 66:293-294, 1968.
58. Burris TE, Nordquist RE, Rowsey JJ: Model of epithelial downgrowth. I. Clinical correlations and light microscopy, *Cornea* 2:277-287, 1983.
59. Burris TE, Nordquist RE, Rowsey JJ: Model of epithelial downgrowth. II. Scanning and transmission electron microscopy of corneal epithelialization, *Cornea* 3:141-151, 1984.
60. Burris TE, Nordquist RE, Rowsey JJ: Model of epithelial downgrowth. III. Scanning and transmission electron microscopy of iris epithelialization, *Cornea* 4:249-255, 1985.
61. Burris TE: Cryopexy of epithelial downgrowth, *Cornea* 5:173-180, 1986.
62. Calhoun FP Jr: The clinical recognition and treatment of epithelialization of the anterior chamber following cataract extraction, *Trans Am Ophthalmol Soc* 47:498-553, 1949.
63. Bruner WE, Green WR, Stark WJ: A case of epithelial ingrowth primarily involving the lens capsule, *Ophthalmic Surg* 17:483-485, 1986.
64. Brown SI: Results of excision of advanced epithelial downgrowth, *Ophthalmology* 86:321-328, 1979.
65. Samples JR, Van Buskirk EM: Epithelial ingrowth on an intraocular lens, *Ophthalmic Surg* 15:869-870, 1984.
66. Schaeffer AR, Nalbandian RM, Brigham DW et al: Epithelial downgrowth following wound dehiscence after extracapsular cataract extraction and posterior chamber lens implantation: surgical management, *J Cataract Refract Surg* 15:437-441, 1989.
67. Smith RE, Parrett C: Specular microscopy of epithelial downgrowth, *Arch Ophthalmol* 96:1222-1224, 1978.
68. Laing RA, Sandstrom MM, Leibowitz HM et al: Epithelialization of the anterior chamber: clinical investigation with the specular microscope, *Arch Ophthalmol* 97:1870, 1979.
69. Chiou AGY, Kaufman SC, Kaz K et al: Characterisation of epithelial downgrowth by confocal microscopy, *J Cataract Refract Surg* 25:1172-1174, 1999.
70. Verhoeff A: In discussion of Vail D: Epithelial downgrowth into the anterior chamber following cataract extraction arrested by radiation treatment, *Trans Am Ophthalmol Soc* 33:306, 1935.
71. Calhoun FP: An aid to the clinical diagnosis of epithelial downgrowth into the anterior chamber following cataract extraction, *Am J Ophthalmol* 61:1055-1059, 1966.
72. Verrey F: Cytologie de l'humeur aqueuse et invasion epitheliale de la chambre antérieure, *Ophthalmologica* 154:310, 1967.
73. Iwamoto T, Srinivasan BD, DeVoe AG: Electron microscopy of epithelial downgrowth, *Ann Ophthalmol* 9:1095-1110, 1977.
74. Bernadino VB, Kim JC, Smith TR: Epithelialization of the anterior chamber after cataract extraction, *Arch Ophthalmol* 82:742-750, 1969.
75. Matsuda H, Smelser GK: Electron microscopy of corneal wound healing, *Exp Eye Res* 16:427-442, 1976.
76. Smith P, Stark WJ, Maumenee AE et al: Epithelial, fibrous, and endothelial proliferation. In Ritch R, Shields MB, Krupin T, eds: *The glaucomas,* St Louis, 1989, Mosby, pp 1299-1335.
77. Küchle M, Naumann GOH: Mucogenic secondary open-angle glaucoma in diffuse epithelial ingrowth treated by block-excision, *Am J Ophthalmol* 111:230-234, 1991.
78. Handmann M: Disparition complète d'un Kyste traumatique de l'iris après roentgenthérapie, *Klin Monatsld Augenheilkd* 72:111, 1924.
79. Pincus MH: Epithelial invasion of the anterior chamber following cataract extraction: effect of radiation therapy, *Arch Ophthalmol* 43:509, 1950.
80. Maumenee AE: Epithelial invasion of the anterior chamber, *Trans Am Acad Ophthalmol Otolaryngol* 61:51-57, 1957.
81. Sullivan GL: Epithelization of the anterior chamber following cataract extraction: a new approach to treatment, *Trans Am Ophthalmol Soc* 56:606-654, 1958.
82. Long JC, Tyner GS: Three cases of epithelial invasion of the anterior chamber treated surgically, *Arch Ophthalmol* 58:396-400, 1957.
83. Brown SI: Treatment of advanced epithelial downgrowth, *Trans Am Acad Ophthalmol Otolaryngol* 77:618-622, 1973.
84. Friedman AH: Radical anterior segment surgery for epithelial invasion of the anterior chamber: report of three cases, *Trans Am Acad Ophthalmol Otolaryngol* 83:216-223, 1977.
85. Stark WJ, Michels RG, Maumenee AE et al: Surgical management of epithelial ingrowth, *Am J Ophthalmol* 85:772, 1978.
86. Fish LA, Heuer DK, Baerveldt G et al: Molteno implantation for secondary glaucomas associated with advanced epithelial ingrowth, *Ophthalmology* 97:557-561, 1990.
87. Bacin F, Kantelip B: Tentative de traitement des complications de l'invasion epitheliale par la valve de Krupin-Denver, *Bull Soc Ophtalmol Fr* 83:519-521, 1983.
88. Lai MM, Haller JA: Resolution of epithelial ingrowth in a patient treated with 5-fluorouracil. *Am J Ophthalmol* 133:562-564, 2002.

89. Shaikh AA, Damji KF, Mintsioulis G et al: Bilateral epithelial downgrowth managed in one eye with intraocular 5-fluorouracil. *Arch Ophthalmol* 120:1396-1398, 2002.
90. Loane ME, Weinreb RN: Glaucoma secondary to epithelial downgrowth and 5-fluorouracil, *Ophthalmic Surg* 21:704-706, 1990.
91. Henderson T: A histological study of the normal healing of wounds after cataract extraction, *Ophthalmol Rev* 26:127, 1907.
92. Collins ET: Discussion on post-operative complications of cataract extractions, *Trans Ophthalmol Soc UK* 34:18-44, 1914.
93. Levkoieva E: The regeneration of wounds of external membrane of the eye in the light of new pathologicoanatomical results, *Br J Ophthalmol* 31:336-361, 1947.
94. Allen JC: Epithelial and stromal ingrowths, *Am J Ophthalmol* 65:179-182, 1968.
95. Swan KC: Fibroblastic ingrowth following cataract extraction, *Arch Ophthalmol* 89:445-449, 1973.
96. McDonnell PJ, de la Cruz ZC, Green WR: Vitreous incarceration complicating cataract surgery, *Ophthalmology* 93:247, 1986.
97. Brown SI, Kitano S: Pathogenesis of the retrocorneal membrane, *Arch Ophthalmol* 75:518-525, 1966.
98. Sherrard ES, Rycroft PV: Retrocorneal membranes. I. Their origin and structure, *Br J Ophthalmol* 51:379-386, 1967.
99. Bettman JW: Pathology of complications of intraocular surgery, *Am J Ophthalmol* 68:1037-1050, 1969.
100. Bloomfield SE, Jakobiec FA, Iwamoto T: Fibrous ingrowth with retrocorneal membrane, *Ophthalmology* 88:459-465, 1981.
101. Waring GO, Laibson PR, Rodrigues M: Clinical and pathologic alterations of Descemet's membrane: with emphasis on endothelial metaplasia, *Surv Ophthalmol* 18:325, 1974.
102. Waring GO: Posterior collagenous layer of the cornea: ultrastructural classification of abnormal collagenous tissue posterior to Descemet's membrane in 30 cases, *Arch Ophthalmol* 100:122-134, 1982.
103. Waring GO, Bourne WM, Edelhauser HF et al: The corneal endothelium: normal and pathologic structure and function, *Ophthalmology* 89: 531-590, 1982.
104. Swan KC: Some contemporary concepts of scleral disease, *Arch Ophthalmol* 45:630-644, 1951.
105. Duke-Elder S: A system of ophthalmology, vol XIV, *injuries,* St Louis, 1958, Mosby, 1958, p 335.
106. Mandelcorn M, Men G: Viscoelastic displacement of fibrous ingrowth: a new surgical approach to retrocorneal membranes. *Can J Ophthalmol* 36:341-343, 2001.
107. Friedman AH, Henkind P: Corneal stromal overgrowth after cataract extraction, *Br J Ophthalmol* 54:528-534, 1970.

Macular Causes of Poor Postoperative Vision: Cystoid Macular Edema, Epiretinal Fibrosis, and Age-Related Macular Degeneration

47

Richard D. Pesavento, MD

With modern cataract surgery techniques, fewer operative complications are encountered. However, disappointing cases in which poor visual outcomes follow uncomplicated cataract surgery still occur. When this poor result cannot be attributed to a corneal irregularity, a lens implant problem, or an opacity of the ocular media (i.e., capsule, cornea, or vitreous), the problem often lies with a macular disease or neurologic dysfunction. This chapter deals with those problems involving the macula.

Some macular conditions may be undetected preoperatively. Others may have been suspected preoperatively, but the extent to which they contribute to the visual deficit was underestimated. Those macular conditions that are detected postoperatively can develop with a confusing array of presentations. The onset can be insidious or acute and can follow immediately after surgery or be delayed for a year or more. Diagnosis can be difficult, but a systematic approach can help to narrow the differential diagnosis and, more importantly, alert the surgeon as to which conditions are potentially treatable and which require urgent evaluation and treatment.

Table 47-1 lists many of the common macular conditions that can affect surgical outcome. The list is not comprehensive, but it is useful in categorizing the majority of patients with suspected macular dysfunction. This chapter covers three of these conditions in depth—*cystoid macular edema (CME)*, *age-related macular degeneration (ARMD)*, and *epiretinal fibrosis*—and provides guidelines for diagnosing many of the most common problems.

Clues to the Diagnosis

Knowing the characteristic patterns of presentation for some of the more common macular diseases can be helpful in guiding the clinician's workup and decision making regarding the need for and urgency of treatment. It is useful to think of these patterns in terms of historical findings, characteristic features on examination, and special adjunctive tests. A finely focused history and examination will often pin down a diagnosis even before the tests are completed.

History

Onset

Onset of symptoms can be categorized as immediate, delayed, and late onset. Conditions that present immediately postoperatively may have been present but undetected, unsuspected, or underestimated preoperatively. These would include ARMD, myopic macular degeneration, macular holes, vitreofoveal traction, retinal vein occlusions, ischemic optic neuropathy, and scarring conditions such as toxoplasmosis, histoplasmosis, and trauma. Intraoperative lesions also present immediately after surgery. These would include subretinal hemorrhages, choroidal detachments, perforation of the globe, light toxicity, and accidental intraocular injection with gentamicin.

Delayed onset of symptoms presents within a few weeks of surgery. This is characteristic of CME. At times this can be associated with a more demonstrative iritis or uveitis, especially if there is retained lens material. Subacute endophthalmitis caused by anaerobic organisms such as *Propionibacterium acnes* must be a consideration in this setting. Choroidal neovascularization and retinal detachments occur during this period. A filtering bleb or wound leak can lead to hypotony with choroidal detachments, folds, and serous detachment of the macula.

Late-onset symptoms occur months and even up to several years after surgery. There is a subgroup of patients in whom CME develops in this late period.[1] This can occur even in the absence of complications. It may be associated with neodymium: yttrium-aluminum-garnet (Nd:YAG) posterior capsulotomy in some cases.[2] Epiretinal fibrosis and choroidal neovascularization also should be considered.

Scotomata and Central Blurring

A central area of darkened or absent vision frequently represents a central scotoma. The sudden onset of such a symptom should make one suspect that a choroidal neovascular membrane (CNVM) may be developing. In the elderly, this most often results from ARMD. If a subretinal hemorrhage results from the neovascularization, the patient may see a red scotoma.

TABLE 47-1

Common Macular Diseases Found After Cataract Surgery

Inflammatory or infectious conditions	Cystoid macular edema (CME)
	Serpiginous choroiditis
	Toxoplasmosis
	Histoplasmosis
	Any preexisting uveitis
Degenerative disorders	Age-related macular degeneration (ARMD)
	Pathologic myopia
Vitreomacular/vitreoretinal interface disorders	Rhegmatogenous retinal detachment
	Macular holes
	Vitreofoveal traction
Proliferative disorders	Epiretinal fibrosis
Vascular diseases	Retinal vein occlusions
	Choroidal neovascularization
	Anterior ischemic optic neuropathy
	Temporal arteritis
	Retinal arterial occlusion
	Idiopathic perifoveal telangiectasis
	Central serous choroidopathy
Systemic diseases	Diabetic retinopathy
	Hypertensive retinopathy
	Angioid streaks
Toxic maculopathies	Light toxicity
	Intraocular gentamicin
	Hydroxychloroquine (Plaquenil)
	Thioridazine (Mellaril)
Hypotensive maculopathies	Choroidal detachment
	Choroidal macular folds
	Exudative serous detachment of macula
Traumatic maculopathies	Perforated globe (retrobulbar injection)
	Choroidal rupture and scarring

A macular hole may present as an acute or subacute central area of visual distortion. This is usually followed within a few weeks or months by a well-defined central scotoma. This is most often seen in elderly women.

Patients with central or branch retinal artery occlusions can be suddenly stricken with a rather poorly defined but dense central scotoma. They can sometimes describe a red-tinged altitudinal type of field loss with a branch or hemiretinal vein occlusion.

The symptoms arising from CME and central retinal vein occlusions are often described as a more diffuse central blurring rather than a distinct central blind spot.

Metamorphopsia and Micropsia

Distortion of the central visual field that develops suddenly following cataract surgery most likely represents choroidal neovascularization or a retinal pigment epithelial detachment secondary to ARMD. A more protracted onset may be seen with epiretinal fibrosis, although sudden contraction of the membrane can induce acute symptoms. Less commonly this symptom may signal the development of an impending macular hole or vitreofoveal traction. In a younger age group, usually under age 55, vaguely distorted central images or the perception that an image is smaller in the affected than in the fellow eye (micropsia) should suggest central serous choroidopathy. In diabetic retinopathy, postoperative macular edema sometimes causes metamorphopsia.

These symptoms are frequently confused with tilting of an undistorted visual image, which often represents an extraocular muscle dysfunction.

Altitudinal Visual Field Defects

A scotoma that develops acutely and involves the superior or inferior half of the central visual field may be seen in anterior ischemic optic neuropathy, retinal detachments, and branch retinal artery or vein occlusions. Patients will frequently report a "veil covering over my vision" with a vitreous detachment, but when questioned further, they will admit that they can see through it.

Photopsias

Flashing lights in the peripheral vision are a well-known symptom of vitreous detachments, retinal holes, retinal detachments, and migraine syndromes. Photopsias caused by retinal traction by the vitreous are usually brief, lasting less than a second, and recurrent in the peripheral visual field. They are seen best in dim illumination. In contrast, migraine syndromes have visual auras that last for minutes or more and usually have a geometric pattern of some sort, such as jagged edges. This is sometimes associated with an enlarging scotoma that resolves completely. In contrast, patients with CME often complain of central photopsias, which they describe as a "pinwheel" or a "four leaf clover." This symptom may persist and even worsen during the resolution phase of CME and disappears when the edema is no longer present. Central photopsias with colored lights are sometimes reported by patients with choroidal neovascularization in the macula secondary to ARMD.

Nyctalopia

Poor vision in subdued lighting always brings to mind the specter of rod-cone degeneration. However, this symptom is more commonly encountered in patients with ARMD. A patient's description that progressively more intense light is needed to make out any visual detail is the usual complaint, and usually this must be elicited by prompting the patient.

Examination

Most of the macular diseases outlined in this chapter provide their clues to diagnosis in the funduscopic exam. This is described further in the discussions of the individual diseases. There are a few valuable observations to be made anterior to the retina.

Examination of the pupils before dilation may reveal irregularity caused by posterior synechiae. This can result from anterior chamber inflammation in response to retained lens material or other uveitic processes that can be aggravated by implantation of an intraocular lens. A peaked pupil is more likely to be due to prolapse of vitreous into the anterior chamber with incarceration of iris or vitreous in the wound. An elliptical pupil may be due to iris tuck by one of the lens haptics or damage to the iris or iris sphincter during lens removal. All of these pupillary signs should raise concerns about CME, which is seen more often in complicated cataract extractions.

Macular lesions do not generally result in an afferent pupillary defect (APD), so when an APD is present, an optic nerve lesion such as ischemic optic neuropathy is a likely diagnosis.

The slit lamp examination can provide a few valuable clues in the diagnosis of macular problems. Strands and sheets of vitreous in the anterior chamber, often incarcerated in the wound, suggest CME. These may be seen best on gonioscopy. Anterior chamber cells and flare may also accompany this condition. Undetected diabetic retinopathy or retinal vein occlusions with significant retinal ischemia can induce iris neovascularization, especially if there is breach of the lens capsule. A shallow anterior chamber may occur if significant choroidal detachments develop. Pigment granules in the anterior vitreous are very commonly seen in retinal tears and detachments.[3]

Macular Diseases Resulting in Reduced Postoperative Vision

Cystoid Macular Edema

Although 16% to 30% of patients who have undergone uncomplicated extracapsular cataract surgery will show signs of CME on fluorescein angiography, few will experience a significant effect on their vision, and less than 2.5% will suffer a permanent visual deficit as a result.[4,5] Still, CME is the most common cause of unexpected poor vision following cataract surgery. The debate as to whether Nd:YAG capsulotomy increases this risk remains unsettled. There are studies to support both viewpoints.[6-8] There is general agreement, however, that complicated cataract surgery does increase the risk of CME. Table 47-2 enumerates the complications that contribute to the development of CME. Of these, incarceration of iris tissue in the wound has been shown to be the strongest predictor of a poor visual outcome.[9]

TABLE 47-2
Signs of Surgical Complications Contributing to CME

Iris incarceration in the wound
Anterior vitreous adhesions or incarceration
Pupil irregularity
Pupillary capture of IOL
Iris distortion by IOL (tuck)
Iris retraction by vitreous adhesions
Anterior chamber inflammation
Posterior capsule rupture

CME, Cystoid macular edema; *IOL, intraocular lens.*

Although some debate continues regarding the role of vitreous traction and inflammatory mediators in the genesis of CME, most investigators think that inflammation is the most important factor in pseudophakic cases. Numerous mediators take part in the inflammatory response,[10,11] but the prostaglandins seem to have the actions most consistent with those observed in intraocular inflammations.[12,13] For this reason, treatment has focused primarily on control of prostaglandin activity.

DIAGNOSIS

Macular edema often can be diagnosed on funduscopic examination. Using a contact lens or a handheld slit lamp fundus lens with a thin, angled slit beam, cystic thickening of the macula is often apparent. Small perifoveal splinter hemorrhages (Figure 47-1) and subtle wrinkling of the surface of the macula can sometimes be seen even with indirect ophthalmoscopy. Frequently the perifoveal area will take on a slight pallor, accentuating the yellow foveal xanthophyll coloration (Figure 47-2 and Table 47-3).

It is often very difficult, and sometimes impossible, to distinguish between pseudophakic CME and macular edema resulting from epiretinal fibrosis. Therapeutic outcomes can be very favorable if the correct diagnosis is made. The differential features of epiretinal fibrosis are described in a later section. If the diagnosis cannot be made with certainty, a therapeutic trial of medications for pseudophakic CME is advisable before surgical intervention for epiretinal fibrosis.

Although fluorescein angiography is necessary in most cases to diagnose CME, the extent of staining on the angiogram does not correlate well with the patient's visual deficit.[14] The extent of macular thickening seen on funduscopic exam is a much better predictor of visual function. Nonetheless, fluorescein angiography is probably the easiest and certainly the most dramatic way of demonstrating CME for most ophthalmologists. Mild CME may just produce a faint halo of hyperfluorescence around the fovea. Clinically significant CME will show pinpoint spots of staining

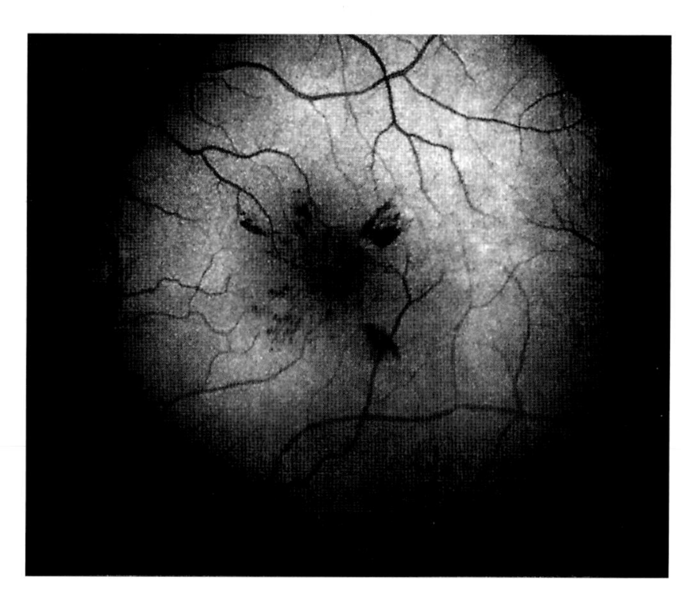

FIGURE 47-1 Perifoveal flame-shaped hemorrhages in pseudophakic CME.

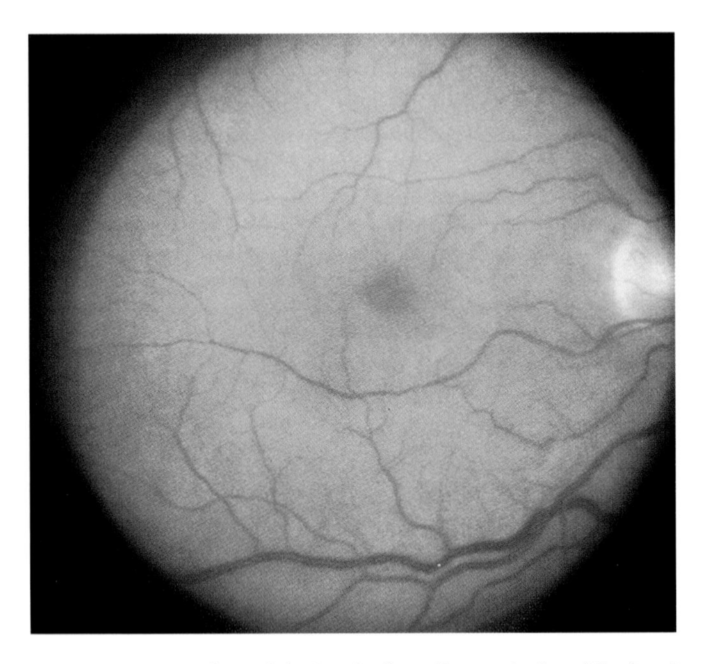

FIGURE 47-2 Loss of the foveal reflex with accentuation of the foveal xanthophyll pigment and relative pallor of the perifoveal area in a patient with pseudophakic CME.

in the perifoveal area as fluorescein oozes from the macular capillaries in the early frames. Later these areas coalesce into the classic "petaloid" staining pattern, sometimes with a dark or bright central cyst in the fovea (Figure 47-3). The optic disc is frequently hyperfluorescent in these cases as well. There is a widespread breakdown of the blood-aqueous barrier in the macula of these patients.[13] The late frames often show a diffuse hazy hyperfluorescence as the dye leaks into the aqueous and vitreous cavities.

TABLE 47-3
Clinical Signs of CME

Clinical Signs of CME
Cystic thickening of the macula
Perifoveal splinter hemorrhages
Central foveal cyst
Subtle surface wrinkling of the macula
Accentuation of the yellow xanthophyll pigment by perifoveal pallor

CME, Cystoid macular edema.

Ultimately cellular damage to the retina will occur.[15] This will result in irreversible visual loss. The goal of treatment is resolution of the macular edema before irreversible cellular damage occurs. There is no method of conclusively determining when a patient with CME will develop irreversible cellular damage. Many patients with CME will spontaneously improve within the first 6 months.[16]

The differential diagnosis includes epiretinal fibrosis, macular edema overlying a CNVM, diabetic maculopathy, a branch retinal vein occlusion, and vitreofoveal traction.

TREATMENT

Opinions vary as to when treatment for CME should begin. Some experts suggest waiting for at least 6 months before treatment, and others advocate starting sooner.[17] The severity

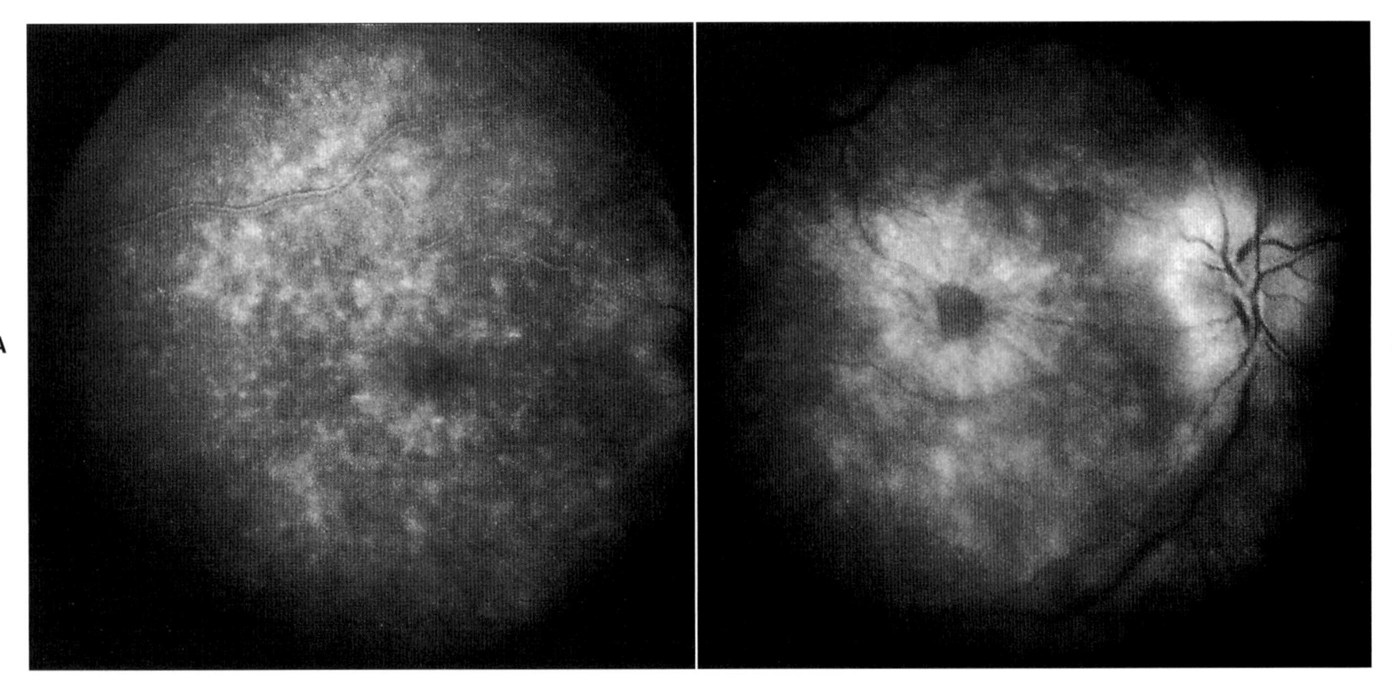

FIGURE 47-3 A, Focal leakage of fluorescein from perifoveal capillaries in early frames of angiogram of a patient with CME. **B,** Classic angiographic pseudophakic CME or Irvine-Gass syndrome with late petaloid staining of the macula, hyperfluorescence of the disc, and a central hypofluorescent cyst.

TABLE 47-4
Therapeutic Agents in the Treatment of CME

CORTICOSTEROIDS	
Topical	Prednisolone acetate 1% qid
	Prednisolone sodium phosphate 1% qid
	Dexamethasone 0.1% qid
	Rimexolone (Vexol) 1% qid
	Loteprednol etabonate (Lotemax) 0.5% qid
Peribulbar	Triamcinolone (Kenalog) 40 mg (1 ml) every 3-6 weeks
	Methylprednisolone (Depo-Medrol) 20 mg every 3-6 weeks
Oral	Prednisone 1-1.5 mg/kg/day
NONSTEROIDAL ANTIINFLAMMATORY DRUGS	
Topical	Diclofenac sodium 0.1% qid (Votaren)
	Ketorolac tromethamine 0.5% qid (Acular)
CARBONIC ANHYDRASE INHIBITORS	
Oral	Acetazolamide (Diamox) 500 mg once daily

CME, Cystoid macular edema.

of the condition seems to be a reasonable starting point for making a therapeutic decision. If there is extensive thickening of the macula with a visual acuity of 20/50 or less, earlier treatment within the first 2 to 3 months should be considered on the assumption that cellular death may be more imminent. However, treatment with topical agents usually poses a small risk as long as the patient is adequately followed. Treatment of patients that are significantly symptomatic is not unreasonable even if the visual acuity is better than 20/50.

Treatment modalities can be classified as either medical or surgical. Table 47-4 summarizes the medical therapeutics that are described here and lists specific agents.

MEDICAL TREATMENT

Corticosteroids. This was the first class of drugs to be used to treat CME, and they still play an important role.[5]
Mechanism of action. These drugs block the release of arachidonic acid from cell membranes. Arachidonic acid is the precursor of a number of inflammatory mediators, including prostaglandins.[12]
Mode of delivery. This has an important effect on the therapeutic efficacy. Topical corticosteroids penetrate the anterior chamber well and have the lowest potential for serious systemic adverse effects. Because irritation to the iris is thought to be the most important factor in the production of inflammatory mediators,[11] the lack of effective penetration into the posterior chamber is less important than one would expect. Peribulbar injection of corticosteroids delivers a higher concentration of the drug closer to the macula, but the risk of perforation of the globe, prolonged elevation of the intraocular pressure, and orbital complications is higher. Systemic corticosteroids provide a more consistently sustained antiinflammatory effect at higher doses, but the side effects are significant with prolonged therapy.
Adverse effects. Prolonged treatment with topical corticosteroids are well known to cause cataracts[18] and increased intraocular pressure[19] in some patients. Suppression of the external immunologic defenses can predispose to infections, including herpes keratitis and corneal ulcers. Peribulbar injections pose many of the same risks; however, the commonly used drugs are depo-corticosteroids, which release slowly over 4 to 6 weeks and commit the patient (even steroid responders) to the effects for this length of time. Proptosis and extraocular muscle fibrosis can develop with repeated injections. Commonly reported side effects of systemic corticosteroids in the treatment of CME are hyperglycemia, hypertension, and psychiatric symptoms,[9] although gastric symptoms (including peptic ulcers) and early cushingoid symptoms are also occasionally experienced.

Nonsteroidal antiinflammatory drugs. Within this group of drugs the cyclooxygenase (COX) inhibitors have been the focus of treatment trials for CME.
Mechanism of action. COX inhibitors block the action of the enzyme cyclooxygenase, which is a necessary step in the conversion of arachidonic acid to prostaglandins.
Mode of delivery. Topical COX inhibitors have been shown to be effective at improving visual acuity in established CME.[20-22] The antiinflammatory effect may even be superior to corticosteroids in inhibiting the breakdown of the blood-aqueous barrier.[23] Oral nonsteroidal antiinflammatory drugs have not been shown to have any therapeutic effect on CME. Studies have shown better ocular penetration with topical than with systemic administration.[24]
Adverse reactions. Fortunately few adverse effects have been reported with topical administration. Some burning on instillation is common.

Carbonic anhydrase inhibitors. A nonrandomized study has shown an improvement in CME while the drug is being administered in some patients.[25] Unfortunately there is a propensity for CME to recur when the drug is discontinued.
Mechanism of action. The ability of the retinal pigment epithelium (RPE) to pump excess fluid out of the macula is probably stimulated by acetazolamide.[26] No effect on the underlying inflammation has been postulated.
Mode of delivery. In the treatment of CME the oral route appears to be most effective. Attempts to use topical carbonic anhydrase inhibitors have not shown as much effect on CME associated with retinitis pigmentosa as oral administration.[27]
Adverse reactions. The most common reactions include paresthesias, such as tingling in the extremities, loss of appetite, taste alterations, and gastrointestinal symptoms. A history of allergic reactions to the sulfonamide group of drugs, of which carbonic anhydrase inhibitors are a member, is a contraindication to their use. Like the sulfonamides, these agents are suspected to be the source of some rare but serious reactions, such as Stevens-Johnson syndrome, aplastic anemia,[28] and other blood dyscrasias.

TREATMENT RECOMMENDATIONS

There is reasonably good evidence that medical treatment of CME has a favorable effect on the natural course and long-term outcome of CME.[29] Reducing the severity of the macular thickening and cystic changes will most likely mitigate cellular damage by delaying it until the underlying pathologic process runs its course.

The following regimen for the treatment of CME is one of many that can be formulated based on the preceding infor-

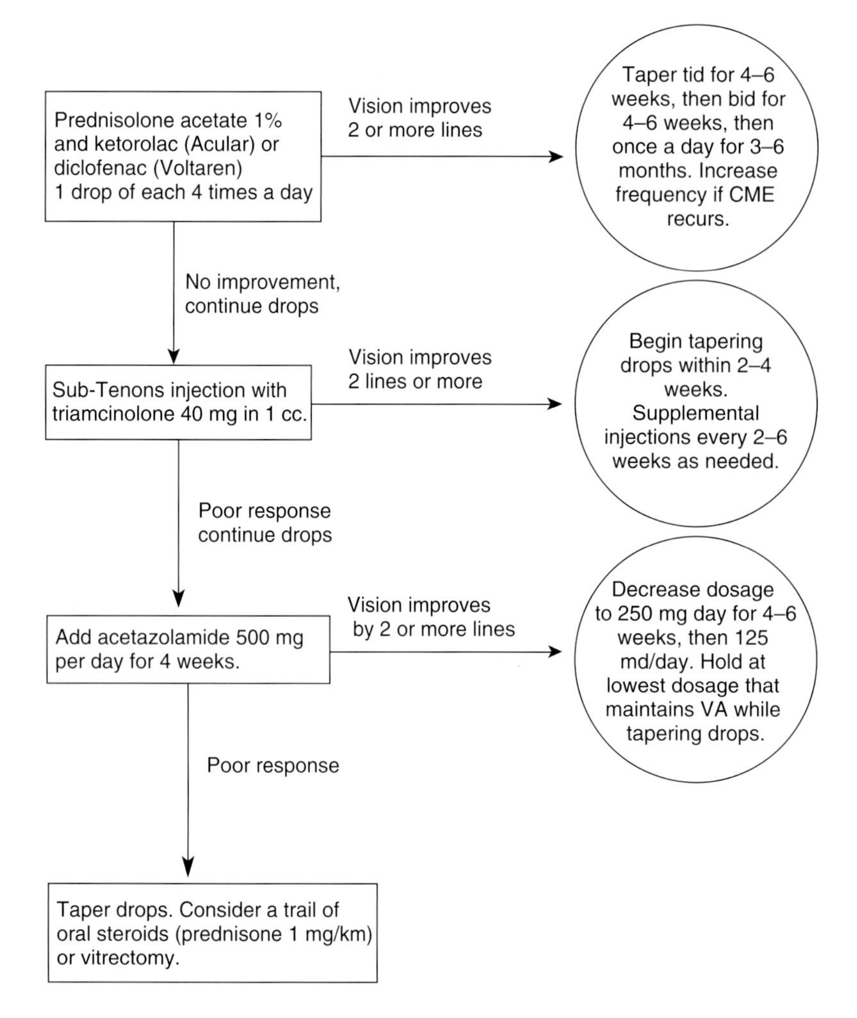

FIGURE 47-4 Flow chart of pharmacologic treatment for cystoid macular edema *(CME). VA,* Visual acuity.

mation. Corticosteroids and COX inhibitors both work synergistically to suppress the production of prostaglandins by inhibiting different steps in its production, justifying their concomitant use at the outset.

The treatment is conducted in a stepwise manner. The therapy is instituted and continued without change for 6 to 8 weeks. If no progress is made toward resolution, the next therapeutic step is taken *without* changing or discontinuing the previous step. If the patient starts to respond favorably at any point, the patient can be slowly tapered off of the medications. If rebound occurs and the vision falls, the therapy can be increased up to the previous level (Figure 47-4).

1. ***Prednisolone acetate 1% (Pred Forte) and diclofenac (Voltaren) or ketorolac (Acular) 1 drop of each four times daily for 6 to 8 weeks***

Good response. If the patient responds with two or more lines of visual improvement, decrease the frequency of both drops to three times a day for 4 to 6 weeks, and then twice a day for 4 to 6 weeks if the improvement continues or persists. Keep the patient on one drop of each per day for 3 to 6 months before completely discontinuing. If the patient responds to topical steroids with increased intraocular pressure, loteprednol etabonate 0.5% (Lotemax) or rimexolone 1% (Vexol) can be used in place of prednisolone.

No response. Proceed to the next step.

2. ***Sub-Tenon's steroid injection (triamcinolone or methylprednisolone) 40 mg (1 ml)***

Good response. Begin tapering topical medication within 2 to 4 weeks. If there is a good response to the initial injection, this may require supplementation with additional injections every 3 to 6 weeks if the vision declines. A total of three or four injections can be given. If there is no response to one or two injections, it is not advisable to give additional injections.

Poor response. Procede to next step.

3. ***Add acetazolamide (Diamox) 500 mg sequels, one tablet per day for 4 weeks***

Good response. Decrease the dosage to 250 mg/day, then after 4 to 6 weeks, 125 mg/day if vision is stable. Maintain this dosage while tapering the drops.

Poor response. Consider a trial of oral or intravitreal steroids.

Because of their potentially serious adverse effects in elderly patients, and because systemic corticosteroid treatment may be required for an extended period in resistant CME, they are rarely indicated. If the patient will not tolerate sub-Tenon's injections or if they are contraindicated for some reason, a trial of prednisone may help. Start with 60 mg/day in a single dose and taper down weekly to 40, 20, and then 10 mg. In smaller, frail, or very elderly patients, calculate a starting dose of 1 to 1.5 mg/kg. If the patient shows improvement, then maintenance at 10 or 20 mg every other day for several months may show some long-term benefit. If the patient begins to respond but then shows some deterioration when the dose is dropped, increase the dose slightly and hold there a little longer. This is only a reasonable treatment if the patient can be maintained at a very low dose.

Intravitreal injections with triamcinolone have been tried with some measure of success but require more study.

Unfortunately some cases of CME are refractory to treatment. It is not advisable to treat a patient with CME with a prolonged course of high-dose systemic steroids because the risk of side effects is known to be high and the efficacy of the treatment has not been firmly established.

SURGICAL TREATMENT

Surgery is probably most effective in the presence of any of the complications of cataract surgery listed in Table 47-2.[30] One study showed a median visual improvement from 20/200 to 20/60 following vitrectomy in patients with chronic CME unresponsive to medical therapy even in the absence of any visible surgical complications.[31]

Nd:YAG vitreolysis. Severing sheets of vitreous that have formed abnormal adhesions to anterior segment structures or have been incarcerated in the cataract wound is possible using the Nd:YAG laser. Although no controlled trials have been performed, convincing reports have associated resolution of CME with successful transection of these adhesions.[32] This can occur in patients who have been treated unsuccessfully for months with medical therapy, suggesting that this treatment should be considered as a first line of therapy in patients with obvious adhesions.

Vitreous adhesions should be suspected when an irregular or peaked pupil is present following cataract surgery. The diagnosis can be confirmed with gonioscopy. Often more vitreous is present than is appreciated even on gonioscopy. The technique of cutting vitreous adhesions is detailed in Chapter 45.

Vitrectomy. Vitreous adhesions may also form to the posterior surface of the iris, causing irritation to the anterior uveal structures. The goal of vitrectomy is to remove all of the vitreous adhesions. The only randomized controlled study performed to date looked at aphakic patients with incarceration of vitreous in the wound.[30] A significant benefit was demonstrated in patients who underwent vitrectomy.

Removal of vitreous via a posterior approach offers advantages over anterior vitrectomy. Adhesions to the posterior surface of the iris are more easily accessible, and less traction to the anterior retina is likely to occur.

Age-Related Macular Degeneration

CME is the most common postoperative complication causing reduced vision after cataract extract, whereas ARMD is the most likely preexisting condition to result in disappointing postoperative vision. ARMD is the most common cause of irreversible vision loss in the elderly population. Cataracts and ARMD very often coexist in these patients.[33] The cataract surgeon faces two challenges in the preoperative evaluation. One is to diagnose ARMD through a hazy medium, and the other is to estimate the relative contribution of the cataract and the macular disease to the visual deficit. If ARMD is suspected as the cause of poor vision after cataract surgery, the diagnosis may be equally difficult through a cloudy lens capsule. It is important here to determine whether there has been a recent, acute change in vision suggesting choroidal neovascularization, which is the only potentially treatable complication of ARMD.

DIAGNOSIS

The diagnosis of ARMD in the presence of a significant media opacity is not always straightforward. Take, for example, the case of a patient with a moderately hazy cataract or lens capsule and a very lightly pigmented fundus. This patient may have extensive RPE atrophy in the central macula, which can drop vision to the level of 20/200 or worse, and this can still be missed on a routine funduscopic examination.

Any sudden change of vision, especially if it is associated with metamorphopsia or a central scotoma, should raise the suspicion of an exudative lesion. Patients who experience a short-term improvement in vision postoperatively followed by a gradual drop in vision are more likely to have a lens capsule opacity or CME. Those that never achieve any visual improvement may have had preexisting ARMD that was underestimated. Poor vision in dim light is also a frequent complaint in ARMD.

It is important to establish the absence of an optic nerve lesion with careful pupillary testing before examining the macula. Defective color vision may help in establishing the presence of a macular or optic nerve lesion, especially with dense media opacification, but it does not help in predicting postoperative visual acuity.

The funduscopic examination should be performed with both the indirect ophthalmoscope and fundus slit lamp lens or contact lens. The indirect ophthalmoscope provides a superior view through hazy media and a wider field of view. This is helpful in visualizing broad areas of RPE atrophy. The slit lamp fundus lenses and the contact lens provide a much more detailed view of the surface contour and depth of fundus lesions. This provides more information on the fine irregularities of the RPE and their location relative to the fovea. The key diagnostic features on exam are drusen, pigment aggregation and hypertrophy, areas of RPE atrophy, subretinal blood, and serous or lipid exudation. Table 47-5 lists some of the high-risk features that suggest that macular dysfunction is significant and should be studied further with fluorescein angiography.

A fluorescein angiogram can be invaluable at sharply enhancing the visualization of a macular pathologic condition in ARMD. Transmission of choroidal fluorescence through thin or atrophic RPE, commonly known as "window defects," presents as sharply delineated areas of early, uniform hyperfluorescence that fade in the late-phase photographs. If the area appears to involve the fovea, the prognosis should be considered extremely guarded. RPE detachments will also stain uniformly, but more slowly, and the hyperfluorescence will persist into the late phase of the study. Large, soft drusen have the same staining characteristics but are smaller, irregular, and often confluent.[34] If any of these

TABLE 47-5
Risk Factors in ARMD That May Warrant Preoperative Fluorescein Angiography

A sudden decrease in vision by history
A history of visual distortion (metamorphopsia)
Visual deficit out of proportion to the media opacity
Multiple soft coalescent drusen involving fovea
Lightly pigmented fovea with suspected atrophic ARMD
An irregular "lumpy" RPE with pigment clumps and atrophy
Atrophic areas in the central macula
RPE detachment in the central macula
Unexplained lipid or subretinal blood in the macula
Localized serous detachment of the macula
Subretinal discolored lesion suggesting CNVM

ARMD, Age-related macular degeneration; *CME,* cystoid macular edema; *CNVM,* choroidal neovascular membrane; *RPE,* retinal pigment epithelium.

TABLE 47-6
Signs of a Poorly Defined and Occult CNVMs on Fluorescein Angiography

Early ill-defined hyperfluorescence with late diffuse oozing
Cystoid macular edema
A "notched" RPE detachment
Late, "stippled" hyperfluorescence
Serous detachment of the macula
Lipid exudation
Subretinal blood
An RPE detachment with a "hot spot"

CNVMs, Choroidal neovascular membranes; *RPE,* retinal pigment epithelium.

lesions involve the fovea, a significant macular dysfunction may exist. Small, hard drusen may demonstrate punctate areas of hyperfluorescence beginning early in the angiogram, or they can block fluorescence as a result of dense deposits of lipofuscin showing punctate areas of hypofluorescence.

A cataract extraction performed when a coexistent CNVM is present can result in an intraoperative subretinal hemorrhage. Presumably the sudden drop in intraocular pressure results in the rupture of fragile neovascular capillaries. On fluorescein angiography, a classic, well-delineated CNVM appears early in the angiogram, during the choroidal or arterial filling phase, and roughly resembles all or part of a spoked wheel with fine capillaries radiating from the central point of penetration through the RPE to the peripheral arc of surrounding vessels. These vessels leak fluorescein and produce a fog bank of dye in the late-phase photographs, which blurs the capillary detail (Figure 47-5). Any area of hyperfluorescence, however, that develops early and shows late, hazy appearing leakage should be considered a possible CNVM. More frequently than not, CNVMs are poorly defined, demonstrating no individual capillaries that can be discriminated. Occult CNVMs are hidden under the RPE, often underlying a pigment epithelial detachment. Signs of poorly defined and occult CNVMs are listed in Table 47-6.

ESTIMATING MACULAR DYSFUNCTION

Most experienced ophthalmologists can estimate fairly accurately the visual deficit attributable to an opacified lens. However, when the opacity of the lens does not appear consistent with the

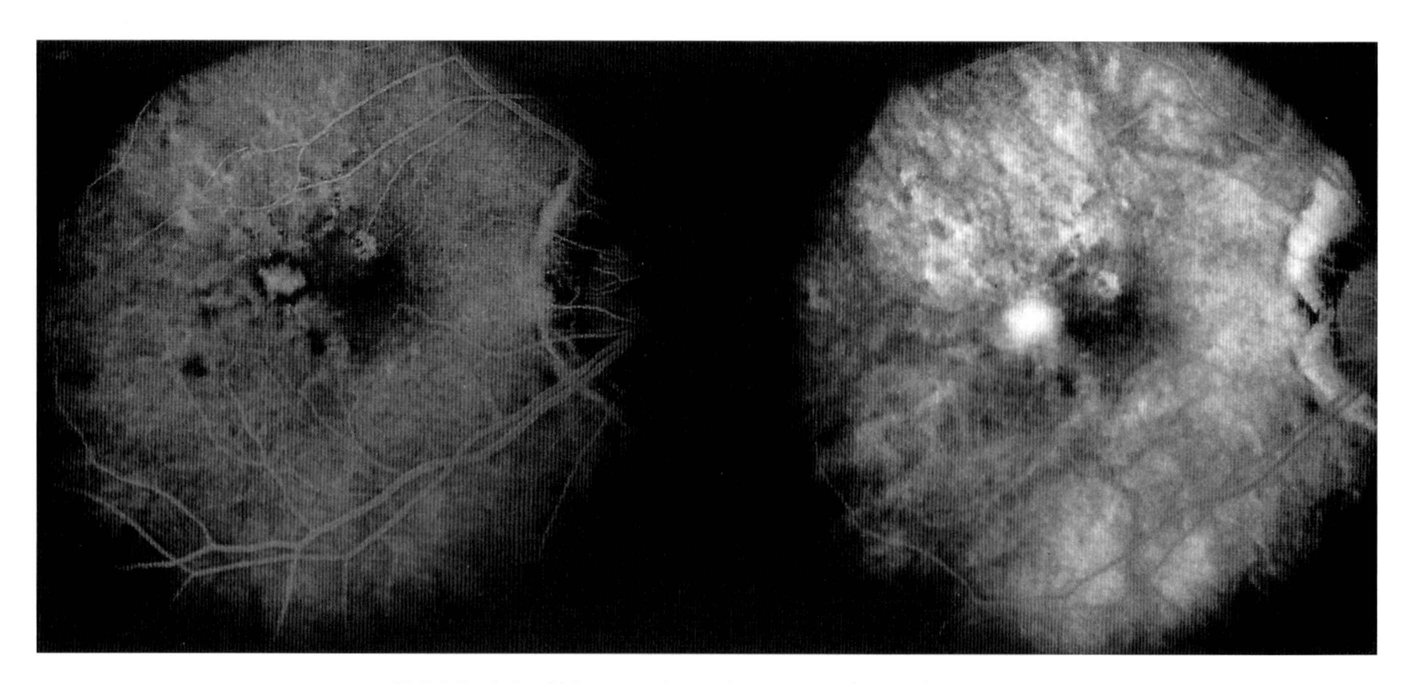

FIGURE 47-5 Well-defined choroidal neovascular membrane temporal to the fovea in a patient with moderate nuclear sclerosis and 20/60 vision. The early photograph *(left)* shows a hyperfluorescent plaque temporal to the central fovea, and the late photograph *(right)* shows hazy leakage of dye into the overlying retina.

level of visual loss, an estimate must be made of the functional status of the macula. Assuming that optic nerve lesions have been ruled out, principally with pupillary testing and visual fields when appropriate, an experienced clinical evaluation of the fundus is often the most accurate means of predicting postoperative outcome.[35] The use of indirect and slit lamp funduscopy together with accurately interpreted fundus photography and fluorescein angiography can yield correct estimates of postoperative vision much more frequently than technological means of prediction alone.

Potential acuity meters and laser interferometers have been shown to be unreliable in predicting postoperative vision, especially when the predicted vision is 20/50 or less.[36] Some authors have discouraged the use of any technological means of estimating the potential acuity in the preoperative evaluation.[37] However, there is evidence that estimates of potential vision with the potential acuity meter or laser interferometer may be up to 90% accurate when the predicted vision is 20/40 or better. Visual evoked potentials, although less accessible to most ophthalmologists, have shown some success in predicting visual outcome.[38] Technological studies are not advocated for the routine workup of all patients with macular disease, but selective testing can be helpful when the clinical evaluation yields ambiguous results.

When the cataract and the macular lesion together do not appear consistent with the visual loss, it is important to rule out a central nervous system lesion with careful visual fields, followed by imaging studies such as magnetic resonance imaging with contrast if the visual fields suggest a central nervous system disorder.

TREATMENT

Visual loss resulting from atrophic or pigmentary changes is irreversible. Laser treatment for drusen to decrease the risk of neovascularization and slow vision loss is under investigation, but it is not advocated at this time. Laser photocoagulation of well-delineated CNVMs has been shown by the Macular Photocoagulation Study Group[39] to be beneficial to patients with ARMD, although a high rate of recurrence has been reported. The treatment consists of photocoagulating the CNVM with overlapping, heavy white spots 200 μm to 500 μm in size, which extend at least 100 μm beyond the visible margin of the lesion and 0.2 seconds or more in duration.

With extrafoveal and juxtafoveal lesions, the risk of experiencing severe vision loss of six lines or more was 1.5 times greater in the untreated group. This persisted through 5 years of follow-up.[40] A 54% rate of recurrences was seen, with 80% of these developing in the first year. Recurrences were seen more frequently in smokers[41] and in patients treated with krypton red rather than argon green laser.[42] Overall, photocoagulation seems to delay the onset of severe vision loss on average for approximately 18 months.[40] Patients must be monitored very closely, especially during the first year following laser treatment, to detect recurrences.

Patients with well-defined subfoveal neovascular lesions have also been shown to benefit from treatment. In the Macular Photocoagulation Study,[43] patients with new neovascular lesions less than 3.5 disc areas in size and with vision better than 20/320 experienced severe vision loss of six lines or greater in 20% of the treated group and 37% of those untreated after 2 years of follow-up. They also retained better contrast threshold for large letters on the acuity chart with treatment. This benefit also held true for patients with recurrent subfoveal neovascularization 6 disc areas or less in size and sparing some retina within 1500 mm of the center of the fovea.[44] However, the incidence of immediate drop in vision within the first 3 months after treatment was twice as high in the treated group, prompting many ophthalmologists to treat only after the visual acuity falls below 20/100.

Photodynamic therapy with verteporfin has been shown to have an advantage over conventional laser photocoagulation for patients with predominantly classical subfoveal CNVMs. In the subgroup of patients with wet macular degeneration in which the CNVM is subfoveal and is at least 50% "classic" and in which the greatest linear diameter of the lesion is 5400 mm or less, photodynamic therapy was found to stabilize the vision in 61.2% as opposed to 46.4% of controls. Vision improved in a smaller number of patients, by at least one line in 16% of the treated group versus 7% of controls.[45] The vision is rarely seen to decrease immediately following therapy. Patients with occult subfoveal neovascularization have also been found to have a significantly reduced risk of moderate to severe vision loss with verteporfin therapy over controls (67% vs. 54%) but to a lesser extent than in patients with a 50% or greater classic component.[46]

Treatment of poorly defined CNVMs is more problematic. Almost 90% involve the fovea at presentation, and the natural course shows a high rate of severe vision loss within the first 2 years.[47] Delineating the margins of the area to be treated is often impossible, and this predisposes to a potentially high rate of recurrence, which may lead to severe vision loss even more rapidly with treatment than the natural course. Treatment judgments are best left to an experienced retinal specialist.

The Age-Related Eye Disease Study demonstrated that the risk of severe vision loss can be reduced in patients with moderate to severe macular degeneration by nutritional supplementation. Patients with moderate to advanced AMD taking 15 mg beta-carotene and 80 mg zinc oxide daily showed a 25% reduction in their risk of severe vision loss (compared to controls) over 5 years. This is currently the only treatment for dry macular degeneration with proven efficacy.[48] Strong evidence has shown that smoking accelerates the rate of vision loss in ARMD.[49]

Epiretinal Fibrosis

Proliferation of a fibrous membrane over the surface of the macula is common in the elderly population. Twelve percent of all autopsied elderly eyes[50] and 20% of eyes in patients over 75 years of age have epiretinal membranes to some degree, making this a frequently coexistent condition with cataracts.[51] Epiretinal membranes are associated with posterior vitreous detachments; vascular, inflammatory, or traumatic injuries; vitreous hemorrhages; and retinal holes.[52-54] Often they are idiopathic.[55] Importantly, they have been found following most types of intraocular surgery, including cataract extraction.[51] It can be easy to confuse postoperative epiretinal fibrosis with pseudophakic CME. Because the treatment is different for the two conditions, this is an important distinction to make.

DIAGNOSIS

The most common symptoms associated with epiretinal membranes are blurring and visual distortion. These usually develop slowly, but the onset can be more acute if there is an abrupt contraction of the membrane.

Membranes can be translucent with a wrinkled cellophane appearance or can have varying degrees of opacity. Retinal striae are common. This is associated with contraction of the membranes, which have been found to contain actin filaments and have myofibroblast-like properties.[56] At times this can lead to a shallow tabletop traction detachment of the macula. Rarely, membranes can spontaneously peal from the surface of the macula.[57] Tractional forces can pull the fovea into an ectopic location and can abnormally straighten or distort retinal vessels. In some instances an opacified membrane can be seen crossing over vessels. Traction on retinal vessels can result in vascular leakage and CME. These features can be seen with the slit lamp fundus lens or contact lens (Table 47-7). Pseudophakic CME lacks most of these features.

Contraction of a membrane around the fovea can produce the appearance of a macular hole.[58] These pseudoholes can be distinguished from true macular holes in several ways. Retinal tissue can be seen in the base of the pseudohole, and a layer of translucent tissue can sometimes be seen covering the pseudohole in the plane of the inner retinal surface on slit lamp fundus exam. A narrow slit beam directed through the lesion will be seen by the patient with a central distortion, not a central scotoma as with a true hole. The very distinct and well-delineated hyperfluorescence in the central macula seen on fluorescein angiography with a macular hole is very subtle or absent with pseudoholes.

TABLE 47-7
Funduscopic Features of Epiretinal Fibrosis of the Macula

Surface wrinkling or retinal striae
Opaque membrane
Whitened vascular crossover points
Shallow traction detachment of macula
Foveal ectopy
Vascular tortuosity or straightening
Macular thickening or CME
Macular pseudohole

CME, Cystoid macular edema.

Fluorescein angiography may show macular staining that looks like classic CME. However, the staining is much more irregular and asymmetric than in pseudophakic CME (Figure 47-6) and often lacks the usual petaloid staining pattern of CME.[59] Vascular tortuosity and straightening, surface irregularities, and the opacified points where thickened membranes cross over blood vessels are often best seen on the red-free photographs.

TREATMENT

As a general rule, most patients with epiretinal fibrosis do not require treatment. Seventy percent present with a vision of 20/30 or better,[60] and only 10% to 25% will progress within the first 2 years.[61,62] However, many patients find the visual distortion disabling even when their acuity is good.

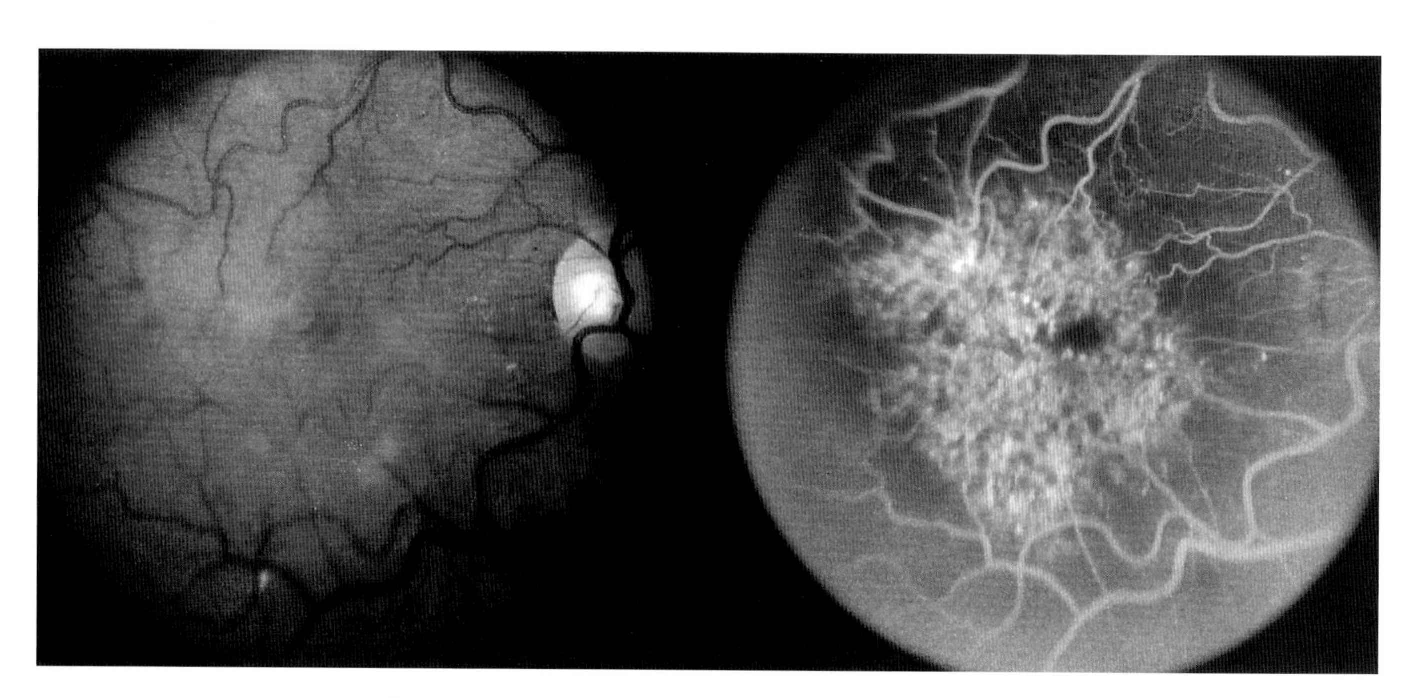

FIGURE 47-6 Epiretinal fibrosis. The red-free photographs show tortuosity of the vessels with pale areas of fibrosis overlying the macula, one of which can be seen overlying an inferonasal vessel *(left).* Extensive, moderately asymmetric cystoid staining of the macula in the late phase of the angiogram is present *(right).*

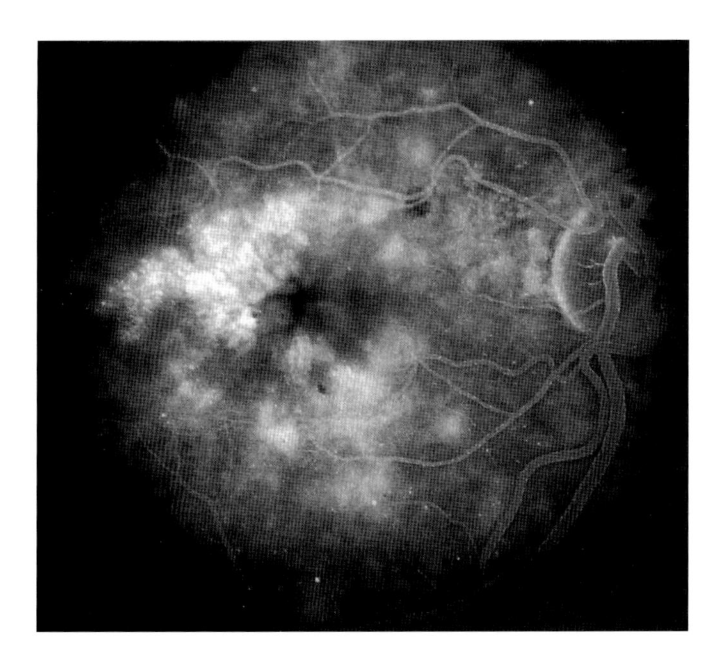

FIGURE 47-7 CME developing in a patient with nonproliferative diabetic retinopathy following cataract surgery. The edema did not respond favorably to medical treatment for pseudophakic CME but did improve with focal laser treatment.

Definitive treatment consists of performing a core vitrectomy and peeling the membrane[52,63] from the surface of the macula. Significant visual improvement occurs in 60% to 90% of patients, usually within the first year of follow-up.[64] Although patients with preoperative vision worse than 20/100 show more lines of visual improvement postoperatively, overall they achieve a better final visual acuity if preoperative vision is better than 20/80 and if symptoms have been present for 6 months or less.[65] Some studies suggest that CME associated with epiretinal fibrosis may be a bad prognostic sign,[52,55,65] but this has been contradicted by others.[63,64] If there is any confusion in differentiating between pseudophakic CME and that secondary to epiretinal fibrosis, a 6- to 8-week trial of pharmacologic treatment for pseudophakic CME may help to clarify the diagnosis.

Diabetic Retinopathy

There is reasonably good evidence that cataract extraction can accelerate the progression of nonproliferative diabetic retinopathy in some patients (Figure 47-7). Jaffe et al.[66] showed a 74% rate of progression of nonproliferative retinopathy in operated eyes compared with a 37% rate of progression in the nonoperated fellow eye. It is not known whether surgical technique or lens implant style have any affect on the risk of progression. More advanced stages of diabetic retinopathy and retinopathy that is inadequately treated before surgery portend poor visual results.[67] Patients without macular edema who have minimal nonproliferative retinopathy or quiescent proliferative retinopathy after PRP have the best chance of attaining a postoperative visual acuity of 20/40 or better, whereas those with significant nonproliferative diabetic maculopathy or active proliferation have the worse chance.[68]

Patients with diabetic retinopathy should have a thorough retinal examination before cataract surgery and should receive treatment for clinically significant macular edema and/or proliferation before surgery.

Other Macular Diseases

Other conditions involving the macula can result in a poor visual outcome. Some of the more common ones are summarized in Table 47-8.

TABLE 47-8

Differential Diagnosis of Other Macular Diseases Causing Poor Postoperative Vision

	Macular-Hole	Retinal Vein Occlusion	Diabetic Maculopathy	Light Toxicity	Intraocular Gentamicin	Hypotensive Maculopathy	Vitreofoveal Traction
Symptoms	Early: distortion, blurring Late: central scotoma	Central blurring "Red" scotoma	Central blurring Floaters Metamorphopsia	Central blurring	Decreased postoperative vision (often severe)	Decreased vision Sometimes pain	Central blurring Occasional distortion
Clinical signs	Round, smooth central hole No tissue over or in base of hole Scotoma seen in slit beam through hole Surrounding perifoveal detachment	Venous dilation, tortuosity Multiple flame hemorrhages Macular edema Retinal and iris neovascularization	Microaneurysms Lipid exudate Retinal hemorrhages Macular edema Cotton wool infarcts Retinal neovascularization	RPE pigment mottling and subtle atrophy	Intraretinal hemorrhages Edematous retina Cotton wool infarcts Arteriolar narrowing Venous beading Neovascularization	Choroidal detachment Shallow anterior chamber Macular choroidal folds Shallow macular detachment Disc swelling	Central pseudocyst Fovea elevated above macula Anterior-posterior vitreous traction
Fluorescein angiogram	Distinct central hyperfluorescence	Blocked fluorescence (blood and ischemia) Macular staining (edema) Disc staining Vascular dilation, tortuosity Neovascularization	Fluorescent microaneurysms Blocked fluorescence (blood) Capillary nonperfusion Macular staining (diffuse or focal) Leakage of dye from neovascularization	"Window" defect through RPE lesion Occasional filament pattern RPE defect	Severe retinal ischemia	Curvilinear fluorescent streaks (folds) Disc staining	Perifoveal staining Disc may stain Bright or dark pseudocyst
Treatment	Vitrectomy, gas exchange	CRVO: Laser for retinal neovascular and neovascular glaucoma BRVO: Laser for retinal neovascular and macular edema Systemic workup	Laser: PRP, focal or grid macular treatment	None	None	Increase intraocular pressure	Vitrectomy to release vitreous traction

BRVO, Branch retinal vein occlusion; *CRVO,* central retinal vein occlusion; *PRP,* panretinal photocoagulation; *RPE,* retinal pigment epithelium.

REFERENCES

1. Weene LE: Delayed onset of aphakic cystoid macular edema, *Ann Ophthalmol* 16:774-775, 1984.
2. Albert DW, Wade EC, Parrish RK 2d et al: A prospective study of angiographic cystoid macular edema one year after Nd:YAG posterior capsulotomy, *Ann Ophthalmol* 22:139-143, 1990.
3. Shafer DM: General discussion. In Schepens CL, Regan CDJ, editors: *Controversial aspects of the management of retinal detachment,* Boston, 1965, Little, Brown & Co, p 51.
4. Wright PL, Wilkinson CP, Balyeat HD et al: Angiographic cystoid macular edema after posterior chamber lens implantation, *Arch Ophthalmol* 10:740, 1988.
5. Gass JDM, Norton EWD: Follow-up study of cystoid macular edema following cataract extraction, *Trans Am Acad Ophthalmol Otolaryngol* 73:665, 1969.
6. Steinert RF, Puliafito CA, Kumar SR et al: Cystoid macular edema, retinal detachment, and glaucoma after Nd:YAG laser posterior capsulotomy, *Am J Ophthalmol* 112:373, 1991.
7. Jampol LM: Cystoid macular edema following cataract surgery, *Arch Ophthalmol* 106:894, 1988 (letter).
8. Lewis H, Singer TR, Hanscom TA et al: A prospective study of cystoid macular edema after neodymium:YAG posterior capsulotomy, *Ophthalmology* 94:478, 1987.
9. Spaide RF, Yannuzzi LA: Post-cataract surgery cystoid macular edema, *Clinical Signs in Ophthalmology* XIII(4), 1992.
10. Miyake K, Mibu H, Horiguchi M et al: Inflamatory mediators in post-operative aphakic and pseudophakic baboon eyes, *Arch Ophthalmol 108:1764, 1990.*
11. Yannuzzi LA: A perspective on the treatment of aphakic cystoid macular edema, *Surv Ophthalmol* 28(suppl):540, 1984.
12. Jampol LM: Pharmacologic therapy of aphakic cystoid macular edema: a review, *Ophthalmology* 80:891, 1982.
13. Miyake K: Indomethacin in the treatment of postoperative cystoid macular edema, *Surv Ophthalmol* 28(suppl):554, 1984.
14. Nussenblatt RB, Kaufman SC, Palestine AG et al: Macular thickening and visual acuity: measurement in patients with cystoid macular edema, *Ophthalmology* 94:1134, 1987.
15. Tso MOM: Pathology of cystoid macular edema, *Ophthalmology* 89:902, 1982.
16. Jampol LM: Cystoid macular edema following cataract surgery, *Arch Ophthalmol* 106:894, 1988 (letter).
17. Flach AJ: Cystoid macular edema following cataract surgery, *Arch Ophthalmol* 107:166, 1989 (letter).
18. Spaeth GL, von Sallman: Corticosteroids and cataracts, *Int Ophthalmol Clin* 6:915, 1966.
19. Becker B: Intraocular pressure response to topical corticosteroids, *Invest Ophthalmol* 4:198, 1965.

20. Miyake K: Indomethacin in the treatment of postoperative cystoid macular edema, *Surv Ophthalmol* 28(suppl):554, 1984.
21. Burnett J, Tessler H, Isenberg S et al: Double-masked trial of fenoprofen sodium: treatment of chronic aphakic cystoid macular edema, *Ophthalmic Surg* 14:150, 1983.
22. Flach AJ, Jampol LM, Weinberg D et al: Improvement in visual acuity in chronic aphakic and pseudophakic cystoid macular edema after treatment with topical 0.5% ketorolac tromethamine, *Am J Ophthalmol* 112:514, 1991.
23. Kraff MC, Sanders DR, McGuigan L et al: Inhibition of blood-aqueous barrier breakdown with diclofenac: a fluorophotometric study, *Arch Ophthalmol* 108:380, 1990.
24. Flach AJ: Cyclo-oxygenase inhibitors in ophthalmology, *Surv Ophthalmol* 36:259, 1992.
25. Cox SN, Hay E, Bird AC: Treatment of chronic macular edema with acetazolamide, *Arch Ophthalmol* 106:1190, 1988.
26. Marmor MF, Maack T: Enhancement of retinal adhesion and subretinal fluid absorption by acetazolamide, *Invest Ophthalmol Vis Sci* 23:121, 1982.
27. Grover S, Fishman GA, Fiscella RG et al: Efficacy of dorzolamide hydrochloride in the management of chronic cystoid macular edema in patients with retinitis pigmentosa, *Retina* 17:222-231, 1997.
28. Shapiro S, Fraunfelder FT: Acetazolamide and aplastic anemia, *Am J Ophthalmol* 113:328, 1992.
29. Heier JS, Topping TM, Bauman W et al: Ketorolac versus prednisolone versus combination therapy in the treatment of acute pseudophakic cystoid macular edema, *Ophthalmology* 107:2034-2038, 2000.
30. Fung WE: Vitrectomy for chronic aphakic cystoid macular edema: results of a national, collaborative, prospective, randomized investigation, *Ophthalmology* 92:1102, 1985.
31. Pendergast SD, Margherio RR, Williams GA et al: Vitrectomy for chronic pseudophakic cystoid macular edema, *Am J Ophthalmol* 128:317-323, 1999.
32. Steinert RF, Wasson PJ: Neodymium:YAG laser anterior vitreolysis for Irvine-Gass cystoid macular edema, *J Cataract Refract Surg* 15:304, 1989.
33. West SK, Rosenthal FS, Bressler NM et al: Exposure to sunlight and other risk factors for age related macular degeneration, *Arch Ophthalmol* 107:875, 1989.
34. Gass JDM: *Stereoscopic atlas of macular diseases, diagnosis and treatment,* ed 4, St Louis, 1997, Mosby, pp 72-78.
35. Miller ST, Graney MJ, Elam JT et al: Prediction of outcome from cataract surgery in elderly persons, *Ophthalmology* 95:1125, 1988.
36. Graney MJ, Applegate WB, Miller ST et al: A clinical index for predicting visual acuity after cataract surgery, *Am J Ophthalmol* 105:460, 1988.
37. O'Day DM and the Cataract Management Guideline Panel of the Agency for Health Care Policy and Research: Management of cataracts in adults: quick reference guide for clinicians, *Arch Ophthalmol* 111:453, 1993.
38. Cavender SA, Hobson RR, Chao G et al: Comparison of preoperative 10-Hz visual evoked potentials to contrast sensitivity and visual acuity after cataract extraction, *Documenta Ophthalmologica* 81:181, 1992.
39. Macular Photocoagulation Study Group: Argon laser photocoagulation for senile macular degeneration: results of a randomized clinical trial, *Arch Ophthalmol* 100:912, 1982.
40. Macular Photocoagulation Study Group: Argon laser photocoagulation for neovascular maculopathy: three year results from randomized clinical trials, *Arch Ophthalmol* 104:694, 1986.
41. Macular Photocoagulation Study Group: Recurrent choroidal neovascularization after argon laser photocoagulation for neovascular maculopathy, *Arch Ophthalmol* 104:503, 1986.
42. Macular Photocoagulation Study Group: Persistent and recurrent neovascularization after krypton laser photocoagulation for neovascular lesions of age related macular degeneration, *Arch Ophthalmol* 108:825, 1990.
43. Macular Photocoagulation Study Group: Laser photocoagulation of subfoveal neovascular lesions in age-related macular degeneration, *Arch Ophthalmol* 109:1220, 1992.
44. Macular Photocoagulation Study Group: Laser photocoagulation of subfoveal recurrent neovascular lesions in age related macular degeneration, *Arch Ophthalmol* 109:1232, 1991.
45. Treatment of Age-related Macular Degeneration with Photodynamic Therapy (TAP) Study Group: Photodynamic therapy of subfoveal choroidal neovascularization in age-related macular degeneration with verteporfin: one-year results of 2 randomized clinical trials. TAP report 1, *Arch Ophthalmol* 117:1329-1345, 1999.
46. Verteporfin in Photodynamic Therapy Study Group: Verteporfin therapy of subfoveal choroidal neovascularization in age-related macular degeneration: two-year results of a randomized clinical trial including lesions with occult with no classic choroidal neovascularization. Verteporfin in photodynamic therapy report 2, *Am J Ophthalmol* 131:541-560, 2001.
47. Bressler NM, Frost LA, Bressler SB et al: Natural course of poorly defined choroidal neovascularization associated with macular degeneration, *Arch Ophthalmol* 106:1537, 1988.
48. Age-Related Eye Disease Study Research Group: A randomized, placebo-controlled, clinical trial of high-dose supplementation with vitamins C and E, beta carotene, and zinc for age-related macular degeneration and vision loss. AREDS Report no. 8. *Arch Ophthalmol* 119:1417-1436, 2001.
49. The Eye Disease Case-Control Study Group: Risk factors for neovascular age-related macular degeneration, *Arch Ophthalmol* 110:1701, 1992.
50. Roth AM, Foos RY: Surface wrinkling retinopathy in eyes enucleated at autopsy, *Trans Am Acad Ophthalmol Otolaryngol* 75:1047, 1971.
51. McDonald HR, Schatz H: Introduction to epiretinal membranes. In Ryan S, editor: *Retina,* St Louis, Mosby, 1989, pp 789-795.
52. Michels RG: Vitreous surgery for macular puckers, *Am J Ophthalmol* 92:628, 1981.
53. Carney MD, Jampol LM: Epiretinal membranes in sickle cell retinopathy, *Arch Ophthalmol* 105:214, 1987.
54. Lobes LA, Burton TC: The incidence of macular pucker after retinal detachment surgery, *Am J Ophthalmol* 85:72, 1978.
55. Hirokawa H, Jalkh AE, Takahashi M et al: Role of the vitreous in idiopathic preretinal macular fibrosis, *Am J Ophthalmol* 101:166, 1986.
56. Jiang DY, Hiscott PS, Grierson I et al: Growth and contractility of cells from fibrocellular epiretinal membranes in primary tissue culture, *Br J Ophthalmol* 72:116, 1988.
57. Greven CM, Slusher MM, Weaver RG: Epiretinal membrane release and posterior vitreous detachment, *Ophthalmology* 95:902, 1988.
58. Allen A, Gass J: Contraction of a perifoveal Epiretinal membrane simulating a macular hole, *Am J Ophthalmol* 82:684-691, 1976.
59. Ciulla TA, Pesavento RD: Epiretinal fibrosis, *Ophthalmic Surg Lasers* 28:670, 1997.
60. Wise GN: Preretinal macular fibrosis (an analysis of 90 cases), *Trans Ophthalmol Soc U K* 92:131-140, 1972.
61. Gass JDM: *Stereoscopic atlas of macular diseases,* St Louis, 1987, Mosby. pp 694-712.
62. Akiba J, Yoshida A, Trempe CL: Prognostic factors in idiopathic preretinal macular fibrosis, *Graefe's Arch Clin Exp Ophthalmol* 229:101, 1991.
63. McDonald HR, Verre WP, Aaberg TM: Surgical management of idiopathic epiretinal membranes, *Ophthalmology* 93:978, 1986.
64. Pesin SR, Olk RJ, Grand MG et al: Vitrectomy for premacular fibroplasia: prognostic factors, long-term follow-up, and time course of visual improvement, *Ophthalmology* 98:1109, 1991.
65. Rice TA, DEBustros S, Michels RG et al: Prognostic factors in vitrectomy for epiretinal membranes of the macula, *Ophthalmology* 93:602, 1986.
66. Jaffe GJ, Burton TC, Kuhn E et al: Progression of nonproliferative diabetic retinopathy and visual outcome after extracapsular cataract extraction and intraocular lens implantation, *Am J Ophthalmol* 114:448, 1992.
67. Dowler JGF, Hykin PG, Lightman SL et al: Visual acuity following extracapsular cataract extraction in diabetics: a meta-analysis, *Eye* 9:313-317, 1995.
68. Hykin PG, Gregson RMC, Stevens JD et al: Extracapsular cataract extraction in proliferative diabetic retinopathy, *Ophthalmology* 100:394, 1992.

Postoperative Endophthalmitis

48

Robert I. Park, MD
Trexler M. Topping, MD

Postoperative endophthalmitis is a rare but much feared complication of cataract surgery. The potential sequelae of untreated or late treated endophthalmitis include loss of vision, severe ocular damage, and, in some cases, phthisis bulbi or enucleation. However, early detection and treatment of endophthalmitis may limit damage, and patients may regain good vision. Early identification and prompt treatment or referral of endophthalmitis cases are thus crucial factors in salvaging a patient's vision.

The following chapter addresses the issue of post–cataract extraction endophthalmitis and should not be extrapolated to cases of trauma or glaucoma filtration–related endophthalmitis because the mode of infection and the causative organisms are very different. Emphasis is placed on the results of the Endophthalmitis Vitrectomy Study (EVS), a randomized, prospective, multicenter trial evaluating the treatment of endophthalmitis following cataract surgery (see later description).

Epidemiology

A number of retrospective studies have been undertaken to define the incidence of endophthalmitis following cataract extraction.[1-5] The overall results appear in Table 48-1. The incidence of endophthalmitis has been reported to be between 0.07% to 0.22%.[1-5] The most comprehensive review was performed by Javitt et al.,[4] who reviewed billing records for approximately 50% of all Medicare beneficiaries over the age of 65 who underwent cataract extraction in 1984. The incidence of endophthalmitis was found to be 0.17% for intracapsular cataract extraction and 0.12% for extracapsular cataract extraction. The primary criticism of Javitt's study is that it was based on a review of Medicare billing records. Although the results are likely to be unbiased, clinical information about each case was limited; that is, no data regarding the organisms or culture positivity or negativity were available. Although the exact incidence of endophthalmitis varied from study to study, all reported the incidence of endophthalmitis to be well below 1% following cataract surgery.

A number of factors that increase the risk for postoperative endophthalmitis have been identified. Diabetes mellitus, chronic alcoholism, complicated surgery, wound complications, intracapsular vs. extracapsular cataract extraction, capsular rupture, amount and duration of instrumentation, history of prior surgery, vitreous loss, and intraocular lens (IOL) type have been implicated in an increased rate of endophthalmitis.[6-10] Of particular note is data from Javitt's review of the Medicare database in 1991, which demonstrated that the incidence of endophthalmitis after cataract extraction with anterior vitrectomy was significantly higher than for cataract surgery alone (0.58% for cataract extraction with anterior vitrectomy vs. 0.13% for cataract surgery alone, $p < 0.0001$).[4]

Clinical Presentation

A high level of clinical suspicion must be maintained during the examination of postoperative patients. A detailed history including the time course of onset of symptoms and a careful examination may increase the rate of early detection of endophthalmitis. Patients should be well informed of the signs of possible infection on the day of surgery, as well as during the postoperative visit, and should be instructed to contact the surgeon's office immediately should they develop postoperative problems. Early detection by patients may give the best hope for a good outcome. The surgeon should not fear overdiagnosis because the sequelae of a missed diagnosis are severe.

Symptoms

Blurred vision, a red eye, and pain are common complaints in patients developing endophthalmitis. Counterintuitively, blurred vision and a red eye were more common than pain as the presenting symptom in the EVS.[11] Table 48-2 summarizes the presenting symptoms in the EVS.

The median time to presentation was 6 days after cataract extraction, with a majority presenting within 2 weeks of cataract extraction. However, a significant number of patients (22%) presented after 2 to 6 weeks. Table 48-3 shows the distribution of time to presentation in the EVS.

Previous studies demonstrate a similar time course, with a majority presenting within 3 days of surgery and 88% presenting within 6 weeks of surgery.[12,13] Late endophthalmitis is discussed later in the chapter.

TABLE 48-1
Incidence of Endophthalmitis After Cataract Surgery

Year	Author	Number of Charts	Overall Incidence	Culture (+) Incidence	Location
1998	Aaberg et al[1]	41,654	0.082%	NA	Miami, FL
1991	Menikoff et al[2]	24,105	0.22%	0.17%	New York, NY
1991	Kattan et al[3]	30,002	0.089%	0.072%	Miami, FL
1991	Javitt et al[4]	338,141	0.13%	NA	Medicare database
1974	Allen and Mangiaracine[5]	36,000	NA	0.086	Boston, MA

NA, Not applicable.

TABLE 48-2
Patients Presenting with Type of Symptom in Endophthalmitis Vitrectomy Study[11]

Symptom	Percentage
Blurred vision	94.3%
Red eye	82.1%
Pain	74.3%
Swollen lid	34.5%

Examination

A thorough ocular examination should be performed. Common presenting signs in the EVS are listed in Table 48-4. Anterior segment examination may reveal conjunctival injection or chemosis, significant anterior segment inflammation, a hypopyon, an afferent pupillary defect, and a loss of red reflex. Corneal ring ulcers may be present in infections with streptococci, clostridia, and bacilli; in rare cases of *Clostridium* endophthalmitis, a gas bubble may be seen in the anterior chamber. Any abnormalities of the surgical wound(s) should be noted, that is, wound gaping, vitreous wick, wound leaks (check with Seidel's test), or torn or broken sutures, because they have been found to be associated with endophthalmitis.[14-18] Examination of the retina should be performed to assess the clarity of the ocular media and to determine the status of the retina. If no view of the retina is possible, ultrasound examination should be performed to assess for retinal detachment, retained lens fragments, choroidal thickening, or vitreous membranes.

Differential Diagnosis

A number of conditions may present with clinical findings similar to endophthalmitis, and the distinction between early endophthalmitis and other entities may be difficult. Retained nuclear fragments or a posteriorly displaced lens nucleus may cause severe intraocular inflammation.[19] The surgeon is generally aware of dislocation of any lens fragments; however, in the case of inadvertent lens particle dislocation, intraocular pressure may be useful in distinguishing lens particle inflammation from endophthalmitis. The intraocular pressure is more often elevated with lens particle retention than with endophthalmitis. Careful examination of the retina and vitreous for retained lens fragments, either by visualization or ultrasound, must be performed. Other causes of intraocular inflammation must be considered. Severe anterior segment inflammation and a hypopyon may accompany corneal ulcers without endophthalmitis (Figure 48-1). Incarceration of vitreous in the surgical wound may cause an intraocular inflammation that is generally less severe than endophthalmitis but may be mistaken for early endophthalmitis. Intraocular blood may be mistaken for inflammation. Reaction to IOL materials and processing chemicals is rare today but must be considered; during the early days of IOLs, reactions to residual polishing compounds and sterilizing agents were reported.[20,21]

TABLE 48-3
Patients Presenting at Given Periods After Cataract Extraction in Endophthalmitis Vitrectomy Study

Number of Days Post–cataract Extraction	Percentage of Endophthalmitis Patients
0-3 days	24%
4-7 days	37%
8-13 days	17%
2-6 weeks	22%

Data from Endophthalmitis Vitrectomy Study Group: Results of the endophthalmitis vitrectomy study: a randomized trial of immediate vitrectomy and of intravenous antibiotics for the treatment of postoperative bacterial endophthalmitis, *Arch Ophthalmol* 113:1479-1496, 1995.

TABLE 48-4
Incidence of Ocular Signs in Endophthalmitis Vitrectomy Study

Sign	Incidence
Hypopyon	85.7%
Red eye	82.1%
No view of retinal vessel	79.1%
Loss of red reflex	68.0%
Corneal infiltrate or ring ulcer	4.8%

Data from Endophthalmitis Vitrectomy Study Group: Results of the endophthalmitis vitrectomy study: a randomized trial of immediate vitrectomy and of intravenous antibiotics for the treatment of postoperative bacterial endophthalmitis, *Arch Ophthalmol* 113:1479-1496, 1995.

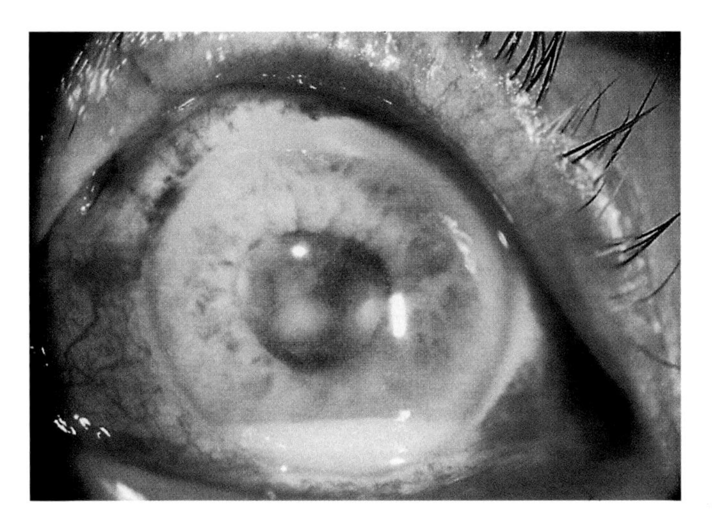

FIGURE 48-1 Hypopyon in patient with postoperative endophthalmitis.

Alternative sources of endophthalmitis must also be considered during history taking. Concurrent infections, including dental abscesses, and previous surgery, especially glaucoma filtration surgery, are potential sources of seeding of bacteria into the eye and have broad implications regarding the infecting organism and potential clinical course.

Unfortunately, there is no specific combination of signs and symptoms that a surgeon may use to definitively diagnose endophthalmitis, especially early cases. Given the severity of the damage that may be inflicted by endophthalmitis, questionable cases should be treated empirically as endophthalmitis.

Endophthalmitis Vitrectomy Study

The EVS[11] was a National Eye Institute–funded multicenter, prospective, randomized trial evaluating the effectiveness of immediate vitrectomy and intravenous antibiotics in the treatment of postoperative bacterial endophthalmitis. Specifically, the EVS looked at 420 cases of endophthalmitis occurring after cataract extraction. Patients were randomized to either pars plana vitrectomy or vitreous needle biopsy and intravenous antibiotics or no intravenous antibiotics. Study end points were media clarity and visual acuity. All patients received the following:

1. Intravitreal vancomycin (1 mg/0.1 ml) and amikacin (0.4 mg in 0.1 ml)
2. Subconjunctival vancomycin (25 mg/0.5 ml), ceftazidime (100 mg/0.5 ml), and dexamethasone sodium phosphate (6 mg in 0.25 ml). Subconjunctival amikacin (25 mg/0.1 ml) was substituted for ceftazidime if the patient was allergic to penicillin.
3. Topical vancomycin, 50 mg/ml; amikacin, 20 mg/ml; cycloplegic; and prednisolone acetate 1%.
4. Oral prednisone, 30 mg bid, for 5 to 10 days.

Patients randomized to the intravenous antibiotic arm received the following:

1. Ceftazidime, 2 g q8h, or ciprofloxacin, 750 mg PO bid, if allergic to penicillin.
2. Amikacin, 7.5 mg/kg IV loading dose and then 6 mg/kg every 12 hours. Doses were adjusted to keep peak and trough levels within an acceptable level.

The EVS demonstrated several important points:

1. There was no difference in final visual acuity or media clarity whether or not intravenous antibiotics were used. The findings were consistent across all subsets of patients.
2. Patients with light perception vision who received pars plana vitrectomy had a threefold increase in the likelihood of achieving 20/40, a twofold chance of achieving 20/100 vision, and a 50% decrease in the likelihood of severe visual loss as compared with patients receiving vitreous needle biopsy.
3. Patients with hand-motions vision or better demonstrated no significant difference in final visual acuity or media clarity whether or not immediate vitrectomy was performed.

The EVS should be used as a general guide to the care of postoperative endophthalmitis patients. Clinical judgment should, however, be used to determine care on a case-by-case basis. Coverage of the details of the EVS is beyond the scope of this chapter; for more information, see EVS journal articles.[11,22-27]

Organisms

Identification of the infectious organism has been reviewed in a number of studies. The distribution of organisms causing endophthalmitis in the EVS appears in Table 48-5.[22] Microbiologic culture growth was demonstrated in 69.3% of samples, and gram-positive coagulase-negative organisms predominated.

Although the exact percentages of organisms causing endophthalmitis varies through other smaller studies, the trends seen in the EVS are upheld.[13,14,28,29] Gram-positive, coagulase-negative bacteria, *Staphylococcus aureus,* and *Streptococcus* species are reported to be the three leading infecting organisms in post–cataract extraction endophthalmitis.

Late-onset endophthalmitis associated with glaucoma filtration surgery presents a very different microbiologic spectrum. Several studies have reported a predominance of *Streptococcus* and gram-negative bacteria in bleb-associated

TABLE 48-5

Incidence of inciting Organisms in Endophthalmitis Vitrectomy Study

Organism	Incidence
Gram positive, coagulase negative *(Staphylococcus epidermidis)*	70.0%
Staphylococcus aureus	9.9%
Streptococcus	9.0%
Miscellaneous gram positive	3.1%
Enterococcus	2.2%
Gram negative	5.9%

Data from Han DP, Wisniewski SR, Wilson LA et al: Spectrum and susceptibilities of microbiologic isolates in the Endophthalmitis Vitrectomy Study, *Am J Ophthalmol* 122:1–17, 1996.

endophthalmitis.[29-31] Because of the virulence of the causative organisms, patients with bleb-associated endophthalmitis carry a much poorer visual prognosis than early post–cataract extraction endophthalmitis. Fungal endophthalmitis is generally uncommon but must be considered as a potential cause.

Treatment

Once the clinical diagnosis of endophthalmitis has been made, anterior chamber and vitreous samples should be obtained for Gram staining and culture because the results from the vitreous and anterior chamber biopsies will guide antibiotic selection during postoperative treatment. Vitreous samples have been demonstrated to show growth at a greater rate than anterior chamber samples.[32] However, in early cases of endophthalmitis with an intact capsule and posterior chamber (PC) IOL, anterior chamber biopsies have been found to show growth even with no growth from vitreous biopsies.[33]

The EVS guidelines should be followed, although with some caveats. Patients presenting with hand-motions vision or better may receive anterior chamber and vitreous needle biopsy with an injection of intravitreal antibiotics. Patients with light perception or nonlight perception vision should receive an anterior chamber biopsy with pars plana vitrectomy and intravitreal antibiotics. Clinical judgment, however, must be used to temper the decision to perform or not perform pars plana vitrectomy. Patients with a rapidly worsening clinical picture should be considered for immediate vitrectomy because the etiologic organism may be extremely virulent. A low threshold for vitrectomy should be used for diabetic and immunocompromised patients. In the EVS, diabetic patients with endophthalmitis demonstrated a nonstatistically significant trend toward better outcome with pars plana vitrectomy than with needle biopsy.[27] The samples size, however, was small; a larger study is required to further investigate this trend.

TABLE 48-6

Treatment of Endophthalmitis: Anterior Chamber and Vitreous Biopsy and Injection of Antibiotics

NEEDLE BIOPSY

Anterior chamber

1. Make a peripheral keratotomy using a Wheeler or 15-degree blade. Avoid previous surgical incisions.
2. Insert 25-gauge needle attached to a tuberculin syringe.
3. Withdraw 0.1 ml aqueous solution.

Vitreous chamber

1. Insert a 25-gauge, ½-inch needle into the midvitreous chamber through a point 3.5 mm posterior to the limbus.
2. Gently withdraw 0.2-0.3 ml fluid.
3. If the yield is poor, proceed to three-port vitrectomy.
4. Otherwise, inject antibiotics through a 25-gauge, ½-inch needle into the midvitreous through a point 3.5 mm posterior to the limbus.
5. Check intraocular pressure and repeat anterior chamber paracentesis to relieve pressure, if necessary.

PARS PLANA VITRECTOMY

Prepare a three-port pars plana vitrectomy using a 6-mm infusion cannula.

Anterior chamber

1. Make a limbal keratotomy using a Wheeler or 15-degree blade. Avoid any previous surgical incisions.
2. Insert 25-gauge needle attached to a tuberculin syringe.
3. Withdraw 0.1 ml aqueous solution.

Vitreous chamber

1. Perform a core vitrectomy.
2. Close two of three sclerotomies.
3. Inject antibiotics and then close final sclerotomy.
4. Check intraocular pressure and perform anterior chamber paracentesis, if necessary, to relieve pressure.

Collection and Antibiotic Injection

NEEDLE BIOPSY

Needle biopsy samples may be taken in the operating room or in the office setting if the appropriate equipment is available. Most samples may be taken under local anesthesia; only in rare cases of severe periorbital inflammation is general endotracheal anesthesia required. Generally, a retrobulbar or subconjunctival block with 2% lidocaine is performed. The eye is then prepared in the usual sterile fashion, and a lid speculum is placed. Conjunctival cultures are generally not taken. Next, several drops of 5% povidone-iodine are instilled into the fornices, and the eye is not disturbed for several minutes to allow antimicrobial action by the povidone-iodine.

Table 48-6 lists the steps taken in obtaining samples. A 25- or 27-gauge needle is inserted into the anterior chamber through the peripheral clear cornea, and 0.1 ml of fluid is aspirated into a tuberculin syringe. Care is taken to avoid any previous surgical incisions. If a capsule or PC IOL is present, a pars plana needle biopsy may be obtained by passing a 25-gauge needle 3.5 mm posterior to the limbus into the midvitreous. In either case, 0.2 to 0.3 ml should be gently aspirated. If a sample cannot be obtained during vitreous biopsy, the patient should receive a standard three-port pars plana vitrectomy. Otherwise, antibiotics should be injected into the midvitreous through a 25-gauge, ½-inch needle placed 3.5 mm posterior to the limbus. The intraocular pressure is checked, and a second anterior chamber paracentesis is performed if the pressure is elevated. The anterior chamber and vitreous samples are set for Gram staining and culture.

PARS PLANA VITRECTOMY

Pars plana vitrectomy should be performed in the operating room under local or general anesthesia. Generally, a retrobulbar block with 2% lidocaine and 0.75% bupivacaine is performed. The eye is then prepared in the usual sterile fashion, and a lid speculum is placed. Conjunctival cultures are not routinely taken. Table 48-6 lists the steps taken in obtaining samples.

The eye is prepared for a standard three-port vitrectomy. A 6-mm infusion cannula is placed because the view into the vitreous is often very poor. To obtain anterior chamber samples, a 25- or 27-gauge needle is inserted into the anterior chamber at the limbus, and 0.1 ml of fluid is aspirated into a tuberculin syringe. Care is taken to avoid any previous surgical incisions. The pars plana vitrectomy is performed. On completion of a core vitrectomy, the infusion is clamped, and an additional 0.2 to 0.3 ml of fluid is withdrawn. Two of the three sclerotomies are closed, and antibiotics are injected before closure of the final sclerotomy. All surgical wound abnormalities from the initial surgery, including wound gape, exposed sutures, vitreous wick, and so on, should be corrected before antibiotic injection and closure. The anterior chamber sample and cassette are sent for concentration, culture, and Gram staining.

Culture

Specimens obtained from anterior chamber aspiration and vitreous needle biopsy or pars plana vitrectomy should be cultured and stained separately. Cassette washings from pars plana vitrectomy should be concentrated by centrifuge or filtration before culture and staining. Samples should be plated on blood agar, chocolate agar, Sabouraud, and thioglycolate broth and should be cultured in aerobic and anaerobic conditions. Samples should be placed on slides and stained using Gram and Giemsa stains. A positive culture result is defined as growth on two or more media or confluent growth on one solid medium at the site of inoculation.

Treatment

INITIAL TREATMENT

Initial treatment is directed toward sterilization of the eye using intravitreal, topical, and oral antibiotics. Most vitreoretinal surgeons agree that intravitreal antibiotics are crucial for maximizing chances for a good outcome. We choose to inject two antibiotics: vancomycin (1 mg in 0.1 ml) and ceftazidime (2 mg in 0.1 ml). In cases of penicillin or cephalosporin allergy, we inject vancomycin (1 mg in 0.1 ml) and amikacin (0.4 mg in 0.1 ml). Table 48-7 summarizes the combination of medications recommended.

Dilutions must be performed carefully, especially in the case of amikacin because higher concentrations may be toxic to the eye or may cause systemic complications. Although dilutions may be performed by the surgeon, evidence exists that dilutions may be safer when performed by the pharmacist.

CHOICE OF ANTIBIOTICS

Controversy exists regarding the choice of antibiotics for intravitreal injection. The EVS used a combination of antibiotics, including intravitreal vancomycin and amikacin, subconjunctival vancomycin, ceftazidime (amikacin if patients were allergic to penicillin or cephalosporin), and dexamethasone, and topical vancomycin and amikacin postoperatively.

Vancomycin is very effective in the treatment of endophthalmitis for a number of reasons. First, vancomycin has been found to be active against most gram-positive organisms found in endophthalmitis. Second, vancomycin is cleared from the eye anteriorly, resulting in a long half-life. Data from rabbit studies demonstrated a vitreal half-life of 20 to 40 hours in uninfected rabbit eyes and 38 to 54 hours in infected rabbit eyes.[34-36] Vancomycin appears to be well tolerated by ocular structures.

TABLE 48-7
Initial Therapeutic Regimen for Endophthalmitis

INTRAVITREAL INJECTION FOR ENDOPHTHALMITIS

1. Vancomycin 1 mg in 0.1 ml normal saline
2. Ceftazidime 2 mg in 0.1 ml normal saline
3.
4. Substitute amikacin 0.4 mg in 0.1 ml water for ceftazidime in patients allergic to penicillin or cephalosporin

TOPICAL REGIMEN

1. Vancomycin 50 mg/ml hourly
2. Ciprofloxacin 0.3% hourly
3. Scopolamine 0.25% twice daily
4. Add prednisolone acetate 1% hourly when improvement is apparent

ORAL REGIMEN

Ciprofloxacin 750 mg twice daily

The choice of an agent for coverage of gram-negative organisms remains controversial. Although the EVS used amikacin, an aminoglycoside, a number of vitreoretinal surgeons have advocated the use of other antibiotics. The potential benefits of amikacin include a good gram-negative spectrum of coverage, a long half-life, a synergistic effect with vancomycin against gram-positive cocci, and a concentration-dependent bactericidal activity.[37] Potential problems are ocular toxicity (including macular infarction), ototoxicity, and nephrotoxicity.[38]

Intravitreal ceftazidime (a beta-lactam) has also been used for treatment of endophthalmitis. Ceftazidime has a similar spectrum of coverage and a similar half-life as amikacin.[39] Although ceftazidime does not have the synergistic effect with vancomycin against gram-positive cocci that amikacin has, it does not carry the potential risk of ocular and systemic toxicity.

Ciprofloxacin, a fluoroquinolone, has been considered for intravitreal injection. Ciprofloxacin has a similar spectrum of coverage to amikacin and ceftazidime, but several problems preclude its use in intravitreal injection. Doses higher than 100 μg injected into rabbit vitreous have been demonstrated to cause retinal and corneal toxicity,[40] and the half-life of ciprofloxacin is short (~2 hours in the rabbit).[41]

On the basis of the preceding evidence, our choice is to inject vancomycin and ceftazidime. We do not routinely treat for fungal endophthalmitis and limit antifungal agents to culture-proven cases.

INTRAVITREAL STEROID INJECTION

Controversy exists concerning the use of intravitreal injection of steroids. A number of studies have been performed in animal models, as well as in humans. Some studies demonstrate an improvement in clinical inflammation and visual outcome with concurrent intravitreal injection of steroids and antibiotics,[42-45] whereas others demonstrate worsened inflammation and visual outcome.[46-48] Histopathologic studies have shown similarly contradictory results for intravitreal steroids.[42,43,46] The study designs, including type of antibiotic, dose of steroid injected, and type of bacterium injected (in the animal models), were not consistent across studies; therefore comparison of results is difficult. On the basis of the existing studies, we do not support the injection of intravitreal steroids at the time of antibiotic injection but await a comprehensive evaluation of the efficacy of intravitreal steroids in endophthalmitis.

ADJUVANT TREATMENT

The EVS used subconjunctival antibiotics for eradication of any anterior segment infection, and many surgeons advocate their use in the treatment of endophthalmitis. We believe that the application of subconjunctival antibiotics is redundant when an aggressive postoperative topical antibiotic regimen is planned and do not generally use subconjunctival antibiotics or steroids.

Our recommendations for postoperative treatment with topical and systemic antibiotics are based on bioavailability studies. Topical vancomycin is used to treat any gram-positive anterior segment inflammation, whereas topical and oral ciprofloxacin (750 mg bid) is used to cover gram-negative organisms and to give some additional gram-positive coverage. Rabbit studies have demonstrated that the combination of oral and topical ciprofloxacin gives aqueous and vitreous concentrations above the MIC for many common infecting organisms in endophthalmitis.[49] On the basis of EVS data, no intravenous antibiotics are recommended.

Aggressive postoperative administration of prednisolone acetate 1% is started 1 day after surgery. Oral prednisone, 30 to 60 mg, may additionally be started if the patient has no contraindications to steroid use, but we rarely use it. Cycloplegic drops are used postoperatively to relieve discomfort and synechiae formation.

Clinical Course

The clinical course varies on a case-by-case basis. Often, the clinical appearance is worse 1 day after surgery than on the day of surgery. Generally speaking, 2 days after surgery, the eye should appear clinically improved, although a hypopyon and media opacities may be present. Although the eye may be sterilized, aggressive antiinflammatory therapy is imperative to prevent late sequelae. It is important to evaluate and reevaluate the anterior and posterior segments for development of complications such as posterior synechiae with iris bombé, vitreous membranes, retinal traction, and retinal detachment. The surgeon should not hesitate to bring the patient back to the operating room should further complications develop or should a persistent infection be suspected.

Prognosis

The final outcome depends on a number of factors, including appearance at presentation, the inciting organism, and the baseline medical condition. Patients infected with coagulase-negative *Staphylococcus* generally have the best outcome, whereas those with streptococcal infections have a worse prognosis. Gram-negative endophthalmitis carries a poor prognosis. Recent data from the EVS demonstrate a trend toward worsened outcomes for diabetic patients; the surgeon should consider earlier, more aggressive intervention for diabetics. Early detection and treatment may be the best hope for a good outcome.

Prevention

Evidence exists that the use of topical 5% povidone-iodine applied to the ocular surface preoperatively decreases the incidence of culture-positive endophthalmitis,[50] and we advocate its use. There has been a recent trend toward the use of antibiotics within the irrigating solution. Recent studies involving animal models and retrospective chart reviews have not definitively demonstrated a benefit to the use of antibiotics within irrigating solutions during cataract surgery.[51-54] We do not advocate or oppose the use of irrigating solution antibiotics but caution the surgeon that some antibiotics carry the risk of ocular damage or systemic side effects.

Chronic Postoperative Endophthalmitis

Although most of this chapter has focused on early postoperative endophthalmitis, the surgeon should be aware of the signs of chronic postoperative endophthalmitis. A number of weakly virulent organisms may produce a late, chronic infection that may mimic a chronic uveitis. Organisms that have been reported to produce such a reaction include *Propionibacterium acnes, Staphylococcus epidermidis,* and fungi, such as *Candida* species.

P. acnes is a commensal anaerobic diphtheroid bacterium that is found on the skin. *P. acnes* endophthalmitis has been reported to present with a an equatorial white plaque on the lens capsule after extracapsular cataract extraction, low-grade chronic inflammation (often steroid responsive), granulomatous keratic precipitates, fibrin strands or beaded infiltrates in the anterior vitreous, and an intermittent hypopyon.[55-57] Our experience has been that *P. acnes* generally produces a chronic low-grade inflammation with a white plaque seen within the capsular bag but without hypopyon or other changes. Patients have often been treated chronically with steroids, which may mask the development of classic findings.

A number of treatments for patients with *P. acnes* endophthalmitis have been used, including various combinations of topical, intravenous, and intraocular antibiotics with or without vitrectomy.[57] We generally perform a pars plana vitrectomy, partial capsulectomy, to remove the intracapsular colony, and injection of vancomycin (1 mg in 0.1 ml) as a first step. If this treatment is unsuccessful in eradicating the *P. acnes,* a repeat pars plana vitrectomy with IOL extraction, capsular removal, and vancomycin injection is performed. The patient is left aphakic with a planned secondary IOL placement after complete resolution of the endophthalmitis. In all cases, the vitreous washings and capsular remnant are sent for culture and staining.

Patients with suspected chronic late endophthalmitis that is not believed to be *P. acnes* are treated with a pars plana vitrectomy, anterior chamber biopsy, and injection of intravitreal antibiotics. We elect to use intravitreal vancomycin, 1 mg in 0.1 ml, and ceftazidime, 2 mg in 0.1 ml. Postoperatively, patients receive vancomycin and ciprofloxacin drops and ciprofloxacin, 750 mg PO bid. We do not start antifungal therapy until cases are culture proven.

Conclusion

Postoperative endophthalmitis is a greatly feared complication of cataract surgery with potentially devastating results. However, early diagnosis and prompt treatment of endophthalmitis can result in the preservation of good vision. Surgeons should remain vigilant during their evaluation of the postoperative patient and should treat or refer the patient for immediate treatment if endophthalmitis is suspected.

REFERENCES

1. Aaberg TM Jr, Flynn HW Jr, Schiffman J et al: Nosocomial acute-onset postoperative endophthalmitis survey: a 10-year review of incidence and outcomes, *Ophthalmology* 105:1004-1010, 1998.
2. Menikoff JA, Speaker MG, Marmor M et al: A case-control study of risk factors for postoperative endophthalmitis, *Ophthalmology* 98:1761-1768, 1991.
3. Kattan HM, Flynn HW, Pflugfelder SC et al: Nosocomial endophthalmitis survey: current incidence of infection after intraocular surgery, *Ophthalmology* 98:227-238, 1991.
4. Javitt JC, Vitale S, Canner JK et al: National outcomes of cataract surgery: endophthalmitis following inpatient cataract surgery, *Arch Ophthalmol* 109:1085-1089, 1991.
5. Allen HF, Mangiaracine AB: Bacterial endophthalmitis after cataract extraction. II. Incidence in 36,000 consecutive operations with special reference to topical preoperative antibiotics, *Arch Ophthalmol* 91:3-7, 1974.
6. Haiman MH, Burton TC, Brown CK: Epidemiology of retinal detachment, *Arch Ophthalmol* 100:289-292, 1982.
7. Wilkinson CP, Anderson LS, Little JH: Retinal detachment following phacoemulsification, *Ophthalmology* 85:151-156, 1978.
8. Smith PW, Stark WJ, Maumenee et al: Retinal detachment after extracapsular cataract extraction with posterior chamber intraocular lens, *Ophthalmology* 94:495-504, 1987.
9. Javitt JC, Vitale S, Canner JK et al: National outcomes of cataract extraction. I. Retinal detachment after inpatient surgery, *Ophthalmology* 98:895-902, 1991.
10. Steinert RF, Puliafito CA, Kumar SR et al: Cystoid macular edema, retinal detachment, and glaucoma after Nd:YAG laser posterior capsulotomy, *Am J Ophthalmol* 112:373-380, 1991.
11. Endophthalmitis Vitrectomy Study Group: Results of the endophthalmitis vitrectomy study: a randomized trial of immediate vitrectomy and of intravenous antibiotics for the treatment of postoperative bacterial endophthalmitis, *Arch Ophthalmol* 113:1479-1496, 1995.
12. Rowsey JJ, Jensen H, Sexton DJ: Clinical diagnosis of endophthalmitis, *Int Ophthalmol Clin* 27:82-88, 1987.
13. Weber DJ, Hoffman KL, Thoft RS et al: Endophthalmitis following intraocular lens implantation: a report of 30 cases and review of the literature, *Rev Infect Dis* 8:12-20, 1986.
14. Driebe WT Jr, Mandelbaum S, Forster RK et al: Pseudophakic endophthalmitis: diagnosis and management, *Ophthalmology* 93:442-448, 1986.
15. Lindstrom RL, Doughman DJ: Bacterial endophthalmitis associated with vitreous wick, *Ann Ophthalmol* 11:1775-1778, 1979.
16. Gelender H: Infectious endophthalmitis following cutting of sutures after cataract surgery, *Am J Ophthalmol* 94:528-533, 1982.
17. Stonecipher KG, Parmley VC, Jensen H et al: Infectious endophthalmitis following sutureless cataract surgery, *Arch Ophthalmol* 109:1562-1563, 1991.
18. Cinfino J, Brown SI: Bacterial endophthalmitis associated with exposed monofilament sutures following corneal transplantation, *Am J Ophthalmol* 99:111-113, 1985.
19. Irvine WE, Flynn HW, Murray TG et al: Retained lens fragments after phacoemulsification manifesting as marked inflammation with hypopyon, *Am J Ophthalmol* 114:610-614, 1992.
20. Meltzer DW: Sterile hypopyon following intraocular lens surgery, *Arch Ophthalmol* 98:100-104, 1980.
21. Stark WJ, Rosenblum P, Maumenee AE et al: Postoperative inflammatory reactions to intraocular lenses sterilized with ethylene oxide, *Ophthalmology* 87:385-389, 1980.
22. Han DP, Wisniewski SR, Wilson LA et al: Spectrum and susceptibilities of microbiologic isolates in the Endophthalmitis Vitrectomy Study, *Am J Ophthalmol* 122:1-17, 1996.
23. Johnson MW, Doft BH, Kelsey SF et al: The Endophthalmitis Vitrectomy Study: relationship between clinical presentation and microbiologic spectrum, *Ophthalmology* 104:261-272, 1997.
24. Barza M, Pavan PR, Wisniewski SR et al: Evaluation of the microbiological diagnostic techniques in postoperative endophthalmitis in the Endophthalmitis Vitrectomy Study, *Arch Ophthalmol* 115:1142-1150, 1997.
25. Doft BH, Kelsey SF, Wisniewski SR, the EVS Study Group: Additional procedures after the initial vitrectomy or tap-biopsy in the Endophthalmitis Vitrectomy Study, *Ophthalmology* 105:707-716, 1998.
26. Han DP, Wisniewski SR, Kelsey SF et al: Microbiologic yields and complication rates of vitreous fine needle aspiration vs mechanized vitreous biopsy in the Endophthalmitis Vitrectomy Study, *Retina* 19:98-102, 1999.
27. Doft BH, Wisniewski SR, Kelsey SF et al: Diabetes and postoperative endophthalmitis in the Endophthalmitis Vitrectomy Study, *Arch Ophthalmol* 119:650-656, 2001.
28. Stern GA, Engel HM, Driebe WT: The treatment of postoperative endophthalmitis: results of differing approaches to treatment, *Ophthalmology* 96:62-67, 1989.
29. Puliafito CA, Baker AS, Haaf J et al: Infectious endophthalmitis: review of 36 cases, *Ophthalmology* 89:921-929, 1982.
30. Ciulla TA, Beck AD, Topping TM et al: Blebitis, early endophthalmitis, and late endophthalmitis after glaucoma filtering surgery, *Ophthalmology* 115:986-995, 1997.
31. Mandelbaum S, Forster RK, Gelender H et al: Late onset endophthalmitis associated with filtering blebs, *Ophthalmology* 92:964-972, 1985.
32. Mandelbaum S, Forster RK: Postoperative endophthalmitis, *Int Ophthalmol Clin* 27:95-106, 1987.
33. Beyer TL, O'Donnell RE, Goncalves V et al: Role of posterior capsule in the prevention of postoperative bacterial endophthalmitis: experimental primate studies and clinical implications, *Br J Ophthalmol* 69:841-846, 1985.
34. Homer P, Peyman GA, Koziol J et al: Intravitreal injection of vancomycin in experimental staphylococcal endophthalmitis, *Acta Ophthalmol* 53:311-320, 1975.
35. Smith MA, Sorensen JA, Lowy FD et al: Treatment of experimental methicillin resistant *Staphylococcus epidermidis* endophthalmitis with intravitreal vancomycin, *Ophthalmology* 93:1328-1335, 1986.
36. Smith MA, Sorenson JA, Smith C et al: Effects of intravitreal dexamethasone on concentration of intravitreal vancomycin in experimental methicillin resistant *Staphylococcus epidermidis* endophthalmitis, *Antimicrob Agents Chemother* 35:1298-1302, 1991.
37. Doft BH, Barza MB: Optimal management of postoperative endophthalmitis and results of the Endophthalmitis Vitrectomy Study, *Curr Opin Ophthalmol* 7:84-94, 1996.
38. Campochiaro PA, Lim JI: Aminoglycoside toxicity in the treatment of endophthalmitis (the Aminoglycoside Toxicity Study Group), *Arch Ophthalmol* 112:48-53, 1994.
39. Meridith TA: Antimicrobial pharmacokinetics in endophthalmitis treatment: studies of ceftazidime, *Trans Am Ophthalmol Soc* 91:653-699, 1993.
40. Stevens SX, Fouraker BD, Jensen HG: Intraocular safety of ciprofloxacin, *Arch Ophthalmol* 109:1737-1743, 1991.
41. Pearson PA, Hainsworth DP, Ashton P: Clearance and distribution of ciprofloxacin after intravitreal injection, *Retina* 13:326-330, 1993.
42. Meredith TA, Aguilar HE, Trabelsi A et al: Comparative treatment of experimental *Staphylococcus epidermidis* endophthalmitis, *Arch Ophthalmol* 108:857-860, 1990.
43. Maxwell DP, Brent BD, Diamond JG et al: Effect of intravitreal dexamethasone on ocular histopathology in a rabbit model of endophthalmitis, *Ophthalmology* 98:1370-11376, 1991.
44. Park SS, Samly N, Ruoff K et al: Effect of intravitreal dexamethasone in treatment of pneumococcal endophthalmitis in rabbits, *Arch Ophthalmol* 113:1324-1329, 1995.
45. Jett BD, Jensen HG, Atkuri RV et al: Evaluation of therapeutic measures for treating endophthalmitis caused by isogenic toxin producing and non-toxin producing *Enterococcus faecalis* strains, *Invest Ophthalmol Vis Sci* 36:9-15, 1995.
46. Meredith TA, Aguilar HE, Drews C et al: Intraocular dexamethasone produces a harmful effect on treatment of experimental *Staphylococcus aureus* endophthalmitis, *Trans Am Ophthalmol Soc* XCIV:241-252, 1996.
47. Das T, Jalali S, Gothwal VK et al: Intravitreal dexamethasone in exogenous bacterial endophthalmitis: results of a prospective randomized study, *Br J Ophthalmol* 83:1050-1055, 1999.

48. Shah GK, Stein JD, Sharma S et al: Visual outcomes following the use of intravitreal steroids in the treatment of postoperative endophthalmitis, *Ophthalmology* 107:486-489, 2000.
49. Ozturk F, Kortunay S, Kurt E et al: Penetration of topical and oral ciprofloxacin into the aqueous and vitreous humor in inflamed eyes, *Retina* 19:218-222, 1999.
50. Speaker MG, Menikoff JA: Prophylaxis of endophthalmitis with topical povidone-iodine, *Ophthalmology* 98:1769-1775, 1991.
51. Beigi B, Westlake W, Chang B et al: The effect of intracameral, per-operative antibiotics on microbial contamination of anterior chamber aspirates during phacoemulsification, *Eye* 12:390-394, 1998.
52. Gritz DC, Cevallos AV, Smolin G et al: Antibiotic supplementation of intraocular irrigating solutions: an in vitro model of antibacterial action, *Ophthalmology* 103:1204-1208, 1996.
53. Adenis JP, Robert PY, Mounier M et al: Anterior chamber concentrations of vancomycin in the irrigation solution at the end of cataract surgery, *J Cataract Refract Surg* 23:111-114, 1997.
54. Feys J, Salvanet-Bouccara A, Edmond JP et al: Vancomycin prophylaxis and intraocular contamination during cataract surgery, *J Cataract Refract Surg* 23:894-897, 1997.
55. Meisler DM, Palestine AG, Vastine DW et al: Chronic *Propionibacterium acnes* endophthalmitis after extracapsular cataract extraction and intraocular lens implantation, *Am J Ophth* 102:733-739, 1986.
56. Meisler DM, Mandelbaum S: *Propionibacterium acnes* associated endophthalmitis after extracapsular cataract extraction: review of reported cases, *Ophthalmology* 96:54-61, 1989.
57. Zambrano W, Flynn HW, Pflugfelder SC et al: Management options for *Propionibacterium acnes* endophthalmitis, *Ophthalmology* 96:1100-1105, 1989.

Retinal Detachment

49

Jay S. Duker, MD

Retinal detachment (RD) represents the physical separation of the neurosensory retina from its underlying retinal pigment epithelium (RPE) by an accumulation of fluid. This separation results in dysfunction of the photoreceptors and is clinically manifested by a scotoma corresponding to the area of detached retina.

Generally speaking, RD can be divided into three varieties on the basis of etiology: rhegmatogenous RD (RRD), exudative RD, and tractional RD. It is the first type, RRD, that under certain circumstances is pathophysiologically related to cataract surgery. RRD is therefore the focus of this chapter.

With current techniques, most cases of RRD (>95%) can be eventually repaired, that is, the retina returned to its normal anatomic position, juxtaposed to the RPE. However, visual recovery does not necessarily mirror anatomic appearance. Because the presence or absence of submacular fluid is the most important preoperative factor correlating to visual recovery, early diagnosis and prompt therapy before macular detachment occurs can preserve sight. In this regard, education of the postcataract patient concerning the symptoms of RD, with instructions to seek immediate attention if symptoms should develop, is paramount.

Pathophysiology

The current understanding of the pathophysiology of primary RRD hinges on the basic tenet that a posterior vitreous detachment (PVD) is the inciting event in most, if not all, cases of acute primary RRD.[1,2] In susceptible individuals, the PVD creates one or more retinal tears via associated abnormal vitreoretinal traction. These tears, in turn, allow the passage of vitreous fluid into the subretinal space and eventual RRD. The relationship between RRD and cataract surgery can therefore be reduced to a study of the relationship between cataract surgery and the induced alterations in the vitreous gel that eventually culminate in PVD. Barring rare instances of direct surgical trauma to the posterior segment resulting in a secondary RD (e.g., globe perforation from the anesthetic needle), it is currently believed that cataract surgery is a risk factor for RD only so far as cataract surgery is a risk factor for earlier onset PVD. When a PVD ensues, pseudophakic eyes do not appear to be at any more risk than phakic eyes for retinal tears.

Following removal of the crystalline lens by any method, structural changes in the vitreous have been documented to occur. Loss of hyaluronic acid, increased vitreous gel mobility, and progressive vitreous syneresis together result in the development of PVD. These alterations occur sooner in aphakic and pseudophakic globes than in eyes in which the crystalline lens remains intact.

The status of the posterior capsule is also important. Laboratory and epidemiologic data suggest that the presence of an intact posterior capsule delays the onset of these vitreous changes compared with eyes with open posterior capsules (Table 49-1). The hyaluronic acid concentration in the vitreous cavity is reduced in aphakic eyes, whereas eyes in which the posterior capsule is intact show minimal loss of hyaluronic acid.[3] PVD has been noted to occur more commonly in aphakic eyes when compared with phakic eyes.[4] In aphakic or pseudophakic eyes with intact posterior capsules, however, the rate of PVD appears to be less than when the posterior capsule is interrupted.[5] When PVD does develop, aphakic eyes do not appear to be any more susceptible to retinal tear formation than are phakic eyes.[6]

Controversy does exist over whether anterior manipulation of the vitreous results in earlier PVD. RRD does appear to be more common in eyes that have undergone cataract surgery complicated by vitreous loss. Improperly performed vitrectomy with undue traction on the vitreous base or aggressive intraoperative traction on the vitreous base in the setting of dislocated nuclei and intraocular lenses (IOLs) can certainly cause direct trauma to the retina, resulting in a secondary RRD. Fortunately, this is rare.

Incidence, Timing, and Risk Factors

Over 40% of all patients with acute RRD are either pseudophakic or aphakic. Therefore previous cataract surgery represents the most important risk factor for patients undergoing surgical repair of RRD.[7] Other risk factors are well known: high myopia, lattice degeneration, blunt trauma, familial history of RD, and certain systemic diseases such as Stickler's syndrome and Marfan's disease.

In pseudophakic eyes operated on with an extracapsular technique, the overall incidence of subsequent RD is between

TABLE 49-1

Prevention and Prophylaxis of Postcataract Retinal Detachment

- Keep posterior capsule intact.
- Perform careful preoperative dilated fundus examination before both cataract surgery and Nd:YAG laser capsulotomy.
- Perform frequent dilated fundus examinations in the first year after surgery.
- Educate the patient.

1% and 2%.[8-10] In one large retrospective series of Medicare recipients rehospitalized for RD over a 4-year period following cataract surgery, the incidence following extracapsular surgery was found to be 0.9%, whereas it was 1.55% for intracapsular surgery.[10] In this study, initial vitrectomy increased the risk of RD to 5%. Other authors have documented a higher rate of RRD in complicated cases that were associated with vitreous loss. Wilkinson, Anderson, and Little[8] found an incidence between 7% and 14%. In such eyes, persistent anterior traction on the vitreous base from vitreous adherence to the wound, IOL, or anterior segment structures may result in an increased risk for traction-induced peripheral retinal tears.

As already stated earlier, the status of the posterior capsule is an important determinant of the onset of PVD and therefore the risk of RRD. Any maneuver that interrupts the posterior capsule is likely to accelerate the loss of hyaluronic acid and culminate in premature PVD. With the advent of neodymium: yttrium-aluminum-garnet (Nd:YAG) laser capsulotomy, extracapsular surgery rapidly became the method of choice for cataract extraction. Nd:YAG laser, however, increases the risk of RRD compared with eyes with intact posterior capsules.[11-13] The incidence of RRD following capsulotomy with the Nd:YAG laser has been estimated to be between 0.1% and 3.6%. In another large retrospective study of Medicare patients undergoing laser capsulotomy following cataract surgery, the incidence of subsequent RD was 1.6%.[14] It was 0.8% for those patients not requiring capsulotomy. Younger age, male sex, and white race all were increased risk factors for RRD. This study was flawed, however, in that it did not differentiate between eyes. Therefore patients undergoing rehospitalization for RRD in a contralateral eye were counted as an RRD after capsulotomy. Axial myopia appears to increase the risk of RRD following laser capsulotomy as well. Neither the size of the capsulotomy nor the amount of energy delivered appears to be a significant risk factor for RRD.[11] It is not believed that the Nd:YAG laser produces retinal tears directly.

Most cases of pseudophakic RRD occur within 1 year after the cataract removal.[8,9] Following laser capsulotomy, the typical time for RRD is within 6 months of the procedure.[14,15] It is rare for RRD to be seen in the immediate postoperative period following cataract surgery. A recent retrospective review of 215 aphakic and pseudophakic cases of RRD found that only 13% occurred within 3 months of cataract surgery.[16] Presumably this time course pattern is due to the timing of PVD following cataract surgery.

Examination Techniques

Retinal tear and/or RRD is a clinical diagnosis made with the indirect ophthalmoscope when the media is clear. Scleral depression should be used as an adjunct. Although other posterior segment viewing systems (direct ophthalmoscopy, noncontact slit lamp lenses) can also be employed to diagnose RRD, none give the wide-field, stereoscopic view obtained with the binocular indirect ophthalmoscope. With the addition of scleral depression, none of the other techniques can match indirect ophthalmoscopy for the examination of the ora serrata region either.

Indirect ophthalmoscopy should be preformed preoperatively on all patients scheduled for cataract surgery. In the commonly encountered scenario in which the lens opacity precludes adequate view to the anterior retina, repeat indirect examination as soon as it is practical following cataract surgery should be performed.

In the postoperative period, the onset of flashes, floaters, visual field loss, or any unexplained drop in central visual acuity should prompt an immediate posterior segment examination through a pharmacologically dilated pupil. Up to 50% of patients with acute RRD do not complain of previous flashes and floaters before presentation for detached retina.

If the media is not clear, ultrasonography is invaluable to rule out the presence of RRD. When the media is too cloudy secondary to the cataract to obtain an adequate view to the posterior pole, B-scan ultrasonography should be performed before cataract surgery. This examination is sensitive and specific for RD but is less helpful in the identification of occult retinal breaks.

In the postcataract surgery patient who complains of acute flashes, floaters, or other symptoms of PVD/RRD, the presence of pigment granules in the anterior vitreous (tobacco dust) in the setting of an intact posterior capsule nearly always means that an open retinal break is present. Similarly, the finding of vitreous hemorrhage with a symptomatic PVD implies a greater than 70% chance that a retinal tear is present. Acute flashes and floaters in an eye that lacks any pigment or red blood cells in the vitreous are associated with an acute retinal tear in less than 5% of cases.

Prophylactic Treatment

Whenever possible, retinal lesions that represent a significant risk for RRD should be identified and treated before cataract surgery and/or laser capsulotomy. Although controversy still exists concerning the appropriateness of prophylactic treatment for certain lesions (e.g., asymptomatic lattice degeneration without breaks in the fellow eye of an individual whose contralateral eye had a RRD), all agree that more worrisome lesions should be treated with retinopexy.

The same guidelines for prophylactic treatment hold true for patients about to undergo Nd:YAG capsulotomy. In fact, some authors believe that laser capsulotomy carries anywhere from 2 to 4 times greater risk for subsequent RRD than does uncomplicated extracapsular cataract surgery alone.

In the asymptomatic patient about to undergo cataract surgery or Nd:YAG laser capsulotomy, the following lesions should be considered for prophylactic treatment: (1) any tear

TABLE 49-2
Treatment of Suspicious Retinal Lesions

ASYMPTOMATIC

- Any tear with greater than 1 disc diameter of fluid (subclinical RRD)
- Horseshoe or flap tears with fluid
- Horseshoe or flap tear in contralateral eye of patients with previous RRD

SYMPTOMATIC

- Any tear with greater than 1 disc diameter of fluid (subclinical RRD)
- All horseshoe or flap tears
- Most operculated tears
- Atrophic holes in contralateral eye of patients with previous RRD

RRD, Rhegmatogenous retinal detachment.

with significant subretinal fluid (more than 1 disc diameter), (2) horseshoe or flap tears in the contralateral eye of a patient who already had RRD, (3) lattice degeneration with holes and/or subretinal fluid in the contralateral eye of a patient who already had RRD (Table 49-2).[17]

Asymptomatic flap tears with pigment, round holes, and atrophic holes probably do not need prophylactic treatment. Asymptomatic lattice degeneration does not require prophylactic treatment.

Treatment of Symptomatic Lesions

If the patient has symptoms of ongoing vitreous traction, then the threshold for treating observed retinal pathologic conditions should be lowered. Attention should be directed especially to the superior retina because approximately 80% of pseudophakic retinal tears will be found in the superior clock hours.[18] In about 50% of eyes, PVD-induced tears will be multiple. In acutely symptomatic eyes, flap or horseshoe tears, operculated tears, and atrophic holes with fluid may all be considered for retinopexy.

Laser or cryotherapy retinopexy should be performed with 24 to 48 hours of the identification of symptomatic retinal tears. Which modality to use is based on the size of tear, its location, and the availability of the different modalities. There is no direct clinical evidence that one is preferential. Theoretically, laser retinopexy is preferred whenever possible because an immediate, albeit incomplete, adhesion is obtained and fewer RPE cells are liberated.[19,20] Laser indirect ophthalmoscope units, both argon and diode, have revolutionized the treatment of postoperative eyes because a noncontact lens laser treatment can be performed.

Patients requiring retinopexy for symptomatic retinal lesions need careful posttreatment follow-up. Up to 22% may require additional treatment, and 5% will need treatment in the fellow eye.[21]

Differential Diagnosis

In the setting of an acute visual field defect with an examination showing a corresponding area of retinal elevation accompanied by an open retinal tear, the diagnosis of RRD is confirmed. When the view to the posterior segment is poor because of media opacity or a small pupil, or when no open break can be found, than the diagnosis may be less clear. In this case, certain ancillary testing can be helpful.

The most likely entity to be confused with RRD in the immediate postoperative period is localized choroidal detachment and/or choroidal hemorrhage. Usually seen in the setting of hypotony, choroidal detachment appears as a dark, solid multilobular mass or masses. Its development may be delayed by hours or days after surgery and may be heralded by the onset of acute pain. Often the ora serrata is elevated, allowing for its visualization without scleral depression. Associated findings to rule out include a leaking wound, filtering bleb, or posterior perforation from the anesthetic needle or bridle suture. Exudative RD may develop overlying the choroidal detachment. This usually resolves spontaneously. B-scan ultrasonography is often diagnostic for choroidal detachment.

Central serous chorioretinopathy can result in a serous RD involving the posterior pole. Rarely such an RD can extend into the interior retina. No open retinal break will be visible, and retinal pigment epithelial alterations in the posterior pole may be apparent. Intravenous fluorescein angiography can usually confirm the diagnosis.

Cystoid macular edema is one of the most common causes of decreased vision in the postcataract patient. Rarely it can be confused with RRD.[22] It may result in clinical thickening of the central macula but should not be associated with subretinal fluid to any significant degree. Intravenous fluorescein angiography can confirm the diagnosis.

A variety of underlying choroidal, retinal, or scleral disorders can result in secondary exudative RD. Differentiation from RRD can be a daunting clinical challenge. Shifting fluid that pools inferiorly; the absence of fixed folds; the lack of a full-thickness retinal tear; the presence of intraocular inflammation; and/or scleral, choroidal, or retinal inflammatory, infiltrative, or tumorous lesions all point toward an exudative RD.

Immediate Management of Retinal Detachment

If an acute RRD is diagnosed with the macula threatened, all efforts should be made to repair the retina as soon as possible. If a delay is unavoidable, bedrest with bilateral patching can slow the accumulation of subretinal fluid. Once the macula is involved, the timing of surgical intervention is less critical. Recent evidence suggests that macula-off RRD repaired within 5 to 7 days has no different visual outcome than those operated on within 1 to 2 days.[23] If the macula has been off for a longer interval, elective surgery is appropriate.

Surgical Management

Scleral buckling surgery remains the treatment of choice for the majority of pseudophakic and aphakic RDs. Most surgeons advocate encirclement of the entire globe via a circumferential buckling element in eyes that have undergone previous cataract surgery to reduce the risk of failure caused by new or missed retinal breaks. Recent data indicate that this approach may reduce the risk of reoperation by 3%.[24] Overall, 85% of all cases of pseudophakic RRD can be fixed with one operation.[25]

Pneumatic retinopexy can be used for RRD following cataract surgery, but the success rate is lower than that in phakic eyes. New or missed breaks account for most of the failed cases. Proliferative vitreoretinopathy does not appear to be any greater in eyes treated with pneumatic retinopexy.

Recently, some posterior segment specialists have investigated pars plana vitrectomy with laser, gas injection, and internal drainage of subretinal fluid without scleral buckling in selected cases of pseudophakic RRD. This approach is less painful, and some of the risks associated with scleral buckling (extrusion, diplopia) and side effects (altered refractive error) are eliminated. In one large, prospective, nonrandomized trial (294 eyes), pars plana vitrectomy with fluid-gas exchange and endolaser without scleral buckling reattached pseudophakic RRD in 88% of the patients with one operation.[26]

Summary

RRD subsequently develops in 1% to 2% of all patients undergoing cataract extraction by an extracapsular technique. Interruption of the posterior capsule either intraoperatively or postoperatively increases the risk for RRD. Before both cataract extraction and Nd:YAG laser capsulotomy, a dilated examination should be performed to identify lesions at risk. Because the majority of RRD cases occur within 1 year following cataract extraction, patients should be screened relatively frequently with dilated examinations during this period.

Most importantly, all postcataract patients must be educated about the signs and symptoms of RRD and instructed to seek medical attention immediately if any such changes develop.

REFERENCES

1. Michels RG, Wilkinson CP, Rice TA: *Retinal detachment,* St Louis, 1990, Mosby.
2. Benson WE: *Retinal detachment: diagnosis and management.* Philadelphia. 1988, JB Lippincott.
3. Kangro M, Osterlin S: Hyaluronate concentration in the vitreous of the pseudophakic eye, *Invest Ophthalmol Vis Sci* 26(suppl):28, 1985.
4. Heller MD, Straatsma BR, Foos RY: Detachment of the posterior vitreous in phakic and aphakic eyes, *Mod Probl Ophthalmol* 10:23-26, 1972.
5. McDonnell PJ, Patel A, Green WR: Comparison of intracapsular and extracapsular cataract surgery: histopathologic study of eyes obtained postmortem, *Ophthalmology* 92:1208-1225, 1985.
6. Friedman Z, Neumann E: Posterior vitreous detachment after cataract surgery in non-myopic eyes and the resulting retinal lesions, *Br J Ophthalmol* 59:451-454, 1975.
7. Haiman MH, Burton TC, Brown CK: Epidemiology of retinal detachment, *Arch Ophthalmol* 100:289-292, 1982.
8. Wilkinson CP, Anderson LS, Little JH: Retinal detachment following phacoemulsification, *Ophthalmology* 85:151-156, 1978.
9. Smith PW, Stark WJ, Maumenee AE et al: Retinal detachment after extracapsular cataract extraction with posterior chamber intraocular lens, *Ophthalmology* 94:495-504, 1987.
10. Javitt JC, Vitale S, Canner JK et al: National outcomes of cataract extraction. I. Retinal detachment after in patient surgery, *Ophthalmology* 98:895-902, 1991.
11. Steinert RF, Puliafito CA, Kumar SR et al: Cystoid macular edema, retinal detachment, and glaucoma after Nd:YAG laser posterior capsulotomy, *Am J Ophthalmol* 112:373-380, 1991.
12. Ober RR, Wilkinson CP, Fiore JV et al: Rhegmatogenous retinal detachments after neodymium-YAG laser capsulotomy in aphakic and pseudophakic eye, *Am J Ophthalmol* 101:81-87, 1986.
13. Rickman-Barger L, Florine CW, Larson RD et al: Retinal detachment after neodymium-YAG laser posterior capsulotomy, *Am J Ophthalmol* 107:531-536, 1989.
14. Javitt JC, Tielsch JM, Canner JK et al: National outcome of cataract extraction: increased risk of retinal complications associated with Nd:YAG laser capsulotomy, *Ophthalmology* 99:1486-1498, 1992.
15. Yoshida A, Ogasawara H, Jalkh AE et al: Retinal detachment after cataract surgery, *Ophthalmology* 99:453-459, 1992.
16. Duker JS, Sabates NR, Thomas GJ et al: Retinal detachment following recent cataract extraction (in press).
17. *Preferred Practice Pattern. Retinal detachment,* American Academy of Ophthalmology, San Francisco, 1990.
18. Jungschaffer OH: Retinal detachment after intraocular lens implants, *Arch Ophthalmol* 95:1203-1204, 1977.
19. Yoon YH, Marmor MF: Rapid enhancement of retinal adhesion by laser photocoagulation, *Ophthalmology* 95:1385-1388, 1988.
20. Campochiaro PA, Kaden IH, Vidaurri-Leal J et al: Cryotherapy enhances intravitreal dispersion of viable retinal pigment epithelial cells, *Arch Ophthalmol* 103:434- 436, 1985.
21. Smiddy WE, Flynn HW, Nicholson DH et al: Results and complications in treated retinal breaks, *Am J Ophthalmol* 112:623-631, 1991.
22. Lakhanpal V, Schocket SS: Pseudophakic and aphakic retinal detachment mimicking cystoid macular edema, *Ophthalmology* 94:785-791, 1987.
23. Ross WH, Kozy DW: Visual recovery in macula-off rhegmatogenous retinal detachments, *Ophthalmology* 105:2149-2153, 1998.
24. O'Malley P, Swearingen K: Scleral buckling with diathermy for simple retinal detachments, *Ophthalmology* 99:269-277, 1992.
25. Greven CM, Sanders RJ, Brown GC et al: Pseudophakic retinal detachments, *Ophthalmology* 99:257-262, 1992.
26. Campo RV, Sipperley JO, Sneed SR et al: Pars plana vitrectomy without scleral buckle for pseudophakic retinal detachments, *Ophthalmology* 106:1811-1816, 1999.

Prolonged Intraocular Inflammation

50

Michael B. Raizman, MD

The most feared and severe form of inflammation after cataract surgery is acute endophthalmitis. Occurring within days of surgery, acute endophthalmitis often results in rapid loss of vision (see Chapter 48). This chapter concentrates on a more insidious form of postoperative inflammation. Chronic inflammation may begin weeks, months, or even years after cataract surgery and can last as long as endophthalmitis. This inflammation is often caused by infection with organisms of low virulence that are sequestered in the capsular bag. However, other causes must also be considered, including the lens implant, retained lens material, and coincidental uveitis unrelated to the surgery.[1] This chapter reviews the practical aspects of diagnosis and management of prolonged intraocular inflammation after cataract surgery.

The incidence and degree of inflammation after cataract surgery have decreased significantly in recent years. Modern instrumentation, better surgical techniques, and improved intraocular lens (IOL) designs are all responsible for this advance. Perhaps more important is the common use of surgical techniques that minimize iris manipulation and reduce the amount of transected vascular tissue. The elimination of iridectomy and the use of smaller incisions in the cornea and/or sclera are good examples of such techniques. Placement of the IOL in the capsular bag certainly reduces contact with the vascularized and pigmented ocular tissues. Phacoemulsification contributes to the ability to minimize ocular manipulation; hence, it reduces inflammation. With phacoemulsification it is usually possible to avoid contact with the iris. Although manual expression of the nucleus can be performed with minimal iris manipulation in most cases (and with minimal resultant inflammation), some stretching of the iris is unavoidable.

Fortunately, improvements in IOL design have also reduced inflammation. Early versions of IOLs incited inflammation in a variety of ways. A few lenses were contaminated during manufacture or packaging with substances toxic to the eye. Some lenses were poorly finished, with rough surfaces that induced inflammation. Others, such as closed-loop anterior chamber IOLs, caused inflammation because of their shape and design. Any lens that led to increased contact with the iris or cocoons of uveal tissue around haptics was liable to induce inflammation. The uveitis-glaucoma-hyphema (UGH) syndrome is one that is rarely encountered today because of improved lens design.

A better understanding of the tolerance and physiology of ocular tissues led to the development of better irrigating solutions, intraocular viscoelastics, and intraocular medications. Together these limit the amount of inflammation induced by the cataract extraction procedure. It is interesting to note that little development of new pharmacologic agents for the treatment of postoperative inflammation has occurred, although our understanding of the application of existing medications has proved beneficial. Implantable sustained-release drug delivery systems may prove useful.[2,3]

Recognition of Abnormal Inflammation

Acute endophthalmitis in the first week after cataract surgery is discussed in Chapter 48. Many of the conditions discussed in this chapter may also cause acute inflammation and should be considered in that context. Abnormal chronic inflammation is cellular activity in the eye of a greater degree and a longer duration than generally expected. Some inflammation is inevitable after any cataract extraction. After routine phacoemulsification and lens implantation, the lack of significant inflammation may be remarkable. Many of these eyes would probably do well without postoperative antiinflammatory therapy, although few surgeons would be willing to take this risk, considering the current medicolegal atmosphere. With low-dose topical corticosteroids, most of these eyes have little inflammation after 1 or 2 weeks and are free of inflammation after 2 to 3 weeks. On the other side of the spectrum, a case of complicated manual expression of a nucleus, with iris sphincterotomies, peripheral iridectomy, and vitreous loss, may cause inflammation for 6 to 8 weeks. Therefore inflammation lasting more than 3 to 8 weeks, depending on the clinical setting, should raise concerns about infection or other causes of abnormal inflammation. Of equal concern is inflammation that does not respond to aggressive topical corticosteroids, the development of a hypopyon at any time, and an increase in vitreous cellular infiltrate.

Causes of Prolonged Inflammation

Patients with preoperative uveitis are at increased risk of excessive postoperative inflammation (see Chapter 23). Diabetics usually display more inflammation, and some surgeons in the Far East

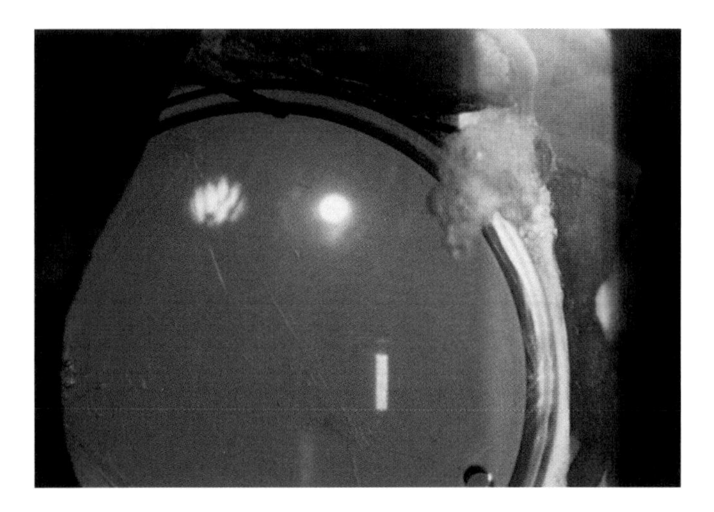

FIGURE 50-1 Cortical material, shown adjacent to the posterior chamber IOL, may harbor bacteria and incite postoperative inflammation.

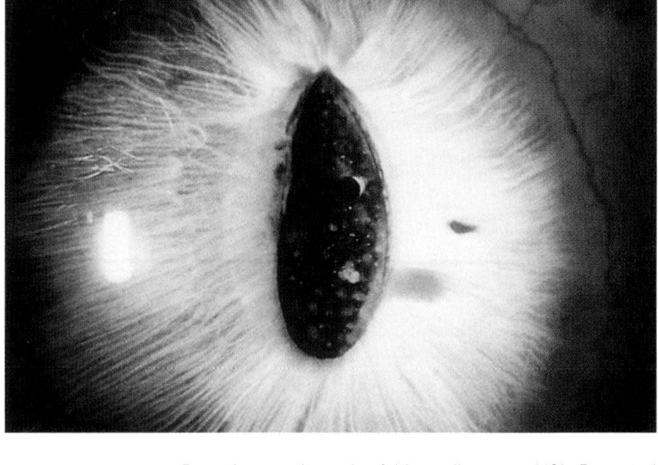

FIGURE 50-2 Deposits coat the optic of this pupil-captured IOL. Repeated neodymium: yttrium-aluminum-garnet laser cleaning of the lens optic surface provided only transient effect. (See also Figure 45-13.)

believe that Asians are more prone to inflammation, especially from retained lens epithelium. As mentioned previously, intraoperative factors such as manipulation of the iris, vitrectomy, and prolonged surgical times may contribute to increases in postoperative vascular leakage and inflammation. Residual cortical material induces inflammation in many cases by inducing attempts by phagocytes to clear the material and perhaps by stimulating cytokine release in the anterior chamber, with subsequent recruitment of inflammatory cells. Cortical material may also harbor organisms that induce an inflammatory response (Figure 50-1). Retained nuclear material commonly causes inflammation and elevated intraocular pressure. Iris to the wound is especially likely to induce inflammation and cystoid macular edema (CME).

Debate continues about the role of lens materials in inducing inflammation. Polymethylmethacrylate seems to induce less complement activation than does polypropylene (Prolene),[4] but the clinical relevance of this finding is not certain. Epidemiologic studies suggest the Prolene haptics are more often associated with endophthalmitis than are polymethylmethacrylate haptics,[5] perhaps because of differences in bacterial adhesion. Surface modification of lens implants with heparin may reduce postoperative inflammation.[6] As noted previously, improvements in lens design over the past 15 years have dramatically reduced the incidence of excessive postoperative inflammation.

When the IOLs are responsible for prolonged inflammation, it is generally their misplacement that is to blame. Anterior chamber lenses are most likely to induce inflammation because they necessarily contact the angle structures. This is rarely a problem unless the lens is too long (causing pressure or even erosion), too short (leading to excessive movement), anteriorly displaced (inducing corneal endothelial damage), or posteriorly displaced (causing iris trauma, iris tuck, or cocooning). Posterior chamber IOLs (PC IOLs) that are placed in the capsular bag rarely cause inflammation. One or both haptics in the sulcus are almost always well tolerated. On occasion, haptics may abrade or erode uveal tissue, producing inflammation and recurrent hemorrhage.[7-10] Capture of the lens optic by the pupil is often associated with iritis and with deposition of inflammatory cells and debris on the optic surface from repeatedly traumatized iris tissue (Figure 50-2).

Uveitis unrelated to the surgery may present for the first time any time after cataract surgery. This coincidental appearance can cause a delay in diagnosis. Sympathetic ophthalmia after modern cataract extraction is exceedingly rare.[11] Latanoprost and newer prostaglandin analogues can induce intraocular inflammation and CME.[12] Miotic agents and other glaucoma medications can do the same.

Examination of the Eye

The examination should be directed at those conditions outlined previously. The patient should be asked about localized pain, which may suggest an offending IOL haptic contacting uveal tissue. Keratic precipitates (Figure 50-3) and anterior chamber

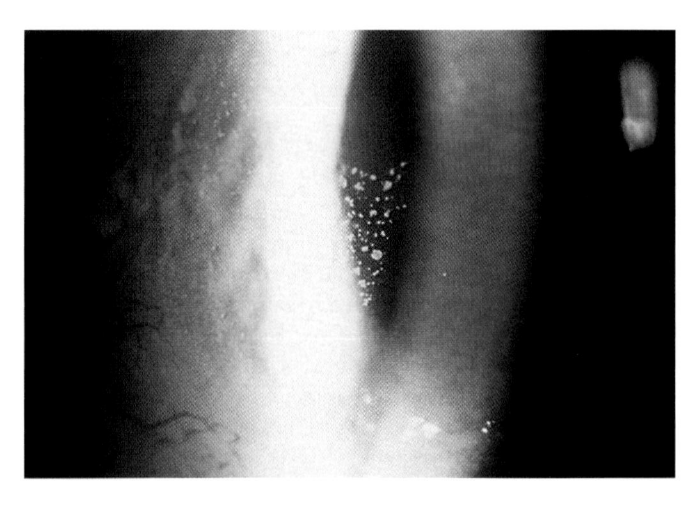

FIGURE 50-3 Granulomatous keratic precipitates in a case of chronic postoperative endophthalmitis from *Propionibacterium acnes.*

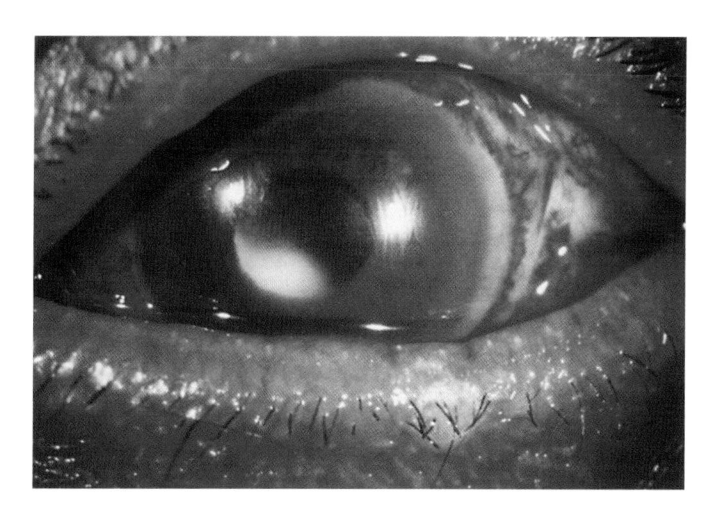

FIGURE 50-4 Posterior capsular abscess containing *Staphylococcus epidermidis* developed in this case about 1 year after cataract extraction.

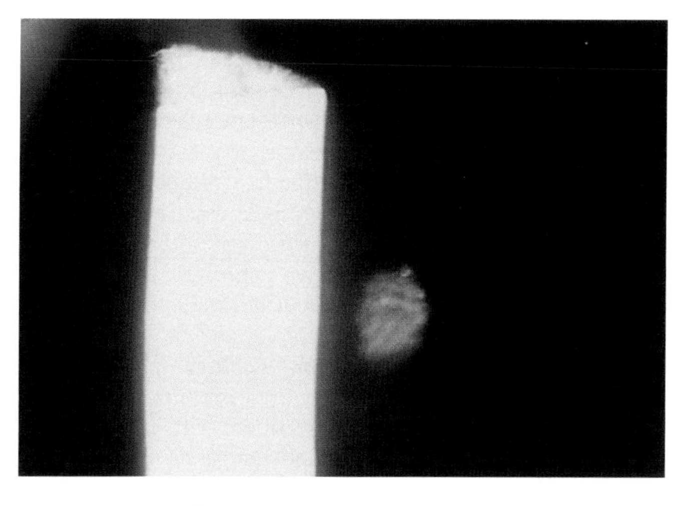

FIGURE 50-5 Posterior capsular plaque in a case of presumed *P. acnes* endophthalmitis. In this case, vitreous culture revealed no organisms, but gram-positive rods were found on the capsule in the region of the plaque.

cell and flare should be quantified to allow accurate comparisons from one visit to the next. A widely dilated pupil should allow better visualization of the PC IOL implant to determine position, of the capsular bag to visualize residual cortex and abscesses (Figure 50-4), and of the posterior capsule to detect plaques of anaerobic organisms (Figure 50-5). Gonioscopy is useful to view the angle for synechiae, iris to the wound, and haptic position; the mirror also assists in the posterior chamber evaluation. Gonioscopy can allow visualization of a greater portion of the peripheral capsule and PC IOL. The vitreous should be examined at the slit lamp examination to grade any vitreous infiltrate. CME is best seen with a contact lens or with a 78- or 90-diopter lens at the slit lamp examination. Indirect ophthalmoscopy allows visualization of retained lens material and inflammation in the vitreous.

Management

Any obvious cause of excessive inflammation should be corrected where possible and when indicated. Some low-grade inflammation from IOL misplacement may not reduce vision or cause discomfort and may be controllable with low doses of corticosteroids. Such cases may be followed without surgical intervention. Inflammation may disappear weeks or months later. If glaucoma therapy is suspected as a contributing factor to the inflammation, the drops should be stopped as a trial. Eyes with visual loss (usually below 20/40), uncontrollable inflammation, glaucoma, hyphema, or CME may require appropriate surgical intervention, that is, lens reposition or exchange, removal of residual cortex from the anterior chamber, or release of iris from the wound. The presence of an abscess or plaque on the capsule suggests endophthalmitis and requires antibiotic and/or surgical therapy, as discussed in Chapter 48.

In many cases, no obvious cause of inflammation is apparent, or the inflammation may be considered consistent with operative trauma. In such cases, topical corticosteroids may be given frequently, up to every hour. A significant reduction in inflammation should be seen. If little or no response is noted, it is often helpful to try an intraorbital injection (through the lower lid and orbital septum) of triamcinolone (Kenalog), 40 mg in 1 ml. If little or no response is seen following the injection, endophthalmitis must be seriously considered. On occasion, the inflammation responds nicely but relapses when corticosteroids are tapered. Failure to control the inflammation by these techniques should raise the possibility of chronic endophthalmitis.

Several series of cases have been published on the use of subconjunctival or intraocular tissue plasminogen activator (tPA). tPA is a naturally occurring enzyme that induces fibrinolysis by converting plasminogen into plasmin; plasmin is responsible for the degradation of fibrin. Its use is still considered experimental, but it seems to be a safe method of reducing or eliminating fibrin clots in situations where this must be accomplished quickly (e.g., obstructed filtering blebs or pupillary block glaucoma). The ideal dose has not been determined, but current formulations of tPA, created for other clinical and laboratory uses, need to be diluted. The cost is quite high, and the use of tPA for treating ocular fibrin must be considered experimental pending the performance of larger-scale studies.[13-16] Topical use of tPA is ineffective.[17]

Propionibacterium and Other Chronic Endophthalmitis

When all noninfectious causes of chronic postoperative inflammation have been addressed and ruled out, infection with *Propionibacterium* species or other organisms must be presumed. Chronic endophthalmitis may be present in many ways, but characteristic features have been recognized: chronic, often mild granulomatous or nongranulomatous uveitis; white plaques on the lens capsule; and onset of inflammation months (or, rarely, years) after surgery. Cases appearing after neodymium: yttrium-aluminum-garnet capsulotomy suggest that organisms may be sequestered in the capsular bag. Patients may or may not complain of pain. Blurry vision is a common symptom. Conjunctival hyperemia, keratic precipitates, hypopyon, and vitritis are variable signs. In unusual cases of *Propionibacterium acnes* endophthalmitis, the onset of severe inflammation may be acute. The average time to onset is about 4 months after cataract extraction. The inflammation may respond transiently to topical corticosteroids. Although most cases are caused by the gram-positive anaerobic *P. acnes* rod, other offending organisms include *Staphylococcus* species, *Actinomyces, Achromobacter, Corynebacterium, Propionibacterium granulosum,* and fungi.[18]

All suspected cases deserve at least a culture of the vitreous and injection of vancomycin (1 mg in 0.1 ml) into the vitreous cavity. One report of successful treatment with systemic and topical (but no intraocular) antibiotics suggests that this may be a feasible alternative, but the literature contains multiple cases of failure with such an approach.[19-21] Recurrence of endophthalmitis after simple culture and injection of vancomycin has been reported, prompting some investigators to recommend more aggressive surgery. Among the additional interventions needed in some cases are partial capsulectomy and total capsulectomy with lens explantation.[22-24]

Based on the literature, the following guidelines are suggested: the combined techniques of pars plana vitrectomy with culture; partial capsulectomy, including capsule-containing plaques or abscesses; and injection of vancomycin. Cases with extensive areas of capsular infection probably require full capsulectomy. If inflammation recurs after partial capsulectomy, then removal of the entire capsule is recommended. This usually necessitates removal of any PC IOL. Concurrent IOL exchange is reasonable in most cases, with a replacement IOL either sutured in the posterior chamber or placed in the anterior chamber. Removal of the capsular bag may be facilitated by the use of chymotrypsin. Iris hooks or pupil expanders may aid visualization when pupillary dilation is inadequate.

In addition to the routine culture, vitreous specimens should be cultured under anaerobic conditions for 14 days to increase the chances of recovering the *P. acnes* organisms. Culture-negative cases of chronic inflammation may represent infections that failed to grow in the laboratory. It has been suggested that culturing the vitrectomy cassette contents may be more rewarding than culturing an initial vitreous aspirate.[25] It is probably prudent to do both. It may also be helpful to stain and culture the excised portion of the posterior capsule, as this may demonstrate organisms when vitreous cultures do not (see Figure 50-5).

As with all rare conditions, suspicion is the key to diagnosis. All cases of chronic inflammation after cataract extraction should be considered infectious until proven otherwise. The rewards of such a diagnosis are great because good vision is the rule after appropriate treatment.[26]

REFERENCES

1. Berrocal AM, Davis JL: Uveitis following intraocular surgery, *Ophthalmol Clin North Am* 15:357-364, 2002.
2. Tan DTH, Chee SP, Lim L et al: Randomized clinical trial of a new dexamethasone drug delivery system (Surodex) for treatment of post-cataract surgery inflammation, *Ophthalmology* 106:223-231, 1999.
3. Chang DF, Garcia IH, Hunkeler JD et al: Phase II results of an intraocular steroid delivery system for cataract surgery, *Ophthalmology* 106:1172-1177, 1999.
4. Mondino BJ, Nagata S, Glovsky MM: Activation of the alternative complement pathway by intraocular lenses, *Invest Ophthalmol Vis Sci* 26:905-908, 1985.
5. Menikoff JA, Speaker MG, Marmor M et al: A case-control study of risk factors for post-operative endophthalmitis, *Ophthalmology* 98:1761-1768, 1991.
6. Trocme SD, Li H: Effect of heparin-surface-modified intraocular lenses on postoperative inflammation after phacoemulsification: a randomized trial in a United States patient population: Heparin-Surface-Modified Lens Study Group, *Ophthalmology* 107:1031-1037, 2000.
7. Percival SP, Das SK: UGH syndrome after posterior chamber lens implantation, *J Am Intraocul Implant Soc* 19:200-201, 1983.
8. Van Liefferinge T, Van Oye R, Kestelyn P: Uveitis-glaucoma-hyphema syndrome: a late complication of posterior chamber lenses, *Bull Soc Belge Ophthalmol* 252:61-66, 1994.
9. Aounuma H, Matsushita H, Nakajima K et al: Uveitis-glaucoma-hyphema syndrome after posterior chamber intraocular lens implantation, *Jpn J Ophthalmol* 47:98-100, 1997.
10. Masket S: Pseudophakic posterior iris chafing syndrome, *J Cataract Refract Surg* 1986;12:252-256, 1986.
11. Lubin JR, Albert DM, Weinstein M: Sixty-five years of sympathetic ophthalmia: a clinicopathologic review of 105 cases (1913-1978), *Ophthalmology* 87:109, 1980.
12. Miyaki K, Ota I, Maekubo K et al: Latanoprost accelerates disruption of the blood brain barrier and the incidence of angiographic cystoid macular edema in early postoperative pseudophakia, *Ophthalmology* 117:34-40, 1999.
13. Snyder RW, Lambrou FH, Williams GA: Intraocular fibrinolysis with recombinant human tissue plasminogen activator, *Arch Ophthalmol* 105:1277-1280, 1987.
14. Piltz JR, Starita RJ: The use of subconjunctivally administered tissue plasminogen activator after trabeculectomy, *Ophthalmic Surg* 25:51-53, 1994.
15. Wedrich A, Menapace R, Ries E et al: Intracameral tissue plasminogen activator to treat severe fibrinous effusion after cataract surgery, *J Cataract Refract Surg* 873-877, 1997.
16. Helingenhaus A, Steinmetz B, Lapuente R et al: Recombinant tissue plasminogen activator in cases with fibrin formation after cataract surgery: a prospective randomized multicentre study, *Br J Ophthalmol* 82:810-815, 1998.
17. Zwaan J, Latimer WB: Topical tissue plasminogen activator appears ineffective for the clearance of intraocular fibrin, *Ophthalmic Surg Lasers 29:476-483, 1998.*
18. Meisler DM, Mandelbaum S: *Propionibacterium*-associated endophthalmitis after extracapsular cataract extraction: review of reported cases, *Ophthalmology* 96:54-61, 1989.
19. Meisler DM, Zakov ZN, Bruner WE et al: Endophthalmitis associated with sequestered intraocular *Propionibacterium acnes, Am J Ophthalmol* 104:428-429, 1987 (letter).
20. Brady SE, Cohen EJ, Fischer DH: Diagnosis and treatment of chronic postoperative bacterial endophthalmitis, *Ophthalmic Surg* 19:580-584, 1988.
21. Sawusch MR, Michels RG, Stark WJ et al: Endophthalmitis due to *Propionibacterium acnes* sequestered between IOL optic and posterior capsule, *Ophthalmic Surg* 20:90-92, 1989.
22. Winward KE, Pflugfelder SC, Flynn HW et al: Postoperative *Propionibacterium* endophthalmitis: treatment strategies and long-term results, *Ophthalmology* 100:447-451, 1993.
23. Clark WL, Kaiser PK, Flynn Jr. HW et al: Treatment strategies and visual acuity outcomes in chronic post-operative *Propionibacterium acnes* endophthalmitis, *Ophthalmology* 106:1665-1670, 1999.
24. Aldave AJ, Stein JD, Deramo VA et al: Treatment strategies for postoperative *Propionibacterium* endophthalmitis, *Ophthalmology* 106:2395-2401, 1999.
25. Donahue SP, Kowalski RP, Jewart BH et al: Vitreous cultures in suspected endophthalmitis: biopsy or vitrectomy, *Ophthalmology* 100:452-455, 1993.
26. Zambano W, Flynn HW, Pflugfelder SC et al: Management options for *Propionibacterium acnes endophthalmitis, Ophthalmology* 96:1100-1105, 1989.

Lasers in Cataract Surgery

51

Jack M. Dodick, MD
Julia D. Katz, MD

Over 30 years ago Kelman[1] revolutionized the field of cataract surgery by introducing not only a radically different surgical technique, ultrasound phacoemulsification, but also the concept of small-incision cataract surgery. Small-incision cataract surgery, in turn, spurred the development of new lens technology, namely the foldable intraocular lens (IOL). With further refinement over the intervening years, clear corneal phacoemulsification has become the procedure of choice among cataract surgeons[2] because it greatly enhances patient outcomes by decreasing wound complications, minimizing induced astigmatism, and enabling quicker rehabilitation. Phacoemulsification, however, is not without its problems. Issues of safety related to the release of excess energy at the probe tip and the inadvertent effects on nontarget tissues, such as the cornea, iris, and posterior capsule, remain a concern. The excessive heat generated around the phaco probe tip necessitates a cooling irrigation sleeve to minimize the risks of a corneal burn or wound distortion. To date, the technology is limited to an incision size of 2.2 to 3.2 mm. Just as Kelman was driven to improve the accepted standard of care when he introduced ultrasound phacoemulsification, so there still exists the need to continually improve current technology and techniques to circumvent our current limitations.

Evolution of Lasers in Cataract Surgery

In 1975, Krasnov[3] reported the first laser procedure for cataract removal, laser phacopuncture. With a Q-switched ruby laser, microperforations were made in the anterior capsule, thus enabling the gradual release and reabsorption of the lens material over time. This technique had very limited applications; it was effective only for very soft cataracts, such as congenital cataracts, and patients were maintained on dilation drops to prevent closure of the puncture sites, as well as steroids for the treatment of induced uveitis for extended postoperative periods.

In the ensuing years, interest shifted to four ultraviolet wavelengths: 193 nm (argon fluoride), 248 nm (krypton fluoride), 308 nm (xenon chloride), and 351 nm (xenon fluoride).[4-6] Of these, the 308-nm laser appeared to be the most promising for both its transmissibility through fiber optics and its ablation profile: the threshold for ablation of the lens capsule was significantly higher than that of the lens nucleus and cortex, an appealing characteristic for endocapsular emulsification.[4] The cataractogenic effects of the 308-nm laser, however, as well as questions of possible retinal toxicity and carcinogenic effects, posed potential threats to the eyes of both patient and surgeon.[7-10] These concerns led further investigation away from these excimer lasers and toward the infrared wavelengths, namely the erbium:yttrium-aluminum-garnet (Er:YAG)[11-14] and the neodymium:yttrium-aluminum-garnet (Nd:YAG)[15-17] lasers. In 1980, Aron-Rosa et al.[18] and others reported the use of the Nd:YAG (1064-nm) laser for performing posterior capsulotomy,[19-20] peripheral iridotomy,[20-22] and cutting of pupillary membranes. These developments laid the groundwork for the next use of lasers in cataract surgery: laser anterior capsulotomy.[23] However, due to its potential complications, including a rise in intraocular pressure, inflammation, and poor mydriasis after laser treatment (which required the surgery to be performed promptly after the laser treatment), as well as the conversion of cataract surgery from a one-step to a two-step procedure, Nd:YAG laser anterior capsulotomy never gained widespread acceptance.[24,25]

These attempts to broaden the use of lasers in cataract surgery led to laser photofragmentation,[26-30] a technique that involved using the Nd:YAG laser to photodisrupt the lens nucleus and thereby soften it before phacoemulsification. Although several studies confirmed the use of shorter phaco time and less phaco power required when using this combination method, the procedure carried the increased risk of inadvertent perforations of the anterior and posterior capsules and thus the increased risk of intraoperative complications. Also, similar to laser anterior capsulotomy, laser photofragmentation carried the additional inconvenience of converting a one-stage surgery into two stages.

Nd:YAG Laser Systems

Dodick Laser Photolysis (ARC Lasers)

The Dodick laser Photolysis system (Figure 51-1), currently the only laser unit approved for cataract removal by the Food and Drug Administration (FDA), transfers laser energy in a Q-switched mode from a laser source, via a 300-μm quartz-clad

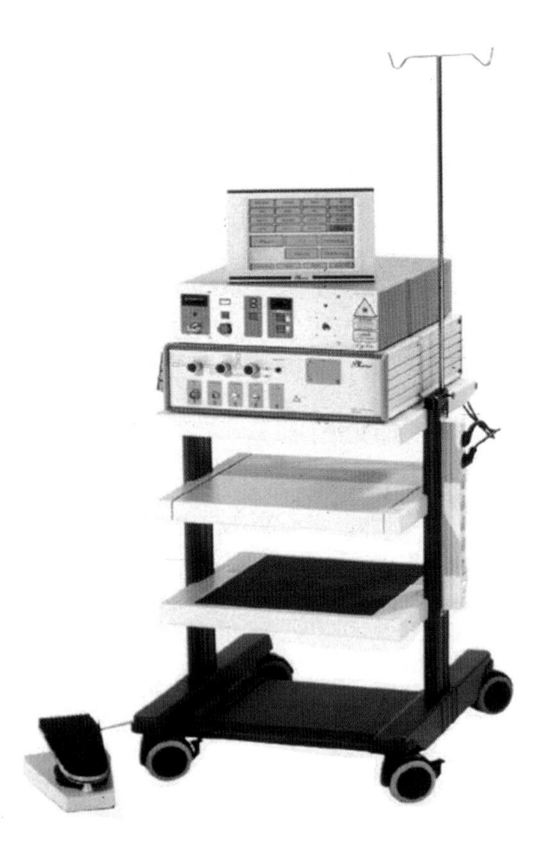

FIGURE 51-1 Dodick Photolysis system.

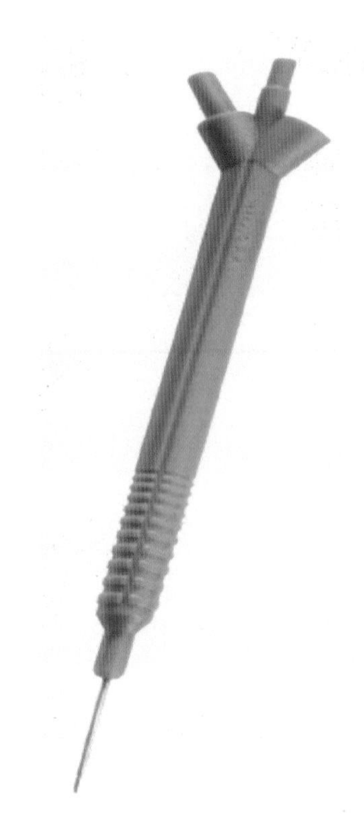

FIGURE 51-2 Dodick photolysis laser-aspiration probe for disruption and removal of cataract material.

fiber optic, to a titanium plate, generating a shock wave. In contrast to phacoemulsification, which generates heat by transforming electrical energy into mechanical energy with the subsequent generation of emulsifying shock waves,[1] the laser probe produces no significant heat[31] and therefore requires no irrigation cooling sleeve. This lack of heat production provides two clear advantages: (1) it eliminates the risk of a corneal burn, which can result in significant astigmatism, corneal endothelial cell compromise, and, in severe cases, a penetrating keratoplasty; and (2) it allows for the separation of the irrigation port from the emulsifying needle. This second advantage is responsible for the reduced diameter of the handpiece and explains how laser technologies are able to use much smaller wound sizes than are possible with current phacoemulsification devices.

The laser-aspiration handpiece (Figure 51-2), which is similar to the aspiration probe of a standard bimanual irrigation-aspiration instrument, transmits the laser beam and ultimately directs it onto a titanium plate that resides just within the tip of the probe (Figure 51-3). This titanium target allows optical breakdown of the laser energy to occur at a greatly reduced threshold than would otherwise be required without such a target and therefore allows plasma formation to occur at a much lower energy level. Plasma formation results in shock waves emanating from the tip of the laser probe. These shock waves emulsify the cataract material, which is subsequently aspirated through the same probe[32] (Figure 51-4). In addition, the titanium target shields the nontarget tissues such as the endothelium and the retina, as well as the surgeon's eyes, from direct laser light.[33,34]

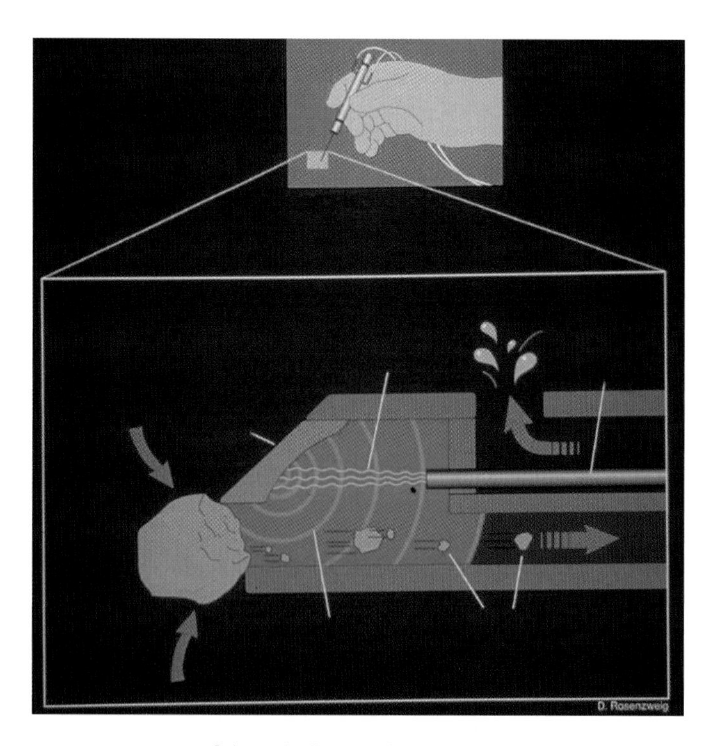

FIGURE 51-3 Schematic diagram of the photolysis mechanism. Nd:YAG laser beam is transmitted through the probe and strikes a titanium plate housed within the tip of the probe. Optical breakdown and plasma formation result in shock waves emanating from the mouth of the probe, which break up the cataract material. The cataract fragments are then aspirated through the same probe.

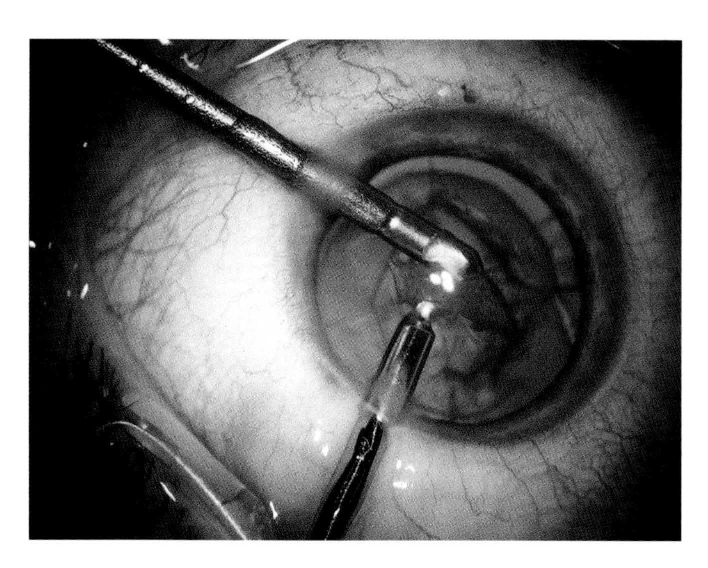

FIGURE 51-4 Dodick photolysis cataract surgery. Laser-aspiration probe *(top left)* disrupts lens material presented to it by the irrigation probe *(below)*. Both probes currently fit through 1.4-mm incisions.

Since the early 1990s, Dodick had been studying the use of the Q-switched, pulsed 1064-nm Nd:YAG laser for one-stage photolysis of cataractous lenses. In 1991, Dodick and Christiansen[17] developed a method of high-speed photography to study the formation and propagation of shock waves created after the Nd:YAG laser pulses strike the titanium target. They demonstrated that within 205 nanoseconds after firing the laser, a shock wave formed on the inside surface of the titanium target, and a weaker one formed on the outside surface. The shock wave was shown to propagate toward the mouth of the aspiration port, and only attenuated shock waves emanated outside of the probe. This method was subsequently used to modify the target configuration to maximize shock waves up to but not beyond a focal point while minimizing propagation beyond the tip of the probe.

After initial and promising studies on cataractous cadaveric lenses,[15,16] the first animal studies were performed to evaluate the safety of Nd:YAG photolysis.[35,36] One eye each of 14 New Zealand white rabbits was exposed to Nd:YAG laser energy levels far in excess of that required for the cadaveric cataracts; the nonoperated fellow eyes served as controls. Examination of the eyes using specular microscopy, ultrasonic pachymetry, and light microscopy revealed no damage to the corneal endothelium, trabecular meshwork, or retina of the rabbit eye. In 1991, following an Investigational Device Exemption (IDE) granted by the FDA, the first laser lens ablation of a nuclear sclerotic cataract in a 60-year-old woman was performed without complication.[16] Less than 4 minutes of laser time was required, and postoperatively there was minimal inflammation and endothelial cell loss.

Following the treatment of this initial patient, an IDE was granted to Dodick to treat 50 patients. The results of this series were reported at the 1999 American Society of Cataract and Refractive Surgery (ASCRS) meeting. For lenses of 1 to 3+ density, an average of 450 laser shots, at 10 mJ/shot, were used, translating into an average of 4.5 joules (J) per case. When compared with studies on the energy delivered by phacoemulsification, the difference is striking: in a study comparing "phaco chop" to "divide and conquer," DeBry, Olson, and Crandall[37] noted that the former technique reduced the mean energy delivered by phacoemulsification from a mean of 3264 ± 1218 J to 782 ± 446 J—a significant reduction. More recently, Fine, Packer, and Hoffman[38] reported using power modulations and altered phacoemulsification techniques to deliver lower ultrasound energy, which is estimated to be as low as the single digits. These latter numbers, albeit estimated, certainly rival the early statistics of photolysis.

Kanellopoulos et al.[39] reported results from a multicenter series of 100 consecutive patients, measuring outcome by visual acuity, endothelial cell loss, change in intraocular pressure, total energy used, and intraoperative and postoperative complications. Lens density ranged from 1 to 4+. Mean visual acuity improved from 20/46.5 (0.43) to 20/26.6 (0.75), and endothelial cell loss was 7.55%, comparable to that found with phacoemulsification. There was no significant change in preoperative and postoperative intraocular pressure. Average intraocular energy released by the laser was 6.7 J. Posterior capsule rupture occurred in three cases, but only one occurred during photolysis; one tear occurred after a 4+ nuclear sclerotic lens required the conversion from photolysis to phacoemulsification, and one tear occurred during the placement of the IOL implant. The investigators concluded that the 1 to 2+ nuclear sclerotic cataracts removed with the Dodick Photolysis technology resulted in comparable surgical times when compared with phacoemulsification, but denser nuclei required longer operative time.

In a follow-up prospective multicenter study of 1000 consecutive cases, Kanellopoulos et al.[40] measured outcome by visual acuity improvement, total energy used, mean operative time, and intraoperative and postoperative complications. Lens density again ranged from 1 to 4+ density. Mean visual acuity improved from 20/70.2 to 20/24.4, with a mean intraocular energy of 5.65 J per case, reduced from the earlier study. Average photolysis time again was again comparable to phaco time for 1 to 2+ nuclear sclerotic cataracts, but the mean time for 3+ lenses was 9.8 minutes. Of the 1000 cases, there were 16 cases of intraoperative capsular ruptures (4 without vitreous loss) and 2 cases of brief intraoperative hyphema. Postoperatively, there was 1 case of cystoid macular edema in a patient who had undergone anterior vitrectomy and placement of a sulcus posterior chamber lens implant, 1 case of pseudophakic bullous keratopathy in a patient who had also undergone anterior vitrectomy, and 1 case of a subluxated IOL, again in a patient who had undergone anterior vitrectomy and placement of a sulcus posterior chamber implant. The authors concluded that photolysis is a safe and effective alternative to phacoemulsification in softer cataracts.

In a separate prospective clinical trial using the Dodick Photolysis system, Huetz and Eckhardt[41] reported 100 cases with a 6-month follow-up. The Lens Opacities Classification III (LOCS III) system was used to divide patients into groups I to III depending on the density of nuclear sclerosis. The mean total energy used was 1.97 ± 1.43 J in group I, 3.37 ± 1.59 J in group II, and 7.7 ± 2.09 J in group III. There was no significant difference in preoperative and postoperative pachymetry in groups I and II; group III had a 1.84% increase on postoperative day 2, but at 6 months there was no significant difference from the preoperative value.

The Dodick Photolysis system uses a Venturi pump system to generate aspiration, with a range of 0 to 650 mm Hg. In addition, a continuously pressurized infusion system is adjustable from 0 to 200 mm Hg. The laser output can be set at 8 or 10 mJ per pulse, and the pulse rate can be set at 1 to 20 Hz, although the majority of photolysis surgeons report that settings of 1 to 5 Hz are sufficient for emulsification. The external probe diameter is 1.2 mm, with an internal probe opening of 0.75 mm, although newer probe designs (0.9 mm external diameter) are currently undergoing clinical testing and would require 1-mm wound incisions. At present, two 1.4-mm paracentesis ports are required: one for the laser-aspiration probe and one for the separate irrigation probe. The quartz-clad fiber and the titanium targets are relatively inexpensive, allowing for handpieces to be disposable. The same tips may be used for irrigation-aspiration removal of cortical material or may be switched for specially designed, wound size–matched irrigation-aspiration handpieces.

At present, no IOLs are available that can be inserted through a 1.4-mm incision. Certain lenses are currently under investigation and are being combined with laser photolysis to minimize wound enlargement. Kanellopoulos et al.[40] reported implanting a dehydrated, prefolded, acrylic posterior chamber IOL (model H44-1C-1, Acritec, Berlin, Germany) in three cases using the Dodick Photolysis system. The lens was prefolded to an external diameter of 1.2 to 1.3 mm and ultimately implanted through the original photolysis wound incision; it was noted to be fully unfolded within the capsular bag less than 30 minutes postoperatively. The further development of these prefolded IOLs, or perhaps new implant materials altogether, is now mandated to take advantage of laser technology's ultrasmall-incision surgery.

Photon (Paradigm Medical Industries)

The Photon is an Nd:YAG system that is partnered with the company's conventional ultrasonic phaco system. The probe consists of a titanium tip with a fused silica fiber. It currently has a repetition rate of 10 to 50 Hz, which will eventually be increased above 50 Hz to improve its ability to fragment tissue. Its fluidics system also allows for surge control at all vacuum levels up to 500 mm Hg. It is a unimanual unit, incorporating the irrigation-aspiration system into the laser probe. The probe has a tip diameter ranging from 1.2 to 1.7 mm and passes through a 3- to 3.5-mm incision. The unit uses a peristaltic system with up to 500 mm Hg of vacuum. Clinical trials are currently underway.

Erbium:YAG Systems

Another laser of interest since the 1980s for the removal of cataracts is the Erbium:YAG, first investigated by Peyman and Katoh[13] and Tsubota.[14] Er:YAG emits energy in the midinfrared region (2940 nm) and may be transmitted through a 150-μm fiber optic probe. Like the Nd:YAG laser, Er:YAG offers a potentially safer medium than ultrasound phacoemulsification because of its lower energy requirements and lack of heat production.[42] One advantage of the Er:YAG system is that the 2940-nm wavelength corresponds to the maximum peak of water absorption, allowing low penetration (approximately 1 μm); excess energy is absorbed by water without dispersion to surrounding nontarget tissues. The laser is focused directly into the lens nucleus; subsequent optical breakdown results in microfractures of the lens material with no generation of heat. Lin, Stern, and Puliafito[43] showed that higher pulse frequencies lead to the creation of longitudinal chains of cavitation bubbles forming at the tip of the probe. These cavitation bubbles may extend up to 1 mm in nuclear material and allow the laser energy to travel farther and increase the depth of penetration than if fired in water, where the energy would be absorbed. The accumulation of these bubbles thus facilitates emulsification of denser nuclei, but with the added risk of damage to adjacent structures.

Phacolase MCL-29 (Asclepion-Meditec)

The MCL-29, an Erbium:YAG-based laser system, was introduced by Asclepion-Meditec in 1997 and received approval in 1988 for cataract surgery in Europe after undergoing multicenter clinical studies. The MCL-29 uses a zirconium fluoride–based optical fiber; because of the toxic properties of this material when degraded, it must be connected to a nontoxic silica tip.[43] The distal end of the fiber, housed within the laser handpiece, is composed of quartz, and may be replaced after every four to five surgeries. Although quartz is less efficient in transmitting the infrared radiation, this part of the fiber is extremely short, and so the attenuation of the energy is minimal.[44] The MCL-29 handpiece requires a 3.2-mm incision, as it is a unimanual device, coupling both infusion and aspiration (Figure 51-5).

Hoh and Fischer[45] reported the results of 40 cases using the MCL-29, 36 of which were completed with the laser and 4 of which required conversion to an alternate surgical technique because of prolonged surgical time in 3 cases and a ruptured posterior capsule in 1 case. The mean total energy applied in

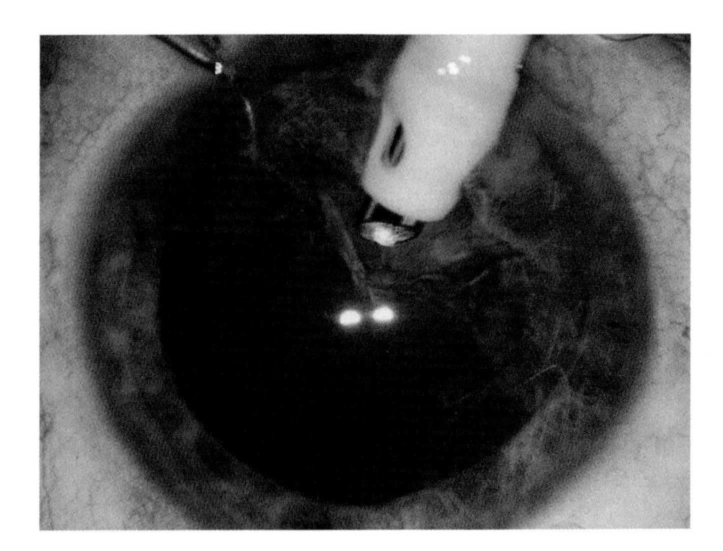

FIGURE 51-5 Evacuation of nuclear lens material with MCL-29 Er:YAG probe.

those 36 cases was 38.5 J, and the mean laser emulsification time was 3 minutes. Endothelial cell count decline was 0.96%, below that commonly seen with phacoemulsification.

Francini[47] reported the results of 35 patients with nuclear density ranging from 1 to 4+ who underwent Er:YAG laser cataract surgery with the MCL-29 system. Two additional patients with extremely dense lenses required conversion to phacoemulsification and were excluded from the study. The overall average amount of energy used per case was 62.74 J, and the average emulsification time was about 9 minutes (9'23"). At 6 months' follow-up, the endothelial cell loss averaged 5.15%, with the ultrasound phacoemulsification control group averaging 6.19%. On the first postoperative day, the laser patients had a 6.1% increase in corneal thickness, whereas the ultrasound patients had a 9.1% increase in corneal thickness.

The MCL-29 evolved into the Phacolase MCL-29 (Figure 51-6). The pulse energy of the Phacolase ranges from 5 to 50 mJ, and the frequency ranges from 10 to 100 Hz. It has a pulse duration of 200 microseconds. The surgeon may choose to work either in the energy mode, which delivers a fixed frequency that allows for the adjustment of the amount of energy delivered, or in the frequency mode, which will alternatively alter the frequency of the pulses while leaving the amount of energy per pulse fixed. The Phacolase is coupled to a Megatron irritation-aspiration pump, which is a peristaltic-based system with a Venturi-like effect.[48]

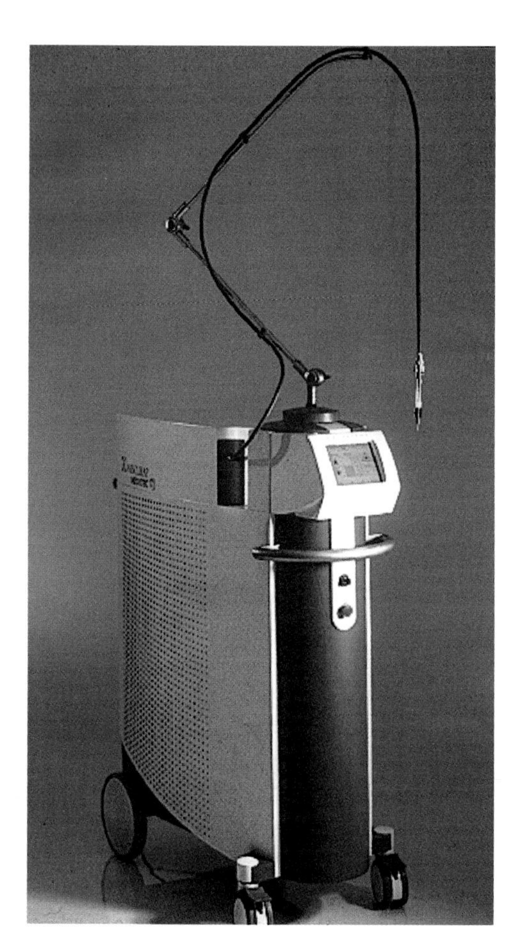

FIGURE 51-6 Phacolase Er:YAG system.

Francini[46] conducted a prospective study using the Phacolase MCL-29 in 58 cases. A bimanual technique was employed, with the laser-aspiration probe through one 1- to 1.5-mm clear corneal wound and an irrigation probe through another 1- to 1.5-mm clear corneal wound. Nuclear density ranged from 1 to 4+. The average energy used was 31.1865 J, and the average emulsification time was almost 5 minutes (4'48"). Two patients were noted to have an elevated intraocular pressure on postoperative day 1, but it returned to within normal limits by postoperative day 4. Endothelial cell loss at 12 months' follow-up was 2.12%. Corneal thickness on postoperative day 1 increased by 5.82%, slightly lower than the 6.19% reported with the unimanual technique[47] although not statistically significant.

Conclusion

Where are these new technologies leading us? Although it is unlikely to replace ultrasound phacoemulsification in the near future, laser cataract surgery offers several advantages over ultrasound. Most notably, the potential for increased safety promises the biggest reward for cataract patients. With the lack of any clinically significant heat reported in studies using both the Nd:YAG and the Er:YAG devices, the threat of corneal burns is eliminated. Furthermore, the comparable or potential decrease in endothelial cell loss is certainly reassuring.

Unlike ultrasound phacoemulsification handpieces, the laser probes do not contain motors and vibrating needles, both of which are subject to wear and tear with repeated use and sterilization. In addition to being lighter and easier to handle, the components of these laser probes are relatively inexpensive, thus allowing for disposable handpieces.

The biggest limitation of the current laser systems is the challenge of denser cataracts. Given the rapidly evolving refinements and advances made in the technology to date, however, it is likely that this problem will be overcome.

What does the future hold? Perhaps, by making ultra–small-incision cataract surgery a reality, laser cataract surgery has opened the door to true endocapsular surgery. Maybe the probes of the future will allow for anterior capsule *puncture,* and on completion of lens removal, perhaps the capsular bag will be reinflated with an injectable lens, allowing for the preservation of accommodation. One can only guess at the directions this rapidly advancing technology will take, but one thing is sure: lasers are expanding the frontier of cataract surgery.

REFERENCES

1. Kelman CD: Phaco-emulsification and aspiration: a new technique of cataract removal—a preliminary report, *Am J Ophthalmol* 64:23-35, 1967.
2. Leaming DV: Practice styles and preferences of ASCRS members: 1999 survey, *J Cataract Refract Surg* 26:913-921, 2000.
3. Krasnov MM: Laser phakopuncture in the treatment of soft cataracts, *Br J Ophthalmol* 56:96-98, 1975.
4. Maguen E, Martinez M, Grundfest W et al: Excimer laser ablation of the human lens at 308 nm with a fiber delivery system, *J Cataract Refract Surg* 15:409-414, 1989.
5. Nanevicz T, Prince MR, Gawande AA et al: Excimer laser ablation of the lens, *Arch Opthalmol* 104:1825-1829, 1986.
6. Puliafito CA, Steinert RF, Deutsch TF et al: Excimer laser ablation of the cornea and lens: experimental studies, *Ophthalmology* 92:741-748, 1985.

7. Marshall J, Sliney DH: Endoexcimer laser intraocular ablative photodecomposition, *Am J Ophthalmol* 101:130-131, 1986 (letter).
8. Zuclich JA: Ultraviolet-induced photochemical damage in ocular tissues, *Health Phys* 56:671-682, 1989.
9. Borkman RF: Cataracts and photochemical damage in the lens, *Ciba Found Symp* 106:88-109, 1984.
10. Kochevar IE: Cytotoxicity and mutagenicity of excimer laser radiation, *Lasers Surg Med* 9:440-445, 1989.
11. Colvard DM: Erbium:YAG laser removal of cataracts. Presented at the American Society of Cataract and Refractive Surgery Annual Meeting, Seattle, May 1993.
12. Margolis TI, Farnath DA, Destro M et al: Erbium-YAG laser surgery on experimental vitreous membranes, *Arch Ophthalmol* 107:424-428, 1989.
13. Peyman GA, Katoh N: Effects of an erbium:YAG laser in ocular ablation, *Int Ophthalmol* 10:245-253, 1987.
14. Tsubota K: Application of erbium:YAG laser in ocular ablation, Ophthalmologica 200:117-122, 1990.
15. Dodick JM: Laser phacolysis of the human cataractous lens, *Dev Ophthalmol* 22:58-64, 1991.
16. Dodick JM, Sperber LTD, Lally JM et al: Neodymium-YAG laser phacolysis of the human cataractous lens, *Arch Ophthalmol* 111:903-904, 1993.
17. Dodick JM, Christiansen J: Experimental studies on the development and propogation of shock waves created by the interaction of short Nd:YAG laser pulses with a titanium target: possible implication for Nd:YAG laser phacolysis of the cataractous human lens, *J Cataract Refract Surg* 17:794-797, 1991.
18. Aron-Rosa D, Aron J, Griesemann M et al: Use of the neodymium:YAG laser to open the posterior capsule after lens implant surgery: a preliminary report, *J Am Intraocul Implant Soc* 6:352-354, 1980.
19. Dodick JM: Nd:YAG laser treatment of the posterior capsule, *Trans New Orleans Acad Ophthalmol* 36:169-178, 1988.
20. Fankhauser F, Roussel P, Steffen J et al: Clinical studies on the efficiency of high power laser radiation upon some structures of the anterior segment of the eye: first experiences of the treatment of some pathological conditions of the anterior segment of the human eye by means of a Q-switched laser system. *Int Ophthalmol Clin* 3:129-139, 1981.
21. Fankhauser F: The Q-switched laser: principles and clinical results. In Trokel SL, editor: *YAG laser ophthalmic microsurgery,* Norwalk, Conn, 1983, Appleton-Century-Crofts, pp 101-146.
22. Klapper RM: Q-switched neodymium:YAG laser iridotomy, *Ophthalmology* 91:1017-1021, 1984.
23. Fankhauser F, Rol P: Microsurgery with the Nd:YAG laser: an overview, *Int Ophthalmol Clin* 25:55-58, 1985.
24. Aron-Rosa D: Use of a pulsed neodymium-YAG laser for anterior capsulotomy before extracapsular cataract extraction, *J Am Intraocul Implant Soc* 7:332-333, 1981.
25. Aron-Rosa DS, Aron JJ, Cohn HC: Use of a pulsed picosecond Nd:YAG laser in 6,654 cases, *J Am Intraocul Implant Soc* 10:35-39, 1984.
26. Chambless WS: Neodymium:YAG laser anterior capsulotomy and a possible new application, *J Am Intraocul Implant Soc* 11:33-34, 1985.
27. Chambless WS: Neodymium:YAG laser phacofracture: an aid to phacoemulsification, *J Cataract Refract Surg* 14:180-181, 1988.
28. L'Esperance FA Jr: *Ophthalmic lasers,* vol 2, ed 3, St Louis, 1989, Mosby, p 1032.
29. Levin ML, Wyatt KD: Prospective analysis of laser photophacofragmentation, *J Cataract Refract Surg* 16:96-98, 1990.
30. Ryan EH Jr, Logani S: Nd:YAG laser photodisruption of the lens nucleus before phacoemulsification, *Am J Ophthalmol* 104:382-386, 1987.
31. Zelman J: Photophaco fragmentation, *J Cataract Refract Surg* 13:287-289, 1987.
32. Alzner E, Grabner G: Dodick laser phacolysis: thermal effects, *J Cataract Refract Surg* 25:800-803, 1999.
33. Dodick JM: Can cataracts be removed using laser technology? *Ophthalmol Clin North Am* 4:355-364, 1991.
34. Dodick JM, Lally JM, Sperber LTD: Lasers in cataract surgery, *Curr Opin Ophthalmol* 4:107-109, 1993.
35. Dodick JM, Sperber LTD: The future of cataract surgery, *Int Ophthalmol Clin* 34:201-210, 1994.
36. Sperber LTD: Nd:YAG laser lens ablation in a rabbit model, *J Cataract Refract Surg* 22:485-489, 1996.
37. DeBry P, Olson RJ, Crandall AS: Comparison of energy required for phacochop and divide and conquer phacoemulsification, *J Cataract Refract Surg* 24:689-692, 1998.
38. Fine IH, Packer M, Hoffman RS: Use of power modulations in phacoemulsification: choo-choo chop and flip phacoemulsification, *J Cataract Refract Surg* 27:188-197, 2001.
39. Kanellopoulos AJ, Dodick JM, Brauweiler P et al: Dodick photolysis for cataract surgery: early experience with the Q-switched neodymium:YAG laser in 100 consecutive patients, *Ophthalmology* 106:2197-2202, 1999.
40. Kanellopoulos AJ: Laser cataract surgery: a prospective clinical evaluation of 1000 consecutive laser cataract procedures using the Dodick Photolysis neodymium:YAG system. *Ophthalmology* 108:649-654, 2001.
41. Huetz WW, Eckhardt HB: Photolysis using the Dodick-ARC laser system for cataract surgery, *J Cataract Refract Surg* 27:208-212, 2001.
42. Berger JW, Talamo JH, LaMarche KJ et al: Temperature measurements during phacoemulsification and erbium:YAG laser phacoablation in model systems, *J Cataract Refract Surg* 22:372-378, 1996.
43. Lin CP, Stern D, Puliafito CA: High-speed photography of Er:YAG laser ablation in fluid: implications for laser vitreous surgery, *Invest Ophthalmol Vis Sci* 32:2546-2550, 1990.
44. Neubaur CC, Steven G: Erbium:YAG laser cataract removal: role of fiberoptic delivery system, *J Cataract Refract Surg* 25:514-520, 1999.
45. Hoh H, Fischer E: Pilot study on erbium laser phacoemulsification, *Ophthalmology* 107:1053-1062, 2000.
46. Francini A: The bimanual erbium laser phacoemulsification. Personal communication.
47. Francini A, Galarati BZ: The Er:YAG laser emulsification: clinical results. Personal communication.
48. Packer M, Fine IH, Hoffman RS: Cataract surgery with the Er:YAG laser. Personal communication.

New Phacoemulsification Technologies*

52

I. Howard Fine, MD
Mark Packer, MD
Richard S. Hoffman, MD

New technology brings challenges and opportunities to the anterior segment surgeon. The drive toward less traumatic surgery and more rapid visual rehabilitation after cataract surgery has spawned various modalities for reducing incision size and decreasing energy use.

Although ultrasonic phacoemulsification allows relatively safe removal of cataractous lenses through astigmatically neutral small incisions, current technology still has its drawbacks. In ultrasonic phacoemulsification, piezoelectric crystals convert electrical energy into mechanical energy, which emulsifies the lens material by means of tip vibration. Ultrasonic tips create both heat and cavitational energy. A conventional phaco tip moves at ultrasonic frequencies of between 25 and 62 kHz. The amount of heat generated is directly proportional to the operating frequency. In addition, cavitational effects from the high-frequency ultrasonic waves generate even more heat.

Because of the liberation of heat, phacoemulsification needles have required an irrigation sleeve for cooling. This irrigation sleeve carries heat away from the tip and necessitates an incision size larger than the tip alone would require. Nevertheless, standard ultrasonic phacoemulsification with an irrigation sleeve still carries with it the potential for thermal injury to the cornea in case of diminished flow. Flow and aspiration problems may be caused by compression of the irrigation sleeve at the incision site, kinking of the sleeve during manipulation of the handpiece, tip clogging by nuclear or viscoelastic material, and inadequate flow rate or vacuum settings.[1] Heating of the tip can create corneal incision burns.[2] When incisional burns develop in clear corneal incisions, there may be a loss of self-sealability, corneal edema, and severe induced astigmatism.[3]

Cavitational energy results from pressure waves emanating from the tip in all directions. Although increased cavitational energy can allow for phacoemulsification of dense nuclei, it can also damage the corneal endothelium and produce irreversible corneal edema in compromised corneas with preexisting endothelial dystrophies. Reduction in average phaco power and effective phaco time has been correlated with improved patient outcomes after cataract surgery.[4] Low-power phaco technology will have an important advantage in minimizing intraoperative damage to ocular structures and maximizing the level and rapidity of visual rehabilitation of the patient.

The last decade has given rise to some of the most profound advances in both phacoemulsification technique and technology. Techniques for cataract removal have moved from those that use mainly ultrasound energy to emulsify nuclear material for aspiration to those that use greater levels of vacuum and small quantities of energy for lens disassembly and removal. Advances in phacoemulsification technology and fluidics have made this ongoing change in technique possible by allowing greater amounts of vacuum to be used safely and by providing power modulations that use ultrasound energy more efficiently with greater safety for the delicate intraocular environment.[5]

Elimination of the frictional heat produced during ultrasound phacoemulsification and reduction of the power required for cataract extraction represent important steps toward the goal of atraumatic surgery. Laser technology, including the erbium: yttrium-aluminum-garnet (Er:YAG) (Phacolase, Zeiss-Meditec) and neodymium (Nd):YAG (Photon PhacoLysis, Paradigm, and Dodick Photolysis, ARC), offers one approach to the elimination of thermal energy and reduction of power during phacoemulsification. The sonic phacoemulsification system (STAAR Wave, STAAR Surgical) demonstrates another new approach to elimination of heat and the danger of thermal injury to the cornea. Modification of ultrasound energy through refinement of power modulation offers yet another route leading to elimination of heat and reduction of incision size (White Star, Allergan). The introduction of innovative oscillatory tip motion in coordination with power modulation permits further reduction of average phaco power and effective phaco time (NeoSoniX, Alcon). Other new modalities under investigation, which promise low-energy, nonthermal cataract extraction, include vortex phacoemulsification (Avantix, Bausch & Lomb) and Aqualase (Alcon), a fluid-based cataract extraction system.

Erbium:YAG Laser Phacoemulsification

Laser phacoemulsification represents an emerging technology in cataract surgery. As a method for cataract extraction, it has

*Modified and reprinted from Fine IH, Packer M, Hoffman RS: New phacoemulsification technologies, *J Cataract Refract Surg* 28:1054-1060, 2002.

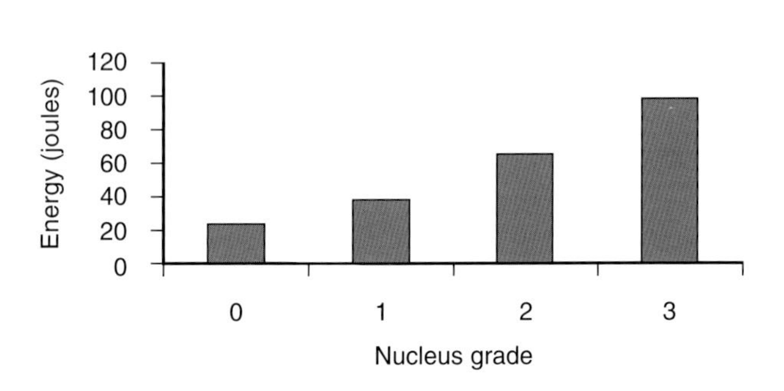

FIGURE 52-1 Mean Er:YAG laser energy in joules by nucleus grade.

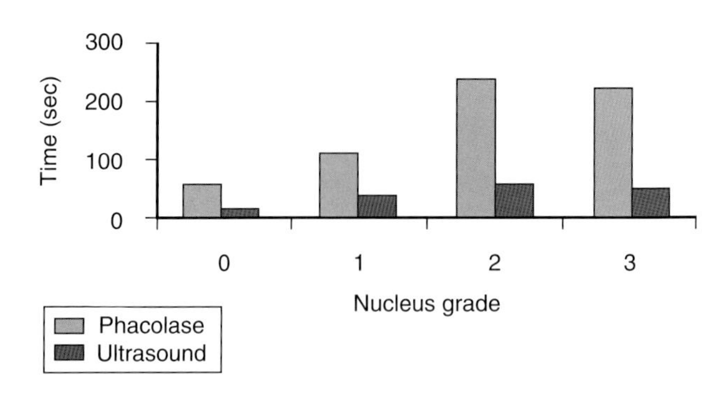

FIGURE 52-2 Time required for Er:YAG phacoemulsification as compared with ultrasound phacoemulsification by nucleus grade.

several potential advantages over ultrasound, including relative reduction in the energy requirement for cataract extraction and the absence of any potential for thermal injury to the cornea. However, investigation has demonstrated that the efficacy of laser is limited to extraction of grades 0 to 3 nuclear sclerosis and that phacoemulsification time with the laser, although certainly dependent on the surgeon's level of experience, tends to be longer than with ultrasound.

The Er:YAG laser produces a wavelength of 2.94 μm, which lies in the infrared spectrum and is highly absorbed by water. In water, cavitation bubbles form and collapse instantaneously. However, in the nuclear material of the lens, the collapse of the bubbles occurs more slowly. The laser beam can travel across the first bubble and form a second bubble in line with the first. If a third bubble forms, it increases the effective range of the laser to 3 mm. Direct concussive effects of the laser energy propagation wave disrupt the lens material, creating an emulsate that is aspirated from the eye.

As mentioned previously, one of the principal advantages of laser cataract extraction in general and of the Er:YAG system in particular is the absence of thermal energy. Because the tip of the erbium laser system does not produce relevant heating effects, the risk of corneal burn is eliminated, and the potential for reduced incision size is created.[6]

The Phacolase Er:YAG laser features a variable pulse energy from 5 to 50 mJ, as well as a variable frequency from 10 to 100 Hz. In its present form the Phacolase system is coupled to a Megatron irrigation-aspiration pump (Geuder, Heidelberg). The Megatron has a peristaltic pump with Venturi-like effect. The Phacolase handpiece incorporates the laser fiber inside the aspiration port. A bidirectional foot switch is employed, which separates infusion and aspiration from laser energy. Moving the foot pedal laterally increases the repetition rate in a linear fashion. Pushing the pedal down provides linear control of vacuum.

One method of nuclear disassembly with the Phacolase involves prechopping the nucleus with the device developed by Takayuki Akahoshi. This prechopper can be used to segment the nucleus before phacoemulsification with the Phacolase. For denser grades of nuclei, prechopping provides an advantage in reduced total operating time. Further evolution of technique will likely emphasize separation of irrigation from aspiration and laser in the development of a bimanual technique. Because of the absence of risk from thermal injury, the incision size may effectively be reduced to 1 mm. However, at present, all systems are limited by the incision sizes necessary for intraocular lens (IOL) implantation.

Food and Drug Administration (FDA) phase III clinical trials are currently ongoing in the United States. Preliminary data from the multicenter, randomized comparison of Er:YAG and ultrasound phacoemulsification were reported by Packer[7] at the European Society of Cataract and Refractive Surgery Congress in Amsterdam.

At the time of this writing, a total of 101 eyes of 72 patients have been enrolled in the study at seven treatment centers, with 78 eyes randomized to laser phacoemulsification. Intraoperative performance parameters have revealed mean energy requirements ranging from 24.7 J for extraction of grade 0 nuclei to 99.1 J for extraction of grade 3 nuclei (Figure 52-1). The mean laser phacoemulsification time varied from 56.1 seconds for grade 0 to 222.5 seconds for grade 3 nuclei (Figure 52-2).

In summary, Er:YAG laser phacoemulsification represents an emerging technology with several promising attributes. These include reduction of energy required for phacoemulsification, absence of risk from thermal injury, and potential reduction of incision size.

Neodymium:YAG Laser Phacoemulsification

Dodick Photolysis

Dodick[8] introduced the pulsed Q-switched Nd:YAG laser in 1991. The United States FDA has approved the laser for cataract extraction. This Nd:YAG laser (1064 nm) system employs plasma formation and shock wave generation to produce photolysis of lens material. The shock wave results from the impact of laser radiation on a titanium plate. Alzner[9] has demonstrated that there is no heat production at the laser tip. As with the other nonthermal modalities discussed here, the Nd:YAG laser does not require a cooling sleeve and therefore permits cataract extraction through a 1.25-mm incision (Figure 52-3).

In the Dodick system, laser light does not emerge from the tip. Rather, the shock waves are produced by a titanium block within the tip. Therefore the eye is not directly exposed to laser energy.

Nd:YAG photolysis represents a low-energy modality for cataract extraction. Kanellopoulos[10] reported a mean intraocular energy use of 5.65 J per case. This level of energy compares favorably with values previously reported for ultrasound

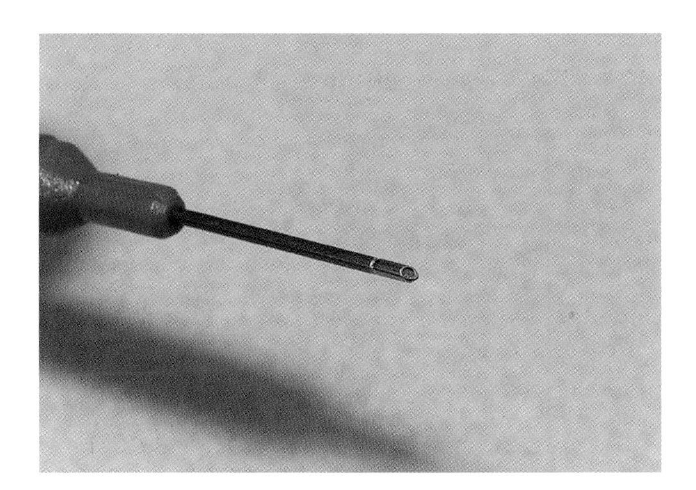

FIGURE 52-3 Dodick Photolysis laser tip.

phacoemulsification and approximates the level of energy reported for the choo-choo chop and flip phacoemulsification technique using power modulations.[11]

Surgeons generally use a groove and crack technique with the laser, sculpting in a bimanual fashion and cracking as soon as possible. Alternatively, a prechopping technique may be employed, as taught by Kammann and Dodick. Residual fragments are then removed by laser emulsification. The total time that the tip is in the eye varies with the grade of nucleus, from 2.15 minutes for 1+ nuclear sclerosis to 9.8 minutes for 3+ nuclear sclerosis.

The absence of thermal energy and the consequent ability to extract a cataract through an incision of less than 2 mm await the development of IOLs capable of insertion via smaller incisions to achieve a real advantage.

Photon Laser PhacoLysis

The Paradigm Medical Photon Laser PhacoLysis system employs an Nd:YAG 1064-nm laser to produce photoacoustic ablation of cataract material under aspiration. The ski-shaped distal tip of the probe curves up to provide the laser light emitted from the optical fiber (Figure 52-4). The aspiration inlet is placed in the face of the tip, creating a photon trap. Thus all rays of laser photons that enter the aspiration port are internally reflected and kept within the probe tip. Although some minimal heating of tissue occurs, the heat is rapidly removed by aspiration, and the temperature of the probe tip only rises about 1° C.

The peak intensity of the Photon Laser PhacoLysis system is more than 10 thousand times below that required for the onset of plasma generation, the operative action during posterior capsulotomy. Therefore PhacoLysis represents an exceptionally safe modality in terms of capsular integrity. In the wet lab, using pig eyes, one can actually place the anterior lens capsule directly in the line of the laser beam and fire repeatedly without causing any discernible damage to the capsule.

A pilot study with the Paradigm PhacoLysis system has shown promising results, and a clinical study protocol is now underway in the United States. The laser is coupled to the Mentor SIStem peristaltic irrigation-aspiration pump. The study is

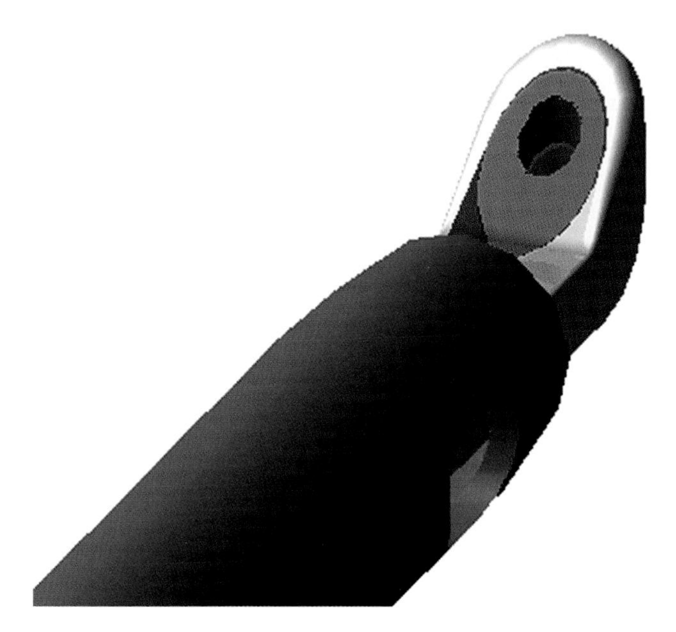

FIGURE 52-4 Paradigm Photon PhacoLysis ski-shaped distal tip.

restricted to the softer grades of nuclear sclerosis for which this technology is most advantageous.

Sonic Phacoemulsification

Sonic technology offers an innovative way of removing cataractous material without the generation of heat or cavitational energy by means of sonic rather than ultrasonic technology. Its operating frequency is in the sonic range, between 40 and 400 Hz. In contrast to ultrasonic tip motion, the sonic tip moves back and forth without changing its dimensional length. The tip of an ultrasonic handpiece can exceed 500° C, whereas the tip of the STAAR Wave handpiece in sonic mode barely generates any frictional heat. In addition, the Sonic tip does not generate cavitational effects, and thus fragmentation, rather than emulsification or vaporization, of material takes place.

The same handpiece and tip can be used for both sonic and ultrasonic modes. The surgeon can alternate between the two modes using a toggle switch on the foot pedal when more or less energy is required. The modes can also be used simultaneously with varying percentages of both sonic and ultrasonic energy. We have found that we can use our same chopping cataract extraction technique in sonic mode as we used in ultrasonic mode with no discernable difference in efficiency.

The STAAR Wave also allows improved stability of the anterior chamber with coiled SuperVac tubing, which increases vacuum capability to up to 650 mm Hg (Figure 52-5). The key to chamber maintenance is a positive fluid balance between infusion flow and aspiration flow. When occlusion is broken, vacuum previously built in the aspiration line generates a high aspiration flow that can be higher than the infusion flow. This results in anterior chamber instability. The coiled SuperVac tubing limits surge flow resulting from occlusion breakage in a dynamic way. The continuous change in direction of flow through the coiled tubing

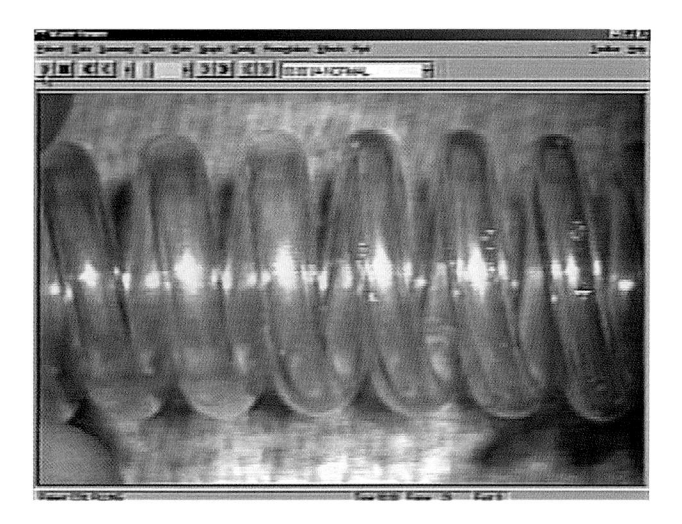

FIGURE 52-5 Coiled "SuperVac" tubing available with the STAAR Wave system.

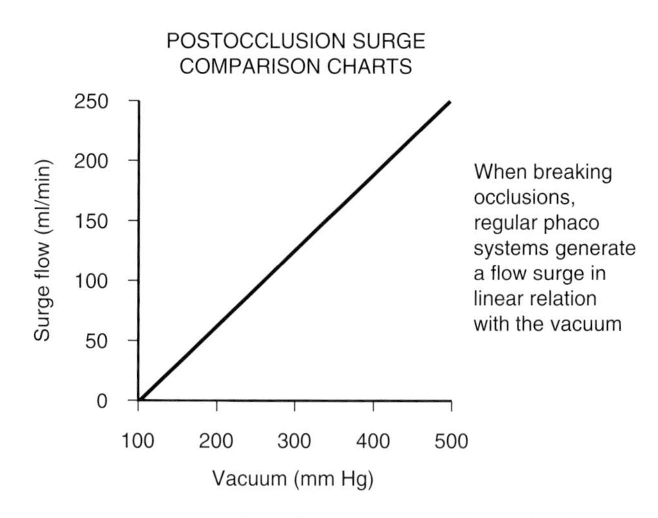

FIGURE 52-6 Surge flow versus vacuum for regular tubing.

increases resistance through the tubing at high flow rates, such as on clearance of occlusion of the tip (Figures 52-6 and 52-7). This effect only takes place at high flow rates (greater than 50 ml/min). The fluid resistance of the SuperVac tubing increases as a function of flow, and unoccluded flow is not restricted (Alex Urich, personal communication, STAAR Surgical).[12]

The STAAR Wave combines important innovations in phacoemulsification technology, which satisfy the demands of nonthermal, low-power cataract extraction.

NeoSoniX Phacoemulsification

NeoSoniX technology (Alcon) represents a hybrid modality involving low-frequency oscillatory movement that may be used alone or in combination with standard high-frequency ultrasonic phacoemulsification (Figure 52-8). Softer grades of nuclear sclerosis may be completely addressed with the low-frequency modality, whereas denser grades will likely require the addition of ultrasound.

In the NeoSoniX mode, the phaco tip has a variable rotational oscillation up to 2 degrees, at 120 Hz. As with sonic phacoemulsification, this lower frequency does not produce significant thermal energy and so minimizes the risk of thermal injury.

The Legacy may be programmed to initiate NeoSoniX at any desired level of ultrasound energy. Thus the surgeon may use the low-frequency mode to burrow into the nucleus for stabilization before chopping by setting the lower limit of NeoSoniX to 0% phaco power. This approach works best with a straight tip, which acts like an apple corer to impale the nucleus. Alternatively, NeoSoniX may be initiated as an adjunct to ultrasound at the 10% or 20% power level.

We have found NeoSoniX most effective at 50% amplitude with a horizontal chopping technique in the AdvanTec burst mode at 50% power, 45 ml/min linear flow, and 450 mm Hg vacuum. A 0.9-mm microflare straight ABS tip rapidly impales and holds nuclear material for chopping. During evacuation of nuclear segments the material flows easily into the tip, with very little tendency for chatter and scatter of nuclear fragments. With refinement of our parameters, we have found a 57% reduction

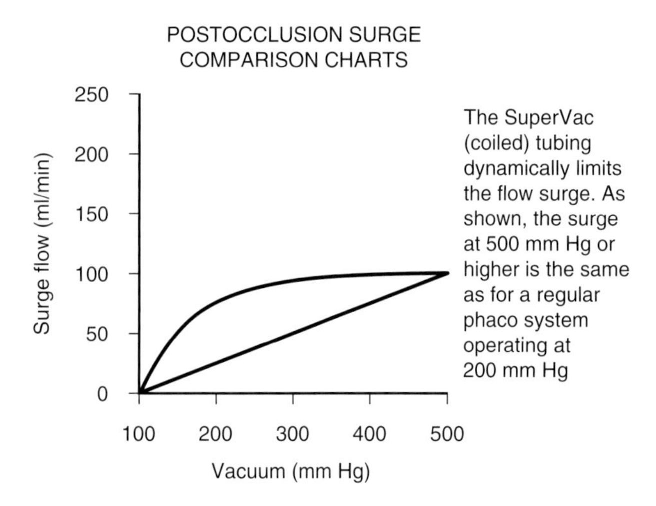

FIGURE 52-7 Surge flow versus vacuum for coiled tubing.

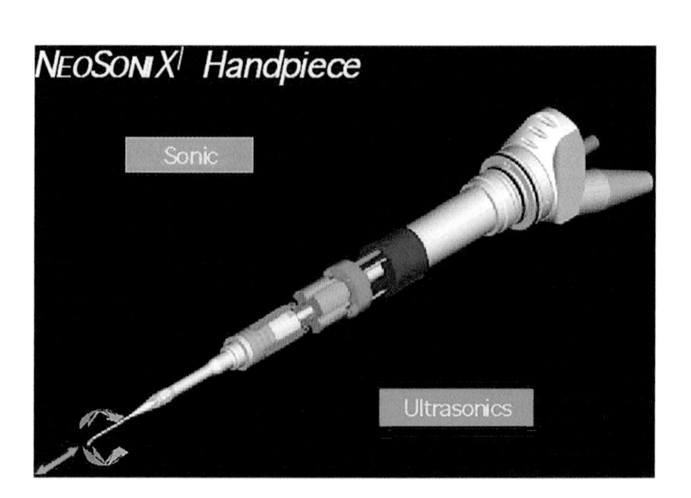

FIGURE 52-8 Schematic diagram of NeoSoniX handpiece.

in average phaco power, and an 87% reduction in effective phaco time, compared with the data we previously published with the Legacy system.[13]

NeoSoniX has permitted further reduction in the application of ultrasonic energy to the eye when used in conjunction with ultrasound and has allowed nonthermal cataract extraction when used alone. It represents an important new modality in phacoemulsification technology.

White Star Technology

White Star (Sovereign, Allergan) represents a new power modulation within ultrasonic phacoemulsification that virtually eliminates the production of thermal energy. Analogous to the ultrapulse mode familiar to users of carbon dioxide lasers, White Star extrapolates pulse mode phacoemulsification to its logical limit. As the duration of the energy pulse is reduced, it eventually becomes less than the thermal relaxation time of ocular tissue. Thus it is theoretically impossible to produce a corneal wound burn.

White Star technology sets the stage for bimanual cataract extraction with the Sovereign phacoemulsification machine. The absence of thermal energy obviates the need for an irrigation sleeve on the phaco tip, thus permitting reduction of incision size and allowing irrigation through a second instrument, such as an irrigating chopper, placed through the side port. With an incision size for cataract extraction less than 1 mm, the challenge becomes production of IOLs capable of insertion through such microphaco incisions.

Olson and Soscia[14] and Packard[15] have reported exciting results using a 21-gauge irrigating chopper and a 21-gauge bare phaco needle with the bimanual technique. Olson's study of cadaver eyes has demonstrated that thermal injury does not occur even in the absence of aspiration with 100% power for 3 minutes. Packard reported an absence of wound burns with excellent surgical ease and efficiency via incisions less than 2 mm in size.

The White Star technology demonstrates important advantages in improved safety and efficiency of cataract extraction, whether used in standard fashion or with the microphaco technique.

Avantix

Vortex phacoemulsification involves placement of a tiny rotary impeller inside the capsular bag through a 1-mm capsulorhexis. The impeller rotates at 60 kHz and causes expansion of the capsular bag with rotation of the nuclear complex, thus allowing extraction of the cataract from a nearly intact lens capsule. Expansion of the capsular bag minimizes risk of capsular rupture.

The tiny circular capsulorhexis is constructed with a round diathermy instrument, thus reducing the technical demands of such a surgical feat. The irrigation-aspiration tube containing the rotary impeller is placed over the capsulorhexis while hydrodissection is performed with gentle irrigation. The tube is then inserted into the capsular bag through the 1-mm capsulorhexis before initiation of rotation, thus completely isolating the anterior chamber from the activity of cataract extraction. Nuclear material is effectively removed from the capsular bag with vortex action, after which cortex is actually stripped away and extracted.

The advantages of leaving nearly the entire capsular bag in situ following cataract extraction will not be realized until an injectable artificial crystalline lens becomes available and the problem of capsular opacification is eliminated. Okahiro Nishi[16] and others are currently investigating these devices and may soon have a prototype available. See Chapter 51 for a complete discussion of endocapsular vortex emulsification.

Aqualase

Research at Alcon has led to the development of a fluid-based cataract extraction system. Another nonthermal modality, Aqualase, employs pulses of balanced salt solution at 50 to 100 Hz to dissolve the cataract. This method may potentially demonstrate advantages in terms of safety and prevention of secondary posterior capsular opacification. Still early in its development, Aqualase represents an innovative and potentially advantageous means for cataract extraction.

Conclusion

Since the time of Charles Kelman's inspiration in the dentist's chair (while having his teeth ultrasonically cleaned), incremental advances in phacoemulsification technology have produced ever-increasing benefits for patients with cataracts. The modern procedure simply was not possible even a few years ago, and until recently, prolonged hospital stays were common after cataract surgery.

The competitive business environment and the wellspring of human ingenuity continue to demonstrate synergistic activity in the improvement of surgical technique and technology. Future advances in cataract surgery will continue to benefit our patients as we develop new phacoemulsification technology.

REFERENCES

1. Sugar A, Schertzer RIO: Clinical course of phacoemulsification wound burns, *J Cataract Refract Surg* 25: 688-692, 1999.
2. Majid MA, Sharma MK, Harding SP: Corneoscleral burn during phacoemulsification surgery, *J Cataract Refract Surg* 24:1413-1415, 1998.
3. Sugar A, Schertzer RM: Clinical course of phacoemulsification wound burns, *J Cataract Refract Surg* 25: 688-692, 1999.
4. Fine IH, Packer M, Hoffman RS: Use of power modulations in phacoemulsification, *J Cataract Refract Surg* 27:188-197, 2001.
5. Fine IH: The choo choo chop and flip phacoemulsification technique, *Operative Techniques Cataract Refractive Surg* 1:61-65, 1998.
6. Berger JW, Talamo JH, La Marche KJ et al: Temperature measurements during phacoemulsification and Er:YAG laser phacoablation in model systems, *J Cataract Refract Surg* 22:372-378, 1996.
7. Packer M: *Safety and efficacy of the Er yttrium aluminum garnet (Er:YAG) laser for cataract extraction,* XIX Congress of the ESCRS, Amsterdam, September 1, 2001.
8. Dodick JM: Laser phacolysis of the human cataractous lens, *Dev Ophthalmol* 22:58-64, 1991.
9. Alzner E, Grabner G: Dodick laser phacolysis: thermal effects, *J Cataract Refract Surg* 25:800-803, 1999.
10. Kanellopoulos AJ: Laser cataract surgery, *Ophthalmology* 108:649-655, 2001.

11. Fine IH, Packer M, Hoffman RS: Use of power modulations in phacoemulsification, *J Cataract Refract Surg* 27:188-197, 2001.
12. Fine IH, Hoffman RS, Packer M: The Staar wave. In Kohnen T, editor: Modern cataract surgery update, *Dev Ophthalmol,* Basel, Karger, 2002, vol 34, pp 32-40.
13. Fine IH, Packer M, Hoffman RS: Use of power modulations in phacoemulsification, *J Cataract Refract Surg* 27:188-197, 2001.
14. Olson RJ, Soscia WL: *Safety and efficacy of bimanual phaco chop through two stab incisions with the Sovereign,* XIII Congress of the European Society of Ophthalmology, Istanbul, June 3-7, 2001.
15. Packard R: *Evaluation of a new approach to phacoemulsification: bimanual phaco with the Sovereign system rapid pulse software,* XIII Congress of the European Society of Ophthalmology, Istanbul, June 3-7, 2001.
16. Nishi O, Nishi K: Accommodation amplitude after lens refilling with injectable silicone by sealing the capsule with a plug in primates, *Arch Ophthalmol* 116: 1358-1361, 1998.

Endocapsular Vortex Emulsification for Cataract Removal

53

Richard L. Lindstrom, MD

Endocapsular vortex emulsification (EVE) is a new technology in which the cataract is emulsified by a high-speed rotary impeller. Research on eyes from animals and human eye bank suggests it may be a viable alternative to phacoemulsification. Optex Ophthalmologics and Richard P. Kratz, MD, first presented the concept at the 1998 meeting of the American Society of Cataract and Refractive Surgery under the name *Catarex*. The future trade name has yet to be determined, so subsequent references here to the procedure use the acronym *EVE*.

As an enabling technology, EVE may provide additional stimulus for future development of injectable accommodating lenses. Until then, EVE potentially offers an important alternative to ultrasound phacoemulsification. EVE appears to be less challenging to learn and less difficult to perform; animal studies suggest it may provide several safety advantages and clinical benefits compared with ultrasound phacoemulsification.

Distinct Differences

EVE and ultrasound phacoemulsification share certain similarities. Both technologies deliver energy to the eye via a probe that emulsifies the lens and cortex for removal by aspiration. Both systems are software driven and include touch screen panels that enable preset parameters and active feedback throughout the procedure.

Some distinct differences, however, clearly set EVE apart from current cataract removal technology. EVE is a true endocapsular procedure.

Following a standard clear corneal incision, the nucleus and cortex are removed through a 1-mm capsulotomy in a single-handed, one-step process that takes place entirely within the capsular bag, which remains functionally intact. There is no sculpting, cracking, or chopping and very little movement of the probe within the bag.

Ultrasound phacoemulsification typically depends on carefully choreographed movements and procedures, as well as the complex balance and interplay among flow, vacuum, and power to attract, hold, and then emulsify the cataract.

In contrast, EVE creates two separate and distinct flows and does not rely on tip occlusion and vacuum holding force. The first flow type, called endocapsular vortex flow, recirculates within the bag and draws the cataract to the probe tip, where it is reduced by the mechanical action of a high-speed impeller. This vortex flow also keeps the bag fully inflated and hydrodissects the cortex from the capsule.

The second type is a typical irrigation-aspiration flow, but unlike in phaco, in EVE the irrigation and aspiration do not function to attract lens material to the tip. The sole purpose of EVE irrigation-aspiration flow is to gently remove the emulsified cataract from the eye. Although the speed of endocapsular vortex flow is greater than conventional irrigation-aspiration flow in phacoemulsification, the irrigation-aspiration flow rate for EVE is significantly less—approximately 5 ml/min. This reduced irrigation-aspiration flow requires less vacuum and lower bottle heights, drastically reducing the potential for post-occlusion surge. In animal studies, no significant movement of the anterior or posterior capsule has been observed.

Compared with ultrasound phacoemulsification, the capsular bag not only appears more stable but also confines most of the energy needed to remove the cataract, effectively isolating it from the anterior chamber. This may protect the corneal endothelium and trabecular meshwork from high flow, cataract debris, and radiated energy typical of ultrasound phacoemulsification. Animal studies and Miyake view observations also suggest that the EVE procedure may exert less stress on the capsule and zonules because the bag remains totally inflated and vacuum is not used to "pull" on nucleus or cortex. Also, in a controlled simulation the EVE procedure was shown to pose no significant thermal risk, even with irrigation and aspiration turned off.

Complex Design, Simple Use

The core mechanical component of the EVE technology is the single-use handpiece that contains a 1.37-mm-diameter impeller-tipped probe. Fluid, vacuum, and pneumatic lines attach to modular units on the main console (Bausch & Lomb Millennium) and supply irrigation, aspiration, and pneumatic power to the turbine-driven handpiece.

The stainless steel impeller is contained within a translucent protective sleeve and is deployed or retracted using the foot pedal. The pneumatic turbine spins the impeller at speeds between 20,000 and 100,000 rpm (Figure 53-1). It is similar to the turbine systems that power dental drills except that those typically run above 400,000 rpm and do not function smoothly

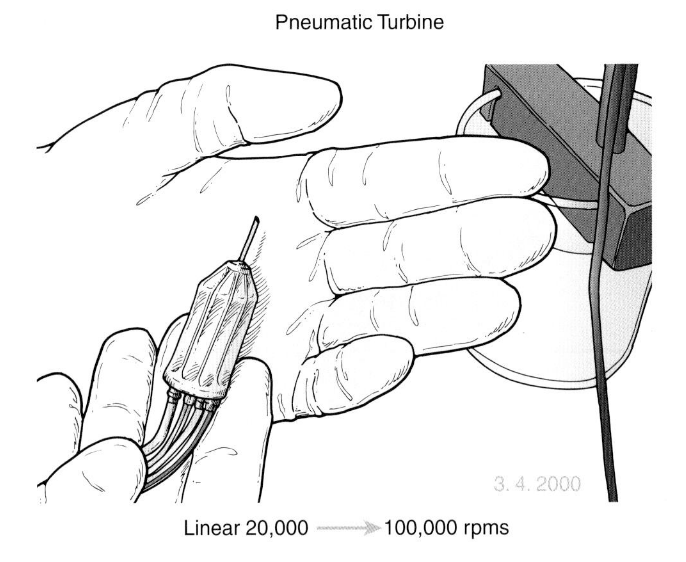

FIGURE 53-1 Pneumatic turbine spins the impeller at speeds between 20,000 and 100,000 rpm.

at slower speeds. EVE engineers have developed a proprietary means of controlling pneumatic input pressure that ensures true smooth operation throughout the entire speed range.

The high-speed impeller has three struts that radiate from the shaft like the spokes of a wheel. Each strut has a horizontal and vertical component. The horizontal struts are pitched like a propeller and create the endocapsular vortex flow (Figure 53-2).

This vortex flow brings the nucleus to the impeller, where the vertical struts emulsify it. The impeller is partially shielded by a beveled protective sleeve that also includes the irrigation ports.

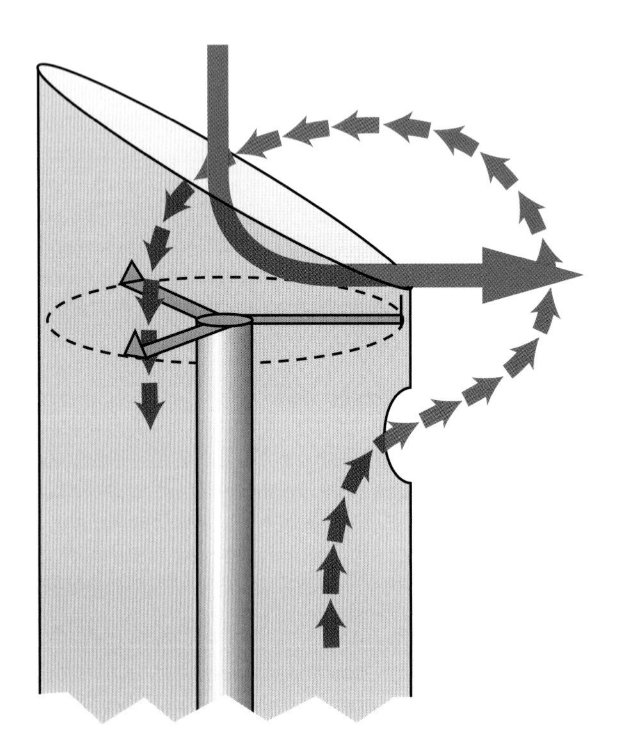

FIGURE 53-2 High-speed impeller has struts that rotate from the shaft like the spokes of a wheel and when rotating create the endocapsular vortex flow.

Procedure

One key to performing true endocapsular surgery is the ability to produce a round capsulotomy of 1 mm or less. This is now easily and reproducibly accomplished with a proprietary electrosurgical device that uses a differential current density to produce a 1-mm capsulotomy (Figure 53-3). A disposable 21-gauge circular tip is affixed to a reusable shielded probe and is then placed on the lens capsule through a clear corneal incision. (Bausch & Lomb is currently developing the disposable version of the probe featuring the proprietary technology patented by Optex. A bipolar version may be available in the future.)

The capsulotomy is usually placed tangentially to allow a carousel-type movement of the nucleus (Figure 53-4). A dispersive pad placed in contact with the patient's skin completes the necessary circuit.

Power is engaged by means of the foot pedal for approximately 1 or 2 seconds, and the resulting edges are consistently round and smooth.

In multiple wet labs, there have been no occurrences of the radial tears that sometimes can occur with a larger capsulorhexis produced by hand.

Hydrodissection is performed using a specially sized curved cannula that fits over the capsulorhexis and generally requires only a single, gentle infusion to produce a complete fluid wave.

The surgical probe is then inserted through the clear corneal incision (a scleral or limbal incision is also suitable) and approximately 1 mm into the capsular bag, slightly stretching the capsulotomy. The surgeon must visually confirm that the irrigation ports of the probe are within the capsular bag. The beveled tip of the probe is angled slightly toward the anterior lens capsule, but no more than 45 degrees relative to the iris plane. The impeller is advanced using the foot pedal.

Once the impeller is activated, a vortex flow builds within the bag, which provides a slight but very stable centrifugal pressurization of the capsular bag, hydrodissects the cortex from the capsule, and draws the nucleus and cortical material to the probe tip. The direction of the vortex fluid movement within the capsular bag is determined, in part, by the bevel of the protective sleeve and the peripheral placement of the handpiece

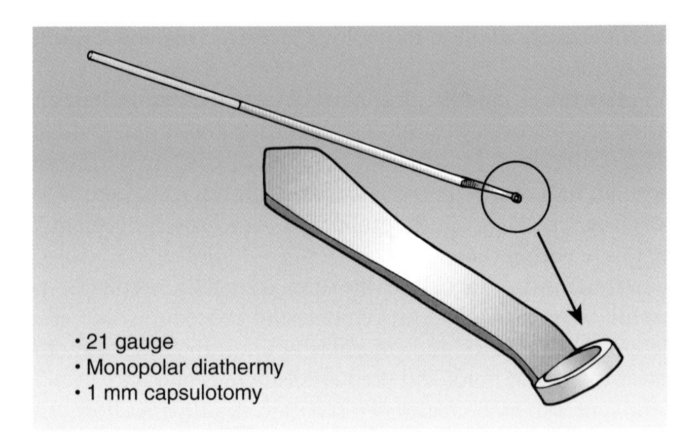

FIGURE 53-3 Round 1-mm anterior capsulotomy is performed with a reusable shielded electrosurgical diathermy probe.

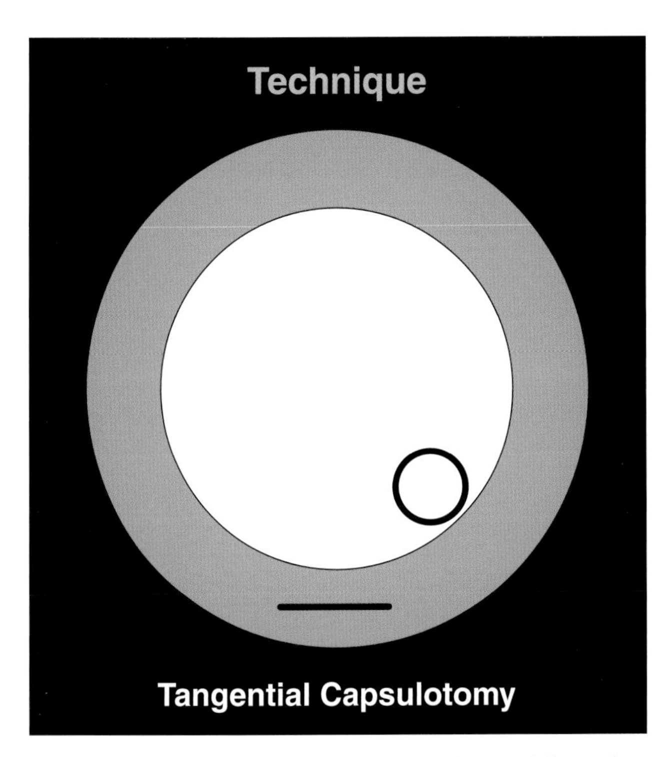

FIGURE 53-4 Capsulotomy is usually placed tangentially to allow a carousel-type movement of the nucleus.

tip relative to the center of the capsular bag. Vortex fluid discharges from the bevel toward the capsular walls, where it recirculates back to the probe.

This explains why there is very little movement of the EVE handpiece in the eye. The sculpting-type movements commonly used with phacoemulsification would be counterproductive and interfere with the creation of the recirculating vortex flow essential to the EVE process. Only slight rotations of the bevel and changes in the impeller speed are usually needed to control "followability."

Unlike ultrasound phacoemulsification, the nucleus and lens cortex are usually removed in a single step in the EVE procedure. The vortex action may also reduce the incidence of retained nuclear fragments for two reasons.

First, all lens particles remain within the capsular bag and cannot become lodged behind the iris, where they would be hidden from the surgeon's view. The endocapsular procedure should also reduce the risk of debris in the trabecular meshwork.

Second, in working with human eyes from eye banks, 3+ nuclear cataracts were easily emulsified, and in contrast to traditional ultrasound phacoemulsification, no nucleus chips were created. Instead, the emulsified lens material was extremely fine, taking on a "dust cloud" appearance.

Once the lens and cortex have been removed, the surgeon can perfectly visualize the capsular bag, and a bright red reflex facilitates the secondary capsulorhexis before insertion of the intraocular lens. It may well be that the "empty bag" secondary capsulorhexis is less prone to uncontrolled tears or extensions because all tension has been removed from the anterior capsule.

Possible Benefits

There is virtually no learning curve when it comes to using the capsulotomy device. Once the surgeon depresses the foot pedal, the software initiates a preprogrammed pause, then activates the device up to a maximum preset time limit. The surgeon then simply removes the deactivated probe from the eye, taking care not to depress the foot pedal again.

Compared with ultrasound phacoemulsification, the EVE procedure is easier to learn. Experienced phacoemulsification surgeons, however, may at first find the rotation and relative lack of movement of the handpiece tip a bit counterintuitive.

Certain surgeons may be tempted to "do phaco in the bag," moving the tip toward a piece of nuclear material or cortex that they want to attract. With EVE, however, "followability" is produced by the vortex flow, not the irrigation-aspiration flow; so rotating the bevel away from the nucleus and varying the revolutions per minute will often attract the nucleus more efficiently.

When the impeller is first activated, it takes a few seconds for the vortex flow to develop, and this may be perceived as a "lag time" when nothing happens. In fact, the vortex is separating the cataract from the capsule and overcoming inertia. With the probe held stationary, the lens will soon begin to spiral within the bag and be conveyed to the tip for emulsification. Surgeons learn quickly to let the vortex develop and bring the nucleus toward the handpiece tip. Although it may seem to take a while for the emulsification of the lens to begin, the entire process is generally completed in 1 to 3 minutes and has proven effective in lab tests on human eye bank cataracts from 1+ to 3+ nuclear sclerosis. So far, 4+ nuclear sclerotic cataracts have not been tested.

Compared with ultrasound phacoemulsification, the entire EVE procedure appears more controlled and less variable from case to case. Ultrasound phacoemulsification uses the opposing forces of flow and ultrasonic power that must be carefully balanced with the vacuum through complex technology and surgeon control. Failing to do so can result in postocclusion surge, chamber collapse, and torn capsules. Although EVE must also maintain fluidic balance, the vortex flow works in harmony with the impeller's power to emulsify the lens and serves to inflate the capsular bag rather than impose a risk of collapse.

Extremely low irrigation-aspiration flow and vacuum further reduce the risk of capsule movement. There is little handpiece movement, fewer steps, reduced bottle heights, and the efficient transfer of energy into the creation of a single vortex flow—all contained within the lens capsular bag. The final result may eventually be a viable alternative means of removing cataracts that potentially may be as safe or safer than traditional ultrasound phacoemulsification. EVE may well provide enhanced protection for the corneal endothelium, reduced risk of capsular rupture, and no chance of thermal injury.

Index

Page numbers followed by "t" indicate tables, "f" indicate figures, "b" indicate boxes.

2457631924576319245763192